Opiate Receptors and Antagonists

For other titles published in this series, go to
www.springer.com/series/7626

Reginald L. Dean III • Edward J. Bilsky
S. Stevens Negus
Editors

Opiate Receptors and Antagonists

From Bench to Clinic

Humana Press

Editors
Reginald L. Dean, III, M.S.
Life Sciences/Toxicology
Alkermes, Inc.
Cambridge, MA 02139
USA

Edward J. Bilsky, Ph.D.
Department of Pharmacology
University of New England
College of Osteopathic Medicine
Biddleford ME 04005
USA

S. Stevens Negus, Ph.D.
Department of Pharmacology
and Toxicology
Virginia Commonwealth University
Richmond, VA 23298
USA

ISBN: 978-1-58829-881-2 e-ISBN: 978-1-59745-197-0
DOI: 10.1007/978-1-59745-197-0

Library of Congress Control Number: 2008941670

Printed on acid-free paper

springer.com

Preface

The evolution in our understanding of opioid receptors and their subtypes is intimately linked to the development of new pharmacological treatments for diseases/ disorders as diverse as addiction, self-injurious behavior, pain, cancer, inflammation, eating disorders, traumatic injury, pruritis, and movement disorders. These potential treatments involve both novel chemical entities and classic opioid antagonists with improved drug delivery systems. The contributions contained in *Opioid Receptors and Antagonists: From Bench to Clinic* represent the efforts from some of the leading international scientists and clinicians making use of the latest information emerging from the study of the opioid receptor system. Given the number of researchers currently active in this and related fields of study, it would be inappropriate to suggest that the entire range of activities is fully reflected in this single volume. Instead, a variety of experimental and clinical approaches involving the fields of neuroscience, molecular biology, biochemistry, anatomy, pharmacology, psychology, and psychiatry have been chosen to illustrate rapidly developing experimental and therapeutic areas.

Opioid Receptors and Antagonists: From Bench to Clinic opens with a forward describing, from first-hand knowledge of the author, the history behind the clinical development of the classic opioid antagonist naltrexone. The book is subsequently organized into seven sections. The first section contains four chapters characterizing the opioid receptor. The second section contains six chapters describing the chemistry and pharmacology of opioid antagonists of different subtypes of receptors. The next four sections concentrate on the therapeutic areas for opioid antagonists. These sections provide support for the use of opioid antagonists for substance abuse (seven chapters), alcohol and ingestive behaviors (four chapters), behavioral disorders (four chapters), and medical indications, supported by nonclinical and clinical evidence (nine chapters). Finally, the seventh section provides five chapters which concentrate on the development of exciting and innovative drug-delivery approaches that are being used with opioid antagonists.

It is hoped that this volume will serve as a useful reference while also stimulating continued research on the opioid receptor system and its interactions with hormonal and other transmitter systems. The ultimate goal of these efforts is to assist in the development of treatments for "brain reward" disorders and for other medical indications that may be responsive to opioid receptor antagonists.

Reginald L. Dean III
S. Stevens Negus
Edward J. Bilsky

Foreword

Opiate Receptors and Antagonists

It would have been very difficult to predict the scope of this volume in the early 1970s when the race to learn about the functions of the newly discovered endogenous opioid system began. The first clinical studies of naltrexone were published by Bill Martin and Don Jasinski based on studies done in heroin addicts living in the USPHS Prison Hospital in Lexington, Kentucky (Martin et al 1973). Founded in the 1930s, this research unit was the forerunner of the NIH intramural program which for NIDA is now located in Baltimore. The Lexington unit at that time was one of the few places in the world doing scientific studies of addiction.

After reading the results of naltrexone studies in Lexington, several groups began trials of the medication as a new treatment for heroin addiction. My original IND for naltrexone dates to 1973 when this medication created great excitement as the antagonist with better properties than cycloazine and fewer side effects. This was a very exciting time for both basic and clinical research on the opioid system. Naltrexone was being hailed as the perfect medication. It was non-addicting with few side effects but it blocked virtually all of the effects of heroin and other opioids.

Of course, we now know that naltrexone as a treatment for opioid addiction appeals to few patients. Thus, compliance of the oral form is very low. After several clinical trials in which naltrexone was tested against placebo, it was found that classic, double-blind studies did not work with this drug (Hollister 1978). If the patient tested the blockade, they immediately knew which drug they were on and they often would simply stop the medication in order to get high. If they failed to test with a trial dose of heroin-, it made no difference whether they were on placebo or naltrexone. In fact, those on placebo would have a tendency to do better because there were fewer but not zero side effects from placebo. When naltrexone was finally approved by the FDA in 1984 as a treatment for heroin addiction, approval was based on its pharmacology and not on clinical trials. Still, the Dupont Company celebrated it as a major treatment advance. All of the scientists who had been studying naltrexone, however, had warned the company that naltrexone (Trexan®) was not appealing to patients and therefore it would likely sell very poorly. In fact that prediction came true and a disappointed Dupont Merck rapidly lost interest in the product.

Basic scientists, however, continued to study the opioid system and a major method for determining its function was to block it utilizing specific antagonists such as naloxone or naltrexone. One of the earliest workers in this field was Larry Reid who showed that both opiate agonists and opiate antagonists influenced alcohol drinking (Reid and Hunter 1984). Clear evidence of a role for opiate antagonists in blocking self administration of alcohol was first published by Hal Altshuler of Houston, Texas who presented a paper at the CPDD Meeting in 1979 showing a dose-related naltrexone effect on suppression of intravenous alcohol self-administration in 8 of 22 Rhesus monkeys (Altshuler et al 1980). This work led me to propose naltrexone as potentially useful in the treatment of alcoholism. I sent a protocol to the FDA and eventually received an IND in 1983 to study naltrexone in alcoholics. I tested it in an open trial with alcoholics, some of whom seemed to do very well. I was encouraged enough to begin a double-blind trial in our Veterans Administration day treatment center for alcoholism. The subjects were 70 male alcoholics with an average of 20 years of alcoholic drinking and numerous relapses after detoxification. The treatment program involved intensive psychotherapy including 12-step/Alcoholics Anonymous groups plus family therapy and 5 days per week (25 hours) in the day hospital program.

Recruitment of subjects was very difficult because of outright hostility by counselors who were often recovering alcoholics themselves and were opposed to the use of medication. The first postdoctoral fellow who was assigned to this study was able to recruit only a handful of subjects over a year but the next post-doctoral fellow, Joe Volpicelli, was convinced that naltrexone was potentially useful because he had also conducted animal studies with the drug (Volpicelli et al 1986). His enthusiasm and determination convinced the counselors to give the study a chance and we recruited a total of 70 male alcoholics. Half were randomized to 50 mg per day of naltrexone, a dose selected because this was what we used for the treatment of heroin addiction. The other half received an identically appearing placebo. Efforts to obtain funding for this study were completely unsuccessful but because we had a VA Research Center and a Postdoctoral Research Training Program, we were able to devote some resources to this effort.

The initial results were positive and we began to report them at various meetings but having the paper published was difficult (Volpicelli et al 1990; 1992). Fortunately, Stephanie O'Malley at Yale attempted to replicate our work and found almost identical results in a population that included both males and females and less intensive psychotherapy (O'Malley et al 1992).

This sequence of testing a laboratory finding in a clinical population points to the validity of animal models in the study of addiction. The history of new medications for the treatment other psychiatric disorders is usually the reverse: an effect is noticed by an astute clinician prescribing the drug for a different reason and laboratory studies come later.

The diversity among the chapters in this volume is a testimony to the widespread influences of the endogenous opioid system. The role in alcoholism seems to be important at least for a subset of alcoholics which could be the first biologically defined endophenotype for this disorder. Since we initially began trying naltrexone as a treatment in patients more than three decades ago, great progress has been made. The future, in my opinion, lies in pharmacogenetics. All clinical trials henceforth should include a request for DNA from the participants. Well-characterized patients including information on treatment response can be extremely useful in the future if DNA is preserved. Using such retrospective analysis, we found that a functional allele of the gene for the μ receptor predicts good response to naltrexone (Oslin et al 2003). Another group led by Ray Anton recently reported the same finding in their sample (Anton R 2006). A very recent analysis of the sub-sample of the VA multisite failed to show a correlation between polymorphism and treatment outcome (Gelernter et al 2007).Family history plays a major role in alcoholism and it is likely that other genetic variations will be discovered that have consistent treatment relevance. A prospective study of the A118G allele certainly should be accomplished. Future studies will also have the advantage of using the extended release naltrexone preparation so that the medication compliance variable can be more effectively managed (Pettinati et al 2000).

We have come a long way since 1973 and I predict that a specific drug such as naltrexone will become even more important as we become more specific in our genetic diagnoses. We still do not know the relative contribution of antagonism at μ, κ and δ receptors on the therapeutics effects of naltrexone. Recent research on the nociception-orphanon receptor will likely yield even more therapeutic potential as medications targeting those receptors are discovered. The up to date reviews in this volume will give the reader a chance to catch up on the recent advances in knowledge of the endogenous opioid system and provide clues to the future as research continues.

Charles P. O'Brien, M.D., Ph.D.
University of Pennsylvania Health System
Penn Behavioral Health
Charles O'Brien Center of Addiction Treatment
Philadelphia, PA

References

Altshuler HL, Phillips PA, Feinhandler DA (1980): Alteration of ethanol self-administration by naltrexone. *Life Sciences* 26:679-688.

Anton R OMS, Couper D, Swift R, Pettinati H, Goldman D, Oraczi G (2006): Does a common variant of the mu opiate receptor gene predict response to naltrexone in the treatment of alcoholism? Results from the COMBINE study. *Neuropsychopharmacology* 31 Suppl 1:S24.

Gelernter J, Gueorguieva R, Kranzler HR, Zhang H, Cramer J, Rosenheck R, Krystal JH (2007): Opioid receptor gene (OPRM1, OPRK1, and OPRD1) variants and response to naltrexone treatment for alcohol dependence: results from the VA Cooperative Study. *Alcohol Clin Exp Res* 31:555-563.

Hollister L (1978): Clinical evaluation of naltrexone treatment of opiate-dependent individuals. *Arch Gen Psychiatry* 35:335-340.

Martin W, Jasinski D, Mansky P (1973): Naltrexone, an antagonist for the treatment of heroin dependence. *Arch Gen Psych* 28:784-791.

O'Malley SS, Jaffe AJ, Chang G, Schottenfeld RS, Meyer RE, Rounsaville B (1992): Naltrexone and coping skills therapy for alcohol dependence: a controlled study. *Arch Gen Psychiat* 49:881-887.

Oslin DW, Berrettini W, Kranzler HR, Pettinati H, Gelernter J, Volpicelli JR, O'Brien CP (2003): A functional polymorphism of the mu-opioid receptor gene is associated with naltrexone response in alcohol-dependent patients. *Neuropsychopharmacology* 28:1546-1552.

Pettinati HM, Volpicelli JR, Pierce JD, Jr., O'Brien CP (2000): Improving naltrexone response: an intervention for medical practitioners to enhance medication compliance in alcohol dependent patients. *J Addict Dis* 19:71-83.

Reid LD, Hunter GA (1984): Morphine and naloxone modulate intake of ethanol. *Alcohol* 1(1):33-37.

Volpicelli JR, Alterman AI, Hayashida M, O'Brien CP (1992): Naltrexone in the treatment of alcohol dependence. *Archives of General Psychiatry* 49:876-880.

Volpicelli JR, Davis MA, Olgin JE (1986): Naltrexone blocks the post-shock increase of ethanol consumption. *Life Sciences* 38:841-847.

Volpicelli JR, O'Brien CP, Alterman AI, Hayashida M (1990): Naltrexone and the treatment of alcohol dependence: initial observations. In: Reid LB editor. *Opioids, Bulimia, Alcohol Abuse and Alcoholism*. New York: Springer-Verlag, pp 195-214.

Contents

Contributors

Subramaniam Ananthan
Organic Chemistry Department, Southern Research Institute, Birmingham, AL 35255

Raymond F. Anton
Center for Drug and Alcohol Programs, Medical University of South Carolina, Charleston, SC 29425

Stan L. Banks
AllTranz, Inc., Lexington, KY 40536

Cécile Béguin
Molecular Pharmacology Laboratory, Department of Psychiatry, Harvard Medical School, McLean Hospital, Belmont, MA 02478

Nora V. Bergasa
Department of Medicine, Metropolitan Hospital Center, New York, NY 10029

Edward J. Bilsky
Department of Pharmacology, University of New England College of Osteopathic Medicine, Biddeford, ME 04005

Richard J. Bodnar
Department of Psychology, Queens College, City University of New York, Flushing, NY 11367

Colin Brewer
The Stapleford Centre, London SW1W 9NP, United Kingdom

Jonathan M. Brotchie
Toronto Western Research Institute, Toronto Western Hospital, Toronto, ON M5T 2S8, Canada

Lindsay H. Burns
Preclinical Development, Pain Therapeutics, Inc., San Mateo, CA 94404

William A. Carlezon, Jr.
Behavioral Genetics Laboratory, Department of Psychiatry, Harvard Medical School, McLean Hospital, Belmont, MA 02478

Ching-Ping Chang
Department of Biotechnology, Southern Taiwan University of Technology, Tainan, Taiwan 710, Republic of China

Sheng-Hsien Chen
Obstetrics and Gynecology, Chi-Mei Medical Center, Yung-Kang City, Tainan, Taiwan 710, Republic of China

Simon F.J. Clarke
Emergency Department, Frimley Park NHS Foundation Trust, Camberley, Surrey, United Kingdom GU16 7UJ

Bruce M. Cohen
Molecular Pharmacology Laboratory, Department of Psychiatry, Harvard Medical School, McLean Hospital, Belmont, MA 02478

Sandra D. Comer
Division on Substance Abuse, Department of Psychiatry, Columbia University, New York, NY 10032

Lauren C. Costantini
Titan Pharmaceuticals, Inc., South San Francisco, CA 94080

Alan Cowan
Department of Pharmacology and Center for Substance Abuse Research, Temple University School of Medicine, Philadelphia, PA 19140

Paul I. Dargan
Guy's and St. Thomas' Poisons Unit, Guy's and St Thomas' NHS Foundation Trust, London, United Kingdom

Reginald L. Dean, III
Life Sciences/Toxicology, Alkermes, Inc., Cambridge, MA 02139

Paul Dietze
Turning Point Alcohol and Drug Centre, Monash Institute of Health Services Research, Clayton, Victoria 3168, Australia

Beatriz Fioravanti
Department of Pharmacology and Anesthesiology, College of Medicine at the University of Arizona, Tucson, AZ 85724

Bernard Le Foll, MD PhD CCFP
Head, Translational Addiction Research Laboratory, CAMH. Associate Professor, University of Toronto. Centre for Addiction and Mental Health, Toronto, Canada M5S 2S1

Susan H. Fox
Division of Neurology, University of Toronto, Toronto, ON M5V 2S8, Canada

Gantt Galloway
Addiction Pharmacology Research Laboratory, California Pacific Medical Center Research Institute, St. Luke's Hospital, San Francisco, CA 94110

Brenda J. Gehrke
Integrative Neuroscience Section, NIH/NIDA Intramural Research Program, Baltimore, MD 21224

Steven R. Goldberg
Preclinical Pharmacology Section, Behavioral Neuroscience Research Branch, NIDA, NIH, Department of Health and Human Services, Baltimore, MD 21224

Jon E. Grant
Department of Psychiatry, University of Minnesota Medical School, Minneapolis, MN 55454

Mark K. Greenwald
Substance Abuse Research Division, Department of Psychiatry and Behavioral Neurosciences, Wayne State University School of Medicine, Detroit, MI 48207

Dana C. Hammell
Department of Pharmaceutical Sciences, University of Kentucky College of Pharmacy, Lexington, KY 40536

Richard D. Howells
Department of Biochemistry and Molecular Biology, University of Medicine and Dentistry of New Jersey, New Jersey Medical School, Newark, NJ 07103

Gary K. Hulse
Unit for Research and Education in Drugs and Alcohol, School of Psychiatry and Clinical Neurosciences, The University of Western Australia, Western Australia 6009, Australia

Saadet Inan
Department of Pharmacology and Center for Substance Abuse Research, Temple University School of Medicine, Philadelphia, PA 19140

Robert J. Israel
Progenics Pharmaceuticals, Inc., Tarrytown, NY 10591

Tom H. Johnston
Toronto Western Research Institute, Toronto Western Hospital, Toronto, ON M5T 2S8, Canada

Alison L Jones
Australian and Clinical Toxicology Unit, Mater Misericordiae Hospital, New Castle, New South Wales, Australia

Zuzana Justinova
Preclinical Pharmacology Section, Behavioral Neuroscience Research Branch, NIDA, NIH, Department of Health and Human Services, Baltimore, MD 21224

Anne-Maree Kelly
Joseph Epstein Centre for Emergency Medicine Research, Department of Emergency Medicine, Western Hospital and The University of Melbourne, Victoria 3021, Australia

Debra Kerr
Joseph Epstein Centre for Emergency Medicine Research, The University of Melbourne, Victoria 3021, Australia

Andrea King
Department of Psychiatry and Behavioral Neuroscience, University of Chicago, Chicago, IL 60637

Paul K. Kiptoo
Department of Pharmaceutical Sciences, University of Kentucky College of Pharmacy, Lexington, KY 40536

Thomas R. Kosten
Department of Psychiatry, Michael E. DeBakey VA Medical Center, Baylor College of Medicine, Houston, TX 77030

David Koval
Department of Psychiatry, Wayne State University, Detroit, MI 48202

Suchitra Krishnan-Sarin
Department of Psychiatry, Yale University School of Medicine, New Haven, CT 06519

Francesco Leri
Department of Psychology, University of Guelph, Guelph, ON N1G2W1, Canada

Mao-Tsun Lin
Department of Medical Research, Chi-Mei Medical Center, Yung-Kang City, Tainan, Taiwan 710, Republic of China.

Paolo Lissoni
Divisione di Radioterapia Oncologica, Ospedale San Gerardo, 20052 Monza, Italy

Liangming Liu
State Key Laboratory of Trauma, Burns and Combined Injury, The Second Department of Research Institute of Surgery, Daping Hospital, The Third Military Medical University, Chongqing 400042, People's Republic of China

Elliot D. Luby
Wayne State University Schools of Medicine and Law, Detroit, MI 48202

Nancy K. Mello
Alcohol and Drug Abuse Research Center, McLean Hospital-Harvard Medical School, Belmont, MA 02478

Jack H. Mendelson
Alcohol and Drug Abuse Research Center, McLean Hospital-Harvard Medical School, Belmont, MA 02478

John Mendelson
Addiction Pharmacology Research Laboratory, California Pacific Medical Center Research Institute, St. Luke's Hospital, San Francisco, CA 94110

Jonathan P. Moorman
Department of Internal Medicine, James H. Quillen College of Medicine, East Tennessee State University, Johnson City, TN 36714

S. Stevens Negus
Department of Pharmacology and Toxicology, Virginia Commonwealth University, Richmond, VA 23298

Mary C. Olmstead
Department of Psychology, Queen's University, Kingston, ON K7L 3N6, Canada

Stephanie O'Malley
Department of Psychiatry, Yale University School of Medicine, New Haven, CT 06519

Kalpana S. Paudel
Department of Pharmaceutical Sciences, University of Kentucky College of Pharmacy, Lexington, KY 40536

R. Reddy Pinninti
Department of Pharmaceutical Sciences, University of Kentucky College of Pharmacy, Lexington, KY 40536

Mark Pletcher
Department of Epidemiology and Biostatistics, University of California at San Francisco, San Francisco, CA 94143

Larry D. Reid
Laboratory for Psychopharmacology, Rensselaer Polytechnic Institute, Troy, NY 12180

Richard B. Rothman
Clinical Psychopharmacology Section, IRP, NIDA, NIH, DHHS, Baltimore, MD 21224

Curt Sandman
Department of Psychiatry and Human Behavior; Women and Childrens' Health and Well-Being Project, University of California-Irvine, Orange, California 92868

Peter Selby
Addiction Program, Centre for Addiction and Mental Health, University of Toronto, Toronto, ON M5S 2S1, Canada

Kevin A. Sevarino
VA Connecticut Healthcare System, Department of Psychiatry, Newington, CT 06111

Toni S. Shippenberg
Integrative Neuroscience Section, NIH/NIDA Intramural Research Program, Baltimore, MD 21224

Marcello Solinas
Institut de Biologie et Physiologie Cellulaires, Centre National de la Recherche Scientifique-6187, University of Poitiers, 86022 Poitiers, France

Caren L. Steinmiller
Substance Abuse Research Division, Department of Psychiatry and Behavioral Neurosciences, Wayne State University School of Medicine, Detroit, MI 48207

Audra L. Stinchcomb
Department of Pharmaceutical Sciences, University of Kentucky College of Pharmacy, Lexington, KY 40536

Caroline Strasinger
Department of Pharmaceutical Sciences, University of Kentucky College of Pharmacy, Lexington, KY 40536

Emmanuel Streel
Universite Libre de Bruxelles, ISEPK, B-1020 Bruxelles, Belgium

Maria A. Sullivan
Division on Substance Abuse, Department of Psychiatry, Columbia University, New York, NY 10032

Gianluigi Tanda
Psychobiology Section, Medications Discovery Research Branch, Intramural Research Program, NIDA, NIH, Department of Health and Human Services, Baltimore, MD 21224

Rachel Torello
The Chicago School of Professional Psychology, Chicago, IL 60610

Rob Török
Emergency Department, Dorset County Hospital, NHS Foundation Trust, London, United Kingdom

Ellen M. Unterwald
Department of Pharmacology and Center for Substance Abuse Research, Temple School of Medicine, Philadelphia, PA 19140 and The Rockefeller University, Biology of Addictive Diseases Laboratory, New York, NY 10021

Todd W. Vanderah
Department of Pharmacology, College of Medicine, University of Arizona Health Sciences Center, Tucson, AZ 85724

Ellen A. Walker
Department of Pharmaceutical Sciences and Center for Substance Abuse Research, Temple University School of Pharmacy, Philadelphia, PA 19140

Hoau-Yan Wang
Department of Physiology and Pharmacology, City University of New York Medical School, New York, NY 10031

Zhi Qiang Yao
Department of Internal Medicine, James H. Quillen College of Medicine, East Tennessee State University, Johnson City, TN 36714

Deling Yin
Departments of Internal Medicine and Pharmacology, James H. Quillen College of Medicine, East Tennessee State University, Johnson City, TN 36714

Chun-Su Yuan
Committee on Clinical Pharmacology, Department of Anesthesia and Critical Care, Pritzker School of Medicine, The University of Chicago, Chicago, IL 60637

Part I
Opioid Receptors

Chapter 1
Ultra-Low-Dose Opioid Antagonists Enhance Opioid Analgesia and Reduce Tolerance

Lindsay H. Burns, Todd W. Vanderah, and Hoau-Yan Wang

Abstract Ultra-low-dose opioid antagonists have been shown to enhance opioid analgesia and attenuate the tolerance to analgesic effects normally seen with chronic opioid administration. This chapter reviews the early work with ultra-low-dose opioid antagonists starting with electrophysiological recordings of dorsal root ganglion neurons and continuing to antinociception in rodents. These pharmacological findings have not adhered to typical dose response curves and have instead been reported to occur at wide ranges of extremely low doses of several opioid antagonists as well as with the rare opioid agonist. Optimal dose ranges have also been reported to vary with sex and strain of rat. Translation into small clinical studies has been met with varied results, related to variations in dose, route of administration, and antagonist selected. Nevertheless, the clinical studies that have demonstrated enhanced analgesia or opioid sparing effects have utilized opioid antagonist doses in lower dose ranges than the studies that failed to demonstrate efficacy. Furthermore, a large double-blind, placebo- and active-controlled clinical trial demonstrated enhanced opioid analgesia with the extremely low dose of 2 μg naltrexone/patient/day. Preclinical data also extend the effects of ultra-low-dose opioid antagonists to neuropathic pain, which is comparatively resistant to opioid treatment and, interestingly, to cannabinoid analgesia. The mechanism of action has been shown to be the prevention of a chronic opioid-induced mu opioid receptor–G protein coupling switch that is associated with analgesic tolerance and dependence. Finally, recent data shows that this G protein coupling switch is controlled by filamin A and that a high-affinity interaction of naloxone or naltrexone with this scaffolding protein mediates their prevention of the altered coupling.

Keywords: Naloxone; Naltrexone; Neuropathic pain; G protein coupling; Filamin A

L.H. Burns (✉), T.W. Vanderah, and H.-Y. Wang
Pain Therapeutics, Inc., Preclinical Development, 2211 Bridgepointe Parkway, Suite 500, San Mateo, CA 94404
e-mail: lburns@paintrials.com

R. Dean et al. (eds.), *Opiate Receptors and Antagonists*,

1.1 Introduction

Opioid analgesics are widely used to manage moderate or severe pain, yet their use is hampered by unwanted side effects, tolerance to their analgesic effects, and physical dependence. The fact that patients often balance analgesia with side effects illustrates the narrow therapeutic window of opioids. Side effects range from nausea, constipation, somnolence, and pruritis to the more serious respiratory depression. Chronic pain patients need analgesia over prolonged or indefinite time periods, yet these patients very often experience a loss of analgesic potency with continued use. Finally, physicians and patients alike are wary of initiating opioid therapy due to the fears or stigma around opioid dependence and even the potential for addiction. As a consequence, the field of pain management is in great need of improved analgesic therapies that provide adequate analgesia for moderate-to-severe pain with fewer adverse effects and minimal potential for tolerance, dependence, and addiction.

One such therapy involves the combination of opioid agonists with "ultra-low-dose" opioid antagonists. In contrast to the typical blockade of opioid receptor functions by higher concentrations of opioid antagonists, ultra-low-dose opioid antagonist cotreatment enhances and prolongs opioid analgesia and also prevents or reverses opioid analgesic tolerance. These phenomena have been demonstrated by preclinical data and have now randomized double-blind, controlled clinical trial data. This chapter will review the effects of ultra-low-dose opioid antagonists on analgesia, tolerance, and the hyperalgesia and allodynia in a model of neuropathic pain, while the attenuation of physical dependence and the addictive properties of opioids will be reviewed in Chapater 13. This chapter will also provide a historical overview of studies probing the mechanism of action for these effects from the initial electrophysiology findings to more recent molecular pharmacology data and identification of the high-affinity binding site. These studies indicate that chronic opioid administration causes alterations in the G protein system associated with mu opioid receptors (MORs) and that ultra-low-dose naloxone (and perhaps other opioid antagonists) suppresses these aberrant signaling changes via a picomolar interaction with filamin A.

1.2 Preclinical Evidence of Enhanced Opioid Analgesia and Reduced Tolerance

The history of ultra-low-dose opioid antagonists starts with electrophysiology studies on dorsal root ganglion (DRG) cell cultures. Crain and Shen first observed that while opioid agonists normally inhibit, or shorten, the action potential duration of DRG cells, lower doses of opioid agonists induce an opposite, excitatory effect – a prolongation of the action potential (39, 9). These researchers noted that prolonged exposure to an opioid agonist would also produce this prolongation of action potentials, and they theorized that these excitatory effects of opioids contributed to opioid tolerance (10). This same publication proposed a regulation by GM1 ganglioside, since exogenous administration of GM1 ganglioside mimicked the prolonged opioid exposure. The hypothesis that excitatory effects of opioids are mediated by opioid receptors coupling to the excitatory G protein Gs rather than the usual inhibitory G proteins, Gi or Go, was suggested by a blockade of the action potential prolongation by administration of cholera toxin-A, an agent that blocks Gs from being activated by receptor stimulation (40).

Using their in vitro model of action potential prolongation by low concentrations of morphine, Crain and Shen (11) showed that ultra-low-dose naloxone blocked the action potential prolongation when added at low picomolar concentrations. In the same 1995 publication, Crain and Shen showed that ultra-low-dose naltrexone (10 ng/kg, s.c.) also enhanced and prolonged morphine's antinociceptive potency in mice. This seminal report also included data demonstrating that cotreatment with ultra-low-dose naltrexone dramatically attenuated morphine withdrawal after an acute high dose of morphine or after a 4-day, twice daily, progressively increasing morphine dosing schedule. Finally, an assessment of tolerance was made in the mice receiving the escalating 4-day morphine treatment, by comparing subsequent antinociception to that of naïve mice. Tolerance was partially prevented by ultra-low-dose naltrexone.

A subsequent study by a different lab extended the work of Crain and Shen, demonstrating enhanced morphine antinociception by ultra-low-dose naltrexone administered either systemically or intrathecally to rats (36). This study also demonstrated that coadministration of ultra-low-dose naltrexone (0.05 ng) prevents analgesic tolerance over 7 days of daily intrathecal administration of morphine (15 μg). An even lower intrathecal dose of naltrexone (0.005 ng) as well as i.p. administration of both drugs was less effective. Using rats instead of mice, these data demonstrated enhanced morphine analgesia, a complete prevention of tolerance over a 7-day treatment period, a lower end of an effective ultra-low-dose range by intrathecal administration, and a spinal site of action. Data also showed that established morphine tolerance could be reversed, at least partially.

Crain and Shen also followed up their earlier work by demonstrating that both analgesic tolerance and precipitated withdrawal-associated hyperalgesia in mice could be prevented by ultra-low-dose naltrexone combined with either morphine (45) or oxycodone (44). In a further extension of their in vitro data, Crain and Shen demonstrated that acute hyperalgesia elicited by a low dose of an opioid agonist, referred to clinically as "paradoxical hyperalgesia" (27,29), could be reversed by ultra-low-dose naltrexone coadministration, yielding a strong analgesic effect (15).

While the early in vitro work primarily utilized naloxone, ultra-low doses of the kappa opioid antagonist nor-binaltorphamine (nor-BNI) and the mu opioid antagonist beta-funaltrexamine (β-FNA) (Crain and Shen, personal communication), as well as the nonselective opioid antagonist diprenorphine (41), have also enhanced the inhibitory effects of opioid agonists in vitro. While most published in vivo work was initially limited to naltrexone, ultra-low-dose naloxone was also recently used in vivo to prevent analgesic tolerance (53; Fig. 1.1). In addition, ultra-low doses of naloxone and nalmefene have demonstrated beneficial effects in clinical studies discussed below. Perhaps more surprisingly, ultra-low doses of the opioid agonists

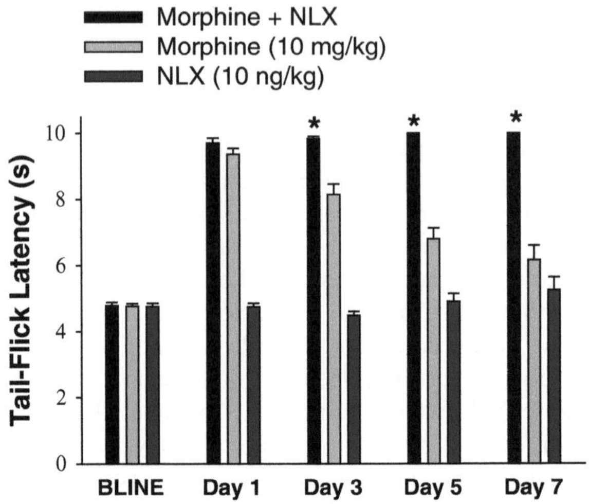

Fig. 1.1 Co-treatment with ultra-low-dose NLX (10ng/kg) prevented the antinociceptive tolerance caused by chronic morphine (10mg/kg, s.c., twice daily for 7 days). Rats treated with morphine+NLX showed stable tail-flick latencies over the week of treatment, while tail-flick latencies of rats receiving morphine alone declined to a level not significantly different from NLX alone. $*p<0.05$ and $**p<0.01$ for morphine+NLX versus morphine. *BLINE* predrug baseline, *NLX* naloxone. Reprinted from Wang et al. (53), with permission from Elsevier

etorphine and dihydroetorphine (41) and of [des-Tyr] fragments of the endogenous opioids dynorphin A-(1–13) and β-endorphin (1–27) (42) also enhance the inhibitory effects of opioid agonists in vitro. Further, ultra-low-dose etorphine enhances morphine's potency in vivo (43). Together, these findings hinted that these phenomena are not unique to naloxone or naltrexone and are also not dependent on opioid antagonist activity.

1.3 Dose Effects and Dependency on Strain and Sex

Ultra-low-dose opioid antagonist effects do not follow a typical dose-response pattern, but typically span several log units without conforming to bell-shaped curves. A wide range of doses has been used successfully. Although some initial studies tested antagonist:agonist ratios rather that discrete antagonist doses, the much narrower effective dose range for agonists than for ultra-low-dose antagonists in enhancing agonist effects suggests that the antagonist dose is independent of agonist dose. This method was likely initiated for ease of calculating antagonist dose. An examination of the antinociceptive effects of various ratios of naltrexone:oxycodone ($1{:}10^9$, $1{:}10^7$, and $1{:}10^5$) combined with a range of oxycodone doses (0.03–3 mg/kg) in male Swiss Webster mice illustrates the wide range of effective doses of naltrexone (Fig. 1.2). Whereas all naltrexone:oxycodone dose ratios examined enhanced the areas under the curve (AUCs) of tailflick latencies

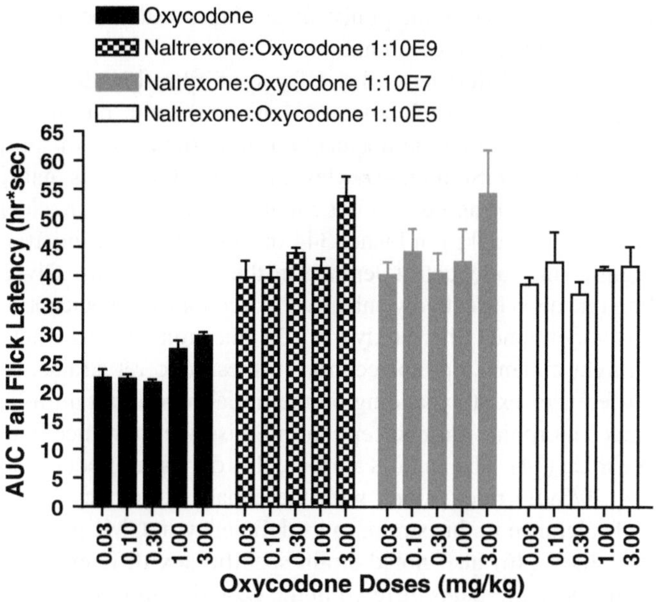

Fig. 1.2 Dose-response of ultra-low-dose naltrexone:oxycodone ratios in enhancing oxycodone antinociception in the 52°C hot water immersion tail-flick tests in male Swiss Webster mice. Three different naltrexone:oxycodone ratios (1:10^9, 1:10^7, and 1:10^5) were superimposed onto a dose-response of oxycodone (0.03, 0.1, 0.3, 1, and 3 mg/kg, s.c.). These naltrexone:oxycodone ratios enhanced the effects of all doses of oxycodone, although the 1:10^9 and 1:10^7 ratios more potently enhanced the antinociceptive effect of the 3 mg/kg oxycodone dose than did the 1:10^5 dose ratio. Data are means ± SEM., $n = 3$. Reprinted from (2) in *Recent Developments in Pain Research*, with permission from Research Signpost

of the oxycodone doses, the strongest antinociceptive effects were obtained with the 3 and 300 pg/kg naltrexone doses, which appear to enhance the antinociceptive effects of 3 mg/kg oxycodone to a greater extent than a 30 ng/kg dose.

While wide antagonist dose ranges have been used effectively, the optimal doses of antagonist vary with both the opioid agonist it is combined with as well as the sex of the animal. The prevention of tolerance and withdrawal-associated hyperalgesia by ultra-low-dose naltrexone was demonstrated at 0.3, 3, 300, and 3,000 ng/kg naltrexone when combined with 3 mg/kg morphine (45) and at 1 pg/kg or 1 ng/kg naltrexone when combined with oxycodone (44). The higher naltrexone doses used in these studies were used in males, suggesting males are less sensitive to ultra-low-dose antagonist effects. Interestingly, although these studies used the same morphine dose for males and females, a tenfold *lower* dose of oxycodone was administered to males, confirming the previously described increased sensitivity to opioid analgesic effects in male rodents (28). Hence, while male rodents may be more sensitive to opioid analgesia, female rodents appear to be more sensitive to ultra-low-dose naltrexone, suggesting some degree of dissociation between the two. In addition, low doses of oxycodone elicited a greater degree of hyperalgesia in male than in female rats (23), while the reverse was reported with morphine-induced hyperalgesia (22). These findings likely contribute to the variations in optimal ultra-low-dose opioid antagonist dose ranges noted both with sex of the animal and the opioid used in combination.

In addition to sex differences, the effects of ultra-low-dose naltrexone on morphine antinociception and tolerance can also vary with rat strain (46). While the enhancement of morphine antinociception and attenuation of morphine tolerance was observed in both Sprague–Dawley and Long–Evans rats, naltrexone at the dose range tested (0.1–100 ng/kg) did not enhance morphine antinociception over a range of doses (2.5–7.5 mg/kg) in Fisher 344 or Lewis rats, nor did 10 or 100 ng/kg naltrexone significantly attenuate tolerance in these two strains. Given that pg/kg doses of naltrexone most effectively enhanced oxycodone antinociception in females in the previously mentioned Shen study (44), the question remains whether this even lower range might enhance antinociception in these two rat strains. Nevertheless, clear strain differences exist expanding on the initial report that ultra-low-dose naltrexone enhances morphine antinociception in Swiss Webster mice but antagonizes it in 129/SvEv mice (14). The authors attribute this opposite effect of ultra-low-dose naltrexone in 129/SvEv mice, along with the enhanced potency of morphine and general lack of tolerance in this strain, to its deficiency in GM1 ganglioside.

The Terner study (46) also noted strain-specific sex differences. In Sprague–Dawley rats, males and females differed in the dose that most effectively enhanced antinociception, with the best effect in males observed at 10 ng/kg and the highest efficacy in females occurring at the lowest dose tested at 0.1 ng/kg. This greater sensitivity to ultra-low-dose naltrexone in female Sprague–Dawley rats, despite the females being less sensitive to the opioid itself, concurs with the findings by Shen and colleagues in Swiss Webster mice (44, 45). An additional strain-dependent sex difference was revealed in the Terner study; 10 ng/kg naltrexone significantly reversed established morphine tolerance only in female Long–Evans rats. In a separate study examining age and sex effects, morphine antinociception was enhanced by low-dose naltrexone in mature female but not in mature male rats (18–22 weeks) and was negligible in younger rats (21). However, the naltrexone dose range used in that study was again comparatively high (0.002–2 μg/kg), and the effect in mature females was "inversely related to dose."

1.4 Ultra-Low-Dose Naltrexone Effects on Neuropathic Pain and Cannabinoid Analgesia

Although opioids are not typically very effective in neuropathic pain, recent preclinical data has shown that ultra-low-dose naltrexone enhances the antihyperalgesic and antiallodynic effects of morphine (49) or oxycodone (30) in the L5/L6 spinal nerve ligated rats. The antihyperalgesic effects of intrathecal delivery of these opioids combined with naltrexone at 0.33 ng were complete, though some tolerance developed after 10 days of twice daily administration. Further, while intrathecal morphine did not elicit any antiallodynic effect in this model, its combination with ultra-low-dose naltrexone produced a moderate though transient antiallodynic effect. With twice daily oral delivery in this rat model of neuropathic pain, ultra-low-dose naltrexone (0.3–3 μg/kg) combined with oxycodone produced strong antihyperalgesic and antiallodynic effects. Tolerance to these effects was dramatically reduced compared to the more rapid tolerance that developed with oral oxycodone alone. The oral 0.3 μg/kg naltrexone dose combination produced an antihyperalgesic effect that showed no tolerance over this time period. Notably, the enhanced antihypersensitivity effects of the opioids in these studies occurred at slightly higher doses of naltrexone than those shown to enhance antinociception in intact rats. Moreover, these preclinical data suggest that ultra-low-dose naltrexone may augment opioid effects in neuropathic pain and minimize the development of tolerance to them.

Further extending the area of research with ultra-low-dose opioid antagonists, a recent study showed ultra-low-dose naltrexone to enhance cannabinoid-induced analgesia (35). This finding may reflect the well-established interaction of the opioid and cannabinoid systems (32), rather than a specific interaction of naltrexone's binding site on filamin A with cannabinoid receptors. The complete abolition of the analgesic effect of the cannabinoid agonist/naltrexone combination by a cannabinoid antagonist suggests that this analgesia is dependent on the cannabinoid system with any opioid effects upstream. The fact that a high dose of naltrexone only slightly (and nonsignificantly) enhanced here the cannabinoid-induced analgesia suggests that that the potentiation of cannabinoid analgesia by ultra-low-dose naltrexone has some opioid component but does not exclusively rely on opioid receptors.

1.5 Clinical Studies of Ultra-Low-Dose Opioid Antagonist Effects in Analgesia

Clinical experience with ultra-low-dose opioid antagonists has grown from case reports and small clinical studies to blinded, randomized, controlled clinical trials. In contrast to preclinical reports that mostly use naltrexone, clinical studies have reported benefits with ultra-low-doses of naloxone, naltrexone, and also nalmefene. In addition, "ultra-low" doses, dosing schedules, and settings have varied along with results. Most small clinical studies assessed postoperative analgesia and used i.v. (intravenous) administration, while current clinical trials have examined analgesia and dependence and have used oral delivery over 3 weeks or 3 months. While no published clinical studies or clinical trials have been able to assess ultra-low-dose opioid antagonist effects on analgesic tolerance, a case report noted strong analgesia in a severely opioid tolerant diabetic neuropathy patient from ultra-low-dose naltrexone (1 μg orally, b.i.d.) combined with methadone (16). This patient reported a pain intensity reduction from 9 to 3 within 24 h that persisted through a 1-month follow-up.

In a postoperative setting, the first clinical study showed that ultra-low-dose naloxone in a continuous i.v. infusion of 0.25 μg/kg/h, but not 1 μg/kg/h, produced an opioid-sparing effect of morphine delivered by patient-controlled analgesia (PCA) following hysterectomy (18). In another study in women undergoing lower abdominal surgery, a single dose of 15 or 25 μg nalmefene administered before morphine PCA decreased severity of pain 24 h later and also decreased the need for antiemetics and antipruritics (26).

A subsequent study using morphine PCA with or without naloxone at an estimated dose of 0.57 followed by 0.19 μg/kg/h failed to demonstrate enhanced analgesia or opioid-sparing effects (4). Reducing the i.v. naloxone dose tenfold in a later study to an estimated 0.05 followed by 0.006 μg/kg/h, Cepeda again did not demonstrate opioid-sparing effects or enhanced morphine analgesia but reported decreased nausea and pruritis (5). It should be noted that in both studies, PCA doses were increased by 20% when pain intensity exceeded 4 and again at 6 on a 0–10 scale, and a rescue dose 2.5 times the PCA solution was administered when pain intensity reached 6, so accurate assessment of doses is difficult. However, the PCA solution contained 6 μg/cc in the first study and 0.6 μg/cc in the second.

A small randomized, double-blind clinical trial of 156 patients presenting to the emergency department with acute, severe pain did not demonstrate any greater analgesic efficacy of a single i.v. bolus of morphine (0.1 mg/kg) combined with one of three different doses of naloxone (0.1, 0.01, or 0.001 ng/kg) compared to the morphine alone (1). In contrast to the only other study that used a single i.v. bolus of an ultra-low-dose opioid antagonist, that is nalmefene administered prior to morphine PCA postoperatively and assessed pain scores 24 h later (26), the present study gave one combined bolus and assessed pain intensity over the next 4 h. Possibly refers to confounding the results of the study were additional doses of morphine or other opioids administered within the 4 h period. While 13 patients in the morphine-only group received additional morphine, 8, 10, and 14 patients in the 0.1, 0.01, and 0.001 ng/kg naloxone groups required additional morphine, respectively. Although, this data may suggest an opioid-sparing effect at the 0.1 ng/kg naltrexone level these differences were not significant due to the small group sizes. Besides the small group sizes in this study, the diversity of pain conditions and changing rates of pain in patients presenting to the emergency department may have hindered this trial. Nevertheless, this study was unable to demonstrate an effect of ultra-low-dose naloxone in the dose range of 0.001–0.1 ng/kg in augmenting opioid analgesia in acute, severe pain.

The first large, randomized, double-blind clinical trial assessed oxycodone and ultra-low-dose naltrexone (Oxytrex™) versus oxycodone alone delivered orally in 350 osteoarthritis patients with pain ≥5 on a 0–10 scale for 3 weeks (7). Naltrexone was formulated with oxycodone at 1 μg per tablet, so that the Oyxtrex b.i.d. dose group received 2 μg/day while the Oxytrex q.i.d. group received 4 μg/day. Both were compared to placebo and oxycodone alone administered q.i.d. in an immediate-release formulation. All active treatment groups received the same daily dose of oxycodone escalating from a starting dose of 10–40 mg/day in the final week. The Oxytrex b.i.d. treatment, with 2 μg/day naltrexone, provided significantly greater analgesia than both placebo and oxycodone by the end of week 2, with the strongest differences seen at the end of week 3. Neither oxycodone itself nor Oxytrex q.i.d., with 4 μg/day naltrexone, separated from placebo in reduction of pain intensity, a result not inconsistent with prior clinical trials of oxycodone at these doses (37, 33). Although this trial included mostly female patients, a sub-analysis by gender illustrated a stronger treatment effect in males, and a stronger separation

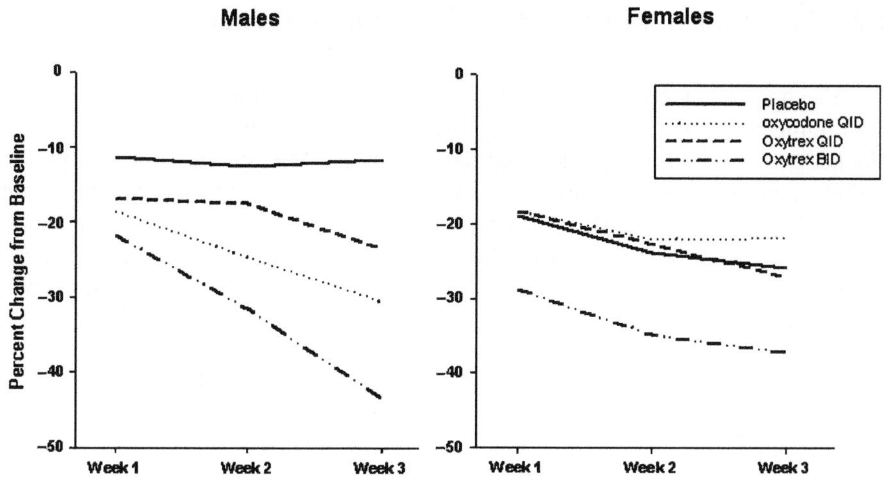

Fig. 1.3 Reduction in pain intensity in males and females. Oxytrex b.i.d. provided the greatest reduction in pain intensity scores in both males and females. At week 3, Oxytrex b.i.d. was significantly better than placebo in males and significantly better than oxycodone in females. Reprinted from Chindalore et al. (7) with permission from American Pain Society

of Oxytrex b.i.d. from placebo in males and a statistical separation of Oxytrex b.i.d. only from oxycodone in females, possibly due to a greater placebo effect in females (Fig. 1.3). Moreover, this first clinical trial demonstrated both enhanced analgesia and the ability to dose b.i.d. without any extended release mechanism, illustrating the prolonged duration of effect seen preclinically. In addition, the enhanced analgesic efficacy of the treatment regimen containing 2 but not 4 μg/patient/day of naltrexone, combined with its ~20% bioavailability by oral delivery, may shed light on earlier studies using i.v. naloxone at higher doses.

A subsequent clinical trial in 750 low-back pain patients showed that Oxytrex b.i.d. provided equivalent analgesia from a significantly lower total average daily dose compared to oxycodone q.i.d. (54). In this trial, patients titrated their dose to a pain score ≤2 or to tolerable side effects up to a maximum of 80 mg/day before being fixed for 12 weeks on their individual doses. Oxytrex b.i.d. also significantly reduced the number of moderate-to-severe events of constipation, somnolence, and pruritis seen with oxycodone alone.

To summarize clinical experience with ultra-low-dose opioid antagonists, some studies may have failed due to "ultra-low" doses that are too high, possibly impeding the effect of the opioid by classical receptor antagonism. In addition, differences in efficacy were observed between studies in postoperative or acute pain and chronic pain populations, possibly suggesting greater efficacy in chronic pain, though one demonstrated enhanced efficacy of morphine intra-operatively. Gender differences in sensitivity to ultra-low-dose opioid antagonists have not emerged clinically, though two positive studies were performed in females. Finally, while some positive studies noted enhanced analgesia, others noted opioid-sparing effects or decreased side effects.

1.6 Mechanism of Ultra-Low-Dose Opioid Antagonists

The mechanism of action of ultra-low-dose opioid antagonists in enhancing and prolonging analgesia and preventing tolerance has long been hypothesized as a blockade of excitatory signaling opioid receptors. Mu opioid receptors preferentially couple to pertussis toxin-sensitive G proteins, Gi and Go, to inhibit the adenylyl cyclase/cyclic AMP (cAMP) pathway (31, 8). Since the in vitro excitatory effects of low doses of opioids (the shortening instead of prolongation of the action potential duration) could be pharmacologically blocked by cholera toxin-A, a compound that blocks activation of the "excitatory" G protein Gs by their associated receptors (40), Crain and Shen hypothesized that the excitatory response to opioids, whether from low doses or prolonged exposure, was mediated by MORs coupling to Gs (12). While Gi and Go proteins are known to inhibit adenylyl cyclase and subsequent production of cAMP from ATP, Gs stimulates this enzyme causing the opposite effects on the cell. Based on their electrophysiology work, Crain and Shen also hypothesized that opioid antagonists selectively antagonized such "excitatory opioid receptors" that signal via Gs proteins (13).

Much of the controversy over this initial hypothesis arose from earlier research suggesting that observable excitatory effects of opioids were not due to a G protein coupling partner novel to MOR, that is, a switch in G protein coupling, but were simply due to altered signaling of the Gβγ dimer contained in the original Gi or Go proteins (20). The Gβγ dimer of the heterotrimeric G proteins coupling to the MOR are thought to contribute to the analgesic effects of opioids by signaling to ion channels and inhibiting cellular activities by hyperpolarization (24, 38). A Gβγ activation of adenylyl cyclase instead would counteract analgesia as would stimulation of adenylyl cyclase by a Gs protein.

Molecular pharmacology work has demonstrated a decrease in MOR Gi and Go coupling concurrent with a striking appearance of Gs coupling in central nervous system (CNS) tissues of rats treated with morphine (10 mg/kg, s.c.) twice daily for 7 days, and an attenuation of these changes by cotreatment with ultra-low-dose naloxone (10 μg/kg, s.c.) (53). A morphine-induced association of MOR with Gs was also demonstrated in Chinese hamster ovary (CHO) cells and in spinal cord (6) by the group who initially demonstrated morphine-induced adenylyl cyclase activation by Gβγ. The development of Gs coupling by MORs may also contribute to the hypersensitivities to thermal and tactile stimuli noted to occur after chronic morphine administration (47, 48). Wang et al. (2005) used a previously established coimmunoprecipitation procedure (50, 25, 55, 56, 3) with antibodies to various Gα proteins to separately isolate each Gα protein along with its associated receptor proteins under basal and morphine-stimulated conditions. Subsequently, the relative amounts of MOR protein associated with each Gα protein were detected via Western blots with a selective antibody directed against an N-terminal epitope of MOR. These relative quantities demonstrated treatment-associated changes in levels of MOR coupling to Gi, Go, and Gs without discernible effects on the expression of either MORs or G proteins (Fig. 1.4). The specificity of antibodies was rigorously demonstrated, and the instatement of Gs coupling with chronic morphine treatment

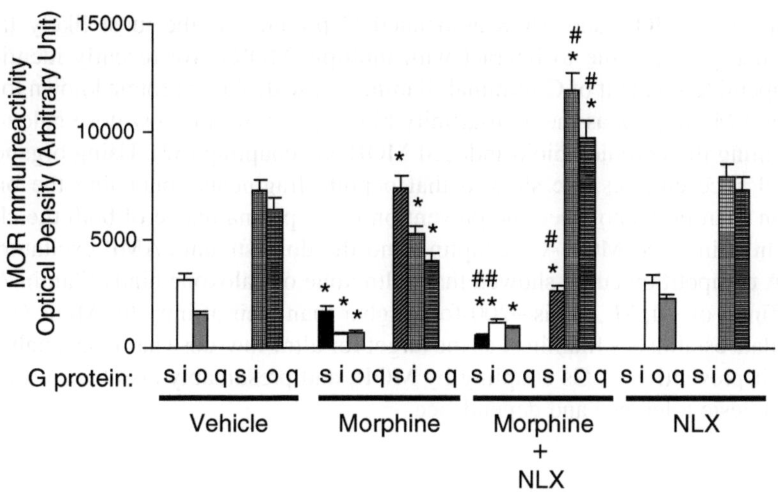

Fig. 1.4 Densitometric quantifications of Western blots showing that chronic morphine-induced Gs–Mu opioid receptor (*MOR*) coupling is attenuated by cotreatment with ultra-low-dose naloxone (*NLX*). MOR protein is detected in immunoprecipitates of Gαi, Gαo and Gαs of spinal cord from rats treated twice daily for 7 days with saline, morphine (10 mg/kg, s.c.), morphine + NLX (10 ng/kg, s.c.) or NLX (10 ng/kg, s.c.). Data are means ± s.e.m. derived from four individual rats in each of the treatment groups that were processed individually ($n = 4$). Solid bars indicate basal coupling, and hatched bars indicate coupling after receptor stimulation by in vitro morphine.*$p < 0.05$ versus same Gα protein in vehicle and NLX-treated groups.**$p < 0.05$ versus same Gα protein in morphine group. Morphine-stimulated coupling was significantly greater ($p < 0.01$) than basal coupling of each Gα protein within each treatment group. Reprinted from Wang et al. (53), with permission from Elsevier

and its attenuation by cotreatment with ultra-low-dose naloxone were confirmed using tritiated DAMGO instead of the MOR antibody.

Wang et al. (53) also examined the interaction of Gβγ with adenylyl cyclase using a similar coimmunoprecipitation procedure using CNS tissues from the same morphine, morphine and naloxone or vehicle-treated rats. Chronic morphine instated an interaction of the MOR-associated Gβγ with adenylyl cyclase types II and IV, and these Gβγ–adenylyl cyclase interactions were similarly attenuated by ultra-low-dose naloxone cotreatment. These treatment-mediated changes in association between Gβγ and adenylyl cyclase type II and IV also occurred without alterations in expression levels of these signaling molecules. We have also demonstrated that the Gβγ that interacts with adenylyl cyclase after chronic morphine treatment originates from a Gs protein that couples to the MOR as opposed to its native G protein (51).

Ultra-low-dose opioid antagonists were initially thought to preferentially bind a subset of MORs (13), and a Gs-coupling MOR subpopulation was again recently proposed (6). However, since naloxone prevents MOR–Gs coupling at concentrations well below its affinity for MOR and since our coimmunoprecipitation data showed it to alter the coupling behavior of MOR, we considered proteins that interact with MOR and MOR-associated G proteins as the most likely targets, particularly those able to interact with multiple MORs. We recently identified a pentapeptide segment of C-terminal filamin A, a scaffolding protein known to interact with MOR (34), as the high-affinity binding site of ultra-low-dose naloxone in preventing the chronic opioid-induced MOR–Gs coupling (52). Using organotypic striatal slice cultures, we showed that peptide fragments containing the binding site on filamin A abolished the prevention by 10 pM naloxone of both the chronic morphine-induced MOR–Gs coupling and the downstream cAMP excitatory signal. A competition curve showed that naltrexone or naloxone binds filamin A with an affinity of ~4pM, that is ~200-fold higher than their affinity for MOR (17, 19). This data establishes filamin A as the target for ultra-low-dose naloxone, naltrexone in their prevention of Gs coupling by MOR, and presumably also their prevention of analgesic tolerance and dependence.

1.7 Conclusions

This chapter has provided an overview of ultra-low-dose opioid antagonist research from the initial discovery of preventing opioid excitatory effects observed by electrophysiology in vitro to preclinical findings of enhanced and prolonged analgesia and reduced analgesic tolerance in vivo. The dose–response relationship spans several log units and does not conform to a bell-shaped curve, although dramatic sex and strain effects have been noted within various dose ranges. This chapter reviewed preclinical and clinical studies conducted with a variety of doses and opioid agonist/antagonist combinations in a variety of settings. The recent identification of the high-affinity interaction binding by naloxone or naltrexone to filamin A may partially explain the varied results seen clinically with various opioid antagonists, doses, and routes of administration, on top of the different patient populations, conditions, and endpoints between studies. Further, the observed sex and strain differences could potentially reflect differences in filamin A levels. Although, a few studies have failed to demonstrate benefits of ultra-low-dose opioid antagonists, most of the available evidence, including results of the larger clinical trials, clearly indicates that certain combinations can substantially improve opioid therapy available today. The effects of ultra-low-dose naltrexone on physical dependence and addictive properties of opioids are reviewed in the Chapter 13.

References

1. Bijur PE, Schechter C, Esses D, Chang AK, Gallagher EJ (2006) Intravenous bolus of ultra-low-dose naloxone added to morphine does not enhance analgesia in emergency department patients. J Pain 7:75–81.
2. Burns, LH (2005) Ultra-low-dose opioid antagonists enhance opioid analgesia while decreasing tolerance, dependence and addictive properties. In: Recent Developments in Pain Research, Anna Capasso (Ed.), pp 115–136.

3. Cai G, Wang H-Y, Friedman E (2002) Increased dopamine receptor signaling and dopamine receptor–protein coupling in denervated striatum. J Pharmacol Exp Ther 302:1105–1112.
4. Cepeda MS, Africano JM, Manrique AM, Fragoso W, Carr DB (2002) The combination of low dose naloxone and morphine in PCA does not decrease opioid requirements in the postoperative period. Pain 96:73–79.
5. Cepeda MS, Alvarez H, Morales O, Carr DB (2004) Addition of ultra low dose naloxone to postoperative morphine PCA: unchanged analgesia and opioid requirement but decreased incidence of opioid side effects. Pain 107:41–46.
6. Chakrabarti S, Regec A, Gintzler AR (2005) Biochemical demonstration of mu-opioid receptor association with Gsα: enhancement following morphine exposure. Mol Brain Res 135:217–224.
7. Chindalore VL, Craven RA, Butera PG, Yu KP, Burns LH, Friedmann N (2005) Adding ultra-low-dose naltrexone to oxycodone enhances and prolongs analgesia. J Pain 6:392–399.
8. Connor M, Christie MD (1999) Opioid receptor signalling mechanisms. Clin Exp Pharmacol Physiol 26:493–499.
9. Crain SM, Shen K-F (1990) Opioids can evoke direct receptor-mediated excitatory effects on sensory neurons. Trends Pharmacol Sci 11:77–81.
10. Crain SM, Shen K-F (1992) After chronic opioid exposure sensory neurons become supersensitive to the excitatory effects of opioid agonists and antagonists as occurs after acute elevation of GM1 ganglioside. Brain Res 575:13–24.
11. Crain SM, Shen K-F (1995) Ultra-low concentrations of naloxone selectively antagonize excitatory effects of morphine on sensory neurons, thereby increasing its antinociceptive potency and attenuating tolerance/dependence during chronic cotreatment. Proc Natl Acad Sci USA 92:10540–10544.
12. Crain SM, Shen K-F (1998) Modulation of opioid analgesia, tolerance and dependence by Gs-coupled, GM1 ganglioside-regulated opioid receptor functions. Trends Pharmacol Sci 19:358–365.
13. Crain SM, Shen K-F (2000a) Antagonists of excitatory opioid receptor functions enhance morphine's analgesic potency and attenuate opioid tolerance/dependence liability. Pain 84: 121–131.
14. Crain SM, Shen K-F (2000b) Enhanced analgesic potency and reduced tolerance of morphine in 129/SvEv mice: evidence for a deficiency in GM1 ganglioside-regulated excitatory opioid receptor functions. Brain Res 856:227–235.
15. Crain SM, Shen K-F (2001) Acute thermal hyperalgesia elicited by low-dose morphine in normal mice is blocked by ultra-low-dose naltrexone, unmasking potent opioid analgesia. Brain Res 888:75–82.
16. Cruciani RA, Lussier D, Miller-Saultz D, Arbuck DM (2003) Ultra-low dose oral naltrexone decreases side effects and potentiates the effect of methadone. J Pain Symptom Management 25:491–494.
17. Emmerson P, Liu M, Woods J, Medzihradsky F (1994) Binding affinity and selectivity of opioids at mu, delta and kappa receptors in monkey brain membranes. J Pharmacol Exp Ther 271:1630–1637.
18. Gan TJ, Ginsberg B, Glass PSA, Fortney J, Jhaveri R, Perno R (1997) Opioid-sparing effects of a low-dose infusion of naloxone in patient-administered morphine sulfate. Anesthesiology 87:1075–1081.
19. Gharagozlou P, Demirci H, Clark J, Lameh J (2003) Activity of opioid ligands in cells expressing cloned μ opioid receptors. BMC Pharmacology 3:1471–2210.
20. Gintzler AR, Chakrabarti S (2001) Opioid tolerance and the emergence of new opioid receptor-coupled signaling. Mol Neurobiol 21:21–33.
21. Hamman SR, Malik H, Sloan JW, Wala EP (2004) Interactions of "ultra-low" doses of naltrexone and morphine in mature and young male and female rats. Recept Chan 10:73–81.
22. Holtman JR and Wala EP (2005) Characterization of morphine-induced hyperalgesia in male and female rats. Pain 114:62–70.
23. Holtman JR and Wala EP (2006) Characterization of the antinociceptive effect of oxycodone in male and female rats. Pharmacol Biochem Behav 83:100–108.

24. Ikeda K, Kobayashi T, Kumanishi T, Niki H, Yano R (2000) Involvement of G-protein-activated inwardly rectifying K + (GIRK) channels in opioid-induced analgesia. Neurosci Res 38:113–116.
25. Jin LQ, Wang H-Y, Friedman E (2001) Stimulated D(1) dopamine receptors couple to multiple G-alpha proteins in different brain regions. J Neurochem 78:981–990.
26. Joshi GP, Duffy L, Chehade J, Wesevich J, Gajraj N, Johnson ER (1999) Effects of prophylactic nalmefene on the incidence of morphine-related side effects in patients receiving intravenous patient-controlled analgesia. Anesthesiology 90:1007–1011.
27. Kayser V, Besson JM, Guilbaud G (1987) Paradoxical hyperalgisic effect of exceedingly low doses of systemic morphine in an animal model of persistent pain (Freund's adjuvant-induced arthritis rats). Brain Res 414:155–157.
28. Kest B, Sarton E, Dahan A (2000) Gender differences in opioid-mediated analgesia. Anesthesiology 93:539–547.
29. Kiyatkin EA (1989) Morphine: some puzzles of a well-known substance. Int J Neurosci 45:231–246.
30. Largent-Milnes TM, Guo W, Wang H-Y, Burns LH, Vanderah T (2008) Oxycodone + ultra-low-dose naltrexone attenuates neuropathic pain and associated mu opioid receptor–Gs coupling. J Pain 9:700–713.
31. Laugwitz KL, Offermanns S, Spicher K, Schultz G (1993) Mu and delta opioid receptors differentially couple to G protein subtypes in membranes of human neuroblastoma SH-SY5Y cells. Neuron 10:233–242.
32. Maldonado R, Valverde O (2003) Participation of the opioid system in cannabinoid-induced antinociception and emotional like responses. Eur Neuropsychopharmacol 13:401–410.
33. Matsumoto A, Ma T, Babul N, Ahdieh H, Lee D (2002) Oxymorphine ER (20 mg and 40 mg) provides superior efficacy compared with placebo and oxycontin (20 mg) in pain associated with osteoarthritis: results of a randomized, controlled trial. In: 10th World Congress of Pain. San Diego, CA.
34. Onoprishvili I, Andria M, Kramer H, Ancevska-Taneva N, Hiller J, Simon E (2003) Interaction between the μ opioid receptor and fliamin A is involved in receptor regulation and trafficking. Mol Pharmacol 64:1092–1100.
35. Paquette J, Olmstead M (2005) Ultra-low dose naltrexone enhances cannabinoid-induced antinociception. Behav Pharmacol 16:597–603.
36. Powell KJ, Abul-Husn NS, Jhamandas A, Olmstead MC, Beninger RJ, Jhamandas K (2002) Paradoxical effects of the opioid antagonist naltrexone on morphine analgesia, tolerance, and reward in rats. J Pharmacol Exp Ther 300:588–596.
37. Roth SH, Fleischmann RM, Burch FX, Dietz R, Bockow B, Rapoport RJ, Rutstein J, Lacouture PG (2000) Around-the-clock, controlled-release oxycodone therapy for osteoarthritis-related pain. Arch Intern Med 160:853–860.
38. Saegusa H, Kurihara T, Zong S, Minowa O, Kazuno A, Han W, Matsuda Y, Yamanaka H, Osanai M, Noda T, Tanabe T (2000) Altered pain responses in mice lacking α1E subunit of the voltage-dependent Ca2 + channel. Proc Natl Acad Sci USA 97:6132–6137.
39. Shen KF, Crain SM (1989) Dual opioid modulation of the action potential duration of mouse dorsal root ganglion neurons in culture. Brain Research 491:227–242.
40. Shen K-F, Crain SM (1990) Cholera toxin-A subunit blocks opioid excitatory effects on sensory neuron action potentials indicating mediation by Gs-linked opioid receptors. Brain Research 525:225–231.
41. Shen KF, Crain SM (1994) Antagonists at excitatory opioid receptors on sensory neurons in culture increase potency and specificity of opiate analgesics and attenuate development of tolerance/dependence. Brain Res 636:286–297.
42. Shen KF, Crain SM (1995) Specific N- or C-terminus modified dynorphin and beta-endorphin peptides can selectively block excitatory opioid receptor functions in sensory neurons and unmask potent inhibitory effects of opioid agonists. Brain Res 673:30–38.

43. Shen KF, Crain SM (1997) Ultra-low doses of naltrexone or etorphine increase morphine's antinociceptive potency and attenuate tolerance/dependence in mice. Brain Res 757: 176–190.
44. Shen K-F, Crain SM, Moate P, Boston R, de Kater AW, Schoenhard GL (2002a) PTI-801, a novel formulation of oxycodone, shows absence of tolerance, physical dependence and naloxone-precipitated withdrawal effects in mice. J Pain 3:49.
45. Shen K-F, Crain SM, Moate P, Boston R, de Kater AW, Schoenhard GL (2002b) PTI-555, reverses and prevents morphine-induced tolerance and naloxone-precipitated withdrawal in mice chronically treated with morphine. J Pain 3:50.
46. Terner JM, Barrett AC, Lomas LM, Negus SS, Picker MJ (2006) Influence of low doses of naltrexone on morphine antinociception and morphine tolerance in male and female rats of four strains. Pain 122:90–101.
47. Vanderah TW, Gardell LR, Burgess SE, Ibrahim M, Zhong C-M, Ossipov MH, Lai J, Malan Jr. TP, Porreca F. (2000) Repeated spinal opioid administration produces abnormal pain and antinociceptive tolerance which is reversed by dynorphin antiserum. J Neurosci., 20: 7074–7079.
48. Vanderah TW, Suenaga NMH, Ossipov MH, Malan Jr. TP, Lai J, Porreca F. (2001) Descending facilitation from the rostral ventromedial medulla mediates opioid-induced abnormal pain and antinociceptive tolerance. J Neurosci 21:279–286.
49. Vanderah TW, Burns LH (2004) Ultra-low-dose naltrexone plus morphine blocks thermal hyperalgesia and attenuates mechanical hypersensitivity in a neuropathic pain model. In: 2nd Joint Meeting of the American and Canadian Pain Societies, Vancouver, BC.
50. Wang H-Y, Friedman E (1999) Effects of lithium on receptor-mediated activation of G proteins in rat brain cortical membranes. Neuropharmacology 38:403–414.
51. Wang H-Y, Burns LH (2006) Gβγ that interacts with adenylyl cyclase in opioid tolerance originates from a Gs protein. J Neurbiol 66:1302–1310.
52. Wang H-Y, Frankfurt M, Burns LH (2008) High-affinity naloxone binding to filamin A prevents mu opioid receptor - Gs coupling underlying opioid tolerance and dependence. PLoS One 3:e1554.
53. Wang H-Y, Friedman E, Olmstead MC, Burns LH (2005) Ultra-low-dose naloxone suppresses opioid tolerance, dependence and associated changes in Mu opioid receptor–G protein coupling and Gβγ signaling. Neuroscience 135:247–261.
54. Webster LR, Butera PG, Moran LV, Wu N, Burns LH, Friedmann N (2006) Oxytrex minimizes physical dependence while providing effective analgesia: a randomized controlled trial in low-back pain. J Pain 7:937–946.
55. Zhang S-P, Wang H-Y, Lovenberg T, Codd E (2001) Functional studies of bradykinin receptors in Chinese hamster ovary cells stably expressing the human B2 bradykinin receptor. Internat Immunopharmacol 1:955–965.
56. Zhen X, Torres C, Wang H-Y, Friedman E (2001) Protein phosphatase 1 regulates brain D1A dopamine receptor phosphorylation: role in dopaminergic dysfunction after in utero cocaine exposure. J Neurosci 21:9160–9167.

Chapter 2
Upregulation of Opioid Receptors

Ellen M. Unterwald and Richard D. Howells

Abstract It is well established that chronic exposure to opioid receptor antagonists can result in opioid receptor upregulation. The phenomenon of antagonist-induced receptor upregulation is not unique to the opioid system but is common to many receptor systems including adenergic, cholinergic, serotinergic, and dopaminergic receptors. Chronic administration of naloxone or naltrexone reliably produces increases in binding to opioid receptors both in vivo and in vitro. This receptor upregulation is associated with functional supersensitivity to subsequent agonist administration. Thus, the analgesic potency of morphine is increased following prior exposure to opioid receptor antagonists. The three opioid receptor types show different degrees of upregulation in response to in vivo antagonist administration, with μ opioid receptors showing the largest increases in binding in response to any given dose of naloxone or naltrexone, followed by more modest increases in δ and κ receptors. Antagonist-induced receptor upregulation appears to vary between brain regions, and the reason for this is not clear. Although the first demonstration of antagonist-induced opioid receptor upregulation occurred more than 30 years ago, the mechanisms mediating this effect remained elusive for much of this time. Recent data have provided new insights into potential molecular mechanisms of opioid receptor upregulation. Data are presented that support the hypothesis that naloxone and naltrexone are acting as pharmacological chaperones, stabilizing intracellular receptor protein molecules and facilitating their trafficking and insertion into the cell membrane. Finally, heterologous opioid receptor upregulation occurs in response to repeated exposure to cocaine and ethanol, and the resulting opioid receptor regulation may play an important role in craving and reinforcement induced by these agents. Given the multiple potential clinical uses of opioid receptor antagonists described in other chapters of this volume, opioid receptor upregulation and the accompanying functional supersensitivity that results from antagonist exposure needs to be further explored in the clinical setting.

E.M. Unterwald (✉) and R.D. Howells
Department of Pharmacology, Temple University School of Medicine,
3420 North Broad Street, Philadelphia, PA 19140
e-mail: ellen.unterwald@temple.edu

R. Dean et al. (eds.), *Opiate Receptors and Antagonists*,

Keywords: Upregulation; Opioid receptors; Opioid antagonist; Naltrexone; Naloxone

2.1 Introduction

Opioid receptor upregulation following exposure to opioid receptor antagonists is one of the most well-documented phenomena in the field. It was first characterized over 30 years ago in nervous tissue of rodents. One of the earliest reports of opioid receptor upregulation following opioid receptor antagonist administration came from Loh and colleagues (1) as part of a larger study on the regulation of opioid receptor binding by morphine. Binding to opioid receptors in mouse brain was significantly increased 2 and 3 days after implantation of naloxone-containing pellets. Chronic administration of opioid receptor antagonists also produce functional opioid receptor supersensitivity, and this was first reported by Tang and Collins (2) who demonstrated that long-term administration of naloxone results in enhanced morphine-induced analgesia which is accompanied by an increase in the number of [^{3}H]-naloxone binding sites (3). Shortly thereafter, Herz and colleagues (4) found that chronic exposure of guinea pigs to naloxone for 1–2 weeks caused an increase in the sensitivity to opioids in the electrically stimulated longitudinal muscle-myenteric plexus ileum preparation. Once again, the enhanced inhibitory properties of opioid agonists were associated with elevations in the number of opioid receptors as measured by [^{3}H]-etorphine binding in both the guinea pig ileum and the brainstem.

The finding that exposure to opioid receptor antagonists in rodents can increase the number of opioid receptors and enhance the pharmacological effects of opioid receptor agonists has since been replicated in cell lines expressing opioid receptors. Despite the appreciation and reproducibility of this phenomenon, the mechanisms involved in opioid receptor upregulation remain elusive. Recently, new data have provided insights into potential molecular mechanisms involved in antagonist-induced opioid receptor upregulation. This chapter will review the pharmacological characteristics of antagonist-induced opioid receptor upregulation, the accompanying functional supersensitivity, and potential mechanisms involved. In addition, upregulation of opioid receptors following administration of nonopioid drugs will also be discussed.

2.2 Opioid Receptor Upregulation Following Opioid Receptor Antagonist Administration

2.2.1 In Vivo Studies

The initial reports of naloxone-induced opioid receptor supersensitivity and upregulation were followed by more detailed characterization of this phenomenon. Antagonist-induced opioid receptor upregulation occurs following chronic administration of either naloxone or naltrexone, and the antagonists are most often administered to rodents by implanting drug-containing pellets or minipumps into the subcutaneous (sc) space. It is interesting to note that antagonist-induced upregulation of opioid receptor binding sites is observed consistently following continuous sc infusion of naloxone or naltrexone for 7 days, but not after intermittent sc injection (every 24h for 7 days) of the same daily dose (5). Another group, however, reported that intraperitoneal (ip) injection of rats with 10mg/kg of naltrexone for 15 days results in a significant increase in [^{3}H]-[D-Ala^2-MePhe^4-Gly(ol)^5] enkephalin (DAMGO) binding to μ receptors in the striatum (6).

Radioligand binding has been the most commonly used technique to measure opioid receptor upregulation. Increases in binding of nonselective opioid receptor ligands such as [^{3}H]-etorphine (7, 8) and [^{3}H]-naloxone (8), as well as some semi-selective opioid receptor ligands like [^{3}H]-dihydromorphine (μ ligand) (8), [^{3}H]-[D-Ala^2-D-Leu^5]enkephalin (DADLE, δ ligand) (8, 9), and [^{3}H]-ethylketocyclazocine (κ ligand) (7) occur following continuous exposure to naloxone or naltrexone. In all cases, increases in receptor number (B_{max}) rather than increases in receptor affinity (K_d) are apparent (7, 8, 10–14). Antagonist-induced receptor upregulation is stereospecific, as it is produced by the (–), but not the inactive (+) isomer of naloxone, indicating that the effect of naloxone is mediated by a specific interaction with opioid receptors (15). In addition, the sensitivity of agonist binding to inhibition by guanyl nucleotides (GTP) is increased significantly following chronic naltrexone administration suggesting augmented receptor coupling to heterotrimeric guanine nucleotide binding proteins (G-proteins) (8), although this has not been replicated in all studies (16). Zukin and colleagues reported that opioid binding reaches a maximum 8 days after naltrexone pellet implantation and is maintained at that level with continued exposure for up to 4 weeks (8). However, Giordano et al. (17) found that opioid receptor binding continues to increase for up to 60 days following naltrexone pellet implantation. Following withdrawal from chronic naltrexone, elevated opioid receptor levels return to control levels after 6 days (7).

With the advent of more selective opioid radioligands came better characterization of the regulation of the three individual opioid receptor types. Results using highly selective radioligands indicate that μ opioid receptors are most affected by naloxone or naltrexone administration, followed by δ opioid receptors (17–21). Naltrexone treatment increases the density of μ opioid receptors as measured by the μ receptor-selective ligand, [^{3}H]-DAMGO, by 80–100% in whole brain minus cerebellum, without altering receptor affinity (14, 16, 17). This is illustrated in Fig. 2.1 which shows a Scatchard plot analysis of the binding of [^{3}H]-DAMGO to membranes prepared from whole brain minus cerebellum from rats treated with saline or naltrexone for 7 days (Unterwald, unpublished data). In comparison to an 81% increase in μ receptors, binding to δ receptors in the same tissue sample is increased by 31% following naltrexone (17). Kappa opioid receptors are more resistant to regulation during naloxone or naltrexone administration (10, 19, 20). Thus, μ receptors are upregulated in response to lower doses of naloxone or naltrexone than are δ and κ opioid receptors (18, 22), and the degree of upregulation to any given dose of antagonist is greatest for μ and lowest for κ opioid receptors (18–20, 22). This may be due to differences in the molecular mechanisms involved in the regulation of the three types of opioid receptors (see Sect. 4) or rather due to the relative affinity of naloxone and naltrexone

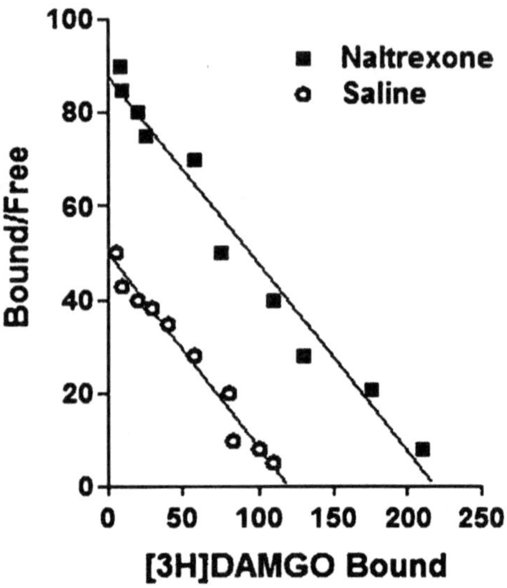

Fig. 2.1 Scatchard analysis of the binding of [^{3}H]-[D-Ala^2-MePhe^4-Gly(ol)^5] enkephalin (*DAMGO*) to mu receptors in whole brain (*minus cerebellum*) of rats exposed to saline (*open circles*) or naltrexone (8 mg/kg/day; *closed squares*) by osmotic minipumps for 7 days. Results demonstrate an 81% increase in B_{max} (120 vs 218 fmol/mg protein) following naltrexone administration. Methods are similar to those previously published (14)

for the three opioid receptors. Naloxone and naltrexone have higher affinity for μ opioid receptors than the other two opioid receptors, although their affinity at κ sites is generally reported to be greater than that for δ receptors (23, 24).

Regional analysis of naltrexone-induced opioid receptor upregulation has been performed using quantitative receptor autoradiography. Mu opioid receptors show widespread upregulation in animals exposed chronically to naltrexone or naloxone (18, 20, 25, 26). Although μ receptor upregulation occurs in most brain regions, reports are contradictory as to which areas show the greatest increase in receptor number. For example, Tempel et al. (25) report that the greatest increases in μ opioid receptor number following naltrexone administration to rats were found in brain areas associated with the A9/A10 dopamine pathway such as the nucleus accumbens, lateral septum, the patches of the striatum, amygdala, substantia nigra pars compacta, and ventral tegmental area, as well as certain nuclei in the hypothalamus and thalamus, Layer I of the neocortex and the central gray. Mu receptors were found to be elevated two- to threefold in these brain regions (25). These results are in partial agreement with those of others, with the hypothalamus, central gray, and ventral tegmental area consistently showing large increases in μ receptor binding (18, 26). However, the absolute rank order of μ receptor upregulation varies between these three papers (18, 25, 26). Chronic naltrexone exposure in the mouse results in increases in binding of the selective μ opioid receptor agonist [^{3}H]-DAMGO throughout the brain with the largest increases found in somatosensory and visual areas of the cortex. Following the cortex, the greatest increases in μ receptor binding occur in the mouse olfactory tubercle, globus pallidus, ventral pallidum, hippocampus, and hypothalamus (20).

In comparison to μ opioid receptors, upregulation of δ receptors occurs in fewer brain regions and is smaller in magnitude. In the rat, chronic naloxone produces the largest upregulation of δ opioid receptors as measured by binding of [^{3}H]-DADLE in the amygdala, striatum, claustrum, and frontal cortex (18). In the mouse brain, upregulation of δ opioid receptor as measured by [^{3}H]-deltorphin-1 binding is widespread with the largest increases noted in the lateral septum, superior colliculus, and pontine nucleus (20). In contrast, consistent upregulation of κ opioid receptors as measured by [^{3}H]-CI-977 binding is found only in cortical brain regions of the mouse and the magnitude of this response is lower than that for μ or δ receptors (20). In the rat, κ receptors as labeled by [^{3}H]-bremazocine under conditions in which binding to μ and δ receptors is suppressed were found to be upregulated in the spinal cord, hippocampus, central gray, and frontal cortex following chronic administration of a high dose of naloxone but not lower doses (18). Comparison of the effects of chronic naltrexone on μ, δ, and κ opioid receptor binding in mouse brain is shown in Fig. 2.2. In their study, quantitative receptor autoradiography was carried out using selective radioligands for the three opioid receptors on adjacent tissue sections from the same mice. Results demonstrate once again that μ receptor upregulation is most robust and widespread and κ receptors are more resistant to upregulation.

Antagonist-induced μ receptor upregulation has also been measured using immunohistochemistry by Unterwald et al. (26). Adjacent brain sections from rats exposed continuously for 7 days to naltrexone were processed for measurement of μ opioid receptors by immunohistochemistry and by receptor autoradiography with [^{3}H]-DAMGO. In agreement with other autoradiography studies (18, 25), increased binding to μ opioid receptors was widespread and occurred in the central gray, hypothalamus, interpeduncular nucleus, ventral tegmental area, amygdala, thalamus, hippocampus, and globus pallidus. However, significant increases in μ receptor

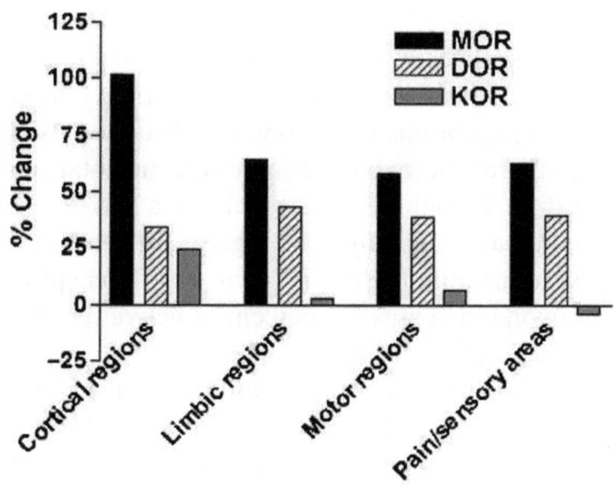

Fig. 2.2 Changes in μ (MOR), δ (DOR), and κ (KOR) opioid receptor binding in brain regions from mice exposed to naltrexone (15 mg pellet sc) for 8 days as compared with placebo pelleted controls. Receptor levels were measured by quantitative receptor autoradiography from tissue obtained 24 h after pellet removal. Results indicate that μ receptors undergo the largest upregulation in response to naltrexone treatment, whereas κ receptors were only significantly upregulated in cortical brain regions. Data adapted from Lesscher et al. (20)

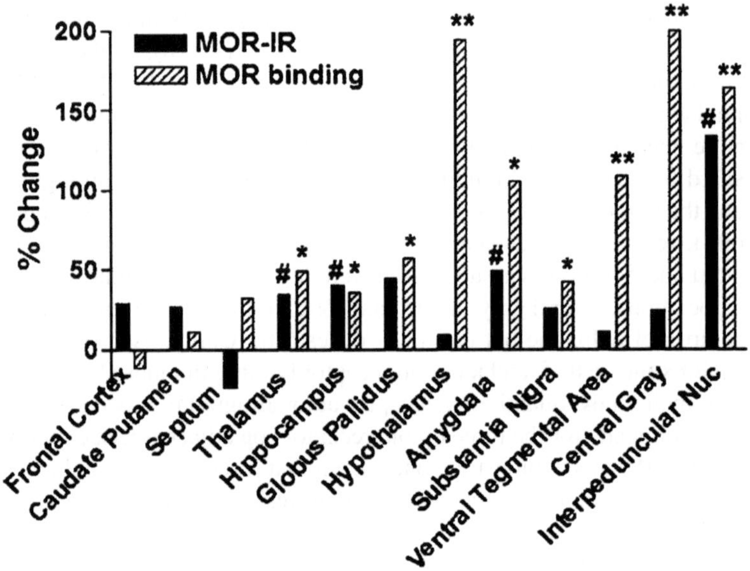

Fig. 2.3 Changes in μ receptors in various regions of rat brain following administration of naltrexone (8 mg/kg/day). Mu receptors were measured by immunoreactivity (*black bars*) or [^{3}H]-[D-Ala^2-MePhe^4-Gly(ol)^5] enkephalin (*DAMGO*) binding (*hatched bars*) on adjacent tissue sections from the same animals. Results show that increases in [^{3}H]-DAMGO binding occur in more brain regions and are generally larger in magnitude than changes in μ receptor immunoreactivity. # indicates values are significantly different from control MOR-IR levels, $p < 0.05$; * indicates values are significantly different from control MOR binding, $p < 0.05$; ** $p < 0.01$. Data adapted from Unterwald et al. (26)

immunoreactivity were limited to the interpeduncular nucleus, amygdala, hippocampus, and thalamus. Comparisons between μ receptor binding and μ receptor immunoreactivity following chronic naltrexone are illustrated in Fig. 2.3. The results indicate that chronic naltrexone exposure increases the total number of μ opioid receptors as measured by immunoreactivity only in a few brain regions, whereas μ receptor binding is increased in many brain regions. Increases in immunoreactivity are also more modest in magnitude than the increases in receptor binding, suggesting that chronic naltrexone increases the percent of active receptors without a large change in the total number of receptor molecules (26).

Opioid receptor upregulation has been well-characterized following administration of naloxone and naltrexone. In addition to these two drugs, other opioids also have been shown to produce opioid receptor upregulation in vivo. For example, Morris and Herz (27) exposed rats continuously for 7 days to bremazocine or nalorphine. Bremazocine is reported to be an agonist at κ receptors and an antagonist at μ and δ receptors (28), and nalorphine is a partial agonist at κ receptors and an antagonist at μ receptors (29, 30). Chronic administration of bremazocine results in upregulation of μ receptors, downregulation of κ receptors, and no change in δ receptors. Nalorphine produces a doubling of μ receptors and no changes in κ receptor density (27). These data demonstrate that opioid receptor upregulation and downregulation can occur simultaneously. In addition, regulation of opioid receptor expression depends on the intrinsic activity and relative receptor selectivities of the ligand.

2.2.2 *In Vitro Studies*

Upregulation of opioid receptors following antagonist exposure not only occurs in vivo, but it has also been demonstrated in vitro. In neuroblastoma-glioma NG108-15 cells which endogenously express δ opioid receptors, receptor upregulation has been found although inconsistently. For example, NG108-15 cells cultured for 48 h with naloxone showed increases in opioid receptor binding in discrete cell membrane fractions (31, 32). In contrast, Law et al. (33) found no changes in opioid receptor binding following 24-h incubation with naloxone. Binding to upregulated δ opioid receptors in naloxone-treated NG108-15 cells reported by Barg et al. was not affected by guanyl nucleotides (32). Increases in [^{3}H]-DADLE and [^{3}H]-diprenorphine binding was also found by Belcheva et al. (34) following exposure of NG108-15 cells for 48 h to naltrexone or the δ receptor antagonist ICI174864. Similar to the findings in brain, receptor number in NG108-15 cells increases without changes in receptor affinity. Upregulation of opioid receptors has been documented in the human neuroblastoma cell line SH-SY5Y which expresses μ and δ receptors at a ratio of 1.4 to 1 (35). Naloxone increases both μ and δ opioid receptor densities in a dose-dependent manner in SH-SY5Y cells (35, 36). The selective μ receptor antagonist D-Phe-Cys-Tyr-D-Trp-Arg-Thr-Pen-Thr-NH2 (CTAP) increases μ and decreases δ opioid receptor densities in these cells, whereas ICI174864 upregulates δ and to a lesser extent μ receptors (35). It has been reported that CTAP at high concentrations has intrinsic agonist activity at the δ receptor in the mouse vas deferens (37) and this might explain the downregulation of δ opioid receptors following CTAP. CTAP-induced downregulation of δ receptors is blocked by ICI174864 (35).

Antagonist-induced opioid receptor upregulation has been studied in transfected cell lines. Human embryonic kidney 293 (HEK293) cells stably expressing the murine μ opioid receptor showed significant increases in surface μ receptors using flow cytometic analysis (38). One-h treatment with naloxone produces a 16% increase in surface receptor staining and an 18-h exposure produces a 39% increase in staining. Buprenorphine, a weak partial μ agonist, also causes an upregulation of μ receptors in these cells, although the magnitude is lower than that produced by equivalent concentrations of naloxone. Addition of pertussis toxin augments the increase in surface receptor staining caused by 18 h of naloxone from 39% to 70%. Thus, pertussis toxin which inhibits the activation of Gi/Go proteins by the receptor (39) modulates the ability of the antagonist to regulate surface receptors (38). In Chinese hamster ovary (CHO) cells stably expressing the rat μ opioid receptor, naloxone increases receptor binding in whole-cell preparations in a concentration- and time-dependent manner, reaching a plateau of about 45% above control levels at

72 h (40). These data indicate that opioid receptors expressed in cell lines undergo upregulation in response to exposure to opioid receptor antagonists with similar pharmacological properties as those in the whole animal.

2.3 Functional Supersensitivity

Chronic exposure to opioid receptor antagonists not only produces an increase in the number of opioid receptor binding sites but also increases the subsequent response to opioid receptor agonists. This was first reported by Tang and Collins (2) who found that long-term treatment with naloxone results in enhanced morphine-induced analgesia and that the enhanced analgesic response is associated with an increase in receptor binding (3). Likewise, Herz and colleagues (4) found that chronic exposure of guinea pigs to naloxone for 1–2 weeks increases the sensitivity to opioids in the electrically stimulated longitudinal muscle-myenteric plexus ileum preparation. The enhanced inhibitory properties of opioid agonists occur together with elevations in the number of opioid receptors as measured by [^{3}H]-etorphine binding in both the guinea pig ileum and the brainstem.

These initial observations were followed by many other reports of functional supersensitivity to opioid receptor agonists after chronic antagonist administration. Long-term exposure to naloxone or naltrexone results in supersensitivity to morphine analgesia as demonstrated by a leftward shift in the morphine analgesic dose-response curve (10, 12, 22, 41). In agreement with the receptor binding data (7), sensitivity to morphine on analgesic tests returns to baseline levels 6 days after cessation of naltrexone administration (10, 22). Supersensitivity to other opioid analgesics also occurs including methadone, etorphine, fentanyl, meperidine, and oxycodone (13). The degree of receptor upregulation coincides with changes in agonist potency. Thus, μ and δ receptor bindings are increased by 81% and 31%, respectively, in mouse whole brain following 8 days of naltrexone administration. Consistent with the binding changes, the potency of morphine administered intracerebroventricularly (icv) to produce analgesia is increased by threefold, whereas the potency of DADLE is increased by 1.7-fold (17). In contrast to the functional supersensitivity to morphine following systemic antagonist administration, it has been shown that chronic spinal infusion of naloxone or naltrexone fails to influence the antinociceptive effect of subsequent intrathecal morphine administration on the hot plate test in rats (42).

Other effects of opioid agonists are also exaggerated following antagonist administration. Six injections of naloxone over 3 days are sufficient to produce an increase in locomotor response to subsequent morphine administration in C57Bl6 mice (43). Likewise, the hyperthermic response to acute morphine administration is enhanced following chronic naltrexone (12). Neurons in the locus coeruleus of chronic naltrexone-treated rats exhibit enhanced inhibitory responses to morphine (44). Augmented morphine withdrawal signs are seen when the morphine treatment is preceded by chronic naloxone (45). The lethality of morphine is increased 2.5-fold following chronic naltrexone treatment in the mouse (46). The ability of μ opioid receptors to activate G-proteins and subsequently inhibit cAMP production is also enhanced. Activation of G-proteins by μ opioid receptor agonists as measured by [^{35}S]GTPγS binding is augmented in mouse spinal cord following 7 days of naloxone injections (47), indicating enhanced receptor G-protein coupling. Chronic naltrexone also augments the efficacy of opioid receptor agonists to inhibit adenylyl cyclase activity (16). Taken together, these results indicate that chronic exposure to opioid receptor antagonists leads to an increase in opioid receptor number and an increase in functional opioid receptors.

2.4 Studies of the Molecular Mechanisms Involved in Antagonist-Induced Opioid Receptor Upregulation

Chronic administration of morphine or other opioid drugs for pain relief results in tolerance to the analgesic effects, and physical dependence which becomes evident in the characteristic opioid withdrawal syndrome upon abrupt cessation of drug use (48). In contrast, chronic blockade of opioid receptors with opioid antagonists such as naloxone or naltrexone does not result in physical dependence, and was shown nearly 30 years ago to be associated with supersensitivity to the analgesic actions of morphine using the tail shock-vocalization test in rats (2). As discussed above, continuous infusion of naloxone for 4 weeks in rats causes a 40% increase in the number of [^{3}H]-naloxone binding sites with no change in affinity, indicating that the enhanced analgesic effects of morphine are correlated with an increase in the number of opioid receptor binding sites (3, 4).

Opioid receptor activation regulates the activity of adenylyl cyclase, potassium channels, calcium channels, and mitogen-activated protein kinase in a pertussis toxin-sensitive manner (via G_i/G_o heterotrimeric guanine nucleotide binding proteins), therefore it was of obvious interest to determine whether antagonist-induced opioid receptor upregulation was also inhibited by the toxin. Yoburn and colleagues (49) treated mice chronically for 8 days with naltrexone with and without pertussis toxin, and the increase in [^{3}H]-DADLE binding to δ receptors and [^{3}H]-DAMGO to μ receptors was not altered in animals pretreated with pertussis toxin. Supersensitivity to morphine analgesia following naltrexone treatment, however, was blocked by pertussis toxin pretreatment, suggesting that morphine analgesia requires opioid receptor coupling to G_i/G_o heterotrimeric guanine nucleotide binding proteins while the antagonist-induced upregulation of opioid binding sites does not.

Following the molecular cloning of μ, δ, and κ opioid receptors, it became feasible to determine whether the increase in opioid binding sites following chronic antagonist treatment is associated with an increase in the steady-state level of opioid receptor mRNA. Unterwald et al. (14) found that 7-day infusion of naltrexone significantly upregulates μ opioid receptor binding rat brain; however, μ opioid receptor mRNA levels are not significantly altered in any brain region. Similar results regarding the lack of an effect of antagonist treatment on μ opioid receptor mRNA levels were reported subsequently by others (6). Jenab and Inturrisi (50) reported that treatment of NG108-15 cells (that express the δ opioid receptor endogenously) with 1 μM naloxone for 24 or 48 h causes a twofold increase in the level of δ opioid receptor mRNA as measured by solution hybridization or Northern blot analysis. Work from our laboratory, however, has not confirmed this result in NG108-15 cells using similar protocols (Wannemacher et al., submitted). Chronic treatment of mice with naltrexone for 7 days results in an eightfold increase in the antinociceptive potency of [D-Ala^2]deltorphin II as measured by the tail-flick test but does not change the levels of δ opioid receptor mRNA in any brain area tested (51). Thus, it appears that posttranscriptional mechanisms are involved in antagonist-induced opioid receptor upregulation, and that changes in the steady-state level of opioid receptor mRNAs do not occur in response to chronic antagonist treatment, either as a result of increased transcription or decreased degradation of the receptor transcripts.

A large number of human diseases, including cystic fibrosis, emphysema, and several neurological disorders, are due to inefficient protein folding resulting from amino acid substitutions, deletions, or insertions that arise from genetic mutations (52, 53). It has been observed that glycerol and other "chemical chaperones" can facilitate proper folding of the mutant cystic fibrosis transmembrane conductance regulator (54), mutant α1-antitrypsin (55), temperature-sensitive folding mutants of p53 (56), prion proteins (57), and defective aquaporin-2 associated with nephrogenic diabetes insipidus (58). It has also been found that a competitive inhibitor of lysosomal α-galactosidase A is able to accelerate the transport and maturation of the mutant form of this protein associated with Fabry disease (59).

There are also several examples in which mutant forms of G protein-coupled receptors are responsible for human diseases. Mutant rhodopsins cause retinitis pigmentosa (60), mutated forms of the luteinizing hormone receptor cause several endocrine disorders in males and females (61), mutant gonadotropin-releasing hormone receptors cause hypogonadotropic hypogonadism (62), and a large number of mutations in the vasopressin V2 receptor are responsible for X-linked nephrogenic diabetes insipidus (63). Many of these mutations cause improper folding during synthesis of the G protein-coupled receptor, and expression levels are reduced as a result of proteolysis by the endoplasmic reticulum quality control system (64). In this system, misfolded membrane proteins are deglycosylated, ubiquitinated, and then degraded by the 26S proteasome.

In an elegant study by Morello et al. (65), it was reported that selective nonpeptidic V2 vasopressin receptor antagonists increase cell-surface expression and can rescue the function of several mutant forms of the receptor that cause human X-linked nephrogenic diabetes insipidus by promoting proper folding and maturation. A cell impermeant V2 receptor antagonist is inactive in this regard, and does not block the rescue activity of the cell-permeable antagonist. The authors suggest that the active antagonists acted intracellularly as "pharmacological chaperones," by binding to and stabilizing the newly synthesized mutant receptors, thereby promoting proper folding, maturation, exit from the endoplasmic reticulum, and trafficking to the cell surface. Interestingly, the cell-permeable, active antagonist does not increase the cell surface expression of the wild-type V2 vasopressin receptor. More recently, it has been found that pharmacological chaperones can rescue mutant forms of gonadotropin-releasing hormone receptors causing hypogonadotropic hypogonadism in humans (62).

The rhopopsin family of G protein-coupled receptors, which the opioid receptors are members of, has an invariant (D/E)RY amino acid sequence located on the cytoplasmic surface of the third transmembrane domain. Substitution of the D/E in this motif with other amino acids results in constitutively active mutants of rhodopsin (66), the α_{1B}- (67) and β_2-adrenergic receptors (68), and the μ opioid receptor (69). Substitution of the aspartic acid in the DRY sequence of the μ opioid receptor with glutamine, histidine, methionine, or tyrosine completely abolishes [^{3}H]diprenorphine binding and reduces receptor expression to undetectable levels in transfected HEK293 and CHO cells; however, inclusion of naloxone in the cell culture media for 96 h greatly enhances the mutant receptor binding activity and expression levels (69). In that study, it was reported that naloxone has little or no effect on wild-type μ receptor binding or immunoreactivity in transfected HEK293 or CHO cells. The authors concluded that naloxone is acting as an inverse agonist to block the agonist-independent constitutive downregulation of the mutant receptor, and naloxone also decreases the rate of denaturation of the mutant receptor binding site (69). Liu-Chen and colleagues subsequently reported that naloxone increased [^{3}H]-diprenorphine binding and protein expression of the D164Q μ opioid receptor without affecting its mRNA level (40). Coexpression of dominant negative forms of GRK2, arrestin, dynamin, rab5A, and rab7 partially prevents the decline in [^{3}H]-diprenorphine binding following removal of naloxone from the culture media of CHO cells transfected with the mutant, and protease inhibitors also partially block the loss of [^{3}H]-diprenorphine binding after naloxone removal. It was concluded that naloxone upregulated the mutant D164Q μ receptor by stabilizing its binding site and inhibiting constitutive internalization and downregulation (40). Mutation of the analogous amino acid, D148A, in the vasopressin V_{1a} receptor also results in a misfolded but nonfunctional intracellular receptor, and the nonpeptide antagonist, SR49059, dramatically increases the cell surface expression and functionality of the mutant receptor (70). The rescue does not involve de novo receptor synthesis or preventing constitutive activity or internalization.

It has been reported that a large fraction (30%) of newly synthesized proteins are degraded by the proteasome as a result of targeting by the endoplasmic reticulum quality control system (71). Thus, not only are mutated, misfolded proteins recognized and degraded by the endoplasmic reticulum quality control, but other "normal" proteins that are intrinsically difficult and slow to fold properly during and shortly after synthesis are also subject to quality control. Studies of δ opioid receptor expression in transfected HEK293 cells reveal that as little as 40% of the newly synthesized receptors are exported out of the endoplasmic reticulum (72), and receptors retained in the endoplasmic reticulum are subsequently ubiquitinated and targeted to the proteasome (73). Chaturvedi et al. (74) demonstrated that the proteasome is also involved in both basal turnover and agonist-induced downregulation of μ and δ opioid receptors expressed in transfected HEK293 cells, and δ opioid receptors expressed endogenously in NG108-15 cells. Using pulse-chase analysis to follow newly synthesized receptors, Bouvier and colleagues found that cell-permeable opioid receptor agonists and antagonists can promote maturation and exportation of δ opioid receptors expressed in HEK293 cells from the endoplasmic reticulum through the Golgi network to the plasma membrane (75). The cell-impermeable peptide, leu-enkephalin, does not increase the efficiency of receptor maturation, and does not inhibit the action of naltrexone when administered together, suggesting that naltrexone acts intracellularly. Further evidence for an intracellular site of action for opioid receptor agonists and antagonists was provided in experiments using brefeldin A, which blocks intracellular trafficking of proteins from the Golgi apparatus to the plasma membrane (76). When transfected HEK293 cells are pulse-chased and incubated with opioid alkaloid agonists and antagonists in the presence of brefeldin A, the cell-permeable ligands stimulate the accumulation of a labeled receptor intermediate in an intracellular compartment. Bouvier and colleagues also found that the D95A substitution in the second transmembrane domain of the δ receptor results in significant retention of the receptor precursor in the endoplasmic reticulum, and that cell-permeable antagonists increase maturation and exit of the receptor from the endoplasmic reticulum and increase the cell surface expression of the mutant (75).

Chaipatikul et al. (77) report that a variety of hydrophobic antagonists and agonists can increase the cell surface expression of mutant μ opioid receptors. Deletion of the RLSKV sequence in the third intracellular loop or the KRCFR sequence in the proximal C-terminus of the rat μ opioid receptor leads to low levels of expression in transfected HEK293 cells. Naloxone causes a time- and concentration-dependent three- to fourfold increase in cell-surface expression and a fivefold increase in [^{3}H]-diprenorphine binding to the mutant receptors but has no effect on cell surface expression or binding to the wild-type μ receptor. In this study (+)-naloxone, the inactive isomer, and naloxone methiodide, the positively charged quaternary analog, lack the ability to increase cell surface expression of the mutant and wild-type μ opioid receptors (77). CTOP, the selective μ receptor peptide antagonist, has no effect on surface expression of the wild-type or mutant receptors. DAMGO, the selective μ receptor peptide agonist, morphine, and etorphine decrease the cell surface expression of the wild-type receptor, and morphine and etorphine, but not DAMGO, increase the surface expression of the μ mutant receptors. The ability of morphine to decrease the cell surface expression of the wild-type μ receptor was unexpected, since it has often been observed that morphine, unlike most other μ receptor agonists, does not stimulate internalization of the μ opioid receptor (78). With the use of confocal immunofluorescence microscopy, it was shown that the mutant μ receptors colocalize with the endoplasmic reticulum chaperone protein, calnexin, while in the presence of naloxone or etorphine, the mutated receptors are located predominantly on the cell surface (77). Brefeldin A completely blocks the action of naloxone to increase the cell surface expression of the mutant receptors, providing further evidence that the antagonist is affecting intracellular trafficking of the mutant receptors. Agonist activation of the mutant μ receptor with the RLSKV deletion does not inhibit adenylyl cyclase activity efficiently even after transfected cells are treated with naloxone; however, naloxone treatment increases the maximal inhibition of the KRCFR-deleted mutant significantly. Since the KRCFR-deleted mutant is capable of signaling to an effector upon agonist stimulation, it is not clear why that mutant receptor did not downregulate following 48-h treatment with potent agonists like etorphine, levorphanol, and methadone (77). Deletion of the RLSKV or KRCFR sequences from the μ opioid receptor do not cause the mutant receptors to become constitutively active, hence the mechanism for the mutant receptor upregulation has to differ from that proposed by Liu-Chen and colleagues (40), and Chaipatikul et al. (77) proposed that the hydrophobic μ ligands were acting like chaperones to promote intracellular trafficking of the mutant receptors.

Howells and colleagues studied antagonist-induced upregulation of the mouse δ opioid receptor using transfected HEK293 cells stably expressing FLAG-tagged receptors (79, 80). Following 24-h incubation with either naltrexone or naloxone, the B_{max} of the δ-expressing cells increases twofold as assessed by [^{3}H]-diprenorphine binding, with no apparent change in affinity. Western blot analysis following antagonist treatment revealed that there is no increase in the main immunoreactive δ receptor species migrating at 60kDa, and the level of a minor receptor form migrating at 40kDa is decreased. The 60kDa δ receptor species contains complex N-glycans, and is most likely responsible for high-affinity ligand binding. Cell surface biotinylation assays show that the 40kDa δ receptor band is located entirely intracellularly. Naltrexone does not have any affect on δ receptor mRNA as assessed by quantitative real-time PCR, or δ receptor translational efficiency as determined by [^{35}S]-methionine and cysteine incorporation. From these observations, we propose that opioid receptor antagonists facilitate the folding of a low-affinity desensitized pool of δ receptors resulting in increased binding without an increase in total immunoreactive receptor protein.

We also studied ligand-induced regulation of the FLAG-tagged rat κ opioid receptor in transfected HEK293 cells (79, 81). Receptor levels were determined following agonist or antagonist treatment by saturation analysis using [^{3}H]-diprenorphine or by Western blotting with the anti-FLAG M1 monoclonal antibody for detection. Treatment of cells expressing the κ opioid receptor with naltrexone produces a time-dependent increase in the κ opioid receptor B_{max} with no apparent change in K_d, with a maximal threefold increase at 8h. Following exposure for 24h with 1μM dynorphin A 1–13, a selective κ receptor peptide agonist, or 1μM U69593, a selective κ receptor arylacetamide agonist, κ opioid receptor levels were unaffected when determined by binding assays or Western blotting. Thus, the rat κ opioid receptor is unusual in that long-term agonist treatment does not cause receptor downregulation, as previously reported (82). To our surprise, incubation of cells with etorphine or cyclazocine, both κ receptor alkaloid agonists, *increased* κ opioid receptor immunoreactivity (81). Similar results were obtained following incubation with the antagonists, naltrexone, and naloxone. Western blot analysis revealed a time-dependent increase in a 52kDa κ opioid receptor immunoreactive species that was similar in magnitude to the increase as assessed by ligand binding. In addition, a 42kDa κ opioid receptor immunoreactive species was decreased in a time-dependent manner following treatment with these ligands. Both κ opioid receptor bands accumulate in the presence of MG132, a proteasome inhibitor, indicating that the proteasome is involved in turnover of the κ receptor. We found that the 52 kDa band bound tightly to wheat germ agglutinin-agarose, whereas the smaller species did not, indicating the larger species contains terminal N-acetylglucosamine residues. Enzymatic digestion with PNGase F and endoglycosidase H indicated that the 52 kDa κ opioid receptor species contains complex N-glycans while the 42 kDa κ opioid receptor species contains N-glycans of the high mannose type, suggesting the 42 kDa κ opioid receptor species is a precursor to the 52 kDa species, and pulse-chase analysis confirmed this (81). Naltrexone did not have any effect on κ opioid receptor mRNA as assessed by quantitative real-time PCR, or κ opioid receptor translational efficiency as determined by [^{35}S]-methionine and cysteine incorporation. Naltrexone treatment does, however, more than double the rate of conversion of the 42 kDa precursor to the mature 52 kDa species, as determined by pulse-chase analysis. Cotreatment of κ opioid receptor cells with naltrexone and brefeldin A, an inhibitor of the secretory pathway, caused the stabilization of an intracellular 46 kDa κ opioid receptor intermediate. Taken together, these results suggest that naltrexone and other select ligands upregulate κ opioid receptor by entering the cell and enhancing the rate of receptor maturation through the secretory pathway and by protecting the receptor from degradation by the proteasome. Cellular uptake studies confirm that [^{3}H]-naloxone and [^{3}H]-U69593 are cell permeable (81). Dynorphin A(1–13) cannot upregulate the κ receptor, presumably because it cannot enter the cell due to its peptidic nature; however, cell permeability is not sufficient for ligand-induced upregulation since U69593 enters the cell but does not stimulate receptor upregulation. To further confound the situation, we found that incubation of κ opioid receptor cells with naloxone methiodide, a quaternary analog of naloxone that is positively charged, increased the κ opioid receptor B_{max} to a similar extent as naloxone (81). Moreover, dynorphin did not block the upregulation induced by naloxone methiodide, suggesting that naloxone methiodide can actually enter the cell despite the common assumption that it does not.

Liu-Chen and colleagues recently published studies on ligand-induced regulation of the human κ opioid receptor expressed in CHO cells (83). It was reported that 4-h exposure to the peptide agonists, dynorphin A and B, downregulates the mature 55 kDa form of the human κ receptor by 70%, while several other nonpeptide agonists tested such as U50488H cause downregulation but to a lesser extent (20–30%). In contrast, the nonpeptide ligands etorphine (a full agonist), pentazocine (a partial agonist), and the antagonists, naloxone and norbinaltorphimine, cause a 15–25% increase in the 55 kDa κ receptor species. Pulse-chase experiments indicate that naloxone slightly increases the extent of conversion of a 45 kDa precursor to the 55 kDa mature form, with no apparent effect on the stability of the mature form following an 8-h chase. Following metabolic labeling in the presence of brefeldin A, naloxone increases the level of a 51 kDa intracellular human κ receptor intermediate. All nonpeptide agonists tested also increase the level of the 51 kDa species that appears in the presence of brefeldin, demonstrating that these agonists can also enter the cell and promote the maturation of the human κ opioid receptor. It was proposed that nonpeptide agonists cause less downregulation of the human κ opioid receptor than peptide agonists due to their pharmacological chaperone activity counteracting the extent of downregulation, although it was not clear why etorphine had such low efficacy in downregulating the receptor, particularly in the presence of brefeldin A.

Long-term exposure to nicotine elicits upregulation of nicotinic acetylcholine receptors in rodent brain and in human cigarette smokers (84–86). Sallette et al. (87) recently reported that in transfected HEK293 cells expressing human α4β2 nicotinic receptors, high mannose, glycosylated subunits mature and assemble into pentamers in the endoplasmic reticulum and only pentameric receptors reach the plasma membrane following carbohydrate processing. Nicotine was found to act intracellularly to increase assembly of pentamers. Kuryatov et al. (88) expressed human nicotinic acetylcholine receptor α4 subunits or mutant α4 subunits found in autosomal-dominant nocturnal frontal lobe epilepsy in HEK cells and studied their sensitivity to activation, rate of desensitization, and ligand-induced upregulation. Upregulation was due to an increase in assembly of nicotinic receptors from pools of subunits and from a fivefold increase in the lifetime of receptors at the cell surface. Nicotine and less permeable quaternary amine cholinergic ligands act as pharmacological chaperones in the endoplasmic reticulum to facilitate the assembly of pentameric receptors. In contrast, Green and colleagues reported that the four- to sixfold increase in binding to α4β2 nicotinic receptors following nicotine exposure does not correspond to an increase in receptors at the cell surface or a change in the assembly, trafficking or turnover of receptors at the cell surface (89). They propose that nicotine slowly stabilizes the α4β2 receptor in a high-affinity state that is more easily activated and slower to desensitize.

Taken together, the opioid receptor studies indicate that the molecular mechanism involved in ligand-induced δ and κ receptor upregulation is not associated with an increase in receptor mRNA or an increase in the efficiency of mRNA translation. Antagonists apparently act as pharmacological chaperones to facilitate the folding of a low-affinity desensitized pool of δ receptors resulting in increased binding without an increase in total cellular immunoreactive protein. Further, our results suggest that naltrexone and other select κ ligands upregulate κ opioid receptors by entering the cell and enhancing the folding and rate of receptor maturation through the secretory pathway and by protecting the receptor from degradation by the proteasome, resulting in an increase in the number of κ receptor binding sites and an increase in the level of κ receptor immunoreactive protein at the cell surface, as shown in the model displayed in Fig. 2.4.

2.5 Opioid Receptor Upregulation Induced by Nonopioid Drugs

Upregulation of opioid receptor number and function following chronic opioid receptor antagonist administration is well documented, as described in the preceding sections. Other classes of drugs have also been shown to produce an upregu-

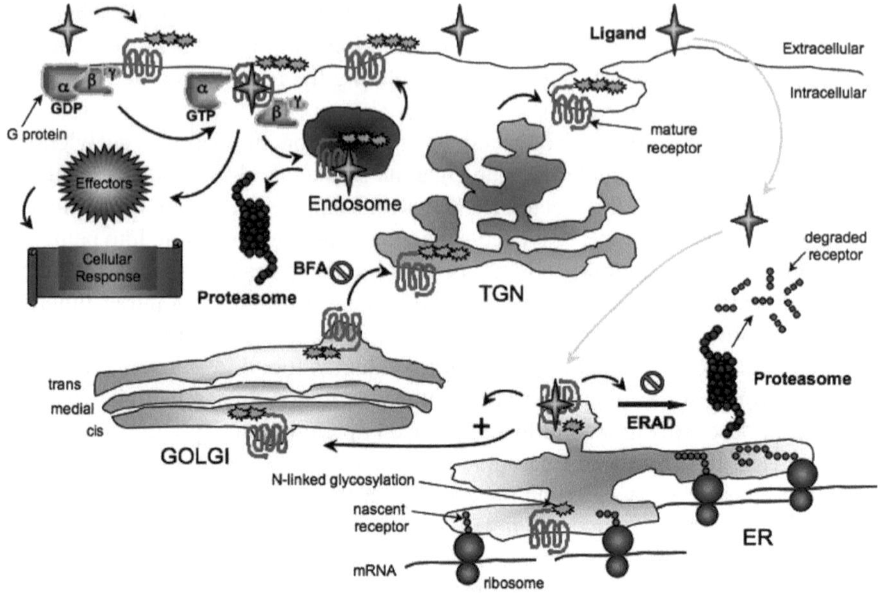

Fig. 2.4 Ligand-induced regulation of the kappa opioid receptor. The kappa opioid receptor is synthesized and partially glycosylated in the rough endoplasmic reticulum (*ER*). Proper receptor folding is monitored in the ER, and misfolded receptors are removed by the proteasome-dependent endoplasmic reticulum-associated degradation (*ERAD*) machinery. Evidence suggests that receptor upregulation is mediated by kappa ligands that enter the cell and engage incompletely processed receptor intermediates in the ER, thereby stimulating proper folding and transport to the Golgi, and limiting proteolysis by ERAD. Correctly folded receptors traverse the Golgi where they are further processed, then pass to the trans-Golgi network (*TGN*) where receptor maturation is completed, before vesicle-mediated insertion in the plasma membrane. Brefeldin A (*BFA*) inhibits transport from the Golgi apparatus to the TGN, and causes fusion of the Golgi and ER compartments. Mature receptors on the cell surface interact with kappa agonists to stimulate G-protein activation and effector regulation, leading to altered cellular responses. Activated receptors undergo endocytosis and are subsequently either recycled back to the plasma membrane or are degraded (receptor downregulation)

lation of opioid receptors, including dopaminergic agents. For example, in vivo administration of cocaine can profoundly affect the expression and function of opioid receptors. Cocaine administered to rats for 14 days results in an increase in μ and κ opioid receptors as measured by quantitative receptor autoradiography (90–92). Unlike the effects of naltrexone or naloxone, cocaine-induced opioid receptor upregulation is regionally confined, such that cocaine causes an increase in μ opioid receptors only in the basolateral amygdala, the rostral aspects of the cingulate cortex, caudate putamen, and nucleus accumbens. Kappa opioid receptors are significantly increased in the cingulate cortex, rostral caudate putamen, caudal olfactory tubercle, and ventral tegmental area. In contrast, significant regulation of δ opioid receptors does not occur following chronic cocaine administration (91). The brain regions that show the greatest regulation of opioid receptors following cocaine administration are regions that contain major dopaminergic pathways. Since cocaine inhibits the reuptake of dopamine thereby acting as an indirect agonist at dopamine receptors, these results suggest that alterations in dopaminergic neurotransmission may play a role in the regulation of μ and κ opioid receptors. In support of this, chronic administration of the D2 dopamine receptor agonist quinpirole also produces an upregulation of μ, but not δ opioid receptors in mouse striatum, whereas chronic administration of the selective D1 receptor agonist SKF38393 is ineffective in altering opioid receptor binding (93). Conversely, administration of a D2 receptor antagonist can reduce levels of striatal μ opioid receptors (94), possibly due to an increase in striatal enkephalin (95, 96). Immunohistochemistry at the electron microscope level has demonstrated that μ opioid and D2 dopamine receptors are coexpressed in individual neurons of the striatum (97), permitting the possibility of an intracellular mechanism for μ receptor regulation by D2 receptor activation.

Cocaine-induced μ receptor upregulation is both dose-dependent and time-dependent with time course studies indicating that chronic administration of cocaine (7 or, in most cases 14 days) is needed to produce an upregulation in μ opioid receptor binding (92) and that acute cocaine is without effect (92, 98). Interestingly, however, increases in μ receptor function as measured by activation of G-proteins, is seen earlier, after only 3 days of binge-pattern cocaine administration in the striatum (99). The upregulation of μ opioid receptors following binge-pattern cocaine persists for at least 14 days after cocaine cessation (100).

The schedule of cocaine administration can influence the extent of opioid receptor regulation. Comparison of 30 mg/kg cocaine given as a single daily injection versus two 15 mg/kg injections spaced 12 h apart versus three 10 mg/kg injections given at 1-h intervals (binge-pattern) demonstrated that cocaine administered in a binge-pattern produced the greatest degree of opioid receptor upregulation (101), suggesting that frequency of administration is important to the degree of receptor regulation. It has been shown that continuous administration of cocaine delivered by subcutaneously implanted minipumps also increases μ opioid receptor binding in rat brain (102, 103). The pattern of receptor regulation across brain regions varies with the dose and method of drug delivery, although upregulation of μ opioid receptors in the nucleus accumbens appears to be a consistent finding.

In addition to occurring in rodents, opioid receptor upregulation following cocaine exposure also occurs in humans and may play a role in cocaine addiction. Binding to μ opioid receptors was measured in cocaine-dependent men and nonaddicted control subjects using positron emission tomography (PET) with the selective μ receptor ligand [^{11}C]-carfentanil (104, 105). Results from these studies show that μ opioid receptor binding is significantly increased in several brain regions of the cocaine-addicted persons when studied 1–4 days after their last use of cocaine. Binding to μ opioid receptors is increased in the caudate nucleus, thalamus, cingulate cortex, frontal cortex, and temporal cortex. Interestingly, self-reports of craving for cocaine collected at the time of the PET scan were positively correlated with μ receptor binding in the amygdala, anterior cingulate cortex, frontal cortex, and temporal cortex (104). After an additional 4 weeks of monitored drug abstinence, μ receptor binding remained increased in most brain regions, although there was no longer a significant correlation with cocaine craving (104). Elevations in μ receptor binding in the anterior cingulate and anterior frontal cortex are still evident after 12 weeks of cocaine abstinence (105). Binding to μ opioid receptors is significantly correlated with the percentage of days of cocaine use and amount of cocaine used per day during the 2 weeks before the first scan and also with urine cocaine metabolite (benzoylecgonine) concentrations at the time of the first scan (105), suggesting a significant dose–response relationship between cocaine and μ receptor changes.

Tissue from postmortem human brains has been used to investigate the regulation of opioid receptors in cocaine-exposed individuals. In contrast to the findings from the PET studies, Hurd and Herkenham (106) report decreases in binding to μ opioid receptors in the caudate nucleus and putamen of persons who have died with positive urine toxicologies for cocaine. The disparate findings between the two studies could be due to methodological issues in measuring binding to μ receptors in living humans versus postmortem tissue. Differences may also be attributed to the differences in duration of cocaine use and amount of cocaine used, as it was found that these factors are significantly correlated with μ receptor upregulation (105). Another potential confound is that many of the postmortem samples came from persons who also tested positive for other drugs such as ethanol (106) which is known to influence the endogenous opioid system (107; 98; see discussion below). In another study using postmortem human brain tissue, binding to κ_2 receptors in the nucleus accumbens and other limbic brain regions was found to be twofold higher in fatal cocaine overdose victims than in age-matched and drug-free control subjects (108). The authors suggest that upregulation of κ opioid receptors may underlie in part the dysphoric mood and psychological distress associated with abrupt withdrawal of cocaine. Similar increases in binding to κ opioid receptors in striatum of human cocaine addicts were reported by Hurd and Herkenham (106). Taken together, these studies demonstrate that opioid receptors can be modulated by cocaine exposure and suggest a potential role of the endogenous opioid system in cocaine addiction.

Heterologous opioid receptor upregulation has also been shown to occur in response to ethanol both in animals and in cell lines. In contrast to the effects of cocaine, ethanol appears to have its greatest effects on δ opioid receptors. Early studies demonstrated that brains obtained from mice fed an ethanol-containing diet for 5 days had altered binding of [^{3}H]-DADLE, without a change in [^{3}H]-naloxone binding (109). In the mouse neuroblastoma-rat glioma hybrid cell line, NG108-15, exposure to high concentrations of ethanol (200 mM) increases opioid receptor binding after 18–24 h, whereas lower concentrations (25–50 mM) produces similar changes after 2 weeks. Opioid receptor density increases by twofold without a change in receptor affinity (110). Ethanol-induced opioid receptor upregulation is accompanied by an increase in receptor function, as shown by a 3.5-fold increase in the potency of etorphine for inhibiting phenylisopropyladenosine-stimulated cAMP accumulation (111). Subsequent studies found that δ opioid receptor mRNA transcript levels in NG108-15 cells are increased two- to threefold after exposure to

200 mM ethanol (50, 112). Delta opioid receptor mRNA levels peak at 24–48 h after ethanol exposure (50).

More recent work in rodents had yielded mixed results. Increases in binding of the selective δ receptor agonist, [^{3}H]-[D-Pen2, D-Pen5]-enkephalin (DPDPE), have been reported in rats exposed to acute ethanol. Using quantitative receptor autoradiography with [^{3}H]-DPDPE, δ opioid receptor upregulation was found in dopaminergic brain regions 1–2 h after acute ethanol administration by the oral route (2.5 g/kg) (113). In contrast, using receptor autoradiography Rosin and colleagues (98) found no changes in [^{3}H]-deltorphin-I binding to δ receptors 3 h after an acute administration of ethanol by the ip route (2 g/kg) (98). Other studies have shown that chronic exposure to ethanol, for example, given in the drinking water for 1 week to 1 month, does not alter δ receptor binding in the striatum of rat brain (114) or brain or spinal cord of the mouse (115). Changes in opioid receptor function, however, have been noted including a 1.6- to 2-fold decrease in the analgesic potency of morphine and the δ opioid receptor agonist DSLET in the mouse talk flick assay (115), as well as alterations in DADLE-inhibited adenylyl cyclase activity (116). However, others have found no changes in δ receptor-mediated G-protein activity in rats allowed to self-administer ethanol for 1 month (117). Using the alternative approach of measuring opioid receptors by immunohistochemical analysis on brain sections, Saland et al. (118) noted increases in immunoreactive δ opioid receptors in the hippocampus of rats that consumed ethanol in their diet, whereas μ opioid receptors were decreased in multiple brain regions (118). The disparate results may lie in the method used to measure opioid receptor levels, that is, radioligand binding versus immunohistochemisty. In any case, this topic will continue to receive attention because the endogenous opioid system has been implicated in playing a role in high ethanol consumption and ethanol reinforcement (119, 120) and the opioid receptor antagonist, naltrexone, is approved by the FDA for the treatment of alcoholism (121).

2.6 Summary and Conclusions

Opioid receptor upregulation induced by chronic administration of opioid receptor antagonists is robust and reproducible. Chronic exposure to opioid receptor antagonists increases the number of opioid receptor binding sites without altering receptor affinity. Mu opioid receptors show the largest degree of upregulation following any given dose of naloxone or naltrexone followed by δ opioid receptors, whereas κ receptor are more resilient to antagonist-induced upregulation. Opioid receptor upregulation appears to mediate the behavioral supersensitivity to subsequent opioid receptor agonist administration. There is an increase in potency of morphine and other opioid agonists including etorphine, fentanyl, meperidine, methadone, and oxycodone to produce analgesia following chronic exposure to naloxone or naltrexone. Many other effects of morphine are also increased following chronic antagonist administration including lethality, respiratory depression, inhibition of locus coeruleus neurons, and stimulation of locomotor activity. The increase in morphine potency on these behavioral and physiological measures following opioid receptor antagonist exposure indicates that the upregulated receptors are fully functional and physiologically relevant. Further, the degree of upregulation of μ and δ receptors parallels the shift in analgesic potency of μ and δ receptor agonists.

Despite the long-held appreciation that opioid receptor antagonists can produce receptor upregulation and functional supersensitivity, elucidation of the molecular mechanisms responsible for this upregulation has proven to be more difficult. Both in brain and in cells lines that express opioid receptors, antagonist-induced opioid receptor upregulation does not appear to be mediated by increases in transcription, as there are no changes in the steady-state levels of opioid receptor mRNAs in response to chronic antagonist treatments. Therefore, it appears that posttranscriptional mechanisms are involved in antagonist-induced opioid receptor upregulation. Recent data generated in cell lines support the hypothesis that opioid receptor antagonists act as pharmacological chaperones that bind to and stabilize newly synthesized or internalized receptors (75, 77, 81, 83). This promotes proper protein folding, maturation, exit from the endoplasmic reticulum, and trafficking to the cell surface. We have shown that κ receptor upregulation is associated with an increase in receptor binding sites and an increase in receptor immunoreactivity; however, upregulation of the δ opioid receptor differs: there is an increase in δ receptor binding sites without a concomitant increase in receptor immunoreactivity. Further work is necessary to elucidate the mechanisms involved in upregulation of the δ receptor.

Drugs other than opioid receptor antagonists can also produce opioid receptor upregulation. It has been established that chronic exposure to cocaine can increase μ opioid receptor number in specific brain regions. This occurs not only in animal models but also in human cocaine abusers. Importantly, PET studies in humans have demonstrated that the level of μ opioid receptor binding in specific brain regions is positively correlated to the degree of craving for cocaine. These results suggest that chronic cocaine use in humans can influence the endogenous opioid system and that these changes may be related to cocaine-induced craving and reinforcement. Ethanol can also produce changes in opioid receptor binding. Studies in animals and cell lines indicate that ethanol can increase delta opioid receptor binding, and studies in alcohol-dependent humans suggest a link between opioid receptor levels and craving for alcohol.

As reviewed in other chapters of this book, opioid receptor antagonists have the potential to be used for a variety of clinical indications. If used chronically, opioid receptor upregulation is a possible sequelae of treatment with such agents. With receptor upregulation, functional supersensitivity to subsequent opioid agonist exposure may occur, and this should be considered when designing treatment regimens for the clinical use of opioid receptor antagonists.

Acknowledgments We thank the editors, Drs. Dean, Bilsky, and Negus, for their efforts in assembling this vast volume of scientific literature. E. M. Unterwald acknowledges Dr. Mary Jeanne Kreek for her role in many of the studies presented herein. R. D. Howells acknowledges the contributions of Kenneth Wannemacher and Prem Yadav to the research performed in his laboratory. This work was supported in part from grants from NIH/NIDA, P50 DA05130 (MJK), DA09580 (EMU), and DA09113 (RDH).

References

1. Hitzemann RJ, Hitzemann BA, Loh HH. Binding of 3H-naloxone in the mouse brain: effect of ions and tolerance development. Life Sci. 1974;14:2393–2404.
2. Tang AH, Collins RJ. Enhanced analgesic effects of morphine after chronic administration of naloxone in the rat. Eur. J. Pharmacol. 1978;47:473–474.
3. Lahti RA, Collins RJ. Chronic naloxone results in prolonged increases in opiate binding sites in brain. Eur. J. Pharmacol. 1978;51:185–186.
4. Schulz R, Wuster M, Herz A. Supersensitivity to opioids following the chronic blockade of endorphine action by naloxone. Naunyn Schmiedebergs Arch. Pharmacol. 1979;306:93–96.
5. Yoburn BC, Purohit V, Patel K, Zhang Q. Opioid agonist and antagonist treatment differentially regulates immunoreactive μ-opioid receptors and dynamin-2 in vivo. Eur. J. Pharmacol. 2004;498:87–96.
6. Castelli MP, Melis M, Mameli M, Fadda P, Diaz G, Gessa GL. Chronic morphine and naltrexone fail to modify μ-opioid receptor mRNA levels in the rat brain. Mol. Brain Res. 1997;45:149–153.
7. Tempel A, Zukin RS, Gardner EL. Supersensitivity of brain opiate receptor subtypes after chronic naltrexone treatment. Life Sci. 1982;31:1401–1404.
8. Zukin RS, Sugarman JR, Fitz-Syage ML, Gardner EL, Zukin SR, Gintzler AR. Naltrexone-induced opiate receptor supersensitivity. Brain Res. 1982;245:285–292.
9. Yoburn BC, Nunes FA, Adler B, Pasternak GW, Inturrisi CE. Pharmacodynamic supersensitivity and opioid receptor upregulation in the mouse. J. Pharmacol. Exp. Ther. 1986;239:132–135.
10. Tempel A, Gardner EL, Zukin RS. Neurochemical and functional correlates of naltrexone-induced opiate receptor up-regulation. J. Pharmacol. Exp. Ther. 1985;232:439–444.
11. Attali B, Vogel Z. Characterization of kappa opiate receptors in rat spinal cord-dorsal root ganglion co-cultures and their regulation by chronic opiate treatment. Brain Res. 1990;517: 182–188.
12. Bhargava HN, Matwyshyn GA, Reddy PL, Veeranna. Effects of naltrexone on the binding of [3H]D-Ala2, MePhe4, Gly-ol5-enkepahlin to brain regions and spinal cord and pharmacological responses to morphine in the rat. Gen. Pharmacol. 1993;24:1351–1357.
13. Yoburn BC, Shah S, Chan K, Duttaroy A, Davis T. Supersensitivity to opioid analgesics following chronic opioid antagonist treatment: relationship to receptor selectivity. Pharmacol. Biochem. Behav. 1995;51:535–539.
14. Unterwald EM, Rubenfeld JM, Imai Y, Wang J-B, Uhl GR, Kreek MJ. Chronic opioid antagonist administration upregulated mu opioid receptor binding without altering mu opioid receptor mRNA levels. Mol. Brain Res. 1995;33:351–355.
15. Tempel A, Crain SM, Peterson ER, Simon EJ, Zukin RS. Antagonist-induced opiate receptor upregulation in cultures of fetal mouse spinal cord-ganglion explants. Dev. Brain Res. 1986;25:287–291.
16. Cote TE, Izenwasser S, Weems HB. Naltexone-induced upregulation of mu opioid receptors on 7315c cell and brain membranes: enhancement of opioid efficacy in inhibiting adenylyl cyclase. J. Pharmacol. Exp. Ther. 1993;267:238–244.
17. Giordano AL, Nock B, Cicero TJ. Antagonist-induced up-regulation of the putative epsilon opioid receptor in rat brain: comparison with kappa, mu and delta opioid receptors. J. Pharmacol. Exp. Ther. 1990;255:536–540.
18. Morris BJ, Millan MJ, Herz A. Antagonist-induced opioid receptor up-regulation. II. Regionally specific modulation of mu, delta and kappa binding sites in rat brain revealed by quantitative autoradiography. J. Pharmacol. Exp. Ther. 1988;247:729–736.

19. Yoburn BC, Luke MC, Pasternak GW, Inturrisi CE. Upregulation of opioid receptor subtypes correlates with potency changes of morphine and DADLE. Life Sci. 1988;43:1319–1324.
20. Lesscher HMB, Bailey A, Burbach JPH, van Ree JM, Kitchen I, Gerrits MAFM. Receptor-selective changes in μ-, δ- and κ-opioid receptors after chronic naltrexone treatment in mice. Eur. J. Neurosci. 2003;17:1006–1012.
21. Hummel M, Ansonoff MA, Pintar JE, Unterwald EM. Genetic and pharmacological manipulation of μ opioid receptors in mice reveals a differential effect on behavioral sensitization to cocaine. Neurosci. 2004;125:211–220.
22. Millan MJ, Morris BJ, Herz A. Antagonist-induced opioid receptor up-regulation. I. Characterization of supersensitivity to selective mu and kappa agonists. J. Pharmacol. Exp. Ther. 1988;247:721–728.
23. Goldstein A, Naidu A. Multiple opioid receptors: ligand selectivity profiles and binding site signatures. Mol. Pharmacol. 1989;36:265–272.
24. Raynor K, Kong H, Chen Y, Yasuda K, Yu L, Bell GI, Reisine T. Pharmacological characterization of the cloned kappa-, delta-, and mu-opioid receptors. Mol. Pharmacol. 1994; 45:330–334.
25. Tempel A, Gardner EL, Zukin RS. Visualization of opiate receptor upregulation by light microscopy autoradiography. Proc. Natl. Acad. Sci. USA 1984;81:3893–3897.
26. Unterwald EM, Anton B, To T, Lam H, Evans CJ. Quantitative immuno-localization of mu-opioid receptors: regulation by naltrexone. Neuroscience 1998;85:897–905.
27. Morris BJ, Herz A. Control of opiate receptor number in vivo: simultaneous κ-receptor down-regulation and μ-receptor up-regulation following chronic agonist/antagonist treatment. Neuroscience 1989;29:433–442.
28. Corbett AD, Kosterlitz HW. Bremazocine is an agonist at κ-opioid receptors and an antagonist at μ-opioid receptors in the guinea-pig myenteric plexus. Br. J. Pharmacol. 1986; 89:245–249.
29. Miller L, Shaw JS, Whiting EM. The contribution of intrinsic activity to the action of opioids in vitro. Br. J. Pharmacol. 1986;87:595–601.
30. Hayes A, Kelly A. Profile of activity of κ receptor agonists in the rabbit vas deferens. Eur. J. Pharmacol. 1985;111:317–322.
31. Baram D, Simantov R. Enkephalins and opiate antagonists control calmodulin distribution in neuroblastoma-glioma cells. J. Neurochem. 1983;40:55–63.
32. Barg J, Levy R, Simantov R. Up-regulation of opiate receptors by opiate antagonists in neuroblastoma-glioma cell culture: the possibility of interaction with guanosine triphosphate-binding proteins. Neurosci. Lett. 1984;50:133–137.
33. Law PY, Hom DS, Loh HH. Opiate receptor down-regulation and desensitization in neuroblastoma X glioma NG108-15 hybrid cells are two separate cellular adaptation processes. Mol. Pharmacol. 1983;24:413–424.
34. Belcheva MM, Barg J, McHale RJ, Gao XM, Chuang DM, Coscia CJ. Up-regulation of delta opioid receptors in neuroblastoma hybrid cells: evidence for differences in the mechanisms of action of sodium butyrate and naltrexone. J. Pharmacol. Exp. Ther. 1991;259:302–309.
35. Zadina JE, Harrison LM, Ge LJ, Kastin AJ, Chang SL. Differential regulation of mu and delta opiate receptors by morphine selective agonists and antagonists and differentiating agents in SH-SY5Y human neuroblastoma cells. J. Pharmacol. Exp. Ther. 1994;270:1086–1096.
36. Zadina JE, Chang SL, Ge LJ, Kastin AJ. Mu opiate receptor down-regulation by morphine and up-regulation by naloxone in SH-SY5Y human neuroblastoma cells. J. Pharmacol. Exp. Ther. 1993;265:254–262.
37. Kramer T, Shook J, Kazmierski W, Ayres E, Wire W, Hruby V, Burks T. Novel peptidic mu opioid antagonists: pharmacologic characterization in vitro and in vivo. J. Pharmacol. Exp. Ther. 1989;249:544–548.
38. Zaki PA, Keith DE, Brine GA, Carroll FI, Evans CJ. Ligand-induced changes in surface μ-opioid receptor number: relationship to G protein activation. J. Pharmacol. Exp. Ther. 2000;292:1127–1134.

39. Kurose H, Katada T, Amano T, Ui M. Specific uncoupling by islet-activating protein, pertussis toxin, of negative signal transduction via α-adrenergic, cholinergic, and opiate receptors in neuroblastoma x glioma hybrid cells. J. Biol. Chem. 1983;258:4870–4875.
40. Li J, Chen C, Huang P, Liu-Chen LY. Inverse agonist up-regulates the constitutively active D3.49(164)Q mutant of the rat μ-opioid receptor by stabilizing the structure and blocking constitutive internalization and down-regulation. Mol. Pharmacol. 2001;60:1064–1075.
41. Yoburn BC, Sierra V, Lutfy K. Chronic opioid antagonist treatment: assessment of receptor upregulation. Eur. J. Pharmacol. 1989;170:193–200.
42. Stevens CW, Yaksh TL. Chronic antagonist infusion does not increase morphine antinociception in rat spinal cord. Brain Res. 1987;425:388–390.
43. Volterra BN, DiGiulio AM, Cuomo V, Racagni G. Modulation of opioid system in C57 mice after repeated treatment with morphine and naloxone: biochemical and behavioral correlates. Life Sci. 1984;34:1669–1678.
44. Bardo MT, Bhatnagar RK, Gebhart GF. Chronic naltrexone increases binding in brain and produces supersensitivity to morphine in the locus coeruleus of the rat. Brain Res. 1983; 289:223–234.
45. Suzuki T, Fukagawa Y, Misawa M. Enhancement of morphine withdrawal signs in the rat after chronic treatment with naloxone. Eur. J. Pharmacol. 1990;178:239–242.
46. Yoburn BC, Nunes FA, Adler B, Pasternak GW, Inturrisi CE. Pharmacodynamic supersensitivity and opioid receptor upregulation in the mouse. J. Pharmacol. Exp. Ther. 1986;239: 132–135.
47. Narita M, Mizoguchi H, Nagase H, Suzuki T, Tseng LF. Up-regulation of spinal μ-opioid receptor function to activate G-protein by chronic naloxone treatment. Brain Res. 2001;913: 170–173.
48. McQuay H. Opioids in pain management. Lancet 1999;353:2229–2232.
49. Chang SC, Lutfy K, Sierra V, Yoburn BC. Dissociation of opioid receptor upregulation and functional supersensitivity. Pharmacol. Biochem. Behav. 1991;38:853–859.
50. Jenab S, Inturrisi CE. Ethanol and naloxone differentially upregulate delta opioid receptor gene expression in neuroblastoma hybrid (NG108-15) cells. Mol. Brain Res. 1994;27:95–102.
51. Jenab S, Kest B, Inturrisi CE. Assessment of delta opioid antinociception and receptor mRNA levels in mouse after chronic naltrexone treatment. Brain Res. 1995;691:69–75.
52. Thomas PJ, Qu B, Pederson PI. Defective protein folding as a basis of human disease. Trends Biochem. Sci. 1995;20:456–459.
53. Welch WJ, Howard M. Antagonists to the rescue. J. Clin. Invest. 2000;105:853–854.
54. Sato S, Ward CL, Krouse ME, Wine JJ, Kopito RR. Glycerol reverses the misfolding phenotype of the most common cystic fibrosis mutation. J. Biol. Chem. 1996;271:635–638.
55. Burrows JA, Willis LK, Perlmutter DH. Chemical chaperones mediate increased secretion of mutant alpha 1-antitrypsin (alpha 1-AT) Z: a potential pharmacological strategy for prevention of liver injury and emphysema in alpha 1-AT deficiency. Proc. Natl. Acad. Sci. USA 2000;97:1796–1801.
56. Brown CR, Hong-Brown LQ, Welch WJ. Correcting temperature-sensitive protein folding defects. J. Clin. Invest. 1997;99:1432–44.
57. Tatzelt J, Prusiner SB, Welch WJ. Chemical chaperones interfere with the formation of scrapie prion protein. EMBO J. 1996;15:6363–6373.
58. Tamarappoo BK, Verkman AS. Defective aquaporin-2 trafficking in nephrogenic diabetes insipidus and correction by chemical chaperones. J. Clin. Invest. 1998;101:2257–2267.
59. Fan J-Q, Ishii S, Asano N, Suzuki Y. Accelerated transport and maturation of lysosomal α-galactosidase A in Fabry lymphoblasts by an enzyme inhibitor. Nat. Med. 1999;5(1):112–115.
60. Sung C-H, Schneider BG, Agarwal N, Papermaster DS, Nathans J. Functional heterogeneity of mutant rhodopsins responsible for autosomal dominant retinitis pigmentosa. Proc. Natl. Acad. Sci. USA 1991;88:8840–8844.
61. Latronico AC, Segaloff DL. Naturally occurring mutations of the luteinizing hormone receptor: lessons learned about reproductive physiology and G protein-coupled receptors. Am. J. Hum. Genet. 1999;65:949–958.

62. Leanos-Miranda A, Ulloa-Aguirre A, Janovick JA, Conn PM. In vitro coexpression and pharmacological rescue of mutant gonadotropin-releasing hormone receptors causing hypogonadotropic hypogonadism in humans expressing compound heterozygous alleles. J. Clin. Endocrinol. Metab. 2005;90:3001–3008.
63. Oksche A, Rosenthal W. The molecular basis of nephrogenic diabetes insipidus. J. Mol. Med. 1998;76:327–337.
64. Ellgaard L, Helenius A. Quality control in the endoplasmic reticulum. Nat. Rev. Mol. Cell. Biol. 2003;4:181–191.
65. Morello J-P, Salahpour A, Laperriere A, Bernier V, Arthus M-F, Lonergan M, Petaja-Repo U, Angers S, Morin D, Bichet DG, Bouvier M. Pharmacological chaperones rescue cell-surface expression and function of misfolded V2 vasopressin receptor mutants. J. Clin. Invest. 2000; 105:887–895.
66. Cohen GB, Yang T, Robinson PR, Oprian DD. Constitutive activation of opsin: influence of charge at position 134 and size at position 296. Biochemistry 1993;32:6111–6115.
67. Scheer A, Fanelli F, Costa T, De Benedetti PG, Cotecchia S. Constitutively active mutants of the α_{1B}-adrenergic receptor: role of highly conserved polar amino acids in receptor activation. EMBO J. 1996;15:3566–3578.
68. Rasmussen SGF, Jensen AD, Liapakis G, Ghanouni P, Javitch JA, Gether U. Mutation of a highly conserved aspartic acid in the β_2-adrenergic receptor: constitutive activation, structural instability, and conformational rearrangement of transmembrane segment 6. Mol. Pharmacol. 1999;56:175–184.
69. Li J, Huang P, Chen C, de Riel JK, Weinstein H, Liu-Chen LY. Constitutive activation of the μ opioid receptor by mutation of D3.49(164), but not D3.32(147): D3.49(164) is critical for stabilization of the inactive form of the receptor and for its expression. Biochemistry 2001;40:12039–12050.
70. Hawtin SR. Pharmacological chaperone activity of SR49059 to functionally recover misfolded mutations of the vasopressin V_{1a} receptor. J. Biol. Chem. 2006;281:14604–14614.
71. Schubert U, Anton LC, Gibbs J, Norbury CC, Yewdell JW, Bennink JR. Rapid degradation of a large fraction of newly synthesized proteins by the proteasome. Nature 2000;404:770–774.
72. Petaja-Repo UE, Hogue M, Laperriere A, Walker P, Bouvier M. Export from the endoplasmic reticulum represents the limiting step in the maturation and cell surface expression of the human δ opioid receptor. J. Biol. Chem. 2000;275:13727–13736.
73. Petaja-Repo UE, Hogue M, Laperriere A, Bhalla S, Walker P, Bouvier M. Newly synthesized human δ opioid receptors retained in the endoplasmic reticulum are retrotranslocated to the cytosol, deglycosylated, ubiquitinated and degraded by the proteasome. J. Biol. Chem. 2001;276:4416–4423.
74. Chaturvedi K, Bandari P, Chinen N, Howells RD. Proteasome involvement in agonist-induced down regulation of mu and delta opioid receptors. J. Biol. Chem. 2001;276:12345–12355.
75. Petaja-Repo UE, Hogue M, Bhalla S, Laperriere A, Morello JP, Bouvier M. Ligands act as pharmacological chaperones and increase the efficiency of δ opioid receptor maturation. EMBO J. 2002;21:1628–1637.
76. Lippincott-Schwartz J, Yuan LC, Bonifacino JS, Klausner RD. Rapid redistribution of Golgi proteins into the ER in cells treated with brefeldin A: evidence for membrane cycling from Golgi to ER. Cell 1989;56:801–813.
77. Chaipatikul V, Erickson-Herbrandson LJ, Loh HH, Law P-Y. Rescuing the traffic-deficient mutants of rat μ-opioid receptors with hydrophobic ligands. Mol. Pharmacol. 2003;64:32–41.
78. Keith DE, Anton B, Murray SR, Zaki PA, Chu PC, Lissin DV, Montellet-Agius G, Stewart PI, Evans CJ, von Zastrow M. μ-Opioid receptor internalization: opiate drugs have differential effects on conserved endocytic mechanism in vitro and in the mammalian brain. Mol. Pharmacol. 1998;53:377–384.
79. Wannemacher K, Yadav P, Doligosa M, Howells RD. Antagonist-induced opioid receptor up-regulation. Soc. Neurosci. Abst. Prog. No. 490.15, online; 2005.
80. Wannemacher K, Yadav P, Howells RD. Opioid antagonists up-regulate delta opioid receptor binding without increasing immunoreactive receptor protein. Int. Narcotic Res. Conf. abstract Th-42, p. 65; 2006.

81. Wannemacher K, Yadav P, Howells RD. A select set of opioid ligands induce up-regulation by promoting the maturation and stability of the rat kappa opioid receptor in human embryonic kidney 293 cells. J. Pharmacol. Exp. Ther. 2007; 323:614–625, eprint DOI:10.1124/jpet.107.125500.
82. Li J-G, Benovic JL, Liu-Chen LY. Mechanisms of agonist-induced down-regulation of the human κ opioid receptor: internalization is required for down-regulation. Mol. Pharmacol. 2000;58:795–801.
83. Chen Y, Chen C, Wang Y, Liu-Chen L-Y. Ligands regulate cell surface level of the human κ opioid receptor (hKOR) by activation-induced down-regulation and pharmacological chaperone-mediated enhancement: differential effects of non-peptide and peptide agonists. J. Pharmacol. Exp. Ther. 2006;319:765–775.
84. Schwartz RD, Keller KJ. Nicotinic cholinergic receptor binding sites in the brain: regulation in vivo. Science 1983;220:214–216.
85. Benwell ME, Balfour DJ, Anderson JM. Evidence that tobacco smoking increases the density of (–)-[^{3}H]nicotine binding sites in human brain. J. Neurochem. 1988;50:1243–1247.
86. Perry DC, Davila-Garcia MI, Stockmeier CA, Keller KJ. Increased nicotinic receptors in brains from smokers: membrane binding and autoradiography studies. J. Pharmacol. Exp. Ther. 1999;289:1545–1552.
87. Sallette J, Pons S, Devillers-Thiery A, Soudant M, Prado de Carvalho L, Changeux J-P, Corringer PJ. Nicotine upregulates its own receptors through enhanced intracellular maturation. Neuron 2005;46:595–607.
88. Kuryatov A, Luo J, Cooper J, Lindstrom J. Nicotine acts as a pharmacological chaperone to up-regulate human alpha4beta2 acetylcholine receptors. Mol. Pharmacol. 2005;68: 1839–51.
89. Vallejo YF, Buisson B, Bertrand D, Green WN. Chronic nicotine exposure upregulates nicotinic receptors by a novel mechanism. J. Neurosci. 2005;25:5563–5572.
90. Unterwald EM, Horne-King J, Kreek MJ. Chronic cocaine alters brain mu opioid receptors. Brain Res. 1992;584:314–318.
91. Unterwald EM, Rubenfeld JM, Kreek MJ. Repeated cocaine administration upregulates kappa and mu, but not delta, opioid receptors. NeuroReport 1994;5:1613–1616.
92. Unterwald EM. Regulation of opioid receptors by cocaine. Ann. N. Y. Acad. Sci. 2001;937:74–92.
93. Chen JF, Aloyo VJ, Weiss B. Continuous treatment with the D2 dopamine receptor agonist quinpirole decreases D2 dopamine receptors, D2 dopamine receptor messenger RNA and proenkephalin messenger RNA, and increases mu opioid receptors in mouse striatum. Neuroscience 1993;54:669–680.
94. Chen JF, Aloyo VJ, Qin ZH, Weiss B. Irreversible blockade of D2 dopamine receptors by fluphenazine-N-mustard increases D2 dopamine receptor mRNA and proenkephalin mRNA and decreases D1 dopamine receptor mRNA and mu and delta opioid receptors in rat striatum. Neurochem. Int. 1994;25:355–366.
95. George SR, Kertesz M. Met-enkephalin concentrations in striatum respond reciprocally to alterations in dopamine neurotransmission. Peptides 1987;8:487–492.
96. Steiner H, Gerfen CR. Enkephalin regulates acute D2 dopamine receptor antagonist-induced immediate-early gene expression in striatal neurons. Neuroscience 1999;88:795–810.
97. Ambrose LM, Unterwald EM, Van Bockstaele EJ. Ultrastructural evidence for co-localization of dopamine D2 and mu opioid receptors in the rat dorsolateral striatum. Anat. Rec. 2004;279A:583–591.
98. Rosin A, Kitchen I, Georgieva J. Effects of single and dual administration of cocaine and ethanol on opioid and ORL1 receptor expression in rat CNS: an autoradiographic study. Brain Res. 2003;978:1–13.
99. Schroeder JA, Niculescu M, Unterwald EM. Cocaine alters mu but not delta or kappa opioid receptor-stimulated in situ [35S]GTPγS binding in rat brain. Synapse 2003;47:26–32.
100. Bailey A, Gianotti R, Ho A, Kreek MJ. Persistent upregulation of mu-opioid, but not adenosine, receptors in brains of long-term withdrawn escalating dose "binge" cocaine-treated rats. Synapse 2005;57:160–166.

101. Unterwald EM, Kreek MJ, Cuntapay M. The frequency of cocaine administration impacts cocaine-induced receptor alterations. Brain Res. 2001;900:103–109.
102. Hammer RP. Cocaine alters opiate receptor binding in critical brain reward regions. Synapse 1989;3:55–60.
103. Izenwasser S, Heller B, Cox BM. Continuous cocaine administration enhances mu- but not delta-opioid receptor-mediated inhibition of adenylyl cyclase activity in nucleus accumbens. Eur. J. Pharmacol. 1996;297:187–91.
104. Zubieta JK, Gorelick DA, Stauffer R, Ravert HT, Dannals RF, Frost JJ. Increased mu opioid receptor binding detected by PET in cocaine-dependent men is associated with cocaine craving. Nat. Med. 1996;2:1225–1229.
105. Gorelick DA, Kim YK, Bencherif B, Boyd SJ, Newson R, Copersino M, Endres CJ, Dannals RF, Frost JJ. Imaging brain mu-opioid receptors in abstinent cocaine users: time course and relation to cocaine craving. Biol. Psychiatry 2005;57:1573–1582.
106. Hurd YL, Herkenham M. Molecular alterations in the neostriatum of human cocaine addicts. Synapse 1993;13:347–369.
107. Bencherif B, Wand GS, McCaul ME, Kim YK, Ilgin Nm Dannais RF, et al. Mu-opioid receptor binding measured by [11C]carfentanil positron emission tomography is related to craving and mood in alcohol dependence. Biol. Psychiatry 2004;55:255–262.
108. Staley JK, Rothman RB, Rice KC, Partilla J, Mash DC. Kappa2 opioid receptors in limbic areas of the human brain are upregulated by cocaine in fatal overdose victims. J. Neurosci. 1997;17:8225–8233.
109. Hynes MD, Lochner MA, Bemis KG, Hymson DL. Chronic ethanol alters the receptor binding characteristics of the delta opioid receptor lignad, D-Ala^2-D-Leu^5 enkephalin in mouse brain. Life Sci. 1983;33:2331–2337.
110. Charness ME, Gordon AS, Diamond I. Ethanol modulation of opiate receptors in cultured neural cells. Science 1983;222:1246–1248.
111. Charness ME, Querimit LA, Diamond I. Ethanol increases the expression of functional delta-opioid receptors in neuroblastoma x glioma NG108-15 hybrid cells. J. Biol. Chem. 1986;261:3164–3169.
112. Charness ME, Hu G, Edwards RH, Querimit LA. Ethanol increases delta-opioid receptor gene expression in neuronal cell lines. Mol. Pharmacol. 1993;44:1119–1127.
113. Mendez M, Morales-Mulia M, Leriche M. [3H]DPDPE binding to δ opioid receptors in the rat mesocorticolimbic and nigrostriatal pathways is transiently increased by acute ethanol administration. Brain Res. 2004;1028:180–190.
114. Turchan J, Przewlocka B, Toth G, Lason W, Borsodi A, Przewlocki R. The effect of repeated administration of morphine, cocaine and ethanol on mu and delta opioid receptor density in the nucleus accumbens and striatum of the rat. Neuroscience 1999;91:971–999.
115. Shah S, Duttaroy A, Sehba F, Chen B, Philippe J, Monderson T, Lau-Cam C, Carroll J, Yoburn BC. The effect of ethanol drinking on opioid analgesia and receptors in mice. Alcohol 1997;14:361–366.
116. Shen J, Chan KW, Chen BT, Philippe J, Sehba F, Duttaroy A, Carroll J, Yoburn BC. The effect of in vivo ethanol consumption on cyclic AMP and delta-opioid receptors in mouse striatum. Brain Res. 1997;770:65–71.
117. Sim-Selley LJ, Sharpe AL, Vogt LJ, Brunk LK, Selley DE, Samson HH. Effect of ethanol self-administration on mu- and dalta-opioid receptor-mediated G-protein activity. Alcohol. Clin. Exp. Res. 2002;26:688–694.
118. Saland LC, Hastings CM, Abeyta A, Chavez JB. Chronic ethanol modulates delta and mu-opioid receptor expression in rat CNS: immunohistochemical analysis with quantitative confocal microscopy. Neurosci. Lett. 2005;381:163–168.
119. Herz A. Endogenous opioid systems and alcohol addiction. Psychopharmacology 1997;129:99–111.
120. Gianoulakis C. Endogenous opioids and addiction to alcohol and other drugs of abuse. Curr. Top. Med. Chem. 2004;4:39–50.
121. Volpicelli JR, Alterman AI, Hayashida M, O'Brien CP. Naltrexone in the treatment of alcohol dependence. Arch. Gen. Psychiatry 1992;49:876–880.

Chapter 3
Imaging Human Brain Opioid Receptors: Applications to Substance Use Disorders

Mark K. Greenwald and Caren L. Steinmiller

Abstract Three types of opioid receptors (ORs: *mu* [μ], *kappa* [κ], and *delta* [δ]) are differentially distributed throughout the brain. Historically, the μOR has been of greatest clinical interest because it mediates therapeutic effects (e.g., analgesia and cough suppression) and nontherapeutic effects (e.g., abuse and physical dependence) of opioid agonists. This "dual-edged sword" underlies the classical dilemma of balancing safety and efficacy when μOR agonists are administered systemically to human subjects. Preclinical studies suggest that κOR- and δOR-specific agonists and antagonists could be useful in treating human substance use disorders, but the lack of such Food and Drug Administration (FDA)-approved medications significantly limits our understanding of the role of these molecular targets in the clinical setting. However, the μOR-specific radiotracer [^{11}C]-carfentanil has been used with positron emission tomography (PET) to elucidate the function of this endogenous system as it relates to substance use disorders, both with antagonists (e.g., naltrexone) and agonists (e.g., buprenorphine). The δOR-specific tracer [^{11}C]-methyl-naltrindole is also available for human use, but has not yet been applied to substance use disorders, and a κOR-specific tracer has shown promise in preclinical testing. Advances in neuroscience and medication development are likely to yield significant progress that will improve our understanding of these disorders and clinical outcomes in the near future.

Keywords: Opioids; Mu receptors; Kappa receptors; Delta receptors; Agonists; Antagonists; Positron emission tomography; Substance abuse

3.1 Introduction

This chapter selectively reviews in vivo neuroimaging methods used to investigate the role of the endogenous opioid system toward understanding and treating substance use disorders. While opioid receptors (ORs) are centrally involved in acute

M.K. Greenwald (✉) and C.L. Steinmiller
Substance Abuse Research Division, Department of Psychiatry and Behavioral Neurosciences, Wayne State University School of Medicine, Detroit, MI 48207
e.mail: mgreen@med.wayne.edu

and chronic pain states (1–7) and may contribute to other CNS disorders including depression (8) and epilepsy (9, 10), the scope of the present discussion is limited to substance use disorders.

Three types of ORs are widely dispersed throughout the brain: *mu* (μ), *kappa* (κ) and *delta* (δ). The neuropharmacology and therapeutic potential of these binding sites will be addressed here. ORs are G-protein coupled receptors (GPCRs) that interact with numerous intracellular proteins including potassium and calcium channels, adenylyl cyclase, phosphatidyl inositol-3-kinase, and MAP kinase (11). Despite similar sequence homologies among these three OR types, there are substantial differences in pharmacology. In addition, the OR-like 1 (ORL1) GPCR, which binds the endogenous ligand nociceptin, is structurally related to ORs; however, it is sufficiently distinct structurally (12) and functionally (13) so it will not be discussed further.

3.2 Mu Receptors

Studies with laboratory animals clearly indicate that μ-receptors are involved in the reinforcing, physical dependence, and physiological effects of opioids (14–17). For this reason, the μOR has been of greatest clinical interest because it mediates therapeutic effects (e.g., analgesia and cough suppression) and nontherapeutic effects (e.g., abuse, respiratory depression, and physical dependence) of opioid agonists. This "dual-edged sword" underlies the classical dilemma of balancing safety and efficacy when μOR agonists are administered systemically to human subjects. Preclinical studies also indicate that μ-receptors are involved, albeit less directly than for heroin-like opioids, in mediating the effects of other abused substances including alcohol (18–21), cocaine (22–26), and nicotine (27–30).

3.2.1 Ligands with μOR Affinity

Advances in positron emission tomography (PET) and radiochemistry have made it feasible to obtain noninvasive in vivo functional images of human brain μOR availability. Specific binding to human brain μORs is measured indirectly by subtracting tracer radioactivity counts at a nonspecific site that does not contain μORs (occipital cortex; 31) from radioactivity counts in each μOR-containing region of interest (ROI). Endogenous opioids also bind μORs at low levels, further emphasizing the point that this method indirectly measures μOR availability. These studies are conducted under conditions of radiotracer equilibrium. For tracers with short half-lives (measured in minutes), steady state levels can be accomplished by calculating the rate of tracer elimination (i.e., constructing a pharmacokinetic model) then adjusting the rate of infusion to offset this concentration decrease in the CNS compartment. The measure B_{max}/K_d is referred to as the "binding potential" (BP)

Table 3.1 Opioid radiotracers used in PET studies with human research volunteers

Radiotracer	Specific activity	Studies in human substance-abusing populations	Studies in other human subject populations
[^{11}C]-carfentanil	μ (1, 32–34)	Buprenorphine (35, 36, 78); Cocaine (40, 41); Alcohol (1, 42, 43); Nicotine (36, 44)	Healthy controls (6, 37–39) Epilepsy (9, 10, 56) Bulimia (45)
[^{18}F]-cyclofoxy	μ and κ (46–50)	Methadone (51)	Healthy controls (51)
[^{11}C]-diprenorphine	μ, κ, and δ (3, 52, 53)	Methadone (54)	Stroke (4) Healthy controls (31, 149, 150)
[^{11}C]-methyl-naltrindole	δ (55)		Healthy controls (56, 57)

or receptor availability. In some human studies, receptor affinity (K_d) for the tracer is assumed to remain constant within participants; under physiological conditions where this assumption is valid the BP measure is hypothesized to be proportional to in vivo μOR availability.

At this time, three radiotracers with acceptably high μOR affinity, but variable specificity, have been used in PET studies with human substance abusers (see Table 3.1): [^{18}F]-cyclofoxy, an antagonist that nonspecifically labels μORs and κORs (46–50); [^{11}C]-diprenorphine, an antagonist that nonspecifically labels μORs, κORs, and δORs (31, 52, 53); and [^{11}C]-carfentanil, an agonist with a short half-life ($t_{1/2}$ = 20.3 min) that specifically labels μORs (32–34).

3.2.2 *Clinical Studies*

3.2.2.1 Studies of Antagonists to Block Receptors in Healthy Humans

Several experiments conducted with healthy human subjects have investigated the ability of Food and Drug Administration (FDA)-approved opioid antagonists to occupy μORs. All of these medications (naltrexone, nalmefene, and naloxone) are nonselective. However, because the majority of these PET studies used the radiotracer [^{11}C]-carfentanil, it is possible to draw conclusions about the specific binding of these medications at μORs. Here, we limit discussion to those studies with the greatest clinical relevance for substance use disorders.

Lee et al. assessed with PET and [^{11}C]-carfentanil the duration of μOR blockade by the long-acting antagonist naltrexone (58). Regional μOR availability was measured before and 1, 48, 72, 120, and 168 h after acute oral administration of naltrexone 50 mg. The estimated $t_{1/2}$ of naltrexone at brain μORs ranged from 72 to 108 h, which correlates closely with the $t_{1/2}$ (96 h) of the terminal phase of plasma naltrexone clearance and duration of action in blocking heroin effects (59). Furthermore, the data suggest the typical clinical dose of naltrexone that is used to treat opioid dependence (50 mg/day) saturates μORs. At the present time, no clinical investigations have attempted to relate the concentration of naltrexone at μORs with its ability to reduce use of (or craving for) opioids or alcohol among individuals dependent on these substances.

Ingman et al. used [^{11}C]-carfentanil and PET to estimate the time course of μOR occupancy after an acute nalmefene dose (20 mg oral, a standard once-daily dose for treating alcohol-dependent patients) and after 7 days repeated administration of this dose (37). Subjects were scanned before the nalmefene dose and 3, 26, 50, and 74 h after each type of dosing regimen (acute and repeated). Plasma concentrations of nalmefene and its metabolite were measured at the same times in each participant. The half-life of nalmefene remained similar (average $t_{1/2}$ = 13.4 h) under both regimens. Interestingly, both acute and repeated dosing produced high levels of μOR occupancy (83–100% at 26 h) and similar brain kinetics (i.e., rate of decrease in occupancy over time) that were longer lasting than nalmefene plasma concentrations. Nalmefene's extended μOR occupancy in this study is consistent with the idea that 20 mg once daily dosing for reducing alcohol consumption. However, studies have not yet been conducted with alcohol-dependent individuals to determine whether nalmefene brain μOR occupancy is correlated with its efficacy in this clinical population.

Kim et al. compared the ability of naloxone and nalmefene to occupy μORs using PET and [^{11}C]-carfentanil (38). Plasma pharmacokinetic data suggest that nalmefene has a longer duration of action than naloxone. μOR availability was measured for 5 min and 2, 4, 8, and 24 h after the administration of nalmefene (1 mg or 1 μg/kg) or naloxone (2 mg or 2 μg/kg). Brain clearance times were about 21.1 and 3.4 times slower than plasma clearance times for nalmefene and naloxone, respectively. In the emergency department setting, repeated 1–2 mg intravenous (IV) doses of nalmefene have been used to reverse opioid overdose (60) and these doses are equally safe and effective as repeated 2 mg doses of naloxone (61). To the extent that nalmefene dissociates more slowly than naloxone from μORs, however, its prolonged blockade might be preferable to naloxone for reversing opioid overdose (62). Recently, Melichar et al. used PET and the nonselective tracer [^{11}C]-diprenorphine to study OR availability following different IV doses of naloxone (1.5–160 μg/kg) (63). Results indicated that about 13 μg/kg naloxone (~1 mg/80 kg) occupied an estimated 50% of ORs. This finding is consistent with the range of naloxone doses used clinically to reverse opioid overdose (0.4 mg–1.2 mg).

3.2.2.2 Opioid Dependence

Using PET and [^{18}F]-cyclofoxy, Kling et al. examined (μ and κ) OR occupancy in long-term methadone-maintained, heroin-abstinent patients, compared to a control group of healthy age-matched volunteers (51). The investigators also measured methadone plasma concentrations in the patient group at 22 h after the daily dose (the same time at which PET studies were performed), which they correlated with OR availability in brain regions of interest, for example, striatum, anterior cingulate cortex, amygdala, and insula. Methadone decreased OR availability in patients from 19% to 32%, relative to the control group. The investigators suggested that this result is consistent with the idea that methadone, a full agonist at the μOR, exerts its therapeutic effects when occupying a fairly small fraction of this receptor pool. However, the investigators were careful to point out that the modest degree of OR occupancy might not adequately account for methadone's ability to block heroin's effects or normalize physiological function. One alternative explanation for this modest level of occupancy is that [^{18}F]-cyclofoxy is a marker at two receptor populations and the calculated B_{max}/K_d values refer to availability at both sites. Because methadone has higher affinity at μORs than κORs (64), the use of this or any other nonselective tracer will tend to underestimate changes in μOR availability, and this could vary depending on the concentrations of receptor sites in a given brain region. Therefore, the actual percentage changes in μOR availability were likely to have been greater than the measured values. Another alternative explanation of reduced BP in the patient group could involve methadone's ability to facilitate internalization of μORs (65–69). Finally, in this study, patients were maintained on a wide range of doses (30–90 mg/day) and, surprisingly, there was no significant association between maintenance dose and OR availability. This lack of correspondence raises concern about employing [^{18}F]-cyclofoxy in future investigations of ORs in substance use disorders.

Using PET and [^{11}C]-diprenorphine, Melichar et al. investigated (μ, κ, and δ) OR occupancy at 4 h postdose in methadone-stabilized, otherwise drug-abstinent, patients compared to age-matched controls. Although the methadone group tended to show reduced OR BP (consistent with the data of Kling et al., 51), this effect failed to achieve statistically significant levels (54). Interestingly, results from in vitro work (70) suggest that [^{11}C]-diprenorphine can label internalized ORs. Melichar et al. acknowledge that this tracer characteristic could account for the lack of reduction in [^{11}C]-diprenorphine binding in their study (54). Internalized receptors may exist in a low affinity state when they have been activated then decoupled from intracellular effectors. Therefore, antagonists like [^{11}C]-diprenorphine and [^{18}F]-cyclofoxy may not reliably differentiate high and low affinity states of the receptor, whereas agonists should preferentially label the receptor in its high affinity state (71). Thus, there may be disadvantages in developing opioid antagonist radiotracers or, at least, it may be necessary to repeat certain studies using both agonist and antagonist PET ligands to discern whether receptor affinity plays a role in the binding profile of opioid drugs.

Our research team has used the tracer [^{11}C]-carfentanil to examine the ability of buprenorphine (BUP) to occupy μORs in heroin-dependent individuals. BUP is a μOR partial agonist and an antagonist at κORs and δORs (52, 72, 73), with high affinities ($K_i < 1$ nM) for all these OR types (74). Although it has also been reported that BUP is a lower-affinity ($K_i \approx 285$ nM; Huang et al.) agonist at the

ORL1 receptor (75–77), suggesting it could have actions that oppose opioid analgesia and abuse liability, there are presently no pharmacological tools available for human use (medications or tracers) to investigate functional correlations between ORL1 receptor availability and behavior.

In our first study (78), which used the earlier BUP sublingual liquid formulation, volunteers were stabilized first on daily doses of 2 mg, then on 16 mg/day, followed by complete dose tapering to 0 mg/day (placebo) and scanned at 4 h after each daily dose. Each participant lived on a residential unit for 4 days prior to each scan (i.e., volunteers were completely drug-abstinent for at least 4 days under the placebo condition), and had to submit a negative urine drug sample on the day of scanning to ensure that any illegal drug use had cleared. Results showed that, relative to placebo, BUP 2 mg/day decreased μOR availability from 36% to 50% (range across nine ROIs: prefrontal cortex, anterior cingulate cortex, caudate, putamen, thalamus, hypothalamus, amygdala, midbrain, and cerebellum) and 16 mg/day decreased μOR availability from 79% to 95%. There was preliminary evidence for increased μOR availability in frontal regions for opioid-detoxified volunteers relative to healthy controls (see Greenwald, 79). Here we address selected methodological issues emanating from this research program, as it influences interpretation of the therapeutic effects of BUP.

By including a within-subject placebo control condition in this initial study, we could calculate the percent increase in μOR occupancy for each individual. This study design feature presents a technical challenge because physically dependent volunteers must undergo opioid detoxification and tend to be uncomfortable when studied under placebo conditions. (This is not a problem with healthy controls, of course, who were also included in this study.) One opioid withdrawal symptom is restlessness, which can increase motion artifact during scanning. Also, because such scans depend on measuring in vivo competitive binding ability of the radiotracer against the "on-board" maintenance medication, it is not acceptable to administer additional opioid doses to abate withdrawal signs and symptoms. While nonopioid drugs (e.g., clonidine, benzodiazepines, and diphenhydramine) could theoretically be used to control symptoms during the scan, these drugs should generally be avoided because their effects on μOR availability in humans have not been determined. These methodological constraints limit feasibility and explain why the sample size for these within-subject studies is often restricted. However, the μOR availability data are remarkably consistent across individuals, increasing confidence that the obtained results would replicate if more volunteers were tested.

Our second study (35) extended the translational scope of the initial experiment by (a) using the marketed BUP mono tablet (i.e., Subutex™, to avoid any potential μOR binding by naloxone), (b) using a detoxification-type protocol across a wider range of maintenance doses (32, 16, 2, and 0 mg/day), and a longer 12-day period of maintenance on placebo (i.e., more stable baseline) than the first study, (c) measuring BUP plasma concentrations, (d) administering the high affinity, full μ-opioid agonist hydromorphone to determine the extent to which BUP blocked its abuse-related subjective effects, and (e) correlating μOR occupancy (or plasma levels) with pharmacodynamic effects across medication doses. We observed

BUP dose-dependent decreases in µOR availability, which were reliable across volunteers and ROIs. Interestingly, we observed 3.5-fold between-subject variation in percentage occupancy at the lowest active dose (2 mg/day, with least occupancy in the amygdala, and increasing levels in the thalamus, nucleus accumbens, caudate, rostral and subgenual anterior cingulate, and prefrontal cortex), but very little regional variance at the higher doses. While we do not yet understand the clinical importance of this finding, one hypothesis worth exploring is that patients who evince greater µOR occupancy and withdrawal symptom suppression in response to low-dose BUP might have better treatment outcomes than individuals with lower µOR occupancy and withdrawal suppression. Another therapeutically relevant finding was the lack of further increase in µOR availability with BUP 32 mg/day over 16 mg/day when measured 4 h after the daily dose. Put another way, there were diminishing returns of the highest dose, which was safe but exceeds that used as a daily maintenance dose in clinical practice. Finally, BUP-induced µOR availability paralleled opioid withdrawal symptoms, although there were marked individual-subject differences in the slope of this relationship. This finding supports the canonical belief that agonist replacement therapy should suppress withdrawal through increasing occupancy, and reinforces long-standing clinical observations that patients are differentially sensitive to withdrawal symptoms during detoxification (when µOR availability was highest in this study). These individual variations are fascinating, in that they may have implications for tailoring treatment.

In our most recent study (36), we examined in volunteers maintained on 16 mg/day of the BUP mono tablet the effect of a double-blind dose omission (placebo substitution) over 3 days. We obtained repeated measures at 4, 28, 52, and 76 h after the active maintenance dose for a duration-of-action pharmacokinetic profile of µOR availability and BUP plasma concentrations, as well as subjective (e.g., withdrawal and craving) and physiological effects (e.g., carbon dioxide sensitivity). On another week, we re-measured under the same pharmacological conditions the ability of BUP to attenuate the agonist effects of cumulative hydromorphone doses (0, 6, 12, and 24 mg IM). Due to the technical challenges described above, we chose not to measure under placebo conditions in this latest study. Instead, we referenced the time-course µOR occupancy data to the placebo condition of the Greenwald et al. (35) study, which used a similar group of heroin-dependent volunteers and the same PET scanner and tracer infusion protocol. There were clear post-BUP time-dependent increases in µOR availability, which were significantly correlated with plasma concentrations (the best-fit curve was an exponential rather than a linear function in most cases). Perhaps the most clinically significant result was that occupying 50% or more µORs with BUP suppressed withdrawal symptoms and blocked agonist effects from high-dose HYD (24 mg IM). While this novel finding provides a starting point for determining µOR occupancy requirements that underlie effective opioid pharmacotherapy, we remain cautious. First, it is not clear whether this estimate would hold true for the full µ-agonist methadone, which as noted earlier may be able to produce its therapeutic effects at a lower level of µ-occupancy compared to the partial µ-agonist BUP. Second, this research study involved volunteers who were not seeking treatment, and it would be preferable to replicate this finding in a patient population.

Recently, long-acting depot versions of BUP (80, 81) and naltrexone (82) have been evaluated for the treatment of opioid dependence. To date, these studies have measured medication plasma concentrations, symptomatic effects, and blockade of opioid challenges to determine the duration of efficacy over several weeks. Interestingly, Comer et al. found that subjective and/or pupil-constricting effects of heroin challenge (which were repeated each week and initially blocked by naltrexone) recovered once 6-β-naltrexol plasma concentrations had decreased below ~2.0 ng/ml (82). In the future, it would be also useful to measure μOR availability to determine the relationship between brain and peripheral kinetic measures, and whether the rate of decrease in μOR occupancy is associated with – and, relative to plasma concentrations, better predicts – the risk of opioid relapse.

3.2.2.3 Nonopioid Substance Use Disorders

Additional PET studies with [^{11}C]-carfentanil have been published that implicate the μOR system in nonopioid substance use disorders.

Nicotine

The prevalence rate of regular tobacco smoking among heroin abusers is very high, often exceeding 90% (83–87). Chronic nicotine exposure and abstinence influences endogenous opioid function in laboratory animals (30, 88–91) and may alter opioid-mediated human behaviors (92) including postsurgical morphine self-administration (93).

In an exploratory analysis from our most recent BUP study (36), we found significantly (≈60%) lower μOR availability among heavier cigarette smokers (≥20 daily) relative to lighter smokers (≤15 daily); this was a generalized effect across brain regions and within-subject study conditions (i.e., post-BUP omission times). A recent human PET/[^{11}C]-carfentanil study (44) found that overnight nicotine abstinence in regular smokers who then smoked a denicotinized cigarette led to decreased μOR availability relative to a healthy control group, and that smoking a nicotine-containing cigarette reversed this effect. While these preliminary data suggest that the endogenous opioid system could play a role in nicotine intake and/or dependence, treating smokers with opioid antagonists has produced a mixed literature (29, 94–97); therefore, further studies need to be conducted to examine this hypothesis in greater detail.

Alcohol

Substantial evidence indicates that ethanol's reinforcing efficacy is partly mediated by the endogenous opioid system (18, 19, 98), and that chronic intake may lead to neuroadaptations in this system (99, 100). Many preclinical studies have shown that ethanol self-administration is reduced by pretreatment with naloxone (101–105), nalmefene (102), and naltrexone (106–109). Also, μOR-selective (β-funaltrexamine and CTOP) and δOR-selective (naltrindole, naltriben, and ICI174864) antagonists have been shown to block ethanol self-administration in rats and mice (20, 110–114).

Naltrexone has been demonstrated in clinical trials to reduce alcohol intake and relapse in alcoholics (115, 116), although there have also been negative findings (117), and preliminary data have suggested that genetic polymorphisms of the μOR could moderate outcomes during naltrexone treatment for alcohol dependence (118). Interestingly, only recently was it shown that the nonselective antagonists nalmefene and naltrexone can reduce ethanol consumption in the human laboratory setting (119, 120).

On the basis of the hypothesis that endogenous opioid function is altered by chronic ethanol exposure, two recent PET/[^{11}C]-carfentanil studies have investigated whether μOR availability differs in alcoholics. In the first study (42), a cross-sectional (single scan) design was used to compare alcohol-dependent male inpatients undergoing withdrawal with an age- and gender-matched control group. Alcohol craving, withdrawal, and mood measures were also obtained in patients and correlated with the imaging data. Alcoholic patients showed significantly reduced μOR availability compared to controls in two brain regions (right dorsolateral prefrontal and anterior cingulate cortices), and less μOR availability in these ROIs was significantly correlated with more alcohol craving (as measured by the Obsessive Compulsive Drinking Scale [OCDS]). Additional significant negative correlations were found between craving and μOR availability in certain ROIs (left dorsolateral prefrontal, left temporal and parietal cortices) and between depression scores (measured with the Beck Depression Inventory) and μOR availability in other ROIs (right dorsolateral prefrontal, right parietal and left temporoparietal cortices), but positive correlations between depression scores and μOR availability in other ROIs (left thalamus, anterior cingulate). In contrast, alcohol withdrawal scores were not significantly correlated with μOR availability. Bencherif et al. discuss two important alternative explanations for their findings: (a) alcoholics may inherit the tendency toward lower μOR availability, making this an etiological factor along with other family history variables; and (b) reduced μOR availability could be secondary to chronic alcohol use or withdrawal, for example, enhanced endogenous release during abstinence (42). Either or both of these mechanisms could contribute to the obtained findings, and these possibilities merit further systematic investigation.

In another recent experiment, male alcohol-dependent inpatients underwent two PET/[^{11}C]-carfentanil studies, the first after detoxification and the second 5 weeks later, and these findings were compared with a healthy control group (43). These alcoholics displayed increased μOR availability in the ventral striatum following detoxification and 5 weeks later, relative to the control group, which was positively correlated with μOR availability. These findings contrast with Bencherif et al. (42), who reported no effect of alcohol dependence on μOR availability in the ventral striatum, and that alcohol dependence was associated with decreased, not increased, μOR availability in several brain regions. Several methodological factors could have contributed to the difference between these two studies. First, in the study by Heinz et al., the group sizes were larger and the average age was slightly older than in the Bencherif et al. study. Second, the image acquisition methods differed (e.g., different [^{11}C]-carfentanil doses and different time frames over which image data contributed to ROI averages). Third, the time at which μOR availability was first measured in the alcohol-dependent patients varied across studies (5 days vs. 1–3 weeks). However, the single most striking observation is that, in two comparable ROIs (prefrontal/anterior frontal and parietal cortical regions) across studies, the absolute B_{max}/K_d values in the respective control groups were markedly higher in the Bencherif et al. study than the Heinz et al. study. Because change in μOR availability in the patient group is interpreted with reference to the control group, this factor alone could account for the opposing conclusions reached by these two research groups. Until this discrepancy is resolved, significant caution is recommended.

Cocaine

Zubieta et al. used [^{11}C]-carfentanil and PET scans to investigate μOR availability in cocaine-dependent individuals at 1–4 days after their last use and again after 4 weeks of supervised abstinence (40). Mean regional μOR availability was significantly increased in cocaine abusers relative to healthy controls during early cocaine abstinence, reaching significance in the frontal cortex (52%, maximum group difference), anterior cingulate, caudate, thalamus, and temporal cortex, and was not significant in the putamen, amygdala, parietal cortex, or cerebellum. The extent of recent cocaine use (as estimated from quantitative benzoylecgonine levels) was significantly negatively associated with μOR availability. In addition, subjective ratings of cocaine craving/need were significantly positively correlated with μOR availability in several regions. Following 4 weeks of monitored drug abstinence, μOR upregulation in cocaine relative to controls remained significant although mean percent effect decreased for frontal cortex (36%, maximum difference), anterior cingulate, caudate, and thalamus. These findings are consistent with the hypothesis that chronic cocaine use reduces endogenous opioid release (which results in compensatory μOR upregulation) primarily in fronto-striatal-thalamic circuitry and that this neuroadaptation persists following cocaine abstinence and is related to cocaine craving. Given the natural course of relapse to drug use, this alteration of the endogenous opioid system could underlie heightened vulnerability to relapse during the initial period of abstinence.

Gorelick et al. used similar methods to investigate whether μOR upregulation persists until 3 months postabstinence (41). Cocaine-dependent individuals were each scanned at three time points: 1 day, 1 week, and 12 weeks after the last cocaine use, while being monitored on an inpatient unit. Receptor availability data from these scans were referenced to those from a healthy control group. Results of the first scan (1-day abstinence) largely replicated the findings of Zubieta et al. (40): μOR availability increased relative to controls in some of the same brain ROIs (notably frontal, anterior cingulate, and the right temporal and parietal cortex, but not in caudate and thalamus), which again correlated positively with cocaine craving but, unlike Zubieta et al. (40), showed less consistent correlations with recent cocaine use. μOR availability in anterior frontal and anterior cingulate regions remained elevated at 1 and 12 weeks postabstinence. In contrast, initially higher μOR availability in other frontal subdivisions (prefrontal, dorsolateral prefrontal, and inferior frontal), temporal and parietal regions no longer differed significantly from control group values after 1 and 12 weeks abstinence. The investigators note that these data partially replicate μOR binding (autoradiography) results obtained in rats that were administered cocaine in a binge pattern (24, 25, 121), lending further confidence in the cross-species reliability and validity of this finding.

3.3 Kappa Receptors

κORs may be involved in several pathologic conditions of the CNS, including drug dependence (122, 123), hallucinations (124), and seizures (125, 126).

3.3.1 Ligands with κOR Affinity

Talbot et al. reported an initial study of a κOR-specific ligand, [^{11}C]-GR103545 (127). Brain uptake of [^{11}C]-GR103545 was studied in baboons under control conditions and after pretreatment with naloxone (1 mg/kg IV). This novel ligand showed excellent brain penetration and uptake kinetics, and significant washout was observed. Naloxone pretreatment did not alter cerebellar total distribution volume whereas it reduced total distribution volume in other regions to a level comparable to that in the cerebellum. The regional pattern of [^{11}C]-GR103545 BP was consistent with the distribution of κORs in primate brain, with highest levels observed in prefrontal cortex, cingulate cortex, and striatum.

3.3.2 Clinical Studies

At this time, there are no studies using [^{11}C]-GR103545 to ascertain the functional role of κORs in CNS conditions. However, there are significant questions and opportunities to address the role of κORs in substance use disorders.

Rothman et al. (2001) hypothesized that, while the effects of chronic heroin use are mediated through the μ-opioid system, the κOR system might compensate for this exposure (50). Some evidence suggests that the κOR system could counteract the biological effect of chronic heroin use on the μOR system and an "overshoot" phenomenon could manifest itself following opioid detoxification (128, 129). κOR upregulation could contribute to dysphoric and anergic features of the abstinence syndrome. Rothman et al. (2001) reasoned that administering a κOR antagonist after detoxification could counteract this overdrive effect (50). First, it would be important to determine with [^{11}C]-GR103545 and PET whether, in fact, there is evidence of κOR upregulation during opioid abstinence. Second, if this were the case, it would be theoretically informative to establish whether opioid-abstinent individuals are hypersensitive to κOR agonists compared to control subjects. Third, from a therapeutic perspective, it would be useful to know whether a κOR antagonist could alleviate both upregulatory and symptomatic effects of this abstinence state.

In addition, κOR agonists have been proposed to be relevant to the treatment of cocaine abuse, in part, by virtue of their ability to attenuate striatal dopamine activity (128, 130–132) and to reduce cocaine self-administration (133). However, a systematic series of studies with a range of compounds found that the capacity of these drugs to attenuate cocaine self-intake may depend not only on their intrinsic activity and selectivity profiles at κORs, but may be partly autonomous of κORs given insensitivity to blockade by the κOR-specific antagonist nor-binaltorphimine (123). At this time, very few studies have been conducted with human cocaine abusers using current FDA-marketed compounds, and evidence of efficacy is not convincing (134, 135). Unfortunately, none of the available medications have the ideal combination of being long acting and κOR-specific, and having high oral bioavailability and high intrinsic activity at κORs. In light of these limitations and preliminary negative findings, it may be useful to "return to the bench" (in the spirit of this volume) by first investigating κOR availability in cocaine abusers (assuming that [^{11}C]-GR103545 becomes available for human PET studies), analogous to the μOR studies of cocaine abusers discussed above (40, 41), before attempting further clinical application. This would be mechanistically helpful, especially given the tendency of κOR agonists at higher doses to produce side effects such as dysphoria, diuresis, sedation, and visual disturbances (e.g., 134, 136, 137).

3.4 Delta Receptors

δ-receptors are involved in numerous behavioral effects of opioids. δOR agonists can produce antinociceptive effects and modify μ-opioid antinociception without producing respiratory depression (138–140). These agents also appear to have minimal reinforcing effects (141). Recent preclinical data also suggest that δOR-selective agonists may function as novel antidepressant-like agents (142–144) or anxiolytic-like agents (145, 146) at doses that do not produce convulsions (147, 148). Finally, as noted above, δOR antagonists may also be useful for the treatment of alcohol dependence. To our knowledge, no δOR-specific medications are presently available for use in human subjects.

3.4.1 Ligands with δOR Affinity

The Johns Hopkins group, which has been a leader in synthesizing and testing OR ligands, also developed [^{11}C]-methyl-naltrindole (NTI) and demonstrated its high selectivity for δORs in mouse brain (55). At this time, this is the only δOR ligand available for human use.

3.4.2 Clinical Studies

Madar et al. studied the regional distribution of NTI and found that it correlated closely with the in vitro distribution of δOR sites but not with μOR or κOR site densities (56). NTI binding was highest in the neocortex (insular, parietal, frontal, cingulate, and occipital), caudate nucleus, and putamen. Binding was intermediate in the amygdala and lowest in the cerebellum and thalamus. In addition, naltrexone inhibited NTI binding, particularly in δOR-rich regions. In a second human methodological study (57), this tracer showed irreversible binding characteristics during the scanning period, and showed results consistent with the density and distribution of δORs in vitro.

At this time, there are no studies using NTI to ascertain the functional role of δORs in substance abusers. However, as noted above, there are many opportunities to use [^{11}C]-methyl-naltrindole and PET to investigate the role of δORs in relation to abuse-related behavioral effects of μOR agonists and ethanol, as well as mood-related effects during detoxification from these substances.

3.5 Conclusions

The present review has spotlighted advances in molecular neuroimaging of the endogenous opioid system as it relates to substance use disorders. We conclude by indicating some research avenues (in addition to those noted above) that seem worthy of further study.

One observation from the data reviewed here is that abstinence from abused substances may impact the endogenous opioid system differently, either increasing μOR availability (higher B_{max}/K_d values in the case of heroin and cocaine) or decreasing μOR availability (lower B_{max}/K_d values in the case of nicotine); data for alcohol are presently ambiguous. Typical human PET studies do not take the extra methodological steps that could disentangle changes in receptor number from affinity. To the extent that chronic heroin or cocaine use or abstinence leads to decreased endogenous opioid release, this could manifest as a compensatory increase in the number of μORs (B_{max}) rather than a change in affinity (K_d). The reverse could be true for nicotine. Because this remains speculative (i.e., PET cannot directly measure neurochemical release), it would be useful to investigate this hypothesis in the human in vivo situation.

Now that PET radioligands exist that specifically label μ, κ, and δORs, the moment seems ripe to undertake repeated measures studies that use these tracers to investigate the unique roles of these subtypes in both therapeutic effects (e.g., medication efficacy) and nontherapeutic effects (e.g., abuse liability). For instance, we noted above that BUP is a μOR agonist, but also a κOR and δOR antagonist. It would therefore be useful to determine whether any of BUP's therapeutic effects may be attributable to its antagonist actions. Another related research opportunity involves determining whether drug abstinence produces subtype and/or regionally specific alterations in OR availability. For instance, preclinical studies suggest that alcohol exposure may produce μOR and δOR alterations, whereas cocaine exposure may induce alterations in all three OR types. Therefore, it would be useful to characterize the panorama of changes for various abused substances, in conjunction with pharmacodynamic measures (e.g., craving, withdrawal, and mood). This could help to delineate which elements of drug abstinence states are shared versus unique.

Acknowledgments NIH Grant P50 DA00254 and Joe Young, Sr. Funds from the State of Michigan supported the preparation of this chapter.

References

1. Bencherif B, Fuchs PN, Sheth R, Dannals RF, Campbell JN, Frost JJ. Pain activation of human supraspinal opioid pathways as demonstrated by [^{11}C]-carfentanil and positron emission tomography (PET). Pain 2002;99:589–598.
2. Jones AK, Cunningham VJ, Ha-Kawa S, Fujiwara T, Luthra SK, Silva S, Derbyshire S, Jones T. Changes in central opioid receptor binding in relation to inflammation and pain in patients with rheumatoid arthritis. Br J Rheumatol 1994;33:909–916.
3. Jones AK, Watabe H, Cunningham VJ, Jones T. Cerebral decreases in opioid receptor binding in patients with central neuropathic pain measured by [^{11}C]diprenorphine binding and PET. Eur J Pain 2004;8:479–485.
4. Willoch F, Schindler F, Wester HJ, Empl M, Straube A, Schwaiger M, Conrad B, Tolle TR. Central poststroke pain and reduced opioid receptor binding within pain processing circuitries: a [^{11}C]diprenorphine PET study. Pain 2004;108:213–220.
5. Zubieta JK, Smith YR, Bueller J, Xu Y, Kilbourn M, Meyer C, Koeppe R, Stohler C. Regional mu opioid receptor regulation of sensory and affective dimensions of pain. Science 2001;293:311–315.
6. Zubieta JK, Heitzeg MM, Smith YR, Bueller JA, Xu K, Xu Y, Koeppe RA, Stohler CS, Goldman D. COMT val^{158}met genotype affects mu-opioid neurotransmitter responses to a pain stressor. Science 2003;299:1240–1243.
7. Zubieta JK, Bueller JA, Jackson LR, Scott DJ, Xu Y, Koeppe RA, Nichols TE, Stohler CS. Placebo effects mediated by endogenous opioid activity on mu-opioid receptors. J Neurosci 2005;25:7754–7762.
8. Mayberg HS, Ross CA, Dannals RF, Ravert HT, Wagner HN Jr, Frost JJ. Elevated mu opiate receptors measured by PET in patients with depression. J Cereb Blood Flow Metab 1991a;11:S821.
9. Frost JJ, Mayberg HS, Fisher RS, Douglass KH, Dannals RF, Links JM, Wilson AA, Ravert HT, Rosenbaum AE, Snyder SH, Wagner HN Jr. Mu-opiate receptors measured by positron emission tomography are increased in temporal lobe epilepsy. Ann Neurol 1988;23:231–237.

10. Mayberg HS, Sadzot B, Meltzer CC, Fisher RS, Lesser RP, Dannals RF, Lever JR, Wilson AA, Ravert HT, Wagner HN Jr, Brian RN, Cromwell CC, Frost JJ. Quantification of mu and non-mu opiate receptors in temporal lobe epilepsy using positron emission tomography. Ann Neurol 1991b;30:3–11.
11. Chaturvedi K, Christoffers KH, Singh K, Howells RD. Structure and regulation of opioid receptors. Biopolymers 2000;55:334–346.
12. Philip AE, Poupaert JH, McCurdy CR. Opioid receptor-like 1 (ORL1) molecular "road map" to understanding ligand interaction and selectivity. Curr Top Med Chem 2005;5:325–340.
13. Reinscheid RK. The orphanin FQ/nociceptin receptor as a novel drug target in psychiatric disorders. CNS Neurol Disord Drug Targets 2006;5:219–224.
14. Elmer GI, Pieper JO, Goldberg SR, George FR. Opioid operant self-administration, analgesia, stimulation and respiratory depression in mu-deficient mice. Psychopharmacology (Berl) 1995;117:23–31.
15. Maldonado R, Negus S, Koob GF. Precipitation of morphine withdrawal syndrome in rats by administration of mu-, delta- and kappa-selective opioid antagonists. Neuropharmacology 1992;31:1231–1241.
16. Matthes HW, Maldonado R, Simonin F, Valverde O, Slowe S, Kitchen I, Befort K, Dierich A, Le Meur M, Dolle P, Tzavara E, Hanoune J, Roques BP, Kieffer BL. Loss of morphine-induced analgesia, reward effect and withdrawal symptoms in mice lacking the mu-opioid-receptor gene. Nature 1996;383:819–823.
17. Negus SS, Henriksen SJ, Mattox A, Pasternak GW, Portoghese PS, Takemori AE, Weinger MB, Koob GF. Effect of antagonists specific for mu, delta and kappa opioid receptors on the reinforcing effects of heroin in rats. J Pharmacol Exp Ther 1993;265:1245–1252.
18. Oswald LM, Wand GS. Opioids and alcoholism. Physiol Behav 2004;81:339–358.
19. Gianoulakis C. Alcohol-seeking behavior: the roles of the hypothalamic-pituitary-adrenal axis and the endogenous opioid system. Alcohol Health Res World 1998;22:202–210.
20. Froehlich JC. The neurobiology of ethanol-opioid interactions in ethanol reinforcement. Alcohol Clin Exp Res 1996;20:181–186.
21. Gianoulakis C. Characterization of the effects of acute ethanol administration on the release of beta-endorphin peptides by the rat hypothalamus. Eur J Pharm 1990;180:21–29.
22. Bailey A, Gianotti R, Ho A, Kreek MJ. Persistent upregulation of mu-opioid, but not adenosine, receptors in brains of long-term withdrawn escalating dose "binge" cocaine-treated rats. Synapse 2005;57:160–166.
23. Tang XC, McFarland K, Cagle S, Kalivas PW. Cocaine-induced reinstatement requires endogenous stimulation of mu-opioid receptors in the ventral pallidum. J Neurosci 2005;25:4512–4520.
24. Unterwald EM, Kreek MJ, Cuntapay M. The frequency of cocaine administration impacts cocaine-induced receptor alterations. Brain Res 2001;900:103–109.
25. Unterwald EM, Rubenfeld JM, Kreek MJ. Repeated cocaine administration upregulates kappa and mu, but not delta, opioid receptors. Neuroreport 1994;5:1613–1616.
26. Hammer RP Jr. Cocaine alters opiate receptor binding in critical brain reward regions. Synapse 1989;3:55–60.
27. Galeote L, Kieffer BL, Maldonado R, Berrendero F. Mu-opioid receptors are involved in the tolerance to nicotine antinociception. J Neurochem 2006;97:416–423.
28. Walters CL, Cleck JN, Kuo YC, Blendy JA. Mu-opioid receptor and CREB activation are required for nicotine reward. Neuron 2005;46:933–943.
29. Pomerleau OF. Endogenous opioids and smoking: a review of progress and problems. Psychoneuroendocrinology 1998;23:115–130.
30. Davenport KE, Houdi AA, Van Loon GR. Nicotine protects against mu-opioid receptor antagonism by beta-funaltrexamine: evidence for nicotine-induced release of endogenous opioids in brain. Neurosci Lett 1990;113:40–46.
31. Jones AK, Luthra SK, Maziere B, Pike VW, Loch C, Crouzel C, Syrota A, Jones T. Regional cerebral opioid receptor studies with [^{11}C]-diprenorphine in normal volunteers. J Neurosci Methods 1988;23:121–129.

32. Dannals RF, Ravert HT, Frost JJ, Wilson AA, Burns HD, Wagner HN Jr. Radiosynthesis of an opiate receptor binding radiotracer: [^{11}C]-carfentanil. Int J Appl Radiat Isot 1985;36:303–306.
33. Frost JJ, Wagner HNJ, Dannals RF, Ravert HT, Wilson AA, Burns HD, Wong DF, McPherson RW, Rosenbaum AE, Kuhar MJ, Snyder SH. Imaging opiate receptors in the human brain by positron emission tomography. J Comput Assist Tomogr 1985;9:231–236.
34. Titeler M, Lyon RA, Kuhar MJ, Frost JF, Dannals RF, Leonhardt S, Bullock A, Rydelek LT, Price DL, Struble RG. Mu opiate receptors are selectively labelled by [^{3}H]-carfentanil in human and rat brain. Eur J Pharmacol 1989;167:221–228.
35. Greenwald MK, Johanson, CE, Moody DE, Woods JH, Kilbourn MR, Koeppe RA. Effects of buprenorphine maintenance dose on *mu*-opioid receptor binding potential, plasma concentration, and antagonist blockade in heroin-dependent volunteers. Neuropsychopharmacology 2003;28:2000–2009.
36. Greenwald MK, Johanson C-E, Bueller J, Chang Y, Moody DE, Kilbourn MR, Koeppe RA, Zubieta JK. Buprenorphine duration of action: *mu*-opioid receptor availability, pharmacokinetic and behavioral indices. Biol Psychiatry 2007;61:101–110.
37. Ingman K, Hagelberg N, Aalto S, Nagren K, Juhakoski A, Karhuvaara S, Kallio A, Oikonen V, Hietala J, Scheinin H. Prolonged central μ-opioid receptor occupancy after single and repeated nalmefene dosing. Neuropsychopharmacology 2005;30:2245–2253.
38. Kim S, Wagner HN Jr, Villemagne VL, Kao PF, Dannals RF, Ravert HT, Joh T, Dixon RB, Civelek AC. Longer occupancy of opioid receptors by nalmefene compared to naloxone as measured in vivo by a dual-detector system. J Nucl Med 1997;38:1726–1731.
39. Zubieta JK, Dannals RF, Frost JJ. Gender and age influences on human brain mu-opioid receptor binding measured by PET. Am J Psychiatry 1996;156:842–848.
40. Zubieta JK, Gorelick DA, Stauffer R, Ravert HT, Dannals RF, Frost JJ. Increased mu opioid receptor binding detected by PET in cocaine-dependent men is associated with cocaine craving. Nat Med 1996;2:1225–1229.
41. Gorelick DA, Kim YK, Bencherif B, Boyd SJ, Nelson R, Copersino M, Endres CJ, Dannals RF, Frost JJ. Imaging brain mu-opioid receptors in abstinent cocaine users: time course and relation to cocaine craving. Biol Psychiatry 2005;57:1573–1582.
42. Bencherif B, Wand GS, McCaul ME, Kim YK, Ilgin N, Dannals RF, Frost JJ. Mu-opioid receptor binding measured by [^{11}C]carfentanil positron emission tomography is related to craving and mood in alcohol dependence. Biol Psychiatry 2004;55:255–262.
43. Heinz A, Reimold M, Wrase J, Hermann D, Croissant B, Mundle G. Correlation of stable elevations in striatal mu-opioid receptor availability in detoxified alcoholic patients with alcohol craving: a positron emission tomography study using carbon 11-labeled carfentanil. Arch Gen Psychiatry 2005;62:57–64.
44. Scott DJ, Domino EF, Heitzeg MM, Koeppe RA, Ni L, Guthrie S, Zubieta JK. Smoking modulation of μ-opioid and dopamine D2 receptor mediated neurotransmission in humans. Neuropsychopharmacology 2007;32:450–457.
45. Bencherif B, Guarda AS, Colantuoni C, Ravert HT, Dannals RF, Frost JJ. Regional mu-opioid receptor binding in insular cortex is decreased in bulimia nervosa and correlates inversely with fasting behavior. J Nucl Med 2005;46:1349–1351.
46. Burke TR, Rice KC, Pert CB. Probes for narcotic receptor mediated phenomena. II. Synthesis of 17-methyl and 17-cyclopropylmethyl-3,14-dihydroxy-4,5 alpha-epoxy-6-beta-fluoromorphinans (foxy and cyclofoxy) as models of opioid ligands suitable for positron emission transaxial tomography. Heterocycles 1985;23:69–99.
47. Carson RE, Channing MA, Blasberg RG, Dunn BB, Cohen RM, Rice KC, Herscovitch P. Comparison of bolus and infusion methods for receptor quantitation: application to [^{18}F] cyclofoxy and positron emission tomography. J Cereb Blood Flow Metab 1993;13:24–42.
48. Channing MA, Eckelman WC, Bennett JM, Burke TR, Rice KC. Radiosynthesis of [^{18}F] 3-acetylcyclofoxy: a high affinity opiate antagonist. Int J Appl Radiat Isot 1985;36:429–433.
49. Pert CB, Danks JA, Channing MA, Eckelman WC, Larson SM, Bennett JM, Burke TR Rice KC. 3-[^{18}F]Acetylcyclofoxy: a useful probe for the visualization of opiate receptors in living animals. FASEB Lett 1984;177:281–286.

50. Rothman RB, McLean SA. An examination of the opiate receptor subtypes labeled by [^{3}H] cyclofoxy: an opiate antagonist suitable for positron emission tomography. Biol Psychiatry 1988;22:423–458.
51. Kling MA, Carson RE, Borg L, Zametkin A, Matochik JA, Schluger J, Herscovitch P, Rice KC, Ho A, Eckelman WC, Kreek MJ. Opioid receptor imaging with positron emission tomography and [^{18}F]cyclofoxy in long-term, methadone-treated former heroin addicts. J Pharmacol Exp Ther 2000;295:1070–1076.
52. Lewis JW, Husbands SM. The orvinols and related opioids – high affinity ligands with diverse efficacy profiles. Curr Pharm Des 2004;10:717–732.
53. Sadzot B, Price JC, Mayberg HS, Douglass KH, Dannals RF, Lever JR, Ravert HT, Wilson AA, Wagner HN Jr, Feldman MA. Quantification of human opioid receptor concentration and affinity using high and low specific activity [^{11}C]-diprenorphine and positron emission tomography. J Cereb Blood Flow Metab 1991;11:204–219.
54. Melichar JK, Hume SP, Williams TM, Daglish MR, Taylor LG, Ahmad R, Malizia AL, Brooks DJ, Myles JS, Lingford-Hughes A, Nutt DJ. Using [^{11}C]diprenorphine to image opioid receptor occupancy by methadone in opioid addiction: clinical and preclinical studies. J Pharmacol Exp Ther 2005;312:309–315.
55. Lever JR, Scheffel U, Kinter CM, Ravert HT, Dannals RF, Wagner HN Jr, Frost JJ. In vivo binding of N1′-[^{11}C]methyl)naltrindole to δ opioid receptors in mouse brain. Eur J Pharmacol 1992;216:459–460.
56. Madar I, Lever JR, Kinter CM, Scheffel U, Ravert HT, Musachio JL, Mathews WB, Dannals RF, Frost JJ. Imaging of δ opioid receptors in human brain by N1′-([^{11}C]methyl)naltrindole and PET. Synapse 1996;24:19–28.
57. Smith JS, Zubieta JK, Price JC, Flesher JE, Madar I, Lever JR, Kinter CM, Dannals RF, Frost JJ. Quantification of δ-opioid receptors in human brain with N1′-([^{11}C]methyl) naltrindole and positron emission tomography. J Cereb Blood Flow Metab 1999;19:956–966.
58. Lee MD, Wagner HD, Tanada S, Frost JJ, Bice AN, Dannals RF. Duration of occupancy of opiate receptors by naltrexone. J Nucl Med 1988;29:1207–1211.
59. Verebey K, Volavka J, Mule SJ, Resnick RB (1976). Naltrexone: disposition, metabolism, and effects after acute and chronic dosing. Clin Pharmacol Ther 1976;20:315–328.
60. Kaplan JL, Marx JA. Effectiveness and safety of intravenous nalmefene for emergency department patients with suspected narcotic overdose: a pilot study. Ann Emerg Med 1993;22:187–190.
61. Kaplan JL, Marx JA, Calabro JJ, Gin-Shaw SL, Spiller JD, Spivey WL, Gaddis GM, Zhao N, Harchelroad FP Jr. Double-blind, randomized study of nalmefene and naloxone in emergency department patients with suspected narcotic overdose. Ann Emerg Med 1999;34:42–50.
62. Wang DS, Sternbach G, Varon J. Nalmefene: a long-acting opioid antagonist. Clinical applications in emergency medicine. J Emerg Med 1998;16:471–475.
63. Melichar JK, Nutt DJ, Malizia AL. Naloxone displacement at opioid receptor sites measured in vivo in the human brain. Eur J Pharmacol 2003;459:217–219.
64. Kristensen K, Christensen CB, Christup LL. The mu1, mu2, delta and kappa opioid receptor binding profiles of methadone stereoisomers and morphine. Life Sci 1995;56:PL45–PL60.
65. Borgland SL, Connor M, Osborne PB, Furness JB, Christie MJ. Opioid agonists have different efficacy profiles for G protein activation, rapid desensitization, and endocytosis of mu-opioid receptors. J Biol Chem 2003;278:18776–18784.
66. Blake AD, Bot G, Freeman JC, Reisine T. Differential opioid agonist regulation of the mouse μ opioid receptor. J Biol Chem 1997;272:782–790.
67. Celver J, Xu M, Jin W, Lowe J, Chavkin C. Distinct domains of the mu-opioid receptor control uncoupling and internalization. Mol Pharmacol 2004;65:492–495.
68. Haberstock-Debic H, Wein M, Barrot M, Colago EE, Rahman Z, Neve RL, Pickel VM, Nestler EJ, von Zastrow M, Svingos AL. Morphine acutely regulates opioid receptor trafficking selectively in dendrites of nucleus accumbens neurons. J Neurosci 2003;23:4324–4332.
69. Keith DE, Anton B, Murray SR, Zaki PA, Chu PC, Lissin DV, Monteillet-Agius G, Stewart PL, Evans CJ, von Zastrow M. Mu-opioid receptor internalization: opiate drugs have differential

effects on a conserved endocytic mechanism in vitro and in the mammalian brain. Mol Pharmacol 1998;53:377–384.
70. Shapira M, Keren O, Gafni M, Sarne Y. Diverse pathways mediate delta-opioid receptor down regulation within the same cell. Mol Brain Res 2001;96:142–150.
71. Snyder SH, Childers SR. Opiate receptors and opioid peptides. Ann Rev Neurosci 1979;2:35–64.
72. Richards ML, Sadee W. In vivo opiate receptor binding of oripavines to mu, delta and kappa sites in rat brain as determined by an ex vivo labeling method. Eur J Pharmacol 1985;114:343–353.
73. Negus SS, Bidlack JM, Mello NK, Furness MS, Rice KC, Brandt MR. Delta opioid antagonist effects of buprenorphine in rhesus monkeys. Behav Pharmacol 2002;13:557–570.
74. Huang P, Kehner GB, Cowan A, Liu-Chen L-Y. Comparison of pharmacological activities of buprenorphine and nor-buprenorphine: nor-buprenorphine is a potent opioid agonist. J Pharmacol Exp Ther 2001;297:688–695.
75. Wnendt S, Kruger T, Janocha E, Hildebrandt D, Englberger W. Agonist effect of buprenorphine in a nociceptin/OFQ receptor-triggered report gene assay. Mol Pharmacol 1999;56:334–338.
76. Hawkinson JE, Acosta-Burruel M, Espitia SA. Opioid activity profiles indicate similarities between the nociceptin/orphanin FQ and opioid receptors. Eur J Pharmacol 2000;389:107–114.
77. Yamamoto T, Shono K, Tanabe S. Buprenorphine activates mu- and opioid receptor like-1 receptors simultaneously, but the analgesic effect is mainly mediated by mu receptor activation in the rat formalin test. J Pharmacol Exp Ther 2006;318:206–213.
78. Zubieta JK, Greenwald MK, Lombardi U, Woods JH, Kilbourn MR, Jewett DM, Koeppe RA, Schuster CR, Johanson, CE. Buprenorphine-induced changes in *mu*-opioid receptor availability in male heroin-dependent volunteers: a preliminary study. Neuropsychopharmacology 2000;23:326–334.
79. Greenwald MK. Human experimental therapeutic models in opioid dependence: translational research advances and implications. In: McKenna CR (Ed.), Trends in Substance Abuse Research, 2007;1–55. New York: Nova Science Publishers, Inc.
80. Sobel B-F, Sigmon SC, Walsh SL, Johnson RE, Liebson IA, Nuwayser ES, Kerrigan JH, Bigelow GE. Open-label trial of an injection depot formulation of buprenorphine in opioid detoxification. Drug Alcohol Depend 2004;73:11–22.
81. Sigmon SC, Wong CJ, Chausmer AL, Liebson IA, Bigelow GE. Evaluation of an injection depot formulation of buprenorphine: placebo comparison. Addiction 2004;99:1439–1449.
82. Comer SD, Collins ED, Kleber HD, Nuwayser ES, Kerrigan JH, Fischman MW. Depot naltrexone: long-lasting antagonism of the effects of heroin in humans. Psychopharmacology (Berl) 2002;159:351–360.
83. Campbell BK, Wander N, Stark MJ, Holbert T. Treating cigarette smoking in drug-abusing clients. J Subst Abuse Treat 1995;12:89–94.
84. Frosch DL, Shoptaw S, Jarvik ME, Rawson RA, Ling W. Interest in smoking cessation among methadone maintained outpatients. J Addict Dis 1998;17:9–19.
85. Navaratnam V, Foong K. Adjunctive drug use among opiate addicts. Curr Med Res Opin 1990;11:611–619.
86. Stark MJ, Campbell BK. Drug use and cigarette smoking in applicants for drug abuse treatment. J. Subst Abuse 1993;5:175–181.
87. Steinmiller CL, Greenwald MK. Factors associated with non-medical use of prescription opioids among heroin abusing research volunteers. Exp Clin Psychopharmacol 2007;15:492–500.
88. Houdi AA, Dasgupta R, Kindy MS. Effect of nicotine use and withdrawal on brain preproenkephalin A mRNA. Brain Res 1998;799:257–263.
89. Malin DH, Lake JR, Payne MC, Short PE, Carter VA, Cunningham JS, Wilson OB. Nicotine alleviation of nicotine abstinence syndrome is naloxone-reversible. Pharmacol Biochem Behav 1996;53:81–85.
90. Rasmussen DD. Effects of chronic nicotine treatment and withdrawal on hypothalamic proopiomelano-cortin gene expression and neuroendocrine regulation. Psychoneuroendocrinology 1998;23:245–259.

91. Wewers ME, Dhatt RK, Snively TA, Tejwani GA. The effect of chronic administration of nicotine on antinociception, opioid receptor binding and met-enkephalin levels in rats. Brain Res 1999;822:107–113.
92. Krishnan-Sarin S, Rosen MI, O'Malley SS. Naloxone challenge in smokers. Preliminary evidence of an opioid component in nicotine dependence. Arch Gen Psychiatry 1999;56:663–668.
93. Marco AP, Greenwald MK, Higgins MS. A preliminary study of 24-hour post-Cesarean patient-controlled analgesia: postoperative pain reports and morphine requests/utilization are greater in abstaining smokers than non-smokers. Med Sci Monit 2005;11:255–261.
94. Gorelick DA, Rose J, Jarvik ME. Effect of naloxone on cigarette smoking. J Subst Abuse 1988;1:153–159.
95. Karras A, Kane JM. Naloxone reduces cigarette smoking. Life Sci 1980;27:1541–1545.
96. Nemeth-Coslett R, Heningfield JE, O'Keeffe MK, Griffiths RR. Effects of mecamylamine on human cigarette smoking and subjective ratings. Psychopharmacology 1986;88:420–425.
97. Sutherland G, Stapleton JA, Russell MAH. Naltrexone, smoking behaviour and cigarette withdrawal. Psychopharmacology 1995;120:418–425.
98. Reid LD, Delconte JD, Nichols ML, Bilsky EJ, Hubbell CL. Tests of opioid deficiency hypotheses of alcoholism. Alcohol 1991;8:247–257.
99. Gianoulakis C, Chan JS, Kalant H, Chretien M. Chronic ethanol treatment alters the biosynthesis of beta-endorphin by the rat neurointermediate lobe. Can J Physiol Pharmacol 1983;61:967–976.
100. Schulz R, Wuster M, Duka T, Herz A. Acute and chronic ethanol treatment changes endorphin levels in brain and pituitary. Psychopharmacology 1980;68:221–227.
101. Froehlich JC, Harts J, Lumeng L, Li TK. Naloxone attenuates voluntary ethanol intake in rats selectively bred for high ethanol preference. Pharmacol Biochem Behav 1990;35:385–390.
102. Hubbell CL, Czirr SA, Hunter GA, Beaman CM, LeCann NC, Reid LD. Consumption of ethanol solution is potentiated by morphine and attenuated by naloxone persistently across repeated daily administrations. Alcohol 1986;3:39–53.
103. Marfaing-Jallat P, Miceli D, LeMagnen J. Decrease in ethanol consumption by naloxone in naïve and dependent rats. Pharmacol Biochem Behav 1983;18:S537–S539.
104. Samson HH, Doyle TF. Oral ethanol self-administration in the rat: effect of naloxone. Pharmacol Biochem Behav 1985;22:91–99.
105. Weiss F, Mitchiner M, Bloom FE, Koob GF. Free-choice responding for ethanol versus water in alcohol preferring (P) and unselected Wistar rats is differentially modified by naloxone, bromocriptine, and methysergide. Psychopharmacology 1990;101:178–186.
106. Altshuler HL, Phillips PE, Feinhandler DA. Alteration of ethanol self-administration by naltrexone. Life Sci 1980;26:679–688.
107. Kornet M, Goosen C, Van Ree JM. Effect of naltrexone on alcohol consumption during chronic alcohol drinking and after a period of imposed abstinence in free-choice drinking rhesus monkeys. Psychopharmacology 1991;104:367–376.
108. Myers RD, Borg S, Mossberg R. Antagonism by naltrexone of voluntary alcohol selection in the chronically drinking macaque monkey. Alcohol 1986;3:383–388.
109. Volpicelli JR, Davis MA, Olgin JE. Naltrexone blocks the post-shock increase of ethanol consumption. Life Sci 1986;38:841–847.
110. Hyytia P, Kiianmaa K. Suppression of ethanol responding by centrally administered CTOP and naltrindole in AA and Wistar rats. Alcohol Clin Exp Res 2001;25:25–33.
111. Krishnan-Sarin S, Jing SL, Kurtz DL, Zweifel M, Portoghese PS, Li T-K, Froehlich JC. The delta opioid receptor antagonist naltrindole attenuates both alcohol and saccharin intake in rats selectively bred for alcohol preference. Psychopharmacology 1995a;120:177–185.
112. Krishnan-Sarin S, Portoghese PS, Li T-K, Froehlich JC. The delta opioid receptor antagonist naltriben selectively attenuates alcohol intake in rats bred for alcohol preference. Pharmacol Biochem Behav 1995b;52:153–159.
113. Krishnan-Sarin S, Wand GS, Li XW, Portoghese PS, Froehlich JC. Effect of mu opioid receptor blockade on alcohol intake in rats bred for high alcohol drinking. Pharmacol Biochem Behav 1998;59:627–635.

114. Stromberg MF, Casale M, Volpicelli L, Volpicelli JR, O'Brien CP. A comparison of the effects of the opioid antagonists naltrexone, naltrindole, and beta-funaltrexamine on ethanol consumption in the rat. Alcohol 1998;15:281–289.
115. O'Malley SS. Opioid antagonists in the treatment of alcohol dependence: clinical efficacy and prevention of relapse. Alcohol 1996;1:77–81.
116. O'Brien CP, Volpicelli LA, Volpicelli JR. Naltrexone in the treatment of alcoholism: a clinical review. Alcohol 1996;13:35–39.
117. Krystal JH, Cramer JA, Krol WF, Kirk GF, Rosenheck RA. Naltrexone in the treatment of alcohol dependence. N Engl J Med 2001;345:1734–1739.
118. Oslin DW, Berrettini W, Kranzler HR, Pettinati H, Gelertner J, Volpicelli JR, O'Brien CP. A functional polymorphism of the mu-opioid receptor gene is associated with naltrexone response in alcohol-dependent patients. Neuropsychopharmacology 2003;28:1546–1552.
119. Drobes DJ, Anton RF, Thomas SE, Voronin K. A clinical laboratory paradigm for evaluating medication effects on alcohol consumption: naltrexone and nalmefene. Neuropsychopharmacology 2003;28:755–764.
120. O'Malley SS, Krishnan-Sarin S, Farren C, Sinha R, Kreek MJ. Naltrexone decreases craving and alcohol self-administration in alcohol-dependent subjects and activates the hypothalamo-pituitary-adrenocortical axis. Psychopharmacology 2002;160:19–29.
121. Clow DW, Hammer RP Jr, Kirstein CL, Spear LP. Gestational cocaine exposure increases opiate receptor binding in weanling offspring. Brain Res Dev Brain Res 1991;59:179–185.
122. Cowen MS, Lawrence AJ. The role of opioid-dopamine interactions in the induction and maintenance of ethanol consumption. Prog Neuropsychopharmacol Biol Psychiatry 1999;23:1171–1212.
123. Mello NK, Negus SS. Interactions between kappa opioid agonists and cocaine. Preclinical studies. Ann NY Acad Sci 2000;909:104–132.
124. Sheffler DJ, Roth BL. Salvinorin A: the "magic mint" hallucinogen finds a molecular target in the kappa opioid receptor. Trends Pharmacol Sci 2003;24:107–109.
125. Mazarati A, Liu H, Wasterlain C. Opioid peptide pharmacology and immunocytochemistry in an animal model of self-sustaining status epilepticus. Neuroscience 1999;89:167–173.
126. Solbrig V, Adrian R, Baratta J, Lauterborn JC, Koob GF. Kappa opioid control of seizures produced by a virus in an animal model. Brain 2006;129:642–654.
127. Talbot PS, Narendran R, Butelman ER, Huang Y, Ngo K, Slifstein M, Martinez D, Laruelle M, Hwang DR. 11C-GR103545, a radiotracer for imaging kappa-opioid receptors in vivo with PET: synthesis and evaluation in baboons. J Nucl Med 2005;46:484–494.
128. Spanagel R, Herz A, Shippenberg TS. Opposing tonically active endogenous opioid systems modulate the mesolimbic dopaminergic pathway. Proc Natl Acad Sci USA 1992; 89:2046–2050.
129. Trujillo KA, Akil H. Changes in prodynorphin peptide content following treatment with morphine or amphetamine: possible role in mechanisms of action of drugs of abuse. NIDA Res Monogr 1989;95:550–551.
130. DiChiara G, Imperato A. Opposite effects of mu and kappa opiate agonists on dopamine release in the nucleus accumbens and in the dorsal caudate of freely moving rats. J Pharmacol Exp Ther 1988;244:1067–1080.
131. Devine DP, Leone P, Pocock D, Wise RA. Differential involvement of ventral tegmental mu, delta and kappa opioid receptors in modulation of basal mesolimbic dopamine release: in vivo microdialysis studies. J Pharmacol Exp Ther 1993;266:1236–1246.
132. Maisonneuve IM, Archer S, Glick SD. U50,488 a K opioid receptor agonist, attenuates cocaine-induced increases in extracellular dopamine in the nucleus accumbens of rats. Neurosci Lett 1994;181:57–60.
133. Glick SD, Maisonneuve IM, Raucci J, Archer S. Kappa opioid inhibition of morphine and cocaine self-administration in rats. Brain Res 1995;681:147–152.
134. Walsh SL, Geter-Douglas B, Strain EC, Bigelow GE. Enadoline and butorphanol: evaluation of kappa-agonists on cocaine pharmacodynamics and cocaine self-administration in humans. J Pharmacol Exp Ther 2001;299:147–158.

135. Preston KL, Umbricht A, Schroeder JR, Abreu ME, Epstein DH, Pickworth WB. Cyclazocine: comparison to hydromorphone and interaction with cocaine. Behav Pharmacol 2004;15:91–102.
136. Martin WR, Gorodetzky CW, McClane TK. An experimental study in the treatment of narcotic addicts with cyclazocine. Clin Pharmacol Ther 1966;7:455–464.
137. Reece PA, Sedman AJ, Rose DS, Wright R, Dawkins R, Rajagopalan R. Diuretic effects, pharmacokinetics, and safety of a new centrally acting kappa-opioid agonist (CI-977) in humans. J Clin Pharmacol 1994;34:1126–1132.
138. Ananthan S. Opioid ligands with mixed mu/delta opioid receptor interactions: an emerging approach to novel analgesics. AAPS J 2006;8:E118–E125.
139. Gallantine EL, Meert TF. A comparison of the antinociceptive and adverse effects of the mu-opioid agonist morphine and the delta-opioid agonist SNC80. Basic Clin Pharmacol Toxicol 2005;97:39–51.
140. Su YF, McNutt RW, Chang KJ. Delta-opioid ligands reverse alfentanil-induced respiratory depression but not antinociception. J Pharmacol Exp Ther 1998;287:815–823.
141. Negus SS, Gatch MB, Mello NK, Zhang X, Rice KC. Behavioral effects of the delta-selective opioid agonist SNC80 and related compounds in rhesus monkeys. J Pharmacol Exp Ther 1998;286:362–375.
142. Broom DC, Jutkiewicz EM, Folk JE, Traynor JR, Rice KC, Woods JH. Nonpeptidic delta-opioid receptor agonists reduce immobility in the forced swim assay in rats. Neuropsychopharmacology 2002;26:744–755.
143. Tejedor-Real P, Mico JA, Smadja C, Maldonado R, Roques BP, Gilbert-Rahola J. Involvement of delta-opioid receptors in the effects induced by endogenous enkephalins on learned helplessness model. Eur J Pharmacol 1998;31:1–7.
144. Torregrossa MM, Folk JE, Rice KC, Watson SJ, Woods JH. Chronic administration of the delta opioid receptor agonist (+)BW373U86 and antidepressants on behavior in the forced swim test and BDNF mRNA expression in rats. Psychopharmacology (Berl) 2005;183:31–40.
145. Perrine SA, Hoshaw BA, Unterwald EM. Delta opioid receptor ligands modulate anxiety-like behaviors in the rat. Br J Pharmacol 2006;147:864–872.
146. Saitoh A, Kimura Y, Suzuki T, Kawai K, Nagase H, Kamei J. Potential anxiolytic and antidepressant-like activities of SNC80, a selective delta-opioid agonist, in behavioral models in rodents. J Pharmacol Sci 2004;95:374–380.
147. Jutkiewicz EM, Baladi MG, Folk JE, Rice KC, Woods JH. The convulsive and electroencephalographic changes produced by nonpeptidic delta-opioid agonists in rats: comparison with pentylenetetrazol. J Pharmacol Exp Ther 2006;317:1337–1348.
148. Jutkiewicz EM, Rice KC, Traynor JR, Woods JH. Separation of the convulsions and antidepressant-like effects produced by the delta-opioid agonist SNC80 in rats. Psychopharmacology (Berl) 2005;182:588–596.
149. Schreckenberger M, Klega A, Grunder G, Buchholz HG, Scheurich A, Schirrmacher R, Schirrmacher E, Muller C, Henriksen G, Bartenstein P. Opioid receptor PET reveals the psychobiologic correlates of reward processing. J Nucl Med 2008;49: 1257–1261.
150. Sprenger T, Valet M, Boecker H, Henriksen G, Spilker ME, Willoch F, Wagner KJ, Wester HJ, Tolle TR. Opioidergic activation in the medial pain system after heat pain. Pain 2006;122:63–67.

Chapter 4
Opioid Receptor Antagonist-Mediated Signaling in the Immune System

Jonathan Moorman, Zhi Qiang Yao, Edward J. Bilsky, and Deling Yin

Abstract An increased susceptibility to infectious diseases in the setting of opiate use has long been noted. Studies on the specific roles of opiates in immune cells using opioid agonists and antagonists reveal a broad array of effects that include altered T and B cell proliferation, antibody production, natural killer cell activity, and cytokine production. The complexity of these effects in the setting of multiple opioid receptor subtypes has only recently been recognized. Novel, receptor-specific opioid antagonists permit more robust studies on the protean effects of these agents on immune cells. This chapter will emphasize what is known about the biologic and clinical effects of opioids on immune function with a focus on the role of opioid antagonists.

Keywords: Opioids; Immunity; Antagonists; Lymphocyte; Infection

4.1 Introduction

Opiates have long been known to exert significant effects on the immune system. Human studies dating back to the 1960s (50) have shown an increased susceptibility to infections in the setting of opiate use. Subsequent studies using opioid agonists and antagonists in animal models have described protean effects on immune cells (5, 30, 52). These include effects on T and B cell proliferation, antibody production, natural killer (NK) cell activity, and cytokine production. The complexity of these effects in the setting of multiple opioid receptor subtypes has only recently been recognized (10, 59, 86, 94).

Early studies revealing a naloxone-reversible suppressive effect of morphine on T cell rosette formation (105) supported a role for opioid receptor antagonists in studying immune responses to opiates. Following these pivotal reports, both nonselective and selective opioid antagonists targeting the classical opioid receptors (μ, κ, and

J. Moorman (✉), Z.Q. Yao, E.J. Bilsky, and D. Yin
Department of Internal Medicine, James H. Quillen College of Medicine,
East Tennessee State University, Box 70622, Johnson City, TN 36714
e-mail: moorman@etsu.edu

R. Dean et al. (eds.), *Opiate Receptors and Antagonists*,

Table 4.1 Opiate agonists and antagonists commonly used to study effects on immune cells

Endogenous opiate agonists	Receptor preference
β-Endorphin	μ, δ
Met/leu enkephalin	δ > μ
Dynorphin A and B	κ
Endomorphin-1	μ
Exogenous opiate agonists	
Morphine	μ, δ, κ
DAMGO	μ
DPDPE	δ
U69593	κ
U50488	κ
Bremazocine	κ
DADLE	δ
Deltorphin 1	δ
N-methylmorphine	μ, δ, κ
Opiate antagonists	
Naloxone	μ > δ, κ
Naltrexone	μ > δ, κ
β-Funaltrexamine	μ
Norbinaltorphimine	κ
Natrindole	δ
Naltriben	δ
ICI174864	δ
SNC-80	δ
N-methylnaltrexone	μ > δ, κ

δ) emerged as tools to examine opioid signaling mechanisms in the immune system. This chapter will summarize the role of these antagonists in immune signaling.

Opioid ligands are in general characterized as agonists or antagonists, although structural differences in these ligands are often quite minor. While both bind the given opioid receptor with good affinity, antagonists stabilize the receptor in an inactive form and inhibit binding by agonists (27). A summary of many of the commonly employed opioid agonists and antagonists, with their selectivities, is presented in Table 4.1.

4.2 Opioid Receptor Expression in the Immune System

The three classical opioid receptors, μ (μOR), δ (δOR), and κ (κOR) as well as nonclassical opioid-like receptors (such as nociceptin, the orphan receptor) have been found on immune cells in multiple studies using pharmacologic approaches (59, 86). The classical receptors, which are members of the superfamily of G protein-coupled receptors which contain seven transmembrane helices, were cloned in the 1990s. Different properties within these three subtypes were also described, based on radioligand binding assays, and may be a result of splice variants of the three receptors.

Sequence analysis of the μOR, κOR, and δOR derived from immune cells suggests that these receptors are homologous to the classical receptors found in the brain (24–26, 59, 78, 104). Differences in the distribution of these receptors on specific immune cells, however, appear likely. In addition, recent studies suggest that multiple receptor mRNA species may be present in at least some immune cells (1, 4, 7, 106). For example, the R1.1 T cell lymphoma line was found to have several κOR mRNA species, as well as inserted sequences in the 5′-noncoding region of the receptor (7).

Splice variants of the κOR and other opioid receptors have also been noted (39, 101, 106), and could represent a mechanism by which immune cells express opioid receptors with variable binding affinities for agonists and antagonists. A splice variant of nociceptin was found in 40–50% of these receptors in mouse lymphocytes (39).

4.2.1 Opioid Receptors on Lymphocytes

Using naloxone, Mehrishi and Mills found binding to human lymphocytes that was sensitive to competition with morphine (60). This suggested the existence of a classical μ opioid receptor on these cells. Two binding sites with different affinities for naloxone were also described on rat T cells and appeared to be expressed following T cell activation (62). μOR were detected by RT-PCR in human T and B cell lines and CD4 + T cells as well (26).

The murine T cell line, EL-4, appears to have a κOR in studies using the κ agonist bremazocine (32). As noted above, the thymoma cell line, R1.1, appears to have a κOR as well (7). Indirect immunofluorescence techniques have also shown κOR on thymocytes and confirm their presence on both $CD4^+$ and $CD8^+$ cells (45). Fluorescent opioid agonist binding was blocked using the selective κ antagonist norbinaltorphimine (nor-BNI) (11, 45).

Jurkat T cells have a δOR based on studies using enkephalins (3, 40), and δORs have been found on MOLT-4 T cells and IM-9 B cells (20) and B- and T cell-enriched murine splenocytes (19). δOR transcripts were also found in murine splenocytes and certain B, T, and monocyte cell lines (104).

4.2.2 Opioid Receptors on Granulocytes, Monocytes, and Macrophages

A μOR appears to be present on granulocytes and monocytes in several studies employing receptor agonists (49, 54, 55, 60), as well as in studies using RT-PCR (26). Macrophage cell lines such as $P33D_1$ likely have a κOR based on binding with κ-selective agonists, as well as a δOR (20). Human granulocytes appear to have at least two δOR binding sites that are not displaceable with μ- or κ-selective antagonists (33). Human polymorphonuclear leukocytes also have been found to have naloxone (29) and deltorphin binding sites (91).

4.3 Opioid Receptor Antagonists: Effects on Immune Functions

Opioid receptor agonists and antagonists have profound effects on immune cell function. It is important to note the difficulty in determining the direct effects of these agents on a given immune cell population because of the interdependency of immune cells to achieve their functions. As such, an accessory cell population could contribute to the results of functional assays in mixed populations of immune cells. Isolation of specific and pure populations has been attempted in several studies.

4.3.1 Effects on T Cell Growth and Proliferation

T cell proliferative responses to stimuli have in general been shown to be inhibited in response to opioid agonists, but the overall effect may be complex (5, 14, 88, 103). Morphine, considered a nonselective agonist, has been shown to suppress cytokine expression (including interleukin-2 (IL-2), and interferon-γ) (18, 67, 65, 74), inhibit T cell proliferation in response to IL-1 (73), and decrease responsiveness to colony-stimulating factors (72).

It has been recognized that activation of naïve T cells upregulates expression of δOR, perhaps as a mechanism to modulate immune responses (87). In these cells, δOR signaling appears to induce phosphorylation of key mitogen-activated protein kinases (MAPKs), including c-jun kinase (JNK) and extracellular signal-related kinase (ERK) (83, 84). The selective δ antagonist naltrindole was able to inhibit the phosphorylation of c-jun induced by [D-Ala^{2}-D-Leu^{5}]enkephalin (DADLE), a δOR agonist, in these studies (84).

In addition, proliferation of purified populations of CD4^{+} and CD8 + T cells derived from mouse spleens can be inhibited by the δOR agonist [D-Pen2,D-Pen5]-enkephalin (DPDPE), with blockade by the δOR antagonist naltrindole (82). However, the δOR agonist deltorphin enhanced splenocyte proliferation that occurred in response to con A; naltrindole blocked this enhancement (82).

Studies on the role of κOR in lymphocyte signal transduction have been difficult due to the relatively low expression of this receptor on mononuclear cells populations (86). Signaling through κOR does appear to affect antibody synthesis (38) (see below) and may alter cytokine levels (69).

4.3.2 Role in Thymocytes and Effect on Cellular Apoptosis

In vivo, treatment with morphine has been consistently shown to induce thymic atrophy, with a remarkable loss of CD4/CD8 double-positive thymocytes (14, 17, 34, 80).

Naloxone treatment was able to prevent the majority of morphine's effects (34, 79). Apoptosis in response to opioid agonists has also been observed in B cells as well as macrophages derived from multiple origins, including rat, mouse, and human (42, 89). This appears to be a direct induction and is blocked by naloxone. It has been unclear, however, as to whether a morphine-induced glucocorticoid increase might be playing a role in this loss of thymocytes via apoptosis; this possibility was supported by studies showing no apoptotic effect of morphine on thymocytes in culture and by inhibition of morphine's effects using glucocorticoid antagonists (36, 80).

We have examined the role of Fas, a receptor protein that regulates immune responses, in apoptotic signaling by opiates (107). Morphine treatment of a T cell hybridoma, A1.1, as well as human peripheral blood mononuclear cells (PBMCs), led to dramatic increases in Fas expression that was blocked by naloxone. In addition, these cells were primed to undergo Fas-mediated apoptosis when exposed to the natural ligand, Fas ligand (FasL). Splenocytes from mice treated with morphine also had a reduction in cell number that was blocked by naloxone, suggesting that the immunosuppressive effects of morphine occur via an opioid receptor. Our recent finding that stress also induces proapoptotic genes (108) in splenocytes suggests the possibility that multiple triggers and perhaps cross talk might contribute to the ultimate decrease in lymphocyte number, and perhaps affect overall lymphocyte function as well.

Endogenous enkephalins can inhibit fetal thymocyte proliferation in response to con A, limiting spontaneous proliferation as perhaps a means of promoting differentiation within the thymus during gestational development (46). The δOR antagonist naltrindole enhanced fetal thymocyte proliferation in these studies, suggesting a role for δOR signaling in early T cell differentiation.

4.3.3 Effects on Cytokine Signaling

Cytokine signaling by immune cells is clearly affected by modulation of opioid receptor signaling, although studies have often been conflicting. For example, naloxone was able to reverse morphine and β-endorphin-induced suppression of interferon-γ production in PBMCs after con A stimulation (66), but opioid agonists were able to elevate interferon-γ in studies by Brown and van Epps (12) and Mandler (58). Similarly, naloxone was able to block opioid agonist-induced enhancement of IL-2 production by IL-1 in lymphoma cell lines (8), but upon morphine treatment IL-2 was inhibited in studies by Jessop et al. (44), and both IL-2 and interferon-γ were inhibited in studies by Lysle et al. (51). Supporting a suppressive effect of opioid agonists are studies in which naloxone antagonism was able to reverse an increase in transforming growth factor beta (TGF-β) in stimulated PBMCs, since this cytokine is known to be immunosuppressive (22).

Disparities in the role of opioid receptor signaling in cytokine production may also be a function of dose dependency. For example, low-dose morphine increased lipopolysaccharide (LPS)-induced nuclear factor kappa-B (NFκB) production, but high-dose morphine reduced this production (76). Similarly, studies by Shahabi et al. showed decreasing IL-2 levels with increasing deltorphin concentrations (81). The majority of studies using δOR agonists, however, have suggested an elevation in IL-2 gene expression and/or protein production.

4.3.4 Effects on Phagocytic Functions

Studies of the effect of opioid agonists and antagonists on phagocytic functions have led to interesting results. In vivo administration of morphine inhibited neutrophils and macrophages in terms of their ability to phagocytose yeast (63, 97–98), a finding blocked by naltrexone (70). While the μOR appeared to be the primary opioid receptor mediating effects on phagocytosis, selective μOR, κOR, and δOR antagonists were able to block the inhibitory effects of μ, κ, and δ agonists (92). Superoxide production was increased in macrophages in response to κOR-selective agonists and β-endorphin (85), which also modulate the oxidative burst and production of IL-1 in various macrophage cell lines (2, 6, 95).

Results in studies of chemotaxis have been less clear. Morphine appeared to enhance chemotaxis in human monocytes and neutrophils upon treatment with endogenous opioids (57, 77, 100). However, several studies using a variety of agonists showed inhibition of chemotaxis in these same cells (47, 64), with decreased response to chemokines and desensitization of chemokine receptors (e.g., CCR1, CCR2, CXCR1, and CXCR2) (77).

4.3.5 Effects on NK Function

When administered either centrally or peripherally, morphine is able to inhibit cytolytic activity of splenic NK cells (43, 53, 88, 102). Interestingly, this inhibition is likely a function of opioid receptor signaling in the central nervous system (CNS). Intracerebroventricular (ICV) injection of morphine led to decreased NK cell activity that was blocked by naltrexone. However, systemic delivery of *N*-methylmorphine – which cannot cross the blood–brain barrier – had no effect of NK cell cytolytic activity (43, 53). Further studies using opioid antagonists revealed that the caudal aspect of the periaqueductal gray matter was the site of opioid receptor signaling that mediated NK cell activity (43, 53, 88). The role of the CNS in immunomodulation by opioid receptor signaling is discussed in further detail below.

4.3.6 Effects on Antibody Production

Administration of morphine can induce prominent suppression of antibody synthesis that is reversible with naltrexone antagonism (9, 17, 18). Selective opioid receptor antagonists such as nor-BNI have also been shown to block the suppression of T cell-dependent antibody synthesis induced by either morphine, U50488, or U65593 (the latter two being κOR agonists) in splenocytes from BALB/c mice (93). Interestingly, splenocytes from mice that are deficient in μOR still exhibit antibody suppression in response to morphine, but not U50488; strain differences in mice, however, appear to influence in vitro responses to these agents (28, 93).

4.4 The Central Nervous System-Immune System Link

While immunomodulatory signaling through opioid receptors is clearly at play, it remains less clear as to where this signaling is occurring. As noted above, immune cells do variably express opioid receptors that do appear to interact directly with opioid antagonists and agonists to mediate responses. Other studies suggest, however, that these agents may be functioning within the CNS that is bidirectionally linked to the immune system (61, 99).

Several studies have supported a central mechanism of action for opioids in immunomodulation (61, 88). Splenic immune cell functions in particular have been examined and found to be negatively affected following ICV injection of morphine; these include NK cell function and T/B cell proliferation in response to mitogens (53). ICV treatment with *N*-methylnaltrexone (which does not cross the blood–brain barrier) was able to antagonize morphine's effects, but not when administered systemically at doses that could not act centrally (31). Different areas of the brain appeared to mediate these immunomodulatory events (41, 53, 102).

Using selective antagonists and agonists, Nelson et al. demonstrated that rats receiving ICV administration of the μOR-selective agonist [D-Ala^2-MePhe^4-Gly(ol)^5] enkephalin (DAMGO) had a dose-dependent decrease in NK cell activity as well as T cell proliferation in response to con A; these findings were abrogated upon antagonism with *N*-methylnaltrexone before DAMGO treatment (61). Interestingly, neither κOR- nor δOR-selective agonists had any effect on splenocyte function, suggesting that CNS-mediated immunomodulatory effects of opioids occur through μOR signaling pathways. In contrast, Roy et al. used μOR knockout mice and noted that morphine was still capable of reducing both splenic and thymic cell number and proliferation (75).

Another area of interest has been the hypothalamic pituitary axis (HPA). Acute and chronic morphine use can activate this axis and lead to splenic and thymic atrophy (99). Systemic administration of morphine induces an increase in corticosteroid concentrations, with the possibility that some of the effects on opioid signaling may be related to these (in particular apoptotic effects). Antagonism of glucocorticosteroids, however, was not able to block splenic and thymic atrophy seen with morphine – suggesting an immune response that is independent of corticosteroids. In mice injected with morphine, the decrease in NK cell activity was blocked by RU486, a steroid antagonist (13–16, 35, 71).

4.5 Opioid Receptor Signaling and Infection

As described above, opioid receptor signaling appears to have a significant effect on immune cell function and this may translate into effects during host infection. In the 1960s, Louria et al. showed that heroin addicts had an increased susceptibility to infection (50). Heroin addicts also demonstrated decreased T cell proliferation (37). In mice experimentally infected with *Toxoplasma gondii*, morphine increased mortality rates (21).

Perhaps the most interesting clinical scenario in which opioid receptor signaling may play a role is during HIV infection. HIV expression was increased in chronically HIV-infected U1 promonocytes cocultured with fetal brain cells upon dynorphin and U50488 treatment; this was blocked with the κ antagonist nor-BNI (23) and perhaps due to increased expression of tumor necrosis factor alpha (TNF-α) and IL-6. Notably, acutely infected microglial cell cultures demonstrated inhibition of HIV expression upon κ agonist treatment which was reversible with nor-BNI antagonism. μOR signaling via enodmorphin-1 or β-endorphin was also shown to potentiate HIV expression in brain cell cultures (68).

Because opiates often behave in a manner similar to cytokines, their role in HIV chemokine/coreceptor function has been examined. For example, morphine regulates the expression of CCR5 and CXCR4, coreceptors for HIV entry, on human monocytes and T cells (90). The opioid μOR antagonist β-fenaprexamine was able to inhibit upregulation of chemokine receptors (CCR5 and CCR3) on astroglia cells (56). A κOR antagonist was shown to inhibit CXCR4 expression on CD4 cells, decreasing their susceptibility to X4 strains of HIV infection (13, 48, 90).

4.6 Conclusions and Perspectives

In this chapter, we have outlined many of the major effects of opioid receptor signaling on immune cell function. Direct and/or indirect effects on immune cells via the CNS lead to protean changes in immune cell function via classical and nonclassical opioid receptor mechanisms. Opiate agonists and antagonists alter lymphocyte proliferative responses, antibody production, cytokine expression, and apoptosis, among others. The role that this immunomodulation may play in clinical infection remains less clear, although it seems likely that the acute or chronic use of opiates will skew normal host immune responses to pathogenic infections.

Opioid receptor signaling in the immune system likely involves a complex interplay of receptor expression, binding specificity, dose dependence, and cross talk between intracellular signaling pathways. Such realities challenge investigators to use novel approaches to discern specific functions in the setting of opiate use. Opioid receptor antagonists have increasingly played a key role in this discernment and will likely have an expanding role in both experimental and clinical approaches to modulating immune cell responses.

References

1. Alicea, C., Belkowski, S. M., Sliker, J. K., Zhu, J., Liu-Chen, L. Y., Eisenstein, T. K., Adler, M. W., & Rogers, T. J. (1998). Characterization of kappa-opioid receptor transcripts expressed by T cells and macrophages. *J Neuroimmunol,* 91(1–2), 55–62.
2. Apte, R. N., Durum, S. K., & Oppenheim, J. J. (1990). Opioids modulate interleukin-1 production and secretion by bone-marrow macrophages. *Immunol Lett,* 24(2), 141–148.
3. Ausiello, C. M., & Roda, L. G. (1984). Leu-enkephalin binding to cultured human T lymphocytes. *Cell Biol Int Rep,* 8(5), 353–362.
4. Bare, L. A., Mansson, E., & Yang, D. (1994). Expression of two variants of the human mu opioid receptor mRNA in SK-N-SH cells and human brain. *FEBS Lett,* 354(2), 213–216.
5. Bayer, B. M., Daussin, S., Hernandez, M., & Irvin, L. (1990). Morphine inhibition of lymphocyte activity is mediated by an opioid dependent mechanism. *Neuropharmacology,* 29(4), 369–374.
6. Belkowski, S. M., Alicea, C., Eisenstein, T. K., Adler, M. W., & Rogers, T. J. (1995). Inhibition of interleukin-1 and tumor necrosis factor-alpha synthesis following treatment of macrophages with the kappa opioid agonist U50,488H. *J Pharmacol Exp Ther,* 273(3), 1491–1496.
7. Belkowski, S. M., Zhu, J., Liu-Chen, L. Y., Eisenstein, T. K., Adler, M. W., & Rogers, T. J. (1995). Sequence of kappa-opioid receptor cDNA in the R1.1 thymoma cell line. *J Neuroimmunol,* 62(1), 113–117.
8. Bessler, H., Sztein, M. B., & Serrate, S. A. (1990). Beta-endorphin modulation of IL-1-induced IL-2 production. *Immunopharmacology,* 19(1), 5–14.
9. Bhargava, H. N., Thomas, P. T., Thorat, S., & House, R. V. (1994). Effects of morphine tolerance and abstinence on cellular immune function. *Brain Res,* 642(1–2), 1–10.
10. Bidlack, J. M. (2000). Detection and function of opioid receptors on cells from the immune system. *Clin Diagn Lab Immunol,* 7(5), 719–723.
11. Bidlack, J. M., Lawrence, D. M., & Ignatowski, T. A. (1996). Kappa opioid receptors on immune cells as studied by fluorescent ligands. *Adv Exp Med Biol,* 402, 13–22.
12. Brown, S. L., & Van Epps, D. E. (1986). Opioid peptides modulate production of interferon gamma by human mononuclear cells. *Cell Immunol,* 103(1), 19–26.
13. Bryant, H. U., & Roudebush, R. E. (1990). Suppressive effects of morphine pellet implants on in vivo parameters of immune function. *J Pharmacol Exp Ther,* 255(2), 410–414.
14. Bryant, H. U., Bernton, E. W., & Holaday, J. W. (1987). Immunosuppressive effects of chronic morphine treatment in mice. *Life Sci,* 41(14), 1731–1738.
15. Bryant, H. U., Bernton, E. W., & Holaday, J. W. (1988). Morphine pellet-induced immunomodulation in mice: temporal relationships. *J Pharmacol Exp Ther,* 245(3), 913–920.
16. Bryant, H. U., Bernton, E. W., & Holaday, J. W. (1990). Immunomodulatory effects of chronic morphine treatment: pharmacologic and mechanistic studies. *NIDA Res Monogr,* 96, 131–149.
17. Bussiere, J. L., Adler, M. W., Rogers, T. J., & Eisenstein, T. K. (1992). Differential effects of morphine and naltrexone on the antibody response in various mouse strains. *Immunopharmacol Immunotoxicol,* 14(3), 657–673.
18. Bussiere, J. L., Adler, M. W., Rogers, T. J., & Eisenstein, T. K. (1993). Cytokine reversal of morphine-induced suppression of the antibody response. *J Pharmacol Exp Ther,* 264(2), 591–597.
19. Carr, D. J., Kim, C. H., deCosta, B., Jacobson, A. E., Rice, K. C., & Blalock, J. E. (1988). Evidence for a delta-class opioid receptor on cells of the immune system. *Cell Immunol,* 116(1), 44–51.
20. Carr, D. J., DeCosta, B. R., Kim, C. H., Jacobson, A. E., Guarcello, V., Rice, K. C., & Blalock, J. E. (1989). Opioid receptors on cells of the immune system: evidence for delta- and kappa-classes. *J Endocrinol,* 122(1), 161–168.

21. Chao, C. C., Sharp, B. M., Pomeroy, C., Filice, G. A., & Peterson, P. K. (1990). Lethality of morphine in mice infected with Toxoplasma gondii. *J Pharmacol Exp Ther,* 252(2), 605–609.
22. Chao, C. C., Hu, S., Molitor, T. W., Zhou, Y., Murtaugh, M. P., Tsang, M., & Peterson, P. K. (1992). Morphine potentiates transforming growth factor-beta release from human peripheral blood mononuclear cell cultures. *J Pharmacol Exp Ther,* 262(1), 19–24.
23. Chao, C. C., Gekker, G., Hu, S., Sheng, W. S., Portoghese, P. S., & Peterson, P. K. (1995). Upregulation of HIV-1 expression in cocultures of chronically infected promonocytes and human brain cells by dynorphin. *Biochem Pharmacol,* 50(5), 715–722.
24. Chuang, L. F., Chuang, T. K., Killam, K. F., Jr., Chuang, A. J., Kung, H. F., Yu, L., & Chuang, R. Y. (1994). Delta opioid receptor gene expression in lymphocytes. *Biochem Biophys Res Commun,* 202(3), 1291–1299.
25. Chuang, L. F., Chuang, T. K., Killam, K. F., Jr., Qiu, Q., Wang, X. R., Lin, J. J., Kung, H. F., Sheng, W., Chao, C., Yu, L., et al. (1995). Expression of kappa opioid receptors in human and monkey lymphocytes. *Biochem Biophys Res Commun,* 209(3), 1003–1010.
26. Chuang, T. K., Killam, K. F., Jr., Chuang, L. F., Kung, H. F., Sheng, W. S., Chao, C. C., Yu, L., & Chuang, R. Y. (1995). Mu opioid receptor gene expression in immune cells. *Biochem Biophys Res Commun,* 216(3), 922–930.
27. Eguchi, M. (2004). Recent advances in selective opioid receptor agonists and antagonists. *Med Res Rev,* 24(2), 182–212.
28. Eisenstein, T. K., Meissler, J. J., Jr., Rogers, T. J., Geller, E. B., & Adler, M. W. (1995). Mouse strain differences in immunosuppression by opioids in vitro. *J Pharmacol Exp Ther,* 275(3), 1484–1489.
29. Falke, N. E., Fischer, E. G., & Martin, R. (1985). Stereospecific opiate binding in living human polymorphonuclear leucocytes. *Cell Biol Int Rep,* 9(11), 1041–1047.
30. Fecho, K., Maslonek, K. A., Dykstra, L. A., & Lysle, D. T. (1993). Alterations of immune status induced by the sympathetic nervous system: immunomodulatory effects of DMPP alone and in combination with morphine. *Brain Behav Immun,* 7(3), 253–270.
31. Fecho, K., Maslonek, K. A., Dykstra, L. A., & Lysle, D. T. (1996). Assessment of the involvement of central nervous system and peripheral opioid receptors in the immunomodulatory effects of acute morphine treatment in rats. *J Pharmacol Exp Ther,* 276(2), 626–636.
32. Fiorica, E., & Spector, S. (1988). Opioid binding site in EL-4 thymoma cell line. *Life Sci,* 42(2), 199–206.
33. Fowler, C. J., & Fraser, G. L. (1994). Mu-, delta-, kappa-opioid receptors and their subtypes. A critical review with emphasis on radioligand binding experiments. *Neurochem Int,* 24(5), 401–426.
34. Freier, D. O., & Fuchs, B. A. (1993). Morphine-induced alterations in thymocyte subpopulations of B6C3F1 mice. *J Pharmacol Exp Ther,* 265(1), 81–88.
35. Freier, D. O., & Fuchs, B. A. (1994). A mechanism of action for morphine-induced immunosuppression: corticosterone mediates morphine-induced suppression of natural killer cell activity. *J Pharmacol Exp Ther,* 270(3), 1127–1133.
36. Fuchs, B. A., & Pruett, S. B. (1993). Morphine induces apoptosis in murine thymocytes in vivo but not in vitro: involvement of both opiate and glucocorticoid receptors. *J Pharmacol Exp Ther,* 266(1), 417–423.
37. Govitrapong, P., Suttitum, T., Kotchabhakdi, N., & Uneklabh, T. (1998). Alterations of immune functions in heroin addicts and heroin withdrawal subjects. *J Pharmacol Exp Ther,* 286(2), 883–889.
38. Guan, L., Townsend, R., Eisenstein, T. K., Adler, M. W., & Rogers, T. J. (1994). Both T cells and macrophages are targets of kappa-opioid-induced immunosuppression. *Brain Behav Immun,* 8(3), 229–240.
39. Halford, W. P., Gebhardt, B. M., & Carr, D. J. (1995). Functional role and sequence analysis of a lymphocyte orphan opioid receptor. *J Neuroimmunol,* 59(1–2), 91–101.
40. Heagy, W., Teng, E., Lopez, P., & Finberg, R. W. (1999). Enkephalin receptors and receptor-mediated signal transduction in cultured human lymphocytes. *Cell Immunol,* 191(1), 34–48.

41. Hernandez, M. C., Flores, L. R., & Bayer, B. M. (1993). Immunosuppression by morphine is mediated by central pathways. *J Pharmacol Exp Ther,* 267(3), 1336–1341.
42. Hilburger, M. E., Adler, M. W., Rogers, T. J., & Eisenstein, T. K. (1997). Morphine alters macrophage and lymphocyte populations in the spleen and peritoneal cavity. *J Neuroimmunol,* 80(1–2), 106–114.
43. Hoffman, K. E., Maslonek, K. A., Dykstra, L. A., & Lysle, D. T. (1995). Effects of central administration of morphine on immune status in Lewis and Wistar rats. *Adv Exp Med Biol,* 373, 155–159.
44. Jessop, J. J., & Taplits, M. S. (1991). Effect of high doses of morphine on Con-A induced lymphokine production in vitro. *Immunopharmacology,* 22(3), 175–184.
45. Lawrence, D. M., el-Hamouly, W., Archer, S., Leary, J. F., & Bidlack, J. M. (1995). Identification of kappa opioid receptors in the immune system by indirect immunofluorescence. *Proc Natl Acad Sci U S A,* 92(4), 1062–1066.
46. Linner, K. M., Quist, H. E., & Sharp, B. M. (1996). Expression and function of proenkephalin A messenger ribonucleic acid in murine fetal thymocytes. *Endocrinology,* 137(3), 857–863.
47. Liu, Y., Blackbourn, D. J., Chuang, L. F., Killam, K. F., Jr., & Chuang, R. Y. (1992). Effects of in vivo and in vitro administration of morphine sulfate upon rhesus macaque polymorphonuclear cell phagocytosis and chemotaxis. *J Pharmacol Exp Ther,* 263(2), 533–539.
48. Lokensgard, J. R., Gekker, G., & Peterson, P. K. (2002). Kappa-opioid receptor agonist inhibition of HIV-1 envelope glycoprotein-mediated membrane fusion and CXCR4 expression on CD4(+) lymphocytes. *Biochem Pharmacol,* 63(6), 1037–1041.
49. Lolait, S. J., Clements, J. A., Markwick, A. J., Cheng, C., McNally, M., Smith, A. I., & Funder, J. W. (1986). Pro-opiomelanocortin messenger ribonucleic acid and posttranslational processing of beta endorphin in spleen macrophages. *J Clin Invest,* 77(6), 1776–1779.
50. Louria, D. B., Hensle, T., & Rose, J. (1967). The major medical complications of heroin addiction. *Ann Intern Med,* 67(1), 1–22.
51. Lysle, D. T., Coussons, M. E., Watts, V. J., Bennett, E. H., & Dykstra, L. A. (1993a). Morphine-induced alterations of immune status: dose dependency, compartment specificity and antagonism by naltrexone. *J Pharmacol Exp Ther,* 265(3), 1071–1078.
52. Lysle, D. T., Coussons, M. E., Watts, V. J., Bennett, E. H., & Dykstra, L. A. (1993b). Morphine-induced modulation of immune status: evidence for opioid receptor mediation and compartment specificity. *Adv Exp Med Biol,* 335, 53–59.
53. Lysle, D. T., Hoffman, K. E., & Dykstra, L. A. (1996). Evidence for the involvement of the caudal region of the periaqueductal gray in a subset of morphine-induced alterations of immune status. *J Pharmacol Exp Ther,* 277(3), 1533–1540.
54. Madden, J. J., Falek, A., Donahoe, R., Ketelson, D., & Chappel, C. L. (1990). Opiate binding sites on cells of the immune system. *NIDA Res Monogr,* 105, 103–108.
55. Madden, J. J., Whaley, W. L., & Ketelsen, D. (1998). Opiate binding sites in the cellular immune system: expression and regulation. *J Neuroimmunol,* 83(1–2), 57–62.
56. Mahajan, S. D., Schwartz, S. A., Shanahan, T. C., Chawda, R. P., & Nair, M. P. (2002). Morphine regulates gene expression of alpha- and beta-chemokines and their receptors on astroglial cells via the opioid mu receptor. *J Immunol,* 169(7), 3589–3599.
57. Makman, M. H., Bilfinger, T. V., & Stefano, G. B. (1995). Human granulocytes contain an opiate alkaloid-selective receptor mediating inhibition of cytokine-induced activation and chemotaxis. *J Immunol,* 154(3), 1323–1330.
58. Mandler, R. N., Biddison, W. E., Mandler, R., & Serrate, S. A. (1986). Beta-endorphin augments the cytolytic activity and interferon production of natural killer cells. *J Immunol,* 136(3), 934–939.
59. McCarthy, L., Wetzel, M., Sliker, J. K., Eisenstein, T. K., & Rogers, T. J. (2001). Opioids, opioid receptors, and the immune response. *Drug Alcohol Depend,* 62(2), 111–123.
60. Mehrishi, J. N., & Mills, I. H. (1983). Opiate receptors on lymphocytes and platelets in man. *Clin Immunol Immunopathol,* 27(2), 240–249.

61. Nelson, C. J., Schneider, G. M., & Lysle, D. T. (2000). Involvement of central mu- but not delta- or kappa-opioid receptors in immunomodulation. *Brain Behav Immun,* 14(3), 170–184.
62. Ovadia, H., Nitsan, P., & Abramsky, O. (1989). Characterization of opiate binding sites on membranes of rat lymphocytes. *J Neuroimmunol,* 21(2–3), 93–102.
63. Pacifici, R., Di Carlo, S., Bacosi, A., & Zuccaro, P. (1993). Macrophage functions in drugs of abuse-treated mice. *Int J Immunopharmacol,* 15(6), 711–716.
64. Perez-Castrillon, J. L., Perez-Arellano, J. L., Garcia-Palomo, J. D., Jimenez-Lopez, A., & De Castro, S. (1992). Opioids depress in vitro human monocyte chemotaxis. *Immunopharmacology,* 23(1), 57–61.
65. Peterson, P. K., Sharp, B., Gekker, G., Brummitt, C., & Keane, W. F. (1987a). Opioid-mediated suppression of cultured peripheral blood mononuclear cell respiratory burst activity. *J Immunol,* 138(11), 3907–3912.
66. Peterson, P. K., Sharp, B., Gekker, G., Brummitt, C., & Keane, W. F. (1987b). Opioid-mediated suppression of interferon-gamma production by cultured peripheral blood mononuclear cells. *J Clin Invest,* 80(3), 824–831.
67. Peterson, P. K., Molitor, T. W., & Chao, C. C. (1993). Mechanisms of morphine-induced immunomodulation. *Biochem Pharmacol,* 46(3), 343–348.
68. Peterson, P. K., Gekker, G., Hu, S., Lokensgard, J., Portoghese, P. S., & Chao, C. C. (1999). Endomorphin-1 potentiates HIV-1 expression in human brain cell cultures: implication of an atypical mu-opioid receptor. *Neuropharmacology,* 38(2), 273–278.
69. Radulovic, J., Miljevic, C., Djergovic, D., Vujic, V., Antic, J., von Horsten, S., & Jankovic, B. D. (1995). Opioid receptor-mediated suppression of humoral immune response in vivo and in vitro: involvement of kappa opioid receptors. *J Neuroimmunol,* 57(1–2), 55–62.
70. Rojavin, M., Szabo, I., Bussiere, J. L., Rogers, T. J., Adler, M. W., & Eisenstein, T. K. (1993). Morphine treatment in vitro or in vivo decreases phagocytic functions of murine macrophages. *Life Sci,* 53(12), 997–1006.
71. Roy, S., & Loh, H. H. (1996). Effects of opioids on the immune system. *Neurochem Res,* 21(11), 1375–1386.
72. Roy, S., Ramakrishnan, S., Loh, H. H., & Lee, N. M. (1991). Chronic morphine treatment selectively suppresses macrophage colony formation in bone marrow. *Eur J Pharmacol,* 195(3), 359–363.
73. Roy, S., Loh, H. H., & Barke, R. A. (1995). Morphine-induced suppression of thymocyte proliferation is mediated by inhibition of IL-2 synthesis. *Adv Exp Med Biol,* 373, 41–48.
74. Roy, S., Chapin, R. B., Cain, K. J., Charboneau, R. G., Ramakrishnan, S., & Barke, R. A. (1997). Morphine inhibits transcriptional activation of IL-2 in mouse thymocytes. *Cell Immunol,* 179(1), 1–9.
75. Roy, S., Barke, R. A., & Loh, H. H. (1998). MU-opioid receptor-knockout mice: role of mu-opioid receptor in morphine mediated immune functions. *Brain Res Mol Brain Res,* 61(1–2), 190–194.
76. Roy, S., Cain, K. J., Chapin, R. B., Charboneau, R. G., & Barke, R. A. (1998). Morphine modulates NF kappa B activation in macrophages. *Biochem Biophys Res Commun,* 245(2), 392–396.
77. Ruff, M. R., Wahl, S. M., Mergenhagen, S., & Pert, C. B. (1985). Opiate receptor-mediated chemotaxis of human monocytes. *Neuropeptides,* 5(4–6), 363–366.
78. Sedqi, M., Roy, S., Ramakrishnan, S., Elde, R., & Loh, H. H. (1995). Complementary DNA cloning of a mu-opioid receptor from rat peritoneal macrophages. *Biochem Biophys Res Commun,* 209(2), 563–574.
79. Sei, Y., McIntyre, T., Fride, E., Yoshimoto, K., Skolnick, P., & Arora, P. K. (1991). Inhibition of calcium mobilization is an early event in opiate-induced immunosuppression. *Faseb J,* 5(8), 2194–2199.
80. Sei, Y., Yoshimoto, K., McIntyre, T., Skolnick, P., & Arora, P. K. (1991). Morphine-induced thymic hypoplasia is glucocorticoid-dependent. *J Immunol,* 146(1), 194–198.
81. Shahabi, N. A., & Sharp, B. M. (1995a). Antiproliferative effects of delta opioids on highly purified CD4 + and CD8 + murine T cells. *J Pharmacol Exp Ther,* 273(3), 1105–1113.

82. Shahabi, N. A., & Sharp, B. M. (1995b). Delta opioid agonists inhibit proliferation of highlypurified murine CD4 + and CD8 + T-cells. *Adv Exp Med Biol*, 373, 29–36.
83. Shahabi, N. A., McAllen, K., & Sharp, B. M. (2003). Phosphorylation of activating transcription factor in murine splenocytes through delta opioid receptors. *Cell Immunol*, 221(2), 122–127.
84. Shahabi, N. A., McAllen, K., & Sharp, B. M. (2006). Delta opioid receptors stimulate Akt-dependent phosphorylation of c-jun in T cells. *J Pharmacol Exp Ther*, 316(2), 933–939.
85. Sharp, B. M., Keane, W. F., Suh, H. J., Gekker, G., Tsukayama, D., & Peterson, P. K. (1985). Opioid peptides rapidly stimulate superoxide production by human polymorphonuclear leukocytes and macrophages. *Endocrinology*, 117(2), 793–795.
86. Sharp, B. M., Roy, S., & Bidlack, J. M. (1998). Evidence for opioid receptors on cells involved in host defense and the immune system. *J Neuroimmunol*, 83(1–2), 45–56.
87. Sharp, B. M., Li, M. D., Matta, S. G., McAllen, K., & Shahabi, N. A. (2000). Expression of delta opioid receptors and transcripts by splenic T cells. *Ann N Y Acad Sci*, 917, 764–770.
88. Shavit, Y., Depaulis, A., Martin, F. C., Terman, G. W., Pechnick, R. N., Zane, C. J., Gale, R. P., & Liebeskind, J. C. (1986). Involvement of brain opiate receptors in the immune-suppressive effect of morphine. *Proc Natl Acad Sci U S A*, 83(18), 7114–7117.
89. Singhal, P. C., Reddy, K., Franki, N., Sanwal, V., & Gibbons, N. (1997). Morphine induces splenocyte apoptosis and enhanced mRNA expression of cathepsin-B. *Inflammation*, 21(6), 609–617.
90. Steele, A. D., Henderson, E. E., & Rogers, T. J. (2003). Mu-opioid modulation of HIV-1 coreceptor expression and HIV-1 replication. *Virology*, 309(1), 99–107.
91. Stefano, G. B., Melchiorri, P., Negri, L., Hughes, T. K., Jr., & Scharrer, B. (1992). [D-Ala2]deltorphin I binding and pharmacological evidence for a special subtype of delta opioid receptor on human and invertebrate immune cells. *Proc Natl Acad Sci USA*, 89(19), 9316–9320.
92. Szabo, I., Rojavin, M., Bussiere, J. L., Eisenstein, T. K., Adler, M. W., & Rogers, T. J. (1993). Suppression of peritoneal macrophage phagocytosis of Candida albicans by opioids. *J Pharmacol Exp Ther*, 267(2), 703–706.
93. Taub, D. D., Eisenstein, T. K., Geller, E. B., Adler, M. W., & Rogers, T. J. (1991). Immunomodulatory activity of mu- and kappa-selective opioid agonists. *Proc Natl Acad Sci USA*, 88(2), 360–364.
94. Tegeder, I., & Geisslinger, G. (2004). Opioids as modulators of cell death and survival – unraveling mechanisms and revealing new indications. *Pharmacol Rev*, 56(3), 351–369.
95. Tosk, J. M., Grim, J. R., Kinback, K. M., Sale, E. J., Bozzetti, L. P., & Will, A. D. (1993). Modulation of chemiluminescence in a murine macrophage cell line by neuroendocrine hormones. *Int J Immunopharmacol*, 15(5), 615–620.
96. Tubaro, E., Borelli, G., Croce, C., Cavallo, G., & Santiangeli, C. (1983). Effect of morphine on resistance to infection. *J Infect Dis*, 148(4), 656–666.
97. Tubaro, E., Avico, U., Santiangeli, C., Zuccaro, P., Cavallo, G., Pacifici, R., Croce, C., & Borelli, G. (1985). Morphine and methadone impact on human phagocytic physiology. *Int J Immunopharmacol*, 7(6), 865–874.
98. Tubaro, E., Santiangeli, C., Belogi, L., Borelli, G., Cavallo, G., Croce, C., & Avico, U. (1987). Methadone vs morphine: comparison of their effect on phagocytic functions. *Int J Immunopharmacol*, 9(1), 79–88.
99. Vallejo, R., de Leon-Casasola, O., & Benyamin, R. (2004). Opioid therapy and immunosuppression: a review. *Am J Ther*, 11(5), 354–365.
100. van Epps, D. E., & Saland, L. (1984). Beta-endorphin and met-enkephalin stimulate human peripheral blood mononuclear cell chemotaxis. *J Immunol*, 132(6), 3046–3053.
101. Wang, J. B., Johnson, P. S., Imai, Y., Persico, A. M., Ozenberger, B. A., Eppler, C. M., & Uhl, G. R. (1994). cDNA cloning of an orphan opiate receptor gene family member and its splice variant. *FEBS Lett*, 348(1), 75–79.
102. Weber, R. J., & Pert, A. (1989). The periaqueductal gray matter mediates opiate-induced immunosuppression. *Science*, 245(4914), 188–190.

103. Weber, R. J., Ikejiri, B., Rice, K. C., Pert, A., & Hagan, A. A. (1987). Opiate receptor mediated regulation of the immune response in vivo. *NIDA Res Monogr,* 76, 341–348.
104. Wick, M. J., Minnerath, S. R., Roy, S., Ramakrishnan, S., & Loh, H. H. (1996). Differential expression of opioid receptor genes in human lymphoid cell lines and peripheral blood lymphocytes. *J Neuroimmunol,* 64(1), 29–36.
105. Wybran, J., Appelboom, T., Famaey, J. P., & Govaerts, A. (1979). Suggestive evidence for receptors for morphine and methionine-enkephalin on normal human blood T lymphocytes. *J Immunol,* 123(3), 1068–1070.
106. Yakovlev, A. G., Krueger, K. E., & Faden, A. I. (1995). Structure and expression of a rat kappa opioid receptor gene. *J Biol Chem,* 270(12), 6421–6424.
107. Yin, D., Mufson, R. A., Wang, R., & Shi, Y. (1999). Fas-mediated cell death promoted by opioids. *Nature,* 397(6716), 218.
108. Yin, D., Zhang, Y., Stuart, C., Miao, J., Zhang, Y., Li, C., Zeng, X., Hanley, G., Moorman, J., Yao, Z., & Woodruff, M. (2006). Chronic restraint stress modulates expression of genes in murine spleen. *J Neuroimmunol,* 177(1–2), 11–17.

Part II
Opioid Antagonists: Chemistry and Pharmacology

Chapter 5
The Chemistry and Pharmacology of μ-Opioid Antagonists

Jean M. Bidlack and Jennifer L. Mathews

Abstract Opioid analgesics, such as morphine, are used clinically for the treatment of moderate to severe pain. However, the utility of opioid therapy can be limited by side effects including tolerance, physical dependence, respiratory depression, and constipation. Many of these classical side effects associated with the clinical use of opioid agonists are mediated by the mu (μ)-opioid receptor. This dichotomy has warranted extensive research to better understand the functions of each of the opioid receptors, along with synthesis of novel pharmacological tools that would alleviate these unwanted side effects. Because of the association of μ-opioid receptor stimulation with many of the most problematic side effects hindering opioid use, compounds with some μ antagonist properties may offer viable treatment options. The following overview of μ antagonists will address the evolution of these compounds and their utility not only in treating opioid-related side effects but also as pharmacotherapeutics for other disease processes which are associated with the opioid system. In addition, many of these compounds have important functions as tools for the basic scientist in furthering our understanding of the μ-opioid receptor.

Keywords: Mu; Opioid; Antagonist; Clinical; Side effects; Medicinal chemistry

5.1 Introduction

Opioid analgesics, such as morphine, are used clinically for the treatment of moderate to severe pain. However, the utility of opioid therapy can be limited by side effects including tolerance, physical dependence, respiratory depression, and constipation (1). This dichotomy has warranted extensive research to better understand the functions of each of the opioid receptors, along with synthesis of novel pharmacological tools

J.M. Bidlack and J.L. Mathews
Department of Pharmacology and Physiology,
University of Rochester School of Medicine and Dentistry,
601 Elmwood Avenue, Rochester, NY 14642-8711
e-mail: Jean_Bidlack@urmc.rochester.edu

R. Dean et al. (eds.), *Opiate Receptors and Antagonists*,

that would alleviate the unwanted side effects associated with opioid treatment without affecting the analgesic properties.

5.1.1 *Opioid Background*

Opioid receptors are members of the Rhodopsin family of G protein coupled receptors. Molecular cloning resulted in the identification of three opioid receptors, μ, delta (δ), and kappa (κ) (2–4).

The opioid receptors couple to the heterotrimeric G proteins G_i and G_o. Activation of opioid receptors results in several physiological phenomenon including pertussis toxin-sensitive inhibition of adenylyl cyclase activity (5, 6), activation of inwardly rectifying K^+ channels (7, 8), inhibition of voltage-activated Ca^{2+} channels, particularly the N-type and P/Q types (9, 10), and the activation of the mitogen-activated protein (MAP) kinase, Erk-1/2 (11).

5.1.2 *μ Opioid-Related Side Effects*

Many of the classical side effects associated with the clinical use of opioid agonists are mediated by the μ-opioid receptor. A well-known consequence of frequent and repeated administration of opioids is the development of tolerance. Tolerance develops to repeated administration of agonists at all three receptors; however, tolerance to μ-opioid analgesics develops more rapidly (12).

Respiratory depression is a consistent, dose-dependent side effect seen with all opioid analgesics that are currently used. There is general agreement that opioid-induced respiratory depression is caused by activation of μ receptors in the rostrodorsal region of the pons (13).

The most common side effect associated with chronic opioid treatment is constipation, with rates as high as 40–45% (14). In many cases, constipation can be severe enough that opioid therapy must be discontinued (14). Activation of μ receptors, which are located on neural processes that innervate the smooth muscle, reduces excitability by increasing K^+ conductance shortening action potential duration, thus reducing muscle contraction (15).

Because of the association of μ-opioid receptor stimulation with many of the most problematic side effects hindering opioid use, a μ-opioid antagonist offers a viable treatment option. The following overview of μ antagonists will address the evolution of these compounds and their utility not only in treating opioid-related side effects but also as pharmacotherapeutics for other disease processes which are associated with the opioid system. In addition, many of these compounds have important functions as tools for the basic scientist in furthering our understanding of the μ-opioid receptor.

5.2 When Is an Antagonist Called an Antagonist

In vitro analysis of opioid ligands is an important first step in understanding the pharmacological properties of the compound. Radioligand receptor-binding assays give an indication of the affinity of a ligand for the receptor of interest. Compounds with high affinity in the receptor-binding assay are then often tested in the [^{35}S] Guanosine-5'-O-(3-thio)triphosphate ([^{35}S]GTPγS) binding assay to determine if the ligand is an agonist, antagonist, or partial agonist at the receptor of interest.

5.2.1 *The [^{35}S]GTPγS Binding Assay*

G Protein-coupled receptors transduce signals from extracellular stimuli, such as ligand binding, to the intracellular environment through a series of signal transduction events. Upon agonist binding, Gα dissociates from guanosine diphosphate (GDP) and subsequently binds to guanosine triphosphate (GTP). This binding allows for Gα-GTP along with Gβγ to signal to downstream effectors. The heterotrimer is reformed due to the GTPase activity of the Gα subunit. Binding of the nonhydrolyzable GTP analog, [^{35}S]GTPγS, measures the level of G-protein activation following agonist binding, and is a measure of the efficacy of a compound (16–18). If a compound does not stimulate binding of [^{35}S]GTPγS, it may be an antagonist. To determine if a compound is an antagonist, the [^{35}S]GTPγS assay is performed in the presence of a receptor-selective agonist, at a concentration known to stimulate [^{35}S]GTPγS binding. If the compound does not stimulate [^{35}S]GTPγS binding alone, but inhibits agonist-stimulated [^{35}S]GTPγS binding, it is an antagonist in this assay (16). In the experiment represented below, [D-Ala^2,*N*-Me-Phe^4,Gly^5-ol] enkephalin (DAMGO, a μ-selective agonist) stimulated [^{35}S]GTPγS binding (Fig. 5.1a) which was antagonized by cyclazocine, a μ-receptor antagonist (Fig. 5.1b). It is important to note, that although cyclazocine acted as a μ-receptor antagonist in this assay, this compound also had agonist properties at other receptors, therefore, is not classified as a pure antagonist (19).

5.2.2 *From In Vitro Antagonist Characterization to an In Vivo Model*

There is generally a good correlation between the in vitro [^{35}S]GTPγS binding results and the properties of the compound in vivo. To initially characterize the pharmacological properties of an antagonist in vivo, the compound is administered with a receptor-selective agonist. In the graph represented below, cyclazocine, the compound of interest, was administered concomitantly with morphine. All injections were intracerebroventricular (i.c.v.) and antinociception was assessed in the

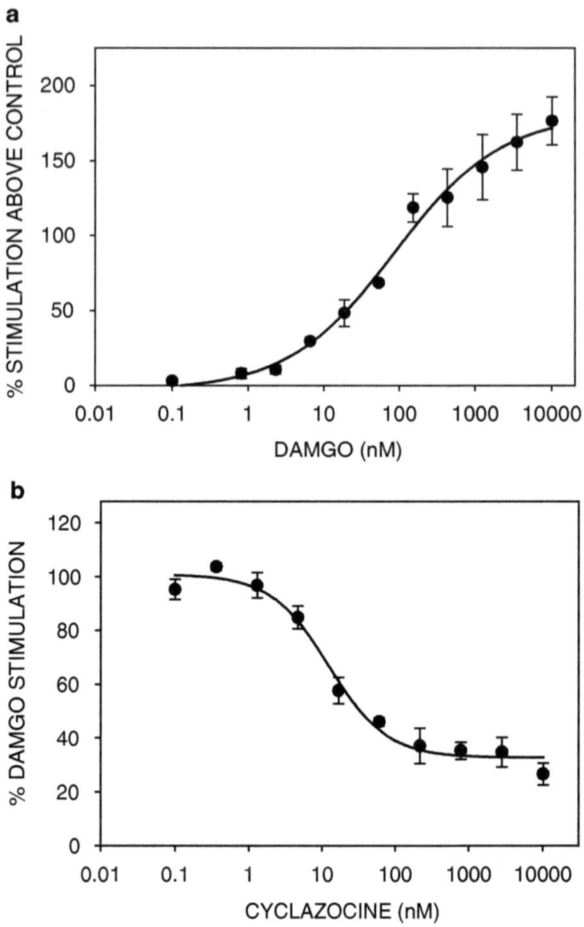

Fig. 5.1 DAMGO ([D-Ala[2],*N*-Me-Phe[4],Gly[5]-ol]enkephalin) stimulated [^{35}S]GTPγS binding to human μ-opioid receptors (**a**). In a final volume of 0.5 ml, 12 different concentrations of compound were incubated with 10 μg of Chinese hamster ovary (*CHO*) cell membranes that stably expressed the human μ-opioid receptor. The assay buffer consisted of 50 mM Tris-HCl, pH 7.4, 3 mM $MgCl_2$, 0.2 mM ethylene glycol tetraacetic acid (*EGTA*), 3 μM guanosine diphosphate (*GDP*), and 100 mM NaCl. The final concentration of [^{35}S]GTPγS was 0.08 nM. Nonspecific binding was measured by inclusion of 10 μM GTPγS. Binding was initiated by the addition of the membranes. After incubation of 60 min at 30°C, the samples were filtered through no. 32 glass fiber filters. To determine if cyclazocine was an antagonist at the μ receptor, the compound was titrated at varying concentrations against the known μ agonist, DAMGO (200 nM) and incubated with 10 μg of CHO cell membranes that stably expressed the human μ-opioid receptor (**b**). The final concentration of [^{35}S]GTPγS was 0.08 nM. Nonspecific binding was measured by inclusion of 10 μM GTPγS. Binding was initiated by the addition of the membranes. After incubation of 60 min at 30°C, the samples were filtered through no. 32 glass fiber filters

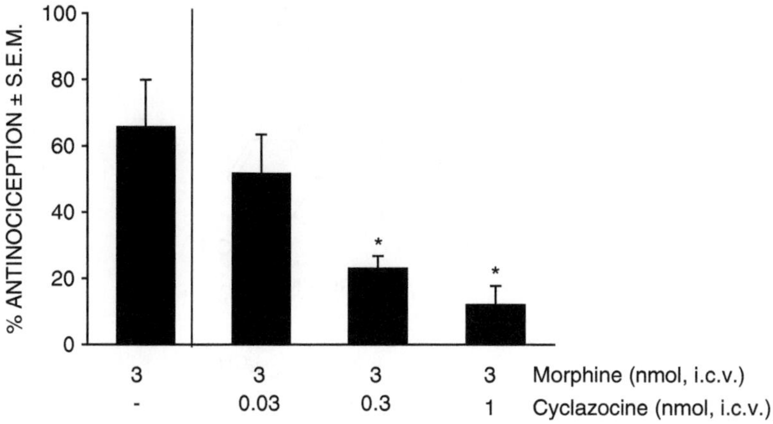

Fig. 5.2 Antinociceptive effects of intracerebroventricular (*i.c.v.*) morphine in mice treated with i.c.v. doses of cyclazocine. Morphine was coinjected with cyclazocine. Antinociception was measured in the mouse 55°C warm-water tail-flick test at 20 min after the injection of compounds. Ten mice were used for each data point.*Significant from morphine alone, $P < 0.05$. Data reproduced from Bidlack et al. (20)

55°C warm-water tail-flick assay. In this experiment, cyclazocine acted as a μ antagonist and inhibited morphine-induced antinociception (20) (Fig. 5.2). These data correlated with the in vitro [^{35}S]GTPγS binding data (Fig. 5.1b).

5.3 Nalorphine, Naloxone, and Naltrexone: A History Lesson

Opioid antagonists are structurally very similar to opioid agonists. In general, the only difference is the moiety attached to the N atom. In opioid agonists, such as morphine, it is a methyl group (21) (Fig. 5.3). Alteration of groups on the nitrogen of the morphine core structure has significant effects on analgesic activity. As the alkyl group on the nitrogen is changed from methyl to ethyl, and then to propyl, the pharmacological profile is drastically changed (21). In opioid antagonists, the most common N substituents are allyl (CH_2=CH–CH_2) and cyclopropylmethyl. The main characteristics of these substituents are their high reactivity, in addition to their bulky size when compared to the methyl group in opioid agonists (21).

Nalorphine is the allyl derivative of morphine, and in the 1940s one of the first compounds to be recognized as an opioid antagonist (22) (Fig. 5.3). Subsequent studies revealed that nalorphine also had analgesic properties, and was thus defined as a mixed agonist/antagonist (21). Further modifications of the morphine core structure resulted in the several other mixed agonist/antagonist molecules: pentazocine, cyclazocine, buprenorphine, nalbuphine, and butorphanol.

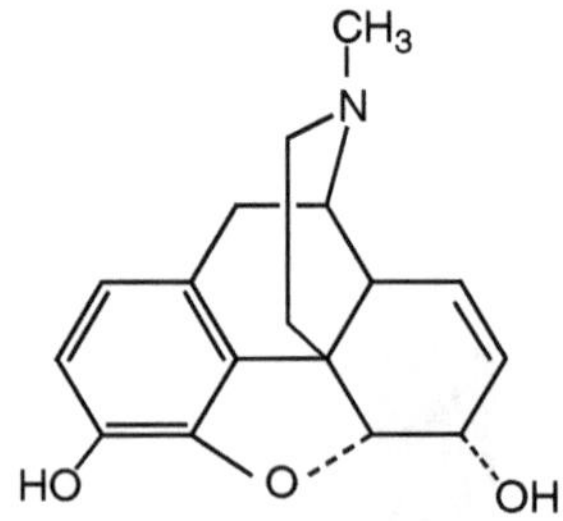

MORPHINE

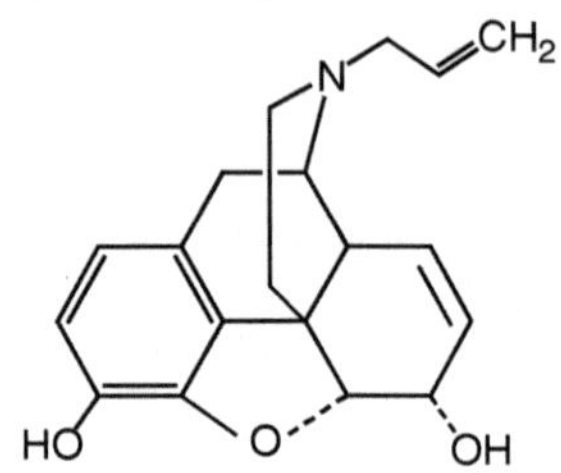

NALORPHINE

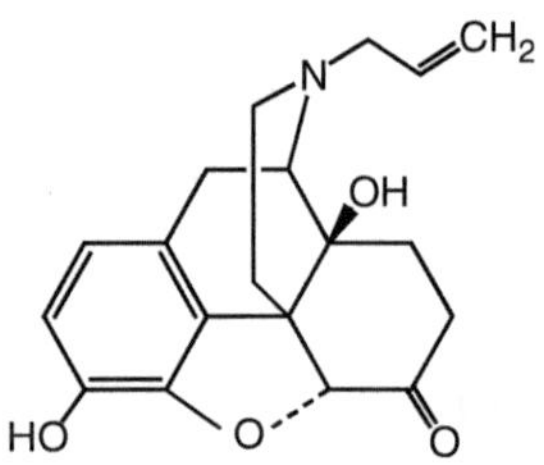

NALOXONE

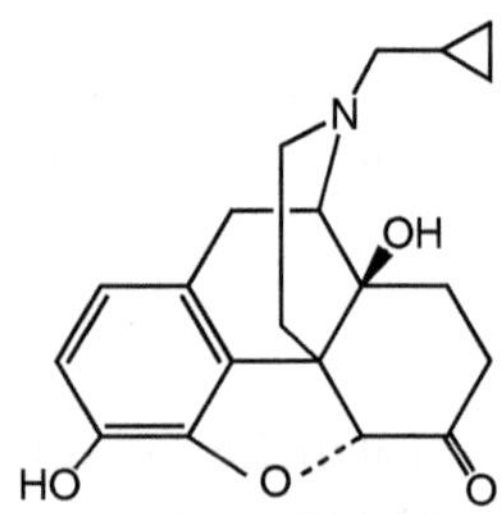

NALTREXONE

Fig. 5.3 The evolution of the first μ-opioid antagonists. Morphine is the prototypic μ-opioid agonist, and many μ antagonists have been based off the morphine core structure. Nalorphine, was characterized as one of the first opioid antagonists in the 1940s. Naloxone was the first pure opioid antagonist synthesized. Naltrexone is an opioid antagonist which has been useful both to scientists and clinicians

The first pure opioid antagonist, naloxone (Narcan) was synthesized in 1963 after further modification of the morphine molecule (Fig. 5.3). Jasinski and colleagues conducted the first human studies on the pharmacological effects of naloxone in 1967 (23). Naloxone is still used frequently in emergency care settings for treatment of opioid-induced respiratory depression and overdose. The synthesis of naltrexone was soon to follow. Naltrexone, a more potent, long-acting, bioactive antagonist was synthesized and described in 1967 (24) (Fig. 5.3). Naltrexone is modestly more μ selective, as an antagonist compared to naloxone (25). For these reasons, naltrexone has been used extensively not only clinically but also as a scaffold for development of new, receptor-selective antagonists, as experimental tools (25).

5.3.1 Clinical Applications for Naltrexone

5.3.1.1 Alcohol

The endogenous opioid system has been implicated in the reinforcing effects of alcohol, suggesting that the use of an opioid antagonist may alleviate these effects and reduce drinking (26). In clinical trials, naltrexone was safe and efficacious in preventing relapse severity in people with alcohol dependence (27, 28).

5.3.1.2 Opioid Detoxification

Naltrexone has been used in opioid-dependent patients to shorten the duration of opioid withdrawal symptoms (29). Naltrexone used in combination with the α2-adrenergic agonist, clonidine, has been shown to shorten detoxification from either heroin or methadone from 2 weeks to only 1 day. Under general anesthesia or heavy sedation (rapid detoxification), naltrexone further shortened the detoxification to 4–6 h (30).

The use of naltrexone for opioid dependence has been hindered by poor compliance (31). Recently, a sustained-release depot formulation of naltrexone was tested in a randomized, placebo-controlled trial. The study found that the treatment was well tolerated and a dose-related increase in treatment retention was observed (31).

5.3.1.3 Feeding Behaviors

Several studies have examined the effects of opioids in mediating feeding behaviors. The opioid receptors and endogenous peptides are expressed in brain regions important for regulation of feeding (32). Administration of the opioid antagonists, naltrexone, or LY255582 both inhibited long-term weight gain in rats (33–35). Interestingly, studies utilizing the μ-opioid receptor knock-out mice suggest that the μ receptor may be of primary importance in feeding behaviors, and antagonists specific for this receptor would have potential as antiobesity agents (36).

As mentioned earlier, naltrexone was also important for development of the new generation of receptor-selective antagonists.

5.4 Irreversible Antagonists

Irreversible opioid antagonists produce long-term antagonism of opioid-induced antinociception. The antagonist forms a permanent, covalent bond with the opioid receptor. This irreversible bond allows for the antagonist to stay bound to the receptor blocking the receptor binding site from other opioids.

5.4.1 β-Funaltrexamine

β-Funaltrexamine (β-FNA) is structurally related to the opioid-antagonist, naltrexone with a fumarate group in the C-6 position. The fumarate side chain is an α,β-unsaturated carbonyl, which acts as a Michael acceptor for nucleophilic attack, allowing for β-FNA to form a covalent bond with the μ receptor. Site-directed mutagenesis studies have revealed that β-FNA and Lys^{233} of the μ receptor are involved in the covalent bond (37). In mouse analgesic assays, β-FNA has been shown to antagonize morphine-induced antinociception up to 72 h (38, 39). It is important to note that the μ-antagonist properties of β-FNA are delayed and the compound must be administered 24 h in advance of testing to avoid the reversible, κ-mediated agonist properties (38).

5.4.2 Dihydromorphinone and Dihydrocodeinone Derivatives

One of the first compounds within this series was 14β-(*p*-chlorocinnamoylamino)-7,8-dihydro-*N*-cyclopropylmethylnormorphinone (C-CAM; clocinnamox), which is a derivative of naltrexone with a chlorocinnamoylamino group at the C-14 position, replacing the 14β-hydroxyl group (40). In the mouse tall-flick assay, C-CAM produced long-term μ-receptor antagonism (40, 41). The mechanism of the long-term antagonism was different than that seen with β-FNA. C-CAM shifted the dose–response curve of morphine downward and rightward, suggesting that C-CAM was producing antagonism through a nonequilibrium mechanism (41,42). Additionally, in Scatchard analysis, C-CAM caused a reduction in the number of binding sites without affecting the K_d value (40). C-CAM is also devoid of agonist activity, unlike β-FNA (40).

Two derivatives of metopon-containing 14β-*p*-nitrocinnamoylamino constituents, 5β-methyl-14β-(*p*-nitrocinnamoylamino)-7,8-dihydromorphinone (MET-CAMO) and its *N*-cyclopropylmethyl derivative, *N*-(cyclopropylmethyl)-14β-(*p*-nitrocinnamoylamino)-7,8-dihydronormorphinone (*N*-CPM-MET-CAMO) selectively antagonized μ-mediated antinociception, in the 55°C tail-flick assay, for up to 72 h through an irreversible covalent interaction with the receptor (43, 44). Similar results were also obtained for the disulfide-containing compound 14α,14′β-[dithiobis[(2-oxo-2,1-ethanediyl)imino]]bis-7,8-dihydro-*N*-(cyclopropylmethyl) normorphinone (*N*-CPM-TAMO) (41).

In addition to work done with the cinnamoyl compounds MET-CAMO, *N*-CPM-MET-CAMO and C-CAM, the dihydrocodeinone derivatives 14β-(*p*-nitrocinnamoylamino)-7,8-dihydrocodeinone (CACO), *N*-cyclopropylmethylnor-14β-(*p*-nitrocinnamoylamino)-7,8-dihydrocodeinone (*N*-CPM-CACO), 14β-(*p*-chlorocinnamoylamino)-7,8-dihydrocodeinone (CAM), and *N*-cyclopropylmethylnor-14β-

(*p*-chlorocinnamoylamino)-7,8-dihydrocodeinone (MC-CAM) produced long-term antagonism of the μ receptor. Pretreatment for 24 h, in mice, produced a dose-dependent antagonism in mouse analgesic assays that lasted for at least 48 h after i.c.v. administration (45).

Further studies with the cinnamoyl derivatives have explored 3-alkyl ethers of C-CAM and MC-CAM. These studies were carried out to address data, which suggested that although C-CAM was an insurmountable μ antagonist, MC-CAM was actually a partial μ agonist, and that the delayed antagonist actions of MC-CAM could be a result of the metabolism of this compound to C-CAM (46). The study included ethers with different levels of metabolic stability but was unable to conclusively establish that the delayed onset of antagonism with MC-CAM was actually due to metabolism to C-CAM (46).

A final modification in this series of compounds was to contrast the importance of the phenolic hydroxyl group, which has been recognized as a key structural feature for binding to the μ receptor, with the cinnamoylamino group. *N*-Cyclopropylmethyl-14-(4-chlorocinnamoylamido)-3-deoxymorphinone (DOC-CAM) did not have a 3-oxygen function to form a hydrogen bond with the receptor, however, retained high affinity μ-antagonist properties similar to C-CAM (47). These studies addressed the importance of the cinnamoyl side chain in the synthesis of irreversible μ antagonists.

5.5 Reversible Antagonists

Unlike irreversible antagonists, which do not display any antagonist effects when coadministered with agonists and always require a longer time before they antagonize opioid-mediated agonist effects, such as antinociception, reversible antagonists immediately show their antagonistic properties when coadministered with an agonist (43, 44). Naloxone and naltrexone were described earlier in the chapter and are the chemical scaffold for a few of the other reversible antagonists that will be discussed. In addition, novel motifs will also be addressed.

5.5.1 Quarternary Antagonists

Quarternary antagonists are derived by utilizing all four of the available bonding sites of the tertiary amine in older generation opioid antagonists (48). These compounds do not cross the blood-brain barrier due to their charged characteristics. The rational for administering a quarternary antagonist is that it would block the undesired peripheral side effects of opioid therapy, such as constipation, while sparing the central nervous system (CNS) effects that is, analgesia (14).

5.5.1.1 Methylnaltrexone

Methylnaltrexone is a quarternary ammonium derivative of the opioid antagonist naltrexone. Yuan and colleagues demonstrated that both intravenous (i.v.) infusion and oral administration of methylnaltrexone induced laxation and reversed oral-cecal transit time in opioid-dependent patients (14, 49). The doses of methylnaltrexone used did not induce an opioid withdrawal syndrome, unlike the tertiary antagonists naltrexone, naloxone, and nalmefene (48, 49). This compound has been tested in several clinical trials with positive results, including 650 healthy volunteers and patients (48). The clinical trials have involved patients with opioid-induced constipation, patients with advanced medical illness (i.e., cancer, AIDS, and heart disease), and patients at risk for postoperative bowel dysfunction (48). Two caveats to methylnaltrexone treatment are its low bioavailability after oral ingestion along with the potential to produce severe diarrhea in patients who are opioid dependent (14, 49).

5.5.1.2 Alvimopan

Alvimopan is a quarternary antagonist structurally related to the μ agonist, fentanyl. This compound has the quarternary amine and is also dipolar, making it a zwitterion (48). Alvimopan has been tested in clinical trials specifically for postoperative ileus which to date have involved over 2,100 patients (48). In patients receiving alvimopan, a reduction in the duration of postoperative ileus was observed. This translated to an accelerated recovery of gastrointestinal function and accelerated hospital discharge (48). Alvimopan, similar to methylnaltrexone, has low systemic absorption and limited oral bioavailability (50).

5.6 Other Structural Motifs as μ Antagonists

5.6.1 Dmt-Tic Analogues

The 2′,6′-dimethyl-L-tyrosine (Dmt)-1,2,3,4-tetrahydroisoquinoline-3-carboxylic acid (Tic) motif had previously been recognized for its importance in conferring potent δ-antagonist properties to ligands, enhancing both affinity and functional bioactivity (51). The dipeptide Dmt-Tic represented the minimal peptide sequence needed for interaction with the receptor, along with potent antagonist activity (52). Modifications to the DMT-Tic pharmacophore, including addition of bulky uncharged hydrophobic groups at the C-terminal enhanced μ-receptor affinity and decreased δ selectivity (53). This finding suggests that the C-terminal portion of the DMT-Tic pharmacophore serves as the “address domain” (52). Further modifications have included a motif containing the 4-amino-1,2,4,5-tetrahydro-2-benzazepine-3-one skeleton as a substitute for the Tic residue. This modification provided the conformational constraint needed for binding of the μ receptor and provided a series of fairly potent μ antagonists (54).

5.6.2 Somatostatin Analogues

D-Phe-Cys-Tyr-D-Trp-Orn-Thr-Pen-Thr-NH_2 (CTOP) and D-Phe-Cys-Tyr-D-Trp-Arg-Thr-Pen-Thr-NH_2 (CTAP) are cyclic, conformationally constrained peptides related to somatostatin (55). The synthesis of this series of antagonists represented a novel approach to finding receptor-selective antagonists. Somatostatin binds to opioid receptors with low affinity, but allowed for a chemical backbone for modification to improve potency and receptor specificity (55, 56). In mouse-analgesic assays neither CTOP nor CTAP showed antinociceptive properties when administered alone, i.c.v., but did display competitive μ antagonism in other analgesic assays (56).

5.6.3 Morphinans

Synthesis of the morphinans demonstrated that the basic five ring structure of morphine did not need to be preserved either to maintain analgesic properties or to design opioid antagonists. Removal of the D ring resulted in levorphanol, a potent agonist, and its *N*-cyclopropylmethyl derivative, cyclorphan, and the *N*-allyl structure, levallorphan, both which are antagonists (21).

5.6.4 Benzomorphans

This group of compounds resulted from the opening of the C and D ring of the morphine core structure. Two benzomorphans that have been used clinically are cyclazocine and pentazocine (Talwin) (Fig. 5.4). Both compounds are mixed agonists/antagonists.

In vitro, cyclazocine had high affinity for both the κ- and μ-opioid receptors. In vivo, including both animal and human studies, cyclazocine was a potent κ agonist, and a long-acting μ antagonist. Human studies demonstrated that as an analgesic 0.25–0.5 mg/70 kg was equivalent to 10 mg/70 kg of morphine (19).

Pentazocine also had high affinity for both the κ- and μ-opioid receptors. Relative to morphine, pentazocine had less analgesic activity and a shorter duration of action, but decreased addiction liability. Dosages of 20–40 mg by subcutaneous, an intramuscular, routes are equivalent to 10-mg morphine (21).

Fig. 5.4 Chemical structures of the benzomorphans–cyclazocine and pentazocine

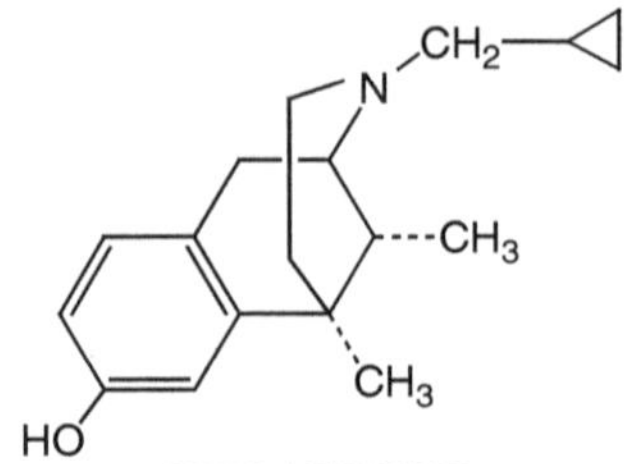

CYCLAZOCINE

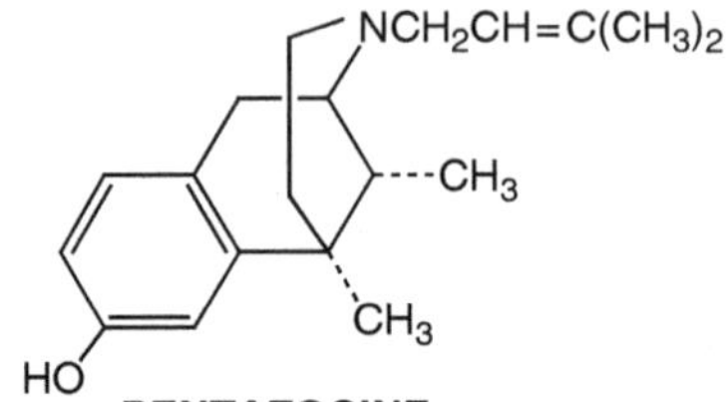

PENTAZOCINE

5.6.5 *Oripavines*

Rigidification is a strategy used to limit the number of conformations a molecule can adopt. Ideally, the active conformation for the receptor would be retained, while eliminating alternative conformations that may bind other targets. The oripavines are a good example of the utility of this strategy (21). The potent agonist etorphine belongs to this class of drugs. Addition of a cyclopropyl group yields the high affinity, general antagonist, diprenorphine. A similar compound is buprenorphine, a mixed agonist/antagonist. Buprenorphine is an alternative treatment to methadone for heroin addicts (57).

5.7 Summary

The importance of μ antagonists both to the basic scientist and clinician are clear. Antagonists have been used as pharmacological tools for studying and characterizing the μ-opioid receptor in vitro, and for addressing agonist-mediated effects in vivo (41, 44, 45). The knowledge that is accrued from these studies can be applied to the patient setting.

Clinically, opioid analgesics are still the gold standard for treatment of moderate to severe pain. However, the side effects and abuse liability associated with their use can become a hindrance both to the patient and clinician. It has been the task of both medicinal chemists and pharmacologists to synthesize and screen novel opioids to find ligands which would allow for the retention of the analgesic potency of currently available agonists, with a much-improved side effect and abuse liability profile.

Our understanding of the μ-opioid receptor and the structure–activity relationship of opioid ligands with the receptor have increased tremendously, allowing fresh perspectives into this problem.

Acknowledgments The authors thank Peter Gareiss and Dr. Brian Fulton for their helpful medicinal chemistry suggestions. Part of these studies was funded by K05-DA00360 and T32 DA07232.

References

1. Ellison NM. Opioid analgesics for cancer pain: toxicities and their treatments. In Pratt RB, ed. Cancer Pain, Philadelphia: J.P. Lipincott, 1993:185–194.
2. Evans CJ, Keith DE, Morrison H, Bagendzo K, and Edwards RH. Cloning of a delta opioid receptor by functional expression. Science 1992;258:1952–1955.
3. Kieffer Bl, Befort K, Gaveriaux-Ruff C, and Hirth CG. The δ-opioid receptor: isolation of a cDNA by expression cloning and pharmacological characterization. Proc Natl Acad Sci USA 1992;89:12048–12052.
4. Chen Y, Mestek A, Liu J, and Yu L. Molecular cloning of a rat κ-opioid receptor reveals sequence similarities to the μ and δ opioid receptors. Biochem J 1993;295:625–628.
5. Childers SR. Opioid receptor-coupled second messenger systems. Life Sci 1991;48:1991–2003.
6. Sharma SK, Klee WA, and Nirenberg M. Opiate-dependent modulation of adenylate cyclase. Proc Natl Acad Sci USA 1977;74:3365–3369.
7. Armstrong DL, White RE. An enzymatic mechanism for potassium channel stimulation through pertussis-toxin-sensitive G proteins. Trends Neurosci 1992;15:403–408.
8. North RA, Williams JT, Surprenant A, and Christie MJ. Mu and delta receptors belong to a family of receptors that are coupled to potassium channels. Proc Natl Acad Sci USA 1987;84: 5487–5491.
9. Moises HC, Rusin KI, and Macdonald RL. Mu- and kappa-opioid receptors selectively reduce the same transient components of high-threshold calcium current in rat dorsal root ganglion sensory neurons. J Neurosci 1994;14:5903–5916.
10. Schroeder JE, Fischbach PS, Zheng D, and McCleskey EW. Activation of mu opioid receptors inhibits transient high- and low-threshold Ca^{2+} currents, but spares a sustained current. Neuron 1991;6:13–20.
11. Law PY, Loh HH, and Wei LN. Insights into the receptor transcription and signaling: implications in opioid tolerance and dependence. Neuropharmacology 2004;4:300–311.
12. Jasinski DR. Human pharmacology of narcotic antagonists. Br J Clin Pharmacol 1979; 7:287S–290S.
13. Rothman RB, Holaday JW, and Porreca F. Allosteric coupling among opioid receptors: evidence for an opioid receptor complex. In Herz A, ed. Handbook of Experimental Pharmacology, Opioids I, Vol. 104. New York: Springer-Verlag, 1993:217–237.
14. Yuan CS, Foss JF, O'Connor M, Osinski J, Roizen MF, and Moss J. Effects of intravenous methylnaltrexone on opioid-induced gut motility and transit time changes in subjects receiving chronic methadone therapy: a pilot study. Pain 1999;83:631–635.
15. Kromer W. Gastrointestinal effects of opioids. In Herz A, ed. Handbook of Experimental Pharmacology, Opioids I, Vol. 104. New York: Springer-Verlag, 1993:163–190.
16. Bidlack JM, Parkhill AP. Assay of G protein-coupled receptor activation of G proteins in native cell membranes using [^{35}S]GTPγS binding. In Smrcka AV, ed. Methods in Molecular Biology: G Protein Signaling Methods and Protocols, Vol. 237. Totowa, NJ: Humana Press, 2004:135–144.
17. Harrison C, Traynor JR. The [^{35}S]GTPγS binding assay: approaches and applications in pharmacology. Life Sci 2003;74:489–508.

18. Selley DE, Liu Q, and Childers SR. Signal transduction correlates of mu opioid agonist intrinsic efficacy: receptor-stimulated [^{35}S]GTPγS binding in mMOR-CHO cells and rat thalamus. J Pharmacol Exp Ther 1998;285:496–505.
19. Archer SA, Glick SD, and Bidlack JM. Cyclazocine revisited. Neurochem Res 1996; 21:1369–1373.
20. Bidlack JM, Cohen DJ, McLaughlin JP, Lou R, Ye Y, and Wentland MP. 8-Carboxyamidocyclazocine: a long-acting, novel benzomorphan. J Pharmacol Exp Ther 2002;302:374–380.
21. Soloway AH. Analgesics. In: Foye WO, ed. Principles of Medicinal Chemistry. Philadelphia, PA: Lea and Febiger, 1974:252–274.
22. Hart ER, McCawley EL. The pharmacology of *N*-allylnormorphine as compared with morphine. J Pharmcol Exp Ther 1944;82:339–348.
23. Jasinksi DR, Martin WR, and Haertzen CA. The human pharmacology and abuse potential of *N*-allylnoroxymorphone (naloxone). J Pharmacol Exp Ther 1967;157:420–426.
24. Gritz ER, Shiffman SM, Jarvik ME, Schlesinger J, and Charuvastra VC. Naltrexone: physiological and psychological effects of single doses. Clin Pharmacol Ther 1976;19:773–776.
25. Takemori AE, Portoghese PS. Selective naltrexone-derived opioid receptor antagonists. Annu Rev Pharmacol Toxicol 1992;32:239–269.
26. Koob GF, Roberts AJ, Schulteis G, Parsons LH, Heyser CJ, Hyytia P, Merlo-Pich E, and Weiss F. Neurocircuitry targets in ethanol reward and dependence. Alcohol Clin Exp Res 1998;22:3–9.
27. Volpicelli JR, Alterman AI, Hayashida M, and O'Brien CP. Naltrexone in the treatment of alcohol dependence. Arch Gen Psychiatry 1992;49:876–880.
28. Volpicelli JR, Rhines KC, Rhines JS, Volpicelli LA, Alterman AI, and O'Brien CP. Naltrexone and alcohol dependence: role of subject compliance. Arch Gen Psychiatry 1997;54:737–742.
29. Bhargava HN, Matwyshyn GA, Gerk PM, Bozek PS, Bailey MD, Ko KH, Simko RJ, and Thorat SN. Effects of naltrexone pellet implantation on morphine tolerance and physical dependence in the rat. Gen Pharmacol 1994;25:149–155.
30. Tai B, Blaine J. Naltrexone: an antagonist therapy for heroin addiction. National Institute on Drug Abuse, National Institutes of Health. November 12–13, 1997: NIDA treatment workgroup.
31. Comer SD, Sullivan MA, Yu E, Rothenberg JL, Kleber HD, Kampman K, Dackis C, and O'Brien CP. Injectable, sustained-release naltrexone for the treatment of opioid dependence: a randomized, placebo-controlled trial. Arch Gen Psychiatry 2006;63:210–218.
32. Will MJ, Franzblau EB, and Kelley AE. Nucleus accumbens μ-opioids regulate intake of high-fat diet via activation of a distributed brain network. J Neurosci 2003;23:2882–2888.
33. Shaw WN. Long-term treatment of obese Zucker rats with LY255582 and other appetite suppressants. Pharmacol Biochem Behav 1993;46:653–659.
34. Marks-Kaufman R, Balmagiya T, and Gross E. Modifications in food intake and energy metabolism in rats as a function of chronic naltrexone infusions. Pharmacol Biochem Behav 1984;20:911–916.
35. Glass MJ, Billington CJ, and Levine AS. Opioids and food intake: distributed functional neural pathways? Neuropeptides 1999;33:360–368.
36. Zhang M, Gosnell BA, and Kelley AE. Intake of high-fat food is selectively enhanced by mu opioid receptor stimulation within the nucleus accumbens. J Pharmacol Exp Ther 1998;285:908–914.
37. Chen C, Yin J, de Riel K, DesJarlais RL, Raveglia LF, Zhu J, and Liu-Chen L-Y. Determination of the amino acid residue involved in [^{3}H]β-Funaltrexamine covalent binding in the cloned rat μ opioid receptor. J Biol Chem 1996;271:21422–21429.
38. Ward SJ, Portoghese PS, and Takemori AE. Pharmacological characterization in vivo of the novel opiate, β-funaltrexamine. J Pharmacol Exp Ther 1982;220:494–498.
39. Ward SJ, Fries DS, Larson DL, Portoghese PS, and Takemori AE. Opioid receptor binding characteristics of the non-equilibrium mu antagonist, β-funaltrexamine (β-FNA). Eur J Pharmacol 1985;85:665–673.

40. Aceto MD, Bowman ER, May EL, Harris LS, Woods JH, Smith CB, Medzinradsky F, and Jacobsen AE. Very long-acting narcotic antagonists: the 14 β-*p*-substituted cinnamoylaminomorphinones and their partial mu agonist codeinone relatives. Arzneim Forsch Drug Res 1989;39:570–575.
41. Comer SD, Burke TF, Lewis JW, and Woods JH. Clocinnamox: a novel systemically active, irreversible opioid antagonist. J Pharmacol Exp Ther 1992;262:1051–1056.
42. Burke TF, Woods JH, Lewis JW, and Medzihradsky F. Irreversible opioid antagonist effects of clocinnamox on opioid analgesia and mu receptor binding in mice. J Pharmacol Exp Ther 1994;271:715–721.
43. Jiang Q, Seyed-Mozaffari A, Archer S, and Bidlack JM. Pharmacological study of 14β-(thioglycolamido)-7,8-dihydro-*N*(cyclopropylmethyl)-normorphinone (*N*-CPM-TAMO). J Pharmacol Exp Ther 1993;264:1021–1027.
44. Jiang Q, Sebastian A, Archer S, and Bidlack JM. 5β-Methyl-14β-(*p*-nitrocinnamoylamino)-7,8-dihydromorphinone and its corresponding *N*-cyclopropylmethyl analog, *N*-cyclopropylmethylnor-5β-methyl-14β-(*p*-nitrocinnamoylamino)-7,8-dihydromorphinone: mu-selective irreversible opioid antagonists. J Pharmacol Exp Ther 1994;268:1107–1113.
45. McLaughlin JP, Hill KP, Jiang Q, Sebastian A, Archer S, and Bidlack JM. Nitrocinnamoyl and chlorocinnamoyl derivatives of dihydrocodeinone: in vivo and in vitro characterization of μ-selective agonist and antagonist activity. J Pharmacol Exp Ther 1999;289:304–311.
46. Husbands SM, Sadd J, Broadbear JH, Woods JH, Martin J, Traynor JR, Aceto MD, Bowman ER, Harris LS, and Lewis JW. 3-Alkyl ethers of clocinnamox: delayed long-term μ-antagonists with variable μ efficacy. J Med Chem 1998;41:3493–3498.
47. Derrick I, Neilan CL, Andes J, Husbands SM, Woods JH, Traynor JR, and Lewis JW. 3-Deoxyclocinnamox: the first high-affinity, nonpeptide μ-antagonist lacking a phenolic hydroxyl group. J Med Chem 2000;43:3348–3350.
48. Sinatra RS. Peripherally acting mu-opioid-receptor antagonists and the connection between postoperative ileus and pain management: the anesthesiologist's point of view. J Perianesth Nurs 2006;21:S16–S23.
49. Yuan C-S, Foss JF, Osinski J, Toledano A, Roizen MF, and Moss J. The safety and efficacy of oral methylnaltrexone in preventing morphine-induced delay in oral-cecal transit time. Clin Pharmcol Ther 1997;61:467–475.
50. Camilleri M. Alvimopan, a selective peripherally acting μ-opioid antagonist. Neurogastroenterol Motil 2005;17:157–165.
51. Balboni G, Guerrini R, Salvadori S, Bianchi C, Rizzi D, Bryant SD, and Lazarus LH. Evaluation of the Dmt-Tic pharmacophore: conversion of a potent δ-opioid receptor antagonist into a potent δ agonist and ligands with mixed properties. J Med Chem 2002;45:713–720.
52. Balboni G, Salvadori S, Guerrini R, Negri L, Giannini E, Bryant SD, Jinsmaa Y, and Lazarus LH. Direct influence of C-terminally substituted amino acids in the Dmt-Tic pharmacophore on δ-opioid receptor selectivity and antagonism. J Med Chem 2004;47:4066–4071.
53. Salvadori S, Guerrini R, Balboni G, Bianchi C, Bryant SD, Cooper PS, and Lazarus LH. Further studies on the Dmt-Tic pharmacophore: hydrophobic substituents at the C-terminus endows δ antagonists to manifest μ agonism or μ antagonism. J Med Chem 1999;42:5010–5019.
54. Van den Eynde I, Laus G, Schiller PW, Kosson P, Chung NN, Lipkowski AW, and Tourwe D. A new structural motif for μ-opioid antagonists. J Med Chem 2005;48:3644–3648.
55. Pelton JT, Kazmierski W, Gulya K, Yamamura HI, and Hruby VJ. Design and synthesis of conformationally constrained somatostatin analogues with high potency and specificity for μ opioid receptors. J Med Chem 1986;29:2370–2375.
56. Kramer TH, Shook JE, Kazmierski W, Ayres EA, Wire WS, Hruby VJ, and Burks TF. Novel peptidic mu opioid antagonists: pharmacological characterization in vitro and in vivo. J Pharmacol Exp Ther 1989;249:544–551.
57. O'Connor PG, Oliveto AH, Shi JM, Triffleman EG, Carroll KM, Kosten TR, and Rounsaville BJ. A randomized trial of buprenorphine maintenance for heroin dependence in a primary care clinic for substance abusers versus a methadone clinic. Am J Med 1998;105:100–105.

Chapter 6
Medicinal Chemistry of Kappa Opioid Receptor Antagonists

Cécile Béguin and Bruce M. Cohen

Abstract The kappa opioid receptor (KOR), a member of the opioid receptor family, was initially studied for its involvement in the mediation of pain. More recently, there has been growing interest in selective KOR agents for their potential effects on mood and reward. In particular, selective KOR antagonists may offer a novel approach to relieve symptoms of depression. In this chapter, we describe the structure–activity relationships (SAR) of nonpeptidic KOR antagonists. Specifically, we review the SAR of norbinaltorphimine (norBNI) and its structurally simplified derivative GNTI. We present the SAR of JDTic and the recently developed MTHQ. The SAR patterns of norBNI have been extensively studied, but there have been relatively fewer studies on the SAR of JDTic and MTHQ. While the overall SAR trends of these structurally distinct agents differ, there appears to be a common requirement for KOR inhibition: the presence of a phenol unit and a basic nitrogen. In the second part of this chapter, we discuss the unusually long duration of action of the available KOR antagonists and make suggestions on possibilities for the design of additional KOR antagonists.

Keywords: Kappa opioid receptors; Structure–activity relationship; Nonpeptidic antagonists; norBNI; GNTI; JDTic; MTHQ

6.1 Introduction

Opium has been used for its analgesic properties for centuries. Morphine (Fig. 6.1, **1**), the primary active ingredient of opium, was isolated in 1805 by the German pharmacist Friedrich Sertürner. Because of the highly addictive properties of morphine, chemists have long searched for analogues with fewer side effects

C. Béguin (✉) and B.M. Cohen
Department of Psychiatry, Harvard Medical School, McLean Hospital, MRC 322A, 115 Mill Street, Belmont, MA 02478
e-mail: cbeguin@mclean.harvard.edu

R. Dean et al. (eds.), *Opiate Receptors and Antagonists*,

Fig. 6.1 Agonist and antagonist with preferential μ-opioid receptor (MOR) affinity

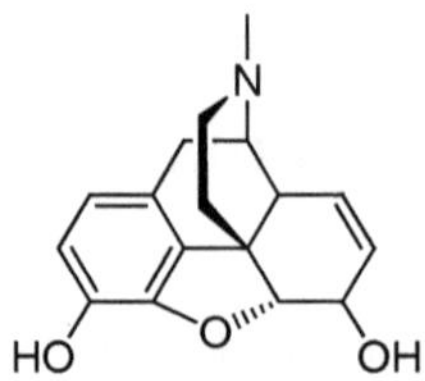

morphine, **1**

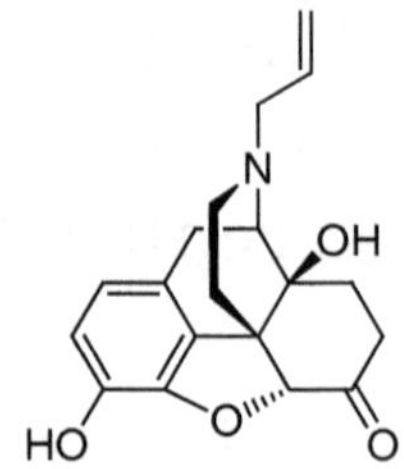

naloxone, **2**

(less tolerance and dependence) and have identified novel opioid agents with diverse chemical and pharmacological profiles. As part of this process, compounds that could antagonize the effects of morphine [e.g., naloxone (Fig. 6.1, **2**)] were identified and, when used in binding studies, made possible the discovery, in 1973, of receptors that mediate the effects of opioid agents (1). In the mid-1970s, the opioid receptors were classified into three subtypes using behavioral studies (2, 3): the κ-opioid receptor (KOR, named after the KOR ligand ketocyclazocine), the μ-opioid receptor (MOR, named after the MOR ligand morphine), and the σ-opioid receptor (named after SKF-10,047). The δ-opioid receptor was characterized in 1977 after the discovery of its endogenous agonist enkephalin (4).

The initial pharmacological characterization of KOR ligands suggested the existence of three KOR subtypes: κ_1, κ_2, and κ_3 (5, 6). However, only one gene encoding the KOR has been cloned (7), calling into question the existence of these subtypes. Alternative reasons may explain the different pharmacological responses observed upon activation of KOR. Some studies suggest the existence of several splice variants for the KOR (8). Additionally, selective KOR agonists may recognize different activated states of the KOR receptor and induce the binding of intracellular proteins involved in distinct secondary signaling pathways (9, 10). More recently, several reports suggested that the KOR may exist in different oligomeric states: the KOR may exist as a homodimer (11), or form a heterodimer with the DOR (11), the MOR (12), or the β_2-adrenergic receptor (13). Finally, the initial identification of several receptor subtypes may have been due, in part, to the nonselectivity of some of the compounds tested. For example, Olianas and coworkers have shown that the prototypic κ_3 agonist naloxone benzoylhydrazone is not a specific KOR agonist, but, rather, a nonselective opioid ligand (14).

In vivo KOR agents affect reward and pain perception, among other CNS effects. KOR agonists are potent antinociceptive drugs. Selective KOR antagonists have been investigated for their potential effect on depression (15), drug addiction (16), and feeding behavior (17).

We will describe in this chapter the structure–activity relationships (SAR) of selective nonpeptidic KOR antagonists. We will then comment on the unusually long duration of action of these agents. Finally, we will discuss some future directions for the design of additional KOR antagonists.

6.2 SAR of Selective Nonpeptidic KOR Antagonists

The earliest work on KOR-specific agents produced agonists, developed for their potential to treat pain and substance abuse. More recently, creative efforts in medicinal chemistry have led to the discovery of several selective KOR antagonists. A few peptidic KOR antagonists such as dynantin (18) and arodyn (19) show both high affinity and high selectivity for the KOR, as are needed for targeted drugs. Similarly, a few nonpeptidic molecules have been developed as selective KOR antagonists. Peptidic and nonpeptidic KOR ligands probably interact with different domains of the KOR (20). We will focus in this chapter on nonpeptidic agents that are likely to cross the blood–brain barrier. Specifically, we will review information on the SAR of the nonpeptidic KOR antagonists norbinaltorphimine (norBNI) (Fig. 6.2, **3**) (21), JDTic (Fig. 6.2, **4**) (22), and MTHQ (Fig. 6.2, **5**) (23). We will show the structures and in vitro pharmacological data for selected analogues of **3** (Figs. 6.3 and 6.4, Table 6.1), **4** (Fig. 6.5, Table 6.2), and **5** (Fig. 6.6, Tables 6.3 and 6.4), choosing compounds that provide information relevant to the SAR of norBNI, JDTic, and MTHQ. Additional information can be found in excellent reviews by Metcalf and Coop (37), and Portoghese and coworkers (38, 39). Tables 6.1–6.5 list in vitro pharmacological data obtained by various research groups. Many factors affect in vitro binding and functional assays, and assay conditions vary among laboratories (see Table 6.5). The data presented in Tables 6.1–6.5 are relative and should be viewed as approximations. In some cases, the binding and functional tests give very different selectivity profiles. Such differences are most likely a consequence of the different conditions of binding and functional assays, as well as differences in the interaction of ligands with receptors and their coeffector molecules in these two categories of assay.

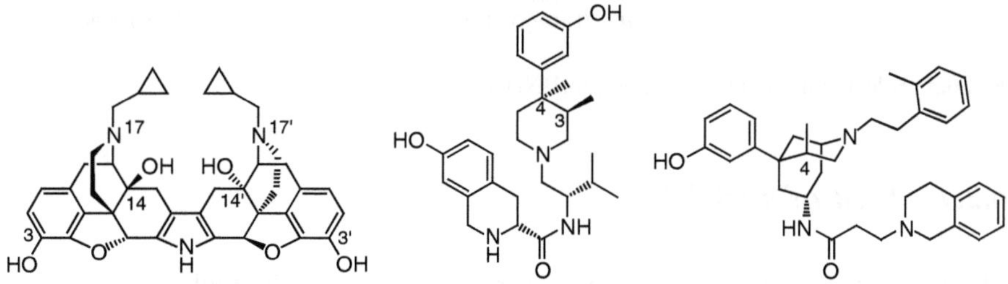

norBNI, **3** JDTic, **4** MTHQ, **5**

Fig. 6.2 Selective nonpeptidic kappa opioid receptor (KOR) antagonists

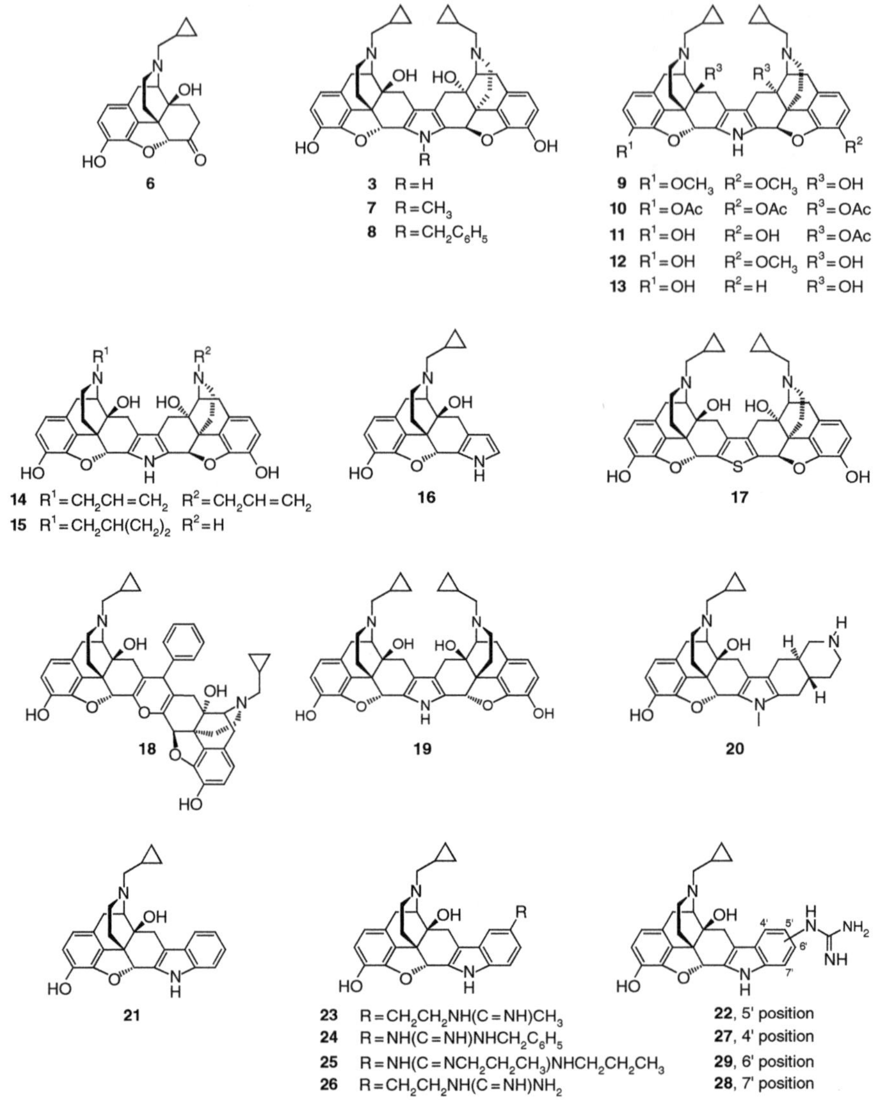

Fig. 6.3 Selected norbinaltorphimine (norBNI) analogues

6.2.1 *SAR of norBNI*

The first selective KOR antagonists were discovered by Portoghese et al. using rational drug design. On the basis of hypothesis that opioid receptors might form homodimers, Portoghese et al. proposed that the distance between the two binding sites of KOR homodimers would differ from that of MOR or DOR homodimers.

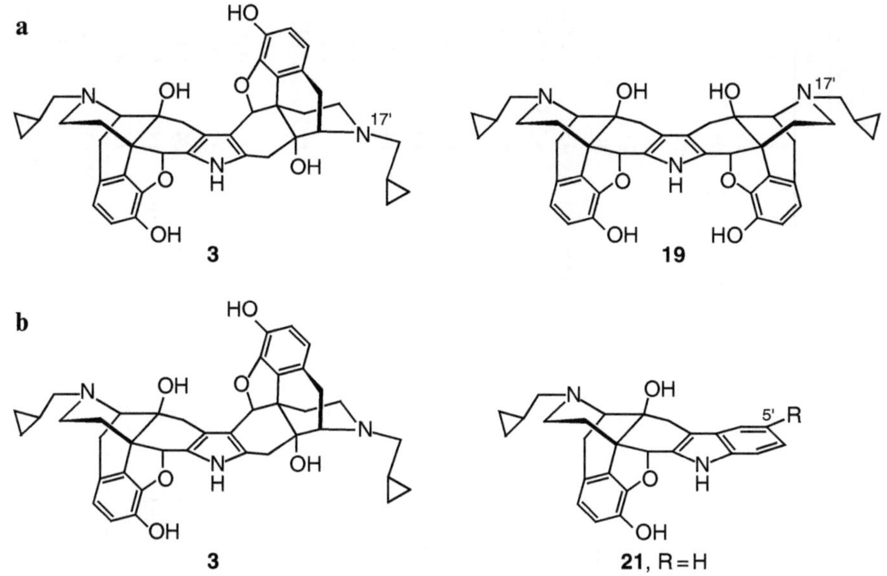

Fig. 6.4 Three-dimensional representation of selected norbinaltorphimine (norBNI) derivatives

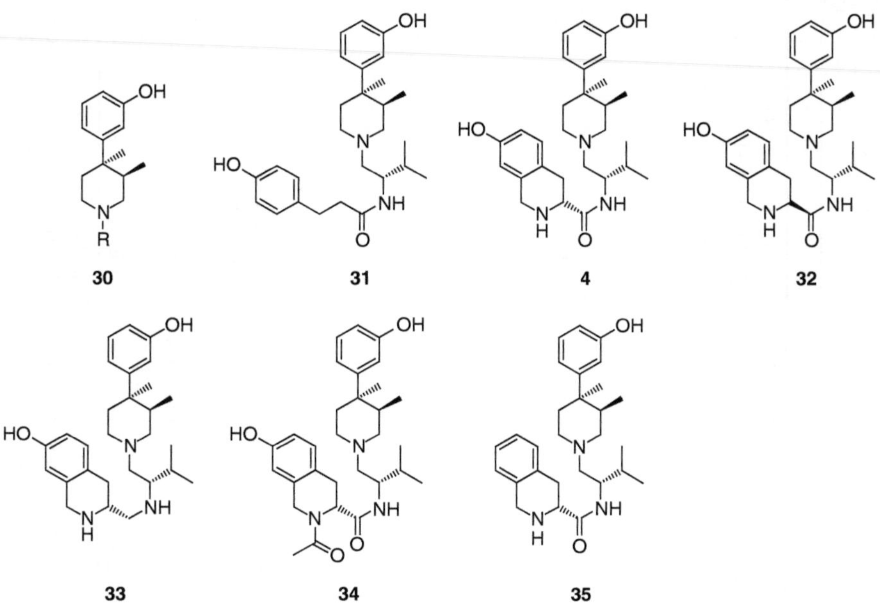

Fig. 6.5 Selected JDTic analogues

Table 6.1 Opioid receptor affinities (K_i) and antagonist potencies (K_e) of norBNI derivatives

	K_i (nM)			K_i ratio		K_e (nM)			K_e ratio	
Compound	μ	δ	κ	μ/κ	δ/κ	μ (GPI)	δ (MVD)	κ (GPI)	μ/κ	δ/κ
3	47 (35–64)[a]	39 (10–153)[a]	0.26 (0.07–0.09 (sic))[a]	181	150	13[b]	20[b]	0.41[b]	32	49
7	18 (1.4–222)[a]	58 (20–170)[a]	0.41 (0.04–4.5)[a]	44	141	11[b]	5.7[b]	0.14[b]	79	41
8[c]	10.0 ± 2.5	8.6 ± 0.7	0.7 ± 0.1	14	12	25.5 ± 2.3	13.3 ± 4.5	0.26 ± 0.085	98	51
9[b]	–	–	–	–	–	–[d]	–[d]	7.1	–	–
10[b]	–	–	–	–	–	–[d]	–[d]	–[d]	–	–
11[b]	–	–	–	–	–	42	12	0.38	111	32
12[b]	–	–	–	–	–	38	45	1.3	29	35
13[e]	8.3 ± 0.4	110.8 ± 10.7	1.33 ± 0.24	6	83	5.55 ± 1.00	>300	0.13 ± 0.01	43	>2307
14[b]	–	–	–	–	–	>250	>143	0.91	>275	>157
15[f]	–	–	–	–	–	111	13	2.5	44	5.2
16[g]	–	–	–	–	–	0.7	3.7	2.1	0.3	1.8
17[a]	189 (105–339)	77 (65–92)	1.4 (1.2–1.6)	135	55	41	33	2.6	16	13
18[a]	29 (12–67)	10 (2.6–42)	2.6 (2.3–2.9)	11	4	39	36	2.6	15	14
19[h]	–	–	–	–	–	1.1	1.3	0.08	14	16
20[i]	–	–	–	–	–	–[d]	1000	2.6	–	385
27[j]	>1000	>1000	>1000			–[d]	263	80	–	3.3
22[j]	99.7 ± 8.7	24.8 ± 11.3	0.14 ± 0.03	712	177	30.3	115	0.16	189	719
29[j]	81.8 ± 20.7	20.3 ± 6.7	1.15 ± 0.39	71	17.7	–[k]	–[d]	–[k]	–	–
28[j]	181 ± 20	2.75 ± 0.48	69.1 ± 25	2.6	0.04	238	0.96	100	2	0.01
23[l]	–	–	–	–	–	7.6	18	0.3	27	65
24[m]	10.47 ± 1.87	26.81 ± 6.47	0.86 ± 0.20	12	31	1.41 ± 0.17	4.09 ± 0.63	0.06 ± 0.01	24	68
25[m]	9.83 ± 0.09	8.52 ± 1.99	2.72 ± 0.39	4	3	4.59 ± 0.80	2.43 ± 0.31	0.26 ± 0.05	18	9
26[l]	33.4 ± 4.7	10.7 ± 3.0	0.507 ± 0.13	66	21	12	3.4	1.7	7.3	2.0

[a]Data from Portoghese et al. (24); [b]Data from Portoghese et al. (25); [c]Data from Chauvignac et al. (26); [d]Not calculated because IC_{50} ratio ≤1; [e]Data from Thomas et al. (27); [f]Data from Portoghese et al. (28); [g]Data from Portoghese et al. (29); [h]Data from Portoghese et al. (30); [i]Data from Lin et al. (31); [j]Data from Sharma et al. (32). K_i values were obtained using cloned opioid receptors; [k]Not calculated due to full agonist activity; [l]Data from Stevens et al. (33); [m]Data from Black et al. (34)

Table 6.2 Opioid receptor affinities (K_i) and antagonist potencies (K_e) of JDTic derivatives[a]

	K_i (nM)			K_i ratio		K_e (nM)			K_e ratio	
Compound	μ	δ	κ	μ/κ	δ/κ	μ	δ	κ	μ/κ	δ/κ
31[b]	171 ± 15	>3400	3.84 ± 0.26	45	>885	7.25 ± 0.52	450 ± 74.1	4.7 ± 0.56	1.5	96
4[b]	3.73 ± 0.17	301 ± 50	0.32 ± 0.05	12	940	2.16 ± 0.75	>300	0.02 ± 0.002	108	>15000
4[c]	0.96 ± 0.01	29.6 ± 11.9	0.41 ± 0.10	2.3	72	3.41 ± 0.36	79.3 ± 9.3	0.01 ± 0.00	341	7930
32[b]	596 ± 29	>4900	9.8 ± 1.6	61	>500	11 ± 0.8	327 ± 35	4.2 ± 0.20	2.6	78
33[b]	107 ± 11	>4900	0.63 ± 0.05	170	>7777	12.8 ± 1.4	>300	0.20 ± 0.03	64	>1500
33[c]	3.80 ± 0.30	83.6 ± 8.09	1.82 ± 0.20	2.1	46	14.3 ± 2.27	427 ± 109	0.14 ± 0.02	102	3100
34[b]	764 ± 66	>4900	146 ± 15	5	>34	17.4 ± 1.2	>300	19.6 ± 1.6	0.9	15
35[b]	775 ± 75	>4900	2.1 ± 0.17	369	>2333	68.6 ± 6.5	147 ± 11	11.5 ± 1	5.9	12.8
35[c]	33.1 ± 0.89	1090 ± 174	2.18 ± 0.12	15	500	8.38 ± 0.30	–	2.95 ± 0.42	2.8	–
3[b]	65 ± 5.6	86 ± 7.2	1.09 ± 0.14	60	79	16.7 ± 1.5	10.2 ± 1.0	0.038 ± 0.005	440	268
3[c]	21 ± 5.0	5.7 ± 0.9	0.2 ± 0.05	105	29	19 ± 1.8	4.4 ± 0.38	0.04	475	115

[a]Data from Thomas et al. (35)

[b]Using brain tissues

[c]In CHO cells with cloned human receptors

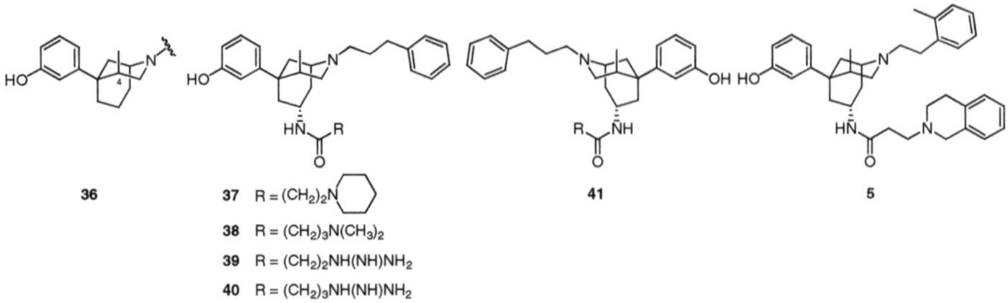

Fig. 6.6 Selected MTHQ analogues

Table 6.3 Opioid receptor affinities (K_i) of MTHQ derivatives[a]

	K_i (nM)			K_i ratio	
Compound	μ	δ	κ	μ/κ	δ/κ
37	147 ± 9.8	>3400	4.3 ± 0.7	34	>790
38	57 ± 4.4	1457 ± 113	12 ± 0.65	5	122
39	5.2 ± 0.3	56.5 ± 3.4	23.3 ± 3	0.2	2
40	87 ± 6.3	1744 ± 98	13.2 ± 1.7	7	132
41	775 ± 55	2184 ± 93	36 ± 5	22	61
3	65.0 ± 5.6	86 ± 7.2	1.09 ± 0.14	60	79

[a]Data from Thomas et al. (36)

Table 6.4 Inhibition of agonist-stimulated [35S]GTPγS binding (K_e) by MTHQ derivatives in CHO cells with cloned human opioid receptors[a]

	K_e (nM)			K_e ratio	
Compound	μ	δ	κ	μ/κ	δ/κ
37	42 ± 4	33 ± 2.7	0.24 ± 0.01	175	138
5	28 ± 9	25 ± 9	0.04 ± 0.01	700	625
4	25 ± 4	76 ± 3	0.02 ± 0.01	1250	3800
3	26 ± 7	29 ± 8	0.05 ± 0.02	520	580

[a]Data from Carroll et al. (23)

Therefore, they hypothesized that selectivity for each receptor subtype might be obtained by designing ligands containing two recognition units separated by an appropriate linker. Varying the length and flexibility of the spacer would provide compounds that preferentially recognize KOR versus MOR or DOR. They chose the nonselective KOR antagonist naltrexone (Fig. 6.3, **6**) as the recognition unit, found that short and rigid spacers led to KOR selectivity (47), and designed the selective KOR antagonist norBNI (**3**) (21) containing two naltrexone units linked by a pyrrole spacer.

Preliminary SAR studies showed that methyl substitution of the pyrrole is tolerated: BNI (Fig. 6.3, **7**) (21) is a potent and selective KOR antagonist in smooth muscle preparations. In a more recent study, Husbands et al. looked at the effect

Table 6.5 Opioid receptor affinities (K_i) and antagonist potencies (K_e) of norBNI (X), GNTI (X12), JDTic (Y), and MTHQ (Z)

	K_i (nM)			K_i ratio			K_e (nM)		K_e ratio		
Compound	μ	δ	κ	μ/κ	δ/κ	μ (GPI)	δ (MVD)	κ (GPI)	μ/κ	δ/κ	References
3	–	–	–	–	–	33	20	0.40	83	50	(21)
3	–	–	–	–	–	13	20	0.41	32	49	(25)
3	–	–	–	–	–	12.5	10	0.41	30	24	(30)
3	47 (35–64)	39 (10–153)	0.26 (0.07–0.09 (sic))	181	150	14	10.6	0.55	25	19	(24, 28)
3	101.9 ± 10.2	–	0.12 ± 0.04	849	–	13.7	10.6	0.56	25	19	(40)
3	70.0 ± 17.9	–	0.13 ± 0.04	538	–	–	–	–	–	–	(41)
3	49.7 ± 6.6	41.5 ± 13	0.244 ± 0.064	204	170	13	11	0.4	33	28	(33)
3	56.6 ± 6.6	41.5 ± 13.0	0.24 ± 0.06	236	173	–	–	–	–	–	(42)
3	–	–	–	–	–	12.5	10.6	0.41	30	26	(32)
3	21.0 ± 5.0	5.7 ± 0.9	0.2 ± 0.05	105	28	18.9 ± 1.8	4.42 ± 0.38	0.039 ± 0.004	484	113	(34, 43–45)
3	1.20 ± 0.2	5.8 ± 0.645	0.4 ± 0.06	3	15	2.38 ± 0.58	5.17 ± 0.73	0.11 ± 0.01	22	47	(26)
3	65.06 ± 5.6	86 ± 7.3	1.09 ± 0.14	60	79	16.7 ± 1.5	10.2 ± 1.0	0.038 ± 0.005	439	268	(22)
3	–	–	–	–	–	19 ± 1.52	4.6 ± 0.39	0.04 ± 0.003	475	115	(36)
3	–	–	–	–	–	26 ± 7	29 ± 8	0.05 ± 0.02	520	580	(23)
22	9.23 ± 1.39	–	0.09 ± 0.01	103	–	30	115	0.14	208	799	(40)
22	22.5 ± 3.9	46.2 ± 5.1	0.180 ± 0.052	125	257	30	–[a]	0.2	193	366	(33, 42)
22	36.9 ± 2.3	70.0 ± 0.3	0.18 ± 0.10	205	389	–	–	–	–	–	(46)
22	99.7 ± 8.7	24.8 ± 11.3	0.14 ± 0.03	712	177	30.3	115	0.16	189	719	(32)
4	3.73 ± 0.17	301 ± 50	0.32 ± 0.05	12	940	2.16 ± 0.75	>300	0.02 ± 0.002	108	>15000	(22)
4	0.96 ± 0.01	29.6 ± 11.9	0.41 ± 0.10	2.3	72	3.41 ± 0.36	79.3 ± 9.3	0.01 ± 0.00	341	7930	(35)
4	–	–	–	–	–	25 ± 4	76 ± 3	0.02 ± 0.01	1250	3800	(23)
5	–	–	–	–	–	28 ± 9	25 ± 9	0.04 ± 0.01	700	625	(23)

[a]Not calculated because IC_{50} ratio ≤1

of pyrrole *N*-benzylation of norBNI (26). In vitro, they found that BnorBNI (Fig. 6.3, **8**) was a potent KOR antagonist with modest partial agonist properties at KOR and MOR at high concentrations. In vivo, it behaved as a short-lasting MOR agonist after subcutaneous (sc) administration and a long-lasting KOR antagonist after intracerebroventricular (icv) administration. It is not known whether this pharmacological profile is due to the unique interaction of **8** with opioid receptors or to its pharmacokinetic properties. Additional evaluation of the SAR of norBNI suggests that at least one of the phenolic OH groups is necessary for in vitro KOR potency (25): methylation (**9** vs **3**) or acetylation (**10** vs **11**) of both phenol OH groups leads to a moderate to significant loss of KOR antagonist activity, while methylation of a single phenolic group gave compound **12** (25) which is only threefold less potent than norBNI in smooth muscle preparations and retains selectivity for the KOR. This SAR characteristic was recently revisited by Carroll et al.: a single phenolic group dehydroxylation leads to compound **13** (35) with moderate loss of KOR binding affinity and a significant drop in KOR selectivity, suggesting that the second phenolic oxygen of norBNI might contribute to KOR selectivity. However, functional assay data do not strongly support these findings. Further evaluation of the SAR of norBNI reveals that (a) the *N*-cyclopropylmethyl groups can be replaced by *N*-allyl substituents (**14** vs **3**) (25); (b) at least one *N*-cyclopropylmethyl unit is necessary for selectivity (e.g., **15** vs **3**) (28); and (c) neither the hydroxyl group at the C-14 nor the C-14′ position is critical for activity (e.g., **11** vs **3**) (25). In addition, Portoghese et al. explored the role of the linker: the pyrrole spacer alone is not responsible for KOR selectivity (**16** vs **3**) (29). In another study, the authors disclosed the influence of various heterocyclic linkers: replacement of the pyrrole with a thiophene gave the bivalent compound **17**, which kept selectivity for KOR in binding studies, while the γ-substituted pyran derivative **18** was not selective in this assay (24). Surprisingly, compounds **17** and **18** had similar potencies at all three opioid receptors in smooth muscle preparations (24). Overall, these data suggest that the pyrrole ring acts as a rigid spacer that holds the two naltrexone pharmacophores in the appropriate positions but does not participate in interactions with the KOR.

To address the roles of the two naltrexone pharmacophores, Portoghese and his group first synthesized the *meso* isomer of norBNI (**19**) (30). In vitro pharmacological evaluation of **19** revealed that it was slightly more potent than norBNI and suggested that only a portion of the second naltrexone molecule was necessary for KOR affinity. The three-dimensional structures of **3** and **19** (Fig. 6.4a) suggest that the basic tertiary nitrogen at the 17′-position is critical for KOR affinity and selectivity. To verify this hypothesis, Portoghese and colleagues then prepared a simplified analogue (Fig. 6.3, **20**) (31) of BNI (**7**), resulting from removal of portions of the second naltrexone pharmacophore. Interestingly, compound **20** retained affinity and high selectivity for KOR.

Chavkin et al. (48) had previously reported that the opioid peptides follow the message address concept introduced by Schwyzer (49). This concept suggests that one portion of a molecule (message) interacts with a binding domain that is common to a family of receptors, while another part of the molecule (address) recognizes a binding pocket that is unique to a specific receptor subtype. In the case of opioid peptides, the conserved amino acid sequence Tyr-Gly-Gly-Phe is responsible for recognition by all opioid receptors (message), while Arg^7 in dynorphin A is believed to act as the address and confer selectivity for KOR. Following this concept, Portoghese et al. suggested that N-17′ of norBNI may mimic Arg^7 of dynorphin and be responsible for KOR selectivity. They proposed that structurally simpler molecules that contain one naltrexone unit and a basic substituent at the right orientation may be selective KOR antagonists. Using a three-dimensional representation of norBNI (Fig. 6.4b, **3**), they designed a series of compounds that contain the selective DOR antagonist NTI (Fig. 6.4b, **21**) as a rigid backbone on which they could attach protonated substituents (alkylamidino and guanidino groups) (50). The most promising compound in this series, 5′-guanidinonaltrindole (GNTI, Fig. 6.3, **22**) (40), has improved binding affinity and antagonist potency compared to norBNI and is more selective for KOR. 5′-acetamidinoethylnaltrindole (ANTI, **23**) (33), an analogue of GNTI with increased lipophilicity, has lower selectivity for the KOR but may be used in experiments that require improved bioavailability (15, 33). The SAR for these compounds follows the SAR observed for norBNI. In particular, the basicity of the 5′ substituent is important for selectivity: guanidine > amidine ~ quaternary ammonium > amine (33). Husbands et al. subsequently reported that guanidine benzylation (e.g., **24** vs **22**) leads to compounds that retain preferential affinity for KOR but are less selective than GNTI (34). Guanidine dialkyl substitution leads to an even greater loss of selectivity (e.g., **25** vs **22**) (34). The position of the indole substituent is also critical: introduction of one to two carbon atom spacers between the 5′-position and the guanidine substituent leads to decreased KOR selectivity (**26** vs **22**). Additionally, substitution at the 4′-position (**27**) or 7′-position (**28**) of the indole leads to loss of KOR selectivity (32). In fact, 7′-GNTI (**28**) is a selective DOR antagonist (32). Interestingly, 6′-GNTI (**29**) converts GNTI from a potent antagonist to a potent KOR agonist in the guinea pig ileum assay (32). Portoghese et al. first proposed that the 6′-substituent may contribute to receptor activation by inducing a conformational change of KOR transmembrane helix 6 (TM6) and inner loop 3 (32), while a recent report by Waldhoer et al. suggests that 6′-GNTI (**29**) may in fact have the unique property of activating KOR/DOR heterodimers but not KOR homomers (51).

Takahashi and colleagues have recently reported the solid phase synthesis of 120 norBNI derivatives in which they altered the pyrrole N-substituent and the N-17 and N-17′ moieties (see Fig. 6.2) (52). The biological data for these compounds have not been reported in the literature but would provide additional information on the SAR of norBNI.

Opioid receptor mutation and chimera studies suggest that N-17 interacts with residue Asp138 of the KOR, and that N-17′ confers selectivity for KOR by ionic interaction with Glu297 located near the extracellular end of TM6 (41, 53). Subsequent studies indicated that the address of dynorphin A interacted through hydrophobic interaction with extracellular loop 2 (EL2) (54). Therefore, the addresses of norBNI and dynorphin A seem to interact with distinct binding pockets of the KOR.

6.2.2 SAR of JDTic

A structurally different selective KOR antagonist was developed by Carroll and colleagues using the 1,3,4-trialkyl-4-phenylpiperidines as lead compounds (55). Early studies showed that *trans*-3,4-dimethyl(3-hydroxyphenyl)piperidines (Fig 6.5, **30**) have opioid antagonist properties and initial modifications of the piperidine N-substituent provided compounds with mixed MOR/KOR antagonist properties (56, 57), or preferential MOR antagonist properties (58). In 1998, Thomas and colleagues reported the synthesis and evaluation of 288 N-substituted *trans*-3,4-dimethyl(3-hydroxyphenyl)piperidine analogues (59). One of these derivatives, RTI-5989-29 (**31**) (59), showed selectivity for KOR over DOR and MOR in in vitro binding assays, but was nonselective in the [^{35}S]GTPγS functional assay. Further structural modifications produced JDTic (**4**) (22), the first 4-phenylpiperidine derivative with high selectivity for KOR in the [^{35}S]GTPγS functional assay (22). Surprisingly, in the binding assay, while JDTic showed high KOR affinity, it was not highly selective for KOR versus MOR in guinea pig (22) or human tissues (35).

In a recent study, Thomas et al. identified key SAR patterns for JDTic (35). Configuration of the tetrahydroisoquinoline amide substituent is critical for receptor potency and selectivity in the [^{35}S]GTPγS assay (**32** vs **4**) (35). The effect is not as pronounced in binding studies. The amide carbonyl group is not essential since **33** (35) shows only a modest loss of potency and selectivity when compared to JDTic in the [^{35}S]GTPγS assay, and has increased selectivity in the binding assay. The basicity of the tetrahydroisoquinoline amino group is important: acetylation of the amino group (**34**) leads to a significant loss of KOR affinity and selectivity. Removal of the tetrahydroisoquinoline OH group shows it to be necessary for KOR selectivity in the [^{35}S]GTPγS functional assay (**35** vs **4**) (27, 35). However, the opposite trend is observed in the binding assay: **35** has greater KOR selectivity than **4**. Finally, Thomas et al. confirmed the importance of the 3*R* and 4*R* configurations.

In analogy with norBNI, Thomas et al. proposed that the *trans*-3,4-dimethyl (3-hydroxyphenyl)piperidine part of JDTic serves as a message that recognizes all opioid receptors, while the piperidine N-substituent confers selectivity for KOR. They suggested that the tetrahydroisoquinoline amino group may be involved in ionic interaction with Glu297 of KOR (35). This hypothesis has yet to be tested by mutagenesis studies.

6.2.3 SAR of MTHQ

In a continuation of their studies with the *trans*-3,4-dimethyl(3-hydroxyphenyl) piperidines, Carroll and colleagues reported the synthesis and in vitro pharmacological evaluation of 4β-methyl-5-(3-hydroxyphenyl)morphan (Fig. 6.6, **36**) derivatives. The 5-(3-hydroxyphenyl)morphans are conformationally restricted analogues of the *trans*-3,4-dimethyl(3-hydroxyphenyl)piperidines and have nonselective opioid antagonist properties (60).

Carroll and coworkers first reported the synthesis and evaluation of seven 4β-methyl-5-(3-hydroxyphenyl)morphan derivatives (36), and identified KAA-1 (**37**) (36) as the first selective KOR antagonist in this series. KAA-1 has a lower KOR over MOR selectivity than norBNI but shows improved KOR over DOR selectivity. Other compounds prepared in this study (**38–40**) (36) resulted in a reduction of KOR selectivity. Configuration at the chiral centers is important for binding affinity (**41** vs **37**). Subsequently, Carroll and coworkers reported the synthesis and evaluation of 17 KAA-1 analogues (23). All compounds displayed preferential KOR antagonist properties. In particular, MTHQ (**5**) (23) was found to be a highly potent and selective KOR antagonist in the [^{35}S]GTPγS assay. Using ligand–receptor interaction models previously proposed by Portoghese and coworkers (61, 62), Carroll et al. (23) compared in this paper the putative binding interactions (Fig. 6.7) between the KOR and the oxymorphone-related compounds (e.g., naltrexone, GNTI), the *trans*-3,4-dimethyl(3-hydroxyphenyl)piperidines (e.g., JDTic), and the 4β-methyl-5-(3-hydroxyphenyl)morphans (e.g., KAA-1, MTHQ). They suggested

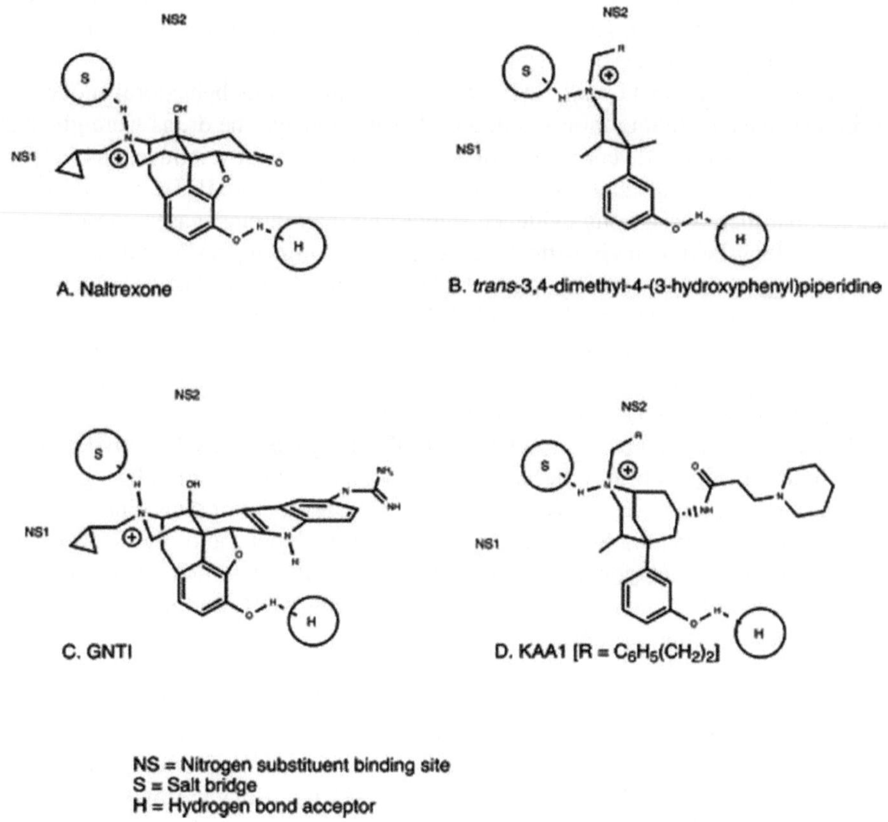

Fig. 6.7 Comparison of kappa opioid receptor binding domains for naltrexone, *trans* 3,4-dimethyl-4(3-hydroxyphenyl) piperidine, GNTI, and KAAI. Figure taken from J Med Chem 2006, 1781–1791

that (a) the phenolic group present in each of these derivatives interacts through hydrogen bonding with a common residue of the KOR, (b) the protonated basic nitrogen is involved in ionic interaction with a common anionic site of the KOR, (c) the basic nitrogen substituents interact with two different binding domains of the KOR.

It is not well understood if structurally diverse selective KOR antagonists bind to the same binding pocket. However, they have common structural features such as a phenolic unit and a basic amino group that may interact with the same KOR residues.

6.3 Unusually Long Duration of Action of Current Selective KOR Antagonists

Here, we will note and comment on the unusually long duration of action of all KOR-specific antagonists that have been evaluated in vivo: norBNI (Fig. 6.2, **3**), GNTI (Fig. 6.3, **22**), ANTI (Fig. 6.3, **23**), and JDTic (Fig. 6.2, **4**). It is unclear at this time if this characteristic is a consequence of the chemistry of the agents or reflects a property of the KOR itself.

norBNI, GNTI, ANTI, and JDTic were tested in various behavioral models in several species, including mouse, rat, and rhesus monkey. The drugs were given at a range of doses using diverse routes of administration [e.g., icv, intravenous (iv), sc] (37). The durations of action of norBNI, GNTI, ANTI, and JDTic varied across studies, but there was strong evidence suggesting that, in most cases, these agents have very long-lasting in vivo effects (up to 56 days following a single dose). Select studies suggest that the less lipophilic GNTI may have shorter-lasting effects than norBNI (63, 64), and that norBNI and JDTic may have similar durations of action (65, 66). Studies designed to determine the durations of action of norBNI, GNTI, ANTI, and JDTic under the exact same experimental conditions have not been done and would provide valuable further information.

There have only been a few selective KOR antagonists tested in vivo and the long duration of action may be an artifact peculiar to these particular agents. In fact, an ongoing study (E. Bilsky and J. Lowery, University of New England, personal communication via S. Negus) indicates that the blockade of the KOR by the nonspecific opioid antagonist naltrexone is short lasting (less than 100 min). This finding suggests that interaction of an antagonist with KOR need not lead to long-lasting blockade or loss of KOR.

It is not clear why the available selective KOR antagonists have such long-lasting effects. None of the functionalities of norBNI, GNTI, ANTI, and JDTic can form covalent bonds with the KOR protein, suggesting that these compounds are not irreversible ligands. By comparison, the antagonist effects of DIPPA [2-(3,4-Dichlorophenyl)-N-methyl-N-[(1S)-1-(3-isothiocyanatophenyl)-2-(1-pyrrolidinyl)ethyl]acetamide], which does bind irreversibly to KOR, only last 2–4 days (67). Furthermore, antagonism produced by norBNI remains competitive (68), a finding inconsistent with irreversible binding. In addition, at least in one study

(69), the time required for norBNI to block the effects of different specific KOR agonists compared head to head varied from 1 day for salvinorin A to 5 days for U69,593, suggesting a dynamic and changing relationship between the antagonist, the KOR and, perhaps, other proteins, and effector molecules.

Portoghese et al. suggested that norBNI dissolves in brain membranes, which may affect the rate of drug excretion (39). This hypothesis could explain why the less lipophilic GNTI has shorter-lasting effects than norBNI. Alternatively, some KOR antagonists may have an unusual interaction with KOR that keeps the receptor in a prolonged inactivated state. For example, KOR inhibition may induce receptor internalization and degradation.

Lipophilic agents can last in tissue for days to weeks at levels high enough to produce receptor blockade (70). A study of the bioavailability of KOR antagonists could help determine if they or their metabolites are retained in tissue for weeks at levels high enough to block KOR. In fact, there is also no published data on the metabolism of norBNI, GNTI, ANTI, and JDTic, and it is not known whether they have active metabolites which might contribute to the long-lasting in vivo effects of these agents.

6.4 Future Directions

The number of available, chemically distinct KOR antagonists is small and it is not yet known if their properties will turn out to be ideal for further development. In vitro JDTic has 12-fold selectivity for KOR versus MOR in guinea pig brain tissue, but only twofold selectivity with cloned human receptors (35). In vivo characterization of norBNI, GNTI, and ANTI has revealed that some of these compounds may not be as selective as predicted by in vitro data. For example, norBNI has short-lasting MOR antagonist properties followed by long-lasting KOR antagonists effects (71, 72). GNTI and JDTic do not seem to share this property but they also

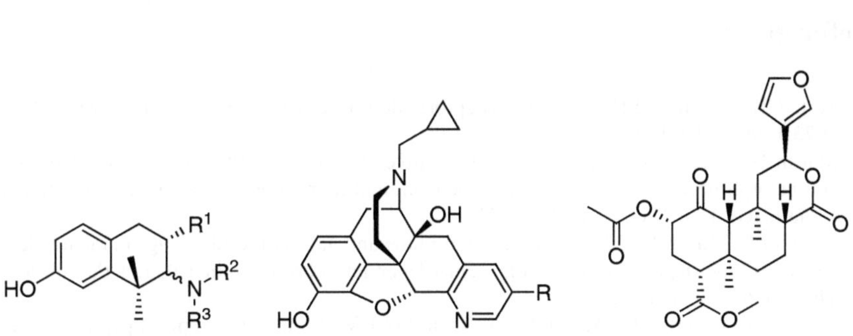

42 **43** **44**

Fig. 6.8 Potential lead compounds for the design of additional selective kappa opioid receptor (*KOR*) antagonists

have not been characterized extensively in vivo. Further studies of the specificity of these agents and the development of additional compounds acting specifically at the KOR would be worthwhile.

The design of norBNI, GNTI, JDTic, and MTHQ resulted from the modification of nonselective opioid antagonists. Husbands and coworkers recently identified the amino tetralins (Fig. 6.8, **42**) as nonselective opioid antagonists, which could be used as a template for the design of additional novel selective KOR antagonists (73). Similarly, the pyridomorphinans (Fig. 6.8, **43**) developed as nonselective opioid antagonists by Ananthan et al. may serve as lead compounds for the design of selective KOR antagonists (74). Alternatively, it may be possible to produce new antagonists by modifying compounds which are KOR agonists. Thus, the selective KOR agonist 6′-GNTI (**29**) can be converted to the selective KOR antagonist 5′-GNTI (**22**) (32) by simple chemical modification, and oxymorphinans can be converted from opioid agonists into antagonists by modification of their *N*-methyl substituent into a *N*-cyclopropylmethyl substituent. We have been studying whether modification of the highly potent and selective KOR agonist salvinorin A (Fig. 6.8, **44**) may produce selective KOR antagonists. Thus far, preliminary work has not produced any analogues with KOR antagonist properties (75, 76). Finally, numerous studies have shown that opioid receptor subtype selectivity may be affected by simple structural modifications. For example, the selective DOR antagonist NTI (Fig. 6.4, **21**) can be converted to the selective KOR antagonist 5′-GNTI (Fig. 6.3, **22**) (33) by addition of a guanidino group to the indole unit. Additional selective KOR antagonists may be obtained from selective MOR or DOR antagonists. Finally, the screening of large libraries of structurally diverse compounds is increasingly being used to find new ligands for known targets. Such screening for the KOR as a target may provide lead compounds for the design of novel selective KOR antagonists. With more compounds available, we could learn more about receptor–ligand interactions and increase the chance of developing useful clinical agents.

References

1. Pert CB, Snyder SH. Opiate receptor: demonstration in nervous tissue. Science 1973;179(77):1011–4.
2. Martin WR, Eades CG, Thompson JA, Huppler RE, Gilbert PE. The effects of morphine- and nalorphine-like drugs in the nondependent and morphine-dependent chronic spinal dog. J Pharmacol Exp Ther 1976;197(3):517–32.
3. Gilbert PE, Martin WR. The effects of morphine and nalorphine-like drugs in the nondependent, morphine-dependent and cyclazocine-dependent chronic spinal dog. J Pharmacol Exp Ther 1976;198(1):66–82.
4. Lord JAH, Waterfield AA, Hughes J, Kosterlitz HW. Endogenous opioid peptides: multiple agonists and receptors. Nature 1977;267(5611):495–9.
5. Zukin RS, Eghbali M, Olive D, Unterwald EM, Tempel A. Characterization and visualization of rat and guinea pig brain kappa opioid receptors: evidence for kappa 1 and kappa 2 opioid receptors. Proc Natl Acad Sci USA 1988;85(11):4061–5.

6. Clark JA, Liu L, Price M, Hersh B, Edelson M, Pasternak GW. Kappa opiate receptor multiplicity: evidence for two U50,488-sensitive kappa 1 subtypes and a novel kappa 3 subtype. J Pharmacol Exp Ther 1989;251(2):461–8.
7. Yasuda K, Raynor K, Kong H, et al. Cloning and functional comparison of kappa and delta opioid receptors from mouse brain. Proc Natl Acad Sci USA 1993;90(14):6736–40.
8. Gaveriaux-Ruff C, Peluso J, Befort K, Simonin F, Zilliox C, Kieffer BL. Detection of opioid receptor mRNA by RT-PCR reveals alternative splicing for the delta- and kappa-opioid receptors. Brain Res Mol Brain Res 1997;48(2):298–304.
9. Rusovici DE, Negus SS, Mello NK, Bidlack JM. Kappa-opioid receptors are differentially labeled by arylacetamides and benzomorphans. Eur J Pharmacol 2004;485(1–3):119–25.
10. Pogozheva ID, Przydzial MJ, Mosberg HI. Homology modeling of opioid receptor-ligand complexes using experimental constraints. AAPS J 2005;7(2):E434–48.
11. Jordan BA, Devi LA. G-protein-coupled receptor heterodimerization modulates receptor function. Nature 1999;399(6737):697–700.
12. Wang D, Sun X, Bohn LM, Sadee W. Opioid receptor homo- and heterodimerization in living cells by quantitative bioluminescence resonance energy transfer. Mol Pharmacol 2005;67(6): 2173–84.
13. Jordan BA, Trapaidze N, Gomes I, Nivarthi R, Devi LA. Oligomerization of opioid receptors with beta 2-adrenergic receptors: a role in trafficking and mitogen-activated protein kinase activation. Proc Natl Acad Sci USA 2001;98(1):343–8.
14. Olianas MC, Concas D, Onali P. Agonist activity of naloxone benzoylhydrazone at recombinant and native opioid receptors. Br J Pharmacol 2006;147(4):360–70.
15. Mague SD, Pliakas AM, Todtenkopf MS, et al. Antidepressant-like effects of kappa-opioid receptor antagonists in the forced swim test in rats. J Pharmacol Exp Ther 2003;305(1):323–30.
16. Prisinzano TE, Tidgewell K, Harding WW. Kappa opioids as potential treatments for stimulant dependence. AAPS J 2005;7(3):E592–9.
17. Jewett DC, Grace MK, Jones RM, Billington CJ, Portoghese PS, Levine AS. The kappa-opioid antagonist GNTI reduces U50,488-, DAMGO-, and deprivation-induced feeding, but not butorphanol- and neuropeptide Y-induced feeding in rats. Brain Res 2001;909(1–2):75–80.
18. Lu Y, Nguyen TM, Weltrowska G, et al. [2′,6′-Dimethyltyrosine]dynorphin A(1–11)-NH2 analogues lacking an N-terminal amino group: potent and selective kappa opioid antagonists. J Med Chem 2001;44(19):3048–53.
19. Bennett MA, Murray TF, Aldrich JV. Identification of arodyn, a novel acetylated dynorphin A-(1-11) analogue, as a kappa opioid receptor antagonist. J Med Chem 2002;45(26): 5617–9.
20. Xue JC, Chen C, Zhu J, et al. Differential binding domains of peptide and non-peptide ligands in the cloned rat kappa opioid receptor. J Biol Chem 1994;269(48):30195–9.
21. Portoghese AS, Lipkowski AW, Takemori AE. Bimorphinans as highly selective, potent kappa opioid receptor antagonists. J Med Chem 1987;30(2):238–9.
22. Thomas JB, Atkinson RN, Rothman RB, et al. Identification of the first trans-(3R,4R)- dimethyl-4-(3-hydroxyphenyl)piperidine derivative to possess highly potent and selective opioid kappa receptor antagonist activity. J Med Chem 2001;44(17):2687–90.
23. Carroll FI, Melvin MS, Nuckols MC, Mascarella SW, Navarro HA, Thomas JB. N-substituted 4beta-methyl-5-(3-hydroxyphenyl)-7alpha-amidomorphans are potent, selective kappa opioid receptor antagonists. J Med Chem 2006;49(5):1781–91.
24. Portoghese PS, Garzon-Aburbeh A, Nagase H, Lin CE, Takemori AE. Role of the spacer in conferring kappa opioid receptor selectivity to bivalent ligands related to norbinaltorphimine. J Med Chem 1991;34(4):1292–6.
25. Portoghese PS, Nagase H, Lipkowski AW, Larson DL, Takemori AE. Binaltorphimine-related bivalent ligands and their kappa opioid receptor antagonist selectivity. J Med Chem 1988;31(4):836–41.
26. Chauvignac C, Miller CN, Srivastava SK, Lewis JW, Husbands SM, Traynor JR. Major effect of pyrrolic N-benzylation in norbinaltorphimine, the selective kappa-opioid receptor antagonist. J Med Chem 2005;48(5):1676–9.

27. Thomas JB, Fix SE, Rothman RB, et al. Importance of phenolic address groups in opioid kappa receptor selective antagonists. J Med Chem 2004;47(4):1070–3.
28. Portoghese PS, Lin CE, Farouz-Grant F, Takemori AE. Structure-activity relationship of N17′-substituted norbinaltorphimine congeners. Role of the N17′ basic group in the interaction with a putative address subsite on the kappa opioid receptor. J Med Chem 1994;37(10):1495–500.
29. Portoghese PS, Sultana M, Nagase H, Takemori AE. Application of the message-address concept in the design of highly potent and selective non-peptide delta opioid receptor antagonists. J Med Chem 1988;31(2):281–2.
30. Portoghese PS, Nagase H, Takemori AE. Only one pharmacophore is required for the kappa opioid antagonist selectivity of norbinaltorphimine. J Med Chem 1988;31(7):1344–7.
31. Lin CE, Takemori AE, Portoghese PS. Synthesis and kappa-opioid antagonist selectivity of a norbinaltorphimine congener. Identification of the address moiety required for kappa-antagonist activity. J Med Chem 1993;36(16):2412–5.
32. Sharma SK, Jones RM, Metzger TG, Ferguson DM, Portoghese PS. Transformation of a kappa-opioid receptor antagonist to a kappa-agonist by transfer of a guanidinium group from the 5′- to 6′-position of naltrindole. J Med Chem 2001;44(13):2073–9.
33. Stevens WC, Jr., Jones RM, Subramanian G, Metzger TG, Ferguson DM, Portoghese PS. Potent and selective indolomorphinan antagonists of the kappa-opioid receptor. J Med Chem 2000;43(14):2759–69.
34. Black SL, Chauvignac C, Grundt P, et al. Guanidino N-substituted and N,N-disubstituted derivatives of the kappa-opioid antagonist GNTI. J Med Chem 2003;46(25):5505–11.
35. Thomas JB, Atkinson RN, Vinson NA, et al. Identification of (3*R*)-7-hydroxy-*N*-((1*S*)-1-[[(3*R*,4*R*)-4-(3-hydroxyphenyl)-3,4-dimethyl-1-piperidinyl]methyl]-2-methylpropyl)-1,2,3,4-tetrahydro-3-isoquinolinecarboxamide as a novel potent and selective opioid kappa receptor antagonist. J Med Chem 2003;46(14):3127–37.
36. Thomas JB, Atkinson RN, Namdev N, et al. Discovery of an opioid kappa receptor selective pure antagonist from a library of N-substituted 4 β-methyl-5-(3-hydroxyphenyl)morphans. J Med Chem 2002;45(16):3524–30.
37. Metcalf MD, Coop A. Kappa opioid antagonists: past successes and future prospects. AAPS J 2005;7(3):E704–22.
38. Takemori AE, Portoghese PS. Selective naltrexone-derived opioid receptor antagonists. Annu Rev Pharmacol Toxicol 1992;32:239–69.
39. Portoghese PS. From models to molecules: opioid receptor dimers, bivalent ligands, and selective opioid receptor probes. J Med Chem 2001;44(14):2259–69.
40. Jones RM, Hjorth SA, Schwartz TW, Portoghese PS. Mutational evidence for a common kappa antagonist binding pocket in the wild-type kappa and mutant mu[K303E] opioid receptors. J Med Chem 1998;41(25):4911–4.
41. Larson DL, Jones RM, Hjorth SA, Schwartz TW, Portoghese PS. Binding of norbinaltorphimine (norBNI) congeners to wild-type and mutant mu and kappa opioid receptors: molecular recognition loci for the pharmacophore and address components of kappa antagonists. J Med Chem 2000;43(8):1573–6.
42. Metzger TG, Paterlini MG, Ferguson DM, Portoghese PS. Investigation of the selectivity of oxymorphone- and naltrexone-derived ligands via site-directed mutagenesis of opioid receptors: exploring the "address" recognition locus. J Med Chem 2001;44(6):857–62.
43. Jales AR, Husbands SM, Lewis JW. Selective kappa-opioid antagonists related to naltrindole. Effect of side-chain spacer in the 5′-amidinoalkyl series. Bioorg Med Chem Lett 2000;10(20):2259–61.
44. Black SL, Jales AR, Brandt W, Lewis JW, Husbands SM. The role of the side chain in determining relative delta- and kappa-affinity in C5′-substituted analogues of naltrindole. J Med Chem 2003;46(2):314–7.
45. Grundt P, Jales AR, Traynor JR, Lewis JW, Husbands SM. 14-amino, 14-alkylamino, and 14-acylamino analogs of oxymorphindole. Differential effects on opioid receptor binding and functional profiles. J Med Chem 2003;46(8):1563–6.

46. RM, Portoghese PS. 5′-Guanidinonaltrindole, a highly selective and potent kappa-opioid receptor antagonist. Eur J Pharmacol 2000;396(1):49–52.
47. Portoghese PS, Larson DL, Sayre LM, et al. Opioid agonist and antagonist bivalent ligands. The relationship between spacer length and selectivity at multiple opioid receptors. J Med Chem 1986;29(10):1855–61.
48. Chavkin C, Sud S, Jin W, et al. Salvinorin A, an active component of the hallucinogenic sage salvia divinorum is a highly efficacious kappa-opioid receptor agonist: structural and functional considerations. J Pharmacol Exp Ther 2004;308(3):1197–203.
49. Schwyzer R. ACTH: a short introductory review. Ann N Y Acad Sci 1977;297:3–26.
50. Olmsted SL, Takemori AE, Portoghese PS. A remarkable change of opioid receptor selectivity on the attachment of a peptidomimetic kappa address element to the delta antagonist, natrindole: 5′-[N2-alkylamidino)methyl]naltrindole derivatives as a novel class of kappa opioid receptor antagonists. J Med Chem 1993;36(1):179–80.
51. Waldhoer M, Fong J, Jones RM, et al. A heterodimer-selective agonist shows in vivo relevance of G protein-coupled receptor dimers. Proc Natl Acad Sci USA 2005;102(25):9050–5.
52. Tanaka H, Moriwaki M, Takahashi T. Efficient solid-phase synthesis of symmetric norbinaltorphimine derivatives. Org Lett 2003;5(21):3807–9.
53. Hjorth SA, Thirstrup K, Grandy DK, Schwartz TW. Analysis of selective binding epitopes for the kappa-opioid receptor antagonist nor-binaltorphimine. Mol Pharmacol 1995;47(6):1089–94.
54. Ferguson DM, Kramer S, Metzger TG, Law PY, Portoghese PS. Isosteric replacement of acidic with neutral residues in extracellular loop-2 of the kappa-opioid receptor does not affect dynorphin A(1–13) affinity and function. J Med Chem 2000;43(7):1251–2.
55. Zimmerman DM, Nickander R, Horng JS, Wong DT. New structural concepts for narcotic antagonists defined in a 4-phenylpiperidine series. Nature 1978;275(5678):332–4.
56. Mitch CH, Leander JD, Mendelsohn LG, et al. 3,4-Dimethyl-4-(3-hydroxyphenyl)piperidines: opioid antagonists with potent anorectant activity. J Med Chem 1993;36(20):2842–50.
57. Zimmerman DM, Leander JD, Cantrell BE, et al. Structure-activity relationships of *trans*-3,4-dimethyl-4-(3-hydroxyphenyl)piperidine antagonists for mu- and kappa-opioid receptors. J Med Chem 1993;36(20):2833–41.
58. Thomas JB, Mascarella SW, Rothman RB, et al. Investigation of the N-substituent conformation governing potency and mu receptor subtype-selectivity in (+)-(3*R*, 4*R*)-dimethyl-4-(3-hydroxyphenyl)piperidine opioid antagonists. J Med Chem 1998;41(11):1980–90.
59. Thomas JB, Fall MJ, Cooper JB, et al. Identification of an opioid kappa receptor subtype-selective N-substituent for (+)-(3*R*,4*R*)-dimethyl-4-(3-hydroxyphenyl)piperidine. J Med Chem 1998;41(26):5188–97.
60. Thomas JB, Zheng X, Mascarella SW, et al. N-Substituted 9β-methyl-5-(3-hydroxyphenyl) morphans are opioid receptor pure antagonists. J Med Chem 1998;41(21):4143–9.
61. Portoghese PS. A new concept on the mode of interaction of narcotic analgesics with receptors. J Med Chem 1965;8(5):609–16.
62. Portoghese PS, Alreja BD, Larson DL. Allylprodine analogues as receptor probes. Evidence that phenolic and nonphenolic ligands interact with different subsites on identical opioid receptors. J Med Chem 1981;24(7):782–7.
63. Butelman ER, Negus SS, Ai Y, de Costa BR, Woods JH. Kappa opioid antagonist effects of systemically administered nor-binaltorphimine in a thermal antinociception assay in rhesus monkeys. J Pharmacol Exp Ther 1993;267(3):1269–76.
64. Negus SS, Mello NK, Linsenmayer DC, Jones R, Portoghese PS. Kappa opioid antagonist effects of the novel kappa antagonist 5′-guanidinonaltrindole (GNTI) in an assay of schedule-controlled behavior in rhesus monkeys. Psychopharmacology 2002;163(3–4):412–9.
65. Carroll I, Thomas JB, Dykstra LA, et al. Pharmacological properties of JDTic: a novel kappa-opioid receptor antagonist. Eur J Pharmacol 2004;501(1–3):111–9.
66. Beardsley PM, Howard JL, Shelton KL, Carroll FI. Differential effects of the novel kappa opioid receptor antagonist, JDTic, on reinstatement of cocaine-seeking induced by footshock stressors vs cocaine primes and its antidepressant-like effects in rats. Psychopharmacology (Berl) 2005;183(1):118–26.

67. Chang AC, Takemori AE, Ojala WH, Gleason WB, Portoghese PS. Kappa opioid receptor selective affinity labels: electrophilic benzeneacetamides as kappa-selective opioid antagonists. J Med Chem 1994;37(26):4490–8.
68. Horan P, Taylor J, Yamamura HI, Porreca F. Extremely long-lasting antagonistic actions of nor-binaltorphimine (nor-BNI) in the mouse tail-flick test. J Pharmacol Exp Ther 1992;260(3): 1237–43.
69. Fantegrossi WE, Kugle KM, Valdes LJ, 3rd, Koreeda M, Woods JH. Kappa-opioid receptor-mediated effects of the plant-derived hallucinogen, salvinorin A, on inverted screen performance in the mouse. Behav Pharmacol 2005;16(8):627–33.
70. Cohen BM, Tsuneizumi T, Baldessarini RJ, Campbell A, Babb SM. Differences between antipsychotic drugs in persistence of brain levels and behavioral effects. Psychopharmacology (Berl) 1992;108(3):338–44.
71. Endoh T, Matsuura H, Tanaka C, Nagase H. Nor-binaltorphimine: a potent and selective kappa-opioid receptor antagonist with long-lasting activity in vivo. Arch Int Pharmacodyn Ther 1992;316:30–42.
72. Broadbear JH, Negus SS, Butelman ER, de Costa BR, Woods JH. Differential effects of systemically administered nor-binaltorphimine (nor-BNI) on kappa-opioid agonists in the mouse writhing assay. Psychopharmacology (Berl) 1994;115(3):311–9.
73. Grundt P, Williams IA, Lewis JW, Husbands SM. Identification of a new scaffold for opioid receptor antagonism based on the 2-amino-1,1-dimethyl-7-hydroxytetralin pharmacophore. J Med Chem 2004;47(21):5069–75.
74. Ananthan S, Kezar HSIII, Saini SK, et al. Synthesis, opioid receptor binding, and functional activity of 5′-substituted 17-cyclopropylmethylpyrido[2′,3′:6,7]morphinans. Bioorg Med Chem Lett 2003;13(3):529–32.
75. Beguin C, Richards MR, Wang Y, et al. Synthesis and in vitro pharmacological evaluation of salvinorin A analogues modified at C(2). Bioorg Med Chem Lett 2005;15(11):2761–5.
76. Beguin C, Richards MR, Li JG, et al. Synthesis and in vitro evaluation of salvinorin A analogues: effect of configuration at C(2) and substitution at C(18). Bioorg Med Chem Lett 2006;16(17):4679–85.

Chapter 7
The Chemistry and Pharmacology of Delta Opioid Antagonists

Beatriz Fioravanti and Todd W. Vanderah

Abstract The cloning of the δ-opioid receptor prompted significant chemical and pharmacological efforts toward the discovery of potent and selective antagonists for this G protein-coupled receptor. The field has advanced with the synthesis of peptide and nonpeptide compounds characterized by in vitro and in vivo assays, which have aided in the understanding of the various physiological roles of the δ-receptor. This chapter provides a review of the development of classical and new δ-opioid receptor antagonists and briefly comments on therapeutic indications for this class of drugs.

Keywords: ICI 174,864; Naltrindole; TIPP; DALCE; 5′-Isothiocyanate; Naltriben; BNTX

7.1 Introduction

Antagonists are useful tools in the investigation of receptor function at both the cellular and the whole animal level. This chapter provides a historical review of the development of δ-opioid receptor (DOR) antagonists and briefly comments on therapeutic indications for this class of drugs. The reader is directed to specific chapters in this book, as well as the primary scientific literature, for more detailed discussion of the potential clinical applications of DOR antagonists and the progress being made in their development.

The idea that opioid analgesics such as morphine acted on specific receptor sites was suggested several decades ago (1–3). The synthesis of many analogs of naturally occurring opiates, as well as unrelated molecular entities that displayed opioid-like activity, was instrumental in the characterization of opioid receptors. The use of various opioid

B. Fioravanti and T.W. Vanderah (✉)
Department of Pharmacology and Anesthesiology,
College of Medicine at the University of Arizona, 1501 N. Campbell Ave,
LSN 567, Tucson, AZ 85724
e-mail: vanderah@email.arizona.edu

agonists and antagonists in classical pharmacological assays, as well as the development of novel techniques, such as radioligand binding assays, provided evidence for at least three distinct types of opioid receptors (4, 5). These receptors were initially named after the proposed prototypic agonists: μ (morphine), κ (ketocyclazine), and σ (SKF-1044) (3). The latter was subsequently identified as a nonopioid receptor (6).

Following the discovery of endogenous opioid peptides (e.g., enkephalins, endorphins, and dynorphins), the DOR was identified by the high potency of enkephalins and β-endorphin in the isolated mouse vas deferens (MVD) tissue compared to morphine. The greater potency of morphine in the guinea pig ileum (GPI) assay and of enkephalins in the MVD suggested that morphine and enkephalins might act on different populations of opioid receptors (7). It is now known that the MVD has all three of the major opioid receptor types (μ, δ, and κ) whereas the GPI lacks functional DORs (8). Thus, selective δ-opioid agonists are always more potent in MVD preparation compared to the GPI assay for this reason.

In 1992, the mouse DOR was cloned from NG-108 cell line by two independent laboratories (9–11). The cloned receptor was designated as DOR. Subsequently, the other two major types of opioid receptors were cloned from human and various rodent species (12). Following the determination of the nucleotide sequences of the three primary opioid receptors (DOR, MOR, and KOR), a number of molecular approaches were employed to study receptor pharmacology. Using site-directed mutagenesis and chimeric, truncated or nonfunctional mutant receptors, the amino acid residues, and protein domains responsible for opioid ligand binding, signal transduction activation, and receptor regulation were investigated. These same molecular techniques were also instrumental in the synthesis and characterization of novel opioid ligands, which display greater subtype selectivity, have more diverse intrinsic efficacies (e.g., inverse agonists, neutral antagonists, or partial agonists), or that demonstrate unique interactions with homo- and heterodimers.

7.2 Classical δ-Opioid Antagonists

7.2.1 N,N-diallyl-Tyr-Aib-Aib-Phe-Leu-OH

A number of δ-selective antagonists have been obtained through diallylation of the N-terminal amino group of enkephalin peptides. This series of compounds has been reviewed previously (13). In 1984, Cotton and colleagues reported on a putative δ-antagonist, *N,N*-diallyl-Tyr-Aib-Aib-Phe-Leu-OH (ICI 174,864) (Aib, α-amino isobutyric acid), an enkephalin analog with restricted conformation. The compound displayed moderate affinity for δ-receptors (K_i^{δ} = 193 nM) and modest selectivity for δ-receptors over μ-receptors (K_i^{μ}/K_i^{δ} = 128) in receptor binding assays (14, 15). The compound was also a moderately potent δ-antagonist in the MVD assay (K_e = 36.4 nM). ICI 174,864 became a useful tool in identifying DOR-mediated effects both in vitro and in vivo. In addition, the compound proved valuable in first demonstrating the concept of basal or constitutive signaling for G protein-coupled receptors. Costa and Herz (16) identified ICI 174,864 as an inverse-agonist at the DOR in NG108-15 neuroblastoma-glioma cells. The negative intrinsic activity of ICI 174,864 was demonstrated by the inhibition of GTPase basal activity present in these cells. Importantly, the inverse agonist effects of ICI 174,864 were blocked by the neutral μ-/κ-antagonist (–)-(1R,5R,9R)-5,9-Diethyl-2-3(-furylmethyl)-2′-hydroxy-6,7-benzomorphan (MR2266) (16).

7.2.2 *Naltrindole*

The first example of a selective nonpeptidic δ-opioid antagonist was presented by Portoghese's group in 1988 (17). The rationale for design of this compound, named 17-cyclopropylmethyl-6,7-dehydro-4,5α-epoxy-3,14-dihydroxy-6,7,2′,3′-indolomorphinan (naltrindole or NTI), was based on the message–address concept. According to this theory, one portion of the ligand mediates signal transduction (message) while another ligand site determines selectivity (address) toward δ-, κ-, or μ-opioid receptors. The use of this approach to develop δ- and κ-selective antagonists has been reviewed previously (18–21). NTI was the most potent member of the series, with a calculated K_e value of 0.1 nM in the MVD using the δ-agonist [D-Ala^2, D-Leu^5]enkephalin (DADLE). In contrast, ICI 174,864 is over 500-times less potent than NTI (19). In terms of binding, NTI (K_i^{δ} = 0.031 nM) displayed an ~1,000-fold greater affinity compared to ICI 174,864. NTI, similarly to ICI 174,864, showed moderate selectivity for δ- over μ-opioid receptor (K_i^{μ}/K_i^{δ} = 127) (17–19).

7.2.3 *H-Tyr-Tic-Phe-Phe-OH*

The results of structure–activity relationship (SAR) studies on opioid peptides led to the discovery of a new class of δ-opioid antagonists known as TIP(P) peptides. The two prototype peptides, TIPP (H-Tyr-Tic-Phe-Phe-OH) and TIP (H-Tyr-Tic-Phe-OH), which contain an L-1,2,3,4-tetrahydroisoquinoline-3-carboxylic acid (Tic) residue in the position 2, displayed potent δ-antagonist activity and good δ-receptor selectivity (Table 7.1). Although as a δ-antagonist TIPP is more potent than ICI 174,864 in vitro and more δ-selective than either ICI 174,864 or NTI, this compound was shown to undergo spontaneous cleavage of the Tic-Phe peptide bond in DMSO and MeOH. Substituting the Tic-Phe bond by a reduced peptide bond originated analogs such as H-Tyr-TicΨ[CH_2NH]Phe-Phe-OH (TIPP[Ψ]) and H-Tyr-TicΨ[CH_2NH]Phe-OH (TIP[Ψ]), which were found to be highly stable against chemical and enzymatic degradation. These compounds also presented high selectivity and antagonist activity to the DOR (26).

Following the development of the parent TIP(P) peptides, a large number of highly potent and δ-opioid selective antagonists were synthesized as a result of extensive

Table 7.1 Classical δ-opioid antagonists: K_e values and binding affinities

		Receptor binding assays			
Compound	MVD K_e [nM][a]	K_i^δ [nM][b]	K_i^μ [nM][c]	K_i^μ/K_i^δ	References
ICI 174,864	36.4	193	24700	128	(14) (15)
	68.0	–	–	–	(17)
Naltrindole (NTI)	0.130	0.031	3.8	127	(17, 19)
	0.270				(17)
	0.636	0.687	12.2	17.8	(22, 23)
TIPP	4.80	1.22	1,720	1,410	(23)
TIP	16.1	9.07	1,280	141	(23)
BNTX	5.3	0.1	13.3	–	(24)
	2.0	10.8	–	–	(24)
Naltriben (NTB)	0.27	0.013	18.8	1,446	(25)
[D-Ala^2, Leu^5, Cys^6] enkephalin (DALCE)					
5′ Isothiocyanate (5′NTII)					

Only IC_{50} values or ratios were found for DALCE and 5′NTII

[a]Mouse vas deferens (MVD) bioassay was used to evaluate the effect of the δ-antagonists in the presence of δ-agonists (DADLE, DSLET, or DPDPE depending on the reference)

[b]Displacement of DADLE, DSLET, or DPDPE from rat or guinea pig brain membranes (depending on the reference)

[c]Displacement of DAMGO from rat or guinea pig brain membranes (depending on the reference)

SAR studies. Schiller and colleagues (22) have provided a comprehensive review on these series. Toth et al. (27) reported on several analogues in which Tyr[1] was replaced by 2′,6′-dimethyltyrosine (Dmt) and Phe[3] by β-methylcyclohexylalanine (β-MeCha). One compound in particular showed subnanomolar δ-antagonist potency ($K_i = 0.48$ nM) and twofold higher selectivity for DOR than the parent TIPP ($K_i^\mu/K_i^\delta = 2800$). Many of the compounds belonging to the TIPP series synthesized thus far present mixed partial μ-agonist/δ-antagonist properties (22, 27). The potential clinical application of these bifunctional compounds is discussed in Chap. 18 of this book. Although these compounds represent important pharmacological tools in opioid research, their potential liability to enzymatic cleavage and restricted blood–brain barrier (BBB) access suggest limited therapeutic applications for these series of antagonists.

More recently, Martin et al. (28, 29) have reported that both TIP(P) and TIP[Ψ] can act as agonists or inverse agonists in cellular models. The inhibition of adenylyl cyclase by TIP(P) and TIP[Ψ], an effect normally demonstrated by agonists, was selective for DOR, concentration-dependent, pertussis-toxin sensitive, and antagonized by the addition of δ-antagonists such as naltriben, naloxone, and ICI 174,864 (28). The same researchers reported in 2002 that TIP(P) exhibited properties of antagonist, agonist, or inverse agonist depending on the step in the signal transduction cascade examined and the assay conditions employed (29).

7.2.4 [D-Ala^2, Leu^5, Cys^6]enkephalin and [D-Ala^2, Leu^5, Ser^6]enkephalin

Bowen et al. (30), in 1987, characterized the peptide [D-Ala^2, Leu^5, Cys^6]enkephalin (DALCE) as a nonequilibrium DOR antagonist. DALCE was reported to bind covalently to DOR by a thiol-disulfide exchange mechanism. Like other enkephalin analogues, DALCE incorporates a D-alanine for aminopeptidase resistance but is unique in that it contains a single cysteine at the C-terminus (30). In the radioligand binding assay, the peptide DALCE showed high affinity to δ-opioid receptor (IC_{50} = 4 nM), moderate affinity to μ-opioid receptor (IC_{50} = 55 nM), and negligible affinity to κ-opioid receptors (KORs) (IC_{50} > 10,000 nM) (30). The noncompetitive (covalent) nature of this peptide was demonstrated by the failure of NaCl and Gpp(NH)p to induce recovery of DOR sites after incubation of rat brain membranes with DALCE (30). The compound also produced long-lasting antagonism in vivo (described below).

Studies by Calcagnetti et al. (31) provided characterization of DALCE in vivo. The results indicated that DALCE produced short-term antinociception at the μ- and δ-receptor following i.c.v. administration in rats; additionally, DALCE acted as a long-lasting and selective δ-opioid antagonist, reversing the analgesia produced by [D-Pen^2, D-Pen^5]enkephalin (DPDPE), but not that by [D-Ala^2, *N*-Me-Phe^4, Gly^5-ol]enkephalin (DAMGO) or trans-3,4-dichloro-*N*-methyl-*N*-[2-(1-pyrrolidinyl)cyclohexyl] benzene-acetamide methane sulfonate (U50488H). Further characterization of DALCE's direct agonist and antagonist properties was reported by Qi et al. (32).

With the development of DALCE, and a few other selective δ-antagonists as described below, additional evidence was collected in vivo to suggest the existence of two functional types of DORs. For example, Jiang and colleagues (33) showed that pretreatment with DALCE produced a dose- and time-related antagonism of the antinociceptive effects of DPDPE (δ_1-agonist), but not of those of deltorphin II (δ_2-agonist) or of μ-agonists.

DALCE has also been a useful tool in studies that aimed the characterization of the proposed types of functional μ–δ complex receptors known as δ_{ncx} and δ_{cx} (34). When a sub-antinociceptive dose of DALCE was coadministered i.c.v. with graded doses of morphine, DALCE did not produce any change in morphine antinociceptive potency or efficacy, which suggests that DALCE binds to the δ_{ncx} site (32). This study also showed that pretreatment of mice with DALCE, at doses that directly antagonized the antinociceptive actions of DPDPE and DALCE, did not prevent the positive modulation of morphine antinociception produced by DPDPE or the negative modulation produced by [Met^5]enkephalin, further supporting a lack of interaction with the putative δ_{cx} receptor (32).

In 1991, the structural analogue of DALCE, [D-Ala^2, Leu^5, Ser^6]enkephalin (DALES), in which serine is substituted for cysteine in position 6, was reported by Mattia et al. The replacement of serine for cysteine at the C-terminus prevented DALES from exhibiting the irreversible profile associated with DALCE. DALES, like DALCE, did not appear to interact with δ_{cx} (35).

7.2.5 5′-Isothiocyanate

The design of 5′-isothiocyanate (5′-NTII), the first nonpeptide δ-opioid antagonist characterized as possessing noncompetitive/nonequilibrium receptor interactions, was based on the attachment of isothiocyanate group to NTI (36). 5′-NTII antagonized DPDPE and DADLE in the MVD bioassay, demonstrated by IC_{50} ratios higher than 1.0. The irreversible antagonism of 5′-NTII was supported by the fact that there were no significant differences between pre- and postwash IC_{50} ratios. When evaluated for its effect in mice, the i.c.v. administration of 5′-NTII produced full blockade of the antinociceptive effects of Tyr-D-Ser-Gly-Phe-Leu-Thr (DSLET) (ED_{50} ratio 52.1), but not morphine or U50488H in the abdominal stretch assay. The time course for antagonism activity indicated that ED_{50} ratio for DSLET peaked at 24 h (52.1) and declined to an ED_{50} ratio of 10 at 48 h.

5′-NTII has been an important compound in differentiating between δ_1- and δ_2-mediates effects. This noncompetitive antagonist was shown to selectively block the antinociceptive effects of deltorphin II (δ_2-agonist), but not those of DPDPE (δ_1-agonist) or of μ- and κ-agonists in mice (33, 37). The DOR antagonists 5′NTII and DALCE were used by Vanderah and colleagues (37) to further investigate the selectivity of DPDPE and deltorphin II for the different DOR subtypes in vivo. In mice pretreated with DALCE, the δ-agonist DPDPE antagonized the antinociceptive effect of deltorphin. However, in 5′NTII pretreated mice, deltorphin had no effect on DPDPE-induced antinociception, suggesting that DPDPE has actions at both δ_1 and δ_2 receptors.

7.2.6 Naltriben

The benzofuran analogue of NTI, Naltriben (NTB), was first reported in 1991 (25, 38). When tested in the MVD and the GPI smooth muscle preparations, NTB robustly antagonized DADLE (K_e = 0.27 nM), but not morphine (K_e = 27 nM) or ethylketazocine (EK) (K_e = 48 nM). In the binding studies employing guinea pig brain membranes, NTB showed high δ-opioid affinity (K_i = 0.013 nM) determined against [^{3}H]DADLE (25).

NTB was further evaluated in vivo for its antagonism of the antinociceptive effect of the δ-receptor agonists DPDPE (δ_1-agonist), DSLET (δ_2-agonist) and DADLE (δ_1-agonist) (38). NTB, given s.c. or i.c.v., significantly increased the antinociceptive ED_{50} of i.c.v. DSLET (ED_{50} ratios 3.6 and 6.7, respectively), however, no antagonism of i.c.v. DPDPE (ED_{50} ratio 1.4) or DADLE (ED_{50} ratios 1.4 and 1.2, respectively) by NTB was observed. Moreover, the potency of NTB was evaluated after i.t. administration of the δ-agonists. NTB, when given s.c. or i.t., efficiently antagonized i.t. DSLET (ED_{50} ratios 12.5 and 7.2, respectively), but not i.t. DPDPE (ED_{50} ratios 1.0 and 0.8, respectively) or DADLE (ED_{50} ratios 0.8 and 1.0, respectively) (38).

Although NTB continues to be an important antagonist to characterize δ_2-mediated effects in vivo, in certain doses this compound can also act as agonist and antagonist at other opioid receptors. At doses higher than those selective for δ_2-selective blockade, NTB produced antinociception (effect typically produced by δ-agonists) following injection i.c.v. or in the ventromedial medulla (VMM) in rats (20, 39). NTB (3 mg/kg, s.c.) induced antinociception, which was blocked by pretreatment with norbinaltorphimine (norBNI), indicating that NTB can act as a κ-agonist (40).

Kim et al.(41), in 2001, examined the effects of NTB on the specific binding of radiolabeled compounds for μ- ([^{3}H]DAMGO) and κ_2- ([^{3}H]diprenorphine) opioid receptors in rat cerebral cortex slices. NTB inhibited the specific binding of [^{3}H]DAMGO and [^{3}H]diprenorphine with K_i values of 19.79 ± 1.12 and 82.75 ± 6.32 nM, respectively (41).

7.2.7 7-Benzylidenenaltrexone

Following the reports that suggested the existence of different subtypes of DORs, and the characterization of DALCE as δ_1-antagonist (33), and 5′-NTII (36) and NTB (25) as δ_2-antagonists, Portoghese's group developed an analogue of naltrexone, 7-benzylidenenaltrexone (BNTX). BNTX displayed high selectivity for δ_1-sites on guinea pig brain membranes (24). When administered i.c.v. in mice, BNTX significantly antagonized DPDPE (ED_{50} ratio 7.2) actions in the tail flick assay, but did not change the ED_{50} values for DSLET, morphine, or U50488H. In another study by the same group (42), BNTX administered s.c. or i.t. increased the antinociceptive ED_{50} value of DPDPE (ED_{50} ratios of 5.9 and 4.0, respectively); however, no significant antagonism of deltorphin II was observed for BNTX (ED_{50} ratio 1.2). In other reports, BNTX did not seem to be any more selective to human δ- over μ-opioid receptors (43, 44).

7.3 New δ-Opioid Antagonists

7.3.1 [(±)-KF4]

Carroll and colleagues (45) have recently reported on the synthesis of a potent and selective δ-opioid antagonist that belongs to the 5-phenylmorphan class of opioids. The compound, (+)-5-(3-hydroxyphenyl)-4-methyl-2-(3-phenylpropyl)-2-azabicyclo-[3.3.1]-non-7-yl-(1-phenyl-1-cyclopentane)carboxamide or (+)-KF4, was evaluated along with the reference δ-antagonists NTI and ICI 174,864. In the [^{35}S]GTPγS functional assay, (+)-KF4 showed K_e value of 0.15 nM against DPDPE, being more potent than ICI 174,864 (K_e = 7.85 nM) and as potent as NTI (K_e = 0.21 nM). In the competition binding assays, the K_i value of (+)-KF4 was 0.96 nM, indicating higher affinity for the δ-receptor than ICI 174,864 (K_i = 19.1 nM), however, less than NTI (K_i = 0.07 nM). There was additional evidence presented indicating that (+)-KF4 may act as an inverse agonist at DOR under some conditions (IC_{50} = 1.8 nM), being more potent than ICI 174,864 (IC_{50} = 83 nM) (45). Additional analogs containing the (+)-phenylmorphan scaffold have been synthesized revealing one compound, termed delmorphan-A, which showed picomolar inhibitory potency (K_e = 0.1 nM) and higher selectivity for DOR (K_i^{μ}/K_i^{δ} = 103) when compared to the parent compound (+)-KF4 (K_i^{μ}/K_i^{δ} = 58) (46). Every analogue of this series was found to have potent negative intrinsic activity, therefore suggesting that these compounds may be valuable tools for the elucidation of DOR's constitutive activity.

7.3.2 Fluorescent δ-Antagonists

Fluorescent opioid ligands can be important probes in the study of opioid receptor distribution, signal transduction, and internalization. Kshirsagar and colleagues (47) designed and synthesized a nonpeptide fluorescent δ-antagonist, NTI4F, which showed high potency (IC_{50} ratio = 31.3 ± 7.6; K_e = 3.30 nM) in the MVD assay against the agonist DADLE and no significant antagonist activity in the GPI test at μ- or κ-receptors. In the binding assay, NTI4F showed K_i value of 1.1 nM, indicating a loss of affinity for the δ-receptor when compared to NTI. Confocal microscopy studies performed in Madin-Darby canine kidney (MDCK) cells transfected with the DOR revealed that NTI4F successfully bound to the δ-receptor and, unlike the δ-agonist DADLE, the antagonist NTI4F did not induce receptor internalization.

In 2004, a fluorescent tripeptide probe derived by coupling fluorescein to the C-terminus of H-Dmt-Tic-Glu-NH_2, which evolved from the TIPP series, was reported by Balboni and colleagues (48). Characterized in the MVD assay as an irreversible δ-receptor antagonist, this compound, H-Dmt-Tic-Glu-NH-(CH_2)5-NH-(C = S)-NH-fluorescein, showed very high binding affinity (K_i = 0.0035 nM) and selectivity (K_i^{μ}/K_i^{δ} = 4,370) for the δ-receptor. Moreover, following incubation of the fluorescent tripeptide with NG108-15 cells, which naturally express DOR, fluorescent δ-receptor sites were visualized by a confocal scanning laser microscope. Preincubation with NTI eliminated the fluorescence bound to DORs.

Fluorescent analogues of the peptide δ-antagonists TIPP and TIP have also been reported (49). 6-Dimethyl-amino-2-acyl-naphthalene (DAN) constitutes a fluorophore that has been incorporated into the side chain of L-alanine, resulting in the fluorescent amino acid β-(6′dimethyl-amino-2′-naphthoyl)alanine (Aladan [Ald]) (50). In the report published by Chen and coworkers, analogues of the peptide δ-antagonists TIPP and TIP containing Ald in the place of Phe^3 were evaluated. In comparison with the TIPP parent peptide (K_e = 4.8 nM), the Ald^3-analogue, H-Tyr-Tic-Ald-Phe-OH, showed twice as higher potency (K_e = 2.03 nM) in the MVD assay, and about half the δ-receptor affinity (K_i = 2.56 nM) in the binding assays. The Ald^3-tripeptide showed similar antagonist potency (K_e = 24.3 nM) and δ-receptor affinity

(K_i = 10.8 nM) to the parent compound TIP. Although fluorescence parameters and molecular mechanics for these analogues were determined, these compounds have not yet been employed in any cellular or tissue study.

7.4 Clinical Applications of δ-Antagonists

As described in various chapters throughout this book, there continues to be interest in developing antagonists/inverse agonists for the DOR not just as tools for elucidating the role of the DOR in physiology/pathology but also as pharmacological treatments for prevention and treatment of disease. Several promising indications are briefly discussed below.

7.4.1 Prevention of Morphine-Induced Antinociceptive Tolerance

Opioids still remain the standard analgesic for the treatment of moderate-to-severe pain. The clinical use of this class of compounds is limited by the severe side effects that include the development of tolerance and physical dependence, respiratory depression, and constipation. Preclinical and clinical data indicate that most of these effects are mediated primarily through the μ-opioid receptor (MOR) (51). For example, both analgesia and tolerance to morphine are abolished in MOR knockout mice, suggesting a major role of the μ-receptor in opioid tolerance (52).

With the goal of limiting the side effects from chronic treatment with opioids, an array of strategies has been attempted. The large body of evidence showing the critical role of DORs in antinociceptive tolerance provides a rationale for the development of dual functional μ-agonist/δ-antagonist compounds. This approach and the specific compounds that display the μ-agonist/δ-antagonist profile are discussed in detail in Chap. 18 of this book.

7.4.2 Antitussive Properties

In a published review, Kamei (53) reports on the relative contributions of μ-, δ-, and κ-opioid receptors to the antitussive activity of opioid receptors, revealing that δ-antagonists produce a potent antitussive effect in animals exposed to a nebulized solution of capsaicin. Systemic administration of NTI in mice, rats, and guinea pigs dose-dependently reduced the number of coughs induced by capsaicin (53). NTI produced a maximum effect and duration of the antitussive action greater than or similar to those produced by morphine.

Also BNTX (δ_1-antagonist) and NTB (δ_2-antagonist) dose-dependently reduced the number of coughs in mice. The effect of BNTX was attenuated by pretreatment with DPDPE. However, deltorphin II, β-funaltrexamine (μ-antagonist), or norBNI (κ-antagonist) showed no effect on the antitussive action of BNTX, which strongly suggests that the antitussive effect of BNTX is mediated by δ_1-opioid receptors. The antitussive effect of NTB, surprisingly, was not affected by pretreatment with DPDPE, deltorphin II, or β-funaltrexamine. Unlike BNTX, norBNI significantly reduced the antitussive effect of NTB, which suggests that the antitussive effect of NTB is mediated through KORs.

7.4.3 Ethanol Addiction

Alcohol abuse and dependence are major health concerns worldwide. In recent years, the urge to understand the neurobiological mechanisms of alcoholism provided a large body of evidence that alcohol affects a variety of neurotransmitters such as dopamine, glutamate, gamma-aminobutyric acid (GABA), β-endorphin, serotonin, cannabinoids, and neuropeptides (54). The rewarding (reinforcing) effects of ethanol are thought to originate from the increase in synaptic dopamine accumulation in the ventral tegmental area (VTA), particularly in the nucleus accumbens (NAC) (55). Since endogenous opioid systems also modulate the mesolimbic dopamine system (56–58), and ethanol can stimulate opioid receptors by several direct and indirect mechanisms (59, 60), it has been suggested that opioid systems mediate at least in part the rewarding properties of ethanol (61, 62).

Reid (Chap. 18) provides behavioral and pharmacological data suggesting a link between the endogenous opioid system and the ethanol consumption, as well as on the use of μ-opioid receptor antagonists (e.g., naloxone and naltrexone). Here, we focus on evidence for the involvement of the DOR and δ-antagonists as potential therapeutic agents in the treatment of alcohol abuse and alcoholism.

The search for the mechanisms through which ethanol interacts with opioid systems has provided evidence that ethanol alters opioid peptide synthesis and secretion. Acute ethanol administration increases β-endorphin gene expression and release in various brain areas (63–66). On the contrary, prolonged ethanol administration generally induces a decrease in endogenous opioid activity (67–69). Ethanol-induced changes on opioid receptors appear to vary depending on the brain region and lineage of the animals used (70). Furthermore, several studies with naturally occurring, as well as selective-bred, rodent lines that are ethanol preferring or nonpreferring, yielded data suggesting a relationship between endorphin and ethanol self-administration (64, 71–74). Variations in μ-, δ-, and κ-opioid receptors expression have also been described in ethanol-preferring and ethanol-avoiding animals (75–77). For a complete review, see Oswald and Wand (78).

The nonselective opioid antagonists naloxone, naltrexone, and nalmefene have been extensively shown to decrease alcohol intake under a variety of experimental conditions in rodents and monkeys (Reid, Chap. 18) (79–81). Following the findings of these preclinical studies, clinical trials were conducted to investigate the efficacy of nonselective opioid antagonists on alcohol drinking behavior in detoxified outpatient alcoholics. The results obtained by Volpicelli (82, 83) and O'Malley (84, 85) indicated that subjects receiving naltrexone had decreased mean number of drinking days, decreased frequency of relapse, decrease subjective craving for alcohol, and a decrease in alcohol-induced "high." In 1995, naltrexone was approved by the Food and Drug administration (FDA) for the treatment of ethanol dependence. Subsequent studies, however, indicated that naltrexone was less effective for treating alcohol dependence and had more adverse effects than was initially suggested (86–91).

Although the importance of MOR in reinforcing effects of alcohol is well established (72, 92, 93), studies employing selective δ-opioid antagonists to investigate the role of the DOR in ethanol consumption have produced divergent findings. Froehlich and colleagues (94) reported that ICI 174,864, a selective δ-opioid antagonist, decreased alcohol consumption in a dose-dependent manner. In this study, systemically administered ICI 174,864 appeared to be more potent than and just as efficacious as naloxone on decreasing voluntary ethanol intake by the high alcohol drinking rats. Moreover, the authors demonstrated that the enkephalinase inhibitor thiorphan, which protects enkephalins from degradation, increased alcohol ingestion during the first 30 min following thiorphan administration. In a short communication, Lê et al. (95) reported that, in C57BL/6 mice in a restricted access paradigm, the selective DOR antagonist NTI reduced ethanol consumption to the same extent as that observed with naltrexone.

In contrast, Hyytiä (92) observed no significant changes in alcohol drinking by the male adjuvant arthritic (AA) rats with i.c.v. administration of ICI 174,864; in females, this compound produced postural abnormalities and barrel rolling. Honkanen (93) demonstrated that blockade of DORs by NTI failed to decrease alcohol consumption in AA rats. Both ICI 174,864 and NTI attenuated alcohol intake (96) in alcohol-preferring P rats; however, NTI displayed a more prolonged duration of action (8 h vs 1 h following drug treatment). Noteworthy, the suppressive effects of NTI were not specific for alcohol, since NTI suppressed the intake of both saccharin solution containing alcohol and the saccharin solution without alcohol, suggesting that ingestion of either alcohol or sweets may activate the endogenous opioid system.

A significant amount of evidence indicates that opioid antagonists are not selective for alcohol as evidenced by the fact that they attenuate the intake of a wide variety of ingesta. For instance, both naloxone and naltrexone have been reported to decrease the intake of alcohol, sweets, fats, food, and water (97–99). With the findings uncovering the existence of two subtypes of δ-receptors, named δ_1- and δ_2-, and that the antagonist NTI blocks both subtypes, Krishnan-Sarin and coworkers (100) proposed to investigate the effects of NTB, a highly potent receptor antagonist with high affinity and selectivity for δ_2-opioid receptors, on alcohol intake. The results showed that NTB significantly suppressed ethanol ingestion without altering water intake or body weight in rats given a free choice between alcohol and water for 8 h daily. Moreover, NTB significantly suppressed intake of the saccharin solution containing alcohol without altering intake of saccharin without alcohol. Although the nonselective antagonist naltrexone was effective in attenuating ethanol intake in AA rats in a 4-h limited access paradigm, acute injections of the selective DOR antagonist Me_2-Dmt-Tic-OH did not reduce voluntary alcohol consumption (62). Selective opioid receptors antagonists have not altered ethanol intake in all rodent strains consistently, which suggests that genotype may modulate their suppressive effects (101).

Despite the large amount of supporting findings that the opioid system plays a major role in ethanol reinforcement, the attempts to treat alcoholism with opioid receptor antagonists, using either selective or nonselective compounds, have not been consistently proven to be efficacious in reducing alcohol intake. The fact is that alcoholism is a much more complex disease, in which the interactions between the endogenous opioid system and the ethanol are not as straightforward as once hoped. If a δ-antagonist (or inverse agonist) makes it into clinical testing, it will be interesting to see if this class of compounds has efficacy in at least a subset of alcoholics.

7.4.4 Cardiovascular Effects

The opioid system promises to be a major target for pharmacological intervention in the treatment of myocardial infarction (102). For a comprehensive review concerning the role of opioid receptors in both acute and delayed ischemic preconditioning (IPC), see review by Gross (103). Although both δ- and κ-receptors have been shown to be present on cardiac myocytes (104, 105), several studies provided evidence that the δ-receptor, and more specifically the δ_1-subtype, is responsible for acute opioid-induced cardioprotection (106–109). Therefore, selective δ-antagonists can be of great value here. For example, Schultz (106) demonstrated that BNTX (δ_1-antagonist), but not NTB (δ_2-antagonist), produced a dose-related blockade of infarct size reduction induced by IPC. Treatment with naloxone or NTI abolished the protective effects of IPC in humans and rats (109, 110).

Studies have indicated that the endogenous opiate system is also activated in patients with heart failure. In animal models of heart failure, nonselective opioid antagonists such as naloxone and nalmefene have been shown to improve systemic hemodynamics and myocardial contractile function (111, 112). Imai (113) attributes the beneficial hemodynamic effects of naloxone to be mediated via an inhibitory action on the δ-receptor, because the selective δ-antagonist ICI 154,129 increased mean aortic pressure, myocardial mechanical function, and cardiac output in a similar way to that produced by naloxone and nalmefene in congestive heart failure.

Maslov et al. (114) recently reported that both δ-agonists and δ-antagonists produced a negative chronotropic effect on isolated and perfused rat heart, suggesting that the examined selective δ-ligands can interact with so-called nonopioid receptors for opioid peptides. A more detailed discussion on the clinical application of DOR antagonists can be found in Chap. 18 of this book.

7.5 Conclusion

Since the cloning of the DOR in 1992, significant chemical and pharmacological efforts have been made toward the discovery of potent and selective antagonists for this G protein-coupled receptor. The field has advanced with the synthesis of peptide and nonpeptide compounds characterized by in vitro and in vivo assays, which have aided in the understanding of the various physiological roles of the δ-receptor. However, 16 years later, many unanswered questions still remain. Firstly, some of the classical δ-antagonists here mentioned have not shown reliable selectivity for DOR across species (e.g., rodent vs human-cloned receptors). Secondly, there is enough behavioral evidence indicating the existence of two subtypes of δ-receptors; however, molecular cloning has not yet found clues for distinguishing between them. Finally, the inverse agonism demonstrated by some ligands strongly suggests constitutive activity of the δ-receptor, although the biological relevance of DOR's tonic activity in many functions has not been fully elucidated. The continuous hope for the future is that truly δ-selective ligands with high antagonistic potency will reveal clinical therapeutic opportunities for this class of compounds.

References

1. Portoghese PS. A new concept on the mode of interaction of narcotic analgesics with receptors. J Med Chem 1965; 8(5):609–16.
2. Pert CB, Snyder SH. Opiate receptor: demonstration in nervous tissue. Science 1973; 179(77):1011–4.
3. Martin WR, Eades CG, Thompson JA, Huppler RE, Gilbert PE. The effects of morphine- and nalorphine- like drugs in the nondependent and morphine-dependent chronic spinal dog. J Pharmacol Exp Ther 1976; 197(3):517–32.
4. Goldstein A. Binding selectivity profiles for ligands of multiple receptor types: Focus on opioid receptors. Trends in Pharmacological Sciences 1987; 8(12):456–459.
5. Pasternak GW. Pharmacological mechanisms of opioid analgesics. Clin Neuropharmacol 1993; 16(1):1–18.
6. Quirion R, Chicheportiche R, Contreras PC et al. Classification and nomenclature of phencyclidine and sigma receptor sites. Trends in Neurosciences 1987; 10(11):444–446.
7. Hughes J, Kosterlitz HW, Leslie FM. Effect of morphine on adrenergic transmission in the mouse vas deferens. Assessment of agonist and antogonist potencies of narcotic analgesics. Br J Pharmacol 1975; 53(3):371–81.
8. Knapp RJ, Yamamura HI. Delta opioid receptor radioligands. Biochem Pharmacol 1992; 44(9):1687–95.
9. Evans CJ, Keith DE, Jr., Morrison H, Magendzo K, Edwards RH. Cloning of a delta opioid receptor by functional expression. Science 1992; 258(5090):1952–5.
10. Kieffer BL, Befort K, Gaveriaux-Ruff C, Hirth CG. The delta-opioid receptor: isolation of a cDNA by expression cloning and pharmacological characterization. Proc Natl Acad Sci U S A 1992; 89(24):12048–52.
11. Kieffer BL, Befort K, Gaveriaux-Ruff C, Hirth CG. The delta-opioid receptor: isolation of a cDNA by expression cloning and pharmacological characterization. Proc Natl Acad Sci U S A 1994; 91(3):1193.
12. Zaki PA, Bilsky EJ, Vanderah TW, Lai J, Evans CJ, Porreca F. Opioid receptor types and subtypes: the delta receptor as a model. Annu Rev Pharmacol Toxicol 1996; 36:379–401.

13. Schiller P.W. Opioid Peptide-Derived Delta Antagonists, Inverse Delta Agonists, and Mixed Mu Agonist/Delta Antagonists. In: Chang K-J, Porreca F, Woods J.H., editors. The Delta Receptor. New York: Marcel Dekker, Inc., 2004: 191–210.
14. Cotton R, Giles MG, Miller L, Shaw JS, Timms D. ICI 174864: a highly selective antagonist for the opioid delta-receptor. Eur J Pharmacol 1984; 97(3–4):331–2.
15. Corbett AD, Gillan MG, Kosterlitz HW, McKnight AT, Paterson SJ, Robson LE. Selectivities of opioid peptide analogues as agonists and antagonists at the delta-receptor. Br J Pharmacol 1984; 83(1):271–9.
16. Costa T, Herz A. Antagonists with negative intrinsic activity at delta opioid receptors coupled to GTP-binding proteins. Proc Natl Acad Sci U S A 1989; 86(19):7321–5.
17. Portoghese PS, Sultana M, Takemori AE. Naltrindole, a highly selective and potent non-peptide delta opioid receptor antagonist. Eur J Pharmacol 1988; 146(1):185–6.
18. Portoghese PS. The bivalent ligand approach in the design of highly selective opioid receptor antagonists. NIDA Res Monogr 1990; 96:3–20.
19. Portoghese PS, Sultana M, Takemori AE. Design of peptidomimetic delta opioid receptor antagonists using the message-address concept. J Med Chem 1990; 33(6):1714–20.
20. Takemori AE, Sultana M, Nagase H, Portoghese PS. Agonist and antagonist activities of ligands derived from naltrexone and oxymorphone. Life Sci 1992; 50(20):1491–5.
21. Daniels D.J., Portoghese P.S. Delta-Selective Ligands Related to Naltrindole. In: Chang K-J, Porreca F, Woods J.H., editors. The Delta Receptor. New York: Marcel Dekker, Inc, 2004: 139–158.
22. Schiller PW, Weltrowska G, Berezowska I et al. The TIPP opioid peptide family: development of delta antagonists, delta agonists, and mixed mu agonist/delta antagonists. Biopolymers 1999; 51(6):411–25.
23. Schiller PW, Nguyen TM, Weltrowska G et al. Differential stereochemical requirements of mu vs. delta opioid receptors for ligand binding and signal transduction: development of a class of potent and highly delta-selective peptide antagonists. Proc Natl Acad Sci U S A 1992; 89(24):11871–5.
24. Portoghese PS, Sultana M, Nagase H, Takemori AE. A highly selective delta 1-opioid receptor antagonist: 7-benzylidenenaltrexone. Eur J Pharmacol 1992; 218(1):195–6.
25. Portoghese PS, Nagase H, MaloneyHuss KE, Lin CE, Takemori AE. Role of spacer and address components in peptidomimetic delta opioid receptor antagonists related to naltrindole. J Med Chem 1991; 34(5):1715–20.
26. Schiller PW, Weltrowska G, Nguyen TM, Wilkes BC, Chung NN, Lemieux C. TIPP[psi]: a highly potent and stable pseudopeptide delta opioid receptor antagonist with extraordinary delta selectivity. J Med Chem 1993; 36(21):3182–7.
27. Toth G, Ioja E, Tomboly C et al. Beta-methyl substitution of cyclohexylalanine in Dmt-Tic-Cha-Phe peptides results in highly potent delta opioid antagonists. J Med Chem 2007; 50(2):328–33.
28. Martin NA, Terruso MT, Prather PL. Agonist Activity of the delta-antagonists TIPP and TIPP-psi in cellular models expressing endogenous or transfected delta-opioid receptors. J Pharmacol Exp Ther 2001; 298(1):240–8.
29. Martin NA, Ruckle MB, VanHoof SL, Prather PL. Agonist, antagonist, and inverse agonist characteristics of TIPP (H-Tyr-Tic-Phe-Phe-OH), a selective delta-opioid receptor ligand. J Pharmacol Exp Ther 2002; 301(2):661–71.
30. Bowen WD, Hellewell SB, Kelemen M, Huey R, Stewart D. Affinity labeling of delta-opiate receptors using [D-Ala2,Leu5,Cys6]enkephalin. Covalent attachment via thiol-disulfide exchange. J Biol Chem 1987; 262(28):13434–9.
31. Calcagnetti DJ, Fanselow MS, Helmstetter FJ, Bowen WD. [D-Ala2,Leu5,Cys6]enkephalin: short-term agonist effects and long-term antagonism at delta opioid receptors. Peptides 1989; 10(2):319–26.
32. Qi JA, Bowen WD, Mosberg HI, Rothman RB, Porreca F. Opioid agonist and antagonist antinociceptive properties of [D-Ala2,Leu5,Cys6]enkephalin: selective actions at the deltanoncomplexed site. J Pharmacol Exp Ther 1990; 255(2):636–41.

33. Jiang Q, Takemori AE, Sultana M et al. Differential antagonism of opioid delta antinociception by [D-Ala2,Leu5,Cys6]enkephalin and naltrindole 5′′-isothiocyanate: evidence for delta receptor subtypes. J Pharmacol Exp Ther 1991; 257(3):1069–75.
34. Rothman RB, Long JB, Bykov V, Jacobson AE, Rice KC, Holaday JW. beta-FNA binds irreversibly to the opiate receptor complex: in vivo and in vitro evidence. J Pharmacol Exp Ther 1988; 247(2):405–16.
35. Mattia A, Vanderah T, Mosberg HI, Omnaas JR, Bowen WD, Porreca F. Pharmacological characterization of [D-Ala2,Leu5,Ser6]enkephalin (DALES): antinociceptive actions at the delta non-complexed-opioid receptor. Eur J Pharmacol 1991; 192(3):371–5.
36. Portoghese PS, Sultana M, Takemori AE. Naltrindole 5′′-isothiocyanate: a nonequilibrium, highly selective delta opioid receptor antagonist. J Med Chem 1990; 33(6):1547–8.
37. Vanderah T, Takemori AE, Sultana M et al. Interaction of [D-Pen2,D-Pen5]enkephalin and [D-Ala2,Glu4]deltorphin with delta-opioid receptor subtypes in vivo. Eur J Pharmacol 1994; 252(2):133–7.
38. Sofuoglu M, Portoghese PS, Takemori AE. Differential antagonism of delta opioid agonists by naltrindole and its benzofuran analog (NTB) in mice: evidence for delta opioid receptor subtypes. J Pharmacol Exp Ther 1991; 257(2):676–80.
39. Thorat SN, Hammond DL. Modulation of nociception by microinjection of delta-1 and delta-2 opioid receptor ligands in the ventromedial medulla of the rat. J Pharmacol Exp Ther 1997; 283(3):1185–92.
40. Stewart PE, Holper EM, Hammond DL. Delta antagonist and kappa agonist activity of Naltriben: evidence for differential kappa interaction with the delta 1 and delta 2 opioid receptor subtypes. Life Sci 1994; 55(4):79–84.
41. Kim KW, Son Y, Shin BS, Cho KP. Pharmacological effects of naltriben as a ligand for opioid mu and kappa receptors in rat cerebral cortex. Life Sci 2001; 68(11):1305–15.
42. Sofuoglu M, Portoghese PS, Takemori AE. 7-Benzylidenenaltrexone (BNTX): a selective delta 1 opioid receptor antagonist in the mouse spinal cord. Life Sci 1993; 52(8):769–75.
43. Payza K. Binding and Activity of Opioid Ligands at the Cloned Human Delta, Mu, and Kappa Receptors. In: Chang K-J, Porreca F, Woods J.H., editors. The Delta Receptor. New York: Marcel Dekker, Inc., 2004: 261–275.
44. Parkhill AL, Bidlack JM. Several delta-opioid receptor ligands display no subtype selectivity to the human delta-opioid receptor. Eur J Pharmacol 2002; 451(3):257–64.
45. Carroll FI, Zhang L, Mascarella SW et al. Discovery of the first N-substituted 4beta-methyl-5-(3-hydroxyphenyl)morphan to possess highly potent and selective opioid delta receptor antagonist activity. J Med Chem 2004; 47(2):281–4.
46. Thomas JB, Zhang L, Navarro HA, Carroll FI. Highly potent and selective phenylmorphan-based inverse agonists of the opioid delta receptor. J Med Chem 2006; 49(18): 5597–5609.
47. Kshirsagar T, Nakano AH, Law PY, Elde R, Portoghese PS. NTI4F: a non-peptide fluorescent probe selective for functional delta opioid receptors. Neurosci Lett 1998; 249(2–3):83–6.
48. Balboni G, Salvadori S, Dal Piaz A et al. Highly selective fluorescent analogue of the potent delta-opioid receptor antagonist Dmt-Tic. J Med Chem 2004; 47(26):6541–6.
49. Chen H, Chung NN, Lemieux C et al. [Aladan3]TIPP: a fluorescent delta-opioid antagonist with high delta-receptor binding affinity and delta selectivity. Biopolymers 2005; 80(2–3): 325–31.
50. Cohen BE, McAnaney TB, Park ES, Jan YN, Boxer SG, Jan LY. Probing protein electrostatics with a synthetic fluorescent amino acid. Science 2002; 296(5573):1700–3.
51. Ellison N. Opioid analgesic for cancer pain: toxicities and their treatments. In: RB P, editor. Cancer Pain. Philadelphia, PA: JB Lippincott Company, 1993: 184–194.
52. Sora I, Elmer G, Funada M et al. Mu opiate receptor gene dose effects on different morphine actions: evidence for differential in vivo mu receptor reserve. Neuropsychopharmacology 2001; 25(1):41–54.
53. Kamei J. Delta-opioid receptor antagonists as a new concept for central acting antitussive drugs. Pulm Pharmacol Ther 2002; 15(3):235–40.

54. Buonopane A, Petrakis IL. Pharmacotherapy of alcohol use disorders. Subst Use Misuse 2005; 40(13–14):2001–20.
55. Di Chiara G, Imperato A. Drugs abused by humans preferentially increase synaptic dopamine concentrations in the mesolimbic system of freely moving rats. Proc Natl Acad Sci U S A 1988; 85(14):5274–8.
56. Koob GF. Drugs of abuse: anatomy, pharmacology and function of reward pathways. Trends Pharmacol Sci 1992; 13(5):177–84.
57. Robinson TE, Berridge KC. The neural basis of drug craving: an incentive-sensitization theory of addiction. Brain Res Brain Res Rev 1993; 18(3):247–91.
58. Cowen MS, Lawrence AJ. The role of opioid-dopamine interactions in the induction and maintenance of ethanol consumption. Prog Neuropsychopharmacol Biol Psychiatry 1999; 23(7):1171–212.
59. Davis VE, Walsh MJ. Alcohol, amines, and alkaloids: a possible biochemical basis for alcohol addiction. Science 1970; 167(920):1005–7.
60. Tabakoff B, Hoffman PL. Alcohol interactions with brain opiate receptors. Life Sci 1983; 32(3):197–204.
61. Herz A. Endogenous opioid systems and alcohol addiction. Psychopharmacology (Berl) 1997; 129(2):99–111.
62. Ingman K, Salvadori S, Lazarus L, Korpi ER, Honkanen A. Selective delta-opioid receptor antagonist N,N(CH3)2-Dmt-Tic-OH does not reduce ethanol intake in alcohol-preferring AA rats. Addict Biol 2003; 8(2):173–9.
63. Gianoulakis C. Characterization of the effects of acute ethanol administration on the release of beta-endorphin peptides by the rat hypothalamus. Eur J Pharmacol 1990; 180(1):21–9.
64. De Waele JP, Papachristou DN, Gianoulakis C. The alcohol-preferring C57BL/6 mice present an enhanced sensitivity of the hypothalamic beta-endorphin system to ethanol than the alcohol-avoiding DBA/2 mice. J Pharmacol Exp Ther 1992; 261(2):788–94.
65. de Waele JP, Gianoulakis C. Effects of single and repeated exposures to ethanol on hypothalamic beta-endorphin and CRH release by the C57BL/6 and DBA/2 strains of mice. Neuroendocrinology 1993; 57(4):700–9.
66. Li XW, Li TK, Froehlich JC. Enhanced sensitivity of the nucleus accumbens proenkephalin system to alcohol in rats selectively bred for alcohol preference. Brain Res 1998; 794(1):35–47.
67. Scanlon MN, Lazar-Wesley E, Grant KA, Kunos G. Proopiomelanocortin messenger RNA is decreased in the mediobasal hypothalamus of rats made dependent on ethanol. Alcohol Clin Exp Res 1992; 16(6):1147–51.
68. Gianoulakis C, de Waele JP. Genetics of alcoholism: role of the endogenous opioid system. Metab Brain Dis 1994; 9(2):105–31.
69. Winkler A, Roske I, Furkert J, Fickel J, Melzig MF. Effects of voluntary ethanol ingestion on the POMC gene expression in the rat pituitary and on the plasma beta-endorphin content. Alcohol Alcohol 1995; 30(2):231–8.
70. Gianoulakis C. Influence of the endogenous opioid system on high alcohol consumption and genetic predisposition to alcoholism. J Psychiatry Neurosci 2001; 26(4):304–18.
71. Gianoulakis C, de Waele JP, Kiianmaa K. Differences in the brain and pituitary beta-endorphin system between the alcohol-preferring AA and alcohol-avoiding ANA rats. Alcohol Clin Exp Res 1992; 16(3):453–9.
72. Krishnan-Sarin S, Wand GS, Li XW, Portoghese PS, Froehlich JC. Effect of mu opioid receptor blockade on alcohol intake in rats bred for high alcohol drinking. Pharmacol Biochem Behav 1998; 59(3):627–35.
73. Jamensky NT, Gianoulakis C. Comparison of the proopiomelanocortin and proenkephalin opioid peptide systems in brain regions of the alcohol-preferring C57BL/6 and alcohol-avoiding DBA/2 mice. Alcohol 1999; 18(2–3):177–87.
74. Marinelli PW, Kiianmaa K, Gianoulakis C. Opioid propeptide mRNA content and receptor density in the brains of AA and ANA rats. Life Sci 2000; 66(20):1915–27.
75. de Waele JP, Kiianmaa K, Gianoulakis C. Distribution of the mu and delta opioid binding sites in the brain of the alcohol-preferring AA and alcohol-avoiding ANA lines of rats. J Pharmacol Exp Ther 1995; 275(1):518–27.

76. de Waele JP, Gianoulakis C. Characterization of the mu and delta opioid receptors in the brain of the C57BL/6 and DBA/2 mice, selected for their differences in voluntary ethanol consumption. Alcohol Clin Exp Res 1997; 21(4):754–62.
77. Jamensky NT, Gianoulakis C. Content of dynorphins and kappa-opioid receptors in distinct brain regions of C57BL/6 and DBA/2 mice. Alcohol Clin Exp Res 1997; 21(8):1455–64.
78. Oswald LM, Wand GS. Opioids and alcoholism. Physiol Behav 2004; 81(2):339–58.
79. Altshuler HL, Phillips PE, Feinhandler DA. Alteration of ethanol self-administration by naltrexone. Life Sci 1980; 26(9):679–88.
80. Myers RD, Borg S, Mossberg R. Antagonism by naltrexone of voluntary alcohol selection in the chronically drinking macaque monkey. Alcohol 1986; 3(6):383–8.
81. Froehlich JC, Harts J, Lumeng L, Li TK. Naloxone attenuates voluntary ethanol intake in rats selectively bred for high ethanol preference. Pharmacol Biochem Behav 1990; 35(2):385–90.
82. Volpicelli JR, Alterman AI, Hayashida M, O'Brien CP. Naltrexone in the treatment of alcohol dependence. Arch Gen Psychiatry 1992; 49(11):876–80.
83. Volpicelli JR, Volpicelli LA, O'Brien CP. Medical management of alcohol dependence: clinical use and limitations of naltrexone treatment. Alcohol Alcohol 1995; 30(6):789–98.
84. O'Malley SS, Jaffe AJ, Chang G, Schottenfeld RS, Meyer RE, Rounsaville B. Naltrexone and coping skills therapy for alcohol dependence. A controlled study. Arch Gen Psychiatry 1992; 49(11):881–7.
85. O'Malley SS. Opioid antagonists in the treatment of alcohol dependence: clinical efficacy and prevention of relapse. Alcohol Alcohol Suppl 1996; 1:77–81.
86. Volpicelli JR, Rhines KC, Rhines JS, Volpicelli LA, Alterman AI, O'Brien CP. Naltrexone and alcohol dependence. Role of subject compliance. Arch Gen Psychiatry 1997; 54(8):737–42.
87. Anton RF, Moak DH, Waid LR, Latham PK, Malcolm RJ, Dias JK. Naltrexone and cognitive behavioral therapy for the treatment of outpatient alcoholics: results of a placebo-controlled trial. Am J Psychiatry 1999; 156(11):1758–64.
88. Chick J, Anton R, Checinski K et al. A multicentre, randomized, double-blind, placebo-controlled trial of naltrexone in the treatment of alcohol dependence or abuse. Alcohol Alcohol 2000; 35(6):587–93.
89. Kranzler HR, Modesto-Lowe V, Van Kirk J. Naltrexone vs. nefazodone for treatment of alcohol dependence. A placebo-controlled trial. Neuropsychopharmacology 2000; 22(5):493–503.
90. Krystal JH, Cramer JA, Krol WF, Kirk GF, Rosenheck RA. Naltrexone in the treatment of alcohol dependence. N Engl J Med 2001; 345(24):1734–9.
91. Gastpar M, Bonnet U, Boning J et al. Lack of efficacy of naltrexone in the prevention of alcohol relapse: results from a German multicenter study. J Clin Psychopharmacol 2002; 22(6):592–8.
92. Hyytia P. Involvement of mu-opioid receptors in alcohol drinking by alcohol-preferring AA rats. Pharmacol Biochem Behav 1993; 45(3):697–701.
93. Honkanen A, Vilamo L, Wegelius K, Sarviharju M, Hyytia P, Korpi ER. Alcohol drinking is reduced by a mu 1- but not by a delta-opioid receptor antagonist in alcohol-preferring rats. Eur J Pharmacol 1996; 304(1–3):7–13.
94. Froehlich JC, Zweifel M, Harts J, Lumeng L, Li TK. Importance of delta opioid receptors in maintaining high alcohol drinking. Psychopharmacology (Berl) 1991; 103(4):467–72.
95. Le AD, Poulos CX, Quan B, Chow S. The effects of selective blockade of delta and mu opiate receptors on ethanol consumption by C57BL/6 mice in a restricted access paradigm. Brain Res 1993; 630(1–2):330–2.
96. Krishnan-Sarin S, Jing SL, Kurtz DL et al. The delta opioid receptor antagonist naltrindole attenuates both alcohol and saccharin intake in rats selectively bred for alcohol preference. Psychopharmacology (Berl) 1995; 120(2):177–85.
97. Maickel RP, Zabik JE. The pharmacology of anorexigenesis. Life Sci 1977; 21(2):173–9.
98. Cooper SJ, McGivern H. Effects of naloxone and naltrexone on the increased water intake and drinking duration in phenobarbitone-treated rats. Psychopharmacology (Berl) 1983; 79(1):25–8.
99. Akkok F, Manha NA, Czirr SA, Reid LD. Naloxone persistently modifies water-intake. Pharmacol Biochem Behav 1988; 29(2):331–4.

100. Krishnan-Sarin S, Portoghese PS, Li TK, Froehlich JC. The delta 2-opioid receptor antagonist naltriben selectively attenuates alcohol intake in rats bred for alcohol preference. Pharmacol Biochem Behav 1995; 52(1):153–9.
101. Hyytia P, Kiianmaa K. Suppression of ethanol responding by centrally administered CTOP and naltrindole in AA and Wistar rats. Alcohol Clin Exp Res 2001; 25(1):25–33.
102. Patel HH, Hsu A, Gross GJ. Attenuation of heat shock-induced cardioprotection by treatment with the opiate receptor antagonist naloxone. Am J Physiol Heart Circ Physiol 2002; 282(6):2011–7.
103. Gross GJ. Role of opioids in acute and delayed preconditioning. J Mol Cell Cardiol 2003; 35(7):709–18.
104. Zukin RS, Zukin SR. Multiple opiate receptors: emerging concepts. Life Sci 1981; 29(26):2681–90.
105. Ventura C, Bastagli L, Bernardi P, Caldarera CM, Guarnieri C. Opioid receptors in rat cardiac sarcolemma: effect of phenylephrine and isoproterenol. Biochim Biophys Acta 1989; 987(1):69–74.
106. Schultz JE, Hsu AK, Gross GJ. Ischemic preconditioning in the intact rat heart is mediated by delta1- but not mu- or kappa-opioid receptors. Circulation 1998; 97(13):1282–9.
107. Tsuchida A, Miura T, Tanno M, Nozawa Y, Kita H, Shimamoto K. Time window for the contribution of the delta-opioid receptor to cardioprotection by ischemic preconditioning in the rat heart. Cardiovasc Drugs Ther 1998; 12(4):365–73.
108. Aitchison KA, Baxter GF, Awan MM, Smith RM, Yellon DM, Opie LH. Opposing effects on infarction of delta and kappa opioid receptor activation in the isolated rat heart: implications for ischemic preconditioning. Basic Res Cardiol 2000; 95(1):1–10.
109. Huh J, Gross GJ, Nagase H, Liang BT. Protection of cardiac myocytes via delta(1)-opioid receptors, protein kinase C, and mitochondrial K(ATP) channels. Am J Physiol Heart Circ Physiol 2001; 280(1):377–83.
110. Tomai F, Crea F, Gaspardone A et al. Effects of naloxone on myocardial ischemic preconditioning in humans. J Am Coll Cardiol 1999; 33(7):1863–9.
111. Sakamoto S, Stone CK, Woolf PD, Liang CS. Opiate receptor antagonism in right-sided congestive heart failure. Naloxone exerts salutary hemodynamic effects through its action on the central nervous system. Circ Res 1989; 65(1):103–14.
112. Himura Y, Liang CS, Imai N, Delehanty JM, Woolf PD, Hood WB, Jr. Short-term effects of naloxone on hemodynamics and baroreflex function in conscious dogs with pacing-induced congestive heart failure. J Am Coll Cardiol 1994; 23(1):194–200.
113. Imai N, Kashiki M, Woolf PD, Liang CS. Comparison of cardiovascular effects of mu- and delta-opioid receptor antagonists in dogs with congestive heart failure. Am J Physiol 1994; 267(3 Pt 2):912–7.
114. Maslov LN, Lishmanov YB, Barzakh EI, Lasukova TV, Rice KK, Oeltgen PR. Negative inotropic and chronotropic effects of delta-opioid receptor antagonists are mediated via non-opioid receptors. Bull Exp Biol Med 2006; 141(4):420–3.

Chapter 8
Novel Opioid Antagonists with Mixed/Dual Selectivity

Richard B. Rothman, Subramaniam Ananthan, and Edward J. Bilsky

Abstract Opioid analgesics are the most effective therapeutic agents available for the treatment of moderate to severe pain. In addition to the well-known opioid side effects of respiratory depression and constipation, tolerance, dependence, and addiction to prescription opioids is a growing problem. These recent trends emphasize the importance of developing new opioid analgesics that do not produce tolerance and dependence and/or have decreased addiction liability. There are several possible strategies for developing opioid analgesic drugs that do not produce tolerance and dependence. Based on observations that co-administration of a delta-opioid receptor antagonist with morphine, a mu-opioid receptor agonist, attenuated the development of morphine tolerance and dependence, we focused our efforts on developing nonpeptide ligands that possess mixed agonist/antagonist activity. We synthesized and evaluated a series of pyridomorphinans derived from the naloxone, oxymorphone, and hydromorphone framework. These efforts led to the identification of hydromorphone-derived pyridomorphinans **3** [formerly **14**] (5′-(4-chlorophenyl)-6,7-didehydro-4,5α-epoxy-3-hydroxy-17-methylpyrido[2′,3′:6,7]morphinan, SoRI 20411) as a compound possessing mu agonist/delta antagonist activity in both the [^{35}S]-GTP-γ-S binding and smooth muscle functional assays. SoRI 20411 produced antinociception (A_{50} potency value of 42.8 nmol in the 55°C warm-water tail-withdrawal assay in mice). The antinociceptive effects were blocked by the mu-selective antagonist β-funaltrexamine (β-FNA). When tested in the tolerance development assays involving repeated injections of the compound for 3 days, SoRI 20411 induced an insignificant shift in the antinociceptive potency (less than 1.1-fold increase in A_{50} value), indicating very little development of tolerance. The identification of SoRI 20411 demonstrates the validity of the hypothesis that nonpeptide opioid ligands with a mixed mu agonist/delta antagonist profile of activity may have diminished propensity to induce tolerance and, therefore, may have therapeutic advantages over mu agonist analgesics for long-term treatment of pain.

R.B. Rothman (✉), S. Ananthan, and E.J. Bilsky
Clinical Psychopharmacology Section, IRP, NIDA, NIH, 5500 Nathan Shock Drive,
Baltimore, MD 21224,
e-mail: rrothman@intra.nida.nih.gov

R. Dean et al. (eds.), *Opiate Receptors and Antagonists*,

Keywords: Opioid; Tolerance; Dependence; Addiction; Morphine; Delta antagonist

8.1 Introduction

Opioid analgesics are the most effective therapeutic agents available for the treatment of moderate to severe pain (9). In addition to the well-known opioid side effects of respiratory depression and constipation, tolerance, dependence, and addiction to prescription opioids is a growing problem. At the outset, it is important to define these terms. Tolerance refers to the need to administer ever-higher doses to produce the same drug effect. Dependence refers to the development of physical dependence on an opioid, such that withdrawal of the opioid, or the administration of an antagonist, such as naloxone, produces a pronounced physical withdrawal syndrome. Addiction refers to a maladaptive behavioral pattern, defined as persistent drug-seeking behavior despite negative consequences to the individual and society. As reviewed elsewhere, recent surveys indicate that among 12th graders ~10% have used Vicodin (acetaminophen and hydrocodone) and ~5% have used OxyContin (oxycodone) (7), and that addiction to prescription opioids is a growing problem (6).

These recent trends emphasize the importance of developing new opioid analgesics that do not produce tolerance and dependence and/or have decreased addiction liability. This goal, of course, has been the "holy grail" driving much of opioid research for many decades. The research we will review in this chapter strongly suggests that the opioid research community may be quite close to developing potent analgesics that do not produce tolerance and physical dependence. Such agents, however, might still have some addictive potential, since it will likely be difficult to completely separate out opioid analgesia and effects that mu agonists have on the limbic system (e.g., positive reinforcement and decreased emotional responses to painful stimuli).

There are several possible strategies for developing opioid analgesic drugs that do not produce tolerance and dependence. The particular strategy we adopted was inspired by the seminal observation that co-administration of the delta-receptor antagonist naltrindole (NTI) prevented the development of morphine tolerance and dependence in mice (1). Subsequent studies confirmed the work of Abdelhamid et al. (1) in rats and also showed that NTI did not prevent the development of tolerance to the respiratory depressant effect of morphine (14). Other studies conducted in the 1990s generally confirmed these basic observations. For example, continuous infusion of the delta-selective antagonist Tyr-Tic-Phe-Phe (TIPP)[Ψ] in parallel with continuous administration of morphine by the subcutaneous (s.c.) route to rats attenuated the development of morphine tolerance and dependence to a large extent (12). The critical role that delta receptors, play in the development of morphine tolerance and dependence was further demonstrated by the use of antisense oligonucleotides to the delta-opioid receptor. These studies showed that knockdown of the delta receptor blocked the development of morphine tolerance and dependence (15, 26). Furthermore, studies with receptor knockout mice have documented the critical role of delta receptors in the development of opioid tolerance. In contrast to wild-type mice, in which the analgesic response to a fixed morphine dose was lost within 5 days, the opioid knockout mice failed to develop tolerance following daily administration of 5 mg/kg of morphine, s.c., for 8 days. After 10 days of chronic morphine dosing, cumulative dose-response curves revealed a significant 2.8-fold shift to the right of the morphine ED_{50} in wild-type mice, whereas the potency of morphine in the receptor knockout mice remained unchanged following chronic morphine administration (31).

Compelling evidence for the involvement of opioid receptors in the development of morphine-induced tolerance was recently obtained using knockin mice, in which the native receptors were replaced by mutant receptors (S196A) (21). This mutant mu receptor permits the antagonist ligand naltrexone to act as a mu agonist. In these animals, acute administration of naltrexone produces antinociception, and chronic administration of naltrexone did not result in tolerance to naltrexone itself or to morphine. This lack of tolerance in these animals was attributed to concurrent blockade of delta-opioid receptors with activation of mu receptors. Further studies using wild-type and knockin mice revealed that inhibition of delta-opioid receptor must occur at the time of mu receptor activation to prevent tolerance development. Tolerance development could therefore be prevented by delta-receptor blockade, but cannot be reversed once it has occurred. These observations clearly indicate that delta-opioid receptors play a major role in the development of morphine tolerance and dependence and provide a rationale for the development of opioid ligands that act as an agonist at the mu receptor and as an antagonist at the delta receptor. Such a mixed mu agonist/delta antagonist would be expected to be an analgesic with low propensity to produce analgesic tolerance and physical dependence. In addition, findings that NTI reversed sufentanil-induced respiratory depression (11) and enhanced colonic propulsion (10) suggests that a mixed mu agonist/delta antagonist may produce less respiratory depression and gastrointestinal side effects compared to a pure mu-opioid analgesic.

8.2 Peptide Ligands Possessing Mixed Mu Agonist/Delta Antagonist Activity

Schiller and coworkers reported for the first time a peptide ligand with mu agonist/delta antagonist properties (24). Among the analogs of the moderately mu-selective β-casomorphin-5, H-Tyr-c[D-Orn-Phe-D-Pro-Gly-], replacement of the Phe^3 residue by 2-naphthylalanine (2-Nal) gave the peptide H-Tyr-c[D-Orn-2-Nal-D-Pro-Gly-]. This peptide which displayed high affinity for both mu and delta receptors, was an agonist in the guinea pig ileum (GPI) smooth muscle assay and a moderately potent antagonist against various delta agonists in the mouse vas deferens (MVD) assay (24). Ligands with a more balanced mu agonist/delta antagonist profile of activity were discovered among analogs of the tetrapeptide amide H-Tyr-Tic-Phe-Phe-NH_2 (TIPP-NH_2). For example, substitution of Dmt for Tyr[1] in TIPP-NH_2 and reduction of the peptide bond between Tic[2] and Phe[3] led to a compound, H-Dmt-TicΨ[CH_2-NH]Phe-Phe-NH_2 (DIPP-NH_2[Ψ]), which showed high mu agonist potency and very high delta antagonist activity in the GPI and MVD bioassays. DIPP-NH_2[Ψ] (administered by the intracerebroventricular or i.c.v. route) produced a potent antinociceptive effect in the rat tail-flick test. DIPP-NH_2[Ψ] produced less tolerance than morphine and no physical dependence when administered chronically at high dose levels. DIPP-NH_2[Ψ], therefore, provided a proof of principle demonstration that a single molecule with mixed mu agonist/delta antagonist actions will produce antinociception while inducing considerably less tolerance and dependence than morphine (23).

8.3 Nonpeptide Ligands that Possess Mixed Agonist/Antagonist Activity

Peptidergic-mixed mu agonist/delta antagonists are unlikely to be developed as therapeutic agents, since most peptides do not readily cross the blood-brain barrier. Thus, we focused our efforts on developing nonpeptide ligands that possess mixed agonist/antagonist activity.

We first synthesized and evaluated a series of NTI analogs possessing phenyl-, phenoxy-, and benzyloxy substituents at putative opioid receptor subtypes. One of the compounds, the 7′-phenoxynaltrindole (**1**, Fig. 8.1) was found to display potent antagonist activity with a K_e of 0.25 nM in the MVD and weak agonist activity, with an IC_{50} of 450 nM, in the GPI (3). The weak mu agonist activity of this compound led us to investigate another series of compounds possessing the pyridomorphinan framework. We identified the first nonpeptide ligand with a mixed antagonist/agonist profile from this series (4).

Table 8.1 reports the K_i values of this series of compounds at opioid receptor subtypes. The naltrexone-derived 4-chlorophenyl substituted pyridomorphinan (**2**, Fig. 8.1) (also referred to as compound **7d** and SoRI 9409) (Table 8.1 and Fig. 8.1), had high affinity for the delta receptor ($K_i = 2.2$ nM) and lower affinity at the mu receptor (51 nM). In functional assays, SoRI 9409 was a potent delta antagonist ($K_e = 0.66$ nM) in the MVD and had moderate potency as a mu agonist in the GPI assay ($IC_{50} = 163$ nM). In antinociceptive evaluations, this compound displayed partial agonist activity in the warm-water tail-withdrawal assay and full agonist activity in the acetic acid writhing assay after i.c.v. or intraperitoneal (i.p.) injections (4, 29). In contrast to morphine, repeated i.c.v. injection of an A_{90} dose of this compound did not produce any significant antinociceptive tolerance (Fig. 8.2).

As reported by Wells et al. (29), to determine the opioid receptor(s) through which SoRI 9409 produces its antinociceptive actions, mice were pretreated with vehicle or a selective mu, delta, or kappa antagonist (Fig. 8.3a). Mice were then injected with an A_{90} i.c.v. dose of SoRI 9409 and antinociception was assessed in

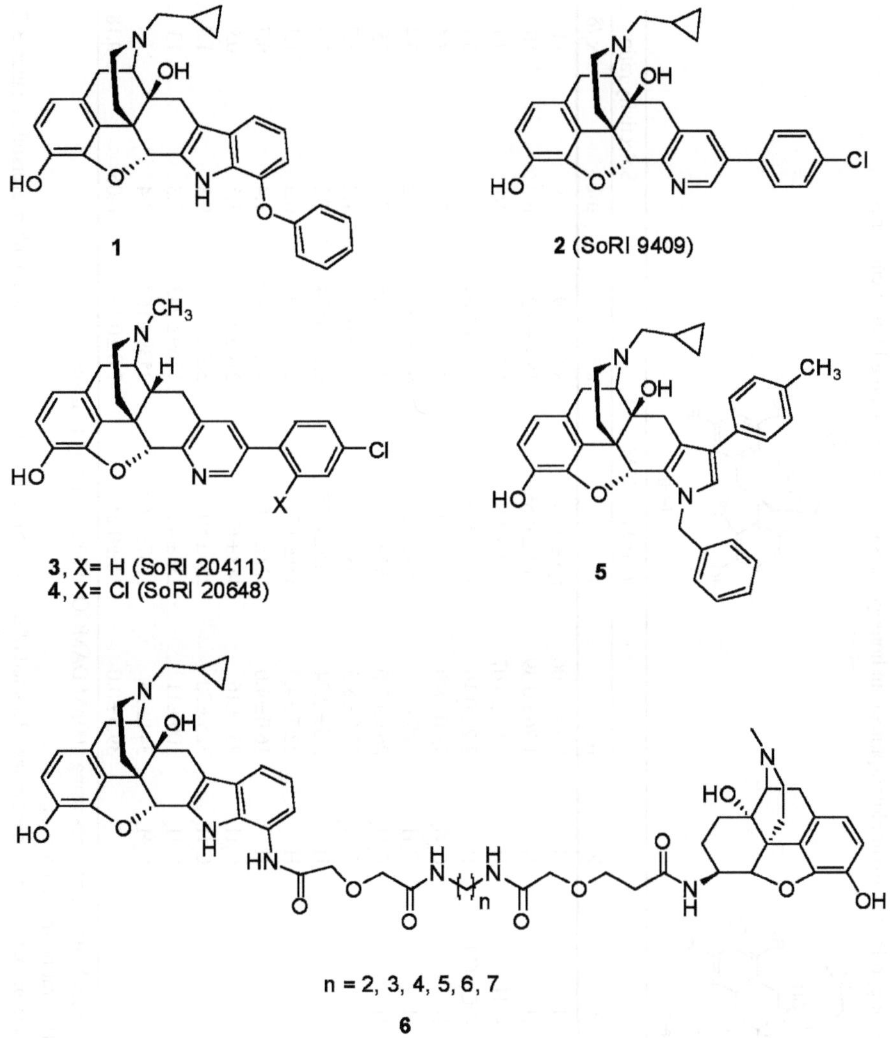

Fig. 8.1 Chemical structures of representative compounds having mixed μ agonist/δ antagonist profiles

the acetic acid writhing assay. An ANOVA of the data depicted in Fig. 8.3 yielded an $F(4,65) = 11.2$, $p < 0.001$. Post hoc analysis using a Scheffe's test indicated that the 30-nmol dose of SoRI 9409 significantly decreased the number of writhes ($p < 0.001$). This effect was blocked by pretreatment with β-FNA ($p < 0.002$) but not by NTI ($p > 0.99$) or nor-binaltorphimine (nor-BNI) ($p > 0.13$). There was also no difference between the vehicle control and nor-BNI group ($p > 0.23$). These experiments established that SoRI 9409 primarily produced antinociception via mu-opioid receptor activation. Other experiments confirmed the delta-selective

Table 8.1 Opioid receptor binding affinities of pyrido- and pyrimidomorphinans in homogenates of rat or guinea pig brain membranes

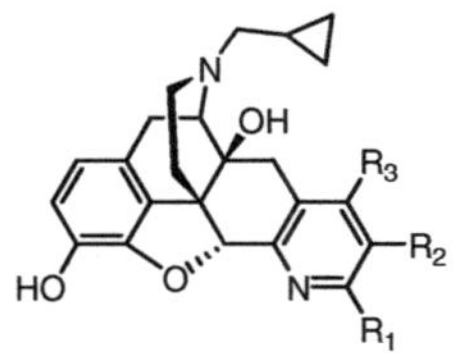

7a-h

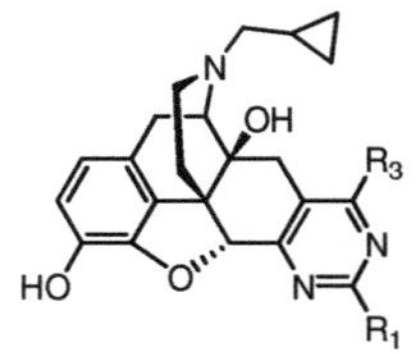

8a-g

				K_i (nM) ± SEM			Selectivity ratio	
Compound	R_1	R_2	R_3	δ[a]	μ[b]	$κ_1$[c]	μ/δ	$κ_1$/δ
7a	H	H	H	0.78±0.06	1.5±0.09	8.8±0.69	1.9	11
7b	C_6H_5	H	H	1.76±0.39	11.0±0.65	18.4±3.2	6.3	10
7c	H	C_6H_5	H	0.87±0.07	13.5±1.0	17.6±1.6	16	20
7d (2)	H	4-Cl–C_6H_4	H	2.2±0.16	51.0±8.0	20.0±1.04	23	9.1
7e	H	H	C_6H_5	73.0±8.0	191±19	264±21	2.6	3.6
7f	CH_3	H	C_6H_5	125±9	154±42	677±63	1.2	5.4
7g	C_6H_5	H	C_6H_5	86.0±9.0	652±71	2116±185	7.6	25
7h	CH=CH–CH=CH		C_6H_5	73.0±8.5	308±31	272±6	4.2	3.7
8a	H		H	3.5±0.24	4.15±0.75	6.24±0.74	1.2	1.8
8b	CH_3		H	22.7±4.0	6.0±0.5	25.0±3.0	0.3	1.1
8c	C_6H_5		H	16.0±4.0	22.0±2.0	11.0±1.4	1.4	0.7
8d	H		C_6H_5	230±16	348±67	216±16	1.5	0.9
8e	CH_3		C_6H_5	325±20	254±50	565±34	0.8	1.7
8f	$CH_2C_6H_5$		C_6H_5	100±11	233±44	1269±243	2.3	13
8g	C_6H_5		C_6H_5	344±38	1167±169	2539±167	3.4	7.4
Naltrexone				39.5±3.0	2.5±0.21	7.0±0.18	0.06	0.18

[a]Displacement of [^{3}H]DADLE (1.3–2.0 nM) in rat brain membranes using 100 nM DAMGO to block binding to μ sites

[b]Displacement of [^{3}H]DAMGO (1.4–2.0 nM) in rat brain membranes

[c]Displacement of [^{3}H]U69, 593 (1.2–2.2 nM) in guinea pig brain membranes depleted of μ- and δ-binding sites by pretreatment with irreversible ligands BIT and FIT. Table adapted from Ananthan et al. (4)

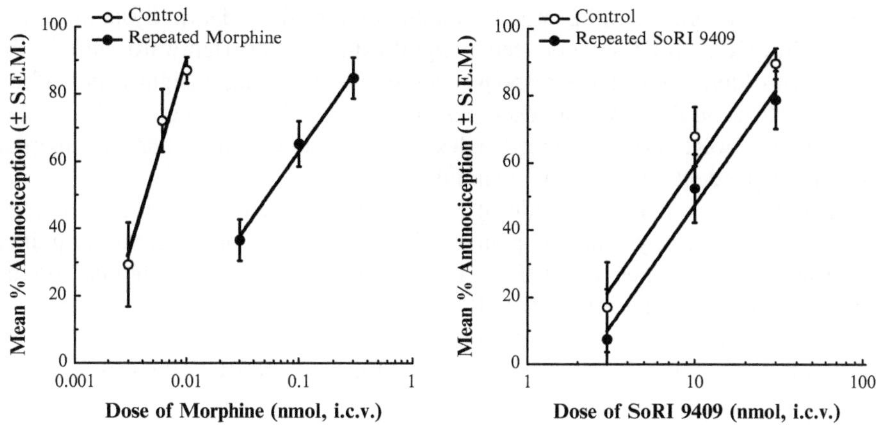

Fig. 8.2 Antinociceptive tolerance studies with morphine (*left panel*) or SoRI 9409 (*right panel*) in the acetic acid writhing assay. Mice received twice daily injections (intracerebroventricular [*i.c.v.*]) of the respective agonists (A_{90} doses) for 3 days. On the morning of day 4, complete dose-response curves were generated and compared to control responses. Repeated morphine administration resulted in a ~12.5-fold rightward shift in the dose-response curve, whereas repeated SoRI 9409 resulted in significantly less tolerance (~1.5-fold rightward shift). Data are adapted from Ananthan et al. (4) and Wells et al. (29)

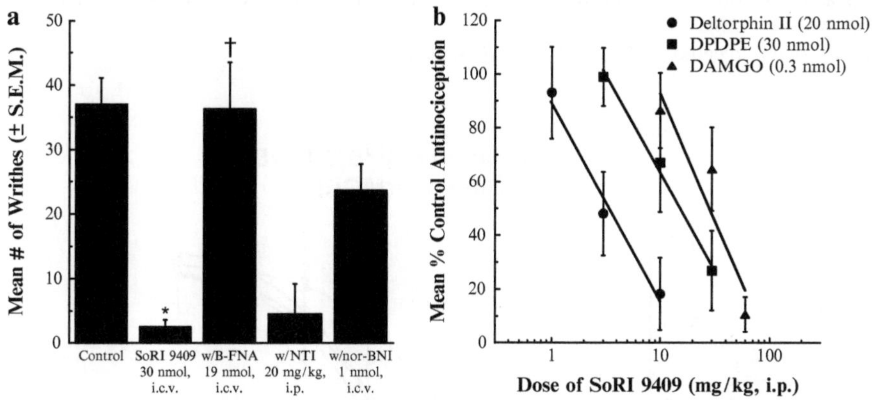

Fig. 8.3 In vivo receptor activity profile of SoRI. The antinociceptive effects of SoRI 9409 (acetic acid writhing assay) were completely blocked by pretreatment with the μ selective antagonist β-funaltrexamine (*β-FNA*), whereas the δ antagonist naltrindole (*NTI*) did not affect the antinociceptive actions of the compound (panel A). In the 55°C tail-flick assay, SoRI 9409 preferentially blocked δ-opioid receptors, whereas higher doses also blocked the μ receptor agonist [D-Ala^2, *N*-Me-Phe^4,Gly^5-ol]enkephalin (*DAMGO*) (panel B). Data are from Wells et al. (29)

antagonist actions of the compound [Fig. 8.3b and Wells et al. (29)]. SoRI 9409 preferentially blocked the antinociceptive effects of delta-opioid agonists in the 55°C tail-flick assay, though the compound was also able to block the μ agonists [D-Ala^2,*N*-Me-Phe^4,Gly^5-ol]enkephalin (DAMGO) and morphine at higher doses

(Fig. 8.3b and Xu, Partilla, and Rothman, unpublished data). Systemic SoRI 9409 (10 mg/kg, i.p.) also produced a significant 8.2-fold rightward shift in the [D-Ala[2],Glu[4]]deltorphin dose–response curve while having insignificant effects (1.5-fold shift) on the DAMGO dose–response curve (29). Wells et al. (29) further showed that SoRI 9409 produced a less severe withdrawal syndrome in mice rendered dependent on morphine than did naloxone.

Paradoxically, when the profile of SoRI 9409 was determined using the [^{35}S] GTP-γ-S binding assays, the compound failed to display agonist activity in guinea pig caudate membranes as well as in cloned cells expressing human opioid receptors (30). The lack of SoRI 9409-induced mu agonist activity prompted us to investigate its actions as an antagonist at cloned mu, delta, and kappa receptors. As reported in Table 8.2 and as shown in Fig. 8.4, SoRI 9409 was a potent

Table 8.2 Antagonist activity of NTI and SoRI 9409 on agonist-stimulated [^{35}S]-GTP-γ-S binding

	K_i (nM ± SD)			Selectivity ratio	
Compound (4)	μ[a] (MOR)	δ[b] (DOR)	κ[c] (KOR)	μ/δ	κ/δ
NTI	4.3 ± 0.5	0.03 ± 0.01	4.7 ± 3.0	143	157
SoRI 9409	8.4 ± 0.9	0.08 ± 0.01	19.3 ± 8.7	105	241

[a] Apparent functional K_i (vs 1 μM DAMGO)
[b] Apparent functional K_i (vs 200 nM SNC80)
[c] Apparent functional K_i [vs 2 μM (−)–U50,488]. Each value is the mean ± SD ($n = 3$). Table taken from Xu et al. (30)
MOR μ-opioid receptor, *NTI* naltrindole, *SD* standard deviation

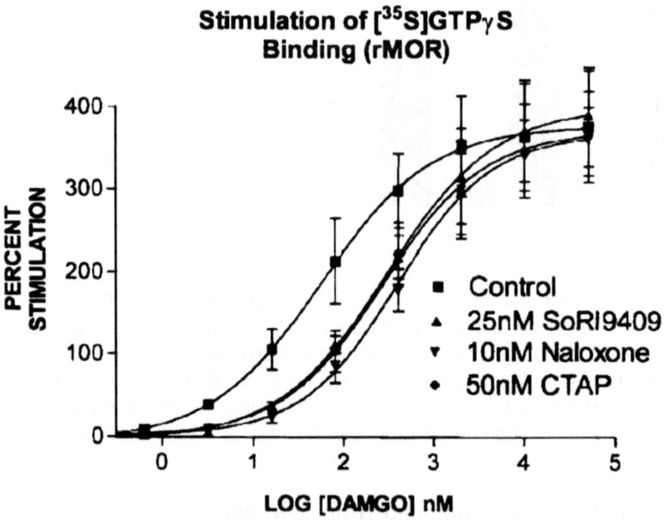

Fig. 8.4 Antagonism by SoRI 9409, naloxone, and CTAP of [^{35}S]-GTP-γ-S binding stimulated by [D-Ala[2],*N*-Me-Phe[4],Gly[5]-ol]enkephalin (*DAMGO*). DAMGO dose-response curves were generated using Chinese hamster ovary (*CHO*) cells stably expressing the human μ-opioid receptor in the absence and presence of test agents. Each value is ±SD ($n = 3$). Data are from Xu et al. (30)

mu receptor antagonist. Moreover, SoRI 9409 was a very potent delta receptor antagonist (K_i = 0.08 nM) with 105- and 241-fold selectivity ratios for mu receptors and kappa receptors, respectively. In comparison, NTI was more selective for mu receptors (143-fold) and less selective for kappa receptors (157-fold). These in vitro data clearly predict that SoRI 9409 should be a mu antagonist in vivo. Although it is possible to speculate that the in vivo analgesic action of SoRI 9409 results from indirect effects, such as active metabolites or release of opioid peptides via nonopioid mechanisms, this hypothesis is unlikely to explain its agonist effects after intracerebroventricular administration or its weak agonist effects in the GPI assay (4, 29). Alternatively, it is possible that SoRI 9409 has partial agonist actions at a splice variant of the mu-opioid receptor (16), or that SoRI 9409 produces antinociception via heterodimers of opioid receptors (13). An explanation of these paradoxical findings with SoRI 9409 remains enigmatic.

In an effort to identify compounds with mu agonist/delta antagonist activity in vitro and in vivo, we synthesized and evaluated an expanded series of pyridomorphinans derived from naloxone, oxymorphone, and hydromorphone framework (Table 8.3) (5). These efforts led to the identification of hydromorphone-derived pyridomorphinans **3** [formerly **14**] (SoRI 20411) and **4** [formerly **15**] (SoRI 20648) as compounds possessing mu agonist/delta antagonist activity in both the [^{35}S]-GTP-γ-S binding and smooth muscle functional assays (Fig. 8.1). In binding assays, both SoRI 20411 and SoRI 20648 had high affinity for the delta receptor, K_i = 4.4 nM and 3.7 nM, respectively, and much lower affinity for mu and kappa receptors. SoRI 20411 (IC_{50} = 177 nM) was more potent in the GPI assay than SoRI 20648 (IC_{50} = 724 nM), but SoRI 20648 (K_e = 5.0 nM) was more potent as a delta antagonist in the MVD assay than SoRI 20411 (K_e = 21.9 nM). In the [^{35}S]-GTP-γ-S assay, the antagonist K_i values for SoRI 20648 (K_i = 1.1 nM) and SoRI 20411 (K_i = 10.9 nM) were similar to the K_e values obtained in the MVD assay. Both SoRI 20648 (EC_{50} = 900 nM) and SoRI 20411 (EC_{50} = 225 nM) were partial mu agonists in the [^{35}S]-GTP-γ-S assay. However, only SoRI 20411 produced antinociception (A_{50} potency value of 42.8 nmol in the 55°C warm-water tail-withdrawal assay in mice). The antinociceptive effects were blocked by the μ-selective antagonist β-FNA (Fig. 8.5a). When tested in the tolerance development assays involving repeated injections of the compound for 3 days, SoRI 20411 induced an insignificant shift in the antinociceptive potency (less than 1.1-fold increase in A_{50} value), indicating very little development of tolerance. This is in contrast to morphine, which in the same paradigm produced a significant 6.4-fold shift in the A_{50} values, indicating the development of tolerance to its antinociceptive effects (Fig. 8.5b). The identification of SoRI 20411 is very significant because it demonstrates the validity of the hypothesis that opioid ligands with a mixed mu agonist/delta antagonist profile of activity may have diminished propensity to induce tolerance and, therefore, may have therapeutic advantages over mu agonist analgesics for long-term treatment of pain.

Compounds possessing delta antagonist and weak mu agonist activity have also been found in other C-ring annulated morphinans such as the pyrrolomorphinans. Among a limited number of such pyrrolomorphinans synthesized and evaluated, it was found that compound **5** [formerly **16**] (Fig. 8.1) possessing a 4-methylphenyl

Table 8.3 Binding affinities of the pyridomorphinans at the opioid δ, μ, and κ receptors in rodent brain membranes

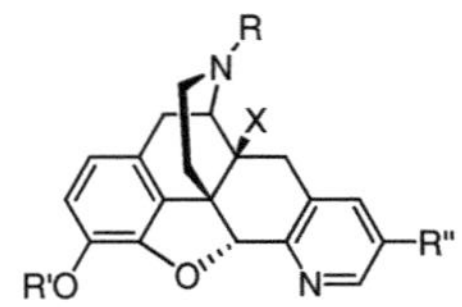

9

Compound	R	X	R′	R″	K_i (nM) ± SEM			Selectivity ratio	
					δ[a]	μ[b]	κ[c]	μ/δ	κ/δ
9a	Allyl	OH	H	4-Chlorophenyl	8.2±0.1	467±19	75±5	57	9
9b	Me	OH	H	H	18±1.4	7.9±0.2	264±18	0.4	15
9c	Me	OH	H	Phenyl	2.9±0.1	26±1.0	360±17	9	124
9d	Me	OH	H	4-Chlorophenyl	3.9±0.2	230±10	468±17	58	120
9e	Me	OH	H	4-Bromophenyl	4.0±0.3	196±4	432±18	49	108
9f	Me	H	H	H	8.0±0.8	13±0.5	66±2	2	8
9g	Me	H	H	Phenyl	1.9±0.1	24±2	81±5	13	43
9h (3)	Me	H	H	4-Chlorophenyl	4.4±0.2	148±9.5	78±13	34	18
9i	Me	H	H	4-Bromophenyl	5.0±0.6	200±11	91±6	40	18
9j	Me	H	H	3,4-Dichlorophenyl	3.7±0.1	93±4	278±7	25	75
9k (4)	Me	H	H	2,4-Dichlorophenyl	1.1±0.1	97±4	403±9	88	366
9l	CPM	H	H	4-Chlorophenyl	2.6±0.1	62±3	6.0±0.3	24	2.3
9m	Me	OH	Me	H	143±9	325±16	6397±353	2.2	45
9n	Me	OH	Me	Phenyl	34±0.6	894±19	>10,000	26	>294
9o	Me	OH	Me	4-Chlorophenyl	21±2	2052±95	>7,100	98	>338
9p	Me	OH	Me	4-Bromophenyl	23±1.3	1887±72	7366±522	82	320
9q	CPM	H	Me	4-Chlorophenyl	41±3	1974±50	539±20	48	13
SNC-80[d]					5.6±0.5	8070±930	8760±710	1440	1,560
DAMGO[d]					469±39	6.1±0.7	5820±540	0.01	12
Morphine[d]					157±11	11.0±1.0	188±20	0.07	1.2
U69593[d]					>5,000	7250±660	4.8±0.5	<1.5	<0.01
Naltrexone[d]					7.5±1.8	2.4±0.3	2.2±0.2	0.3	0.3

[a] Displacement of [^{3}H]DADLE (1.3–2.0 nM) in rat brain membranes using 100 nM DAMGO to block binding to μ sites

[b] Displacement of [^{3}H]DAMGO (1.4–3.0 nM) in rat brain membranes

[c] Displacement of [^{3}H]U69,593 (1.2–2.2 nM) in guinea pig brain membranes

[d] Data included for comparison. Table adapted from Ananthan et al. (5)

DAMGO [D-Ala^2,*N*-Me-Phe^4,Gly^5-ol]enkephalin

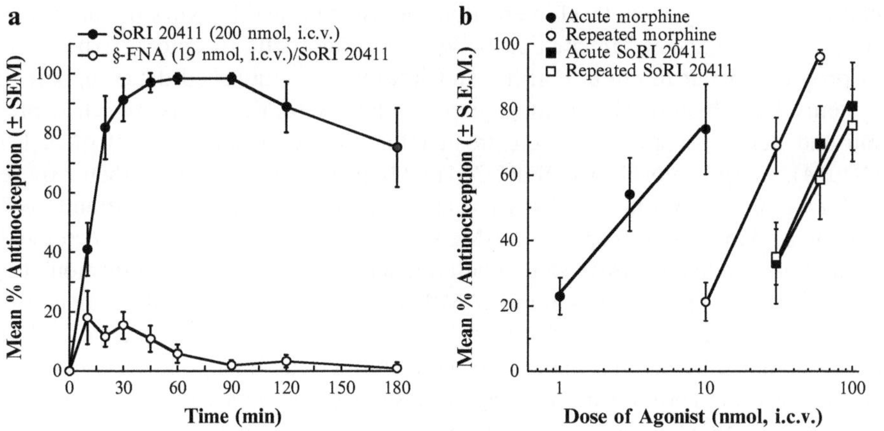

Fig. 8.5 In vivo antinociceptive data with SoRI 20411. Panel A depicts the antinociceptive time–response curve for an A_{90} dose of SoRI20411 (55°C tail-flick assay) in control mice and in mice pretreated with the μ antagonist β-funaltrexamine (*β-FNA*). Panel B represents the tolerance studies with SoRI 20411 compared to morphine. Data are regraphed from Ananthan et al. (5)

substituent on the pyrrole ring displayed delta antagonist activity with a K_e of 14.1 nM and partial mu agonist activity with an EC_{50} of 1,360 nM and an E_{max} of 34% in [^{35}S]-GTP-γ-S binding assays in Chinese hamster ovary (CHO) cells expressing human mu- and delta-opioid receptors (25).

Portoghese and coworkers have, for a long time, pursued the design of bivalent ligands to probe opioid receptor complexes (8, 17–19). The recent demonstration of the existence of receptor hetero-oligomeric complexes has spurred further interest in the design of such bivalent ligands that could potentially interact with these receptor complexes. Of particular interest among such series of bivalent ligands are the bivalent ligands **6** [formerly **17**], which possess a mu agonist and a delta antagonist pharmacophore. These bivalent ligands possess the oxymorphamine unit as the mu agonist pharmacophore and 7′-aminonaltrindole as the delta antagonist pharmacophore connected by spacers of length ranging from 19 Å to 25 Å. These compounds were evaluated in mice for acute antinociception in the tail-flick test and were found to be more potent than morphine and fully efficacious. These were also evaluated for their ability to induce tolerance and dependence. Morphine and the bivalent ligand with the shortest spacer (**5**, $n=2$) promoted the development of tolerance and dependence. The bivalent ligands with slightly longer spacers (**5**, $n=3$ and $n=4$) produced tolerance but not dependence. Ligands with the longest spacers (**5**, $n=5$, 6, and 7) did not produce tolerance or physical dependence (8). The authors interpret this effect as being due to activation of mu–delta heterodimers, pharmacological evidence of which was originally reported in the 1980s (20, 27).

Currently, it is not known if the reduced development of tolerance and dependence produced by chronic administration of mixed mu agonist/delta antagonist compounds results from interactions with distinct and noninteracting mu and delta receptors (systems level interaction) or, as suggested by work of Daniels (8), from a molecular-level interaction between mu and delta receptors. Experiments in progress in our lab (Xu, Partilla, and Rothman, unpublished data) support the systems level hypothesis. In these experiments, SH-SY5Y cells, which express mu and delta receptors (2), were treated for 20 h with morphine (10 μM), NTI (10 μM), morphine/NTI, and SoRI 20411 (10 μM). The cells were then exposed to forskolin (10 μM) in the absence and presence of 10 μM naloxone and cyclic adenosine-3′,5′-monophosphate (cAMP) levels were measured. An increase in forskolin-stimulated cAMP accumulation is termed cAMP "super-activation" (28) and reflects the upregulation of the cAMP system that can occur following chronic morphine administration. A decrease in the level of forskolin-stimulated cAMP accumulation reflects the presence of constitutively active opioid receptors (22). In this case the addition of an antagonist, such as naloxone, results in markedly increased levels of cAMP, termed a cAMP "overshoot," which may be a cellular marker for dependence. In our experiment (Fig. 8.6), we observed that in the SH-SY5Y cells chronic morphine did not produce either a cAMP overshoot or a super-activation. However, treatment of the cells with SoRI 20411 generated constitutively active opioid receptors and a cAMP overshoot. Although preliminary,

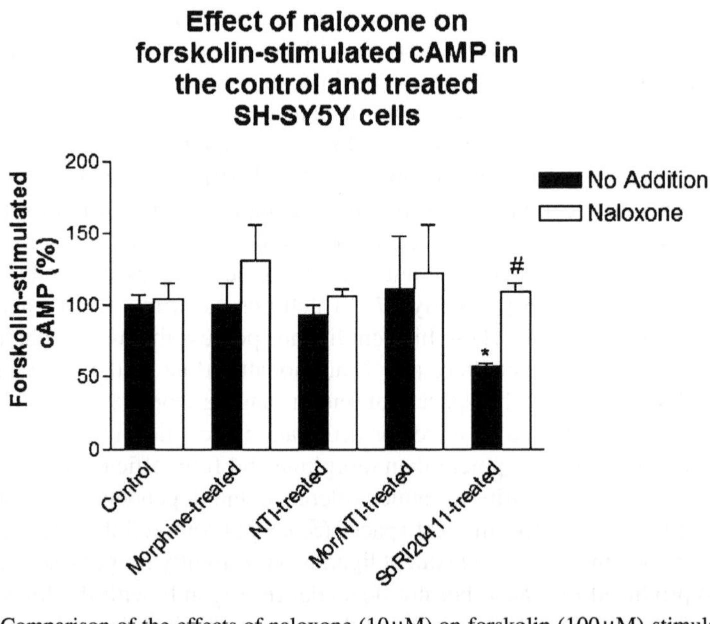

Fig. 8.6 Comparison of the effects of naloxone (10 μM) on forskolin (100 μM)-stimulated cyclic adenosine-3′,5′-monophosphate (*cAMP*) accumulation in the control or pretreated SH-SY5Y cells. Cells were treated for 20 h with morphine (1 μM), naltrindole (*NTI*) (0.1 μM), morphine+NTI, and SoRI 20411 (1 μM). The cells were then exposed to forskolin (10 μM) in the absence and presence of naloxone (10 μM) and cAMP levels were measured. Results are presented as mean ± SEM ($n = 2$). *$p < 0.05$ when compared with control cells; **$p < 0.05$ when compared with no addition group (two-tailed Student's *t*-test). From Xu, Partilla, and Rothman, unpublished data

these results suggest that it will be important to evaluate the actions of mixed mu agonists/delta antagonists in cellular models of tolerance and dependence to complement work being done in whole animals.

8.4 Conclusions

The development of potent opioid analgesics devoid of the limiting side effects has been the goal of considerable research efforts. Recent studies using mixed mu agonist/delta antagonist ligands have provided convincing evidence that there could be clear therapeutic advantages in these agents as compared to mu agonists. Recent successes in the identification of peptide and nonpeptide ligands possessing mixed mu agonist/delta antagonist activities, and the encouraging results obtained in studies with these ligands, is an exciting development in opioid drug discovery. It is likely that the pursuit of this new approach will lead to novel analgesics superior to those currently available for the treatment of pain.

Acknowledgments The authors acknowledge the generous support of the National Institute on Drug Abuse (DA008883), the NIDA Intramural Research Program, as well as the NIDA Drug Supply Program.

References

1. Abdelhamid, EE, Sultana, M, Portoghese, PS, Takemori, AE, Selective blockage of delta opioid receptors prevents development of morphine tolerance and dependence in mice, J Pharmacol Exp Ther, (1991) 258 299–303.
2. Alt, A, Clark, MJ, Woods, JH, Traynor, JR, Mu and delta opioid receptors activate the same G proteins in human neuroblastoma SH-SY5Y cells, Br J Pharmacol, (2002) 135 217–225.
3. Ananthan, S, Johnson, CA, Carter, RL, Clayton, SD, Rice, KC, Xu, H, Davis, P, Porreca, F, Rothman, RB, Synthesis, opioid receptor binding, and bioassay of naltrindole analogues substituted in the indolic benzene moiety, J Med Chem, (1998) 41 2872–2881.
4. Ananthan, S, Kezar III, HS, Carter, RL, Saini, SK, Rice, KC, Wells, JL, Davis, P, Xu, H, Bilsky, EJ, Porreca, F, Rothman, RB, Synthesis, opioid receptor binding, and biological activities of naltrexone-derived pyrido- and pyrimidomorphinans, J Med Chem, (1999) 42 3527–3538.
5. Ananthan, S, Khare, NK, Saini, SK, Seitz, LE, Bartlett, JL, Davis, P, Dersch, CM, Porreca, F, Rothman, RB, Bilsky, EJ, Identification of opioid ligands possessing mixed mu agonist/delta antagonist activity among pyridomorphinans derived from naloxone, oxymorphone, and hydromorphone, J Med Chem, (2004) 47 1400–1412.
6. Cicero, TJ, Inciardi, JA, Munoz, A, Trends in abuse of Oxycontin and other opioid analgesics in the United States: 2002–2004, J Pain, (2005) 6 662–672.
7. Compton, WM, Volkow, ND, Abuse of prescription drugs and the risk of addiction, Drug Alcohol Depend, (2006) 83 Suppl. 1 S4–S7.
8. Daniels, DJ, Lenard, NR, Etienne, CL, Law, PY, Roerig, SC, Portoghese, PS, Opioid-induced tolerance and dependence in mice is modulated by the distance between pharmacophores in a bivalent ligand series, Proc Natl Acad Sci USA, (2005) 102 19208–19213.

9. Ellison, NM, Opioid analgesics for cancer pain: toxicities and their treatments. In R. B. Pratt (Ed.), Cancer Pain, Lippincott, Philadelphia, PA, 1993.
10. Foxx-Orenstein, AE, Jin, JG, Grider, JR, 5-HT4 receptor agonists and delta-opioid receptor antagonists act synergistically to stimulate colonic propulsion, Am J Physiol, (1998) 275 G979–G983.
11. Freye, E, Latasch, L, Portoghese, PS, The delta receptor is involved in sufentanil-induced respiratory depression – opioid subreceptors mediate different effects, Eur J Anaesthesiol, (1992) 9 457–462.
12. Fundytus, ME, Schiller, PW, Shapiro, M, Weltrowska, G, Coderre, TJ, Attenuation of morphine tolerance and dependence with the highly selective delta-opioid receptor antagonist TIPP[psi], Eur J Pharmacol, (1995) 286 105–108.
13. Gomes, I, Jordan, BA, Gupta, A, Trapaidze, N, Nagy, V, Devi, LA, Heterodimerization of mu and delta opioid receptors: a role in opiate synergy, J Neurosci, (2000) 20 RC110.
14. Hepburn, MJ, Little, PJ, Gingras, J, Kuhn, CM, Differential effects of naltrindole on morphine-induced tolerance and physical dependence in rats, J Pharmacol Exp Ther, (1997) 281 1350–1356.
15. Kest, B, Lee, CE, McLemore, GL, Inturrisi, CE, An antisense oligodeoxynucleotide to the delta opioid receptor (DOR-1) inhibits morphine tolerance and acute dependence in mice, Brain Res Bull, (1996) 39 185–188.
16. Pasternak, GW, Multiple opiate receptors: deja vu all over again, Neuropharmacology, (2004) 47 Suppl. 1 312–323.
17. Portoghese, PS, Bivalent ligands and the message-address concept in the design of selective opioid receptor antagonists, Trends Pharmacol Sci, (1989) 10 230–235.
18. Portoghese, PS, Edward E, Smissman-Bristol-Myers Squibb Award Address, The role of concepts in structure-activity relationship studies of opioid ligands, J Med Chem, (1992) 35 1927–1937.
19. Portoghese, PS, From models to molecules: opioid receptor dimers, bivalent ligands, and selective opioid receptor probes, J Med Chem, (2001) 44 2259–2269.
20. Rothman, RB, Westfall, TC, Allosteric coupling between morphine and enkephalin receptors in vitro, Mol Pharmacol, (1982) 21 548–557.
21. Roy, S, Guo, X, Kelschenbach, J, Liu, Y, Loh, HH, In vivo activation of a mutant mu-opioid receptor by naltrexone produces a potent analgesic effect but no tolerance: role of mu-receptor activation and delta-receptor blockade in morphine tolerance, J Neurosci, (2005) 25 3229–3233.
22. Sadee, W, Wang, D, Bilsky, EJ, Basal opioid receptor activity, neutral antagonists, and therapeutic opportunities, Life Sci, (2005) 76 1427–1437.
23. Schiller, PW, Fundytus, ME, Merovitz, L, Weltrowska, G, Nguyen, TM, Lemieux, C, Chung, NN, Coderre, TJ, The opioid mu agonist/delta antagonist DIPP-NH(2)[Psi] produces a potent analgesic effect, no physical dependence, and less tolerance than morphine in rats, J Med Chem, (1999) 42 3520–3526.
24. Schmidt, R, Vogel, D, Mrestani-Klaus, C, Brandt, W, Neubert, K, Chung, NN, Lemieux, C, Schiller, PW, Cyclic beta-casomorphin analogues with mixed mu agonist/delta antagonist properties: synthesis, pharmacological characterization, and conformational aspects, J Med Chem, (1994) 37 1136–1144.
25. Srivastava, SK, Husbands, SM, Aceto, MD, Miller, CN, Traynor, JR, Lewis, JW, 4′-Arylpyrrolomorphinans: effect of a pyrrolo-N-benzyl substituent in enhancing delta-opioid antagonist activity, J Med Chem, (2002) 45 537–540.
26. Suzuki, T, Ikeda, H, Tsuji, M, Misawa, M, Narita, M, Tseng, LF, Antisense oligodeoxynucleotide to delta opioid receptors attenuates morphine dependence in mice, Life Sci, (1997) 61 PL 165–170.
27. Vaught, JL, Rothman, RB, Westfall, TC, Mu and delta receptors: their role in analgesia and in the differential effects of opioid peptides on analgesia, Life Sci, (1982) 30 1443–1455.
28. Waldhoer, M, Bartlett, SE, Whistler, JL, Opioid receptors, Annu Rev Biochem, (2004) 73 953–990.

29. Wells, JL, Bartlett, JL, Ananthan, S, Bilsky, EJ, In vivo pharmacological characterization of SoRI 9409, a nonpeptidic opioid mu agonist/delta antagonist that produces limited antinociceptive tolerance and attenuates morphine physical dependence, J Pharmacol Exp Ther, (2001) 297 597–605.
30. Xu, H, Lu, YF, Rice, KC, Ananthan, S, Rothman, RB, SoRI 9409, a non-peptide opioid mu receptor agonist/delta receptor antagonist, fails to stimulate [^{35}S]-GTP-gamma-S binding at cloned opioid receptors, Brain Res Bull, (2001) 55 507–511.
31. Zhu, Y, King, MA, Schuller, AG, Nitsche, JF, Reidl, M, Elde, RP, Unterwald, E, Pasternak, GW, Pintar, JE, Retention of supraspinal delta-like analgesia and loss of morphine tolerance in delta opioid receptor knockout mice, Neuron, (1999) 24 243–252.

Chapter 9
Experimental Utility and Clinical Potential of Irreversible Opioid Antagonists

Ellen A. Walker and Sandra D. Comer

Abstract In opioid pharmacology, irreversible, insurmountable antagonists have been critical experimental tools to characterize μ-opioid receptors and receptor function with respect to such important concepts of receptor theory as spare receptors, affinity, and efficacy. In the present chapter, we present the specific pharmacological characteristics of four insurmountable antagonists with primary actions at μ-opioid receptors: β-chlornaltrexamine (β-CNA), β-funaltrexamine (β-FNA), buprenorphine, and clocinnamox. After alkylation or long-lasting blockade, fewer receptors are available for agonist interaction, and an agonist may produce a reduced maximum effect. After insurmountable antagonist administration, the method of partial irreversible blockade can be applied to estimate the apparent affinity constant for an agonist (K_A), relative efficacy estimates for agonists, and the fraction of receptors remaining for agonist interaction after alkylation (*o*). Insurmountable antagonists have been exploited to uncover how compounds bind within receptors, to help understand such phenomena as tolerance and dependence, and to determine the rate of turnover of μ-opioid receptors in different species. Probably the most frequent use of opioid insurmountable antagonists has been the estimate of agonist efficacy values with the goal of understanding the relationship of agonist efficacy to functional outcomes. More recently, investigators in clinical experimental pharmacology are using these tools, principles, and results generated from preclinical laboratory animal experiments to understand the role of agonist relative efficacy to behavioral data collected in humans. The development of tools that allow the quantitative assessment of multiple dependent measures (analgesia, reinforcing effects, and respiratory suppression) within and between different medications clearly has important clinical applications.

Keywords: β-Funaltrexamine; Buprenorphine; Clocinnamox; Intrinsic efficacy; μ-Opioid receptor

---

E.A. Walker (✉) and S.D. Comer
Department of Pharmaceutical Sciences, Temple University School of Pharmacy,
3307 North Broad Street, Philadelphia, PA 19140
e-mail: ellen.walker@temple.edu

R. Dean et al. (eds.), *Opiate Receptors and Antagonists*,

9.1 Introduction

Irreversible antagonists are indispensable experimental tools in pharmacology for characterizing receptors and receptor function. In addition, irreversible antagonists have been used to elucidate such important concepts of receptor theory as spare receptors, affinity, and efficacy (1–3). By definition, irreversible antagonists bind covalently and inactivate receptors. For example, β-haloalkylamines form a reactive aziridinium ion that can alkylate proteins easily (1). Irreversible antagonists are difficult to wash off the receptors with drug-free solution in organ-bath assays and theoretically prevent agonist action until new receptors are synthesized. The longer the irreversible antagonist is in contact with the tissue or the greater the dose of irreversible antagonist, the greater the magnitude of antagonism (4). Commonly, a selective irreversible antagonist can simply be used to block the effects of an endogenous or exogenous agonist to investigate receptor selectivity (5–7). Often irreversible antagonists are used to eliminate one receptor from action for the duration of an experiment so that investigators can study another receptor with an agonist that has affinities for multiple receptors (8–10).

The functional consequence of administering an irreversible antagonist is a decreased maximum effect for agonists. This decreased maximum effect for agonists in the presence of an irreversible antagonist is referred to as insurmountable antagonism. Insurmountable antagonism is the defining pharmacological characteristic that distinguishes irreversible antagonists from reversible, surmountable antagonists. However, low doses of irreversible antagonists could produce surmountable antagonism in tissues that are efficiently coupled because in these tissues small proportions of receptors are sufficient to produce a maximal response for agonists. Therefore, to functionally characterize an antagonist as irreversible, a range of irreversible antagonist concentrations or doses must be tested in a given assay (4). Antagonists that do not alkylate receptors also produce insurmountable antagonism by binding tightly to receptors and dissociating very slowly from the receptor. This is the difference between "true" irreversibility and "essentially" irreversible kinetics for an antagonist. Nevertheless, if an insurmountable or "pseudoirreversible" antagonist acts with essentially irreversible kinetics, receptors are still unavailable for agonist interaction within the time constraints of the assay. In general, in this chapter we will refer to all antagonists that alkylate the receptors or produce "essentially" irreversible antagonism as insurmountable antagonists. We will only distinguish between "true" irreversible antagonists and "essentially" irreversible antagonists when necessary.

In the present era of opioid pharmacology, a number of tools exist to characterize receptor function and to study such concepts as affinity and efficacy. One could argue that in the advent of radioligand-binding assays for determining affinity and GTPγS-binding assays for quantifying efficacy (11) in vivo estimates of affinity and efficacy are passé. True, K_A or affinity estimates determined in vivo are not of sufficient accuracy to quantify subtle difference in K_A values with high confidence. However, it is useful from the point of relative classification and to quantify the contributions of affinity to agonist potency and relative contributions of affinity versus efficacy in an entirely functional organism. In this chapter, we will outline the insurmountable antagonists available for studying μ-opioid receptors. Furthermore, we will discuss how these insurmountable antagonists have been exploited to uncover how compounds bind within receptors to determine affinity and efficacy estimates, to help us understand such phenomena as tolerance and dependence in our functional assays, and to determine the rate of turnover of μ-opioid receptors in different species. With this information in hand, we will also explain how the clinical field is using these principles and results from preclinical laboratory animal experiments to understand the same questions in humans and how they may be exploited for use in clinical settings.

9.2 Insurmountable Antagonists Available for μ-Opioid Receptors

The availability of insurmountable antagonists for μ-opioid receptors was a huge advantage in the early studies of receptor characterization, agonist efficacy, and receptor functionality in opioid pharmacology. The insurmountable compounds are introduced here but their experimental utility will be described in detail further on in the chapter (Fig. 9.1).

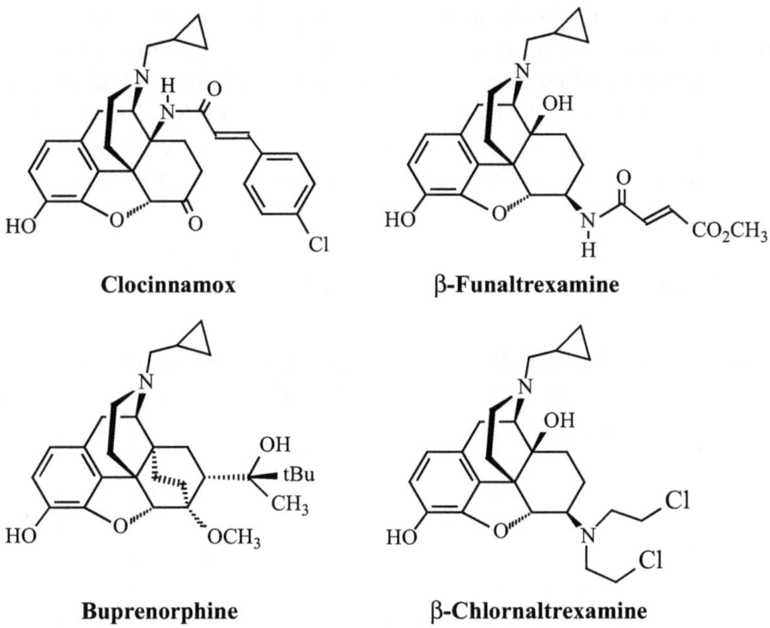

Fig. 9.1 Structures of β-funaltrexamine, β-chlornaltrexamine, clocinnamox, and buprenorphine

9.2.1 *β-Chlornaltrexamine*

The first irreversible antagonist available for alkylating and inactivating μ-, κ-, and δ-opioid receptors was the 6-bis(2-chloroethyl)amine derivative of naltrexone, β-chlornaltrexamine (β-CNA) (12, 13). β-CNA inhibits [^{3}H]naloxone in rat brain homogenates, but this inhibition is resistant to repeated washings. Moreover, β-CNA effects on opioid receptor binding can be prevented by naloxone pretreatment to protect opioid receptors. In smooth muscle functional assays (guinea-pig ileum and mouse vas deferens preparations), β-CNA insurmountably antagonizes the effects of opioid agonists and produces rightward and downward shifts in agonist dose–response curves (13–16). Although poor bioavailability limited the use of β-CNA in vivo, intracerebroventricular (i.c.v.) administration of β-CNA blocked the effects of morphine in mice for at least 3 days (16).

9.2.2 *β-Funaltrexamine*

Shortly after the introduction of β-CNA, β-funaltrexamine (β-FNA) was introduced (17). β-FNA decreases the number of binding sites, B_{max} of [^{3}H]DAMGO, [^{3}H] naltrexone, and [^{3}H morphine binding (18, 19). β-FNA binds to all opioid receptors but reversibly only to κ receptors. At low concentrations, β-FNA binds irreversibly to μ-opioid receptors with high specificity (20–22). β-FNA administered centrally suppresses the maximum analgesic effects of morphine (23) and when administered systemically produces a long-lasting antagonism of the effects of opioid agonists in mice (17), rats (24), and monkeys (25). An experimental limitation of using β-FNA in vivo is that within the first 24 h after administration, β-FNA is a κ agonist and will produce reversible antagonism of μ opioids (19, 26, 27). Therefore, to reduce maximum effect for μ agonists, β-FNA must be administered 24 h prior to testing.

9.2.3 *Buprenorphine*

Around the time β-CNA and β-FNA were being developed and synthesized, buprenorphine was being used in early in vivo studies to estimate K_A and efficacy values for morphine and ethylketocyclazocine in antinociception and gastrointestinal (GI) transit assays (28–30). Although buprenorphine does not alkylate μ-opioid receptors (31–33), buprenorphine does have an unusually long duration of action suggesting a slow dissociation rate from opioid receptors (34–38). Indeed, the rate of dissociation of buprenorphine in binding experiments is slow despite the addition of sodium ions or competing drugs (39), yet see (40). Generally, competitive antagonists can prevent but not reverse the agonist effects of buprenorphine (36, 41, 42) further supporting the notion that buprenorphine could be used as a pseudoirreversible ligand.

Buprenorphine is especially interesting in vivo for a number of reasons. First, buprenorphine produces an U-shaped dose–response curve in rodents, especially in antinociceptive assays (43). More recently, investigators have suggested that this unusual antinociceptive effect is due to buprenorphine's partial agonist activity at ORL1 receptors (44, 45). In assays with lower stimulus intensity, buprenorphine can have agonist effects that last a long time yet at higher stimulus intensities, the same doses will block the effects of higher efficacy opioids (37, 46–48). Buprenorphine in lower doses appears to be reversible and in combination with morphine, oxycodone, hydromorphone, and fentanyl is either additive or supra-additive (49).

9.2.4 Clocinnamox

The cinnamoylamino derivative of naltrexone, clocinnamox, was described as a long-lasting antagonist with little to no agonist effects in vivo (50, 51). In mouse vas deferens, clocinnamox displaces [^{3}H]etorphine and interacts with μ, κ, and δ receptors (51, 52). In other radioligand-binding studies, clocinnamox decreases B_{max} of [^{3}H]DAMGO and [^{3}H]naltrexone without changing affinity (53–55). Clocinnamox displays 20–30-fold μ receptor selectivity over δ and κ receptors in radioligand-binding assays (51, 56, 57). Clocinnamox inhibition of μ receptors is not reversed yet clocinnamox inhibition of δ and κ receptors is time-dependently reversed (56). Clocinnamox does not affect the affinity or density of [^{3}H]U69,593 or [^{3}H]DPDPE binding (54). Although clocinnamox has a cinnamoylamino substituent that can serve as a Michael acceptor for irreversible antagonism, a portion of the binding is still reversible. Time-course studies of [^{3}H]clocinnamox binding indicate that half of the clocinnamox dissociates with a $T_{1/2}$ of 16 min and the other half with a $T_{1/2}$ of 11 h (57). These binding characteristics are similar to data collected with [^{3}H]β-FNA. Most of [^{3}H]β-FNA binding dissociates with a $T_{1/2}$ of 1 min and thereafter, a small portion goes on to form irreversible binding complexes (21). Radioligand binding of clocinnamox parallels the in vivo antagonism of morphine's antinociceptive effects in mice and rats (54, 55).

Recently, clocinnamox was used to examine the binding nature of another insurmountable ligand, buprenorphine (49). In this study, high doses of buprenorphine were difficult to reverse with naloxone and naltrexone; however, clocinnamox time-dependently reversed the antinociceptive effect of buprenorphine in mice whether administered 5 or 60 min after buprenorphine. These results demonstrate that the binding of buprenorphine is pseudoirreversible and can be overwhelmed by the initial reversible and eventual long-lasting effects of clocinnamox. This study underscores the importance of time of onset and duration of action when using insurmountable antagonists as experimental tools.

9.2.5 Others

Other compounds have been designed and synthesized, although fewer studies have exploited these compounds to study μ-opioid receptor. *N*-cyclopropylmethylnor-5β-methyl-14β-(*p*-nitrocinnamoylamino)-7,8-dihydromorphinone (*N*-CPM-MET-CAMO) decreases in vitro binding of [^{3}H]DAMGO and decreases the maximum antinociceptive effects of μ opioids (58). The cinnamoylaminocodeinone congener of clocinnamox is a codeinone derivative of clocinnamox called methoclocinnamox. Methoclocinnamox is partially *O*-demethylated to clocinnamox in human liver homogenates (51, 59). In functional assays, methoclocinnamox is initially a partial agonist but then blocks opioid antinociception and self-administration for hours (59). Methoclocinnamox appears to have a reversible interaction with κ and δ receptors and perhaps reversible interactions with μ-opioid receptors based on partial susceptibility to washout (56). Therefore, the initial partial agonist effects of methoclocinnamox are probably reversible and then after *O*-demethylation to clocinnamox, a longer-lasting antagonism without agonist activity is observed (60, 61).

9.3 Experimental Utility

9.3.1 In Vitro Binding Parameters

In vitro, receptor structure can be elucidated with ligands that form covalent bonds with receptors. These irreversible ligands can be used to determine the molecular mass of the receptor without prior purification and to examine the nature of carbohydrate moieties. Using these ligands as tools, a binding domain can be precisely determined by amino acid sequences of labeled fragments and/or peptide mapping. Because β-FNA is a rigid molecule, it was used for the purpose of molecular modeling of interactions between morphinans and the μ receptor (62, 63). For example, Chen et al. (63) demonstrated that [^{3}H]β-FNA is incorporated into the rat μ-opioid receptor in a specific region of amino acids using peptide mapping of labeled receptor fragments. These authors found that the region from the middle of the third intracellular loop to the C-terminus of the μ receptor is required for β-FNA irreversible binding (62). Also, by comparing a reversible ligand, [^{3}H]diprenorphine, to [^{3}H]β-FNA, IC_{50} values for the reversible ligand were determined to be approximately twofold times the K_i values. These data suggest that diprenorphine and β-FNA may have different reversible binding kinetics (63).

9.3.2 Agonist Affinity and Efficacy Estimates

Early organ-bath studies with irreversible antagonists were integral for determining affinity and efficacy estimates for agonists at a time when radioligand-binding assays were in their infancy. Using multiple concentrations of irreversible antagonists, the affinity constant for an agonist (K_A) could be estimated using the method of partial irreversible blockade. This method requires that an insurmountable or irreversible antagonist blocks a fraction of the receptor population activated by the agonist. After alkylation, fewer receptors are available for agonist interaction and a reduced effect can be observed for an agonist. The K_A value for the agonist is determined by comparing equiactive concentrations of an agonist administered alone and in the presence of an insurmountable antagonist. The reciprocal of these concentrations are plotted on a double reciprocal plot, and the intercept and the slope of this regression line can be used to estimate the agonist K_A and the fraction of receptors remaining for agonist interaction (q) (64). In one of the first papers to describe this technique, dibenamine, an alkylating compound for muscarinic receptors, was used to obtain K_A values for a series of muscarinic agonists such as acetylcholine, methacholine, and pilocarpine in the rat fundus muscle (65).

Theoretically, any depression of the agonist maximum effect should be useful for estimating K_A. Practically, to estimate agonist affinity using irreversible blockade, a reasonably high fraction of the receptor population needs to be inactivated and the maximal response to the agonist depressed. More confident estimates are made when the maximum effect is depressed below 50% (4). The influence of error on the double reciprocal plot can be reduced by using more recent equations and methods for affinity and efficacy estimates such as the operational model of drug agonism (66–68). A key feature of the operational model is the term τ which is a dimensionless proportionality factor that can relate receptor occupancy and receptor stimulus. τ is analogous to Furchgott's efficacy term, since it is a property of the tissue, the assay system, and the receptor system (4, 69). The fraction of receptors available for agonist interaction (q value) is calculated by dividing the τ value obtained after inactivation of the receptors with the insurmountable antagonist by the τ value obtained under control conditions [see, (70)]. Importantly, these in vivo estimates for affinity, efficacy, and q values can be related to more biochemical estimates in vitro. For example, the q values obtained in mouse antinociception experiments were highly correlated to the B_{max} values determined by ex vivo [^{3}H]DAMGO and [^{3}H]naltrexone binding after clocinnamox administration. The similarity of these in vivo and ex vivo estimates of remaining receptors supports the notion that receptor population changes can be investigated with reasonable confidence in the quantitative measurements (57). Probably, the most frequent use of opioid insurmountable antagonists has been the estimate of agonist affinity and efficacy values with the goal of understanding the relationship of these values to agonist action. A secondary goal of these studies is to understand the relationship among in vivo assays and the correlation of the results obtained in in vivo with in vitro assays.

9.3.2.1 Agonist Affinity

The first studies to take advantage of insurmountable antagonism and quantify affinity estimates in vivo were performed with buprenorphine (30). Morphine and ethylketocyclazocine were administered after the agonist effects of buprenorphine were gone, and then equiactive concentrations of morphine in the absence and presence of buprenorphine were determined. Using the method of partial irreversible blockade (Furchgott), K_A estimates were determined for morphine using double reciprocal plots. K_A values were determined for morphine and ethylketocyclazocine in the rat tail-flick assay and GI transit assay. While the K_A values were similar for morphine in antinociceptive assays (but not GI, Table 9.1), the K_A values for ethylketocyclazocine were much smaller in the antinociception assay than in the GI transit assay suggesting that two receptors may be involved in producing the two effects of ethylketocyclazocine (29, 30, 71). In the GI transit assay, morphine's K_A value was slightly lower suggesting that peripheral opioid receptors might be different (29).

Since these initial studies with buprenorphine, affinity estimates for opioid agonists in a variety of behavioral assays have been determined using buprenorphine, β-FNA, and clocinnamox. These studies have used the traditional double reciprocal plot and the operational model of drug agonism and compared the estimates determined using these different methods. The affinity estimates for morphine in these studies are compared across species and assays (Table 9.1). Apparent affinity estimates for morphine have an approximate tenfold range across the assays. However, the affinity of morphine estimated in vivo across mammals appears similar ranging from 18 to78 mg/kg in all assays except the GI transit test (29).

Table 9.1 Comparison of affinity estimates for morphine using insurmountable antagonists in a variety of in vivo assays[a]

Assay	Insurmountable antagonist	Species	Apparent K_A value[b] (mg/kg)	Reference
Antinociception				
Warm-water, tail-withdrawal	Buprenorphine	Rats	25	(30)
Warm-water, tail-withdrawal	Buprenorphine	Rats	22	(71)
Warm-water, tail-withdrawal	Buprenorphine	Rhesus monkeys	60	(37)
Warm-water, tail-withdrawal	Clocinnamox	Rhesus monkeys	22	(72)
Warm-water, tail-withdrawal	Clocinnamox	Rats	50	(73)
Warm-water, tail-withdrawal	β-FNA	Rats	56	(74)[c]
Warm-water, tail-withdrawal	Clocinnamox	Mice	29	(57)
Shock titration	Clocinnamox	Squirrel monkeys	49	(75)
Radiant tail-flick	Clocinnamox	Mice	78	(76)
GI transit	Buprenorphine		7.7	(29)
Operant behavior				
Drug discrimination	Clocinnamox	Rats	18	(77)[c]
Drug discrimination	β-FNA	Pigeons	25	(78)
Drug discrimination	Clocinnamox	Pigeons	10	(78)
Rate-decreasing effects	Clocinnamox	Rats	34	(77)[c]
Rate-decreasing effects	β-FNA	Rats	22	(74)[c]
Self-administration	Buprenorphine	Humans	50	(79)[d]

[a]Updated and modified from Walker et al. (37)
[b]Variance is not reported because the format differs across studies
[c]Value was determined from an original data set but affinity values are not published
[d]Agonist was heroin
β-FNA β-funaltrexamine, *GI* gastrointestinal

Other investigators have used clocinnamox to determine the degree to which efficacy (reflecting differences in receptor reserve) or functional affinity for receptors contributes to potency differences among a group of agonists. In these studies, the major determinant of the antinociception ED_{50} value for morphine, fentanyl, NIH 10741, and etonitazene in mice was the in vivo affinity constant of the agonist as opposed to the in vivo efficacy estimate (57). Although in vivo agonist affinity estimates are informative and should be related to the dose–response curves in some meaningful way, these values are mostly useful as an internal check within an experiment in an era of radioligand-binding assays.

9.3.2.2 Antagonist Affinities

Generally, quantitative in vivo estimates of antagonist potencies are determined through Schild regression analysis to determine apparent pA_2 values (9, 80–83). However, the time-dependent nature of irreversible antagonism indicates a lack of thermodynamic equilibrium and lack of competitive, reversible antagonism which violates the assumptions of the Schild equation (84, 85). Although a pseudoirreversible antagonist would eventually come to true equilibrium, it would be impractical within the time constraints of most experiments with most agonists to measure pseudoirreversible antagonist affinity. Nevertheless, antagonist affinity (K_B) values can be estimated using different equations for such pseudoirreversible antagonists as buprenorphine. Assuming the conditions of hemiequilibrium, estimates for these types of antagonists can be estimated from the double reciprocal regression of 1/[A] against 1/[A′] using the equation $K_B = [B]/(\text{slope} - 1)$. In vivo affinity estimates for buprenorphine as an antagonist were similar in the rhesus monkey (0.15 mg/kg) (37) and rat (0.11 mg/kg) (Walker and Young, unpublished observations) warm-water, tail-withdrawal procedures.

9.3.2.3 Measures of Agonist Efficacy

Agonist efficacy is crucial for drug classification. The definitive measure of agonist efficacy is a functional assay. Tools such as competitive antagonists and insurmountable antagonists are useful to determine receptor selectivity and estimate relative agonist efficacy. High- and low-efficacy agonists are differentially sensitive to irreversible antagonism and this notion forms the basis of agonist classification. Presumably, high-efficacy agonists require fewer receptors to produce an effect whereas lower-efficacy agonists require a higher fraction of the available receptor population to produce an effect. Investigators can contrast the magnitude of irreversible antagonism across a series of opioid agonists to estimate the relative efficacy of the agonists. Although the initial purpose of early studies with β-FNA was to evaluate receptor selectivities for a series of μ and κ agonists, these studies also demonstrated relative efficacy differences among opioid agonists in guinea-pig ileum, mouse vas deferens, and rodent antinociceptive assays (5, 24, 86).

For example, 24 h pretreatment of β-FNA produced about a tenfold shift for higher efficacy agonists fentanyl, l-methadone, and morphine and a 50- to 210-fold shift for lower efficacy agonists nalorphine, cyclazocine, buprenorphine, butorphanol, and nalbuphine (5). Therefore, the magnitude of β-FNA antagonism correlated with the relative efficacy differences for these agonists and not the receptor selectivities.

Researchers use insurmountable inactivation of the receptor population to obtain estimates of agonist efficacy and thus an estimate of the receptor reserve of the system under investigation. For example, the agonists buprenorphine, GPA 1657, morphine, etonitazene, and etorphine all produced dose-dependent antinociception and comparable maximum effects in a warm-water, tail-withdrawal assay in rats. However, these agonists were differentially sensitive to antagonism by clocinnamox. A low dose of 3.2 mg/kg clocinnamox flattened the dose–response curve for buprenorphine and GPA 1657, but produced only a twofold rightward shift in the dose–response curve for morphine without reducing the maximum effect. A higher dose of 10 mg/kg clocinnamox flattened the morphine dose–response curve, but produced only 14- and 4.8-fold rightward shift in the etonitazene and etorphine dose–response curve without reducing their maximum effects. These data suggest that buprenorphine and GPA 1657 may require a larger proportion of the receptor population than morphine, which may require a larger proportion of the receptor population than etonitazene and etorphine to produce antinociception (73). Furthermore, these authors obtained the same rank order of relative efficacy for the five agonists after chronic treatment with etonitazene, morphine, or buprenorphine to rats (87). To compare agonists more quantitatively according to efficacy, the percentage of receptors that remain after administration of a given dose of insurmountable antagonist (q) is calculated. For example, from the data described above, doses of 1, 3.2, and 10 mg/kg clocinnamox eliminate ~48%, 64%, and 94% of the μ-opioid receptor population, respectively. From these estimates of q values, we can compare the relative efficacy requirements for opioid agonists in this assay. Therefore, if 94% of the μ-opioid receptors are unavailable, morphine can no longer produce antinociception in the rat warm-water, tail-withdrawal assay (see Table 9.2). However, etonitazene and etorphine still maintain the capacity to produce full effects demonstrating how strong they are as agonists (73). These q values are useful for understanding the relationship of not only the relative efficacy among agonists but also the relative efficacy requirements for agonists across different procedures (see Table 9.2).

9.3.2.4 Special Considerations

The use of different insurmountable antagonists theoretically should yield similar estimates of agonist affinity and efficacy values within an assay and within a species. For example, β-FNA, buprenorphine, and clocinnamox all produce similar apparent K_A values for morphine in the rat warm-water, tail-withdrawal assay (Table 9.1). Practically, it is more difficult to estimate affinity and efficacy for higher-efficacy agonists using the method of partial irreversible blockade because high doses of the insurmountable antagonist are required to decrease the maximum effect of

Table 9.2 Estimates of the fraction of receptors remaining (q values + 95% C.L.) after CCAM treatment alone (73) or after CCAM in morphine-treated rats in two behavioral procedures

	Tolerance	0.1 mg/kg CCAM	1.0 mg/kg CCAM	3.2 mg/kg CCAM	10 mg/kg CCAM
Antinociception					
CCAM alone				0.44 (0.38–0.52)	0.035 (0.027–0.047)
20 MS + CCAM	0.44 (0.40–0.50)	0.20 (0.14–0.27)	0.062 (0.048–0.082)	0.012 (0.008–0.015)	
Drug discrimination					
CCAM alone					0.19 (0.17–0.43)
20 MS + CCAM	0.36 (0.35–0.37)			0.070 (0.066–0.074)	0.047 (0.041–0.055)

CCAM clocinnamox, 20 MS 20 mg/kg/day morphine

a high-efficacy agonist. For example, although buprenorphine was estimated to reduce the μ-opioid receptor population by greater than 98%, high-efficacy agonists alfentanil and etonitazene still produced a maximum effect (37). Accurate estimates of K_A and therefore efficacy values for an agonist require that the dose–response curve is depressed below 50% to reduce error. The best strategy is to administer multiple doses, including high doses, of insurmountable antagonist and analyze the entire family of dose–response curves (57), but see (88).

9.3.3 Receptor Turnover

Opioid receptor turnover has been quantified using insurmountable antagonists (72, 75). For example, the recovery of μ-opioid receptor binding as measured by [^{3}H]DAMGO was compared to recovery of heroin self-administration in rats (89). After receptor alkylation with β-FNA, the K_D values for [^{3}H]DAMGO were not different for 7 days but then slight increases in affinity were observed from days 9–18. β-FNA decreased receptor numbers for at least 18 days. In the behavioral experiments, β-FNA initially decreased the number of heroin infusions but heroin infusions returned to normal levels by day 10. Therefore, the behavioral indicator of receptor number, self-administration, recovered sooner than the full complement of μ-opioid receptors as measured by radioligand-binding experiments. The authors suggested that recovery of μ-opioid receptors may be more complex than simply the synthesis of new receptors. Perhaps, the residual receptor pool after alkylation compensates for loss of receptor number via an increase in coupling efficiency that may be related to the increased ligand affinity. However, in vitro binding data can be difficult to compare directly to in vivo pharmacology since radioligand-binding studies do not necessarily measure receptors in a state that is related to biochemical or pharmacological function.

The turnover and recovery of μ-opioid receptors may depend on species. Using clocinnamox as the insurmountable antagonist, the $T_{1/2}$ recovery of μ-opioid receptors was estimated to be 6 days in rhesus monkeys (72) but only $T_{1/2}$ of 2–4 days in mice (56). However, in these ex vivo binding experiments in mice, 1/3 of the [^{3}H] DAMGO-binding sites remained inaccessible to the radioligand suggesting the $T_{1/2}$ of clocinnamox elimination in vivo from mouse brain is slower than the $T_{1/2}$ of clocinnamox dissociation from μ receptor (56). Interestingly, a low dose of 0.1 mg/kg clocinnamox reduced [^{3}H]DAMGO binding by ~50% after 24 h but did not alter the morphine dose–response curve for antinociception in rats. However, a higher dose of 1.0 mg/kg clocinnamox, which also reduced binding by ~50% after 24 h, shifted the morphine antinociception dose–response curve tenfold to the right. This antagonism by 1.0 mg/kg clocinnamox of morphine antinociception was still apparent when the rats were tested again 7 days later. Five weeks after a higher dose, 10 mg/kg clocinnamox, neither the morphine sensitivity nor the [^{3}H]DAMGO binding were fully recovered (55). However, as Paronis and Woods (55) point out, the opposite effect is observed with β-FNA: doses of β-FNA that fail to alter [^{3}H]DAMGO binding will antagonize morphine's antinociceptive effects (90–93). Similarly, the reduced B_{max} values for μ-opioid receptors as measured by [^{3}H]DAMGO recovered within hours in rat forebrain membranes using ex vivo binding techniques, yet investigators were still able to detect antagonism in a rat tail-flick model (40). In summary, more experiments are needed that measure both receptor density and functional effects for the insurmountable antagonists to appreciate the relationship between the time course of receptor recovery and actual fully, operational receptor activity.

Alternatively, these discrepancies described above may be due to some unusual pharmacokinetics and pharmacodynamics for clocinnamox or β-FNA. For example, clocinnamox is resistant to washout (52, 56) but [^{3}H]clocinnamox is a fully reversible radioligand with slow dissociation kinetics (57). The observation that the duration of action for clocinnamox in rhesus monkeys is longer than the proposed opioid receptor turnover in rats of 3–6 days (72) suggests that clocinnamox must be able to bind recently synthesized receptors. Therefore, clocinnamox may have a slow clearance rate or some tissue sequestration, and/or active metabolites that contribute to the initial receptor inactivation and then long duration of action (55). On the contrary, in mice, as clocinnamox levels decrease, μ-opioid receptor mRNA levels do not change as μ-opioid receptor density increases. This observation suggests that this recovery of receptors reflects changes in the rate of posttranslational processing such as activation of hidden receptors, and as clocinnamox eventually comes off the receptors, there is still a degree of new receptor synthesis (54).

9.3.4 Underlying Mechanisms of Tolerance and Dependence

Previous studies have exploited the common functional outcomes produced by insurmountable antagonism and chronic treatment to test hypotheses regarding receptor changes during repeated agonist treatments. Specifically, a sufficient dose of insurmountable antagonist or repeated chronic treatment of opioid agonists will produce an initial loss of agonist potency and an eventual decrease in maximal effect for an agonist. When repeated morphine treatment and clocinnamox antagonism are compared for their ability to alter receptor populations, it was found that neither clocinnamox nor repeated morphine treatment altered in vivo affinity estimates for opioid antagonists. These findings suggest that repeated morphine treatment or clocinnamox antagonism does not alter the affinity of antagonists for μ-opioid receptors (53, 94). If both of these pharmacological strategies involve disabling a portion of the receptor population without altering affinity, they can be combined to produce an augmented attack on the receptor population and uncover receptor changes that accompany chronic agonist treatment.

In an early study, the effects of β-CNA were compared in normal and morphine-tolerant guinea-pig ileum myenteric plexus to examine the opioid receptor reserve for normorphine (95). These authors found an apparent reduction in the fraction of spare μ-opioid receptors without any change in the apparent affinity of normorphine for μ receptors. They estimated that in normal ileum, only 10% of the available functional opioid receptors were required for normorphine to produce a maximum effect. However, in morphine-tolerant ileum, 26% of the available functional opioid receptors were required for normorphine to produce a maximum effect. From these results, the authors then concluded that tolerance to opioid agonists might be due to altered postreceptor events so that there is some manner of reduction in the spare receptor fraction. In vivo, using buprenorphine as the insurmountable antagonist, the apparent K_A values for morphine were four times lower in naïve than morphine-tolerant rats yet the efficacy values were similar in the two groups. The slopes of the dose–response curves were different between the naïve and morphine-tolerant rats causing these authors to suggest that tolerance involved both affinity changes and postreceptor event changes (71, 96).

To investigate the role of μ-opioid receptor density on the magnitude of tolerance, mice were injected with clocinnamox and then chronically treated with fentanyl. Although the effects of clocinnamox and chronic fentanyl treatment were additive, as would be expected, the absolute magnitude of tolerance to fentanyl was the same in saline- and clocinnamox-pretreated mice. These authors concluded that fentanyl tolerance appears to be independent of receptor density (97). If ligand efficacy is a determinant of the regulation of μ-receptors and trafficking proteins, as well as changes in opioid agonist potency changes following treatment (98–101), the regulation of μ-opioid receptors and trafficking proteins should coincide with efficacy differences among opioid agonists. For example, lower-efficacy agonists produce more tolerance at equieffective doses than higher-efficacy agonists, but lower-efficacy agonists fail to regulate μ-opioid receptor density or dynamin-2 abundance (102, 103). Recently, in vivo estimates of efficacy for oxycodone, morphine, and etorphine were determined using clocinnamox and correlated to tolerance and regulation of μ-opioid receptor density and dynamin-2 abundance in mice. The apparent efficacy estimates for the agonists predicted the degree of tolerance, the regulation of μ-opioid receptors, and the levels of dynamin-2 abundance (76). Taken together, these studies indicate that agonist efficacy plays an important role in tolerance and regulation of receptors and trafficking proteins.

Combined insurmountable antagonist administration and repeated agonist treatment decrease the maximum effect for higher efficacy agonists to reveal relative efficacy differences and permit estimation of the relative efficacy requirements of different functional assays. For example, high doses of clocinnamox alone fail to decrease the maximum effect for even the lower-efficacy agonists nalbuphine and buprenorphine in a drug discrimination assay, which suggest that the efficacy requirement for this assay is relatively low. However, if the rats are chronically treated for 14 days with 20 mg/kg/day morphine, neither buprenorphine nor nalbuphine substitute greater than 50% for the morphine discriminative stimulus (77). The results of these rat drug discrimination experiments were compared to the results of a series of rat warm-water, tail-withdrawal experiments using the same pharmacological strategy of administering repeated morphine injections and then 14 days later injecting different doses of clocinnamox. In the rat warm-water, tail-withdrawal procedure, in morphine-treated rats, increasing doses of 0.1, 1.0, or 3.2 mg/kg clocinnamox produced a progressive shift to the right and eventual shift downward in the morphine dose–response curve. If the q value is compared after a given dose of clocinnamox before (73) and after repeated morphine treatment, the fractions of receptors remaining can be compared in normal and in morphine-treated rats. For example, in normal rats, 3.2 mg/kg clocinnamox reduces the available receptor population by 56% but after repeated treatment with morphine, 3.2 mg/kg clocinnamox reduces available receptors by 99% (Table 9.2). Essentially these data suggest that a single 24-hour pretreatment of 3.2 mg/kg clocinnamox is equivalent to 1 week of repeated treatment with 20 mg/kg/day morphine. In the rats trained to discriminate morphine from saline in the drug-discrimination procedure, a dose of 3.2 mg/kg clocinnamox produced a parallel shift to the right in the morphine dose–response curve. This same dose of clocinnamox completely abolished the ability of morphine to produce antinociceptive effects in the rat warm-water, tail-withdrawal procedure (Fig. 9.2). Therefore, under conditions of clocinnamox pretreatment in morphine-treated rats, where ~99% of the μ-opioid receptors are unavailable for agonist interaction, morphine can still produce a maximum effect in the drug-discrimination assay but not in the antinociceptive assay. This demonstrates that drug discrimination is an exceedingly sensitive behavioral procedure relative to the warm-water, tail-withdrawal procedure. Future experiments in other assays will continue to fine-tune our understanding of the functional assays used to study and characterize opioid agonists.

9.4 Implications for Clinical Use

9.4.1 Clinical Experimental Utility

Using similar methodology to that reported above, the method of partial irreversible blockade was used in a recent study conducted in human volunteers (79) to determine the apparent in vivo dissociation constant (K_A) and the efficacy estimate (tau, τ)

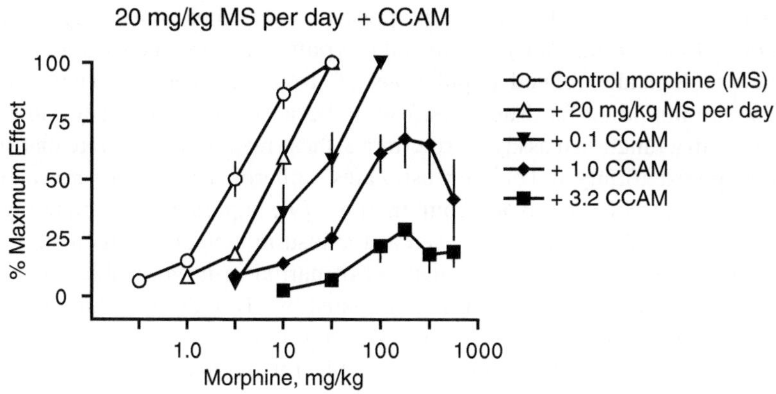

Fig. 9.2 Tolerance and clocinnamox treatment in rat warm-water, tail-withdrawal. Ordinate: the percentage of maximal antinociceptive response (15 sec). Abscissa: dose of morphine in milligrams per kilogram. The control morphine dose–response curve (*circles*, $N = 24$); tolerance alone, that is, the effects of 20 mg/kg/day morphine for 6 days of treatment and then a 24 h pretreatment of saline (*open triangles*, $N = 24$); tolerance plus clocinnamox, that is, six additional days of 20 mg/kg/day of morphine and then 0.1 (*solid inverse triangles*, $N = 8$), 1.0 (*solid diamonds*, $N = 8$), or 3.2 mg/kg (*solid squares*, $N = 8$) clocinnamox

for heroin, as well as the estimated fraction of receptors remaining (q) after treatment with buprenorphine/naloxone. Participants were maintained on 2/0.5, 8/2, and 32/8 mg sublingual buprenorphine/naloxone during an inpatient study and the reinforcing and subjective effects of intranasal heroin were examined. During test weeks, participants first sampled a dose of heroin and $20. During subsequent choice sessions, participants could choose to self-administer heroin and/or money. Participants responded under a modified progressive-ratio schedule (PR 50,…, 2,800) during a ten-trial self-administration task. Heroin break-point values and subjective responses were significantly lower under 8/2 and 32/8 mg buprenorphine/naloxone compared to 2/0.5 mg. The self-administration and subjective effects data for heroin in the presence of buprenorphine/naloxone were compared to a separate control group of recently detoxified participants in order to obtain estimates for the apparent K_A value, efficacy estimates, and the q values for the various doses of buprenorphine/naloxone. The apparent K_A value for heroin ranged from 50 to 126 mg and the efficacy estimate ranged from 13 to 20. The apparent K_A estimates obtained for heroin were remarkably similar to each other across the different behavioral measures. The exact relation of these apparent K_A estimates for heroin determined in human participants (50–126 mg) to those obtained for morphine in rodents and monkeys (11–68 mg/kg) is presently unknown due to the differences in dose measurement units (37, 57, 72, 73, 75, 78). Interestingly, the efficacy estimates for heroin in the present study were comparable to those obtained for morphine in studies conducted in rodents and monkeys (range 9–38). Correspondingly, efficacy estimates for heroin and morphine to produce antinociception in rhesus monkeys were analogous to each other (104) as well as to the estimates obtained in the present study. These data suggest that the behavioral effects produced by heroin and morphine in these studies were mediated by pharmacologically related populations of μ-opioid receptors. These efficacy estimates are important for drug classification because relative efficacy can only be determined in a functional assay. Furthermore, these results demonstrate that similar apparent agonist affinity and efficacy estimates for heroin (morphine) are calculated whether buprenorphine/naloxone combination (79), buprenorphine alone (30, 37), or clocinnamox (72, 73, 75, 78) is used as the insurmountable antagonist.

The investigators then used the method of partial insurmountable blockade to determine the proportion of receptors eliminated by given doses of buprenorphine/naloxone. Doses of 2/0.5, 8/2, and 32/8 mg buprenorphine/naloxone dose-dependently eliminated the receptors available for agonist interaction estimated as a 74%, 83%, and 91% reduction, respectively. A previous study by Greenwald et al. (105) showed similar reductions in whole-brain μ-opioid receptor availability (calculated as changes in binding potential) under maintenance on sublingual buprenorphine as measured with positron emission tomography and [^{11}C]carfentanil (105). This convergence of techniques in humans underscores the importance and validity of asking these questions from multiple angles.

9.4.2 Implications for Therapeutics

Insurmountable antagonists and quantitative procedures may be particularly useful in characterizing the abuse liability of new opioid medications relative to existing medications. For example, one may assume that compounds with higher relative efficacy would possess greater risk for abuse liability taking into account other factors such as formulations and affinity. Similarly, interested researchers can use this methodology to characterize the relative analgesic efficacy of new medications. As described above, testing medications across different assays can characterize the conditions under which these medications may be most or least efficacious. For example, for abuse liability assessments, it will be important to know whether a medication has abuse liability when the organism is opioid dependent versus nondependent. Buprenorphine is a prime example of a drug that serves as a reinforcer in subjects who are not dependent (79, 106–108), but does not serve as a reinforcer in subjects who are dependent (Comer et al., 2008 results) (79, 109). In addition to characterizing the analgesic and reinforcing efficacy of new and existing medications, the methodology may also be useful for assessing safety-related measures such as respiratory suppression. A medication that is an efficacious analgesic with low abuse potential and a high safety margin obviously would be preferable to an equally efficacious analgesic with higher abuse potential and a low margin of safety. The development of a procedure that allows the quantitative assessment of multiple dependent measures (analgesia, reinforcing effects, and respiratory suppression) within and between different medications has important clinical implications.

9.5 Conclusions

Many factors, such as absorption and distribution, can limit the qualitative and quantitative estimates of agonist affinity and efficacy and receptor activity from in vivo, functional studies with insurmountable antagonists. However, the convergence of apparent K_A, τ, and q values across behavioral effects, species, and laboratories lends support to the reliability and validity of the methodology used to understand the relationship between underlying receptor events and observed pharmacological effects. Although modern technology provides us with more precise affinity values from radioligand-binding assays and relative agonist efficacy estimates from GTPγS-signaling assays, truly applicable values can only be obtained in whole, fully functioning organisms. The advent of insurmountable antagonists provided tools to pharmacologists so that they can characterize and study opioid agonists and the receptors on which they act. And, with these tools in hand, we provide convergence of quantitative estimates determined from functional experiments and results from molecular pharmacological approaches, especially with respect to agonist efficacy. Future experiments will continue to exploit insurmountable antagonists to answer questions about drug, receptor, and behavioral events.

Acknowledgment The authors gratefully acknowledge Robert Raffa, Ph.D., for his comments and suggestions.

References

1. Furchgott, R.F., *Dibenamine blockade in strips of rabbit aorta and its use in differentiating receptors*. J Pharmacol Exp Ther, 1954. **111**(3): pp. 265–84.
2. Nickerson, M., *Receptor occupancy and tissue response*. Nature, 1956. **178**: pp. 697–8.
3. Stephenson, R.P., *A modification of receptor theory*. Br J Pharmacol Chemother, 1956. **11**(4): pp. 379–93.
4. Kenakin, T., *Pharmacologic Analysis of Drug–Receptor Interactions*. 1997, Philadelphia, PA: Lippincott-Raven.
5. Zimmerman, D.M., et al., *Use of beta-funaltrexamine to determine mu opioid receptor involvement in the analgesic activity of various opioid ligands*. J Pharmacol Exp Ther, 1987. **241**(2): pp. 374–8.
6. Grider, J.R. and G.M. Makhlouf, *Identification of opioid receptors on gastric muscle cells by selective receptor protection*. Am J Physiol, 1991. **260**(Pt. 1): pp. G103–7.
7. Liu, J.G., M.B. Ruckle, and P.L. Prather, *Constitutively active mu-opioid receptors inhibit adenylyl cyclase activity in intact cells and activate G-proteins differently than the agonist [D-Ala2,N-MePhe4,Gly-ol5]enkephalin*. J Biol Chem, 2001. **276**(41): pp. 37779–86.
8. Jaw, S.P., B. Hoskins, and I.K. Ho, *Opioid antagonists and butorphanol dependence*. Pharmacol Biochem Behav, 1993. **44**(3): pp. 497–500.
9. Garner, H.R., et al., *Butorphanol-mediated antinociception in mice: partial agonist effects and mu receptor involvement*. J Pharmacol Exp Ther, 1997. **282**(3): pp. 1253–61.
10. Ross, F.B. and M.T. Smith, *The intrinsic antinociceptive effects of oxycodone appear to be kappa-opioid receptor mediated*. Pain, 1997. **73**(2): pp. 151–7.
11. Harrison, C. and J.R. Traynor, *The [35S]GTP(gamma)S binding assay: approaches and applications in pharmacology*. Life Sci, 2003. **74**: pp. 489–508.

12. Caruso, T.P., et al., *Chloroxymorphamine, and opioid receptor site-directed alkylating agent having narcotic agonist activity*. Science, 1979. **204**(4390): pp. 316–8.
13. Portoghese, P.S., et al., *6beta-[N,N-Bis(2-chloroethyl)amino]-17-(cyclopropylmethyl)-4,5alpha-epoxy-3,14-dihydroxymorphinan(chlornaltrexamine) a potent opioid receptor alkylating agent with ultralong narcotic antagonist actitivty*. J Med Chem, 1978. **21**(7): pp. 598–9.
14. Portoghese, P.S., et al., *Synthesis and pharmacologic characterization of an alkylating analogue (chlornaltrexamine) of naltrexone with ultralong-lasting narcotic antagonist properties*. J Med Chem, 1979. **22**(2): pp. 168–73.
15. Sayre, L.M., A.E. Takemori, and P.S. Portoghese, *Alkylation of opioid receptor subtypes by alpha-chlornaltrexamine produces concurrent irreversible agonistic and irreversible antagonistic activities*. J Med Chem, 1983. **26**(4): pp. 503–6.
16. Ward, S.J., P.S. Portoghese, and A.E. Takemori, *Pharmacological profiles of beta-funaltrexamine (beta-FNA) and beta-chlornaltrexamine (beta-CNA) on the mouse vas deferens preparation*. Eur J Pharmacol, 1982. **80**(4): pp. 377–84.
17. Ward, S.J., P.S. Portoghese, and A.E. Takemori, *Pharmacological characterization in vivo of the novel opiate, beta-funaltrexamine*. J Pharmacol Exp Ther, 1982. **220**(3): pp. 494–8.
18. Tam, S.W. and L.Y. Liu-Chen, *Reversible and irreversible binding of beta-funaltrexamine to mu, delta and kappa opioid receptors in guinea pig brain membranes*. J Pharmacol Exp Ther, 1986. **239**(2): pp. 351–7.
19. Ward, S.J., et al., *Opioid receptor binding characteristics of the non-equilibrium mu antagonist, beta-funaltrexamine (beta-FNA)*. Eur J Pharmacol, 1985. **107**(3): pp. 323–30.
20. Liu-Chen, L.Y., et al., *[3H] beta-funaltrexamine ([3H] beta-FNA) binds irreversibly to mu opioid receptors in the rat brain: autoradiographic study*. Prog Clin Biol Res, 1990. **328**: pp. 61–4.
21. Liu-Chen, L.Y., S.X. Li, and R.J. Tallarida, *Studies on kinetics of [3H]beta-funaltrexamine binding to mu opioid receptor*. Mol Pharmacol, 1990. **37**(2): pp. 243–50.
22. Liu-Chen, L.Y. and C.A. Phillips, *Covalent labeling of mu opioid binding site by [3H]beta-funaltrexamine*. Mol Pharmacol, 1987. **32**(3): pp. 321–9.
23. Adams, J.U., C.A. Paronis, and S.G. Holtzman, *Assessment of relative intrinsic activity of mu-opioid analgesics in vivo by using beta-funaltrexamine*. J Pharmacol Exp Ther, 1990. **255**(3): pp. 1027–32.
24. Hayes, A.G., M. Skingle, and M.B. Tyers, *Reversal by beta-funaltrexamine of the antinociceptive effect of opioid agonists in the rat*. Br J Pharmacol, 1986. **88**(4): pp. 867–72.
25. Dykstra, L.A., et al., *Kappa opioids in rhesus monkeys. II. Analysis of the antagonistic actions of quadazocine and beta-funaltrexamine*. J Pharmacol Exp Ther, 1987. **242**(2): pp. 421–7.
26. Gmerek, D.E. and J.H. Woods, *Effects of beta-funaltrexamine in normal and morphine-dependent rhesus monkeys: observational studies*. J Pharmacol Exp Ther, 1985. **235**(2): pp. 296–301.
27. Qi, J.A., et al., *Mu antagonist and kappa agonist properties of beta-funaltrexamine (beta-FNA) in vivo: long-lasting spinal analgesia in mice*. J Pharmacol Exp Ther, 1990. **252**(3): pp. 1006–11.
28. Porreca, F., et al., *A comparison of the receptor constants of morphine and ethylketocyclazocine for analgesia and inhibition of gastrointestinal transit in the rat*. Life Sci, 1982. **31**(18): pp. 1955–61.
29. Raffa, R.B., et al., *Morphine-receptor dissociation constant and the stimulus-effect relation for inhibition of gastrointestinal transit in the rat*. Eur J Pharmacol, 1982. **79**(1–2): pp. 11–6.
30. Tallarida, R.J. and A. Cowan, *The affinity of morphine for its pharmacologic receptor in vivo*. J Pharmacol Exp Ther, 1982. **222**(1): pp. 198–201.
31. Boas, R.A. and J.W. Villiger, *Clinical actions of fentanyl and buprenorphine. The significance of receptor binding*. Br J Anaesth, 1985. **57**(2): pp. 192–6.
32. Rothman, R.B., et al., *Ligand selectivity of cloned human and rat opioid mu receptors*. Synapse, 1995. **21**(1): pp. 60–4.
33. Villiger, J.W. and K.M. Taylor, *Buprenorphine: characteristics of binding sites in the rat central nervous system*. Life Sci, 1981. **29**(26): pp. 2699–708.
34. Bullingham, R.E., et al., *Sublingual buprenorphine used postoperatively: ten hour plasma drug concentration analysis*. Br J Clin Pharmacol, 1982. **13**(5): pp. 665–73.

35. Dykstra, L.A., *Behavioral effects of buprenorphine and diprenorphine under a multiple schedule of food presentation in squirrel monkeys*. J Pharmacol Exp Ther, 1983. **226**(2): pp. 317–23.
36. France, C.P., A.E. Jacobson, and J.H. Woods, *Irreversible and reversible narcotic agonists: discriminative and analgesic effects of buprenorphine, oxymorphazone, and morphine*. NIDA Res Monogr, 1984. **49**: pp. 136–42.
37. Walker, E.A., G. Zernig, and J.H. Woods, *Buprenorphine antagonism of mu opioids in the rhesus monkey tail-withdrawal procedure*. J Pharmacol Exp Ther, 1995. **273**(3): pp. 1345–52.
38. Walsh, S.L., et al., *Clinical pharmacology of buprenorphine: ceiling effects at high doses*. Clin Pharmacol Ther, 1994. **55**(5): pp. 569–80.
39. Hambrook, J.M., et al., *Mode of deactivation of the enkephalins by rat and human plasma and rat brain homogenates*. Nature, 1976. **262**(5571): pp. 782–3.
40. Englberger, W., et al., *Reversibility of opioid receptor occupancy of buprenorphine in vivo*. Eur J Pharmacol, 2006. **534**: pp. 95–102.
41. Cowan, A., J.C. Doxey, and E.J. Harry, *The animal pharmacology of buprenorphine, an oripavine analgesic agent*. Br J Pharmacol, 1977. **60**(4): pp. 547–54.
42. Cowan, A., J.W. Lewis, and I.R. Macfarlane, *Agonist and antagonist properties of buprenorphine, a new antinociceptive agent*. Br J Pharmacol, 1977. **60**(4): pp. 537–45.
43. Cowan, A., *Buprenorphine: new pharmacological aspects*. Int J Clin Pract Suppl, 2003(133): pp. 3–8; discussion 23–4.
44. Huang, P., et al., *Comparison of pharmacological activities of buprenorphine and norbuprenorphine: norbuprenorphine is a potent opioid agonist*. J Pharmacol Exp Ther, 2001. **297**(2): pp. 688–95.
45. Lutfy, K., et al., *Buprenorphine-induced antinociception is mediated by mu-opioid receptors and compromised by concomitant activation of opioid receptor-like receptors*. J Neurosci, 2003. **23**(32): pp. 10331–7.
46. Picker, M.J. and L.A. Dykstra, *Discriminative stimulus effects of mu and kappa opioids in the pigeon: analysis of the effects of full and partial mu and kappa agonists*. J Pharmacol Exp Ther, 1989. **249**(2): pp. 557–66.
47. Picker, M.J., et al., *Agonist and antagonist effects of mixed action opioids in the pigeon drug discrimination procedure: influence of training dose, intrinsic efficacy and interanimal differences*. J Pharmacol Exp Ther, 1993. **266**(2): pp. 756–67.
48. Smith, M.A. and M.J. Picker, *Tolerance and cross-tolerance to the rate-suppressing effects of opioids in butorphanol-treated rats: influence of maintenance dose and relative efficacy at the mu receptor*. Psychopharmacology (Berl), 1998. **140**(1): pp. 57–68.
49. Kogel, B., et al., *Interaction of mu-opioid receptor agonists and antagonists with the analgesic effect of buprenorphine in mice*. Eur J Pain, 2005. **9**(5): pp. 599–611.
50. Comer, S.D., et al., *Clocinnamox: a novel, systemically-active, irreversible opioid antagonist*. J Pharmacol Exp Ther, 1992. **262**(3): pp. 1051–6.
51. Lewis, J., et al., *New 14-aminomorphinones and codeinones*. NIDA Res Monogr, 1988. **90**: pp. 136–43.
52. Aceto, M.D., et al., *Very long-acting narcotic antagonists: the 14 beta-p-substituted cinnamoylaminomorphinones and their partial mu agonist codeinone relatives*. Arzneimittelforschung, 1989. **39**(5): pp. 570–5.
53. Burke, T.F., et al., *Irreversible opioid antagonist effects of clocinnamox on opioid analgesia and mu receptor binding in mice*. J Pharmacol Exp Ther, 1994. **271**(2): pp. 715–21.
54. Chan, K., et al., *The effect of the irreversible mu-opioid receptor antagonist clocinnamox on morphine potency, receptor binding and receptor mRNA*. Eur J Pharmacol, 1995. **287**(2): pp. 135–43.
55. Paronis, C.A. and J.H. Woods, *Clocinnamox dose-dependently antagonizes morphine-analgesia and [^{3}H]DAMGO binding in rats*. Eur J Pharmacol, 1997. **337**(1): pp. 27–34.
56. Zernig, G., et al., *Mechanism of clocinnamox blockade of opioid receptors: evidence from in vitro and ex vivo binding and behavioral assays*. J Pharmacol Exp Ther, 1996. **279**(1): pp. 23–31.

57. Zernig, G., et al., *Receptor reserve and affinity of mu opioid agonists in mouse antinociception: correlation with receptor binding*. Life Sci, 1995. **57**(23): pp. 2113–25.
58. Jiang, Q., et al., *5 beta-Methyl-14 beta-(p-nitrocinnamoylamino)-7,8-dihydromorphinone and its corresponding N-cyclopropylmethyl analog, N-cyclopropylmethylnor-5 beta-methyl-14 beta-(p-nitrocinnamoylamino)-7,8-dihydromorphinone: mu-selective irreversible opioid antagonists*. J Pharmacol Exp Ther, 1994. **268**(3): pp. 1107–13.
59. Woods, J.H., et al., *Methoclocinnamox: a mu partial agonist with pharmacotherapeutic potential for heroin abuse*. NIDA Res Monogr, 1995. **147**: pp. 195–219.
60. Briscoe, R.J., et al., *Methoclocinnamox: time course of changes in alfentanil-reinforced responding in rhesus monkeys*. Psychopharmacology (Berl), 2000. **148**(4): pp. 393–9.
61. Broadbear, J.H., et al., *Methocinnamox is a potent, long-lasting, and selective antagonist of morphine-mediated antinociception in the mouse: comparison with clocinnamox, beta-funaltrexamine, and beta-chlornaltrexamine*. J Pharmacol Exp Ther, 2000. **294**(3): pp. 933–40.
62. Chen, C., et al., *Characterization of irreversible binding of beta-funaltrexamine to the cloned rat mu opioid receptor*. J Biol Chem, 1995. **270**(30): pp. 17866–70.
63. Chen, C., et al., *Determination of the amino acid residue involved in [3H]beta-funaltrexamine covalent binding in the cloned rat mu-opioid receptor*. J Biol Chem, 1996. **271**(35): pp. 21422–9.
64. Furchgott, R.F., *Metabolic factors that influence contractility of vascular smooth muscle*. Bull N Y Acad Med, 1966. **42**(11): pp. 996–1006.
65. Furchgott, R.F., *The pharmacological differentiation of adrenergic receptors*. Ann N Y Acad Sci, 1967. **139**(3): pp. 553–70.
66. Black, J.W. and P. Leff, *Operational models of pharmacological agonism*. Proc R Soc Lond B Biol Sci, 1983. **220**(1219): pp. 141–62.
67. Black, J.W., et al., *An operational model of pharmacological agonism: the effect of E/[A] curve shape on agonist dissociation constant estimation*. Br J Pharmacol, 1985. **84**(2): pp. 561–71.
68. Leff, P., *Inverse agonism: theory and practice*. Trends Pharmacol Sci, 1995. **16**(8): p. 256.
69. Kenakin, T., *Efficacy as a vector: the relative prevalence and paucity of inverse agonism*. Mol Pharmacol, 2004. **65**(1): pp. 2–11.
70. Zernig, G., T. Issaevitch, and J.H. Woods, *Calculation of agonist efficacy, apparent affinity, and receptor population changes after administration of insurmountable antagonists: comparison of different analytical approaches*. J Pharmacol Toxicol Methods, 1996. **35**(4): pp. 223–37.
71. Porreca, F., et al., *Estimation in vivo of the receptor constants of morphine in naive and morphine-tolerant rats*. Life Sci, 1982. **31**(20–21): pp. 2355–8.
72. Zernig, G., et al., *In vivo determination of mu opioid receptor turnover in rhesus monkeys after irreversible blockade with clocinnamox*. J Pharmacol Exp Ther, 1994. **269**(1): pp. 57–65.
73. Walker, E.A., G. Zernig, and A.M. Young, *In vivo apparent affinity and efficacy estimates for mu opiates in a rat tail-withdrawal assay*. Psychopharmacology (Berl), 1998. **136**(1): pp. 15–23.
74. Walker, E.A., et al., *Naltrexone and beta-funaltrexamine antagonism of the antinociceptive and response rate-decreasing effects of morphine, dezocine, and d-propoxyphene*. Psychopharmacology (Berl), 1999. **144**(1): pp. 45–53.
75. Pitts, R.C., et al., *Clocinnamox antagonism of the antinociceptive effects of mu opioids in squirrel monkeys*. J Pharmacol Exp Ther, 1998. **285**(3): pp. 1197–206.
76. Pawar, M., et al., *Opioid agonist efficacy predicts the magnitude of tolerance and the regulation of μ-opioid receptors and dynamin-2*. Eur J Pharmacol, 2007 June 1. **563**(1–3): pp. 92–101.
77. Walker, E.A. and A.M. Young, *Clocinnamox distinguishes opioid agonists according to relative efficacy in normal and morphine-treated rats trained to discriminate morphine*. J Pharmacol Exp Ther, 2002. **302**(1): pp. 101–10.
78. Barrett, A.C., E.S. Smith, and M.J. Picker, *Use of irreversible antagonists to determine the relative efficacy of mu-opioids in a pigeon drug discrimination procedure: comparison of beta-funaltrexamine and clocinnamox*. J Pharmacol Exp Ther, 2003. **305**(3): pp. 1061–70.

79. Comer, S.D., E.A. Walker, and E.D. Collins, *Buprenorphine/naloxone reduces the reinforcing and subjective effects of heroin in heroin-dependent volunteers*. Psychopharmacology (Berl), 2005. **181**(4): pp. 664–75.
80. Walker, E.A., et al., *In vivo apparent pA2 analysis for naltrexone antagonism of discriminative stimulus and analgesic effects of opiate agonists in rats*. J Pharmacol Exp Ther, 1994. **271**(2): pp. 959–68.
81. Tallarida, R.J. and R.B. Raffa, *Receptor regulation, competitive antagonism and pA2*. Life Sci, 1992. **51**(7): pp. PL61–5.
82. Negus, S.S., et al., *Effects of opioid agonists selective for mu, kappa and delta opioid receptors on schedule-controlled responding in rhesus monkeys: antagonism by quadazocine*. J Pharmacol Exp Ther, 1993. **267**(2): pp. 896–903.
83. Ko, M.C., et al., *Differentiation of kappa opioid agonist-induced antinociception by naltrexone apparent pA2 analysis in rhesus monkeys*. J Pharmacol Exp Ther, 1998. **285**(2): pp. 518–26.
84. Arunlakshana, O. and H.O. Schild, *Some quantitative uses of drug antagonists*. Br J Pharmacol Chemother, 1959. **14**(1): pp. 48–58.
85. Schild, H.O., *Drug antagonism and pAx*. Pharmacol Rev, 1957. **9**(2): pp. 242–6.
86. Hayes, A.G., M.J. Sheehan, and M.B. Tyers, *Determination of the receptor selectivity of opioid agonists in the guinea-pig ileum and mouse vas deferens by use of beta-funaltrexamine*. Br J Pharmacol, 1985. **86**(4): pp. 899–904.
87. Walker, E.A. and A.M. Young, *Differential tolerance to antinociceptive effects of mu opioids during repeated treatment with etonitazene, morphine, or buprenorphine in rats*. Psychopharmacology (Berl), 2001. **154**(2): pp. 131–42.
88. Van der Graaf, P.H. and M. Danhof, *On the reliability of affinity and efficacy estimates obtained by direct operational model filling of agonist concetration-effect curves following irreversible receptor inactivation*. J Pharmacol Toxicol Meth, 1997. **38**: pp. 81–5.
89. Martin, T.J., S.I. Dworkin, and J.E. Smith, *Alkylation of mu opioid receptors by beta-funaltrexamine in vivo: comparison of the effects on in situ binding and heroin self-administration in rats*. J Pharmacol Exp Ther, 1995. **272**(3): pp. 1135–40.
90. Adams, J.U., et al., *Effects of stress and beta-funal trexamine pretreatment on morphine analgesia and opioid binding in rats*. Life Sci, 1987. **41**(26): pp. 2835–44.
91. Liu-Chen, L.Y., S.X. Li, and M.E. Lewis, *Autoradiographic study of irreversible binding of [3H]beta-funaltrexamine to opioid receptors in the rat forebrain: comparison with mu and delta receptor distribution*. Brain Res, 1991. **544**(2): pp. 235–42.
92. Liu-Chen, L.Y., et al., *Effects of intracerebroventricular beta-funaltrexamine on mu and delta opioid receptors in the rat: dichotomy between binding and antinociception*. Eur J Pharmacol, 1991. **203**(2): pp. 195–202.
93. Liu-Chen, L.Y., et al., *Effect of intracerebroventricular beta-funaltrexamine on mu opioid receptors in the rat brain: consideration of binding condition*. J Pharmacol Exp Ther, 1995. **273**(3): pp. 1047–56.
94. Walker, E.A., T.M. Richardson, and A.M. Young, *In vivo apparent pA2 analysis in rats treated with either clocinnamox or morphine*. Psychopharmacology (Berl), 1996. **125**(2): pp. 113–9.
95. Chavkin, C. and A. Goldstein, *Reduction in opiate receptor reserve in morphine tolerant guinea pig ilea*. Life Sci, 1982. **31**(16–17): pp. 1687–90.
96. Porreca, F. and T.F. Burks, *Affinity of normorphine for its pharmacologic receptor in the naive and morphine-tolerant guinea-pig isolated ileum*. J Pharmacol Exp Ther, 1983. **225**(3): pp. 688–93.
97. Chan, K.W., A. Duttory, and B.C. Yoburn, *Magnitude of tolerance to fentanyl is independent of mu-opioid receptor density*. Eur J Pharmacol, 1997. **319**(2–3): pp. 225–8.
98. Duttaroy, A. and B.C. Yoburn, *The effect of intrinsic efficacy on opioid tolerance*. Anesthesiology, 1995. **82**(5): pp. 1226–36.
99. Patel, M., et al., *Antagonist-induced micro-opioid receptor up-regulation decreases G-protein receptor kinase-2 and dynamin-2 abundance in mouse spinal cord*. Eur J Pharmacol, 2002. **446**(1–3): pp. 37–42.

100. Patel, M.B., et al., *Opioid agonists differentially regulate mu-opioid receptors and trafficking proteins in vivo*. Mol Pharmacol, 2002. **62**(6): pp. 1464–70.
101. Yoburn, B.C., B. Billings, and A. Duttaroy, *Opioid receptor regulation in mice*. J Pharmacol Exp Ther, 1993. **265**(1): pp. 314–20.
102. Hurley, R.W. and D.L. Hammond, *Contribution of endogenous enkephalins to the enhanced analgesic effects of supraspinal mu opioid receptor agonists after inflammatory injury*. J Neurosci, 2001. **21**: pp. 2536–45.
103. Zhang, J., et al., *Role for G protein-coupled receptor kinase in agonist-specific regulation of mu-opioid receptor responsiveness*. Proc Natl Acad Sci USA, 1998. **95**(12): pp. 7157–62.
104. Negus, S.S., et al., *Effects of heroin and its metabolites on schedule-controlled responding and thermal nociception in rhesus monkeys; sensitivity to antagonism by quadazocine, naltrindole and beta-funaltrexamine*. Drug Alcohol Depend, 2003. **70**(1): pp. 17–27.
105. Greenwald, M.K., et al., *Effects of buprenorphine maintenance dose on mu-opioid receptor availability, plasma concentrations, and antagonist blockade in heroin-dependent volunteers*. Neuropsychopharmacology, 2003. **28**(11): pp. 2000–9.
106. Comer, S.D. and E.D. Collins, *Self-administration of intravenous buprenorphine and the buprenorphine/naloxone combination by recently detoxified heroin abusers*. J Pharmacol Exp Ther, 2002. **303**(2): pp. 695–703.
107. Comer, S.D., E.D. Collins, and M.W. Fischman, *Intravenous buprenorphine self-administration by detoxified heroin abusers*. J Pharmacol Exp Ther, 2002. **301**(1): pp. 266–76.
108. Comer, S.D., M.A. Sullivan, and E.A. Walker, *Comparison of intravenous buprenorphine and methadone self-administration by recently detoxified heroin-dependent individuals*. J Pharmacol Exp Ther, 2005. **315**(3): pp. 1320–30.
109. Winger, G. and J.H. Woods, *The effects of chronic morphine on behavior reinforced by several opioids or by cocaine in rhesus monkeys*. Drug Alcohol Depend, 2001. **62**(3): pp. 181–9.
110. Comer, S.D., M.A. Sullivan, R.A. Whittington, S.K. Vosburg, and W.J. Kowalczyk, Abuse liability of prescription opioids compared to heroin in morphine-maintained heroin abusers. Neuropsychopharmacol, 2008. 33:1179–1191.

Chapter 10
Methylnaltrexone: A Peripherally Acting Opioid Antagonist

Chun-Su Yuan and Robert J. Israel

Abstract Opioids are widely used analgesics in patients with moderate or severe pain. Their effectiveness for pain relief is often limited, however, by the most frequently occurring side effect, opioid-induced constipation. Unlike the analgesic effects of opioids, which are centrally mediated, constipation is mediated mainly by peripheral opioid receptors in the gut. Conventional laxatives are often ineffective in treating opioid-inducded constipation. Methylnaltrexone is a novel quaternary derivative of naltrexone that does not cross the blood–brain barrier in humans and acts as a selective peripheral opioid receptor *antagonist*, recently approved by the FDA and other regulatory agencies for the treatment of opioid-induced constipation in patients with advanced illness receiving palliative care. This chapter reviews preclinical studies and data from trials of methylnaltrexone bowel dysfunction induced by opioids. Other potential clinical roles for methylnaltrexone are also briefly presented.

Keywords: Methylnaltrexone peripheral opioid antagonist; Opioid bowel dysfunction; Constipation; Postoperative ileus

10.1 Introduction

Opioids are widely used clinically for relieving both moderate and severe pain. Their use is often limited, however, by opioid-induced constipation, a frequent adverse effect. The adverse effects of opioid treatment which can generally be linked to the opioid receptors outside of the central nervous system, are distressing to patients and therapeutically challenging (1, 2). Opioid antagonists, such as naloxone, naltrexone, and nalmefene, have been studied as a means of antagonizing the undesirable peripheral effects of opioids, but these compounds also enter the central nervous system and reverse analgesia or cause opioid withdrawal symptoms (3–6). Since conventional laxatives are often ineffective in treating

C.-Su. Yuan (✉) and R.J. Israel
Department of Anesthesia & Critical Care, Pritzker School of Medicine,
The University of Chicago, 5841 S. Maryland Avenue, MC 4028, Chicago, IL 60637
e-mail: cyuan@uchicago.edu

R. Dean et al. (eds.), *Opiate Receptors and Antagonists*,

opioid constipation, a selective peripherally acting opioid receptor antagonist may prevent or treat opioid constipation without affecting pain relief.

Methylnaltrexone is a peripheral opioid receptor antagonist with the potential to block or reverse the undesirable effects of opioids without affecting analgesia or precipitating opioid withdrawal symptoms. This chapter reviews preclinical studies and data from clinical trials of opioid bowel dysfunction. Other effects of this compound in clinical practice are also briefly presented.

10.2 Physical and Chemical Properties

N-methylnaltrexone bromide, or methylnaltrexone, is a quaternary derivative of naltrexone (7). Attaching the methyl group to the amine of naltrexone forms methylnaltrexone, a compound with greater polarity and lower lipid solubility than naltrexone. These properties prevent methylnaltrexone from crossing the blood–brain barrier in humans (7, 8). Methylnaltrexone is a white, odorless powder, freely soluble in water. The compound has been formulated for clinical trials as a sterile solution for injection or infusion and as a powder to be administered orally in capsules or tablets.

10.3 Preclinical Development

10.3.1 Receptor Binding Activities

Methylnaltrexone antagonized opioid binding at *mu* opioid receptors (half maximimal inhibitory concentration IC_{50} of 70nM) had a relatively lower affinity for κ opioid receptors (IC_{50} of 575nM) and did not interact with δ opioid or orphanin receptors. It also did not bind significantly to any non-opioid receptors. Methylnaltrexone had no intrinsic opioid agonist activity as measured in standard pharmacological models of analgesia, gastrointestinal motility, or in behavioral tests designed to detect substitutes for narcotics (9–11). Thus, methylnaltrexone can be categorized as a pure antagonist.

In the gastrointestinal tract, methylnaltrexone preferentially selected *mu* receptors. In an in vitro gastric-brainstem preparation, opioid agonists decreased brainstem neuronal firing dose-dependently when the compounds were administered solely to the gastric compartment (12). Methylnaltrexone antagonized the inhibitory effects of morphine and those of the *mu*-selective opioid agonist, DAMGO in a competitive manner, with IC_{50} observed at approximately 300nM. Methylnaltrexone was 18.8-fold less potent as an antagonist of the *kappa*-selective agonist, U-50,488H, and it was ineffective against the *delta*-selective agonist, DPDPE (13).

10.3.2 Acute Toxicity and Demethylation Studies

Methylnaltrexone was administered under a variety of protocols to pigeons, mice, dogs, and rhesus monkeys (7). Toxicity studies over 2 weeks of administration showed a relatively high median lethal dose (LD_{50}) of >100 mg/kg in rats. In other species, including primates, the compound was given in doses up to 50 mg/kg without mortality (7). Animals tolerated doses of methylnaltrexone well above the effective dose range used in human clinical trials.

Demethylation is important, because a tertiary compound, such as naltrexone, has a high affinity for the opioid receptor and more readily crosses the blood–brain barrier, potentially confounding the peripheral selectivity of methylnaltrexone. In rodents, high doses of methylnaltrexone were associated with anti-nociception, suggesting a possible central effect (14). But in a rat model of heroin self-administration, at a high dose of 30 mg/kg, methylnaltrexone did not alter the rate of opioid self-administration (15). Studies of the metabolism of methylnaltrexone showed that there were species-dependent differences in the demethylation of methylnaltrexone to naltrexone. Rats and mice demethylated the compound over time as shown by the exhalation of $^{14}CO_2$ after administration of (^{14}C-methyl) naltrexone methyl bromide (16). This type of conversion was negligible in dogs and primates. In dogs and monkeys, methylnaltrexone 10–50 mg/kg did not penetrate the brain (8, 16) (Fig. 10.1).

10.3.3 Opioid-Induced Emesis

Opioid-induced emesis is peripherally mediated since the chemoreceptor-trigger zone has access to the peripheral circulation (17). Dogs are highly susceptible to morphine-induced emesis and have been used as a model to study this adverse effect. In dogs, methylnaltrexone pretreatment dose-dependently antagonized the emetic effects of morphine (18). The combined administration of methylnaltrexone and morphine reduced both apomorphine- and cisplatin-induced emesis in dogs (19). In a rat model simulating nausea and vomiting, in which the amount of kaolin consumption after morphine reflected the degree of emesis, morphine-induced increase in kaolin ingestion was reduced by methylnaltrexone administration in a dose-dependent manner (20).

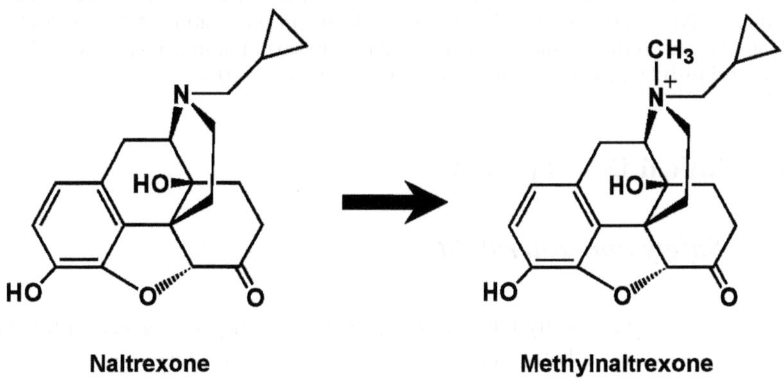

Fig. 10.1 Chemical structure of naltrexone and methylnaltrexone

10.3.4 Gut Motility and Opioids

Morphine and other opioids slow normal gut function (21). The efficacy of methylnaltrexone in the prevention and reversal of opioid-induced inhibition of gastrointestinal motility has been evaluated in animals. Administered subcutaneously to rats, methylnaltrexone antagonized the morphine-induced delay in gut transit time of a charcoal meal (10). Similar findings in rats were reported by other groups (7, 14, 22). In the dog, 0.5 mg/kg methylnaltrexone antagonized the inhibitory effects of morphine on the electrical concomitants of intestinal motor activity (8). In isolated guinea-pig ileum and human small intestine muscle strip preparations, methylnaltrexone reversed morphine-induced inhibition of contraction, indicating its direct action on the bowel (23) (Fig. 10.2).

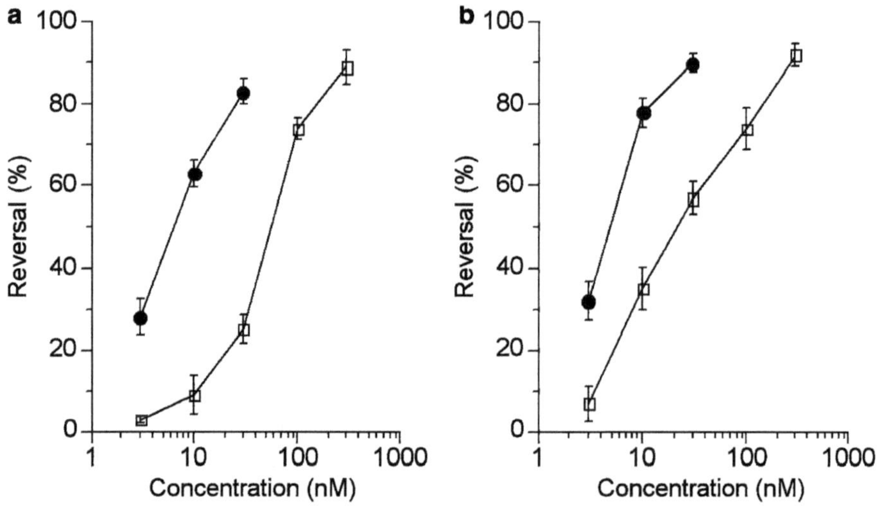

Fig. 10.2 Concentration-related effects of methylnaltrexone (*open square*) and naloxone (*solid circle*) on morphine-induced inhibition of muscle strip contraction. **a** Reversal effects on morphine-induced (300 nM) inhibition in isolated guinea pig ileum preparation. **b** Reversal effects on morphine-induced (100 nM) inhibition in isolated human small intestine preparation. The control is normalized to 100%. Effects of morphine at IC_{70} are treated as 0%

10.4 Clinical Development

10.4.1 Safety and Tolerability

In healthy volunteers, methylnaltrexone up to 0.32 mg/kg was given intravenously without adverse effects. Transient orthostatic hypotension (plasma levels of the drug in excess of 1,400 ng/ml) was observed in some subjects after 0.64–1.25 mg/kg via intravenous bolus (24). This orthostatic hypotension appears unlikely to occur during clinical treatment, since projected therapeutic doses will not exceed 0.45 mg/kg and will be administered subcutaneously or by IV infusion. Additional safety and tolerance data have been generated in other studies at the University of Chicago in over 200 subjects who received intravenous methylnaltrexone from 0.3 to 0.45 mg/kg. No significant subjective or objective adverse effects were observed.

Safety and tolerability following repeated intravenous methylnaltrexone administration were evaluated in 12 normal subjects. During the 72-hour study, subjects received 0.3 mg/kg methylnaltrexone every 6 hours. There were no adverse effects or significant changes in vital signs. Maximum plasma concentrations of methylnaltrexone, determined 2 min post-dose, were 538 ± 237 ng/ml (mean ± S.D.) and 675 ± 180 ng/ml after the first and twelfth doses, respectively. Based on a comparison of the values for the areas under the plasma concentration curve (AUC) after the first and twelfth doses, the accumulation factor at steady state was 1.5 ± 0.5. Thus, there was no clinically significant accumulation of the drug (25).

10.4.2 Absorption, Elimination, and Metabolism

Methylnaltrexone concentrations in plasma or urine can be quantified using solid-phase extraction and reverse-phase high performance liquid chromatography (HPLC) with electrochemical detection (26, 27). A newer method using liquid chromatography and tandem mass spectrometry has been validated (25).

Methylnaltrexone is readily bioavailable after intravenous or subcutaneous administrations in human subjects (28, 29). Plasma levels after subcutaneous doses of 0.1 or 0.3 mg/kg are proportional to dose. Pharamacokinetic data showed that T_{max} was ~20 min. The plasma half-life of methylnaltrexone after parenteral administration has been variously reported in the literature to range between 1.5 and 3 hours (24, 28, 29). Recent investigations suggest a longer terminal half-life of 6–9 hours.

Methylnaltrexone is absorbed from the gastrointestinal tract after oral ingestion (30). Since methylnaltrexone is a charged molecule, gut absorption and peak plasma levels are much lower than after parenteral administration of the drug. Enterically coated forms have been studied in an early clinical trial. The bioavailability of enterically coated methylnaltrexone at oral doses of 3.2 mg/kg and 6.4 mg/kg has been evaluated in normal volunteers (31). Since plasma levels of methylnaltrexone did not correlate with clinical effects, the compound likely has a direct effect on the luminal surface of the intestine. Low doses of enterically coated methylnaltrexone may also treat opioid-mediated gut effects.

The elimination of parenterally administered methylnaltrexone has also been studied in humans. The amount of unchanged compound detected in urine over the period of 0–6 hours after a subcutaneous dose was 52% and 47% for doses of 0.1 or 0.3 mg/kg, respectively (29). A similar fraction was excreted in the urine after IV dosing (24, 28). A significant fraction of administered drug appears to be eliminated in feces. In a study in dogs, samples of urine and feces were collected over a period of 120 hours after an intravenous dose of 2 mg ^{14}C-labeled methylnaltrexone. Cumulative recovered radioactivity amounted to 51% in urine and 32% in feces, the bulk of which was excreted within 24 hours of administration (16).

In studies conducted to date, metabolism of methylnaltrexone does not appear to be important for its elimination. A very small percentage of the compound may undergo hepatic metabolism (possibly glucuronidation) with subsequent biliary, renal, and fecal elimination.

As noted, there are species-dependent differences in the demethylation of methylnaltrexone to naltrexone. Existing data indicate that, although the rate of demethylation is low in rodents, demethylation is not a pathway of methylnaltrexone metabolism in humans (16). In other studies, intravenous methylnaltrexone 0.3 mg/kg did not reverse morphine-induced respiratory depression (32) or opioid-induced miosis (33), suggesting no demethylation of methylnaltrexone to naltrexone in humans.

10.4.3 Activity of Parenteral Methylnaltrexone in Healthy Volunteers

That methylnaltrexone counteracts the gut inhibitory effects of opioids has been demonstrated in a number of studies. In a double-blind, randomized, placebo-controlled trial of 12 healthy volunteers, intravenous morphine at doses of 0.05–0.1 mg/kg delayed oral–cecal transit time as measured by the lactulose hydrogen breath test (34, 35). Delay of gut transit time was effectively prevented by a single intravenous injection of methylnaltrexone 0.45 mg/kg (Fig. 10.3) (28). Morphine significantly increased oral–cecal transit time from a baseline of 104.6 ± 31.1 min to 163.3 ± 39.8 min ($p < 0.01$). In contrast, transit time in subjects given methylnaltrexone plus morphine (106.3 ± 39.8 min) was not significantly different from baseline. The compound thus prevented 97% of morphine-induced changes in oral–cecal transit time ($p < 0.01$ compared to morphine alone). The cold-pressor test (36) also used in this study demonstrated that methylnaltrexone did not reverse morphine-induced analgesia (28).

Even at low doses morphine slows gastric emptying in humans (37). In a controlled trial to evaluate the effects of intravenous methylnaltrexone on the opioid-induced delay in gastric emptying (38), 11 healthy volunteers were given placebo, morphine, or 0.3 mg/kg methylnaltrexone plus morphine on three separate occasions. The rate of gastric emptying was measured by a noninvasive epigastric bioimpedance technique and by the acetaminophen absorption test. The time required for gastric volume to decrease to 50% ($t_{0.5}$) following 500 cc of fluid after placebo was 5.5 ± 2.1 min. Morphine prolonged gastric emptying $t_{0.5}$ to 21 ± 9.0 min ($p < 0.05$). Methylnaltrexone reversed the morphine-induced delay in gastric emptying to $t_{0.5}$ of 7.4 ± 3.0 min ($p < 0.05$). The maximum concentrations of serum acetaminophen and acetaminophen AUC from 0 to 90 min after morphine were significantly different from those of either placebo or morphine administered concomitantly with methylnaltrexone ($p < 0.05$). There was no difference in maximum acetaminophen concentration or AUC between placebo or methylnaltrexone plus morphine, indicating a normalization of gastric emptying by methylnaltrexone.

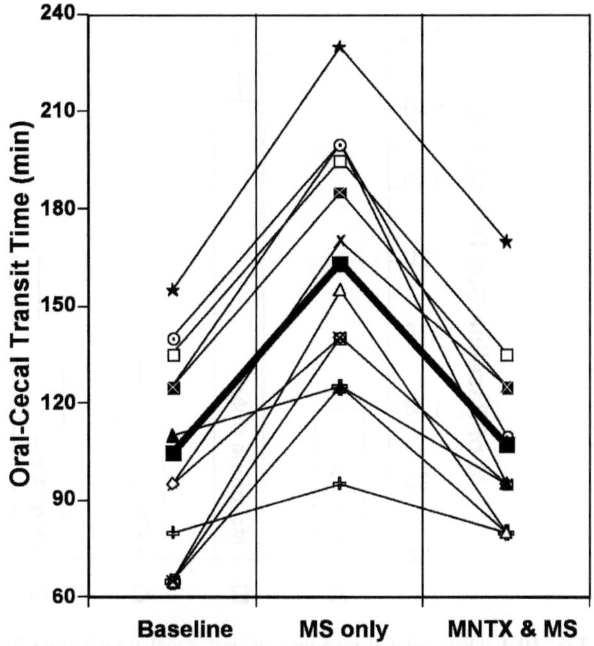

Fig. 10.3 The individual oral–cecal transit time of 12 healthy volunteers after injections. The heavy line represents the mean. *MS* intravenous morphine (0.05 mg/kg). *MNTX* intravenous methylnaltrexone (0.45 mg/kg)

Subcutaneous administration, often a more convenient route of drug delivery than intravenous injection, may be utilized with methylnaltrexone. In a controlled trial, the efficacy of subcutaneous methylnaltrexone in antagonizing morphine-induced delay in oral–cecal transit time was evaluated in 12 normal subjects (29). In the first group ($n = 6$), morphine (0.05 mg/kg intravenously) increased transit time from a baseline level of 85 ± 20.5 min to 155 ± 27.9 min ($p < 0.01$). When 0.1 mg/kg methylnaltrexone was administered subcutaneously at the same time as morphine, the transit time was reduced to 110 ± 41.0 min. In the second group ($n = 6$), morphine increased the transit time from a baseline level of 98 ± 49.1 min to 140 ± 58.2 min ($p < 0.01$). After subcutaneous methylnaltrexone 0.3 mg/kg plus morphine, the transit time was reduced to 108 ± 59.6 min ($p < 0.05$). These data suggest that subcutaneous methylnaltrexone has potential for the treatment of peripheral opioid-induced constipation.

10.4.4 Activity of Oral Methylnaltrexone in Healthy Volunteers

Oral methylnaltrexone has been well tolerated in humans. In 14 healthy subjects, no adverse effects were observed after single oral doses of methylnaltrexone at levels up to 19.2 mg/kg. Oral–cecal transit time was also measured in the study in the presence and absence of co-administered intravenous morphine. Delay of oral–cecal transit time after morphine was effectively prevented by oral methylnaltrexone in a proportional manner to the dose of the antagonist (30) (Fig. 10.4).

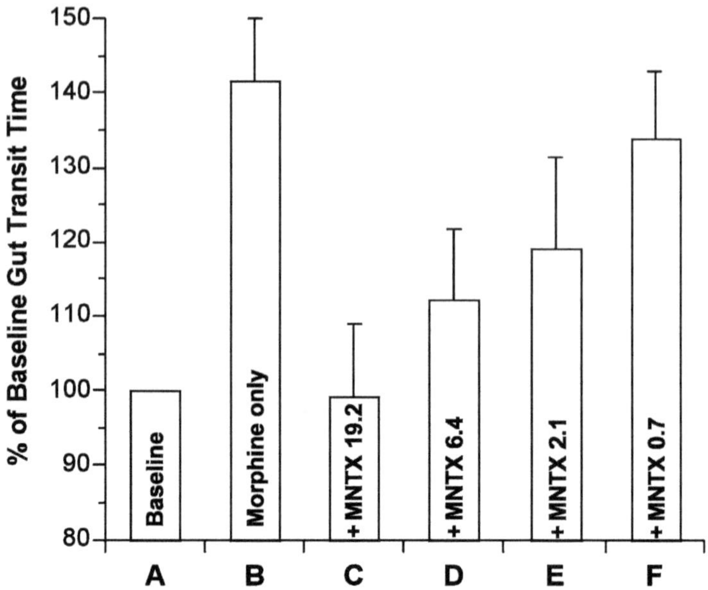

Fig. 10.4 Dose-related response of oral–cecal transit time in 14 healthy volunteers given oral methylnaltrexone. Placebo plus placebo (**a**) is normalized to 100%. Placebo plus intravenous morphine 0.05 mg/kg (**b**) significantly increases transit time. Intravenous morphine (0.05 mg/kg) was administered 20 min after oral methylnaltrexone in **c**–**f**. Changes in oral–cecal transit time after methylnaltrexone doses of 19.2, 6.4, 2.1, 0.7 mg/kg plus morphine are shown in **c**, **d**, **e**, and **f**, respectively. *MNTX* oral methylnaltrexone (mg/kg)

The investigators also observed a rapid initial increase in plasma levels within 5–20 min after administration of regular or uncoated methylnaltrexone, suggesting a correlation to gastric drug absorption (30). Because changes in gastric emptying time do not affect constipation significantly, it was hypothesized that the delivery of relatively higher amounts of methylnaltrexone to the bowel would exert a direct, possibly luminal effect on the intestine. Subsequently, another controlled study was conducted to evaluate the activity of orally administered, enteric-coated methylnaltrexone. The coating prevented degradation or release of drug in the stomach but allowed release in the small and large intestine. Gastric absorption was prevented and lower plasma levels of the compound were achieved. Transit time in subjects was prolonged after morphine administration, and enteric-coated methylnaltrexone 3.2 mg/kg completely prevented morphine-induced increases in oral–cecal transit time. Plasma concentrations after enteric-coated methylnaltrexone at doses of 6.4 mg/kg and 3.2 mg/kg were substantially lower compared to those after administration of the uncoated compound (31). These results suggest a prevailing direct or local effect of enteric-coated methylnaltrexone that the enteric-coated form may exert pharmacological actions on the gut more efficiently than the uncoated form.

10.4.5 Activity of Methylnaltrexone in Chronic Opioid Users

In a survey of 19 methadone-maintained, opioid-dependent volunteers, 58% of subjects reported constipation. The mean oral–cecal transit time of the methadone-maintained individuals was 159 ± 49.2 min, which was significantly longer than the baseline transit time recorded in our previous studies of human volunteers ($p < 0.01$). Tolerance to opioids does not appear to extend to gastrointestinal motility and transit. Subjects taking chronic methadone therapy are therefore a good model in which to evaluate the effects of opioid antagonists (39).

A pilot study was conducted to evaluate the effects of methylnaltrexone in four constipated subjects taking methadone (daily methadone dose, 38–90 mg/kg) (40). All subjects had immediate laxation responses during and after intravenous methylnaltrexone (0.05–0.45 mg/kg). Gut transit times were reduced significantly from baseline levels. At the highest dose (0.45 mg/kg), one subject experienced severe abdominal cramping but showed no other signs of systemic withdrawal such as lacrimation, diaphoresis, mydriasis, or hallucinations. Chronic opioid users were more sensitive to methylnaltrexone than the opioid-naive subjects in our previous trials.

In a subsequent randomized placebo-controlled trial, 22 subjects taking methadone (daily methadone dose, 30–100 mg) who experienced opioid-induced constipation were enrolled (41). For this two-day study with daily intravenous methylnaltrexone (0.1 ± 0.1 mg/kg) administrations, the effects on observed bowel movement (laxation), oral–cecal transit time, and central opioid withdrawal symptoms were determined. The 11 subjects in the placebo group showed no laxation response, whereas the 11 subjects in the methylnaltrexone group had an immediate laxation response after intravenous methylnaltrexone ($p < 0.01$). Most subjects reported mild-to-moderate abdominal cramping after methylnaltrexone, which they described as being similar to a defecation sensation without significant discomfort. Bowel movements, in most cases, were loose and copious. As shown in Fig. 10.5, baseline (predose) oral–cecal transit times for subjects in the methylnaltrexone and placebo groups averaged a little over 2 h (132.3 and 126.8 min, respectively). The average decrease in the methylnaltrexone-treated group was 77.7 ± 37.2 min, a change significantly greater than in the placebo group (−1.4 ± 12.0 min) ($p < 0.01$). Figure 10.6 shows the relationship between effective methylnaltrexone dose and peak plasma concentration. No opioid withdrawal was observed in either group, and no significant side effects were reported by the subjects during the study. The data suggest that low dose methylnaltrexone may have clinical utility in managing opioid-induced constipation.

In one case report, a 70-year-old patient with end-stage cryptogenic cirrhosis and fentanyl patch-induced intractable constipation was successfully treated with methylnaltrexone. Intravenous methylnaltrexone (0.3–0.4 mg/kg/day) induced laxation without affecting analgesia. No significant adverse effects were observed (42).

Oral methylnaltrexone was also investigated in 12 methadone-maintained subjects (43). None of the subjects showed a laxation response to placebo on day 1. On day 2, after receiving 0.3 mg/kg methylnaltrexone, 3 of 4 subjects had a bowel movement, with the time between drug administration and laxation averaging

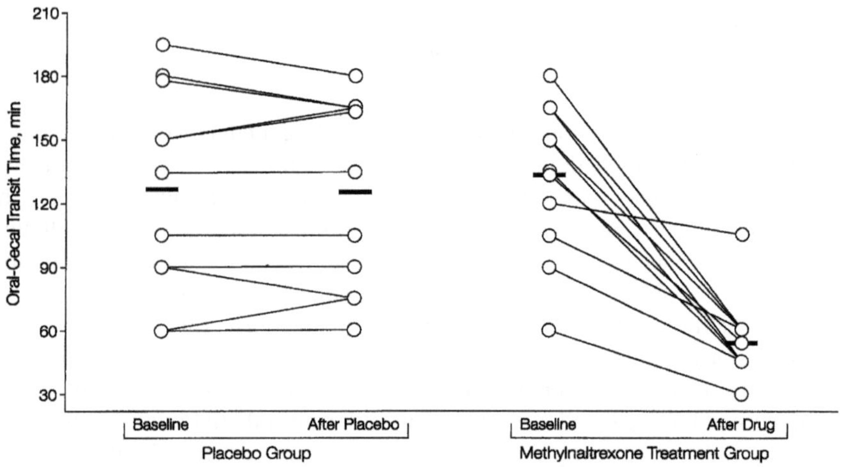

Fig. 10.5 Changes in individual oral–cecal transit times of subjects undergoing long-term methadone treatment. **a** The transit time of 11 subjects in the placebo group from baseline to after placebo injection. **b** The transit time of 11 subjects in methylnaltrexone group from baseline to after study drug administration. The short horizontal bar represents the mean. The average change in the methylnaltrexone group was significantly greater than the average change in the placebo group ($p < 0.01$)

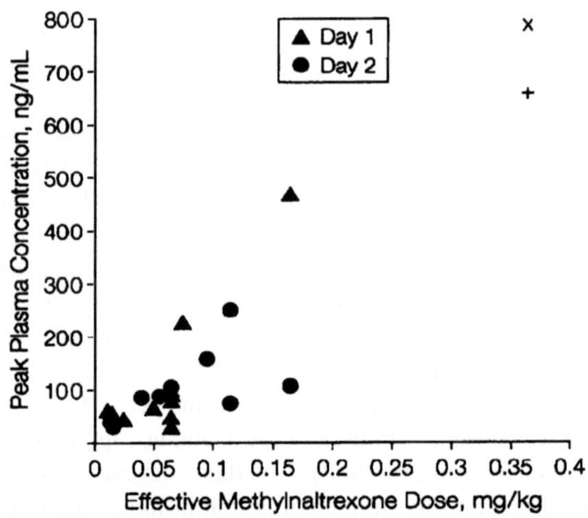

Fig. 10.6 Relationship between effective methylnaltrexone dose and peak plasma concentration in subjects undergoing long-term methadone treatment. Peak plasma concentration (C_{max}) is expressed as a function of the methylnaltrexone dose that induced laxation response on the first day administration (▲) and the second day administration (●). Subject 13 failed to defecate after the maximum dose (0.365 mg/kg) on day 1 (**X**) but responded to the same dose on day 2 (+). The r^2 value for the linear regression of concentration on effective dose is 0.77

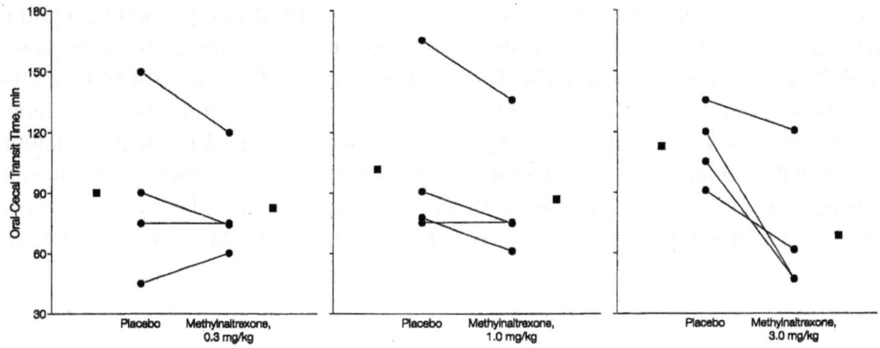

Fig. 10.7 Changes in individual oral–cecal transit times (*ordinate*) of 12 subjects undergoing long-term methodone therapy after placebo or one of three oral methylnaltrexone doses (four subjects in each dose group). Filled squares represent mean values

18.0 ± 8.7h. Higher doses of methylnaltrexone were associated with shorter times to laxation. The four subjects given 1.0mg/kg and the four subjects given 3.0mg/kg had bowel movements at 12.3 ± 8.7 and 5.2 ± 4.5h, respectively, after receiving the oral compound. Dose-related reduction in oral–cecal transit times ($p < 0.05$) is shown in the Fig. 10.7. Plasma drug levels were low or undetectable. There was no opioid withdrawal in any subject, and no adverse effects were reported.

10.4.6 Methylnaltrexone in Long-Term Opioid Users with Advanced Medical Illness (44)

Opioid-induced constipation is an extremely distressing and debilitating problem in patients in advanced stages of disease who require high doses of opioids for pain control (45, 46). In addition to issues of poor mobility and decreased oral intake, such patients may experience constipation from medications, tumor infiltration or bowel hypomotility following chemotherapy or radiation (46, 47). Intravenous methylnaltrexone is not desirable in such poorly mobile patients because it caused laxation very rapidly, often within minutes. Data with subcutaneous administration suggested a less immediate onset of action without the need for intravenous access, a more attractive option in these patients (29).

Patients with a life expectancy of less than six months but greater than one month who also had opioid-induced constipation (2 days without passage of stool) and a constipation distress score of greater than or equal to three (on a five-point scale) were studied. The opioid and laxative regimen was stable, and patients with mechanical bowel obstruction, other constipation-inducing abdominal pathologies, or fecal impaction were excluded.

Patients were randomly allocated to one of four unit doses of methylnaltrexone, 1.0mg, 5.0mg, 12.5mg, or 20mg to be administered subcutaneously every other day (days 1, 3, and 5) before a 3-week open-label period when the drug could be administered as needed. The primary assessments were bowel movements, pain scores, opioid withdrawal and adverse events. The dosing schedule during the double-blind phase was consistent with what the anticipated needs of sick patients with limited oral intake would be, and with bowel hygiene regimens of heavily nursing-dependent populations like spinal cord injury patients. During the open-label period, a subcutaneous dose of 5.0mg was administered and, unlike in the double-blind phase, dose was titrated for effect and tolerability. The aim was to obtain experience with a longer treatment period

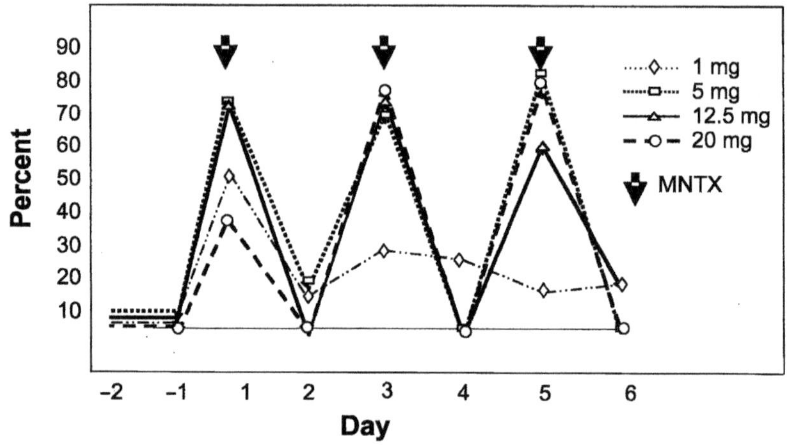

Fig. 10.8 Laxation for four different methylnaltrexone dose groups among 33 advanced medical illness patients with chronic opioid constipation during the double-blind trial period. *MNTX* methylnaltrexone

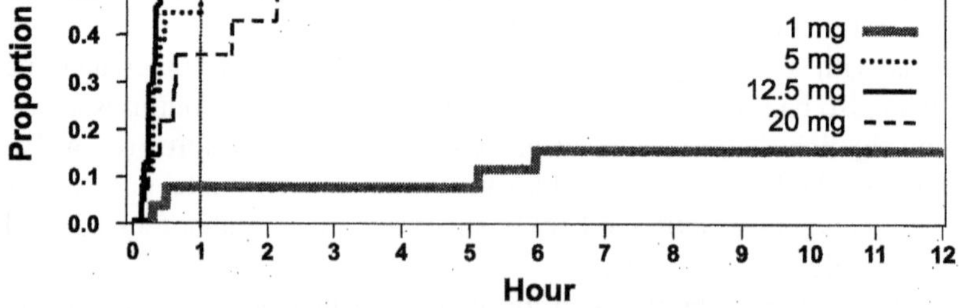

Fig. 10.9 Time to laxation for the groups in Fig. 10.8 during the first 12h of the double-blind trial period

and repetitive dosing and to see how patients and caregivers would use this agent in a clinical setting.

Of 33 patients enrolled, 28 had cancer. The median WHO performance status was 3, the median number of laxatives patients took study start was 2, and the median age was 64 years old. Figure 10.8 shows laxation results by day for each dose group during the double-blind period. In Fig. 10.9, the Kaplan-Meier graph shows that doses ≥5 mg were active, and the median time to laxation following a dose was approximately 1 hour (p = 0.006, log rank). The curves also suggest that nearly all laxation took place within about 4 hours. Thus, doses of at least 5 mg induced laxation in about 60% of patients within 1 hour. Similar results were obtained in the open-label dosing. In general, patients and caregivers elected to continue treatment during the open-label phase, and the drug was needed every other day. No change in pain scores or evidence of opioid withdrawal was reported. The most common adverse events were transient abdominal cramping and flatulence. Methylnaltrexone was well tolerated; there were no drug-related serious adverse events in this study.

10.4.7 Methylnaltrexone for Post-operative Ileus

Ileus after abdominal surgery is common and often unavoidable. It prolongs hospital stay and is associated with a significant increase in morbidity and cost (48). Colonic motility is crucial for the recovery of bowel function following surgery, and surgeries involving colonic anastomoses require especially lengthy recovery periods (49), with a post-operative stay of usually 6–12 days (50).

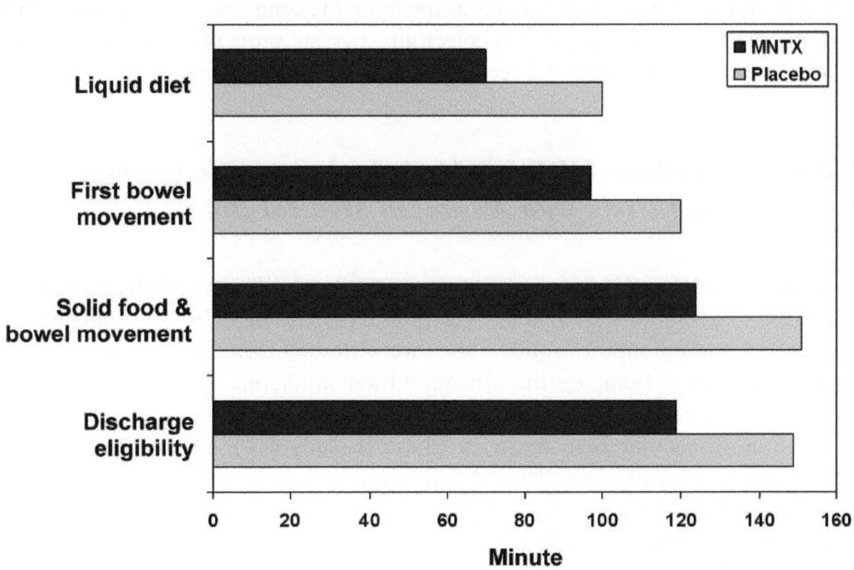

Fig. 10.10 Time to bowel recovery in 65 postoperative patients *MNTX* methylnaltrexone

Table 10.1 Bowel activity-related changes of 65 postoperative patients

	Mean time (h)			p-Value (1-sided)
End point	MNTX	Placebo	Difference	log-rank
First bowel movement	97.965	118.056	20.09	0.019
Discharge eligibility	116.068	148.653	32.59	0.025
First tolerance of full liquids	68.050	97.259	29.21	0.060
Actual discharge	138.329	164.525	26.20	0.080
First tolerance of solids	97.387	123.900	26.51	0.103
Time to solids in solids out[a]	124.064	151.216	27.51	0.062

[a]Time to solids in solids out = time to first tolerance of solids or first bowel movement, whichever occurred first. *MNTX* methylnaltrexone

A controlled trial of intravenous methylnaltrexone was performed in patients following open segmental colonic resection (51). Patients were randomly allocated to receive either placebo or methylnaltrexone 0.3 mg/kg as a 20-min intravenous infusion every 6 hours after surgery. Patients were treated until 24 hours after they tolerated solid foods, were discharged from the hospital, or after 7 full days of treatment.

In the 65 patients enrolled in the study, the most common surgeries were sigmoidectomy and right hemicolectomy. Type and duration of surgery were well balanced between groups. Methylnaltrexone-treated patients recovered bowel function quicker than placebo patients in all measures of upper and lower bowel recovery (Fig. 10.10), and the mean differences in all the parameters of recovery exceeded 1 day (Table 10.1). No differences in opioid use or in mean pain scores were observed. The drug was well tolerated and overall adverse events were similar to these after placebo. Although study suggests that parenteral methylnaltrexone may significantly shorten the duration of ileus after segmental colectomy, two subsequent phase 3 trials did not show improvement in time to GI recovery with methylnaltrexone.

10.4.8 First Phase III Trial: Methylnaltrexone in Chronic Opioid Users with Advanced Medical Illness

In a large phase III trial, to confirm activity and tolerability of methylnaltrexone and to elucidate the relationship of dose to response, patients at 16 hospice and palliative care centers throughout the United States were studied (52). The primary objective of the study was to compare the efficacy of subcutaneous methylnaltrexone with placebo to induce laxation within 4 hours. The secondary objectives were safety and the laxation efficacy at 24 h. As in the phase II study (44), eligible patients had a life expectancy of 1 to 6 months and opioid-induced constipation with no laxation for at least 48 hours with a stable regimen of laxatives and opioids. In addition to placebo, the two doses of methylnaltrexone were 0.15 mg/kg or 0.30 mg/kg in a single, double-blind dose, with assessments at 4 and 24 hours, followed by a 4-week open-label period.

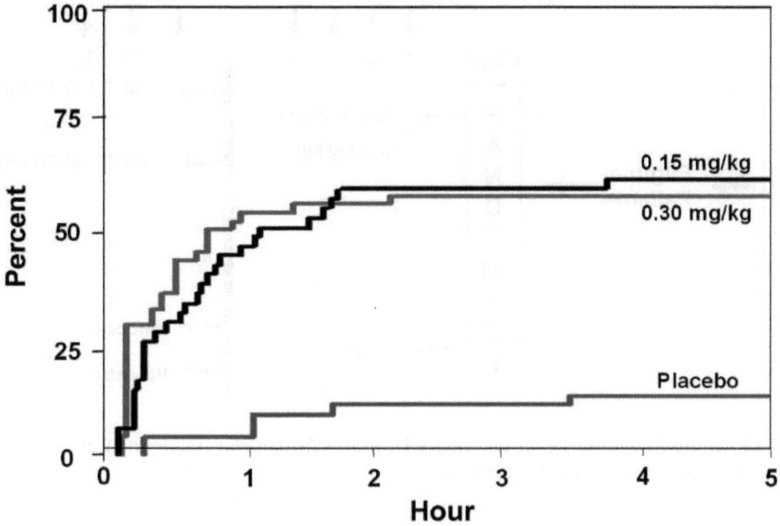

Fig. 10.11 Time to laxation measured over 5 h for two groups given different subcutaneous doses of methylnaltrexone based on body weight and one placebo group among 154 patients with advanced medical illness suffering from chronic opioid-induced constipation

Of the 154 patients with advanced medical illness enrolled, 80% had a primary diagnosis of cancer; others had emphysema, end-stage AIDS, neurologic disease, or cardiovascular disease. As shown in Fig. 10.11, methylnaltrexone had a rapid significant effect at both doses versus placebo ($p < 0.0001$, log rank). Differences remained highly significant at 24 hours. The median time to laxation in the group that received 0.15 mg/kg was 70 min; in those who received 0.30 mg/kg, 45 min. The median time to laxation in the placebo group was greater than 1 day ($p < 0.0001$, log rank). Thus, a single dose of methylnaltrexone induced laxation in about 60% of patients within approximately one hour. The greater single dose did not appear to offer any substantial benefit over the smaller dose.

Similar to the phase II study (44), the most common adverse events were abdominal cramping and flatulence with nausea and dizziness noted with the larger dose, that is, 0.3 mg/kg. Serious adverse events were rare and evenly distributed among the placebo and study drug groups.

10.4.9 Second Phase III Trial: Methylnaltrexone in Chronic Opioid Users with Advanced Medical Illness

This study was designed to replicate the results from the first phase III trial and to confirm the continued activity of methylnaltrexone when administered subcutaneously every-other-day for a more extended period of time (53). A study that includes pla-

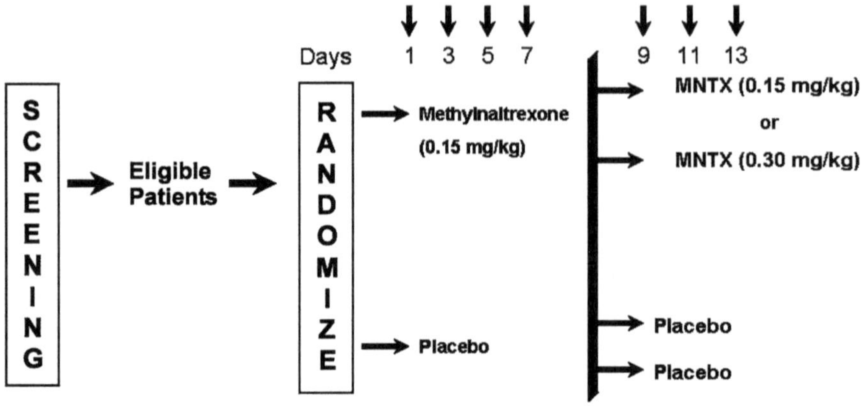

Fig. 10.12 Study design of the second phase III trial, subcutaneous methylnaltrexone in chronic opioid users with advanced medical illness

Fig. 10.13 Graph depicting greater than or equal to two laxation responses within 4 h in the methylnaltrexone group or placebo group for 134 patients with advanced medical illness and opioid-induced constipation. Data were recorded over 1 week after four doses of drug or placebo ($p < 0.0001$, chi-square test)

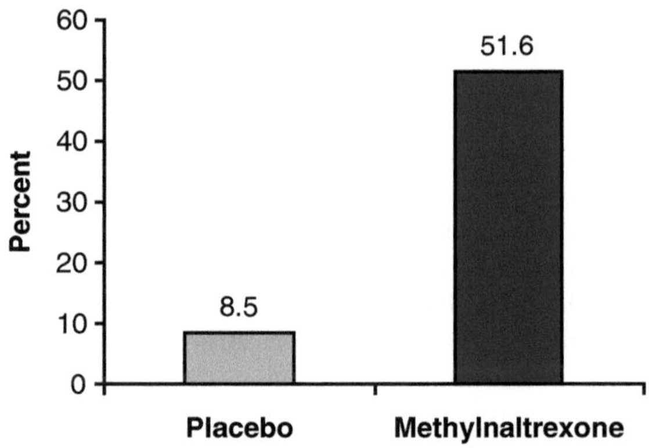

cebo treatment in a population with advanced illness is limited by the medical status of the patients and ethical considerations; therefore, the placebo-controlled treatment period of this phase III trial was limited to 2 weeks. In this trial, patients were given 0.15 mg/kg methylnaltrexone or placebo subcutaneously over 2 weeks-every other day (seven doses on days 1, 3, 5, 7, 9, 11, and 13) (Fig. 10.12). If a patient did not have at least three laxations after the first week, there was the option of increasing the dose of study drug to 0.3 mg/kg or placebo. This was effected by doubling the volume of the injected study medication so as to maintain the blind condition.

The study objectives were to replicate the findings of the first phase III trial following the first dose, to determine the efficacy of the drug over 1 and 2 weeks, and to expand the safety experience in patients with advanced illness (53).

A total of 134 patients were enrolled over 33 palliative care centers and nursing homes. Approximately 60% had a primary diagnosis of cancer, 10% had cardiovascular disease, and 30% had chronic obstructive pulmonary disease or neurologic disease. Within 4 h of the first dose, 48.4% of methylnaltrexone patients laxated

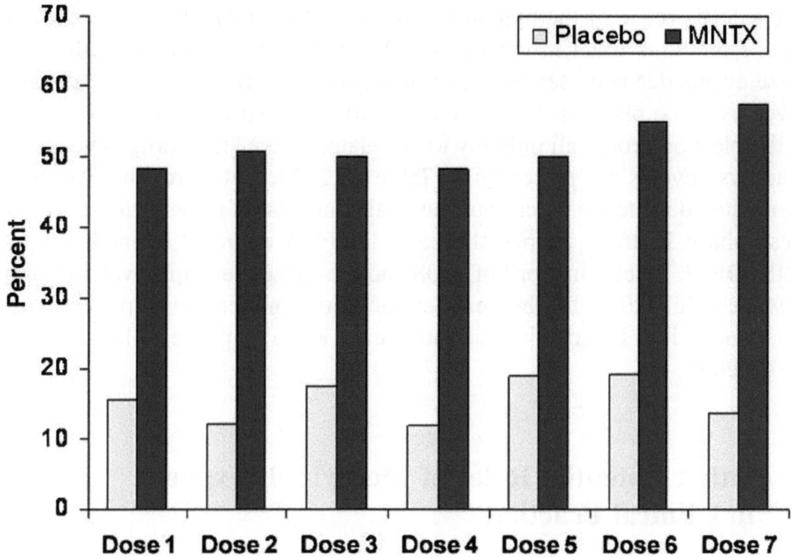

Fig. 10.14 Laxation response within 4h of each dose over seven doses in methylnaltrexone or placebo group (all differences $p < 0.0005$, chi-square test)

Table 10.2 Most common adverse events reported in the second phase III trial by 134 advanced medical illness patients with chronic opioid-induced constipation

	Placebo (n = 71)		Methylnaltrexone (n = 63)	
	n	%	n	%
Abdominal cramping	9	12.7	11	17.5
Flatulence	5	7	8	12.7
Vomiting	9	12.7	8	12.7
Malignant neoplasm progression	9	12.7	7	11.1
Edema peripheral	8	11.3	5	7.9
Nausea	5	7	7	11.1
Pain exacerbated	7	9.9	2	3.2
Asthenia	4	5.6	4	6.3
Lethargy	4	5.6	4	6.3
Fall	7	9.9	1	1.6
Body temperature increased	2	2.8	5	7.9
Dizziness	2	2.8	5	7.9
Diarrhea	3	4.2	4	6.3
Abdominal distension	6	8.5	1	1.6

versus 15% of placebo patients ($p < 0.0001$). Over a week's period (doses 1, 3, 5, and 7), 51.6% of methylnaltrexone patients had greater than or equal to 2 laxations within 2 hours of dosing versus 8.5% in the placebo group (Fig. 10.13).

There was no evidence of diminution of effect over all seven doses of the study (Fig. 10.14) with highly significant differences versus placebo throughout and no change in absolute differences.

The safety profile of methylnaltrexone from this study was consistent with the profile of previous trials in chronic opioid users with advanced medical illness. Adverse events deemed "serious" during the trial occurred in 14 patients on active drug versus 21 on placebo. There were 8 deaths in the methylnaltrexone group and 15 in the placebo group, all unlikely to be related to the study drug. The most common adverse events are presented in Table 10.2. Methylnaltrexone was generally well tolerated despite the precarious medical condition of these patients. The results of these phase III trials formed the basis for FDA approval of methylnaltrexone (RELISTOR™, Wyeth) in April of 2008 and the subsequent approval in Europe by the EMEA in July 2008, for the treatment of opioid-induced constipation in patients with advanced illness receiving palliative care when response to laxatives has not been sufficient.

10.5 Other Potential Roles of Methylnaltrexone in Clinical Practice

10.5.1 Opioid-Induced Delay in Gastric Emptying

Morphine and related opioids delay gastric emptying, even at low doses (37). This opioid effect may be reversed by methylnaltrexone administration (38), and may represent a potential therapeutic use for patients in the intensive care unit if reduced gut motility decreases their ability to be fed enterally. Critically ill patients whose lungs are mechanically ventilated may receive opioids as part of their sedation. Enteric tube feeding provides their nutrition, and the rate-limiting factor for enteral nutrition is often the gastric residual after a feed. Methylnaltrexone appears to have the potential to decrease residuals by enhancing gastric emptying in patients on opioids. Further exploration and clinical confirmation of this activity is warranted.

10.5.2 Opioid-Induced Urinary Retention

One of the troubling adverse effects of opioids, particularly in the posto-perative setting, is urinary retention. Whether central or peripheral mechanisms, or both, control this effect has remained an open question (54). One study showed that continuous infusion of remifentanil caused miosis and profound depression of bladder function in 15 healthy male subjects. Both effects were reversed by naloxone 0.01 mg/kg. Methylnaltrexone 0.3 mg/kg did not affect miosis but reversed the opioid-induced decline in detrussor pressure in 3 of 11 subjects and increased the amount voided in 5 of 11 subjects (33). Thus, opioid effects on the human bladder seem to be at least partially peripherally mediated. Potential clinical application of methylnaltrexone in reversing opioid-induced urinary retention remains to be tested in further studies.

10.5.3 Opioid-Induced Subjective Effects

After opioid administration, dysphoria, dizziness, nausea, and pruritus have been reported. Not all these effects are produced by the action of opioids on the central nervous system. Nausea and vomiting are mediated by receptors located outside of the blood–brain barrier (17, 18). Opioid-induced pruritus also may be peripherally mediated (55). We found that oral methylnaltrexone decreased some subjective effects of morphine, such as nausea and itching, in human volunteers. Plasma methylnaltrexone concentrations at two different oral doses were correlated with its pharmacological effects (56). Thus, methylnaltrexone may have the potential to reduce some undesirable subjective effects associated with opioid medications.

10.5.4 Maintaining the Cough Reflex After Opioids

Coughing is a protective reflex of the airway, especially in post-operative patients. Control of the cough reflex has traditionally been assumed to reside in the central nervous system (57). However, in a study of peripheral agonists, a peripheral site of action for opioids was found (58). Along these lines, methylnaltrexone blocked opioid-induced cough suppression without affecting pain relief in guinea pigs (59). It appears that peripheral opioid receptors may play a role in cough control, and methylnaltrexone may be of potential benefit as an agent to maintain the cough reflex in patients who receive opioids.

10.5.5 Opioid-Induced Immunosuppression

Opioid-induced immunosuppression is a less well-understood adverse effect of opioids (60). Although well described as a laboratory phenomenon in numerous animal experiments and clinical studies (61), its clinical importance as an adverse effect of opioid use has not been generally recognized. There has long been a strong association between the use of opioids and exacerbation of infections, including AIDS. Research data have demonstrated that opioids suppress phagocytic, natural killer, B and T cells. The exact mechanisms of action of opioids on immunomodulation are incompletely understood, but several studies have suggested that these effects might be mediated via mechanisms different from those responsible for analgesia (60). It has been shown that methylnaltrexone antagonized opioid-mediated enhancement of HIV infection of human blood mononuclear phagocytes (62). If peripherally mediated, methylnaltrexone could potentially attenuate opioid-induced immunosuppression while preserving analgesic effect.

10.5.6 Constipation Associated with Functional Bowel Disorders

It has been proposed that endogenous opioids may play a role in gut motility (63). In an experiment on a strip of human small intestine muscle, methylnaltrexone enhanced the force of muscle contractility by up to 30% (23), implying the presence of a background level of endogenous opioid activity in gut tissue. In normal, opioid-naive subjects, when methylnaltrexone alone was given for 3 consecutive days, a trend of accelerated gut transit was observed, further suggesting a role for endogenous opioids in regulating human gut motility (25). Other investigators have found that naloxone was effective in cases of idiopathic constipation (64) and irritable bowel syndrome (65). If a relative or absolute excess of endogenous opioids or an altered opioid receptor affinity contributes to hypomotility, methylnaltrexone may have potential activity in these settings. To our knowledge, these investigations have not been initiated.

10.5.7 Inhibition of Angiogenesis

Angiogenesis, the formation of new blood vessels, promotes the growth and metastatic potential of various cancers. Compounds that inhibit angiogenesis have therapeutic implications in numerous malignancies. A recent study demonstrated the effects of methylnaltrexone on opioid-induced proliferation and migration of human endothelial cells, two key components in angiogenesis (66). In human dermal microvascular cells, opioids and vascular endothelial growth factor (VEGF) induced migration that was inhibited by pretreatment with methylnaltrexone. Proliferation and migration of cells was inhibited via inhibition of VEGF receptor phosphorylation/transactivation, which then inhibited activation of RhoA, a member of the Ras homology family of small GTPases. Inhibition of angiogenesis by methylnaltrexone may be an interesting and important property of this molecule. The clinical relevance of these findings, however, remains to be elucidated.

10.6 Summary

Methylnaltrexone is a peripheral opioid antagonist. Preclinical and clinical studies demonstrate antagonism of many of the peripheral effects of opioids that are often undesirable, such as constipation, urinary retention, pruritus, and others. Data from animal studies and clinical trials with methylnaltrexone are advancing the understanding of a wide variety of actions by opioids in humans. To date, most of the investigations of methylnaltrexone have studied opioid-induced adverse effects in the gastrointestinal tract. Two phase III trials have been conducted in chronic opioid users with advanced medical illness which served as the pivotal trials for the RELISTOR approval. In these patients, constipation has a significant negative impact on quality of life (45), Additional clinical trials are ongoing or planned to show clinical usefulness of methylnaltrexone in other settings. As methylnaltrexone moves to broader marketing approval, the once elusive goal of pain control without adverse effects may soon be achieved.

Conflict of Interest Disclaimer

Methylnaltrexone was originally formulated and subsequently modified by faculty at the University of Chicago. It is currently being developed by Progenics Pharmaceuticals, Inc. and Wyeth Pharmaceuticals. The University of Chicago and Dr. Yuan may benefit financially from the development of methylnaltrexone. Dr. Israel is an employee of Progenics Pharmaceuticals, Inc.

References

1. McCaffrey M, Beebe A. Managing your patients' adverse reactions to narcotics. Nursing 1989;19:166–168.
2. Glare P, Lickiss JN. Unrecognized constipation in patients with advanced cancer: a recipe for therapeutic disaster. J Pain Symptom Manage 1992;7:369–371.
3. Gowan JD, Hurtig JB, Fraser RA, Torbicki E, Kitts J. Naloxone infusion after prophylactic epidural morphine: effects on incidence of postoperative side-effects and quality of analgesia. Can J Anaesth 1988;35:143–148.
4. Culpepper-Morgan JA, Inturrisi CE, Portenoy RK, Foley K, Houde RW, Marsh F, Kreek MJ. Treatment of opioid-induced constipation with oral naloxone: a pilot study. Clin Pharmacol Ther 1992;52:90–95.
5. Cheskin LJ, Chami TN, Johnson RE, Jaffe JH. Assessment of nalmefene glucuronide as a selective gut opioid antagonist. Drug Alcohol Depend 1995;39:151–154.
6. Sykes NP. Using of oral naloxone in the management of opioid bowel dysfunction. In: Handbook of Opioid Bowel Syndrome. Yuan CS (ed). New York: Haworth Medical Press, 2005, pp. 175–195.
7. Brown DR, Goldberg LI. The use of quaternary narcotic antagonists in opiate research. Neuropharmacology 1985;24:181–191.
8. Russell J, Bass P, Goldberg LI, Schuster CR, Merz H. Antagonism of gut, but not central effects of morphine with quaternary narcotic antagonists. Eur J Pharmacol 1982;78:255–261.
9. Woods JH, Medzihradsky F, Smith CB, Young AM, Swain HH. Annual report: evaluation of new compounds for opioid activity (1980). NIDA Res Monogr 1981;34:327–366.
10. Gmerek DE, Cowan A, Woods JH. Independent central and peripheral mediation of morphine-induced inhibition of gastrointestinal transit in rats. J Pharmacol Exp Ther 1986;236:8–13.
11. Walker MJ, Le AD, Poulos CX, Cappell H. Role of central versus peripheral opioid receptors in analgesia induced by repeated administration of opioid antagonists. Psychopharmacology (Berl) 1991;104:164–166.
12. Yuan CS. Gastric effects of mu-, delta- and kappa-opioid receptor agonists on brainstem unitary responses in the neonatal rat. Eur J Pharmacol 1996;314:27–32.

13. Yuan CS, Foss JF. Gastric effects of methylnaltrexone on mu, kappa, and delta opioid agonists induced brainstem unitary responses. Neuropharmacology 1999;38:425–432.
14. Bianchi G, Fiocchi R, Tavani A, Manara L. Quaternary narcotic antagonists' relative ability to prevent antinociception and gastrointestinal transit inhibition in morphine-treated rats as an index of peripheral selectivity. Life Sci 1982;30:1875–1883.
15. Koob GF, Pettit HO, Ettenberg A, Bloom FE. Effects of opiate antagonists and their quaternary derivatives on heroin self-administration in the rat. J Pharmacol Exp Ther 1984;229: 481–486.
16. Kotake AN, Kuwahara SK, Burton E, McCoy CE, Goldberg LI. Variations in demethylation of N-methylnaltrexone in mice, rats, dogs, and humans. Xenobiotica 1989;19:1247–1254.
17. Borison HL, Wang SC. Physiology and pharmacology of vomiting. Pharmacol Rev 1953;5: 193–230.
18. Foss JF, Bass AS, Goldberg LI. Dose-related antagonism of the emetic effect of morphine by methylnaltrexone in dogs. J Clin Pharmacol 1993;33:747–751.
19. Foss JF, Yuan CS, Roizen MF, Goldberg LI. Prevention of apomorphine- or cisplatin-induced emesis in the dog by a combination of methylnaltrexone and morphine. Cancer Chemother Pharmacol 1998;42:287–291.
20. Aung HH, Mehendale SR, Xie JT, Moss J, Yuan CS. Methylnaltrexone prevents morphine-induced kaolin intake in the rat. Life Sci 2004;74:2685–2691.
21. Manara L, Bianchetti A. The central and peripheral influences of opioids on gastrointestinal propulsion. Annu Rev Pharmacol Toxicol 1985;25:249–273.
22. Ferritti P, Tavani A, Manara L. Inhibition of gastrointestinal transit and antinociceptive effects of morphine and FK-33–824 in rats are differently prevented by naloxone and the N-methyl quaternary analog. Res Commun Subst Abuse 1981;2:1–11.
23. Yuan CS, Foss JF, Moss J. Effects of methylnaltrexone on morphine-induced inhibition of contraction in isolated guinea-pig ileum and human intestine. Eur J Pharmacol 1995;276: 107–111.
24. Foss JF, O'Connor MF, Yuan CS, Murphy M, Moss J, Roizen MF. Safety and tolerance of methylnaltrexone in healthy humans: a randomized, placebo-controlled, intravenous, ascending-dose, pharmacokinetic study. J Clin Pharmacol 1997;37:25–30.
25. Yuan CS, Doshan H, Charney MR, O'Connor M, Karrison T, Maleckar SA, Israel RJ, Moss J. Tolerability, gut effects, and pharmacokinetics of methylnaltrexone following repeated intravenous administration in humans. J Clin Pharmacol 2005;45:538–546.
26. Kim C, Cheng R, Corrigall WA, Coen KM. High-perfomance liquid-chromatography with coulometric electochemical detection. Chromatographia 1989;28:359–336.
27. Osinski J, Wang A, Wu JA, Foss JF, Yuan CS. Determination of methylnaltrexone in clinical samples by solid-phase extraction and high-performance liquid chromatography for a pharmacokinetics study. J Chromatogr B Analyt Technol Biomed Life Sci 2002;780:251–259.
28. Yuan CS, Foss JF, O'Connor M, Toledano A, Roizen MF, Moss J. Methylnaltrexone prevents morphine-induced delay in oral-cecal transit time without affecting analgesia: a double-blind randomized placebo-controlled trial. Clin Pharmacol Ther 1996;59:469–475.
29. Yuan CS, Wei G, Foss JF, O'Connor M, Karrison T, Osinski J. Effects of subcutaneous methylnaltrexone on morphine-induced peripherally mediated side effects: a double-blind randomized placebo-controlled trial. J Pharmacol Exp Ther 2002;300:118–123.
30. Yuan CS, Foss JF, Osinski J, Toledano A, Roizen MF, Moss J. The safety and efficacy of oral methylnaltrexone in preventing morphine-induced delay in oral-cecal transit time. Clin Pharmacol Ther 1997;61:467–475.
31. Yuan CS, Foss JF, O'Connor M, Karrison T, Osinski J, Roizen MF, Moss J. Effects of enteric-coated methylnaltrexone in preventing opioid-induced delay in oral-cecal transit time. Clin Pharmacol Ther 2000;67:398–404.
32. Amin HM, Sopchak AM, Foss JF, Esposito BF, Roizen MF, Camporesi EM. Efficacy of methylnaltrexone versus naloxone for reversal of morphine-induced depression of hypoxic ventilatory response. Anesth Analg 1994;78:701–705.

33. Gomery P, Chen T, Stefanovich P, Chandler L, Montgomery E, Rosow C. Antagonism of opioid bladder and pupil effects by methylnaltrexone, naloxone, or placebo. Proc Intl Soc Anesth Pharm 2003;307:1158–1162.
34. Bond JH Jr, Levitt MD, Prentiss R. Investigation of small bowel transit time in man utilizing pulmonary hydrogen (H2) measurements. J Lab Clin Med 1975;85:546–555.
35. Read NW, Al-Janabi MN, Bates TE, Holgate AM, Cann PA, Kinsman RI, McFarlane A, Brown C. Interpretation of the breath hydrogen profile obtained after ingesting a solid meal containing unabsorbable carbohydrate. Gut 1985;26:834–842.
36. Yuan CS, Karrison T, Wu JA, Lowell TK, Lynch JP, Foss JF. Dose-related effects of oral acetaminophen on cold-induced pain: a double-blind, randomized, placebo-controlled trial. Clin Pharmacol Ther 1998;63:379–383.
37. Yuan CS, Foss JF, O'Connor M, Roizen MF, Moss J. Effects of low-dose morphine on gastric emptying in healthy volunteers. J Clin Pharmacol 1998;38:1017–1020.
38. Murphy DB, Sutton JA, Prescott LF, Murphy MB. Opioid-induced delay in gastric emptying: a peripheral mechanism in humans. Anesthesiology 1997;87:765–770.
39. Yuan CS, Foss JF, O'Connor M, Moss J, Roizen MF. Gut motility and transit changes in patients receiving long-term methadone maintenance. J Clin Pharmacol 1998;38:931–935.
40. Yuan CS, Foss JF, O'Connor M, Osinski J, Roizen MF, Moss J. Effects of intravenous methylnaltrexone on opioid-induced gut motility and transit time changes in subjects receiving chronic methadone therapy: a pilot study. Pain 1999;83:631–635.
41. Yuan CS, Foss JF, O'Connor M, Osinski J, Karrison T, Moss J, Roizen MF. Methylnaltrexone for reversal of constipation due to chronic methadone use: a randomized controlled trial. JAMA 2000;283:367–372.
42. Yuan CS, Moss J, Wei G, Maleckar SA, Boyd TA, Israel RJ. Methylnaltrexone for chronic opioid-induced constipation. Am Soc Clin Oncol Proc 2002;21:376a.
43. Yuan CS, Foss JF. Oral methylnaltrexone for opioid-induced constipation. JAMA 2000;284: 1383–1384.
44. Thomas J, Portenoy RK, Moehl M, Von Gunten C, Thielemann P, Stambler N, Tran D, Galasso F, Israel R. A phase II randomized dose-finding trail of methylnaltrexone for the relief of opioid-induced constipation in hospice patients. Am Soc Clin Oncol Proc 2003; 22:2933.
45. Meier DE, Morrison RS, Cassel CK. Improving palliative care. Ann Intern Med 1997;127: 225–230.
46. Abraham JL. A Physician's Guide to Pain and Symptom Management in Cancer Patients. Baltimore: Johns Hopkins University Press, 2000.
47. Mercadante S. Diarrhea, malabsorption, and constipation. In: Palliative Care and Supportive Oncology. Berger AM, Portenoy RK, Weissman DE (eds). Philadelphia: Lippincott, Williams & Wilkins, 2002, pp. 233–249.
48. Bauer AJ, Boeckxstaens GE. Mechanisms of postoperative ileus. Neurogastroenterol Motil 2004;16 Suppl 2:54–60.
49. Huge A, Kreis ME, Zittel TT, Becker HD, Starlinger MJ, Jehle EC. Postoperative colonic motility and tone in patients after colorectal surgery. Dis Colon Rectum 2000;43:932–939.
50. Basse L, Hjort Jakobsen D, Billesbolle P, Werner M, Kehlet H. A clinical pathway to accelerate recovery after colonic resection. Ann Surg 2000;232:51–57.
51. Viscusi E, Rathmell J, Alessandro F, Gan TJ, Israel RJ. A double-blind, randomized, placebo-controlled trial of methylnaltrexone for post-operative bowel dysfunction in segmental colectomy patients. Proc Am Soc Anesth 2005;25:1630.
52. Thomas J, Lipman A, Slatkin N, Wilson G, Moehl M, Wellman C, Zhukovsky D, Stephenson R, Stambler N, Israel RJ. A phase III double-blind placebo-controlled trial of methylnaltrexone (MNTX) for opioid-induced constipation (OIC) in advanced medical illness (AMI). Proc Am Soc Clin Oncol 2005;25:8003.
53. Slatkin N, Karver S, Thomas J, Chamberlain B, Austin-Cooney G, Watt C, Winston JL, Cross K, McGrew D, Stambler N, Israel RJ. A phase III double-blind, placebo-controlled trial

of methylnaltrexone for opioid-induced constipation in advanced illness (MNTX 302). Digest Dis Week 2006;686e.
54. Petersen TK, Husted SE, Rybro L, Schurizek BA, Wernberg M. Urinary retention during i.m. and extradural morphine analgesia. Br J Anaesth 1982;54:1175–1178.
55. Levy JH, Brister NW, Shearin A, Ziegler J, Hug CC, Jr., Adelson DM, Walker BF. Wheal and flare responses to opioids in humans. Anesthesiology 1989;70:756–760.
56. Yuan CS, Foss JF, O'Connor M, Osinski J, Roizen MF, Moss J. Efficacy of orally administered methylnaltrexone in decreasing subjective effects after intravenous morphine. Drug Alcohol Depend 1998;52:161–165.
57. Chakravarty NK, Matallana A, Jensen R, Borison HL. Central effects of antitussive drugs on cough and respiration. J Pharmacol Exp Ther 1956;117:127–135.
58. Adcock JJ, Schneider C, Smith TW. Effects of codeine, morphine and a novel opioid pentapeptide BW443C, on cough, nociception and ventilation in the unanaesthetized guinea-pig. Br J Pharmacol 1988;93:93–100.
59. Foss JF, Orelind E, Goldberg LI. Effects of methylnaltrexone on morphine-induced cough suppression in guinea pigs. Life Sci 1996;59:PL235–PL238.
60. Wei G, Moss J, Yuan CS. Opioid-induced immunosuppression: is it centrally mediated or peripherally mediated? Biochem Pharmacol 2003;65:1761–1766.
61. Eisenstein TK, Hilburger ME. Opioid modulation of immune responses: effects on phagocyte and lymphoid cell populations. J Neuroimmunol 1998;83:36–44.
62. Ho WZ, Guo CJ, Yuan CS, Douglas SD, Moss J. Methylnaltrexone antagonizes opioid-mediated enhancement of HIV infection of human blood mononuclear phagocytes. J Pharmacol Exp Ther 2003;307:1158–1162.
63. Kehlet H. Endogenous morphine—another component and biological modifier of the response to surgical injury? Acta Anaesthesiol Scand 2000;44:1167–1168.
64. Kreek MJ, Schaefer RA, Hahn EF, Fishman J. Naloxone, a specific opioid antagonist, reverses chronic idiopathic constipation. Lancet 1983;1:261–262.
65. Hawkes ND, Rhodes J, Evans BK, Rhodes P, Hawthorne AB, Thomas GA. Naloxone treatment for irritable bowel syndrome – a randomized controlled trial with an oral formulation. Aliment Pharmacol Ther 2002;16:1649–1654.
66. Singleton PA, Lingen MW, Fekete MJ, Garcia JG, Moss J. Methylnaltrexone inhibits opiate and VEGF-induced angiogenesis: role of receptor transactivation. Microvasc Res 2006; 72:3–11.
67. Neary P, Delaney CP. Alvimopan. Expert Opin Investig Drugs 2005;14:479–488.

Part III
Substance Abuse

Chapter 11
Opioid Antagonist Effects in Animal Models Related to Opioid Abuse: Drug Discrimination and Drug Self-Administration

S. Stevens Negus

Abstract Preclinical assays of drug discrimination and drug self-administration are widely used to examine abuse-related drug effects, and opioid antagonists have been extensively studied in these procedures. Studies with opioid antagonists have served two general purposes. First, antagonists selective for mu, kappa and delta receptors have been used as tools to characterize the pharmacological and neuroanatomical mechanisms that underlie the discriminative stimulus and reinforcing effects of opioids. Studies with antagonists have contributed to evidence suggesting that activation of central mu, kappa or delta receptors can mediate robust and receptor-selective discriminative stimulus effects. Conversely, the reinforcing effects of opioids in assays of drug self-administration appear to rely primarily on central mu receptor activation. A second rationale for antagonist studies has been to examine factors that may influence antagonist utility in the treatment of opioid abuse and dependence. In non-dependent animals, opioid antagonists such as naltrexone effectively block the discriminative stimulus and reinforcing effects of abused opioid agonists while producing minimal side effects. However, opioid antagonists themselves produce weak discriminative stimulus effects and do not function as positive reinforcers. In opioid-dependent animals, opioid antagonists precipitate withdrawal, readily function as negative reinforcers that engender avoidance/escape behaviours, and increase the reinforcing efficacy of opioid agonists. These factors likely contribute to the poor compliance with opioid antagonists observed in clinical studies. Compliance could be improved by integrating antagonist treatment into behaviours maintained by other stimuli (e.g. contingency management) or by using very long-acting opioid antagonist formulations to reduce the frequency required for antagonist administration.

Keywords: Opioid antagonist; Drug discrimination; Self-administration; Preclinical; Abuse; Dependence; Withdrawal

---

S.S. Negus
Department of Pharmacology and Therapeutics, Virginia Commonwealth University, Richmond, VA 23298-0613
e-mail: ssnegus@vcu.edu

R. Dean et al. (eds.), *Opiate Receptors and Antagonists*,

11.1 Introduction

Opioid agonists such as morphine, heroin and fentanyl are prominent drugs of abuse, and these drugs also produce characteristic profiles of effects in preclinical assays predictive of abuse liability. The ability of opioid antagonists to block the abuse-related effects of opioid agonists has been extensively studied, and these studies have served two general and related purposes. First, preclinical studies with antagonists have played a key role in delineating the pharmacology and neuroanatomy of receptors that mediate the abuse-related effects of opioid agonists. Second, these studies have informed clinical efforts to use opioid antagonists in the treatment of opioid abuse. The remainder of this chapter will be divided into three general sections. The first section will review basic methodology of three families of procedures that have been used to study the abuse-related effects of opioids and other drugs. The second section will review the effects of opioid antagonists in these procedures. The final section will consider some of the implications of preclinical research for the clinical use of opioid antagonists to treat opioid abuse and dependence.

11.2 Animal Models of Abuse-Related Drug Effects

11.2.1 The 3-Term Contingency

Nearly 70 years ago, B. F. Skinner described a 3-term contingency of operant conditioning (1, 2), and this 3-term contingency has played a key role in guiding the evolution of preclinical procedures that model aspects of drug abuse and dependence. The 3-term contingency can be diagrammed as "$S^D \rightarrow R \rightarrow S^C$", where S^D designates a *discriminative stimulus*, R designates a *response* on the part of the organism, and S^C designates a *consequent stimulus*. The arrows specify the contingency that, in the presence of the discriminative stimulus S^D, performance of the response R will result in the delivery of the consequent stimulus S^C. As a simple and common example from the animal laboratory, a food-restricted rat might be placed into an experimental chamber that contains a stimulus light, a response lever and a food pellet dispenser. Contingencies can be programmed such that, if the stimulus light is illuminated (the discriminative stimulus), then depression of the response lever (the response) will result in delivery of a food pellet (the consequent stimulus). Conversely, if the stimulus light is not illuminated, then responding does not result in the delivery of food pellets. Under these conditions, rats or other animals typically learn to respond when the discriminative stimulus is present. Consequent stimuli that increase responding leading to their delivery are operationally defined as *reinforcers*, whereas stimuli that decrease responding leading to their delivery are termed *punishers*. The rates and patterns of responding are largely determined by the *schedule of reinforcement*. For example, under a fixed-ratio (FR) schedule, a fixed number of X responses is required to produce delivery of the reinforcer (e.g. an FR 10 schedule would require 10 responses). Under a fixed-interval (FI) schedule, a response after an interval of Y seconds is required to produce the reinforcer (e.g. an FI 60-s schedule would require a response after 60 s had elapsed).

Behavioural procedures that employ some version of the 3-term contingency have long been used to generate stable behavioural baselines for the study of drug effects, and an early finding was that drugs of abuse could function as either the discriminative stimulus or as a reinforcing consequent stimulus in the 3-term contingency (3–6). Moreover, the degree to which a given drug produces discriminative or reinforcing stimulus effects has proven useful in predicting abuse liability (7–10). As a result, assays that examine the discriminative or reinforcing stimulus effects of drugs are considered to be assays of "abuse-related" drug effects. By extension, the ability of antagonists to alter the discriminative and reinforcing stimulus effects of a given drug has often been interpreted as evidence of an antagonist-induced modulation of the abuse-related effects of that drug.

11.2.2 Drug Discrimination Procedures

In drug discrimination procedures, a drug injection serves as the discriminative stimulus in the 3-term contingency. In the simplest approach [also referred to as "state-dependent learning" (11)], a rat might receive a set dose of drug or vehicle and then be placed into a chamber equipped with a response lever and food pellet dispenser. Contingencies could be established such that responding produces food delivery if drug was administered before the session, but not if vehicle was administered. After some training under these conditions, a rat might be expected to respond at higher rates after drug injection than after vehicle injection. More recent approaches have improved on this simple design by using *concurrent schedules,* in which two or more sets of 3-term contingencies operate simultaneously (4, 5). For example, the experimental chamber might contain two response levers, and responding on one lever could produce food after treatment with the training drug, whereas responding on the other lever could produce food after treatment with vehicle. Under these conditions, the subject might be expected to respond on the vehicle-appropriate lever after vehicle injections and on the drug-appropriate lever after drug injections. The primary dependent measure in such studies is the allocation of responding across the available choices (e.g. the per cent of responding on the after drug-appropriate lever). Response rates can also be evaluated to provide a measure of non-selective drug effects.

Drug discrimination is useful in the study of abuse-related effects for three reasons (4, 5). First, all known drugs of abuse produce discriminative stimulus effects, which suggests that the ability of a drug to produce discriminative stimulus effects is necessary for abuse. However, many non-abused drugs may also function as discriminative stimuli (e.g. kappa agonists, see Sect.11.3.1 below), so production of discriminative stimulus effects is clearly not sufficient to promote abuse. Second, discriminative stimulus effects display high pharmacological selectivity. In general, drugs share discriminative stimulus effects only with other drugs that act through similar mechanisms of action and that produce similar profiles of other effects. Thus, if a test drug shares discriminative stimulus effects with a known drug of abuse, then it is likely that the test drug possesses an abuse liability similar to that of the known drug. Third, modern drug discrimination procedures that use concurrent schedules of reinforcement yield monotonic dose–effect curves that provide a useful pharmacological baseline for the conduct of studies with putative antagonists. For example, Fig. 11.1a (open circles) shows a heroin dose–effect curve for drug-appropriate responding in rhesus monkeys trained to discriminate heroin from saline using a two-lever, food-reinforced drug discrimination procedure (12).

11.2.3 Drug Self-Administration Procedures

In drug self-administration procedures, the drug serves as the consequent stimulus in the 3-term contingency. For example, a rat equipped with a chronic intravenous catheter might be placed into a chamber with a stimulus light, a lever and a pump for delivering IV injections. Contingencies could be established such that responding produces drug injections only when the stimulus light is illuminated. To date, most drug self-administration studies have used variations on this relatively simple approach, and the principal dependent variable has been the rate of self-administration (expressed as number responses or number reinforcer deliveries

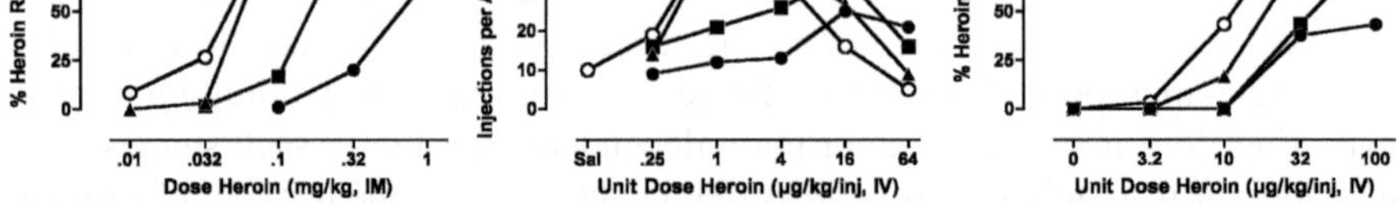

Fig. 11.1 Discriminative stimulus and reinforcing effects of heroin and sensitivity to antagonism by opioid antagonists. (a) Effects of naltrexone on the discriminative stimulus effects of heroin in a two-key, food-reinforced drug discrimination procedure in rhesus monkeys (12). (b) Effects of continuous naltrexone infusion on the reinforcing effects of heroin under a FR1 schedule of reinforcement in rhesus monkeys. In this procedure, the dependent measure was rate of self-administration (injections per access period) (13). (c) Effects of continuous naloxone infusion on the reinforcing effects of heroin under a concurrent-choice schedule of reinforcement in rhesus monkeys. In this procedure, monkeys chose between concurrent schedules of food and heroin delivery, and the dependent measure was per cent heroin choice (14)

per unit time) (3, 6–8). If any dose of drug maintains rates of self-administration higher than rates maintained by vehicle injections, then the drug is considered to function as a reinforcer and to produce reinforcing effects. Most drugs abused by humans also produce reinforcing effects in drug self-administration assays in animals. Figure 11.1b (open circles) shows a heroin self-administration dose–effect curve in rhesus monkeys responding during daily sessions in a simple self-administration procedure in which a single response produced a saline or heroin injection (FR1 schedule) (13). A significant disadvantage of this approach is that drug self-administration dose–effect curves display biphasic, inverted-U-shaped dose–effect curves, which suggests that multiple effects contribute to the dependent measure (15, 16). For example, the reinforcing effects produced by a drug will (by definition) tend to increase self-administration rates, but other effects, such as the sedative effects produced by high doses of opioid agonists, could simultaneously tend to decrease self-administration rates. The potential for response rates to integrate multiple effects poses a problem for the design and interpretation of antagonism studies, because different effects may be differentially sensitive to the antagonist under study.

As with drug discrimination procedures, more sophisticated concurrent schedules of drug self-administration have also been developed, although such procedures are not yet widely used in preclinical research (14, 17–19). In one approach, for example, rhesus monkeys could respond on one key lit with red stimulus lights to receive food pellets, or they could respond on a second, concurrently available key lit with yellow stimulus lights to receive heroin injections (14, 20, 21). In this type of procedure, the reinforcing effects of the drug are indicated by the allocation of responding rather than by the rate of responding, and as a result, non-specific rate-altering effects produced by the self-administered drug or by pretreatment drugs have little effect on the primary dependent measure. Figure 11.1c (open circles) shows the dose–effect curve for heroin choice under a concurrent schedule of heroin and food availability (14). An advantage of this approach is that dose–effect curves display a monotonic shape rather than a biphasic, inverted-U shape, and this type of dose–effect curve is often more amenable than biphasic dose–effect curves to pharmacological analysis of effects with putative antagonists.

11.2.4 Procedures to Study Drug Dependence and Withdrawal

In studies of drug dependence and withdrawal, subjects are exposed to some regimen of drug treatment and then observed for characteristic abstinence signs when the drug is withdrawn. “Spontaneous withdrawal” is achieved by terminating or interrupting the regimen of drug delivery. “Antagonist-precipitated withdrawal” is achieved by administration of a pharmacological antagonist. A wide range of preclinical procedures has been developed to assess both spontaneous and antagonist- precipitated withdrawal in opioid-dependent organisms. These procedures usually involve withdrawal from some regimen of chronic drug treatment, although withdrawal signs can sometimes be demonstrated after even a single acute treatment with an opioid agonist (22). The most commonly measured dependent variables in studies of opioid dependence are overt behavioural signs, such as piloerection or teeth chattering in rats (23–25). Operant procedures have also been used to study aspects of opioid withdrawal. For example, opioid withdrawal may disrupt food-maintained operant responding (26), function as a discriminative stimulus in discrimination procedures (27–29), or increase the reinforcing effects of opioid agonists (14, 30, 31). This chapter will focus on antagonist effects in drug-dependent subjects trained under drug discrimination and drug self-administration procedures.

11.3 Effects of Opioid Antagonists in Assays of Drug Discrimination

11.3.1 Discriminative Stimulus Effects of Opioid Agonists

Three main types of opioid receptors have been pharmacologically characterized and cloned – the mu, kappa and delta opioid receptors (32–34). Numerous studies have demonstrated that agonists acting selectively at each receptor type produce prominent and distinct discriminative stimulus effects. For example, rhesus monkeys have been trained to discriminate vehicle from the mu agonist heroin (35), the delta agonist SNC80 (36) or the kappa agonist U69,593 (37). In heroin-trained monkeys, other mu agonists substituted for the heroin training stimulus, whereas delta and kappa agonists did not. Similarly, in SNC80-trained monkeys, other delta agonists substituted for the SNC80 training stimulus, whereas mu and kappa agonists did not. Lastly, in U69,593-trained monkeys, other kappa agonists substituted for the U69,593 training stimulus, whereas mu and delta agonists did not.

11.3.2 Antagonism of the Discriminative Stimulus Effects of Opioid Agonists

The pharmacological selectivity of opioid discrimination is also apparent in studies with opioid antagonists. The modestly mu-selective and reversible opioid antagonists naloxone (38–40), naltrexone (12, 35, 41–45) and quadazocine (36, 46, 47) displayed differential potencies as antagonists of mu, kappa and delta agonist-induced discriminative stimulus effects in rats, pigeons and rhesus monkeys. As one example, Fig. 11.1a shows naltrexone antagonism of the discriminative stimulus effects of heroin in rhesus monkeys. Antagonist potency can be quantified using apparent pA2 analysis to estimate the -log dose of antagonist (in units of mol/kg) required to produce a twofold rightward shift in agonist dose–effect curves. In rats, the pA2 values for naloxone antagonism of mu agonists ranged from 7.6 to 7.8, whereas the pA2 for antagonism of a kappa agonist was nearly a log unit lower (6.8) (47). Similarly, in pigeons, naltrexone pA2 values were 7.6, 6.8 and 6.3 for antagonism of discriminative stimulus effects produced by mu, kappa and delta agonists, respectively (41). In rhesus monkeys, the pA2 values for quadazocine antagonism of the discriminative stimulus effects of mu, kappa and delta agonists were 7.6–7.9, 5.7–6.4, and <5.5 (36, 46, 47). The potencies of naloxone, naltrexone and quadazocine to antagonize the discriminative stimulus effects of mu, kappa and delta agonists were similar to their potencies in blocking other effects of mu, kappa and delta agonists (e.g. antinociception, rates of schedule-controlled responding) (12, 47–50). Table 11.1 shows illustrative pA2 values for naltrexone in antagonizing the discriminative stimulus, reinforcing and antinociceptive effects of morphine and heroin in different species. Taken together, quantitative analysis of naloxone, naltrexone and quadazocine potencies supports the view that the discriminative stimulus effects of mu, kappa and delta agonists are mediated by pharmacologically distinct populations of receptors.

The pharmacological selectivity of mu, kappa and delta agonist discriminations is also supported by studies with highly selective opioid antagonists. For example, the selective and irreversible mu antagonist β-funaltrexamine (β-FNA) antagonized the discriminative stimulus effects of mu but not kappa agonists in rats, pigeons and non-human primates (53–59). Conversely, the kappa-selective antagonist nor-binaltorphimine (nor-BNI) and the delta-selective antagonist naltrindole selectively antagonized the discriminative stimulus effects of kappa and delta agonists, respectively (36, 41, 53, 57, 60).

In addition to studies of receptor selectivity, antagonism studies in drug discrimination procedures have been used extensively to evaluate other aspects of opioid pharmacology. Four examples will be briefly discussed. First, drug discrimination has been used to study the time course of antagonist actions. For example, oral naltrexone was shown to be more potent and to have a duration of action approximately twice as long as oral naloxone as an antagonist of the discriminative stimulus effects of morphine in rats (61). However, even the antagonist effects of naltrexone lasted only a few hours. By contrast, the kappa antagonist nor-BNI produced a slow-onset and long-acting antagonism of the discriminative stimulus effects of the kappa agonist enadoline, with peak antagonist effects emerging over the first 24 h and lasting for a period of weeks (53).

Second, drug discrimination procedures can be used to examine antagonist effects of mixed-action drugs that act at multiple receptor types. For example, the opioid buprenorphine has similar affinities for mu and kappa opioid receptors and possesses intermediate efficacy at mu receptors but low efficacy at kappa receptors. The potential kappa antagonist effects of buprenorphine in vivo can be masked by its mu agonist effects under some conditions, but in drug discrimination procedures, the mu and kappa receptor-mediated effects of buprenorphine can be effectively evaluated in different groups of animals trained to discriminate a mu and kappa agonist, respectively. Using this approach, buprenorphine was shown to produce mu agonist

Table 11.1 Potency of naltrexone to antagonize the discriminative stimulus, reinforcing and antinociceptive effects of morphine and heroin in rats, pigeons and non-human primates as determined using pA2 analysis

Antagonist (route of admin)	Agonist	Species	Procedure	pA2 or pKB[a]	mg/kg equivalent	Reference
Naltrexone (SC)	Morphine	Rat	Morphine discrimination	7.8	0.0060	(45)
Naltrexone (SC)	Morphine	Rat	Morphine discrimination	7.3	0.019	(50)
Naltrexone (SC)	Morphine	Rat	Morphine discrimination	7.9–8.1[b]	0.0030–0.0048	(42)
Naltrexone (IM)	Morphine	Pigeon	Morphine discrimination	7.3	0.019	(41)
Naltrexone (IM)	Morphine	Squirrel monkey	Morphine discrimination	8.2[c]	0.0024	(44)
Naltrexone (IM)	Morphine	Rhesus monkey	Heroin discrimination	8.0[d]	0.0038	(35)
Naltrexone (IM)	Morphine	Rhesus monkey	Heroin discrimination	8.2	0.0024	(12)
Naltrexone (SC)	Morphine	Rhesus monkey	Reversal of NTX discrimination	8.3[e]	0.0019	(51)
Naltrexone (IM)	Heroin	Rhesus monkey	Heroin discrimination	8.3[f]	0.0019	(35)
Naltrexone (IM)	Heroin	Rhesus monkey	Heroin discrimination	8.2	0.0024	(12)
Naltrexone (IM)	Heroin	Rhesus monkey	Drug self-administration	8.0[d]	0.0038	(52)
Naltrexone (SC)	Morphine	Rat	Thermal antinociception	8.3	0.0019	(50)
Naltrexone (IM)	Morphine	Rhesus monkey	Thermal antinociception	8.2	0.0024	(12)
Naltrexone (IM)	Heroin	Rhesus monkey	Thermal antinociception	7.9	0.0048	(12)

pA2 values show the -log dose of antagonist in mol/kg required to produce a twofold rightward shift in agonist dose–effect curves. pKB values are equivalent but can be determined using a single antagonist dose. For details on calculation of pA2 and pKB values, see (47, 49). The mg/kg equivalent to each pA2 or pKB value is also shown. For all procedures in all species, doses of naltrexone from 0.0019 mg/kg to 0.019 mg/kg were sufficient to produce twofold rightward shifts in morphine and heroin dose–effect curves

[a]All values show pA2 values determined from Schild plots with slopes constrained to −1 except where indicated

[b]Naltrexone pA2 values determined in male and female intact and gonadectomized rats

[c]Shows pA2 value determined from Schild plot with unconstrained slope (slope = −0.63)

[d]Shows pKB value

[e]Shows pA2 value determined from Schild plot with unconstrained slope (slope = −1.04). Experiments were conducted in morphine-dependent subjects discriminating naltrexone from saline

[f]Shows pA2 value determined from Schild plot with unconstrained slope (slope = −1.2)

effects in one set of monkeys (i.e. substitution for a mu agonist training stimulus) at the same doses that produced antagonism of a kappa agonist training stimulus in a second set of monkeys (62). Moreover, the apparent kappa antagonist effects of buprenorphine could not be attributed to its mu agonist effects, because selective mu agonists did not attenuate the discriminative stimulus effects of kappa agonists. A similar approach was used to examine the agonist and antagonist effects of other mixed-action opioids such as metazocine and bremazocine.

Third, studies with β-FNA and clocinnamox (another mu-selective, irreversible mu antagonist) have been used to characterize the relative efficacy of different mu agonists in drug discrimination procedures (63–65). For example, pretreatments with β-FNA or clocinnamox produced greater rightward and/or downward shifts in dose–effect curves for relatively low efficacy mu agonists (e.g. buprenorphine, morphine) than for higher efficacy mu agonists (e.g. fentanyl, etorphine). Using data analytic procedures described elsewhere in this volume, differential degrees of antagonism produced by irreversible antagonists can be quantified to yield quantitative estimates of mu agonist efficacy (66).

Finally, studies with relatively lipid-insoluble antagonists, which do not readily cross the blood–brain barrier, have been used to examine the neuroanatomical location of receptors that mediate the discriminative stimulus effects of opioid agonists (67, 68). Such antagonists can be administered peripherally or centrally to explore the relative contribution of peripheral versus central opioid receptors in mediating discriminative stimulus effects produced by an opioid agonist. In rats, for example, naltrexone methobromide was >500-fold more potent after intracerebroventricular than after peripheral administration in blocking the discriminative stimulus effects of peripherally administered morphine (67). These results were interpreted to suggest that the discriminative stimulus effects of morphine under these conditions were mediated primarily by periventricular opioid receptors in the brain.

11.3.3 Discriminative Stimulus Effects of Opioid Antagonists

Although most studies of opioid discrimination have used opioid agonists as the training stimulus, non-opioid dependent animals can also be trained to discriminate large doses of opioid antagonists (55, 69, 70). For example, high-dose naloxone and naltrexone shared discriminative stimulus effects in non-dependent pigeons trained to discriminate naloxone (30 mg/kg) or naltrexone (10 mg/kg) from vehicle (55, 69, 70). However, it is not clear if these effects are mediated by opioid or non-opioid receptors. The opioid antagonist diprenorphine did not substitute for either naloxone or naltrexone, and β-FNA did not substitute for naltrexone. Moreover, β-FNA doses that antagonized the discriminative stimulus effects of morphine did not alter the discriminative stimulus effects of naltrexone. Finally, doses of naloxone and naltrexone that function as discriminative stimuli in pigeons are much higher than doses that produce mu or even kappa antagonist effects (e.g. see Table 11.1).

In addition to these studies in non-dependent subjects, a great deal of research has been conducted to evaluate the discriminative stimulus effects of opioid antagonists in opioid-dependent animals. This work will be reviewed below in Sect. 11.5.2.

11.4 Effects of Opioid Antagonists in Assays of Drug Self-Administration

11.4.1 Effects of Opioid Agonists As Consequent Stimuli

In general, mu opioid receptor agonists reliably maintain self-administration, whereas kappa agonists do not, and effects with delta agonists are equivocal (71). The earliest studies of drug self-administration in animals employed the prototype mu agonist morphine (72–74). Since then, self-administration has been demonstrated for a host of mu agonists under many schedules of reinforcement (18, 31, 75–81). Mu agonists can maintain self-administration in physically dependent organisms, and mu agonist self-administration itself may sustain or lead to physical dependence if access conditions permit sufficient drug intake; however, physical dependence does not appear to be necessary for mu agonists to function as reinforcers (14, 82). As will be discussed below, the degree of physical dependence may influence antagonist effects on opioid self-administration.

Selective kappa agonists such as U50,488 do not maintain self-administration in either rats or non-human primates (83, 84). Less selective kappa agonists such ketocyclazocine and ethylketocyclazocine also failed to maintain self-administration in non-human primates (85), but these drugs did maintain self-administration in rats (86). This species difference in self-administration may reflect the relatively low proportion of kappa to mu receptors in rats (87). In rhesus monkeys, the addition of a kappa agonist (U69,593) to a mu agonist (fentanyl) reduced the reinforcing effects of the mu agonist (Negus, unpublished results).

Peptidic delta-selective agonists maintained self-administration in rats when the drugs were administered into the ventricles, ventral tegmental area or nucleus accumbens (88–90); however, selective non-peptidic delta agonists have not maintained intravenous self-administration in monkeys (91–93). Moreover, addition of the delta agonist SNC80 to the mu agonist heroin did not enhance heroin's reinforcing effects in rhesus monkeys, although it did enhance heroin's antinociceptive effects (21).

11.4.2 Effects of Opioid Antagonists on Opioid Agonist Self-Administration

The effects of antagonists on opioid self-administration have been studied most often in subjects given relatively limited access to the opioid agonist, and hence, in subjects with little or no physical dependence. This section will focus on antagonist effects in relatively non-dependent animals, and antagonist effects in dependent animals will be discussed in Sect. 11.5.3.

Under conditions of minimal dependence, naloxone, naltrexone and quadazocine typically produce effects consistent with rightward and/or downward shifts in self-administration dose–effect curves (14, 52, 94–103). For example, Fig. 11.1b shows the effects of continuous naltrexone infusion on heroin self-administration maintained under a simple FR procedure, for which the primary dependent measure was rate of self-administration (13). As discussed above in Sect. 11.2.3, this type of procedure typically yields inverted U-shaped dose–effect curves. Naltrexone shifted the heroin self-administration rightward and downward, but notably, naltrexone effects varied dramatically across different unit doses of heroin. Thus, naltrexone dose-dependently *decreased* responding maintained by a low unit dose of 1 μg/kg/inj heroin, dose-dependently *increased* responding maintained by a high dose of 64 μg/kg/inj heroin, and *biphasically increased* self-administration of an intermediate dose of 16 μg/kg/inj heroin. This dependence of naltrexone effect on heroin unit dose likely resulted from the inverted U-shape of the baseline dose-effect curve and the consequences of shifting such a curve to the right. However, as noted in Sect. 11.2.3, self-administration rates integrate multiple effects into a single dependent measure, and one must at least consider the possibility that these multiple effects are differentially sensitive to the antagonist. One could reasonably ask (and many have) whether manipulations that increase high-dose drug self-administration reflect attenuation of the drug's reinforcing effects, attenuation of its rate-suppressing effects, or some combination of these and other effects. These data illustrate the complexity inherent to the design and interpretation of studies that evaluate antagonist effects on opioid self-administration in procedures that use self-administration rate as the principle dependent measure.

For comparison, Fig. 11.1c shows the effects of continuous naloxone treatment in a heroin versus food choice procedure (14). Under these conditions, increasing unit doses of heroin maintained only a monotonic increase in heroin choice, and right shifts in the heroin dose–effect curve were associated with only decreases in heroin choice at different unit doses.

Three other points are also notable from studies with naloxone, naltrexone and quadazocine. First, pA2 analysis has been used to quantify the potency of antagonists in studies using FR or progressive-ratio schedules and examining only the ascending limb of opioid self-administration dose–effect curves (52, 94, 103). In these studies, the potencies of naltrexone and quadazocine to antagonize the reinforcing effects of mu agonists were similar to their potencies to antagonize other mu agonist effects. Thus, these findings suggested that the reinforcing effects of the mu agonists were mediated by populations of mu receptors pharmacologically similar to receptor populations that mediate other mu agonist effects. Second, several studies found that antagonist doses that reliably altered mu agonist self-administration had little or no effect on responding maintained by stimulant drugs (52, 95, 97, 99, 103). Furthermore, when relatively non-dependent monkeys responded for both a mu agonist and for food during alternating components (98, 104) or under a concurrent choice schedule (14), antagonists doses that produced rightward/downward shifts in opioid self-administration dose–effect curves simultaneously increased responding maintained by food. Taken together, these results provide evidence of the selectivity of the antagonist effects and further support the conclusion that the antagonists altered mu agonist self-administration by producing pharmacological antagonism as opposed to non-selective changes in rates of operant responding. Finally, some studies evaluated the effects of relatively long-term treatment with opioid antagonists for 1–8 weeks (13, 14, 97, 99). In all of these studies, antagonist effects were sustained for the duration of the treatment.

Studies with highly selective antagonists have generally confirmed a role for mu receptors in mediating the reinforcing effects of mu agonists. For example, the selective and irreversible mu antagonists β-FNA and clocinnamox antagonized the reinforcing effects of heroin in rats (105, 106) and of alfentanil and nalbuphine in monkeys (107). In contrast, selective doses of the kappa antagonist nor-BNI or the delta antagonist naltrindole did not alter heroin self-administration (106). In one exception to this general finding, ICV injections of the reputed delta-2 antagonist naltrindole isothiocyanate (NTII) produced rightward and downward shifts in heroin self-administration dose–effect curves at NTII doses that did not alter the antinociceptive effects of the mu agonist DAMGO [(D-Ala2, N-Me-Phe4, Gly5-ol)-enkephalin] (108). These latter results suggest that delta-2 opioid receptors may contribute to the reinforcing effects of heroin in rats.

Studies with antagonists have also been employed to examine the neurobiology of opioid reinforcement. For example, a series of studies with a quaternary derivative of naloxone implicated central opioid receptors in nucleus accumbens in mediation of the reinforcing effects of heroin in rats (100, 109, 110). Specifically, methyl naloxone potently produced an antagonist-like increase in heroin self-administration when it was administered ICV or directly into the nucleus accumbens, but not when it was administered systemically even at very high doses. Subsequent studies using intracerebral injections of β-FNA implicated the rostral nucleus accumbens as being especially important in heroin self-administration in the rat (111).

11.4.3 Effects of Opioid Antagonists as Consequent Stimuli

Opioid antagonists do not maintain responding leading to their delivery, and as such, they do not function as positive reinforcers (112, 113). Rather, response-contingent naloxone was more effective than non-contingent naloxone in suppressing codeine self-administration, and these data were interpreted to suggest that naloxone functioned as a punisher under these conditions (104). High doses of opioid antagonists may also function as negative reinforcers in non-dependent animals (114–116). A *negative reinforcer* is a stimulus that maintains responding leading to its termination. For example, monkeys responded under a FR schedule to terminate ("escape from") naloxone infusions delivered at a continuous rate of >0.1 mg/kg/min (114). The effects of opioid antagonists as consequent stimuli have been studied far more extensively in opioid-dependent subjects, and these findings will be reviewed in Sect. 11.5.3.

11.5 Effects of Opioid Antagonists in Opioid-Dependent Subjects

11.5.1 Dependence Associated with Opioid Agonist Treatment

The development of dependence has been studied most extensively with mu opioid agonists, and it is well established that chronic treatment with mu agonists such as morphine can produce physical dependence as indicated by the emergence of abstinence signs upon drug withdrawal (23, 34, 117, 118). Dependence on kappa agonists has also been described in rhesus monkeys (119, 120), but dependence to kappa agonists appears to be weak or absent in rats (121, 122). Delta agonists have not been shown to produce strong signs of dependence in rodents or non-human primates (123–125).

The effects of antagonists in opioid-dependent animals have been extensively studied, and a primary focus has been on elicited behavioural effects. For example, naloxone and naltrexone were among a range of antagonists that precipitated withdrawal signs (e.g. abdominal muscle rigidity, excessive vocalization and apprehension/aggression towards handlers) in morphine-dependent rhesus monkeys (119, 120). Higher doses of these same antagonists also precipitated different withdrawal signs (e.g. yawning, unusual tongue movements and excessive scratching) in rhesus monkeys dependent on the kappa agonist U50,488. Studies with more selective mu, kappa and delta antagonists also generally found that precipitation of opioid withdrawal is pharmacologically selective (25, 120). However, a more detailed review of the massive literature describing elicited signs of antagonist-precipitated withdrawal is tangential to the goals of this chapter. Although withdrawal in mu agonist-dependent subjects is widely considered to be aversive and to contribute to processes underlying addiction (126, 127), the impact of dependence and withdrawal on the abuse-related effects of opioid agonists cannot be easily inferred from a study of elicited withdrawal signs such as abdominal muscle rigidity or excessive vocalization. Accordingly, the next two sections of this chapter will focus on studies that directly evaluated the effects of spontaneous and precipitated withdrawal in assays of drug discrimination and drug self-administration.

11.5.2 Effects of Antagonists in Dependent Subjects: Drug Discrimination Studies

The opioid antagonist naltrexone produces robust discriminative stimulus effects in morphine-dependent rats, pigeons and monkeys (27, 128, 129). The discriminative stimulus effects of opioid antagonists in non-dependent and morphine-dependent subjects differ in three important respects. First, antagonists are much more potent in producing discriminative stimulus effects in morphine-dependent subjects than in non-dependent subjects. For example, naltrexone was 1,000-fold more potent in producing discriminative stimulus effects in morphine-dependent pigeons treated with 10 mg/kg/day morphine than in non-dependent pigeons (70, 128). In addition, the potencies of antagonists to produce naltrexone-like discriminative stimulus effects in morphine-dependent subjects were similar to the their potencies to produce mu antagonist effects under other conditions [(51); also see Table 11.1]. These findings provide one source of evidence to suggest that the discriminative stimulus effects of naltrexone in morphine-dependent subjects are mediated by antagonist effects at mu opioid receptors and not by some other pharmacological effect of naltrexone, as may be the case in non-dependent subjects.

A second distinguishing feature of naltrexone discriminations in morphine-dependent subjects is that the potency, time course and mu agonist reversibility of antagonist-induced discriminative stimulus effects parallels the potency, time course and mu agonist reversibility of other antagonist-precipitated withdrawal signs (28). Moreover, spontaneous withdrawal produces naltrexone-appropriate responding in morphine-dependent subjects (27, 28, 128, 129). These findings suggest that naltrexone-induced discriminative stimulus effects in morphine-dependent animals constitute one of an array of opioid withdrawal signs. To the degree that the discriminative stimulus effects of drugs in animals are concordant with subjective effects in humans (130), naltrexone discriminations in morphine-dependent animals may model subjective effects of opioid withdrawal in humans. The underlying mechanisms of naltrexone-induced discriminative stimulus effects in morphine-dependent subjects have not been extensively investigated, but notably, they can be differentiated from at least some other withdrawal signs. For example, the opioid agonist loperamide, which is peripherally selective after systemic administration, reversed some opioid withdrawal signs in rats (e.g. weight loss), but did not reverse the discriminative stimulus effects of naltrexone (28). Similarly, the alpha-2 adrenergic agonist clonidine reversed several opioid withdrawal signs in rats and monkeys, but it did not reliably reverse naltrexone-induced discriminative stimulus effects (27, 28, 131). These findings suggest that the discriminative stimulus effects of naltrexone in morphine-dependent subjects are independent of (i.e. not caused by) at least a subset of other, overt withdrawal signs.

A final distinguishing feature of naltrexone discriminations in morphine-dependent subjects is that the ability of drugs to substitute for or reverse the discrimination is highly correlated with efficacy at mu opioid receptors (129, 132, 133). Thus, drugs with low efficacy at mu receptors substitute for naltrexone, drugs with high efficacy at mu receptors reverse naltrexone-appropriate responding, and drugs with intermediate efficacy produce variable effects depending on such factors as the degree of dependence. These findings in morphine-dependent subjects contrast with the failure of some low efficacy mu ligands like diprenorphine to substitute for the discriminative stimulus effects of naltrexone in non-dependent subjects.(70) This exquisite sensitivity of naltrexone discriminations in morphine-dependent subjects to mu agonist efficacy has made the procedure extremely useful for characterizing the mu receptor-mediated effects of novel drugs (134–136).

Most antagonist discriminations in opioid-agonist treated subjects have accomplished "agonist treatment" with a chronic regimen of morphine delivery, and they have employed naltrexone as the antagonist. However, variations on these themes have also been explored (22, 137–139). For example, one study evaluated the discriminative stimulus effects of nalbuphine in non-dependent and morphine-dependent pigeons (139). In the non-dependent pigeons, nalbuphine functioned as a weak agonist (e.g. naltrexone did not substitute for nalbuphine and antagonized nalbuphine's effects), but in morphine-dependent pigeons, nalbuphine functioned as an antagonist (e.g. naltrexone substituted for nalbuphine). These results are consistent with the intermediate efficacy of nalbuphine at mu opioid receptors. Another study established a naltrexone discrimination in pigeons chronically treated with the kappa agonist U50,488 (10 mg/kg/day) (138). The discrimination could be trained, but in contrast to the effects of withdrawal in morphine-dependent subjects, spontaneous withdrawal in these U50,488-treated pigeons did not produce substitution for naltrexone. It was concluded that the U50,488 treatment regimen was not sufficient to produce dependence.

11.5.3 Effects of Antagonists in Dependent Subjects: Drug Self-Administration Studies

11.5.3.1 Effects on Self-Administration of Opioid Agonists

Both spontaneous withdrawal and antagonist-precipitated withdrawal increase mu agonist-maintained responding in mu agonist-dependent rats (140, 141) and non-human primates (14, 18, 72, 73, 142, 143). However, this effect differs from antagonist-induced increases in opioid self-administration that are sometimes observed in non-dependent subjects. As noted above, antagonist-induced increases in opioid self-administration in non-dependent subjects are observed only at high agonist doses on the descending limb of agonist self-administration dose-effect curves, and these increases are associated with rightward shifts in inverted-U shaped dose–effect curves. In contrast, withdrawal-induced or antagonist-induced increases in opioid self-administration in dependent subjects are associated with leftward and/or upward shifts in opioid self-administration dose–effect curves.

As one example of the effects of spontaneous withdrawal, Fig. 11.2a shows heroin self-administration dose–effect curves in heroin-dependent rhesus monkeys responding for heroin and food under a concurrent-choice procedure (14). Choice between heroin and food was assessed during daily 2-h choice sessions. Heroin dependence was established and maintained by introducing an additional 21-h supplemental heroin self-administration session each day, and withdrawal was introduced by periodically terminating access to these supplemental heroin self-administration sessions. Under control conditions (i.e. during access to supplemental heroin), heroin maintained a dose-dependent increase in heroin versus food choice. One day of withdrawal from supplemental heroin produced a

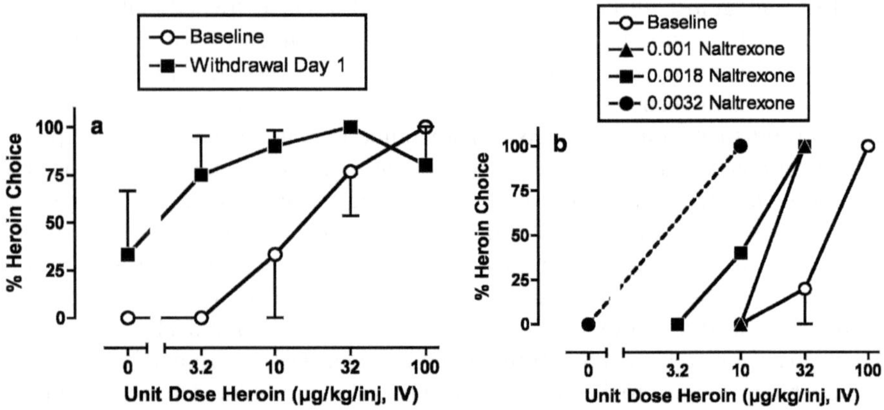

Fig. 11.2 Effects of spontaneous withdrawal and naltrexone on heroin versus food choice in heroin-dependent rhesus monkeys. (a) On day 1 of spontaneous withdrawal, the heroin choice dose–effect curve shifted leftward/upward in a group of three monkeys, indicating an increase in heroin choice and a decrease in food choice (14). (b) Similarly, naltrexone produced a dose-dependent leftward shift in the heroin choice dose–effect curve in one non-withdrawn monkey (S. Negus, unpublished results). In this experiment, naltrexone was administered 30 min before the choice session. The points for 0.0032 mg/kg naltrexone are connected by a dotted line because the subject failed to earn a reinforcer when food and the low dose of 3.2 µg/kg/inj heroin were available. For clarity, only the ascending limb of each dose–effect curve is shown

dramatic leftward/upward shift in the heroin-choice dose–effect curve. Indeed, some monkeys responded on the heroin-associated key even when responding produced no heroin injections (the "0" heroin dose). Withdrawal also resulted in the emergence of typical opioid abstinence signs (data not shown). Figure 11.2b shows that administration of naltrexone produced a similar effect (S. Negus, unpublished results). Specifically, naltrexone produced dose-dependent leftward shifts in the heroin choice dose–effect curve. Notably, these left shifts in the heroin choice dose–effect curve were diametrically opposite to the right shifts in the heroin choice dose–effect curve produced by naloxone in non-dependent monkeys (cf. Fig. 11.1c). Taken together with results of other studies cited in the preceding paragraph, these results suggest that either spontaneous or antagonist-precipitated withdrawal increases the relative reinforcing efficacy of mu agonists.

The mechanisms that underlie withdrawal-associated increases in mu-agonist self-administration are not well understood. However, studies with restricted-distribution antagonists have been conducted to examine potentially important neuroanatomical substrates. For example, injection of methylnaloxonium into regions designated as the "extended amygdala" (the bed nucleus of the stria terminalis and nucleus accumbens shell) in rats selectively reduced heroin self-administration in morphine-dependent rats without affecting heroin self-administration in non-dependent rats (144). These results were interpreted to suggest that these regions may be responsible for the reinforcing effects of opioids in dependent animals, and that activity in these regions may be recruited during the development of dependence.

11.5.3.2 Effects As Consequent Stimuli

Opioid antagonists including naloxone and nalorphine can function as potent negative reinforcers in morphine-dependent monkeys (104, 114, 145–148). In one study, for example, rhesus monkeys self-administered up to 10 mg/kg/day morphine, and once morphine dependence was established, test sessions were introduced during which subjects were exposed to a continuous naloxone infusion in the presence of a blue stimulus light (114). Subjects could terminate the naloxone infusion, extinguish the blue light and initiate a 1-min timeout by responding under a FR20 schedule. Under these conditions, escape from naloxone infusions maintained high rates of responding, with the peak of the naloxone dose–effect curve occurring at infusion rates of 1 μg/kg/min. As noted above in Sect. 11.4.3, naloxone also functioned as a negative reinforcer in non-dependent monkeys; however, in morphine-dependent monkeys, responding could be maintained by naloxone doses 300- to 1,000-fold lower than in non-dependent monkeys. Thus, morphine dependence dramatically increased the potency of opioid antagonists to function as either a discriminative stimulus (see Sect. 11.5.2) or as a consequent stimulus (in this case as a negative reinforcer).

The ability of opioid antagonists to function as negative reinforcers and to increase opioid agonist self-administration in opioid-dependent subjects may be related. In either case, responding is maintained by contingencies that limit antagonist access to opioid receptors and thereby mitigate antagonist effects. In negative-reinforcement procedures, responding limits or prevents antagonist administration. Conversely, in assays of opioid agonist self-administration, responding produces injections of the opioid agonist, and the agonist in turn acts pharmacologically at the level of individual opioid receptors to oppose antagonist effects. The more precise neurobiological mechanisms that underlie these phenomena remain largely unknown. In opioid-dependent subjects, antagonist administration precipitates a host of physiological and behavioural effects mediated by receptors throughout the periphery and neuroaxis, and it is not known which of these effects is necessary or sufficient to mediate the negative reinforcing effects of antagonists or the ability of antagonists to increase opioid agonist self-administration.

One final caveat is also worthy of note. Although opioid antagonists have frequently been demonstrated to function as negative reinforcers in opioid-dependent subjects, they may also function as positive reinforcers under some conditions (104). In this study, two morphine-dependent monkeys were initially trained under an avoidance–escape schedule, in which illumination of a blue light was followed after 30 s by a naloxone infusion. Responding during either the light (avoidance) or the infusion (escape) initiated a 1-min timeout. Once responding under this schedule was established, the schedule was changed to a second-order FR10 (FR30:S) schedule, under which completion of 30 responses produced a brief 1.5-s flash of the blue light, and completion of 10 FR30's produced a naloxone infusion and a 1-min timeout. Naloxone delivery maintained high response rates for ≥16 sessions by both monkeys under this schedule, and when response rates declined, responding could be reinstated by non-contingent naloxone infusions.

These results with naloxone infusions are similar to demonstrations of response-produced shock (149, 150), and together they compellingly demonstrate that effects of a stimulus on behaviour are not inherent to the stimulus, but rather depend on such factors as the behavioural and pharmacological history of the subject and the schedules that govern the consequences of behaviour.

11.6 Summary and Implications for Clinical Studies

Studies with opioid antagonists in preclinical assays of drug discrimination and drug discrimination have been used for two general purposes. First, antagonists have been used as experimental tools to examine the pharmacological and neuroanatomical mechanisms of action that mediate the abuse-related effects of opioid drugs. Studies with antagonists have provided compelling evidence that activation of mu, kappa or delta opioid receptors can generate robust and distinct discriminative stimulus effects. The reinforcing effects of opioids appear to rely primarily on mu receptor activation, although delta receptors may also contribute. Antagonist studies have also provided evidence to suggest that both the discriminative stimulus and reinforcing effects of mu opioids are mediated by opioid receptors in the central nervous system, with a prominent role for rostral nucleus accumbens mu receptors in non-dependent rats and perhaps for mu receptors in the extended amygdala in dependent rats. Further studies to explore the mechanisms of withdrawal-associated increases in the reinforcing effects of opioid agonists are warranted, and antagonists will play an important role in this research.

A second purpose for antagonism studies has been to explore factors that may influence their utility as medications for the treatment of opioid abuse. It is clear that, in non-dependent animals, both modestly selective mu antagonists (naloxone and naltrexone) and highly selective mu-selective antagonists (β-FNA and clocinnamox) produce dose-dependent rightward and/or downward shifts in dose–effect curves for the discriminative stimulus and reinforcing effects of heroin and opioid analgesics with high abuse potential (e.g. morphine, fentanyl and alfentanil). Moreover, the effects of these antagonists on opioid-agonist discrimination and self-administration are sustained during chronic antagonist treatment. Finally, doses of these antagonists that antagonize mu-agonist effects typically do not decrease responding maintained by other reinforcers (e.g. food or non-opioid drug reinforcers) and do not produce other significant untowards effects.

Taken together, these findings suggest that antagonists should be promising treatments for reduction of opioid-taking behaviour with minimal side effects. However, as discussed extensively in the chapter by Sevarino and Kosten in this volume (151), antagonists have relatively limited utility in the treatment of opioid abuse due primarily to poor compliance. Of course, one component of this problem is that pharmacological treatments for opioid abuse and dependence are usually considered only in individuals who have already attained some level of physical dependence, and antagonist administration to physically dependent subjects precipitates withdrawal. As noted above, antagonist-precipitated withdrawal can promote avoidance and escape behaviour that could manifest as either (a) avoidance/escape from stimuli associated with antagonist delivery (e.g. avoidance of or escape from the clinic where the antagonist is delivered), or (b) increased self-administration of opioid agonists. Neither of these outcomes is desirable, and perhaps because of these issues, antagonist administration to dependent subjects virtually requires an inpatient setting where the patient can be monitored and controlled. However, compliance remains poor even after patients have been detoxified and physical dependence has abated. The poor compliance in non-dependent humans agrees with preclinical studies showing that, in non-dependent animals, mu-antagonist doses of opioid antagonists are extremely weak as discriminative or consequent stimuli. In particular, antagonists do not function as positive reinforcers under standard drug evaluation procedures.

Overall, then, neither humans nor animals can be easily coerced into behaviours that result in the delivery of opioid antagonists. At best, these drugs appear to function as weak discriminative or consequent stimuli, and in opioid dependent subjects, they readily engender avoidance/escape behaviour. As a result, the promotion of compliance with antagonist treatments will likely require integration of antagonist delivery into behaviours driven largely by other discriminative and consequent stimuli. This can be achieved pharmacologically. For example, buprenorphine is an intermediate-efficacy mu agonist that can function as a discriminative stimulus and produce sufficient reinforcing effects to maintain responding, but that blocks the effects of higher efficacy mu agonists such as heroin, fentanyl or methadone (152). Antagonists may also be combined with non-opioid drugs that can function as discriminative and reinforcing stimuli, such as the alpha2 adrenergic agonists clonidine or lofexidine (151, 153–155). Alternatively, compliance with antagonist treatments may be enhanced using non-drug stimuli. For example, effective antagonist treatment programmes may benefit from contingency management approaches in which patients receive putative positive reinforcers (e.g. money) for complying with antagonist treatment and/or putative punishers (e.g. revoked privileges, loss of a job) for failing to comply (151). Long-acting formulations of opioid antagonists may also be helpful insofar as they reduce the frequency with which subjects are required to engage in behaviours that result in antagonist delivery (156).

Acknowledgement This work was supported in part by R01-DA11460 from NIDA, NIH.

References

1. Morris EK. The aim, progress, and evolution of behavioral analysis. The Behavior Analyst 1992;15:3–29.
2. Skinner BF. The behavior of orgnaisms. New York: Appleton-Century-Crofts; 1938.
3. Meisch RA, Lemaire GA. Drug self-administration. In: Van Haaren F, ed. Methods in Behavioral Pharmacology. Amsterdam: Elsevier; 1993.
4. Overton DA. Similarities and differences between behavioral control by drug-produced stimuli and by sensory stimuli. Psychopharmacol Ser 1988;4:176–98.

5. Stolerman IP. Drug discrimination. In: Van Haaren F, ed. Techniques in the Behavioral and Neural Sciences: Methods in Behavioral Pharmacology. Amsterdam: Elsevier; 1993:217–43.
6. Young AM, Herling S. Drugs as reinforcers: studies in laboratory animals. In: Goldberg SR, Stolerman IP, eds. Behavioral Analysis of Drug Dependence. Orlando, FL: Academic Press; 1986:9–67.
7. Ator NA, Griffiths RR. Principles of drug abuse liability assessment in laboratory animals. Drug Alcohol Depend 2003;70(3 Suppl):S55–72.
8. Griffiths RR, Balster RL. Opioids: similarity between evaluations of subjective effects and animal self-administration results. Clin Pharmacol Ther 1979;25(5, Pt 1):611–7.
9. Griffiths RR, Brady JV, Bradford LD. Predicting the abuse liability of drugs with animal drug self-administration procedures: psychomotor stimulants and hallucinogens. In: Thompson T, Dews PB, eds. Advances in Behavioral Pharmacology. New York: Academic Press; 1979:163–208.
10. Schuster CR, Johanson CE. The use of animal models for the study of drug abuse. In: Gibbons RJ, ed. Research Advances in Alcohol and Drug Problems. New York: Wiley; 1974:1–31.
11. Overton DA. Experimental methods for the study of state-dependent learning. Fed Proc 1974;33(7):1800–13.
12. Bowen CA, Fischer BD, Mello NK, Negus SS. Antagonism of the antinociceptive and discriminative stimulus effects of heroin and morphine by 3-methoxynaltrexone and naltrexone in rhesus monkeys. J Pharmacol Exp Ther 2002;302(1):264–73.
13. Harrigan SE, Downs DA. Pharmacological evaluation of narcotic antagonist delivery systems in rhesus monkeys. NIDA Res Monogr 1981;28:77–92.
14. Negus SS. Choice between heroin and food in nondependent and heroin-dependent rhesus monkeys: effects of naloxone, buprenorphine, and methadone. J Pharmacol Exp Ther 2006;317(2):711–23.
15. Katz JL. Drugs as reinforcers: pharmacological and behavioural factors. In: Liebman JM, Cooper SJ, eds. The Neuropharmacological Basis of Reward. Oxford: Clarendon Press; 1989:164–213.
16. Zernig G, Wakonigg G, Madlung E, Haring C, Saria A. Do vertical shifts in dose-response rate-relationships in operant conditioning procedures indicate "sensitization" to "drug wanting"? Psychopharmacology (Berl) 2004;171(3):349–51; author reply 52–63.
17. Brady JV, Griffiths RR. Behavioral procedures for evaluating the relative abuse potential of CNS drugs in primates. Fed Proc 1976;35(11):2245–53.
18. Griffiths RR, Wurster RM, Brady JV. Discrete-trial choice procedure: effects of naloxone and methadone on choice between food and heroin. Pharmacol Rev 1975;27(3):357–65.
19. Bergman J, Paronis CA. Measuring the reinforcing strength of abused drugs. Mol Interv 2006;6(5):273–83.
20. Negus SS. Interactions between the reinforcing effects of cocaine and heroin in a drug-vs-food choice procedure in rhesus monkeys: a dose-addition analysis. Psychopharmacology (Berl) 2005;180(1):115–24.
21. Stevenson GW, Folk JE, Rice KC, Negus SS. Interactions between delta and mu opioid agonists in assays of schedule-controlled responding, thermal nociception, drug self-administration, and drug versus food choice in rhesus monkeys: studies with SNC80 [(+)-4-[({alpha}R)-{alpha}-((2S,5R)-4-Allyl-2,5-dimethyl-1-piperazinyl)-3- methoxybenzyl]-N,N-diethylbenzamide] and heroin. J Pharmacol Exp Ther 2005;314(1):221–31.
22. Easterling KW, Holtzman SG. Discriminative stimulus effects of naltrexone after a single dose of morphine in the rat. J Pharmacol Exp Ther 1999;288(3):1269–77.
23. Seevers MH, Deneau GA. Physiological aspects of tolerance and dependence. In: Root WS, Hofmann FG, eds. Physiological Pharmacology I. New York: Academic Press; 1963:565–640.
24. Blasig J, Herz A. Precipitated morphine withdrawal in rats as a tool in opiate research. Curr Dev Psychopharmacol 1977;4:129–49.
25. Maldonado R, Negus S, Koob GF. Precipitation of morphine withdrawal syndrome in rats by administration of mu-, delta- and kappa-selective opioid antagonists. Neuropharmacology 1992;31(12):1231–41.

26. McMillan DE. Effects of narcotics and narcotic antagonists on operant behavior. Adv Biochem Psychopharmacol 1973;8(0):345–59.
27. France CP, Woods JH. Discriminative stimulus effects of naltrexone in morphine-treated rhesus monkeys. J Pharmacol Exp Ther 1989;250(3):937–43.
28. Holtzman SG. Discriminative stimulus effects of morphine withdrawal in the dependent rat: suppression by opiate and nonopiate drugs. J Pharmacol Exp Ther 1985;233(1):80–6.
29. Miksic S, Sherman G, Lal H. Discriminative response control by naloxone in morphine pretreated rats. Psychopharmacology (Berl) 1981;72(2):179–84.
30. Griffiths RR, Wurster RM, Brady JV. Choice between food and heroin: effects of morphine, naloxone, and secobarbital. J Exp Anal Behav 1981;35(3):335–51.
31. Yanagita T. An experimental framework for evaluation of dependence liability of various types of drugs in monkeys. Bull Narcotics 1973;25:57–64.
32. Kieffer BL. Recent advances in molecular recognition and signal transduction of active peptides: receptors for opioid peptides. Cell Mol Neurobiol 1995;15(6):615–35.
33. Lord JA, Waterfield AA, Hughes J, Kosterlitz HW. Endogenous opioid peptides: multiple agonists and receptors. Nature 1977;267(5611):495–9.
34. Martin WR, Eades CG, Thompson JA, Huppler RE, Gilbert PE. The effects of morphine- and nalorphine-like drugs in the nondependent and morphine-dependent chronic spinal dog. J Pharmacol Exp Ther 1976;197(3):517–32.
35. Platt DM, Rowlett JK, Spealman RD. Discriminative stimulus effects of intravenous heroin and its metabolites in rhesus monkeys: opioid and dopaminergic mechanisms. J Pharmacol Exp Ther 2001;299(2):760–7.
36. Brandt MR, Negus SS, Mello NK, Furness MS, Zhang X, Rice KC. Discriminative stimulus effects of the nonpeptidic delta-opioid agonist SNC80 in rhesus monkeys. J Pharmacol Exp Ther 1999;290(3):1157–64.
37. Butelman ER, Ball JW, Kreek MJ. Comparison of the discriminative and neuroendocrine effects of centrally penetrating kappa-opioid agonists in rhesus monkeys. Psychopharmacology (Berl) 2002;164(1):115–20.
38. Herling S, Shannon HE. Discriminative effects of ethylketazocine in the rat: stereospecificity and antagonism by naloxone. Life Sci 1982;31(20–21):2371–4.
39. Krimmer EC, Barry H, 3rd. Measuring naloxone antagonism of discriminative opioid stimulus. Fed Proc 1982;41(7):2319–22.
40. Shannon HE, Cone EJ, Gorodetzky CW. Morphine-like discriminative stimulus effects of buprenorphine and demethoxybuprenorphine in rats: quantitative antagonism by naloxone. J Pharmacol Exp Ther 1984;229(3):768–74.
41. Comer SD, McNutt RW, Chang KJ, De Costa BR, Mosberg HI, Woods JH. Discriminative stimulus effects of BW373U86: a nonpeptide ligand with selectivity for delta opioid receptors. J Pharmacol Exp Ther 1993;267(2):866–74.
42. Craft RM, Heideman LM, Bartok RE. Effect of gonadectomy on discriminative stimulus effects of morphine in female versus male rats. Drug Alcohol Depend 1999;53(2):95–109.
43. Holtzman SG, Cook L, Steinfels GF. Discriminative stimulus effects of spiradoline, a kappa-opioid agonist. Psychopharmacology (Berl) 1991;105(4):447–52.
44. Teal JJ, Holtzman SG. Stimulus effects of morphine in the monkey: quantitative analysis of antagonism. Pharmacol Biochem Behav 1980;12(4):587–93.
45. Young AM, Masaki MA, Geula C. Discriminative stimulus effects of morphine: effects of training dose on agonist and antagonist effects of mu opioids. J Pharmacol Exp Ther 1992;261(1):246–57.
46. Bertalmio AJ, Woods JH. Differentiation between mu and kappa receptor-mediated effects in opioid drug discrimination: apparent pA2 analysis. J Pharmacol Exp Ther 1987;243(2):591–7.
47. Dykstra LA, Bertalmio AJ, Woods JH. Discriminative and analgesic effects of mu and kappa opioids: in vivo pA2 analysis. Psychopharmacol Ser 1988;4:107–21.
48. Ko MC, Butelman ER, Traynor JR, Woods JH. Differentiation of kappa opioid agonist-induced antinociception by naltrexone apparent pA2 analysis in rhesus monkeys. J Pharmacol Exp Ther 1998;285(2):518–26.

49. Negus SS, Burke TF, Medzihradsky F, Woods JH. Effects of opioid agonists selective for mu, kappa and delta opioid receptors on schedule-controlled responding in rhesus monkeys: antagonism by quadazocine. J Pharmacol Exp Ther 1993;267(2):896–903.
50. Walker EA, Makhay MM, House JD, Young AM. In vivo apparent pA2 analysis for naltrexone antagonism of discriminative stimulus and analgesic effects of opiate agonists in rats. J Pharmacol Exp Ther 1994;271(2):959–68.
51. France CP, de Costa BR, Jacobson AE, Rice KC, Woods JH. Apparent affinity of opioid antagonists in morphine-treated rhesus monkeys discriminating between saline and naltrexone. J Pharmacol Exp Ther 1990;252(2):600–4.
52. Rowlett JK, Wilcox KM, Woolverton WL. Self-administration of cocaine-heroin combinations by rhesus monkeys: antagonism by naltrexone. J Pharm Exp Ther 1998;286:61–9.
53. Carey GJ, Bergman J. Enadoline discrimination in squirrel monkeys: effects of opioid agonists and antagonists. J Pharmacol Exp Ther 2001;297(1):215–23.
54. Dykstra LA, Gmerek DE, Winger G, Woods JH. Kappa opioids in rhesus monkeys. II. Analysis of the antagonistic actions of quadazocine and beta-funaltrexamine. J Pharmacol Exp Ther 1987;242(2):421–7.
55. France CP, Woods JH. Beta-funaltrexamine antagonizes the discriminative stimulus effects of morphine but not naltrexone in pigeons. Psychopharmacology (Berl) 1987;91(2):213–6.
56. Holtzman SG. Antagonism of morphine-like discriminative effects by beta-funaltrexamine. Pharmacol Biochem Behav 1997;57(4):771–7.
57. Holtzman SG. Further characterization of the discriminative stimulus effects of spiradoline. Pharmacol Biochem Behav 2000;66(3):517–22.
58. Picker MJ, Dykstra LA. Discriminative stimulus effects of mu and kappa opioids in the pigeon: analysis of the effects of full and partial mu and kappa agonists. J Pharmacol Exp Ther 1989;249(2):557–66.
59. Suzuki T, Mori T, Tsuji M, Misawa M, Nagase H. Discriminative stimulus properties of morphine mediated by mu 1-opioid receptors. Eur J Pharmacol 1995;284(1–2):195–8.
60. Jewett DC, Mosberg HI, Woods JH. Discriminative stimulus effects of a centrally administered, delta-opioid peptide (D-Pen2-D-Pen5-enkephalin) in pigeons. Psychopharmacology (Berl) 1996;127(3):225–30.
61. Shannon HE, Holtzman SG. Blockade of the discriminative effects of morphine in the rat by naltrexone and naloxone. Psychopharmacology (Berl) 1976;50(2):119–24.
62. Negus SS, Picker MJ, Dykstra LA. Interactions between the discriminative stimulus effects of mu and kappa opioid agonists in the squirrel monkey. J Pharmacol Exp Ther 1991;256(1):149–58.
63. Barrett AC, Smith ES, Picker MJ. Use of irreversible antagonists to determine the relative efficacy of mu-opioids in a pigeon drug discrimination procedure: comparison of beta-funaltrexamine and clocinnamox. J Pharmacol Exp Ther 2003;305(3):1061–70.
64. Morgan D, Picker MJ. The mu opioid irreversible antagonist beta-funaltrexamine differentiates the discriminative stimulus effects of opioids with high and low efficacy at the mu opioid receptor. Psychopharmacology (Berl) 1998;140(1):20–8.
65. Walker EA, Young AM. Clocinnamox distinguishes opioid agonists according to relative efficacy in normal and morphine-treated rats trained to discriminate morphine. J Pharmacol Exp Ther 2002;302(1):101–10.
66. Walker EA, Comer SD. Experimental utility and clinical potential of irreversible opioid antagonists. In: Dean R, Bilsky EJ, Negus SS, eds. Opioid Receptors and Antagonists: From Bench to Clinic. New York: Humana Press; 2007.
67. Locke KW, Holtzman SG. Characterization of the discriminative stimulus effects of centrally administered morphine in the rat. Psychopharmacology (Berl) 1985;87(1):1–6.
68. Valentino RJ, Herling S, Woods JH, Medzihradsky F, Merz H. Quaternary naltrexone: evidence for the central mediation of discriminative stimulus effects of narcotic agonists and antagonists. J Pharmacol Exp Ther 1981;217(3):652–9.
69. Carter RB, Leander JD. Discriminative stimulus properties of naloxone. Psychopharmacology (Berl) 1982;77(4):305–8.

70. France CP, Woods JH. Opiate agonist-antagonist interactions: application of a three-key drug discrimination procedure. J Pharmacol Exp Ther 1985;234(1):81–9.
71. Negus SS, Dykstra LA. Neural substrates mediating the reinforcing properties of opioid analgesics. In: Watson RW, ed. Biochemistry and Physiology of Substance Abuse (Vol 1). Boca Raton, FL: CRC Press; 1989:211–42.
72. Spragg SDS. Morphine addiction in chimpanzees. Comp Psychol Mono 1940;15:5–132.
73. Thompson T, Schuster CR. Morphine self-administration, food-reinforced, and avoidance behaviors in rhesus monkeys. Psychopharmacologia 1964;5:87–94.
74. Weeks JR. Experimental morphine addiction: method for automatic intravenous injections in unrestrained rats. Science 1962;138:143–4.
75. Collins RJ, Weeks JR, Cooper MM, Good PI, Russell RR. Prediction of abuse liability of drugs using IV self-administration by rats. Psychopharmacology (Berl) 1984; 82(1–2):6–13.
76. Hoffmeister F. Progressive-ratio performance in the rhesus monkey maintained by opiate infusions. Psychopharmacology (Berl) 1979;62(2):181–6.
77. Johanson CE, Balster RL. A summary of the results of a drug self-administration study using substitution procedures in rhesus monkeys. Bull Narc 1978;30(3):43–54.
78. Sanchez-Ramos JR, Schuster CR. Second-order schedules of intravenous drug self-administration in rhesus monkeys. Pharmacol Biochem Behav 1977;7(5):443–50.
79. Schuster CR, Thompson T. Self administration of and behavioral dependence on drugs. Annu Rev Pharmacol 1969;9:483–502.
80. Woolverton WL, Schuster CR. Behavioral and pharmacological aspects of opioid dependence: mixed agonist-antagonists. Pharmacol Rev 1983;35(1):33–52.
81. Young AM, Swain HH, Woods JH. Comparison of opioid agonists in maintaining responding and in suppressing morphine withdrawal in rhesus monkeys. Psychopharmacology (Berl) 1981;74(4):329–35.
82. Woods JH, Schuster CR. Opiates as reinforcing stimuli. In: Thompson T, Pickens R, eds. Stimulus Properties of Drugs. New York: Apple-Century-Crofts; 1971:163–75.
83. Tang AH, Collins RJ. Behavioral effects of a novel kappa opioid analgesic, U-50488, in rats and rhesus monkeys. Psychopharmacology (Berl) 1985;85(3):309–14.
84. Woods JH, Winger G. Opioid receptors and abuse liability. In: Meltzer HY, ed. Psychopharmacology: Third Generation of Progress. New York: Raven Press; 1987:1555–64.
85. Woods JH, Smith CB, Medzihradsky F, Swain HH. Preclinical testing of new analgesic drugs. In: Beers RF, Bassett EG, eds. Mechanisms of Pain and Analgesic Compounds. New York: Raven Press; 1979:429–45.
86. Young GA, Khazan N. Self-administration of ketocyclazocine and ethylketocyclazocine by the rat. Pharmacol Biochem Behav 1983;19(4):711–3.
87. Mansour A, Khachaturian H, Lewis ME, Akil H, Watson SJ. Anatomy of CNS opioid receptors. Trends Neurosci 1988;11(7):308–14.
88. Belluzzi JD, Stein L. Enkephaline may mediate euphoria and drive-reduction reward. Nature 1977;266(5602):556–8.
89. Goeders NE, Lane JD, Smith JE. Self-administration of methionine enkephalin into the nucleus accumbens. Pharmacol Biochem Behav 1984;20(3):451–5.
90. Devine DP, Wise RA. Self-administration of morphine, DAMGO, and DPDPE into the ventral tegmental area of rats. J Neurosci 1994;14(4):1978–84.
91. Negus SS, Butelman ER, Chang KJ, DeCosta B, Winger G, Woods JH. Behavioral effects of the systemically active delta opioid agonist BW373U86 in rhesus monkeys. J Pharmacol Exp Ther 1994;270(3):1025–34.
92. Negus SS, Gatch MB, Mello NK, Zhang X, Rice K. Behavioral effects of the delta-selective opioid agonist SNC80 and related compounds in rhesus monkeys. J Pharmacol Exp Ther 1998;286(1):362–75.
93. Negus SS, Mello NK, Portoghese PS, Lukas SE, Mendelson JH. Role of delta opioid receptors in the reinforcing and discriminative stimulus effects of cocaine in rhesus monkeys. J Pharmacol Exp Ther 1995;273(3):1245–56.

94. Bertalmio AJ, Woods JH. Reinforcing effect of alfentanil is mediated by mu opioid receptors: apparent pA2 analysis. J Pharmacol Exp Ther 1989;251(2):455–60.
95. Ettenberg A, Pettit HO, Bloom FE, Koob GF. Heroin and cocaine intravenous self-administration in rats: mediation by separate neural systems. Psychopharmacology (Berl) 1982;78(3):204–9.
96. Goldberg SR, Woods JH, Schuster CR. Nalorphine-induced changes in morphine self-administration in rhesus monkeys. J Pharmacol Exp Ther 1971;176(2):464–71.
97. Harrigan SE, Downs DA. Continuous intravenous naltrexone effects on morphine self-administration in rhesus monkeys. J Pharmacol Exp Ther 1978;204(2):481–6.
98. Herling S. Naltrexone effects on food- and codeine-maintained responding in rhesus monkeys. Eur J Pharmacol 1981;73(1):41–9.
99. Killian AK, Bonese K, Schuster CR. The effects of naloxone on behavior maintained by cocaine and heroin injections in the rhesus monkey. Drug Alcohol Depend 1978;3(4):243–51.
100. Koob GF, Pettit HO, Ettenberg A, Bloom FE. Effects of opiate antagonists and their quaternary derivatives on heroin self-administration in the rat. J Pharmacol Exp Ther 1984;229(2):481–6.
101. Martin TJ, Walker LE, Sizemore GM, Smith JE, Dworkin SI. Within-session determination of dose-response curves for heroin self-administration in rats: comparison with between-session determination and effects of naltrexone. Drug Alcohol Depend 1996;41(2):93–100.
102. Weeks JR, Collins RJ. Changes in morphine self-administration in rats induced by prostaglandin E1 and naloxone. Prostaglandins 1976;12(1):11–9.
103. Winger G, Skjoldager P, Woods JH. Effects of buprenorphine and other opioid agonists and antagonists on alfentanil- and cocaine-reinforced responding in rhesus monkeys. J Pharmacol Exp Ther 1992;261:311–7.
104. Woods JH, Downs DA, Carney J. Behavioral functions of narcotic antagonists: response-drug contingencies. Fed Proc 1975;34(9):1777–84.
105. Martin TJ, Dworkin SI, Smith JE. Alkylation of mu opioid receptors by beta-funaltrexamine in vivo: comparison of the effects on in situ binding and heroin self-administration in rats. J Pharmacol Exp Ther 1995;272(3):1135–40.
106. Negus SS, Henriksen SJ, Mattox A, et al. Effect of antagonists selective for mu, delta and kappa opioid receptors on the reinforcing effects of heroin in rats. J Pharmacol Exp Ther 1993;265:1245–52.
107. Zernig G, Lewis JW, Woods JH. Clocinnamox inhibits the intravenous self-administration of opioid agonists in rhesus monkeys: comparison with effects on opioid agonist-mediated antinociception. Psychopharmacology (Berl) 1997;129(3):233–42.
108. Martin TJ, Kim SA, Cannon DG, et al. Antagonism of delta(2)-opioid receptors by naltrindole-5''-isothiocyanate attenuates heroin self-administration but not antinociception in rats. J Pharmacol Exp Ther 2000;294(3):975–82.
109. Vaccarino FJ, Pettit HO, Bloom FE, Koob GF. Effects of intracerebroventricular administration of methyl naloxonium chloride on heroin self-administration in the rat. Pharmacol Biochem Behav 1985;23(3):495–8.
110. Vaccarino FJ, Bloom FE, Koob GF. Blockade of nucleus accumbens opiate receptors attenuates intravenous heroin reward in the rat. Psychopharmacology (Berl) 1985;86(1–2):37–42.
111. Martin TJ, Kim SA, Lyupina Y, Smith JE. Differential involvement of mu-opioid receptors in the rostral versus caudal nucleus accumbens in the reinforcing effects of heroin in rats: evidence from focal injections of beta-funaltrexamine. Psychopharmacology (Berl) 2002;161(2):152–9.
112. Aigner TG, Balster RL. Rapid substitution procedure for intravenous drug self-administration studies in rhesus monkeys. Pharmacol Biochem Behav 1979;10(1):105–12.
113. Woods JH, Young AM, Herling S. Classification of narcotics on the basis of their reinforcing, discriminative, and antagonist effects in rhesus monkeys. Fed Proc 1982;41(2):221–7.

114. Downs DA, Woods JH. Naloxone as a negative reinforcer in rhesus monkeys: effects of dose, schedule, and narcotic regimen. Pharmacol Rev 1975;27(3):397–406.
115. Hoffmeister F, Wuttke W. Negative reinforcing properties of morphine-antagonists in naive rhesus monkeys. Psychopharmacologia 1973;33(3):247–58.
116. Hoffmeister F. Negative reinforcing properties of naloxone in the non-dependent rhesus monkey: influence on reinforcing properties of codeine, tilidine, buprenorphine, and pentazocine. Psychopharmacology (Berl) 1986;90(4):441–50.
117. Martin WR, Wikler A, Eades CG, Pescor FT. Tolerance to and physical dependence on morphine in rats. Psychopharmacologia 1963;4:247–60.
118. Woods JH, Gmerek DE. Substitution and primary dependence studies in animals. Drug Alcohol Depend 1985;14:233–47.
119. Gmerek DE, Woods JH. Kappa receptor mediated opioid dependence in rhesus monkeys. Life Sci 1986;39(11):987–92.
120. Gmerek DE, Dykstra LA, Woods JH. Kappa opioids in rhesus monkeys. III. Dependence associated with chronic administration. J Pharmacol Exp Ther 1987;242(2):428–36.
121. Laorden ML, Milanes MV. Effects of U-50, 488H and U-50, 488H withdrawal on catecholaminergic neurons of the rat hypothalamus. Life Sci 2000;66(9):803–15.
122. Vonvoigtlander PF, Lewis RA. Analgesic and mechanistic evaluation of spiradoline, a potent kappa opioid. J Pharmacol Exp Ther 1988;246(1):259–62.
123. Brandt MR, Furness MS, Rice KC, Fischer BD, Negus SS. Studies of tolerance and dependence with the delta-opioid agonist SNC80 in rhesus monkeys responding under a schedule of food presentation. J Pharmacol Exp Ther 2001;299(2):629–37.
124. Cowan A, Zhu XZ, Mosberg HI, Omnaas JR, Porreca F. Direct dependence studies in rats with agents selective for different types of opioid receptor. J Pharmacol Exp Ther 1988;246(3):950–5.
125. Kovacs GL, Nyolczas N, Krivan M, Gulya K. Analgesic and tolerance-inducing effects of the highly selective delta opioid agonist [D-Pen2, D-Pen5]enkephalin in mice. Eur J Pharmacol 1988;150(3):347–53.
126. Tatum AL, Seevers MH, Collins KH. Morphine addiction and its physiological interpretation based on experimental evidences. J Pharmacol 1929;36:447–75.
127. Koob GF, Ahmed SH, Boutrel B, et al. Neurobiological mechanisms in the transition from drug use to drug dependence. Neurosci Biobehav Rev 2004;27(8):739–49.
128. France CP, Woods JH. Morphine, saline and naltrexone discrimination in morphine-treated pigeons. J Pharmacol Exp Ther 1987;242(1):195–202.
129. Gellert VF, Holtzman SG. Discriminative stimulus effects of naltrexone in the morphine-dependent rat. J Pharmacol Exp Ther 1979;211(3):596–605.
130. Schuster CR, Johanson CE. Relationship between the discriminative stimulus properties and subjective effects of drugs. Psychopharmacol Ser 1988;4:161–75.
131. Katz JL. Effects of clonidine and morphine on opioid withdrawal in rhesus monkeys. Psychopharmacology (Berl) 1986;88(3):392–7.
132. Brandt MR, Cabansag SR, France CP. Discriminative stimulus effects of l-alpha-acetylmethadol (LAAM), buprenorphine and methadone in morphine-treated rhesus monkeys. J Pharmacol Exp Ther 1997;282(2):574–84.
133. Sell SL, McMahon LR, France CP. Relative efficacy of buprenorphine, nalbuphine and morphine in opioid-treated rhesus monkeys discriminating naltrexone. J Pharmacol Exp Ther 2003;306(3):1167–73.
134. France CP, Winger G, Medzihradsky F, Seggel MR, Rice KC, Woods JH. Mirfentanil: pharmacological profile of a novel fentanyl derivative with opioid and nonopioid effects. J Pharmacol Exp Ther 1991;258(2):502–10.
135. France CP, Winger G, Seggel MR, Rice KC, Woods JH. Pharmacological profile of a potent, efficacious fentanyl derivative in rhesus monkeys. Psychopharmacology (Berl) 1992;109(3):291–8.
136. Winger G, France CP, Woods JH, Smith CB, Medzihradsky F, Iorio MA. Opioid and non-opioid effects of novel butyrophenone analogues. Neuropsychopharmacology 1992;7(3):177–87.

137. Brandt MR, France CP. Chronic l-alpha acetylmethadol in rhesus monkeys: discriminative stimulus and other behavioral measures of dependence and withdrawal. J Pharmacol Exp Ther 1998;287(3):1029–37.
138. France CP, Woods JH. U-50, 488, saline and naltrexone discrimination in U-50, 488-treated pigeons. Behav Pharmacol 1993;4(5):509–16.
139. Walker EA, Hawkins ER, Tiano MJ, Picker MJ, Dykstra LA. Discriminative stimulus effects of nalbuphine in nontreated and morphine-treated pigeons. Pharmacol Biochem Behav 1999;64(2):445–8.
140. Carrera MR, Schulteis G, Koob GF. Heroin self-administration in dependent Wistar rats: increased sensitivity to naloxone. Psychopharmacology (Berl) 1999;144(2):111–20.
141. Weeks JR, Collins RJ. Factors affecting voluntary morphine intake in self-maintained addicted rats. Psychopharmacologia 1964;6(4):267–79.
142. Goldberg SR, Woods JH, Schuster CR. Morphine: conditioned increases in self-administration in rhesus monkeys. Science 1969;166(910):1306–7.
143. Yanagita T. Drug dependence studies in laboratory animals. NIDA Res Monogr 1978;19:179–90.
144. Walker JR, Ahmed SH, Gracy KN, Koob GF. Microinjections of an opiate receptor antagonist into the bed nucleus of the stria terminalis suppress heroin self-administration in dependent rats. Brain Res 2000;854(1–2):85–92.
145. Downs DA, Woods JH. Fixed-ratio escape and avoidance-escape from naloxone in morphine-dependent monkeys: effects of naloxone dose and morphine pretreatment. J Exp Anal Behav 1975;23(3):415–27.
146. Goldberg SR, Hoffmeister F, Schlichting U, Wuttke W. Aversive properties of nalorphine and naloxone in morphine-dependent rhesus monkeys. J Pharmacol Exp Ther 1971;179(2):268–76.
147. Kandel DA, Schuster CR. An investigation of nalorphine and perphenazine as negative reinforcers in an escape paradigm. Pharmacol Biochem Behav 1977;6(1):61–71.
148. Tang AH, Morse WH. Termination of a schedule complex associated with intravenous injections of nalorphine in morphine-dependent rhesus monkeys. Pharmacol Rev 1975;27(3):407–17.
149. Kelleher RT, Morse WH. Schedules using noxious stimuli. III. Responding maintained with response-produced electric shocks. J Exp Anal Behav 1968;11(6):819–38.
150. McKearney JW. Maintenance of responding under a fixed-interval schedule of electric shock-presentation. Science 1968;160(833):1249–51.
151. Sevarino K, Kosten T. Naltrexone for initiation and maintenance of opiate abstinence. In: Dean R, Bilsky E, Negus S, eds. Opioid Receptors and Antagonists: From Bench to Clinic. New York: Humana Press; 2007.
152. Negus SS, Woods JH. Reinforcing effects, discriminative stimulus effects, and physical dependence liability of buprenorphine. In: Cowan A, Lewis JW, eds. Buprenorphine: Combatting Drug Abuse with a Unique Opioid. New York: Wiley-Liss; 1995:71–101.
153. Bennett DA, Lal H. Discriminative stimuli produced by clonidine: an investigation of the possible relationship to adrenoceptor stimulation and hypotension. J Pharmacol Exp Ther 1982;223(3):642–8.
154. Weerts EM, Griffiths RR. Evaluation of the intravenous reinforcing effects of clonidine in baboons. Drug Alcohol Depend 1999;53(3):207–14.
155. Woolverton WL, Wessinger WD, Balster RL. Reinforcing properties of clonidine in rhesus monkeys. Psychopharmacology (Berl) 1982;77(1):17–23.
156. Dean R, Gastfriend D, Turncliff R. Preclinical and clinical development of Vivitrol: once-a-month injectable naltrexone microspheres for the treatment of alcohol dependency. In: Dean R, Bilsky E, Negus S, eds. Opioid Receptors and Antagonists: From Bench to Clinic. New York: Humana Press; 2007.

Chapter 12
Naltrexone for Initiation and Maintenance of Opiate Abstinence

Kevin A. Sevarino and Thomas R. Kosten

Abstract Pharmacotherapies for opiate dependence first involve detoxification from physical dependence on opiates and then maintenance of that abstinent state. There are now three agents of distinct pharmacological classes available to achieve both phases: the opiate agonist methadone, the partial opioid agonist buprenorphine, and the opioid antagonist naltrexone. This chapter reviews the role of naltrexone in current opiate detoxification strategies and its use in long-term maintenance of sobriety from opiates.

Keywords: Heroin; Opiate; Naltrexone; Detoxification; Abstinence; Pharmacotherapy

12.1 Overview of Opiate Dependence Pharmacotherapy

The prevalence of opiate dependence is reported to range from 0.1% to 0.3% worldwide, with the annual prevalence in the United States at 0.3% (1, 2). While this places opiate dependence as significantly less common than dependence on nicotine, alcohol, marijuana and cocaine, the severity of opiate withdrawal symptoms and the high incidence of medical and psychiatric comorbidity associated with opiate dependence cause it to account for far greater utilization of medical resources than indicated by its prevalence. For example, in an insured population, opioid abusers compared to nonabusers had 78 times the rates of hepatitis A, B, and C, 36 times the rate of psychiatric illness, and 12 times the rate of inpatient hospitalization (3). Despite clear evidence that methadone maintenance and buprenorphine maintenance can achieve substantial reductions in collateral incidence of hepatitis, HIV, and social and occupational sequelae, maintenance strategies remain utilized

K.A. Sevarino (✉) and T.R. Kosten
VA Connecticut Healthcare System, Newington Campus, Department of Psychiatry 116A3, 555 Willard Avenue, Newington, CT 06111 [KAS] and Department of Psychiatry and Neuroscience, Baylon College of Medicine, Houston, TX and Michael E. DeBakey VA Medical Center Research 151–Bldge 110, Rm 229, 2002 Wolcombe Bolevard Honston, TX 77030 [TRK]
e-mail: kevin.sevarino@va.gov

only by an estimated one-seventh of heroin addicts (4). Use of the competitive opiate antagonist naltrexone has greater availability to addicts, yet also remains underutilized largely because patient adherence is poor. This chapter will focus on the rationale, indications, and limitations of using opiate antagonist therapy both in the initial achievement of opiate abstinence and then in maintaining that state.

12.2 Opiate Detoxification

12.2.1 Range of Pharmacotherapies

Methods of opiate detoxification include (1) methadone taper, (2) buprenorphine with or without taper, (3) symptom amelioration with alpha-2 agonists (clonidine or lofexidine) with ancillary medications for sleep, anxiety, muscle and gastrointestinal symptoms, (4) accelerated withdrawal using opiate antagonists, and (5) ultrarapid detoxification using general anesthesia and antagonist treatment. The use of naltrexone to accelerate opiate detoxification, in combination with other effective detoxification agents, has become a mainstay of current recommendations for detoxification; yet, in practice clonidine-assisted agonist taper without naltrexone acceleration remains the mainstay of inpatient detoxification (KS, personal observation). As we describe below, contrary to expectations the use of an upward titration of naltrexone during the detoxification phase neither increases patients' overall discomfort nor reduces completion rates (5, 6); in fact, the opposite appears true. As a further advantage, the transition to antagonist maintenance in cases where patients have planned to use antagonist rather than agonist maintenance is facilitated by antaganist use during detoxification (7).

12.2.2 Rapid Opiate Detoxification

12.2.2.1 Naltrexone Combined with Alpha-2 Agonists

Although clonidine alone reduces autonomic symptoms of opiate withdrawal, it is less effective at eliminating the subjective, that is, aversive nature of opiate withdrawal (8), and it does not alter the time course of the withdrawal, which typically exceeds 7 days (9). Introducing the opioid antagonist naltrexone during clonidine treatment of opiate withdrawal shortens the duration of withdrawal to about 3 days without increasing patient discomfort (6). In these rapid opiate detoxifications (RODs) induction onto naltrexone typically starts with 12.5 mg of naltrexone on day 1, 25 mg on day 2, and 50 mg on day 3 onwards (5, 10). The dose of clonidine typically is between 0.1 and 0.2 mg every 4 h but is individually determined each day based on the severity of withdrawal symptoms.

In the mid-1980s, Charney et al. (11) first described the use of naltrexone to accelerate detoxification, and Kleber et al. (9) described the first outpatient trial, where 86% of participants utilizing accelerated detoxification completed the study.

Controlled studies comparing naltrexone plus clonidine to clonidine alone or to methadone tapering have found that the former approach was well tolerated and superior in terms of duration of detoxification, treatment retention, and subsequent transition to naltrexone maintenance (5, 7, 10, 12). Vining et al. (13) found that outpatients getting ROD using clonidine plus naltrexone had a completion rate of 75% compared to 40% for methadone taper or clonidine alone. Diazepam 10 mg twice a day on days 1 and 2 was found to be very effective for persistent restlessness and muscle aches during the ROD. Similarly, O'Connor et al. (5) in a randomized double-blind clinical trial showed that 81% of the group treated with the combination of naltrexone plus clonidine were detoxified successfully in comparison with 65% of the participants who received clonidine alone. These findings indicate that naltrexone is an effective and safe addition to clonidine in the management of opiate withdrawal. This study also demonstrated clonidine plus naltrexone shared equal efficacy with buprenorphine for opiate detoxification.

The use of opiate antagonists during detoxification not only may safely reduce the length of the detoxification but also may facilitate greater success in maintaining use of these antagonists beyond the detoxification phase (7). It has been suggested that one mechanism that improves detoxification outcomes is the ability of naltrexone to enhance release of endogenous opioids (14, 15), though these must be acting at non mu-opiate receptors in the presence of the antagonist.

Lofexidine, a centrally acting alpha-2 adrenergic agonist, though not FDA approved for use in the United States for opiate detoxification, appears to have equal efficacy to clonidine (16, 17). Gerra et al. (18) showed equal efficacy for clonidine compared to lofexedine when combined with naloxone and naltrexone for a 3-day rapid detoxification. However, lofexedine had fewer side effects thereby making it more suitable for outpatient settings. This study also allowed oxazepam, baclofen, and ketoprofen to be added during the detoxification, which complicates the study's interpretation.

12.2.2.2 Naltrexone Combined with Buprenorphine

More relevant to current detoxification strategies are the effects of naltrexone when used in combination with buprenorphine. The partial mu-opiate agonist buprenorphine appears to be superior to methadone taper and clonidine for opiate detoxification (19). Gowing et al. (20) reviewed five randomized or quasi-randomized prospective controlled studies comparing buprenorphine to other treatments for managing opiate withdrawal, and found that four of five studies showed buprenorphine superior to (5, 21–23) or equal to (24) clonidine-based strategies for opiate detoxification. In these studies, heroin-dependent candidates were transitioned onto buprenorphine no sooner than 6 h after their last dose of heroin when they generally showed objective signs of opiate withdrawal. Buprenorphine (usually a 4:1 combination of buprenorphine and naloxone available in the United States as Suboxone) typically is started at 4–8 mg SL qd and then is tapered over a 1-week period. There are limited data that more gradual tapers (10–36 days) are superior (21, 25).

Acceleration of the detoxification phase would reduce costs and the treatment burden on providers and patients. Umbricht et al. (23) in a randomized double-blind placebo-controlled trial showed that starting 12.5 mg naltrexone on day 2, 2 h after 12 mg buprenorphine administration, given at least 8 h after the last heroin use, and then performing a cross-titration of increasing doses of naltrexone (daily doses of 12.5, 25, then 50 mg thereafter) and decreasing doses of buprenorphine (daily doses of 8, 4, 2, then 0 mg thereafter) significantly reduced opiate withdrawal symptoms during days 3–5 relative to buprenorphine taper alone. Further, withdrawal signs were abolished by day 5 in the naltrexone-treated group while those who had been treated with buprenorphine taper alone continued to experience moderate withdrawal through 7 days of placebo, and had withdrawal exacerbation on day 8 when 50 mg of naltrexone was administered orally. Overall, withdrawal severity and use of adjunct medications did not differ between the two groups.

In the above study, about one-fifth of patients in the naltrexone arm dropped out on the first day of naltrexone treatment, though opiate withdrawal scores of noncompleters did not differ significantly from those of completers. Thus, dropout may reflect patient aversion not reflected in formal opiate withdrawal rating scales. A significant exacerbation of withdrawal scores was seen 90 min after day 2 naltrexone and peaked in 3 h. On day 3, a much smaller exacerbation was seen, and by day 4 naltrexone administration did not exacerbate withdrawal scores. Others have not found naltrexone addition after buprenorphine induction to result in withdrawal exacerbation (26, 27). This is consistent with the fact that both agents, buprenorphine and naltrexone, share similar high affinities for the mu-opiate receptor, meaning displacement of buprenorphine by naltrexone should be more gradual than displacement of other opiate agonists (28). The more rapid symptom resolution demonstrated by Umbricht et al. (23) suggests that naltrexone in combination with buprenorphine may actually accelerate detoxification *and* reduce withdrawal severity.

12.2.3 Ultrarapid Opiate Detoxification

Ultrarapid opiate detoxification (UROD) using sedatives and anesthetics is a controversial extension of the clonidine-naltrexone combination ROD. Ultrarapid detoxification was first described in 12 opioid-dependent patients who were given naloxone while under general anesthesia (29). While several subsequent advances in anesthetic methodology were reported (e.g., 30–33), studies tended to be small, and did not compare results with other forms of detoxification or examine long-term outcomes. In some studies, withdrawal symptoms persisted for weeks after treatment, though reports of craving were low despite the presence of physical symptoms (34–36). There is some suggestion that this is more the case for subjects detoxifying from methadone compared to heroin or other shorter-acting opiates (37).

It is controversial whether after UROD compliance with naltrexone maintenance, or abstinence in general, is equal to that of other detoxification methods (38).

While Albanese et al. (39) report a 6-month abstinence rate of 55%, this was in a self-pay cohort that was likely to have more support resources at its disposal than is true for most opiate addicts. Further, in this study one method of ascribing abstinence was self-report. Hensel and Kox (37) reported a 68% 1-year abstinence in patients maintained in a naltrexone program following UROD. Conflicting with this, several reports indicate that UROD is no better (40, 41) or less effective (36, 42) there traditional detoxification methods for long-term abstinence rates. In a socially impaired population Bochud et al. (42) reported 14 of 16 patients relapsed after 30 months; Cucchia (36) reported an 80% relapse rate in 6-month follow-up. In perhaps the most informative study to date, Collins et al. (43) compared UROD to buprenorphine/clonidine and clonidine alone and found no benefit of UROD in outcomes compared to the buprenorphine/clonidine group in terms of treatment retention, successful induction onto naltrexone, or opiate-negative urines. Favrat et al. (41) compared UROD to clonidine alone, and found only 30% of the UROD group remained abstinent at 3 months, and less than 5% by 12 months.

UROD requires intensive medical treatment including intubation and artificial ventilation, and because of the medical risks and mortality of anesthesia, its utility and safety has been controversial since its introduction (44, 45). A critical consideration is that untreated opiate withdrawal is not fatal and has no serious medical complications. At least one death during recovery from UROD has been reported (46). In the comparison of UROD with buprenorphine/clonidine and clonidine alone, three life-threatening adverse events occurred in the UROD group and none in the comparison groups (43).

12.3 Naltrexone Maintenance of Opiate Abstinence

12.3.1 Opiate Receptor Antagonists

Naltrexone, an oral, long-acting competitive antagonist of the mu-opiate receptor, is the only available agent approved for use in maintenance of opiate blockade. A daily dose of naltrexone (50 mg) will block the pharmacological effects of 25 mg intravenous heroin for as long as 24 h, and increasing the dose extends its duration of action to 48 h with 100 mg and 72 h with 150 mg (47). Thus, blockade of exogenous opiates lasts longer than might be predicted from the plasma half-life of naltrexone (4 h) or the major active metabolite, 6-beta-naltrexol (12 h). This likely relates to the high affinity of naltrexone for the mu-opiate receptor relative to agonists such as morphine and heroin, consistent with its ability to block opiate receptors even at low blood levels (48). Nalmefene, a similar orally effective antagonist, may be more centrally acting (49, 50) but has yet to receive FDA approval. Naloxone is a short-acting opiate antagonist with relatively low oral bioavailability whose use is restricted to rapid reversal of opiate overdose and intravenous or subcutaneous/intramuscular challenge to determine if physiological opiate dependence is present (see below).

12.3.2 Naltrexone Maintenance

12.3.2.1 Naloxone Challenge, Naltrexone Induction, and Naltrexone Maintenance Dosing

If a detoxification strategy that does not involve placing the patient on naltrexone has been used, then it must be assured that the patient no longer is physiologically dependent on opiates before starting naltrexone. If this is not done severe withdrawal symptoms may occur, which though not life threatening, will adversely affect the patient's subsequent compliance. If opiate withdrawal scores indicate withdrawal symptoms have abated, a subcutaneous or intramuscular injection of naloxone (0.2–0.8 mg) is given. If a withdrawal reaction is elicited, it typically lasts for 60 min or less. Common symptoms include cramps, perspiration, or nausea; if a positive response is elicited, naltrexone is not given that day and the test repeated the next morning. If withdrawal symptoms are not exacerbated by the naloxone challenge, then naltrexone induction typically involves an initial administration of 25 mg on day 1, then 50 mg daily thereafter. It is recommended that doses be observed by a clinician or significant other early in treatment. Once stabilized for 1–2 weeks, patient compliance may be improved by switching to a thrice weekly dosing schedule of 100 mg on Monday, 100 mg on Wednesday, and 150 mg on Friday (5, 47). This schedule provides opiate blockade throughout the week without significant change in side effects. After several months, many clinicians will convert to a twice weekly schedule of 150 mg on Monday and 200 mg on Thursday. While this coverage allows opiate blockade to fall to less than complete by day 4, it is felt patients on this regimen are sufficiently motivated and have an adequate sober support network to maintain abstinence (51). It is vitally important to follow closely those patients who endorse increased drug craving or other signs of imminent relapse. Typically, patients will stop their naltrexone in preparation for such a relapse. Patients must understand that they are no longer tolerant to opiates as they were before detoxification, and if they resume opiate use, they risk serious consequences, including death, from opiate overdose.

12.3.2.2 Safety and Side Effect Profile

Early reports indicated that naltrexone at doses above 200 mg daily were associated with reversible transaminitis (52). After much scrutiny, consensus opinion based on larger studies is that naltrexone, at doses as high as 400 mg per day, does not cause hepatotxicity or elevated liver function tests (LFTs) (15, 53, 54). Nonetheless, it is common clinical practice to evaluate LFTs before starting patients on naltrexone. A general rule of thumb is not to use naltrexone if LFTs are above three to five times normal, though many physicians not experienced in treating addicts avoid naltrexone altogether when any elevation of LFTs is detected. This is unfortunate because this population has a significant incidence of liver disease, for example, 80–90% of methadone clinic patients have hepatitis B or C (55, 56), and a high rate of comorbid alcohol abuse, both of which are associated with elevated liver tests. Indeed, naltrexone has been associated with improvements in LFTs because treatment enhances abstinence from alcohol and improves health in general (57, 58). In general, liver cirrhosis does not affect elimination times for either naltrexone or 6-beta-naltrexol, though the ratio of the parent compound to the metabolite is reduced more slowly in the presence of decompensated cirrhosis (59).

Given its potent antagonist effects at mu-opiate receptors, it is surprising that naltrexone displays so few side effects. As long as physiological dependence has adequately been treated, the most commonly cited complaints are mild headache, nausea, and abdominal pain. Endocrine changes such as elevation of luteinizing hormone and testosterone (60) appear to be clinically insignificant. Naltrexone is not metabolized by the cytochrome P450 system and does not require dosage adjustments when used in conjunction with other medications (61). The one exception appears to be an interaction with thioridazine (now rarely used) where oversedation occurred in two patients on thioridazine when naltrexone was added (62). Dysphoria and depression are commonly cited as side effects in opiate addicts given naltrexone (63), but careful examination supports this as a problem in only a small cohort of those on naltrexone maintenance, at least in those who chose this treatment over agonist maintenance (64, 65).

12.3.2.3 Efficacy in Clinical Use

It is clear that naltrexone will block the reinforcing properties of heroin and other opiates and so should extinguish addictive behavior (47, 51). It is just as clear that because it lacks any positive reinforcing properties itself and because there is no physical withdrawal from it, its clinical use is severely limited by poor adherence compared to agonist-based maintenance. Thus, results have varied regarding the efficacy of oral naltrexone for treatment of opiate dependence. In a multisite controlled trial with random allocation, Hollister (66) examined 170 opiate-dependent patients at 9-month follow-up and found that the group treated with naltrexone had more opiate-free urines and reduced attrition rates. Likewise, Shufman et al. (67) in a double-blind, controlled design evaluated the efficacy of naltrexone in reducing opiate-positive urines during a 12-week trial and found naltrexone to be superior to placebo. Hulse et al. (68) evaluated treatment outcome at 6 months for 100 heroin-dependent patients maintained on naltrexone, defining success either as reduction in periodic heroin use or complete abstinence. At 6 months, 60% of subjects were still on naltrexone although only about half maintained complete abstinence and the rest had returned to periodic heroin use. However, other studies (69–71) have found no differences between treatment groups primarily due to large dropout rates.

To improve the power of analyses in prior studies, several meta-analyses have been reported. In a meta-analysis of randomized control studies evaluating naltrexone, Kirchmayer et al. (72, 73) found insufficient evidence to recommend naltrexone as a treatment of opiate dependence. Only rates of incarceration definitively could be said to be reduced by the combination of naltrexone maintenance and behavioral therapy. In extending this analysis to include studies through 2004 (10 studies, $n = 696$), Minozzi et al. (74) found a reduction in opiate-positive urines in the naltrexone-treated group versus placebo, and naltrexone plus psychosocial treatment versus placebo plus psychosocial treatment. Again, naltrexone treatment was superior to psychosocial treatment in reducing reincarcerations. They found no statistically significant differences between naltrexone treatment and placebo, regardless of behavioral platform, in retention rates, long-term abstinence rates, or side effects. Again, it was concluded that study heterogeneity was too great and treatment effects too small to confirm naltrexone maintenance as a treatment of opiate dependence.

An elegant analysis specifically meant to address whether treatment compliance effects explain lack of naltrexone efficacy in the field was performed by Johansson et al. (75). In this meta-analysis of 9 studies involving 575 patients, the majority of heterogeneity in treatment efficacy (naltrexone vs control) was moderated by treatment retention. In the high-retention groups, opiate-positive urines, opiate craving, rearrests, and psychiatric symptoms were all significantly improved by naltrexone treatment relative to the control group.

A number of explanations are given for the poor compliance to naltrexone. Naltrexone has little or no rewarding effects on its own, though there is limited evidence in animal studies that it can facilitate release of endogenous opioids. However, in the presence of naltrexone, these endogenous opioids could only function through non mu-opioid receptors. Second, besides lacking reward itself, it blocks rewarding effects of opiates such as heroin, and this is a cited reason that opiate addicts choose agonist over antagonist therapy (76). Third, there is no adverse consequence to stopping the medication, in sharp contrast to the withdrawal experienced by patients on opiate agonist therapy.

12.3.2.4 Depot Naltrexone

In order to improve adherence to naltrexone, depot formulations have been developed. These formulations are composed of slow release suspensions of microspheres administered by intramuscular injection, and deliver therapeutic doses over up to 4 weeks after a single injection (77, 78). The actions are identical to those of orally administered naltrexone, including substantial blockade of heroin effects (79). Except for minor, time-limited local reactions, side effects are nearly identical to oral naltrexone. The major focus of research has been on the use of these agents for alcohol dependence, so little experience for opiate-dependent patients has been published. As of this writing, formulations in various stages of testing include Vivitrol by Alkermes and distributed by Cephalon (FDA approved for alcohol dependence, phase 2 for opiate dependence), Depotrex by Biotek, Inc. (phase 2 for opiate dependence), and Naltrel by Drug Abuse Sciences (phase 3 for alcohol dependence, phase 2 for opiate dependence).

The most extensive literature exists for Depotrex. Depotrex is reported to have similar side effect profile to oral naltrexone (80, 81), though clinical trials have focused on its effects on achieving alcohol, not opiate, abstinence. In 2002, Comer and colleagues (78) published the first study examining efficacy of this formulation in heroin dependence. Doses of 192 and 384 mg were tested in 15 heroin-dependent individuals who had undergone opiate detoxification and stabilization on 50 mg oral naltrexone. Two days after the last oral naltrexone dose, depot naltrexone in doses of 192 and 384 mg was administered. Surprisingly, SOWS (Subjective Opiate Withdrawal Scale) scores increased, peaking on day 4 after injection from 11.0 ± 8.2 to 22.5 ± 11.2 in the low-dose group and 18.7 ± 9.0 to 26.3 ± 7.3 in the high-dose group. This may indicate that the mechanism of antagonism may not be entirely identical between the oral and depot formulations of naltrexone. The increase in SOWS was not explained by increased plasma levels resulting from the depot formulation compared to the oral. An oral dose of 50 mg naltrexone results in plasma levels of 30 ng/ml 30 min postdose (82) and 9 ng/ml 60 min postdose (83), while peak levels of 3.8 ± .02 and 8.9 ± 1.4 were achieved 2 h after the low- and high-dose depot naltrexone injection, respectively. A second possibility involves possible sympathetic activity of naltrexone at higher doses, that in itself could mimic or exacerbate withdrawal symptoms. In the Comer study, the high-dose group had higher withdrawal scores throughout the study. Further, they had larger pupil diameters and rated "I want heroin" higher than the low-dose group throughout the study. Interestingly, higher doses of oral naltrexone (120 mg per day) have been associated with increased craving compared to a group receiving 60 mg qd (84).

Complete antagonism of the subjective effects of heroin administered in escalating doses up to 25 mg (roughly equivalent to one "bag" of heroin) was achieved through 5 weeks in the group receiving the 384 mg dose, and 3 weeks in the group receiving 192 mg. It is hypothesized that antagonism of heroin's subjective effects continues even when plasma levels of naltrexone drop to negligible levels. These data are consistent with the experience with oral naltrexone (85, 86). Naltrexone levels fell to less than 1 ng/ml at 22 and 29 days postinjection of the low- and high-dose depot formulation, respectively. The active metabolite 6-beta-naltrexol is present in levels roughly twice that of the parent compound, and peak 24 h postinjection compared to 2 h for the parent compound. This metabolite is likely responsible for the antagonism seen after levels of the parent compound become negligible.

Depotrex again was tested in a randomized, placebo control trial of heroin-dependent patients in 2006 (87). This study was encouraging in that retention in treatment over the 2 months of study was dose related (placebo, 39%, 192 mg, 60% and 384 mg, 68%.). When missing samples were considered positive, the percentage of opiate-negative urine toxicologies, as well as urine toxicologies for cocaine, benzodiazepines, and amphetamines varied significantly with depot naltrexone dose. Unfortunately, the missing urine rates were inversely related to naltrexone dose, so that if missing urines were not considered positive, the relationship of naltrexone treatment to urine toxicologies was lost for all but cocaine-positive urines. At the very least, the data refute the concern that abuse of nonopiates would increase in polysubstance abusers who could no longer experience positive effects of opiates.

Recently, the depot naltrexone formulation Vivitrol, previously known as Vivitrex (Alkermes) was approved for use in alcohol dependence. This preparation consists of naltrexone formulated in microspheres made up of a polyactide-coglycolide polymer (88). Pharmacokinetic studies in humans reveal similar peak and elimination times for equivalent dosages of Vivitrol and Depotrex (89). The ratio of 6-beta-naltrexol to native naltrexone appears lower with this formulation than Depotrex. Dosing does not need to be adjusted, nor is the ratio of 6-beta naltrexol to natrexone altered, in the presence of mild or moderate hepatic impairment (90).

Naltrexone implants represent a second means to obtain sustained release of naltrexone. One gram implants maintain blood levels of naltrexone above 2 ng/ml for 4–5 weeks postinsertion, and this correlates with blockade of opiate agonist effects (91). In this study, two groups totaling 101 patients received implants during UROD and achieved opiate abstinence rates of 74–79% 12 weeks after implantation. Subsequently, Hulse et al. (92, 93) examined implants of 1.7 and 1.8 g produced in Australia (GoMedical Industries). In a small sample of 10 patients, 1.7 g implants maintained naltrexone over 1 ng/ml for 136 days, and 3.4 g implants maintained this level for 297 days; 6-beta-naltrexol levels were maintained above 10 ng/ml for 18 and 83 days, respectively. While clinical trials with this formulation have yet to be reported, in a cohort of 361 opiate-dependent patients, Hulse et al. (94) reported that 21 overdoses involving 20 patients occurred before implant placement, which decreased to 0 overdoses in the 6 months postimplant placement. Waal et al. (95) report an open trial with these implants, in which opiate use was absent for all 13 patients 2–4 months following a single implant, and 5–6.5 months for double implants. Minimal side effects were reported.

12.3.2.5 Pharmacological Adjuncts to Improve Compliance (Lofexidine/Fluoxetine)

To improve the efficacy of naltrexone, new approaches are being developed to address the precipitants of relapse, such as stress. Stress is known to increase drug craving and risk of relapse to drug use (96–99). Lofexidine, an alpha-2 adrenergic agonist, has been shown to attenuate stress-induced reinstatement of opiate seeking behavior in laboratory animals (100, 101). Thus, a pilot safety and preliminary efficacy study was conducted to evaluate the addition of lofexidine to naltrexone treatment of opiate addiction (102). Twenty-five opiate-dependent individuals were recruited immediately following opiate detoxification to participate in a two phase, 8-week study. In phase 1, upon initiation of 50 mg naltrexone daily, subjects were randomly assigned to one of three dosing schedules in an open dosing manner with an induction onto an escalating dose of lofexidine starting at 0.8 mg and titrated to a maximum dose of 2.4 mg daily. Opiate withdrawal symptoms, side effects, blood pressure, and opiate urines were assessed three times weekly. Seventy-two percent of subjects (18/25) completed the 4-week phase 1, and the lofexidine and naltrexone combination was found to be tolerable and without any significant adverse events. In phase 2, subjects were randomized either to remain on lofexidine or be tapered to placebo, in a double-blind placebo-controlled manner, while remaining on 350 mg naltrexone weekly. Lofexidine–naltrexone-treated subjects were significantly more likely to remain opiate free, had higher number of days of compliance with daily naltrexone, and reported lower weekly opiate craving and perceived stress as compared to naltrexone-placebo subjects. These findings suggest that the lofexidine–naltrexone combination is well tolerated and that the combined treatment may enhance opiate treatment outcomes by addressing stress-related relapse. Perhaps related to the ability to tolerate stress, Landabaso et al. (103) examined whether addition of fluoxetine to naltrexone would improve outcomes relative to naltrexone alone. Addition of the antidepressant improved retention at the 6 month time point.

An alternative explanation for the effect of alpha-2 adrenergic agonists such as clonidine and lofexidine is suggested by Negus (104). Clonidine displays discriminative stimulus effects in rats, and lofexidine substitutes fully for the discriminative stimulus effects of clonidine (105). Moreover, clonidine is self-administered by nonhuman primates (106, 107). These discriminative stimulus and reinforcing effects of alpha-2 adrenergic agonists may contribute to the relatively high rates of nonmedicinal clonidine use (clonidine abuse) in opioid-dependent populations (108, 109), and may also contribute to compliance with treatments in which these drugs are delivered in combination with naltrexone.

12.3.2.6 Behavioral Platforms to Improve Compliance

Virtually, all pharmacological approaches in psychiatric treatment should be part of a comprehensive treatment program. This is especially true in substance abuse. Opiate addicts have significant psychiatric and medical comorbidity, and severe disruptions in lifestyle, including checkered social, occupational, and legal histories. Despite this, most programs leave to the wayside funding for case management positions, assuming therapists, nursing, and so on will "pick up" these duties. The therapeutic alliance must be strengthened at as many points as possible to improve compliance with the opiate antagonist approach. Engagement of social work and substance abuse counseling allows for monitored dosing and closer follow-up than the prescribing physician can achieve. Family counseling is critical to improve support and minimize destructive interactions at home. Family can also be engaged in monitoring patient compliance. Finally, many addicts are motivated by court mandate; lose site of this goal, and one usually loses the patient as well, so close work with assigned legal contacts is important.

Two studies of $n = 58$ (110) and $n = 55$ (111) initially showed that contingency management improved naltrexone compliance and treatment retention rates. Following this, a larger study ($n = 127$) confirmed the superiority of contingency management compared to standard naltrexone treatment for treatment retention, naltrexone compliance, and opiate-free urine toxicologies (112). This larger study showed a less robust effect of significant other involvement. Significant other involvement improved opiate use outcomes only where participants attended at least one family counseling session, but improved family functioning in general. The Johansson meta-analysis (75) of these contingency management studies

(3 studies, $n = 240$) confirmed contingency management improved treatment retention, improved naltrexone compliance, and reduced opiate-positive urines.

Fals-Stewart and O'Farrell (113) demonstrated that family counseling was superior to individual counseling for treatment retention, naltrexone compliance, and percentage opiate-positive urines, as well as percent days abstinent. The New York Psychiatric Institute utilizes a combination of significant other involvement, voucher incentives, and motivational and cognitive behavioral therapies called behavioral naltrexone therapy (BNT) (114). They have identified patients exhibiting methadone use and higher than average heroin use as particularly in need of this service platform (115). Compared to a standard treatment of twice weekly manual-guided visits for 6 months called compliance enhancement (CE), BNT improved 6-month treatment retention (22% for BNT compared to 9% for CE), but retention in treatment remained low for both groups (116). These authors postulate that no matter what behavioral platform is applied, a ceiling effect may be reached to improvements in oral naltrexone compliance. They speculate sustained-release formulations will need to reach the field before results can be further improved.

It does not appear counseling has a nonspecific effect on retention. Unspecified behavioral therapy used in the study by Rawson et al. (117) did not improve efficacy of naltrexone. Similarly, group counseling added to naltrexone treatment did not improve treatment retention (118). In summary, to improve treatment retention with oral naltrexone, the best evidence exists for contingency management and then significant other involvement.

12.3.2.7 Patient Selection

A critical decision point in the treatment of opiate dependence is whether to maintain abstinence from opiates or to use opiate agonist substitution therapy. This decision is typically based on several factors. First, the severity and duration of opiate dependence is a factor that must be considered. For example, patients who have been using opiates for less than a year, particularly if they are adolescents, should be encouraged to undergo managed withdrawal with abstinence as the treatment goal, or to be inducted on to naltrexone maintenance. Second, long-term substitution therapy may not be immediately available due to lack of treatment slots and long waiting lists, and to local regulations that restrict this treatment (e.g., some states in the United States do not allow methadone maintenance). While the availability of office-based buprenorphine in France and Australia have addressed successfully this access issue, in the United States there are currently insufficient physicians prescribing buprenorphine to adequately address this problem. Third, patient preference and treatment history are also factors involved in the decision-making process. Recurrent past failures at abstinence-oriented treatments with or without medication strongly suggest that substitution therapy is warranted.

Oral naltrexone maintenance appears most effective in select populations where compliance is strongly reinforced (119). For health professionals, there are often strong psychosocial assets to draw upon, as well as significant peer pressure and career incentives to remain abstinent, and abstinence rates of over 90% have been achieved (120–122). Washton et al. (120) treated 114 business executives with naltrexone, self-help groups, and individual therapy. Of this group, 81% achieved all negative urines for 6 months, and 64% remained in treatment at 12- and 18-month follow-ups. Those with the contingency of job loss did significantly better than those without. Making enrollment in a work release program contingent on naltrexone treatment has greatly reduced the relapse rate of parolees [(123), see O' Brien and Kampman (51)]. Cornish et al. (124) were able to demonstrate a reduction in 6-month reincarceration rates in a group randomized to counseling plus naltrexone compared to those given counseling alone. In general, up to the advent of depot formulations of naltrexone, it has been felt antagonist therapy is likely to work in those with relatively intact social structures and interpersonal skills (51). In part, this may be true because of the greater financial resources available to such individuals, such that they can afford, or have access to, comprehensive treatment that includes individual counseling, compared to the typical platform of 12-step programs and medication management.

12.4 Conclusion

Naltrexone acceleration of opiate detoxification is strongly supported as effective. Use in the maintenance phase, however, has had more variable results, largely because compliance is so poor. While behavioral platforms including contingency management and significant other support will help, addiction services in general have yet to garner the needed financial support to add these services. The development of sustained-release formulations of naltrexone offers the best hope to improve delivery of this treatment modality for opiate dependence.

Acknowledgments This work was supported by the National Institute on Drug Abuse grants K05-DA00454 (TRK), P50-DA12762, R01-DA05626 and the Department of Veterans Affairs, New England MIRECC.

References

1. Sloboda Z. Drug abuse patterns in the United States. In: *Epidemiologic Trends in Drug Abuse. Volume II: Proceeding of the International Epidemiology Work Group on Drug Abuse*. National Institutes of Health, Bethesda, MD, 1999; pp. 89–107.
2. Substance Abuse and Mental Health Services Administration: Summary of Findings from the 2004 National Household Survey on Drug Abuse. (2005) accessed at www.oas.samsha.gov/nsduhlatest.htm
3. White AG, Birnbaum HG, Mareva MN, Daher M, Vallow S, Schein J, Katz N. Direct costs of opioid abuse in an insured population in the United States. *J. Manag. Care Pharm.* 2005; **11**:469–479.
4. Rounsaville BJ, Kosten TR. Treatment for opioid dependence: quality and access. *JAMA* 2000; **283**:1337–1339.

5. O'Connor PG, Carroll KM, Shi JM, Schottenfeld RS, Kosten TR, Rounsaville BJ. Three methods of opioid detoxification in a primary care setting. A randomized trial. *Ann. Intern. Med.* 1997; **127**:526–530.
6. Gowing L, Ali R, White J. Opioid antagonists and adrenergic agonists for the management of opioid withdrawal. *Cochrane Database Syst Rev [computer file]* 2000b; (**2**):CD002021.
7. Gerra G, Zaimovic A, Rustichelli P, Fontanesi B, Zambelli U, Timpano M, Bocchi C, Delsignore R. Rapid opiate detoxification in outpatient treatment: relationship with naltrexone compliance. *J. Subst. Abuse Treat.* 2000; **18**:185–191.
8. Rosen MI, McMahon TJ, Hameedi FA, Pearsall HR, Woods SW, Kreek MJ, Kosten TR. Effect of clonidine pretreatment on naloxone-precipitated opiate withdrawal. *J. Pharmacol. Exp. Ther.* 1996; **276**:1128–1135.
9. Kleber HD, Topazian M, Gaspari J, Riordan CE, Kosten T. Clonidine and naltrexone in the outpatient treatment of heroin withdrawal. *Am. J. Drug Alcohol Abuse* 1987; **13**:1–17.
10. O'Connor PG, Waugh ME, Carroll KM, Rounsaville BJ, Diagkogiannis IA, Schottenfeld RS. Primary care-based ambulatory opioid detoxification: the results of a clinical trial. *J. Gen. Intern. Med.* 1995; **10**:255–260.
11. Charney DS, Heninger GR, Kleber HD. The combined use of clonidine and naltrexone as a rapid, safe and effective treatment of abrupt withdrawal from methadone. *Am. J. Psychiat.* 1986; **143**:831–837.
12. Gerra G, Marcato A, Caccavari R, Fontanesi B, Delsignore R, Fertonani G, Avanzini P, Rustichelli P, Passeri M. Clonidine and opiate receptor antagonists in the treatment of heroin addiction. *J. Subst. Abuse Treat.* 1995; **12**:35–41.
13. Vining E, Kosten TR, Kleber HD. Clinical utility of rapid clonidine-naltrexone detoxification for opioid abusers. *Br. J. Addict.* 1988; **83**:567–575.
14. Foo H, Westbrook RF. Naloxone-induced hypoalgesia: effects of noradrenergic antagonists and agonist. *Pharmacol. Biochem. Behav.* 1991; **39**:795–797.
15. Marrazzi MA, Wroblewski JM, Kinzie J, Luby ED. High-dose naltrexone and liver function safety. *Am. J. Addict.* 1997; **6**:21–29.
16. Kahn A, Mumford JP, Rogers GA, Beckford H. Double-blind study of lofexidine and clonidine in the detoxification of opiate addicts in hospital. *Drug Alcohol Depend.* 1997; **44**:57–61.
17. Lin SK, Strang J, Su LW, Tsai CJ, Hu WH. Double-blind randomised controlled trial of lofexidine versus clonidine in the treatment of heroin withdrawal. *Drug Alcohol Depend.* 1997; **48**:127–133.
18. Gerra G, Zaimovic A, Giusti F, Di Gennaro C, Zambelli U, Gardini S, Delsignore R. Lofexidine versus clonidine in rapid opiate detoxification. *J. Subst. Abuse Treat.* 2001; **21**:11–17.
19. Kosten, TR. Buprenorphine for opioid detoxification. *Addict. Disord. Treat.* 2003; **2**:107–112.
20. Gowing L, Ali R, White J. Buprenorphine for the management of opioid withdrawal. *Cochrane Database Syst Rev [computer file]* 2000a; (**3**):CD002025.
21. Nigam AK, Ray R, Tripathi BM. Buprenorphine in opiate withdrawal: a comparison with clonidine. *J. Subst. Abuse Treat.* 1993; **10**:391–394.
22. Janiri L, Mannelli P, Persico AM, Serretti A, Tempesta E. Opiate detoxification of methadone maintenance patients using lefetamine, clonidine and buprenorphine. *Drug Alcohol Depend.* 1994; **36**:139–145.
23. Umbricht A, Montoya ID, Hoover DR, Demuth KL, Chiang CT, Preston KL. Naltrexone shortened opioid detoxification with buprenorphine. *Drug Alcohol Depend.* 1999; **56**:181–190.
24. Cheskin LJ, Fudala PJ, Johnson RE. A controlled comparison of buprenorphine and clonidine for acute detoxification from opioids. *Drug Alcohol Depend.* 1994; **36**:115–121.
25. Amass L, Bickel WK, Higgins ST, Hughes JR. A preliminary investigation of outcome following gradual or rapid buprenorphine detoxification. *J. Addict. Dis.* 1994; **13**:33–45.
26. Rosen M, Kosten TR. Detoxification and induction onto naltrexone. In: Cowen A and Lewis JW, Eds., *Buprenorphine. Combating Drug Abuse with a Unique Opioid.* Wiley-Liss, New York, New York, 1995; pp. 289–305.
27. O'Connor PG, Kosten TR. Rapid and ultrarapid opioid detoxification techniques. *JAMA* 1998; **279**:229–234.

28. Rothman RB, Ni Q, Xu H. Byprenorphine A review of the binding literature. In: Cowen A and Lewis JW, Eds., *Buprenorphine. Combating Drug Abuse with a Unique Opioid*. Wiley-Liss, New York, New York, 1995; pp. 19–29.
29. Loimer N, Schmid R, Presslich O, Lenz K. Naloxone treatment for opiate withdrawal syndrome. *Br. J. Psychiatry* 1988; **153**:851–852.
30. Loimer N, Schmid R, Lenz K, Presslich O, Grunberger J. Acute blocking of naloxone-precipitated opiate withdrawal symptoms by methohexitone. *Br. J. Psychiatry* 1990; **157**:748–752.
31. Legarda JJ, Gossop M. A 24-h inpatient detoxification treatment for heroin addicts: a preliminary investigation. *Drug Alcohol Depend.* 1994; **35**:91–93.
32. Barttner T, Gooberman LL. Rapid opiate detoxification. *Am. J. Drug Alcohol Abuse* 1996; **22**:489–495.
33. Strang J, Bearn J, Gossop M. Opiate detoxification under anaesthesia. *Br. Med. J.* 1997; **315**:1249–1250.
34. Elman I, D'Ambra MN, Krause S, Breiter H, Kane M, Morris R, Tuffy L, Gastfriend DR. Ultrarapid opioid detoxification: effects on cardiopulmonary physiology, stress hormones and clinical outcomes. *Drug Alcohol Depend.* 2001; **61**:163–172.
35. Scherbaum N, Klein S, Kaube H, Kienbaum P, Peters J, Gastpar M. Alternative strategies of opiate detoxification: evaluation of the so-called ultra-rapid detoxification. *Pharmacopsychiatry* 1998; **31**:205–209.
36. Cucchia AT, Monnat M, Spagnoli J, Ferrero F, Bertschy G. Ultra-rapid opiate detoxification using deep sedation with oral midazolam: short and long-term results. *Drug Alcohol Depend.* 1998; **52**:243–250.
37. Hensel M, Kox WJ. Safety, efficacy, and long-term results of a modified version of rapid opiate detoxification under general anaesthesia: a prospective study in methadone, heroin, codeine and morphine addicts. *Acta Anaesthesiol. Scand.* 2000; **44**:326–333.
38. Rabinowitz J, Cohen H, Tarrasch R, Kotler M. Compliance to naltrexone treatment after ultra-rapid opiate detoxification: an open label naturalistic study. *Drug Alcohol Depend.* 1997; **47**:77–86.
39. Albanese AP, Gevirtz C, Oppenheim B, Field JM, Abels I, Eustace JC. Outcome and six month follow up of patients after Ultra Rapid Opiate Detoxification (UROD). *J. Addict. Dis.* 2000; **19**:11–28.
40. Lawental E. Ultra rapid opiate detoxification as compared to 30-day inpatient detoxification program – a retrospective follow-up study. *J. Subst. Abuse* 2000; **11**:173–181.
41. Favrat B, Zimmermann G, Zullino D, Krenz S, Dorogy F, Muller J, Zwahlen A, Broers B, Besson J. Opioid antagonist detoxification under anaesthesia versus traditional clonidine detoxification combined with an additional week of psychosocial support: a randomized clinical trial. *Drug Alcohol Depend.* 2006; **81**:109–116.
42. Bochud Tornay C, Favrat B, Monnat M, Daeppen JB, Schnyder C, Bertschy G, Besson J. Ultra-rapid opiate detoxification using deep sedation and prior oral buprenorphine preparation: long-term results. *Drug Alcohol Depend.* 2003; **69**:283–288.
43. Collins ED, Kleber HD, Whittington RA, Heitler NE. Anesthesia-assisted vs. buprenorphine- or clonidine-assisted heroin detoxification and naltrexone induction: a randomized trial. *JAMA* 2005; **294**:903–913.
44. San L, Puig M, Bulbena A, Farre M. High risk of ultrashort noninvasive opiate detoxification. *Am. J. Psychiatry* 1995; **152**:956.
45. Pfab R, Hirtl C, Zilker T. Opiate detoxification under anesthesia: no apparent benefit but suppression of thyroid hormones and risk of pulmonary and renal failure. *J. Toxicol. Clin. Toxicol.* 1999; **37**:43–50.
46. Badenoch J. A death following ultra-rapid opiate detoxification: the General Medical Council adjudicates on a commercialized detoxification. *Addiction* 2002; **97**:475–477.
47. Kleber HD. Naltrexone. *J. Subst. Abuse Treat.* 1985; **2**:117–122.
48. Lee MC, Wagner HN Jr., Tanada S, Frost JJ, Bice AN, Dannals RF. Duration of occupancy of opiate receptors by naltrexone. *J. Nucl. Med.* 1988; **29**:1207–1211.

49. Mason BJ, Ritvo EC, Morgan RO, Salvato FR, Goldberg G, Welch B, Mantero-Atienza E. A double-blind, placebo-controlled pilot study to evaluate the efficacy and safety of oral nalmefene HCl for alcohol dependence. *Alcohol Clin. Exp. Res.* 1994; **18**:1162–1167.
50. Jones HE, Johnson RE, Fudala PJ, Henningfield JE, Heishman SJ. Nalmefene: blockade of intravenous morphine challenge effects in opioid abusing humans. *Drug Alcohol Depend.* 2000; **60**:29–37.
51. O'Brien CP, Kampman KM. Opioids: antagonists and partial agonists. In: Galanter M and Kleber HD, Eds., *Textbook of Substance Abuse Treatment, 3rd Edition,* American Psychiatric Publishing Inc., Washington, D.C., 2005; pp. 305–319.
52. Mitchell JE, Morley JE, Levine AS, Hatsukami D, Gannon M, Pfohl D. High-dose naltrexone therapy and dietary counseling for obesity. *Biol. Psychiatry* 1987; **22**:35–42.
53. Croop RS, Faulkner EB, Labriola DF. The safety profile of naltrexone in the treatment of alcoholism: results from a multicenter usage study. The Naltrexone Usage Study Group. *Arch. Gen. Psychiatry* 1997; **54**:1130–1135.
54. Brewer C, Wong VS. Naltrexone: report of lack of hepatotoxicity in acute viral hepatitis, with a review of the literature. *Addict. Biol.* 2004; **9**:81–87.
55. Dhopesh VP, Taylor KR, Burke WM. Survey of hepatitis B and C in addiction treatment unit. *J. Drug Alcohol Abuse.* 2000; **26**:703–707.
56. Hallinan R, Byrne A, Amin J, Dore GJ. Hepatitis C virus prevalence and outcomes among injection drug users on opioid replacement therapy. *J. Gastroenterol. Hepatol.* 2005; **20**:1082–1086.
57. O'Connor PG, Farren CK, Rounsaville BJ, O'Malley SS. A preliminary investigation of the management of alcohol dependence with naltrexone by primary care providers. *Am. J. Med.* 1997; **103**:477–482.
58. Yen MH, Ko HC, Tang FI, Lu RB, Hong JS. Study of hepatotoxicity of naltrexone in the treatment of alcoholism. *Alcohol* 2006; **38**:117–120.
59. Bertolotti M, Ferrari A, Vitale G, Stefani M, Trenti T, Loria P, Carubbi F, Carulli N, Sternieri E. Effect of liver cirrhosis on the systemic availability of naltrexone in humans. *J. Hepatol.* 1997; **27**:505–511.
60. Mendelson JH, Ellinboe J, Kuehnle JC, Mello NK. Heroin and naltrexone effects on pituitary-gonadal hormones in man: interaction of steroid feedback effects, tolerance and supersensitivity. *J. Pharmacol. Exp. Ther.* 1980; **214**:503–506.
61. Porter SJ, Somogyi AA, White JM. Kintetics and inhibition of the formation of 6-beta-naltrexol from nalterexone in human liver cytosol. *Br. J. Clin. Pharmacol.* 2000; **50**:465–471.
62. Manny I, O'Brien CP, Woody G. Interaction between thioridazine and naltrexone. *Am. J. Psychiatry* 1987; **144**:966.
63. Crowley T, Wagner J, Zerbe G, Macdonald M. Naltrexone-induced dysphoria in former opioid addicts. *Am. J. Psychiatry* 1985; **142**:1081–1084.
64. Miotto K, McCann M, Basch J, Rawson R, Ling W. Naltrexone and dysphoria – fact or fiction? *Am. J. Psychiatry* 2002; **11**:151–160.
65. Dean AJ, Saunders JB, Jones RT, Young RM, Connor JP, Lawford BR. Does naltrexone treatment lead to depression? Findings from a randomized controlled trial in subjects with opioid dependence. *J. Psychiatry Neurosci.* 2004; **31**:38–45.
66. Hollister LE. Clinical evaluation of naltrexone treatment of opiate-dependent individuals. Report of the national research council committee on clinical evaluation of narcotic antagonists. *Arch. Gen. Psychiatry* 1978; **35**:335–340.
67. Shufman EN, Porat S, Witztum E, Gandacu D, Bar-Hamburger R, Ginath Y. The efficacy of naltrexone in preventing reabuse of heroin after detoxification. *Biol. Psychiatry* 1994; **35**:935–945.
68. Hulse GK, Basso MR. Reassessing naltrexone maintenance as a treatment for illicit heroin users. *Drug Alcohol Rev.* 1999; **18**:263–269.
69. Curren S, Savage C. Patient response to naltrexone: issues of acceptance, treatment effects, and frequency of administration. *NIDA Res. Monogr.* 1976; **9**:67–69.
70. San L, Pomarol G, Peri JM, Olle JM, Cami J. Follow-up after a six-month maintenance period on naltrexone versus placebo in heroin addicts. *Br. J. Addict.* 1991; **86**:983–990.

71. Lerner A, Sigal M, Bacalu A, Shiff R, Burganski I, Gelkopf M. A naltrexone double blind placebo controlled study in Israel. *Isr. J. Psychiatry Relat. Sci.* 1992; **29**:36–43.
72. Kirchmayer U, Davoli M, Verster A. Naltrexone maintenance treatment for opioid dependence. *Cochrane Database Syst. Rev.* 2001; **2**(CD001333).
73. Kirchmayer U, Davoli M, Verster A. A systematic review on the efficacy of naltrexone maintenance treatment in opioid dependence. *Addiction* 2002; **97**:1241–1249.
74. Minozzi S, Amato L, Vacchi S, Davoli M, Kirchmayer U, Verster A. Oral naltrexone maintenance treatment for opioid dependence. *Cochrane Database Syst. Rev.* 2006; **1**:Art. No. CD001333.pub2. DOI: 10.1002/14651858.
75. Johansson BA, Berglund M, Lindgren A. Efficacy of maintenance treatment with naltrexone for opioid dependence: a meta-analytical review. *Addiction* 2006; **101**:491–503.
76. Greenstein RA, Arndt IC, McLellan AT, O'Brien CP, Evans B. Naltrexone: a clinical perspective. *J. Clin. Psychiatry* 1985; **45**:25–28.
77. Chiang CN, Hollister LE, Gillespie HK, Foltz RL. Clinical evaluation of a naltrexone sustained-release preparation. *Drug Alcohol Depend.* 1985; **16**:1–8.
78. Comer SD, Collins ED, Kleber HD, Nuwayser ES, Kerrigan JH, Fischman MW. Depot naltrexone: long-lasting antagonism of the effects of heroin in humans. *Psychopharmacology* 2002; **159**:351–360.
79. Modesto-Lowe V, Van Kirk J. Clinical uses of naltrexone: a review of the evidence. *Exp. Clin. Psychopharmacol* 2002; **10**:213–227.
80. Alim TN, Tai B, Chiang CN, Green T, Rosse RB, Lindquist T, Deutsch SI. Tolerability of a depot form of naltrexone in substance abusers. In: Harris LS, Ed., *Problems of Drug Dependence 1994, Vol. 2,* NIDA Research Monograph No. 153 (NIH Publication No. 95–3883, U.S. Government Printing Office, Washington, D.C., 1995; p. 253.
81. Kranzler HR, Modesto-Lowe V, Nuwayser ES. Sustained-release naltrexone for alcoholism treatment: a preliminary study. *Alcohol Clin. Exp. Res.* 1998; **22**:1074–1079.
82. Walsh SL, Sullivan JT, Preston KL, Garner JE, Bigelow GE. Effects of naltrexone on response to intravenous cocaine, hydromorphone and their combination in humans. *J. Pharmacol. Exp. Ther.* 1996; **279**:524–538.
83. Meyer MC, Straughn MB, Lo MW, Schary WL, Whitney CC. Bioequivalence, dose-proportionality, and pharmacokinetics of naltrexone after oral administration. *J. Clin. Psychiatry* 1984; **45**:15–19.
84. Judson BA, Carney TM, Goldstein A. Naltrexone treatment of heroin addiction: efficacy and safety in a double-blind safety comparison. *Drug Alcohol Depend.* 1981; **7**:325–346.
85. Preston KL, Bigelow GE. Differential naltrexone antagonism of hydromorphone and pentazocine effects in human volunteers. *J. Pharmacol. Exp. Ther.* 1993; **264**:813–823.
86. Schuh KJ, Walsh SL, Stitzer ML. Onset, magnitude and duration of opioid blockade produced by buprenorphine and naltrexone in humans. *Psychopharmacology* 1999; **145**: 162–174.
87. Comer SD, Sullivan MA, Yu E, Rothenberg JL, Kleber HD, Kampman K, Dackis C, O'Brien CP. Injectable, sustained-release naltrexone for the treatment of opioid dependence. *Arch. Gen. Psychiatry* 2006; **63**:210–218.
88. Johnson BA, Ait-Daoud N, Aubin HJ, Van Den Brink W, Guzzetta R, Loewy J, Silverman B, Ehrich E. A pilot evaluation of the safety and tolerability of repeat dose administration of long-acting injectable naltrexone (Vivitrex) in patients with alcohol dependence. *Alcohol. Clin. Exp. Res.* 2004; **28**:1356–1361.
89. Dunbar JL, Turncliff RZ, Dong Q, Silverman BL, Ehrich EW, Lasseter KC. Single- and multiple-dose pharmacokinetics of long-acting injectable naltrexone. *Alcohol. Clin. Exp. Res.* 2006; **30**:480–490.
90. Turncliff RZ, Dunbar JL, Dong Q, Silverman BL, Ehrich EW, Dilzer SC, Lasseter KC. Pharmacokinetics of long-acting naltrexone in subjects with mild to moderate hepatic impairment. *J. Clin. Pharmacol.* 2005; **45**:1259–1267.

91. Foster J, Brewer C, Steele T. Naltrexone implants can completely prevent early (1-month) relapse after opiate detoxification: a pilot study of two cohorts totaling 101 patients with a note on naltrexone blood levels. Addict. Biol. 2003; 8:211–217.
92. Hulse GK, Arnold-Reed DE, O'Neil G, Chan CT, Hansson R, O'Neil P. Blood naltrexone and 6-beta-naltrexol levels following naltrexone implant: comparing two naltrexone implants. Addict. *Biol.* 2004; **9**:59–65.
93. Hulse GK, Arnold-Reed DE, O'Neil G, Chan CT, Hansson RC. Achieving long-term continuous blood naltrexone and 6-beta-naltrexol coverage following sequential naltrexone implants. *Addict. Biol.* 2004; **9**:67–72.
94. Hulse GK, Tait RJ, Comer SD, Suillivan MA, Jacobs IG, Arnold-Reed D. Reducing hospital presentations for opioid overdose in patients treated with sustained release naltrexone implants. *Drug Alcohol Depend.* 2005; **79**:351–357.
95. Waal H, Frogopsahl G, Olsen L, Christophersen AS, Morland J. Naltrexone implants – duration, tolerability and clinical usefulness. A pilot study. *Eur. Addict. Res.* 2006; **12**:138–144.
96. Kosten TR, Rounsaville BJ, Kleber HD. Relationship of depression to psychosocial stressors in heroin addicts. *J. Nerv. Ment. Dis.* 1983; **171**:97–104.
97. Kosten TR, Rounsaville BJ, Kleber HD. A 2.5 year follow up of cocaine use among treated opiate addicts. Have our treatments helped? *Arch. Gen. Psychiatry* 1987; **44**:281–284.
98. Sinha R, Catapano D, O'Malley SS. Stress-induced craving and stress response in cocaine dependent individuals. *Psychopharmacology (Berl)* 1999; **142**:343–351.
99. Sinha R, Fuse T, Aubin LR, O'malley SS. Psychological stress, drug-related cues and cocaine craving. *Psychopharmacology (Berl)* 2000; **152**:140–148.
100. Shaham Y, Stewart J. Stress reinstates heroin-seeking in drug-free animals: an effect mimicking heroin, not withdrawal. *Psychopharmacology (Berl)* 1995; **119**:334–341.
101. Shaham Y, Highfield D, Delfs J, Leung S, Stewart J. Clonidine blocks stress-induced reinstatement of heroin seeking in rats: an effect independent of locus coeruleus noradrenergic neurons. *Eur. J. Neurosci.* 2000; **12**:292–302.
102. Sinha R, Holtzman K, Hogan I, Meandzija B, Kimmerling A, Scanley BE, Kosten TR. Lofexidine: enhancing naltrexone treatment to prevent stress-related opiate relapse. *Proceedings of College on Problems of Drug Dependence*. 65th Annual Meeting of the College on Problems of Drug dependence, Bal Harbour, Florida, 2003, p. 638.
103. Landabaso MA, Itaugi I, Jiminez-Lerma JM, Sanz J, Fernandez de Corres B, Araluce K, Calle R, Gutierrez-Fraile M. A randomized trial of adding fluoxetine to a naltrexone treatment program for heroin addicts. *Addiction* 1998; **93**:739–744.
104. Negus SS. Opioid antagonist effects in animal models related to opioid abuse: drug discrimination and drug self-administration. In: Dean R, Bilsky E, Negus S, Eds., *Opioid Receptors and Antagonists: From Bench to Clinic*. Humana Press; 2007.
105. Bennett DA, Lal H. Discriminative stimuli produced by clonidine: an investigation of the possible relationship to adrenoceptor stimulation and hypotension. *J. Pharmacol. Exp. Ther.* 1982; **223**:642–648.
106. Woolverton WL, Wessinger WD, Balster RL. Reinforcing properties of clonidine in rhesus monkeys. *Psychopharmacology (Berl)* 1982; **77**:17–23.
107. Weerts EM, Griffiths RR. Evaluation of the intravenous reinforcing effects of clonidine in baboons. *Drug Alcohol Depend.* 1999; **53**:207–214.
108. Beuger M, Tommasello A, Schwartz R, Clinton M. Clonidine use and abuse among methadone program applicants and patients. *J. Subst. Abuse Treat.* 1998; **15**:589–593.
109. Lanford W, Myrick H, O'Bryan E, Gorman J. A severe case of clonidine dependence and withdrawal. *J Psychiatr. Pract.* 2003; **9**:167–170.
110. Preston KL, Silerman K, Umbricht A, Desjens A, Montoya ID, Schuster CR. Improvement in naltrexone treatment compliance with contingency management. *Drug Alcohol Depend.* 1999; **54**:127–135.
111. Carroll KM, Ball SA, Nich C, O'Connor PG, Eagan DA, Frankforter TL, Triffleman EG, Shi J, Rounsaville BJ. Targeting behavioral therapies to enhance naltrexone treatment of opioid

dependence: efficacy of contingency management and significant other involvement. *Arch. Gen. Psychiatry* 2001; **58**:755–761.
112. Carroll KM, Sinha R, Nich C, Babuscio T, Rounsaville BJ. Contingency management to enhance naltrexone treatment for opioid dependence: a randomized clinical trial of reinforcement magnitude. *Exp. Clin. Psychopharmacol.* 2002; **10**:54–63.
113. Fals-Stewart W, O'Farrell T. Behavioral family counseling and naltrexone for male opioid-dependent patients. *J. Consult. Clin. Psychol.* 2003; **71**:432–442.
114. Rothenberg JL, Sullivan MA, Church SH, Seracini A, Collins E, Kleber HD, Nunes EV. Behavioral naltrexone therapy: an integrated treatment for opiate dependence. *J. Subst. Abuse Treat.* 2002; **23**:351–360.
115. Sullivan MA, Rothenberg JL, Bosburg SK, Church SH, Feldman SJ, Epstein EM, Kleber HD, Nunes EV. Predictors of retention in naltrexone maintenance for opioid dependence: analysis of stage I trial. *Am. J. Addict.* 2006; **15**:150–159.
116. Nunes EV, Rothenberg JL, Sullivan MA, Carpenter M, Kleber HD. Behavioral therapy to augment oral naltrexone for opioid dependence: a ceiling on effectiveness? *Am. J. Drug Alcohol Abuse* 2006; **33**:502–517.
117. Rawson RA, Glazer M, Callahan EJ, Lieberman RP. Naltrexone and behavior therapy for heroin addiction. *NIDA Res. Mono gr.* 1979; **25**:289–295.
118. Tucker T, Ritter A, Maher C, Jackson H. A randomized control trial of group counseling in a naltrexone treatment program. *J. Subst. Abuse Treat.* 2004; **27**:277–288.
119. Ward J, Hall W, Mattick RP. Role of maintenance treatment in opioid dependence. *Lancet* 1999; **353**:221–226.
120. Washton AM, Pottash AC, Gold MS. Naltrexone in addicted business executives and physicians. *J. Clin. Psychiatry* 1984; **45**:39–41.
121. Ling W, Wesson DR. Naltrexone treatment for addicted health-care professionals: a collaborative private practice experience. *J. Clin. Psychiatry* 1984; **45**:46–48.
122. Roth A, Hogan I, Farren C. Naltrexone plus group therapy for the treatment of opiate-abusing health care professionals. *J. Subst. Abuse Treat.* 1997; **14**:19–22.
123. Brahen LS, Henderson RK, Capone T, Kordal N. Naltrexone treatment in a jail work-release program. *J. Clin. Psychiatry* 1984; **45**:49–52.
124. Cornish JW, Metzger DM, Woody GE, Wilson D, McLellan AT, Vandergrift B, O'Brien CP. Naltrexone pharmacotherapy for opioid dependent federal probationers. *J. Subst. Abuse Treat.* 1997; **14**:529–534.

Chapter 13
Ultra-Low-Dose Naltrexone Decreases Dependence and Addictive Properties of Opioids

Lindsay H. Burns, Francesco Leri, and Mary C. Olmstead

Abstract Ultra-low-dose opioid antagonist cotreatment was first shown paradoxically to enhance opioid analgesia and to reduce analgesic tolerance and physical dependence. In this chapter, we review data demonstrating that ultra-low-dose naloxone or naltrexone reduces several components of opioid dependence and addiction. While the reduction in opioid dependence, first demonstrated as a reduction in somatic withdrawal signs, might seem merely a correlate of the attenuation in tolerance, the data reviewed here show that ultra-low-dose naltrexone also reduces the "psychological" or negative affective aspect of acute opioid withdrawal. In addition, the acute rewarding properties of opioids are reduced by ultra-low-dose naltrexone. The attenuation of rewarding effects occurs in the same ultra-low dose ranges shown to enhance analgesia, thus dissociating the rewarding or addictive effects of opioids from their analgesic properties. Furthermore, in intravenous self-administration procedures in rats, ultra-low-dose opioid antagonists coadministered with opioids reduced their rewarding potency, reduced motivation to obtain the drug, and reduced "drug-seeking" in the absence of drug availability. Finally, in a Phase III clinical trial, the ultra-low-dose naltrexone component of Oxytrex™ significantly reduced physical signs of opioid dependence after abrupt cessation of treatment, compared to withdrawal from oxycodone alone. Together, the data reviewed in this chapter suggest a reduced potential for opioid dependence and addiction by certain ultra-low-dose opioid antagonists combined with opioids, concurrent with the enhanced analgesia from these opioid agonist/antagonist cotreatments.

Keywords: Place aversion; Place preference; Self-administration; Reinstatement; Withdrawal

---

L.H. Burns (✉), F. Leri, and M.C. Olmstead
Pain Therapeutics, Inc., Preclinical Development, 2211 Bridgepointe Parkway, Suite 500, San Mateo, CA 94404
e-mail: lburns@paintrials.com

13.1 Introduction

Opioid agonists, such as oxycodone or morphine, are commonly used in the clinic to treat moderate to severe pain. Unfortunately, chronic exposure to these drugs typically leads to the development of physical dependence, identified by the presence of somatic or physical withdrawal symptoms that occur upon abrupt cessation of opioid intake. These somatic symptoms include pain, nausea, stomach cramps, muscle spasms, chills, racing heartbeat, muscle tension, aches, yawning, runny eyes, and insomnia.

In “opioid addicts” (9), the somatic symptoms of withdrawal are accompanied by a dysphoric state characterized by depressive-like and anxiety-like symptomatology. The presence of affective withdrawal symptoms often distinguishes the dependent state as “psychological” versus simply “physical” dependence. Avoidance of this negative affective state is believed to contribute to addiction (17,18), defined by NIDA (National Institute on Drug Abuse) as “continued drug use despite potentially harmful consequences.” While pain patients on opioid analgesic therapy commonly develop physical dependence, as evidenced by the need to carefully taper off opioids to avoid withdrawal signs (11), they may also experience drug reward and affective withdrawal to varying degrees. Whether these patients on chronic opioid therapy are at any greater risk for opioid addiction is both unclear and controversial (15, 2). Nevertheless, the wide-scale nonmedical use and abuse of prescription opioids (9) is evidence that these agents are frequently administered for their acute rewarding properties (43).

In this chapter, we discuss the use of ultra-low-dose opioid antagonists, such as naltrexone, to prevent dependence and to reduce the addictive properties of opioids. In addition to data from animal models, we discuss results of a large, well-controlled clinical trial. We focus on three psychopharmacological states that can contribute to opioid addiction: acute drug reward, persistent drug seeking, and adverse somatic and affective symptoms that emerge during acute opioid withdrawal. We will review evidence that ultra-low-dose naltrexone, when co-administered with opioids, suppresses each of these aspects of dependence and addiction. Clearly, higher doses of opioid antagonists will block withdrawal and opioid reward by competitively blocking agonist activation of opioid receptors. The suppressive effects discussed here, however, occur at doses far too low for typical receptor antagonism. These ultra-low dose ranges are the same that were shown paradoxically to *enhance* analgesia and prevent analgesic tolerance, as discussed in the Chapter 1.

13.2 Ultra-Low-Dose Naltrexone or Naloxone Reduces Somatic Withdrawal in Rodents

As mentioned briefly in the Chapter 1, an initial study assessing in vivo effects of ultra-low-dose opioid antagonists demonstrated that naltrexone (10 μg/kg) cotreatment reduces somatic withdrawal symptoms following morphine administration (a single 100 mg/kg dose or 4 days of twice daily, progressively increasing doses of 20–50 mg/kg) in mice (10). Withdrawal was assessed by jumping behavior precipitated by a high dose of naloxone (10 mg/kg). Subsequently, Crain and Shen assessed physical dependence by measuring hyperalgesia precipitated by a lower dose of naloxone (10 μg/kg) that does not induce overt somatic signs. Cotreatment with ultra-low-dose naltrexone (in doses ranging from 1 pg/kg to 3 μg/kg) prevented this withdrawal-associated hyperalgesia after chronic twice-daily treatment with morphine (33) or oxycodone (32). Ultra-low-dose naloxone cotreatment also reduces physical signs of withdrawal in rats, demonstrating that this phenomenon is not limited to naltrexone (38).

In addition to physical withdrawal signs, recent studies have shown a reduction in neurochemical correlates of physical withdrawal. In the first study, intrathecal ultra-low-dose naltrexone coadministered with chronic systemic morphine reduced physical dependence, measured by ptosis, salivation, and jumping behaviors, as well as two spinal indicators of withdrawal (26). Naltrexone cotreatment attenuated a withdrawal-associated increase in spinal *c*-fos expression, an index of neural excitation that correlates with the intensity of opiate withdrawal in various brain regions (5). Ultra-low-dose naltrexone also attenuated a withdrawal-associated decrease of calcitonin gene-related peptide (CGRP) reactivity in the spinal dorsal horn, reflecting dorsal horn release of this sensory neuropeptide previously implicated in opioid physical dependence (36). The intrathecal delivery of naltrexone and its effects on spinal *c*-fos and CGRP in this study suggest a spinal locus as one site of action for naltrexone's reduction of the somatic component of withdrawal.

A subsequent study showed that the suppression of behavioral signs of opioid physical dependence by ultra-low-dose naltrexone was paralleled by a modulation of neurochemical markers of opioid withdrawal in specific brain regions (21). In this study, morphine and ultra-low-dose naltrexone were delivered orally to rats via drinking water. The neurochemical markers *c*-fos, protein kinase A regulatory subunit II (PKA-II), and phosphorylated cyclic adenosine monophosphate response element-binding protein (pCREB) were measured in two brain regions implicated in somatic withdrawal, the locus coeruleus and the nucleus of the solitary tract (28). Ultra-low-dose naltrexone cotreatment attenuated withdrawal-associated increases in these three proteins in these brain regions critical to somatic withdrawal, and also reduced a range of specific withdrawal behaviors. This study also demonstrated the effectiveness of oral delivery of naltrexone at an estimated average dose of 117 μg/day. This dose is much higher than those administered subcutaneously or intraperitoneally in other rodent studies, but comparable (in μg/kg bodyweight) to the estimated 7 μg/day naltrexone delivered to mice via drinking water in an earlier study that showed both enhanced morphine antinociception and reduced physical dependence (31). The effectiveness of this oral dose range in reducing physical dependence underscores the low oral bioavailability of naltrexone (16).

13.3 Ultra-Low-Dose Naltrexone Reduces Affective Withdrawal in Rodents

The studies outlined above examined the effect of ultra-low-dose naltrexone on somatic signs of opioid withdrawal including jumping, teeth chattering, shaking, diarrhea, and salivation. Drug withdrawal is also accompanied by a negative affective state that may occur in the absence of overt physical symptoms. This affective component of withdrawal is revealed in animals using the conditioned place aversion (CPA) paradigm: opioid-dependent rats will avoid a compartment where they previously experienced drug withdrawal. The CPA paradigm provides a reliable and sensitive measure of opiate withdrawal, both naloxone precipitated (1) and spontaneous (4).

In a recent study (24), we investigated whether ultra-low-dose naltrexone coadministration alters motivational withdrawal. Separate groups of rats were treated with morphine (5 mg/kg), morphine plus naltrexone (5 ng/kg), oxycodone (3 mg/kg), or oxycodone plus naltrexone (30 pg/kg) twice daily for 6 days with one injection on day 7. Twenty-four hours after the last drug injections, rats received saline or naloxone (1 mg/kg) and were confined to one compartment of the CPA apparatus; 48 h later, they received the other injection and were confined to the opposite compartment. We chose to use females because our preliminary studies, as well as previous reports (7, 23), suggested that females are more sensitive to conditioned drug effects than males. The use of females allowed a single conditioning session for each injection (naloxone and saline), thereby avoiding the possible confound that withdrawal symptoms would dissipate over time. Animals displayed a robust CPA to naloxone-precipitated withdrawal from either morphine or oxycodone, and coadministration with ultra-low-dose naltrexone blocked the aversive effects (Fig. 13.1). The lack of a CPA suggests that these female rats chronically treated with an opioid combined with ultra-low-dose naltrexone did not experience a negative affective state during withdrawal.

This finding suggests that ultra-low-dose naltrexone not only blocks physical withdrawal signs, as demonstrated previously, but also modulates multiple, independent aspects of opioid dependence. Both pharmacological and neurochemical evidence suggest that somatic and affective symptoms of withdrawal are dissociable. Rats treated chronically with morphine exhibit affective withdrawal (as measured in the CPA paradigm) following low doses of naloxone (7.5 ug/kg) that may last up to 4 months (35). In contrast, somatic withdrawal symptoms are not observed until much higher doses of naloxone are administered (30–120 ug/kg) (13), and the effects typically dissipate within 3–4 weeks. Furthermore, infusions of opioid antagonists in various regions of the rat brain more potently precipitate somatic withdrawal (dorsomedial thalamus), affective withdrawal (nucleus accumbens), or both (locus coeruleus), indicating different neural substrates for affective versus somatic withdrawal [(13, 19)]. The most likely scenario is that affective withdrawal, associated with activation in limited neural sites, occurs in the early stages of opioid treatment and that continued treatment leads to somatic withdrawal as additional neural sites are recruited. In sum, withdrawal from chronic opioid treatment is characterized by overt physical signs as well as by a negative affective state. Preclinical data

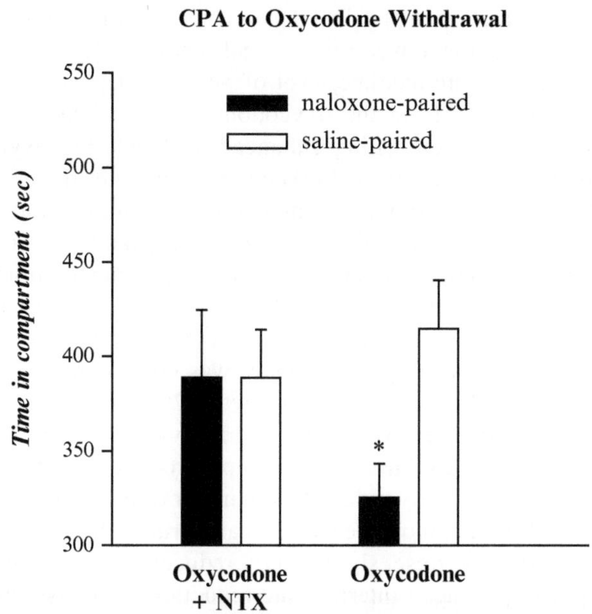

Fig. 13.1 Effect of naltrexone (*NTX*) cotreatment (30 pg/kg, s.c.) on a conditioned place aversion (*CPA*) to naloxone-precipitated withdrawal from chronic oxycodone treatment (3 mg/kg, s.c. twice daily for 7 days). Bars represent the mean (±SEM) amount of time (s) spent in saline- and naloxone-paired compartments on test day. Rats treated with oxycodone alone showed a significant CPA to the naloxone-paired compartment, and cotreatment with NTX blocked this effect. Reprinted from Olmstead and Burns (24) with permission from Springer-Verlag

suggest that both effects are minimized by coadministration with ultra-low-dose naltrexone.

13.4 Reduced Physical Dependence in Clinical Trial of Oxytrex Versus Oxycodone

The effects of ultra-low-dose opioid antagonist cotreatment on physical dependence had not been assessed clinically prior to a recent Phase III clinical trial that compared Oxytrex (oxycodone plus ultra-low-dose naltrexone) to oxycodone in low-back pain patients (39). Compared to oxycodone alone, Oxytrex produced equivalent analgesia at a reduced dose and significantly reduced signs of physical dependence: 55% reduction on the first day after cessation of a 3-month treatment, as assessed by the Short Opioid Withdrawal Scale (SOWS). In this trial, patients were randomized to receive placebo, oxycodone q.i.d., or Oxytrex administered either q.i.d. or b.i.d. Each dose of Oxytrex was formulated to contain 1 μg of naltrexone, so that the q.i.d. treatment group received 4 μg/day and the b.i.d. treatment group received 2 μg/day of naltrexone. All patients titrated their dose to adequate pain relief (a pain intensity score ≤2 on a 0–10 scale) or to a level of tolerable side effects, up to a maximum of 80 mg oxycodone/day.

The significant reduction in physical dependence occurred in the Oxytrex b.i.d. group, which received the lower dose of naltrexone (2 μg/day). The Oxytrex q.i.d. group showed an intermediate level of physical dependence, but this was not significantly different from the oxycodone-alone control group. As in the previous clinical trial demonstrating enhanced analgesia by Oxytrex b.i.d. (8), these results suggest that 2 μg/day naltrexone best replicates the beneficial effects of ultra-low-dose opioid antagonists demonstrated in animal studies. The effectiveness of a b.i.d. treatment also illustrates a prolonged duration of analgesia by Oxytrex without any controlled release mechanism; immediate-release oxycodone is only approved for q.i.d. dosing. This Phase III clinical trial of Oxytrex also suggested enhanced analgesia by Oxytrex b.i.d. compared to oxycodone, since the percent reduction in pain intensity was equivalent but the total average daily dose for the Oxytrex b.i.d. group was 12% lower than for oxycodone q.i.d. The Oxytrex q.i.d. total average daily dose was also significantly reduced by 12%, and all three active treatment groups produced equivalent analgesia. Oxytrex b.i.d. also significantly reduced the number of moderate-to-severe events of constipation by 44%, somnolence by 33%, and pruritis by 51%. Oxytrex q.i.d., with the higher naltrexone dose, significantly reduced moderate-to-severe events of pruritis only, and produced intermediate reductions in constipation and somnolence that were not significant.

An additional finding from this Phase III clinical trial of Oxytrex was that the reduction in physical dependence was more dramatic for patients over 50 years of age. In a subgroup analysis, patients over 50 that received Oxytrex b.i.d. had SOWS scores, the first day after discontinuation, 80.1% lower than aged-matched patients receiving oxycodone q.i.d. Significant reductions in SOWS scores by Oxytrex b.i.d. compared to oxycodone q.i.d. were also seen on days 2 and 4 after discontinuation, with a trend ($p = 0.08$) toward a significant reduction on day 3. This finding echoes an age effect observed in one preclinical study using a fairly high dose range of ultra-low-dose naltrexone (0.002–2 μg/kg delivered systemically) that showed enhanced analgesia by these naltrexone doses in mature female rats, but not in mature male or younger rats (14), even though no sex differences were observed in this clinical trial. Nevertheless, the greater effectiveness of the lower dose of naltrexone observed here and in an earlier clinical trial (8) may suggest that, despite the low oral bioavailability of naltrexone (14), the current 2 μg/day may be on the higher end of an effective dose range.

13.5 Ultra-Low-Dose Naltrexone Reduces the Rewarding Properties of Opioids

In addition to their powerful analgesic properties, opioids induce rewarding effects, which are normally the basis for their nonmedical use or abuse. These rewarding properties may also contribute to continued drug use in opioid-dependent patients. The rewarding effects of drugs are commonly measured in animals using the conditioned place preference (CPP) paradigm: opioids, other abused drugs, as well as natural rewards (e.g., food, sex) induce a CPP in rodents and many other species [for review see (37)]. The development of a CPP to morphine is mediated through opioid receptors in the brain (25) suggesting that the effect may, like analgesia, be modified by ultra-low-dose naltrexone coadministration.

This hypothesis was investigated initially in a study that compared morphine-induced antinociception and reward (27). Using a low, subanalgesic dose of morphine (1.0 mg/kg) to induce a CPP, this study specifically examined whether the duration of reward might be extended by ultra-low-dose naltrexone. To establish a time course for morphine alone, rats were injected with morphine (1 mg/kg) and confined to one CPP compartment at varying delays after the injection. A CPP developed when conditioning sessions started at 0, 30, 60, and 90 min, but not 120 min after the injection. Separate groups of rats were then treated with morphine (1 mg/kg) plus ultra-low-dose naltrexone (10–200 ng/kg) and conditioned 120 min later. Cotreatment with ultra-low-dose naltrexone at 16.7, 20, or 25 ng/kg, but not at 10 or 200 ng/kg, induced a significant CPP after this 2-h delay. This finding implies that, whereas the rewarding effects of morphine have dissipated by 120 min postinjection, ultra-low-dose naltrexone may extend this effect. A prolongation of rewarding effects would resonate with the prolonged antinociception (10) and would also confirm the suggestion that the rewarding and analgesic properties of abused drugs are mediated through common neural substrates (12). Nevertheless, the conclusion that ultra-low-dose naltrexone prolonged the duration of morphine's rewarding effect must be made with caution because this study failed to demonstrate significant differences between the CPP of the morphine-naltrexone groups and that of the morphine-alone group. One must also consider that the four conditioning sessions used in this study may have introduced confounds of tolerance or sensitization, that is, a decrease or increase in reward with repeated drug administration.

A more recent study examined the modulation of opioid-induced reward more directly by testing the effect of ultra-low-dose naltrexone on the CPP to analgesic doses of morphine or oxycodone and with no delay between injection and place conditioning (24). To minimize possible confounds of tolerance and sensitization that may occur with repeated opioid injections, we used single conditioning sessions and female rats because, as noted previously, females were more sensitive to conditioned drug effects. Both morphine (5 mg/kg) and oxycodone (3 mg/kg) produced a robust and significant CPP that was blocked by ultra-low-dose naltrexone coadministration. The dose of naltrexone (5 ng/kg) that eliminated a morphine-induced CPP was two orders of magnitude higher than the doses that blocked the significant CPP to oxycodone (0.03 and 0.3 ng/kg, but not 3 ng/kg; Fig. 13.2). This comparison suggests that oxycodone is more sensitive than morphine to the blockade of opioid reward by ultra-low-dose naltrexone. This finding is in agreement with the demonstration that lower doses of naltrexone are required to reduce oxycodone tolerance and withdrawal than those shown to reduce morphine tolerance and withdrawal (32, 33). Importantly, the doses of naltrexone that blocked a CPP to morphine and oxycodone were the same doses that blocked a CPA to withdrawal from chronic administration of each (24) (see detailed discussion above).

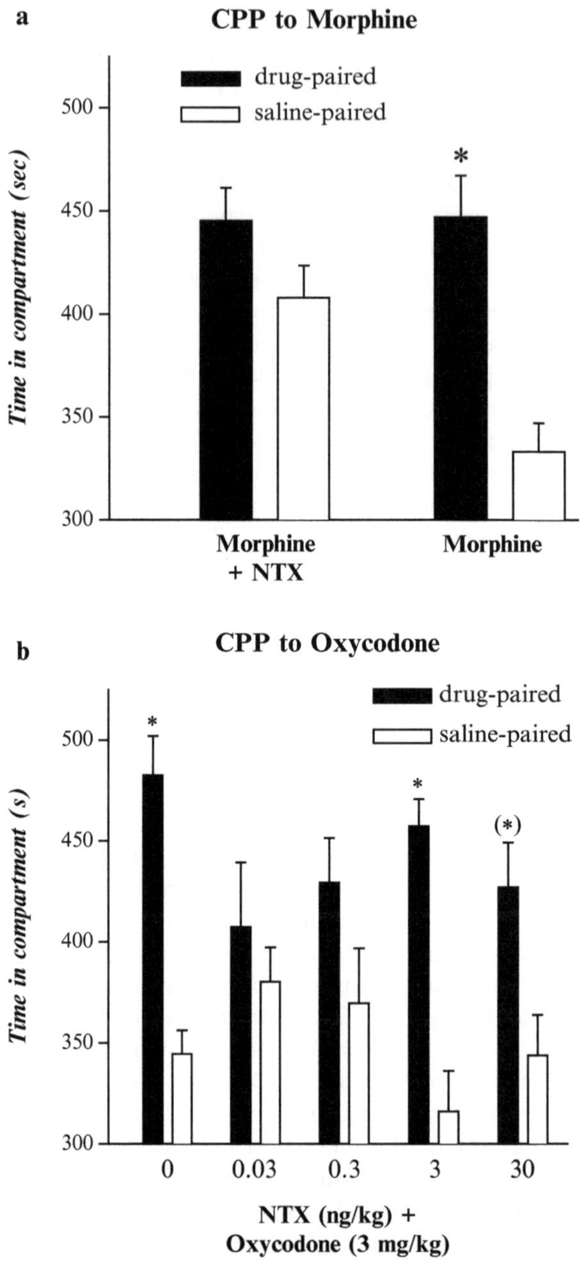

Fig. 13.2 (**a**) Effect of naltrexone (*NTX*) cotreatment (5 ng/kg, s.c.) on a conditioned place preference (*CPP*) to morphine (5 mg/kg, s.c.). Bars represent the mean (±SEM) amount of time (s) spent in saline- and drug-paired compartments on test day. Morphine alone elicited a strong CPP that was blocked by the addition of NTX. (**b**) Dose–response of NTX on a CPP to oxycodone. Bars represent the mean (±SEM) amount of time (s) spent in saline- and drug-paired compartments on test day. Oxycodone (3 mg/kg, s.c.) produced a significant CPP that was blocked by the addition of NTX at 0.03 ng/kg, s.c., or 0.3 ng/kg. In contrast, NTX at 3 ng/kg, s.c. did not block the CPP to oxycodone. Oxycodone combined with the highest dose of NTX, 30 ng/kg, s.c., produced only a trend toward a CPP. Reprinted from Olmstead and Burns (24), with permission from Springer-Verlag

The most recent study (6) examining ultra-low-dose naltrexone effects on the rewarding properties of opiates appears to conflict with the early study (27), but these two studies used very different methodologies and attempted to measure quite different aspects of reward. The first study (27) may have demonstrated a prolongation of the duration of the rewarding effect of a subanalgesic (1 mg/kg) dose of morphine or a prevention of tolerance to this subtle rewarding effect. Both interpretations must take into account the lack of significant difference in the size of the CPP between the morphine alone and morphine plus naltrexone groups. The second study (24) clearly demonstrated a blockade of the CPP to acute administrations of analgesic doses of morphine or oxycodone. It is difficult to imagine that a CPP would emerge in the groups receiving the opiate plus ultra-low-dose naltrexone if the conditioning sessions were delayed by 2 h. In any case, the data described here show that ultra-low-dose naltrexone coadministration blocks the rewarding effects of acute analgesic doses of opioids.

13.6 Ultra-Low-Dose Naltrexone Reduces the Rewarding Potency of Intravenous Oxycodone and Blocks Relapse to Oxycodone Seeking in Rats

The results of three additional studies performed in male rats further support the conclusion that ultra-low-dose naltrexone can effectively reduce the abuse potential of oxycodone (20).

The first study demonstrated that ultra-low-dose naltrexone decreases the rewarding potency of intravenous infusions of oxycodone. This study investigated the effect of ultra-low-dose naltrexone on intravenous self-administration of oxycodone which, like other mu-opioid receptor agonists, promotes and maintains operant behavior in rats (3) and primates (40). The experiments employed fixed-ratio schedules of reinforcement because of their sensitivity to shifts in drug doses: animals increase drug intake when doses are lowered and decrease intake when doses are increased (41, 42). In the first experiment, three different groups of animals self-administered oxycodone alone (0.1 mg/kg/infusion), or oxycodone combined with naltrexone at 100 pg/kg/infusion or 10 pg/kg/infusion. In the second experiment, two groups of animals self-administered oxycodone alone (0.1 mg/kg/infusion) or oxycodone combined with 1 pg/kg/infusion naltrexone. The addition of 10 or 100 pg/kg/ infusion naltrexone did not significantly alter oxycodone self-administration. In contrast, the addition of 1 pg/kg/infusion naltrexone resulted in an increase in drug intake (Fig. 13.3), reflecting a decrease in the rewarding potency of each drug infusion. Interestingly, 1 pg/kg/infusion naltrexone combined with 0.1 mg/kg/infusion of oxycodone corresponds to the naltrexone:oxycodone ratio most effective in enhancing oxycodone analgesia in mice (32) and with the ratio used to block both the CPP to acute oxycodone and the CPA to oxycodone withdrawal (24) (see detailed discussion above).

The second study further indicated that 1 pg/kg/infusion naltrexone attenuates the motivation to obtain infusions of oxycodone (0.1 mg/kg/infusions). In this experiment, two groups of rats self-administered oxycodone alone or combined

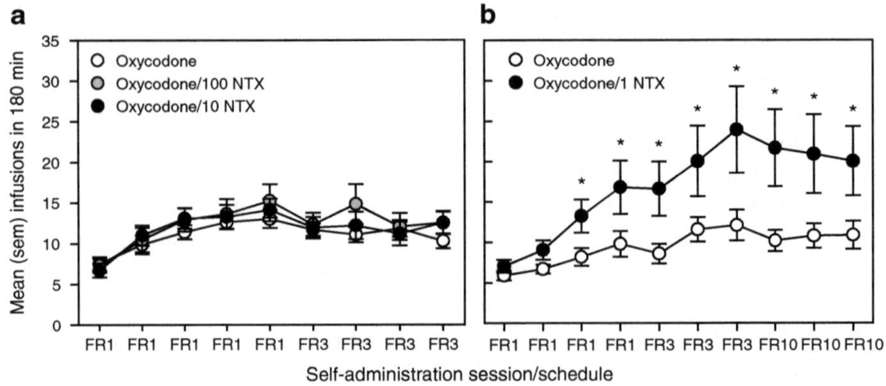

Fig. 13.3 (**a**) There were no group differences in number of infusions during nine sessions of intravenous self-administration on fixed-ratio schedules in rats trained with oxycodone alone (0.1 mg/kg/infusion, $n = 13$) or combined with naltrexone (*NTX*; 100 or 10 ng/kg/infusion; $n = 13$ and $n = 15$, respectively). (**b**) Rats self-administering oxycodone (0.1 mg/kg/infusion) combined with NTX (1 pg/kg/infusion; $n = 14$) took a significantly greater number of drug infusions during ten sessions of self-administration compared to rats self-administering oxycodone alone (0.1 mg/kg/infusion; $n = 10$). *$p < 0.05$ for group comparisons. Reprinted from Leri and Burns (20), with permission from Elsevier

with naltrexone on a progressive ratio (PR) schedule (29, 34). In this schedule, the subjects must meet increasing response requirements for each successive drug infusion. Response requirements continue to increase until subjects reach their "break-point": the ratio at which responding becomes erratic or ceases completely. Although there was no significant group difference in actual break-point responding, rats self-administering the naltrexone–oxycodone combination appeared less motivated than rats administering oxycodone alone to obtain drug infusions. In fact, they displayed a decrease in responding in each PR session (Fig. 13.4), and a larger percentage of rats within this group reached a break-point on the final sessions of testing when the response requirements were most demanding.

In the final study, rats that had self-administered the naltrexone–oxycodone combination showed reduced reinstatement of drug-seeking compared to rats that previously self-administered oxycodone. Relapse vulnerability is an important component of drug addiction (22), and the reinstatement procedure in animals is considered a valid animal model of human relapse (30). In this experiment, rats that self-administered oxycodone alone (0.1 mg/kg/infusion), or oxycodone combined with naltrexone at 100 pg/kg/infusion, 10 pg/kg/infusion, or 1 pg/kg/infusion received extinction sessions in which responding was not reinforced by drug infusions. Following extinction, animals received three different tests of reinstatement of precipitated oxycodone-seeking by reexposure to oxycodone (SC injections: 0.25 mg/kg), reexposure to a conditioned stimulus present during previous drug self-administration, and exposure to stress (15-

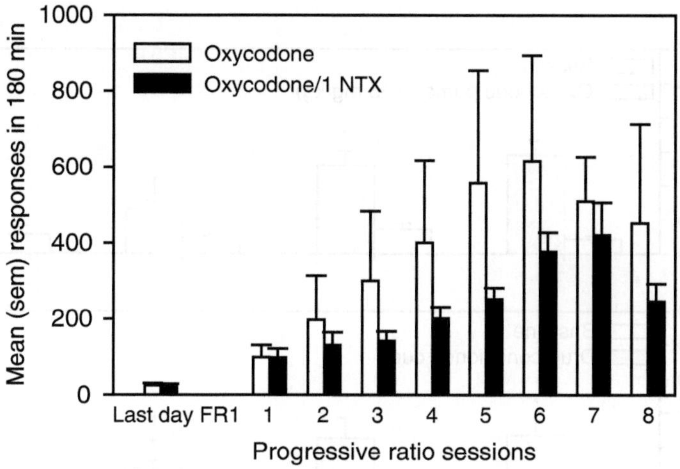

Fig. 13.4 The number of responses on the active lever emitted during the last FR1 session and the eight subsequent sessions of intravenous self-administration on a progressive ratio (*PR*) schedule were lower in rats responding for oxycodone plus naltrexone (*NTX*) (1 pg/kg/infusion; $n = 12$) versus responding for oxycodone alone (0.1 mg/kg/infusion; $n = 14$). Reprinted from Leri and Burns (20), with permission from Elsevier

min period of intermittent foot-shock: 0.5 mA). Rats that had self-administered oxycodone in combination with either 1 pg/kg/infusion or 10 pg/kg/infusion showed no significant reinstatement of responding by priming injections of oxycodone, and all three naltrexone doses prevented stress-induced reinstatement of responding (Fig. 13.5). Responding was significantly reinstated by the stimulus previously paired with oxycodone infusions in all groups, although the level of responding was significantly reduced in rats that had self-administered oxycodone plus naltrexone at the lowest two doses compared to rats that had self-administered oxycodone alone (Fig. 13.5). These results imply that ultra-low-dose naltrexone coadministration may reduce subsequent drug craving compared to that following intake of the opioid alone.

13.7 Conclusions

The findings reviewed here indicate that the addition of ultra-low-dose naltrexone to oxycodone, or to other opioid agonists, diminishes the potential for opioid dependence and addiction. We have reviewed data in rodents showing decreases in both somatic and affective withdrawal, indicating reduced physical and "psychological" dependence. Notably, physical dependence in humans was profoundly decreased in a Phase III clinical trial of chronic pain patients. Preclinical data also demonstrated

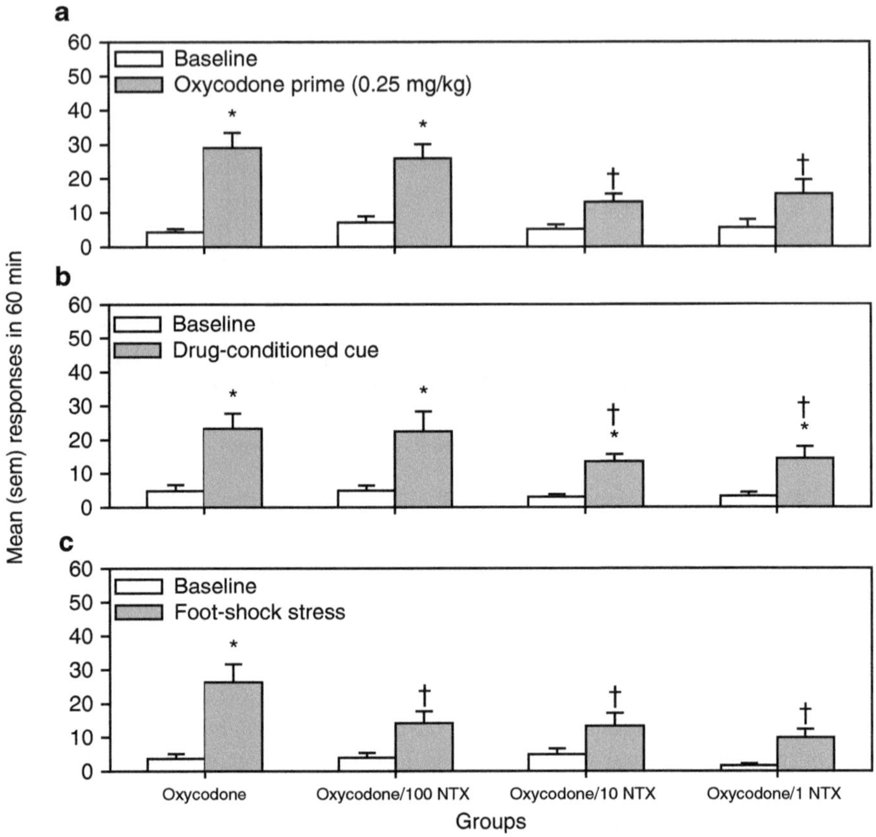

Fig. 13.5 Reinstatement of responding over baseline (extinction) levels precipitated by an oxycodone (0.25 mg/kg, s.c.) priming injection (**a**), the drug-conditioned cue (**b**), or foot-shock stress (**c**), was significantly reduced in rats previously self-administering oxycodone combined with naltrexone (*NTX*) at 10 pg/kg/infusion ($n = 15$) or 1 pg/kg/infusion ($n = 14$) compared to rats that had self-administered oxycodone alone ($n = 23$). Co-self-administration of oxycodone plus NTX at 100 pg/kg/infusion ($n = 13$) also reduced stress-induced reinstatement. *$p < 0.05$ compared to baseline responding within the same group; **$p < 0.05$ compared to oxycodone alone. Reprinted from Leri and Burns (20), with permission from Elsevier

ultra-low-dose naltrexone to decrease acute opioid reward, evidenced by blockade of a CPP to morphine or oxycodone and by alterations in oxycodone self-administration in rats. Further, a decrease in the percentage of rats reaching a "break-point" in final sessions of a PR schedule suggests a diminished motivation to obtain oxycodone if combined with ultra-low-dose naltrexone. Finally, the decreased "drug-seeking" following self-administration of oxycodone plus ultra-low-dose naltrexone predicts a reduced vulnerability to craving or relapse. Together, these findings suggest that oxycodone, or other opioid agonists, formulated with ultra-low-dose naltrexone will have reduced potential for abuse, dependence, and addiction while fully retaining, or even enhancing, analgesic properties.

References

1. Azar MR, Jones BC, Shulteis G (2003) Conditioned place aversion is a highly sensitive index of acute opioid dependence and withdrawal. Psychopharmacology 170:42–50.
2. Ballantyne J, Mao J (2003) Opioid therapy for chronic pain. N Engl J Med 349:1943–1953.
3. Beardsley PM, Aceto MD, Cook CD, Bowman ER, Newman JL, Harris LS (2004) Discriminative stimulus, reinforcing, physical dependence, and antinociceptive effects of oxycodone in mice, rats, and rhesus monkeys. Exp Clin Psychopharmacol 12:163–172.
4. Bechara A, Nader K, van der Kooy D (1995) Neurobiology of withdrawal motivation: evidence for two separate aversive effects produced in morphine-naive versus morphine-dependent rats by both naloxone and spontaneous withdrawal. Behav Neurosci 109:91–105.
5. Beckman A, Matsumoto I, Wilce P (1995) Immediate early gene expression during morphine withdrawal. Neuropharmacology 34:1183–1189.
6. Burns LH, Olmstead MC (2005) Ultra-low-dose naltrexone suppresses rewarding effects of opiates and aversive effects of opiate withdrawal in rats. Psychopharmacology 181:576–581.
7. Chen H, Yang Y, Yeh T, Cherng C, Hsu H, Hsiao S, Yu L (2003) Methamphetamine-induced conditioned place preference is facilitated by estradiol pretreatment in female mice. Chin J Physiol (China) 46:169–174.
8. Chindalore VL, Butera PG, Yu KP, Burns LH, Friedmann N (2005) Adding ultralow-dose naltrexone to oxycodone enhances and prolongs analgesia: A randomized, controlled trial of Oxytrex. J Pain 6:392–399.
9. Compton WM, Volkow ND (2006) Major increases in opioid analgesic abuse in the United States: concerns and strategies. Drug Alcohol Depend 81:103–107.
10. Crain SM, Shen K-F (1995) Ultra-low concentrations of naloxone selectively antagonize excitatory effects of morphine on sensory neurons, thereby increasing its antinociceptive potency and attenuating tolerance/dependence during chronic co-treatment. Proc Natl Acad Sci USA 92:10540–10544.
11. Fne P (2004) Opioid insights: opioid-induced hyperalgesia and opioid rotation. J Pain Palliat Care Pharmacother 18:75–79.
12. Franklin KB (1998) Analgesia and abuse potential: an accidental association or a common substrate? Pharmacol Biochem Behav 59:993–1002.
13. Frenois F, Cador M, Caille S, Stinus L, Le Moine C (2002) Neural correlates of the motivational and somatic components of naloxone-precipitated morphine withdrawal. Eur J Neurosci 16:1377–1389.
14. Hamman S, Wala E, Rebel A, Lock R (2004) Selective antagonism of excitatory opioid receptors: A pilot clinical study demonstrating enhancement of morphine analgesia by low-dose naltrxone in female patients undergoing elective laparotomy. American Society of Anesthesiologists Annual Meeting, Las Vegas, NV
15. Joranson D, Ryan K, Gilson A, Dahl J (2000) Trends in medical use and abuse of opioid analgesics. J Am Med Assoc 283:1710–1714.
16. Kogan MJ, Verebey K, Mule SJ (1977) Estimation of the systemic availability and other pharmacokinetic parameters of naltrexone in man after acute and chronic oral administration. Res Commun Chem Pathol Pharmacol 18:29–34.
17. Koob GF, Le Moal M (1997) Drug abuse: hedonic homeostatic dysregulation. Science 278:52–58.

18. Koob GF, Stinus L, Le Moal M, Bloom FE (1989) Opponent process theory of motivation: neurobiological evidence from studies of opiate dependence. Neurosci Biobehav Rev 13:135–140.
19. Koob GF, Maldonado R, Stinus L (1992) Neural substrates of opiate withdrawal. Trends Neurosci 15:186–191.
20. Leri F, Burns LH (2005) Ultra-low-dose naltrexone reduces the rewarding potency of oxycodone and relapse vulnerability in rats. Pharmacol Biochem Behav 82:252–262.
21. Mannelli P, Gottheil E, Peoples JF, Oropeza VC, Van Bockstaele EJ (2004) Chronic very low dose naltrexone attenuates opioid withdrawal expression. Biol Psychiatry 56:261–268.
22. Marlatt GA, Gordon JR (1985) Relapse Prevention: Maintenance Strategies in the Treatment of Addictive Behavior. New York: Guilford Press.
23. Nazarian A, Russo S, Festa E, Kraish M, Quinones-Jenab V (2004) The role of D(1) and D(2) receptors in the cocaine conditioned place preference of male and female rats. Brain Res Bull 63:295–299.
24. Olmstead MC, Burns LH (2005) Ultra-low-dose naltrexone suppresses rewarding effects of opiates and aversive effects of opiate withdrawal in rats. Psychopharmacology 181:576–581.
25. Olmstead MC, Franklin KBJ (1997) Development of a conditioned place preference to morphine: effects of microinjections into various CNS sites. Behav Neurosci 111:1324–2334.
26. Oxbro K, Trang T, Sutak M, Jhamandas K (2003) The effects of spinal ultra-low doses of an opioid receptor antagonist on systemic morphine dependence. Society for Neuroscience Annual Meeting, New Orleans, LA.
27. Powell KJ, Abul-Husn NS, Jhamandas A, Olmstead MC, Beninger RJ, Jhamandas K (2002) Paradoxical effects of the opioid antagonist naltrexone on morphine analgesia, tolerance, and reward in rats. JPET 300:588–596.
28. Rassmusen K, Beitner-Johnson B, Krystal J, Aghajanian G, Nestler E (1990) Opiate withdrawal and the rat locus coeruleus: behavioral, electrophysiological and biochemical correlates. J Neurosci 10:2308–2317.
29. Roberts DC, Bennett SA (1993) Heroin self-administration in rats under a progressive ratio schedule of reinforcement. Psychopharmacology 111:215–218.
30. Shaham Y, Shalev U, Lu L, de Wit H, Stewart J (2003) The reinstatement model of drug relapse: history, methodology and major findings. Psychopharmacology (Berl) 168:3–20.
31. Shen KF, Crain SM (1997) Ultra-low doses of naltrexone or etorphine increase morphine's antinociceptive potency and attenuate tolerance/dependence in mice. Brain Res 757:176–190.
32. Shen K-F, Crain SM, Moate P, Boston R, de Kater AW, Schoenhard GL (2002a) PTI-801, a novel formulation of oxycodone, shows absence of tolerance, physical dependence and naloxone-precipitated withdrawal effects in mice. Pain 3:49.
33. Shen K-F, Crain SM, Moate P, Boston R, de Kater AW, Schoenhard GL (2002b) PTI-555, reverses and prevents morphine-induced tolerance and naloxone-precipitated withdrawal in mice chronically treated with morphine. Pain 3:50.
34. Stafford D, LeSage MG, Glowa JR (1998) Progressive-ratio schedules of drug delivery in the analysis of drug self-administration: a review. Psychopharmacology (Berl) 139:169–184.
35. Stinus L, Caille S, Koob GF (2000) Opiate withdrawal-induced place aversion lasts for up to 16 weeks. Psychopharmacology 149:115–120.
36. Trang T, Sutak M, Quirion R, Jhamandas K (2002) The role of spinal neuropeptides and prostaglandins in opioid physical dependence. Br J Pharmacol 136:37–48.
37. Tzschentke TM (1998) Measuring reward with the conditioned place preference paradigm: a comprehensive review of drug effects, recent progress, and new issues. Prog Neurobiol 56:613–672.
38. Wang H-Y, Friedman E, Olmstead MC, Burns LH (2005) Ultra-low-dose naloxone suppresses opioid tolerance, dependence and associated changes in Mu opioid receptor-G protein coupling and Gβγ signaling. Neuroscience 135:247–261.
39. Webster LR, Butera PG, Moran LV, Wu N, Burns LH, Friedmann N (2006) Oxytrex minimizes physical dependence while providing effective analgesia: a randomized controlled trial in low-back pain. J Pain 7:937–946.

40. Woods JH, Ko MC, Winger G, France CP, Traynor JR (2002) Evaluation of new compounds for opioid activity. In: NIDA Research Monograph (2003), 183 (Problems of Drug Dependence 2002), Dewey WL, Harris, LS (Eds.), pp 170-190. Baltimore, MD: National Institutes of Health.
41. Yokel RA, Wise RA (1975) Increased lever pressing for amphetamine after pimozide in rats: implications for a dopamine theory of reward. Science 187:547–549.
42. Yokel RA, Wise RA (1976) Attenuation of intravenous amphetamine reinforcement by central dopamine blockade in rats. Psychopharmacology (Berl) 48:311–318.
43. Zacny J, Bigelow G, Compton P, Foley K, Iguchi M, Sannerud C (2003) College on Problems of Drug Dependence taskforce on prescription opioid non-medical use and abuse: position statement. Drug Alcohol Depend 69:215–232.

Chapter 14
Can a Combination Formulation Containing a Neutral Opiate Antagonist Decrease the Abuse of μ-Agonist Opiates

John Mendelson, Mark Pletcher, and Gantt Galloway

Abstract Dependence on and abuse of prescription opiate drugs is now a major health problem with initiation of prescription opiate abuse exceeding cocaine in young people. Coincident with the emergence of abuse and dependence on prescription opiates there has been an increased emphasis on the treatment of pain. Pain is now the "5th vital sign" and physicians face disciplinary action for failure to adequately relieve pain. Thus, physicians are whipsawed between the imperative to treat pain with opiates and the consequences of producing addiction in some patients. Novel approaches are needed to allow appropriate prescribing yet diminish the risk of iatrogenic addiction. In this chapter, we propose a method to develop opioid medications that are resistant to drug abuse and show reduced adverse effects. Among the various strategies to reduce addiction liability, the addition of small doses of an opioid antagonist has received recent attention. This is done with the expectation that the antagonist does not affect the analgesic actions if the combination is given for therapeutic purposes, but will accumulate and then block the opioid effects when the drug is abused – either in high oral doses or by intravenous administration. However, opioid antagonist engender strong adverse effects in opioid-dependent and tolerant subjects. Our method emerges from recent advances in our understanding of the molecular pharmacology of opioid receptors, whereby antagonist can be classified into inverse agonists (e.g., naltrexone) that block basal receptor activity, and neutral antagonists (e.g., 6β-naltrexol) that block only the agonist-stimulated effects – thereby causing less withdrawal effects. Preclinical results indicate that 6β-naltrexol (a main metabolite of naltrexone) has all the desired pharmacokinetic and pharmacodynamic attributes as an ideal candidate for such a combination therapeutic, potentially yielding a significant advance in pain therapy with opiates. In this chapter, we review the evidence for the unfolding prescription opiate epidemic and describe the potential of 6β-naltrexol, a neutral opiate antagonist, in limiting maximal μ-agonist effects of oral opiate analgesics.

J. Mendelson (✉), M. Pletcher, and G. Galloway
Addiction Pharmacology Research Laboratory,
California Pacific Medical Center Research Institute,
St Luke's Hospital, San Francisco, CA 94110
e-mail: mendelje@sutterhealth.org

R. Dean et al. (eds.), *Opiate Receptors and Antagonists*,

Keywords: Prescription opiate abuse; Combination formulation; Neutral opiate antagonist; 6β-naltrexol

14.1 Prescription Opiate Abuse in the United States – An Emerging Epidemic

Abuse of prescription opiate analgesics has emerged as a major public health problem in the United States during the last decade (35). Since 1990, the rate at which young adults initiated abuse of prescription opiates (i.e., use not sanctioned by a physician) has nearly tripled, from 10.2/thousand person-years (1990) to 31.6/thousand person-years (2003) (Fig. 14.1) (7). Generation Rx is the popular name given by the Partnership for a Drug Free America for these teenage and young adult prescription opiate abusers. Each year since 1999, more than 2 million US adults started abusing prescription opiates in the United States (12). Young adults are much more likely to start abusing prescription opiates than they are to start abusing illegal opiates such as heroin, and initiation of prescription opiate abuse is even more common than initiation of cocaine abuse – prescription opiates overtook cocaine in 1996 (7). Among all Americans 12 years and older, 13.2% (nearly 32 million) reported past nonmedical use of prescription opiates in 2004. Eleven million report use in the past year, and 4.4 million during the past month. By comparison, 3.1 million reported ever using heroin (1.6%), 400,000 used in the last year and 166,000 used in the last month. Nearly 1 million of the current (past month) nonmedical users of pain relievers (970,000, 22%) reported physiologic dependence (7); over four times more Americans are dependent on prescription

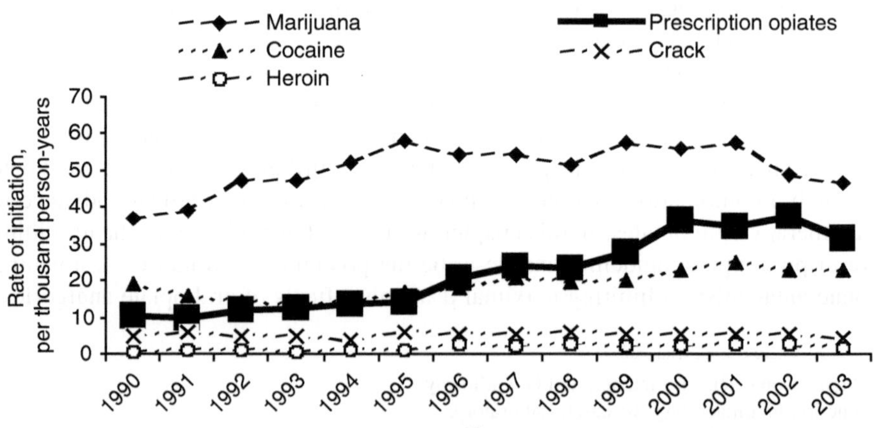

Fig. 14.1 Rates of initiation of illicit drug use per thousand-person years for marijuana, cocaine, heroin, prescription opiates and crack (smoked cocaine)

pain relievers than are dependent on heroin (7). Combined dependence or abuse of opiates is now as common as dependence/abuse of cocaine, and more common than dependence/abuse of any other drug except marijuana (12). Prescription narcotics have more "street value" than marijuana and heroin, and are second only to cocaine, indicating a market has developed in illicit users (25). Because prescription opiates can be legally obtained through a physician, there may be a perception that nonmedical use of these potentially powerful narcotics is less problematic than abuse of illicit substances. However, a parallel rise in the consequences of abuse belies this perception. According to the Drug Abuse Warning Network (DAWN), the estimated number of emergency department (ED) visits involving opiate analgesic abuse in the United States more than doubled from 41,687 to 90,232 between 1994 and 2001 (1). Prescription opiate analgesics were involved in 14% of all drug abuse-related ED visits in 2001. While ED visits involving codeine declined 61%, mentions of all other opiates increased: mentions of hydrocodone (in Vicodin® and other popular schedule 3 analgesics), for example, increased 131%, and mentions of the powerful schedule 2 narcotic oxycodone (in Oxycontin® and others) more than quadrupled (352% increase). Dependence was the most frequently mentioned motive for these ED visits (1).

Persons dependent on prescription opiates are not just presenting emergently to the ED more frequently. According to Treatment Episodes Data Set (TEDS), which collects surveillance data on the numbers of patients admitted for substance abuse treatment, such persons are also seeking substance abuse treatment in record numbers. Between 1992 and 2000, rates of treatment admissions involving opiate analgesics more than doubled from 13 to 27 visits per 100,000 persons aged 12 and over in the United States. In the year 2000, there were 50,000 such visits. While in about half of these visits, opiate analgesics were co-abused with another substance, in the other half an opiate analgesic was the primary substance of abuse (10).

Although the data suggests that nearly 1.3 million Americans aged 12 years and older are highly dependent daily opiate analgesic drug users, it is unknown how many of these patients should be classified as addicted – loosely defined in these data sets as problem use of prescription drugs signifying physiological dependence or heavy daily use. In contrast, there are an estimated 450,000 heroin abusers in the United States (35). Those at greatest risk for developing problematic prescription opiate use include older adults, females, those in poor/fair health, and daily alcohol drinkers (29). Most of these new addicts are prescribed opiates by physicians and purchase their drugs at pharmacies. Although most continue to be "managed" within the health care system, an increasing number are being referred for opiate substitution therapy with buprenorphine and methadone. Brands and coworkers in Toronto found that most of patients presenting for methadone therapy were using prescription opiates in addition to heroin (N = 178, 83%). Surprisingly, in 48% of the patients, prescription opiates were the primary source of opiates (24% used only prescription opiates and an additional 24% started with prescription opiates and migrated to heroin later). In contrast, 35% were primary heroin addicts who also used prescription opiates and only 17% of this sample used heroin exclusively (6). These prescription opiate addicts consumed enormous amounts of short-acting codeine and oxycodone formulations – 23 ± 6 and

21 ± 3 tablets per day of codeine and oxycodone, respectively – equivalent to about 200 mg of morphine per day. About 80% of these patients initiated opiates for the treatment of pain and obtained almost all of their medications from physicians. It is important to note that most were on short-acting opiates that are usually combined with acetaminophen, aspirin, or ibuprofen. Consequently, these patients receive enormous exposures to nephro- and hepatotoxic drugs and metabolites (10–20 g per day of acetaminophen).

The recognition that opiate pain pharmacotherapy can lead to opiate addiction has fueled calls for increased regulation of opiate prescribing. The most common regulatory solution is to increase the DEA schedule (from III, IV, and V to II) of commonly prescribed prescription opiates. Altering the DEA schedule obviously does not alter the pharmacologic effects of opiate analgesics, but can decrease the availability of prescription opiate by increasing the barriers to prescribing. Although decreasing the legitimate supply of prescription opiates might diminish the numbers of new pain patients needing opiate substitution therapy, many patients with chronic pain would be deprived of an essential medicine.

14.1.1 US Trends in Ambulatory Care Opioid Prescribing from 1993 to 2003

Opioid prescribing contributes to the supply of abusable opioids, but little is known about how opioid prescribing patterns have changed during this time. We have studied the contribution of physician prescribing to the rise in prescription opiate dependence. Using 10 years of survey data (from 1993 to 2003) from the National Ambulatory Medical Care Survey (a nationally representative stratified cluster sample of ~30,000 physician office visits per year), we estimated how many US office visits included prescription of an opioid medication (an "opioid visit") to persons aged 12 and over. We calculated rates using US Census denominators and categorized opioid visits by type of opioid in order to explain overall trends. Among the 272,983 evaluated visits we identified 11,327 opioid visits, representing ~32 million office opioid visits per year in the United States, an average rate of 0.142 opioid visits per person per year (95% CI:0.134–0.149). Two pronounced time trends were evident: a significant increase in the visit rate over the decade from 0.126 in 1993 to 0.166 in 2003, a 32% increase ($p < 0.001$ for trend) and a large shift in the types of opioids prescribed. Whereas codeine and propoxyphene visit rates declined (40% and 28% respectively, paralleling a decline in DAWN mentions), visit rates for higher potency opioids such as hydrocodone and oxycodone increased (115% and 156%). Most of the increased opioid visit trend was explained by hydrocodone visits, which increased at a rate of ~1 million additional visits per year from 1993 to 2003 up to a total of 18 million hydrocodone visits in 2003 (95% CI: 14–22 million, 45% of all 2003 opioid visits). These data show that opioid prescribing patterns in ambulatory care have changed markedly in the last decade. Even if all opioid prescribing were appropriate, co-occurring increases in opioid abuse and prescribing suggest the possibility that office visit prescribing is one channel for the supply of abused opioids in the United States. Accordingly, methods that decrease the level of potentially harmful prescribing may have a large impact on prescription opiate dependence.

14.1.2 Opioid Basal Signaling, Inverse Agonists, and Neutral Antagonists

Basal signaling or constitutive activity of G-protein coupled receptor (GPCR) systems has been experimentally measured in numerous receptor systems and the clinical relevance of these phenomena is beginning to be appreciated (30, 23, 17, 5). A series of studies has revealed that basal receptor signaling appears to play a significant role in narcotic addiction. A hallmark of the opioid dependent state is the increasing potency of naloxone to elicit withdrawal with increasing degree of dependence, even in the presence of high agonist concentrations (31, 2, 26). This is paradoxical if one assumes receptor desensitization contributes to opioid tolerance – antagonists should be less potent under these conditions, and would have to compete with agonists at the receptor. Rather, the μ-opiate receptor (MOR) acquires exquisite sensitivity to naloxone, lasting over prolonged time periods. In other chapters, Drs. Sadée and Bilsky explore this paradox in detail. Their work has been echoed by others studying GPCRs in opioid, dopamine, serotonin, and adrenergic systems (5) and support a role for constitutive MOR signaling in addiction (34, 4, 32, 33). Based on these studies in biologically diverse systems a new taxonomy has emerged where ligands are now conceptualized as agonists, inverse agonists or neutral antagonists. In GPCR systems with constitutive activity, agonists increase and inverse agonists decrease the numbers of spontaneously active receptors. Neutral antagonists have little effect on constitutive activity.

Chronic opioid agonist exposure has been demonstrated to increase constitutive activity of opioid receptors in vitro and may account for many of the in vivo observations related to opioid tolerance and dependence, including leftward shifts in opioid antagonist dose–response curves and protean agonism (e.g., naltrexone converting from an antagonist to an inverse agonist) (27). In vivo rodent and canine models of opioid exposure provide additional evidence for the role of constitutive activity and have started to elucidate the molecular and cellular mechanisms that contribute to increases in basal signaling and opioid dependence (13, 15, 26, 28). These findings may extend into humans and have clinical relevance for treating opioid overdose, opioid addiction, and other complications of acute and chronic opioid use. There is, for example, good agreement between animal and human studies with regards to predicting the onset and severity of opioid dependence and the shift in potency of naloxone to precipitate withdrawal as a function of opioid exposure (3, 8). In particular, the acute physical dependence time-courses observed in animals and clinical studies matches well with the observed time-courses for changes in basal signaling measured in animals (16, 4, 26).

Fig. 14.2 Structure of 6-β naltrexone

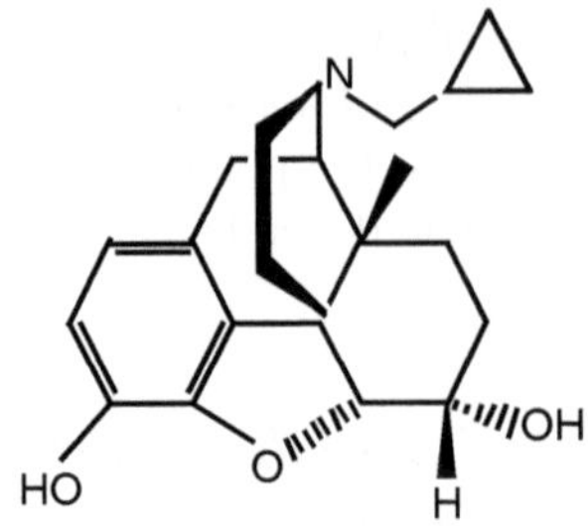

6β-naltrexol is the primary metabolite of naltrexone following oral administration of the parent compound (9, 11) (Fig. 14.2). There is considerable data suggesting that 6β-naltrexol exerts biological and therapeutic effects in humans. On average, 6β-naltrexol plasma levels are approximately ten times higher than naltrexone levels and the half-life of 6β-naltrexol is considerably longer (~12 vs 4 h) (9, 18). When formed from metabolism of naltrexone in the body, it exhibits linear pharmacokinetics with naltrexone doses up to 800 mg [2, 4]. Furthermore, 6β-naltrexol levels have been correlated with the effectiveness of naltrexone therapy in decreasing the subjective effects of alcohol and reducing relapse (24). However, there is substantial variability between individuals with respect to the metabolism of naltrexone into 6β-naltrexol, and this may account in part for the variability in therapeutic response in the treatment of alcoholism/alcohol abuse (24).

In the opioid-dependent state, naloxone and naltrexone act as inverse agonists in a variety of systems (20, 32, 21, 33). Recently, others have confirmed and expanded on these results (20, 22, 21, 14, 15). It is hypothesized that the inverse agonist activity of the compounds contributes to their increased potency/efficacy in precipitating withdrawal, and the severity of the withdrawal syndrome. Moreover, the ability of these inverse agonists to precipitate withdrawal appears not to be competitive with the agonist, so that even small doses of the inverse agonist precipitate withdrawal/aversion by acting selectively on the basally active receptor, while not blocking any of the agonist effects. This could account for the difficulties in finding agonist/antagonist combinations that are not aversive even when opiates are used therapeutically. In contrast, 6β-naltrexol and several other analogs of naloxone and naltrexone with reduced bonds on the 6 position act more like neutral antagonists in the opioid dependent state (32, 33, 26, 28). These neutral antagonists are hypothesized to precipitate less severe opioid withdrawal while still dose-dependently attenuating opioid agonist effects.

These results account for the observation that combination formulations with conventional opiate antagonists (naloxone and naltrexone) are likely to produce significant adverse effects (withdrawal, intestinal cramping, etc.). Sadee and Bilsky have shown that naloxone and naltrexone suppress basal signaling of the MOR in the opioid dependent state (inverse agonism), rather than – or in addition to – blocking the actions of an agonist drug. In contrast, neutral antagonists like 6β-naltrexol appear to block agonist actions at MOR without altering basal signaling – causing significantly less adverse effects.

14.2 Potential Advantages of 6β-naltrexol in Decreasing Abuse of Prescription Opiates

6β-naltrexol has several features that suggest it will work well in combination with short-acting μ-agonists like hydrocodone. In the monkey, 6β-naltrexol has a ~2X lesser affinity for the MOR than naltrexone and is 100-fold less potent than naltrexone in antagonizing alfentanil analgesia (19). In mice, 6β-naltrexol dose-dependently antagonizes morphine analgesia, but only precipitates opiate withdrawal at ~80-fold higher doses (26). In people treated with depo-naltrexone, the 6β-naltrexol AUC exceeds the naltrexone AUC by a factor of 3, suggesting prolonged exposure to modest 6β-naltrexol concentrations is safe.

The long half-life (12–18 h) of 6β-naltrexol in humans, along with the apparent nontoxic and well-tolerated profile as a major metabolite of naltrexone, make 6β-naltrexol attractive as an addition to widely prescribed but also abused short-acting μ-agonists. Hydrocodone, for example, is the most frequently prescribed drug in the United States (~100 million prescriptions per year; enough for 1 Rx for every 3 Americans) and is a major drug of abuse. We predict that a properly formulated combination of 6β-naltrexol and a short-acting μ-agonist (like hydrocodone) will retain analgesic efficacy when used as directed (due to a lack of accumulation of 6β-naltrexol) but, when taken in larger quantities than prescribed, will progressively attenuate reinforcing efficacy (due to kinetic and dynamic differences between 6β-naltrexol and the short-acting opiate) while precipitating only a mild opioid withdrawal and less aversion (due to the drug's neutral antagonist properties), compared to naltrexone or similar analogs (such as the quartenary N-methyl-naltrexone). The combination product should also be abuse-resistant if injected. Moreover, it is also likely that 6β-naltrexol coadministration will decrease some of the limiting side effects of acute and chronic hydrocodone therapy such as nausea, vomiting, and constipation. Based on these data we believe 6β-naltrexol is an outstanding candidate for drug development. If one were developing a highly efficacious μ-inverse agonist 6β-naltrexol would be a poor candidate. However, the lower potency in both blocking μ-agonist effects and much lower propensity to precipitate withdrawal are ideal features for the combination formulation we propose.

6β-Naltrexol is a neutral opiate antagonist that is expected to have intermediate bioavailability while maintaining high affinity for μ-receptors, compared to commonly prescribed μ-opiate analgesics. Preliminary data also suggest that 6β-naltrexol may have a slower clearance than codeine or hydrocodone, suggesting that a combination formulation containing 6β-naltrexol with either of these μ-agonist could limit the maximal dose of the combination by shifting the relative pharmacologic profile from agonist to neutral antagonist. Because of its neutral antagonist profile 6β-naltrexol should interfere with analgesia in nontolerant patients in a well-controlled manner (both time and dose-dependent) but, unlike naltrexone, at low exposures, 6β-naltrexol should not precipitate opiate withdrawal in tolerant/dependent patients. Thus, we predict that pharmacologic differences between potent, short-acting full μ-agonist analgesics and the slowly cleared, neutral antagonist 6β-naltrexol will permit development of a less abusable and less aversive dose formulation of commonly prescribed opiate analgesics.

14.3 Assessing the Neutral Antagonist Properties of 6β-Naltrexol

We plan to conduct a series of experiments directed at establishing the mechanism and exposure (concentration)–response relationship of 6β-naltrexol. Our experiments focus on the hypothesized neutral antagonist mechanism of 6β-naltrexol. Because the functional behavior of 6β-naltrexol is expected to be concentration-dependent, we first define the pharmacokinetics of 6β-naltrexol. At low exposures, we predict 6β-naltrexol will act as a neutral antagonist but at higher exposures, withdrawal-like properties may become evident in severely dependent individuals (similar to what a partial agonist might produce). Because understanding concentration–effect relationships is crucial to predicting individual response to combination formulations containing 6β-naltrexol two studies define bioavailability and pharmacokinetics, permitting dose-selection for tests of mechanism. To gain the fullest understanding of concentration–effect relationships we will make extensive use of population pharmacokinetic modeling and in-silico trial simulation.

Once we understand kinetics we will conduct two mechanistic studies. In our first mechanism study we assess the ability of 6β-naltrexol to precipitate opiate withdrawal in patients highly dependent on μ-opiates (patients on 60–100 mg of daily methadone). If low-modest exposures to 6β-naltrexol do not precipitate withdrawal then a profile of neutral antagonism is supported. In our second mechanistic study, we assess the ability of larger exposures to 6β-naltrexol to attenuate the opiate agonist effects of hydrocodone. If 6β-naltrexol dose-dependently attenuates the μ-agonist effects of hydrocodone at concentrations lower than those that precipitate withdrawal, and in a dose- or concentration-dependent manner, then again, a neutral antagonist mechanism of action is supported.

We will perform a sequential series of studies designed to test the ability of 6β-naltrexol to antagonize the effects of μ-opiate agonists. Critical effort is placed early on to verify and measure the extent of systemic bioavailability and define the single-dose and population pharmacokinetics of 6β-naltrexol. These studies will lay the foundation for properly designed and conducted interaction trials with 6β-naltrexol and hydrocodone. Ultimately, we believe that targeted dosing to optimize pharmacokinetic and profiles of 6β-naltrexol and hydrocodone, in the presence of the other, will improve the chances of successful and efficient development of this combination regimen. Some readers not familiar with the drug development process may wonder why not test the fundamental hypothesis first then proceed to define pharmacokinetics later – if it does not work why go to the substantial effort to define kinetics. We have been guided by industrial experience that shows the risk of progressing too rapidly is that flawed results will be obtained. Before conducting μ-agonist–6β-naltrexol interaction trials it is essential to understand pharmacokinetic variance and expected plasma (and by inference) effect-site concentrations.

Narcotic formulations that lessen the risk of developing dependence and addiction have been sought for more than 100 years. They remain urgently needed. A common clinical problem is self-initiated unsupervised dose-escalation in patients being treated for nonmalignant pain with opiate analgesics. These patients become highly dependent with classic opiate withdrawal symptoms. Many become addicts, meeting most DSM-IV criteria for addiction. Although there is little written about the costs of illicit prescription opiate purchases, some patients in my practice spend up to $200 per day on Internet purchases of Vicodin. These patients have lost all control over drug use and are as addicted as any heroin user. Patients become physically dependent and unable to decrease drug use, even when pain is otherwise well controlled. Our approach of combining an opiate neutral antagonist with an opiate agonist is one possible solution to the rapid rise of prescription opiate addiction.

References

1. American Psychiatric Association (1994). *Diagnostic and statistical manual of mental disorders*. Washington, DC, American Psychiatric Association.
2. Azar, M. R., B. C. Jones, et al. (2003). Conditioned place aversion is a highly sensitive index of acute opioid dependence and withdrawal. *Psychopharmacology (Berl)* **170**(1): 42–50.
3. Azorlosa, J. L. (1994). The effect of chronic naltrexone pretreatment on associative vs non-associative morphine tolerance. *Drug Alcohol Depend* **36**(1): 65–7.
4. Bilsky, E. J., R. N. Bernstein, et al. (1996). Effects of naloxone and D-Phe-Cys-Tyr-D-Trp-Arg-Thr-Pen-Thr-NH_2 and the protein kinase inhibitors H7 and H8 on acute morphine dependence and antinociceptive tolerance in mice. *J Pharmacol Exp Ther* **277**(1): 484–90.
5. Bond, R. A. and A. P. Ijzerman (2006). Recent developments in constitutive receptor activity and inverse agonism, and their potential for GPCR drug discovery. *Trends Pharmacol Sci* **27**(2): 92–6.
6. Brands, B., J. Blake, et al. (2004). Prescription opioid abuse in patients presenting for methadone maintenance treatment. *Drug Alcohol Depend* **73**(2): 199–207.
7. Compton, P., J. Darakjian, et al. (1998). Screening for addiction in patients with chronic pain and "problematic" substance use: evaluation of a pilot assessment tool. *J Pain Symptom Manage* **16**(6): 355–63.
8. Compton, P., K. Miotto, et al. (2004). Precipitated opioid withdrawal across acute physical dependence induction methods. *Pharmacol Biochem Behav* **77**(2): 263–8.
9. Cone, E. J., C. W. Gorodetzky, et al. (1974). The urinary excretion profile of naltrexone and metabolites in man. *Drug Metab Dispos* **2**(6): 506–12.
10. Ferrante, F. M. (1996). Principles of opioid pharmacotherapy: practical implications of basic mechanisms. *J Pain Symptom Manage* **11**(5): 265–73.
11. Ferrari, A., M. Bertolotti, et al. (1998). Serum time course of naltrexone and 6 beta-naltrexol levels during long-term treatment in drug addicts. *Drug Alcohol Depend* **52**(3): 211–20.
12. Fishman, S. M., B. Wilsey, et al. (2000). Adherence monitoring and drug surveillance in chronic opioid therapy. *J Pain Symptom Manage* **20**(4): 293–307.
13. Freye, E. and J. Levy (2005). Constitutive opioid receptor activation: a prerequisite mechanism involved in acute opioid withdrawal. *Addict Biol* **10**(2): 131–7.

14. Guarna, M., A. Bartolini, et al. (2003). Anti-mu opioid antiserum against the third external loop of the cloned mu-opioid receptor acts as a mu receptor neutral antagonist. *Brain Res Mol Brain Res* **119**(1): 100–10.
15. Heinzen, E. L., R. G. Booth, et al. (2005). Neuronal nitric oxide modulates morphine antinociceptive tolerance by enhancing constitutive activity of the mu-opioid receptor. *Biochem Pharmacol* **69**(4): 679–88.
16. June, H. L., M. L. Stitzer, et al. (1995). Acute physical dependence: time course and relation to human plasma morphine concentrations. *Clin Pharmacol Ther* **57**(3): 270–80.
17. Kenakin, T. (2004). Efficacy as a vector: the relative prevalence and paucity of inverse agonism. *Mol Pharmacol* **65**(1): 2–11.
18. King, A. C., J. R. Volpicelli, et al. (1997). Naltrexone biotransformation and incidence of subjective side effects: a preliminary study. *Alcohol Clin Exp Res* **21**(5): 906–9.
19. Ko, M. C., M. F. Divin, et al. (2006). Differential in vivo potencies of naltrexone and 6beta-naltrexol in the monkey. *J Pharmacol Exp Ther* **316**(2): 772–9.
20. Liu, J. G. and P. L. Prather (2001). Chronic exposure to mu-opioid agonists produces constitutive activation of mu-opioid receptors in direct proportion to the efficacy of the agonist used for pretreatment. *Mol Pharmacol* **60**(1): 53–62.
21. Liu, J. G. and P. L. Prather (2002). Chronic agonist treatment converts antagonists into inverse agonists at delta-opioid receptors. *J Pharmacol Exp Ther* **302**(3): 1070–9.
22. Liu, J. G., M. B. Ruckle, et al. (2001). Constitutively active mu-opioid receptors inhibit adenylyl cyclase activity in intact cells and activate G-proteins differently than the agonist [D-Ala2,N-MePhe4,Gly-ol5]enkephalin. *J Biol Chem* **276**(41): 37779–86.
23. Maack, C., B. Cremers, et al. (2000). Different intrinsic activities of bucindolol, carvedilol and metoprolol in human failing myocardium. *Br J Pharmacol* **130**(5): 1131–9.
24. McCaul, M. E., G. S. Wand, et al. (2000). Serum 6-beta-naltrexol levels are related to alcohol responses in heavy drinkers. *Alcohol Clin Exp Res* **24**(9): 1385–91.
25. Parran, T., Jr. (1997). Prescription drug abuse. A question of balance. *Med Clin North Am* **81**(4): 967–78.
26. Raehal, K. M., J. J. Lowery, et al. (2005). In vivo characterization of 6beta-naltrexol, an opioid ligand with less inverse agonist activity compared with naltrexone and naloxone in opioid-dependent mice. *J Pharmacol Exp Ther* **313**(3): 1150–62.
27. Sadee, W., D. Wang, et al. (2005). Basal opioid receptor activity, neutral antagonists, and therapeutic opportunities. *Life Sci* **76**(13): 1427–37.
28. Shoblock, J. R. and N. T. Maidment (2006). Constitutively active mu opioid receptors mediate the enhanced conditioned aversive effect of naloxone in morphine-dependent mice. *Neuropsychopharmacology* **31**(1): 171–7.
29. Simoni-Wastila, L. and G. Strickler (2004). Risk factors associated with problem use of prescription drugs. *Am J Public Health* **94**(2): 266–8.
30. Smit, M. J., R. Leurs, et al. (1996). Inverse agonism of histamine H2 antagonist accounts for upregulation of spontaneously active histamine H2 receptors. *Proc Natl Acad Sci USA* **93**(13): 6802–7.
31. Tulunay, F. C. and A. E. Takemori (1974). The increased efficacy of narcotic antagonists induced by various narcotic analgesics. *J Pharmacol Exp Ther* **190**(3): 395–400.
32. Wang, D., K. M. Raehal, et al. (2001). Inverse agonists and neutral antagonists at mu opioid receptor (MOR): possible role of basal receptor signaling in narcotic dependence. *J Neurochem* **77**(6): 1590–600.
33. Wang, D., K. M. Raehal, et al. (2004). Basal signaling activity of mu opioid receptor in mouse brain: role in narcotic dependence. *J Pharmacol Exp Ther* **308**(2): 512–20.
34. Wang, Z., E. J. Bilsky, et al. (1994). Constitutive mu opioid receptor activation as a regulatory mechanism underlying narcotic tolerance and dependence. *Life Sci* **54**(20): PL339–50.
35. Zacny, J., G. Bigelow, et al. (2003). College on Problems of Drug Dependence taskforce on prescription opioid non-medical use and abuse: position statement. *Drug Alcohol Depend* **69**(3): 215–32.

Chapter 15
Effects of Opioid Antagonists on the Abuse-Related Effects of Psychomotor Stimulants and Nicotine

Brenda J. Gehrke and Toni S. Shippenberg

Abstract Psychomotor stimulant abuse continues to be a major health problem. Despite intensive study, pharmacological therapies for the treatment of stimulant addiction and the prevention of relapse are lacking. Furthermore, although certain individuals may be at greater risk for the development of compulsive drug-seeking behavior, the neural substrates mediating individual differences in sensitivity to the behavioral effects of stimulants are unknown. Opioid receptors and their endogenous ligands are present in high concentrations in brain circuits upon which psychostimulants act to exert control over behavior. Studies in humans and experimental animals have shown that the activity of endogenous opioid systems is altered in response to psychostimulants. It is also apparent that the administration of nonselective opioid receptor antagonists can profoundly affect the responsiveness of an individual to these agents. In the past decade, antagonists selective for the various opioid receptor types have become available. These agents have been used to probe the function of endogenous opioid systems and have provided important insights as to the role of μ-, δ-, and κ-opioid receptor systems in mediating the actions of psychostimulants. This chapter will review preclinical data examining the influence of opioid receptor antagonists on the behavioral and neurochemical effects of psychostimulants. We will provide evidence that opioid receptor antagonists can attenuate or exacerbate several effects of psychostimulants that are linked to their abuse liability. Furthermore, we will show that the effects of opioid receptor antagonists is dependent on the receptor type targeted as well as on the psychostimulant tested, the prior drug history of an individual, and the animal model employed.

Keywords: Opioid antagonists; Mu antagonists; Delta antagonists; Kappa antagonists; Opioid/psychostimulant interactions; Self-administration; CPP; ICSS

B.J. Gehrke and T.S. Shippenberg (✉)
Integrative Neuroscience Section, NIH/NIDA Intramural Research Program,
333 Cassell Drive, Baltimore, MD 21224
e-mail: tshippen@intra.nida.nih.gov

15.1 Introduction

According to the most recent National Survey on Drug Use and Health, nearly 12 million Americans have tried methamphetamine, over 34 million Americans aged 12 and over have reported lifetime use of cocaine, and 7.8 million individuals have used crack (1). Nicotine remains one of the most widely abused substances in the United States with an estimated 70.3 million Americans reporting tobacco use (1). Although substantial progress has been made in identifying the neural substrates mediating the abuse liability of psychoactive drugs, therapeutic agents for the treatment of stimulant addiction are lacking.

Opioid receptors and their endogenous ligands are present in high concentrations in brain regions that subserve mood, incentive motivation, and habit learning. Opposing, tonically active opioid systems regulate neurotransmission in several of these regions (2). Work from various laboratories has shown that the activity of these systems is altered in response to repeated psychostimulant use (3–8). Studies employing opioid receptor antagonists suggest that the dysregulation of opioid peptide systems contributes to the pathogenesis of drug addiction. This chapter will review preclinical data indicating an involvement of endogenous opioid systems in modulating the behavioral and neurochemical effects of psychostimulants. Specifically, we will show that opioid receptor antagonists can, depending on the opioid receptor type targeted, exacerbate or attenuate the responsiveness of an individual to cocaine, amphetamines, and nicotine. The implications of these findings for the treatment of addiction and the prevention of relapse will be discussed.

15.2 Pharmacology of Psychomotor Stimulants

Psychomotor stimulants (stimulants) elicit behavioral activation at doses typically employed for their therapeutic and recreational use. They produce euphoria in humans and rewarding effects in a variety of species. These actions are thought to lead to the initiation of drug abuse. Cocaine binds to and inhibits dopamine (DA), serotonin, and norepinephrine transporters, thereby increasing monoamine transmission at nerve terminals. Amphetamine and methamphetamine enhance monoamine transmission by blocking monoamine reuptake and increasing release. Systemically administered DA receptor antagonists attenuate the rewarding and behavioral-activating effects of stimulants demonstrating that DA transmission is critical for these effects (9–12). Behavioral and neurochemical studies have shown that increased DA transmission within the mesocorticolimbic DA system is essential for the rewarding effects of stimulants and other drugs of abuse. The continued use of these agents produces enduring alterations in the activity of this DA system and in that of its afferent and efferent projections. Increasing evidence suggests that these and other neuroadaptations underlie the transition from drug abuse to the compulsive drug taking and seeking that characterizes addiction.

15.3 Influence of Psychomotor Stimulants on Opioid Gene Expression

The repeated administration of stimulants alters the expression of opioid peptides and their receptors in brain regions comprising the brain's motive circuit. Proenkephalin (PENK) gene expression is increased in the dorsal striatum and nucleus accumbens (Nacc) for some days following the cessation of intravenous (i.v.) cocaine self-administration (13). As abstinence proceeds, expression decreases in the central amygdala, a brain region implicated in mediating drug craving and relapse to addiction (14). Increased PENK expression is also observed during the early phase of abstinence from repeated, noncontingent injections of cocaine (15, 16) and following acute amphetamine administration (17). Amphetamine-evoked increases in PENK expression are attenuated by a δ-opioid receptor (DOPr) antagonist. In contrast, μ-opioid receptor (MOPr) blockade is without effect, indicating mediation by a DOPr mechanism (18).

Postmortem studies of human cocaine addicts have shown that the repeated use of cocaine induces prodynorphin (PDYN) expression in the dorsal striatum (19). Increases in PDYN expression, κ-opioid receptor (KOPr) number and tissue levels of dynorphin are seen in humans and experimental animals with a history of cocaine administration (3, 19). As will become apparent in this chapter, blockade of these endogenous opioid systems by administration of opioid receptor antagonists profoundly affects the behavioral and neurochemical effects of stimulants.

15.4 Animal Models of Addiction

15.4.1 Drug Self-Administration

Procedures in which animals voluntarily self-administer drug provide a framework with which to model the transition from initial drug use to the compulsive drug seeking that is a hallmark of addiction. They have been used to study a variety of issues regarding the rewarding effects of drugs abuse including the relative abuse potential of specific compounds, patterns of drug intake, and the neural mechanisms of drug reinforcement (20). Typically, animals are trained to emit a response (e.g., nose-poke or depression of a lever) to receive a test drug via the oral or i.v. route (21). Different operant reinforcement schedules can be employed. Fixed ratio (FR) schedules require an animal to emit a specified number of responses to receive drug, while fixed interval (FI) schedules require animals wait a particular amount of time before emitting a response. Acquisition of self-administration is assessed by determining the number of sessions required to reach a particular criterion of performance or by measuring responding over a set number of days (e.g., the first 5 days of self-administration). The effects of a treatment on the maintenance of self-administration are assessed once stable operant responding for drug is obtained.

A progressive ratio (PR) schedule of reinforcement is commonly used to assess the reinforcing efficacy of a drug (20, 21). In this procedure, the response requirements for drug delivery increase systematically until the performance of the animal fails to meet a set criterion. The point at which responding ceases represents the break point, and reflects the maximum effort an animal will exert to receive drug (22).

15.4.2 Reinstatement of Drug Seeking

Reinstatement procedures are used to model relapse to addiction in experimental animals. As described above, animals are initially trained to self-administer drug. Once stable performance is achieved, responding is extinguished by substituting delivery of vehicle for drug. Reinstatement of responding produced by presentation of a priming injection of drug (drug-primed reinstatement), stimuli that previously signaled drug availability (cue-induced reinstatement) or a stressor is then assessed (21, 23). Although these procedures provide a useful model of relapse, it is important to note that human addicts do not typically achieve abstinence by extinction of drug self-administration. Rather, abstinence typically results from an active decision to abstain from drug or through forced abstinence.

15.4.3 Conditioned Place Preference

In humans, environmental stimuli (e.g., paraphernalia associated with drug-taking) become associated with the unconditioned effects of a drug through Pavlovian conditioning (24). Subsequent exposure to these stimuli elicits drug craving and can precipitate relapse to drug-taking despite prolonged periods of abstinence (24, 25). Operant models such as cue-induced reinstatement of drug self-administration provide one method with which to evaluate the conditioned rewarding effects of drugs. Conditioned place preference (CPP) procedures, which are based on Pavlovian conditioning, permit evaluation of the approach or avoidance that develops to a particular environment previously associated with experimenter-administered drug. In CPP experiments, a distinct set of contextual cues is paired with drug injection and another set with injection of vehicle. Preference for the drug- or vehicle-paired place is assessed by allowing uninjected animals free access to both contexts and measuring the time spent in contact with each (26). Increased time spent in the drug-paired context, relative to control levels (e.g., to scores before conditioning or to scores of animals that receive vehicle in each of the contexts), is indicative of conditioned rewarding effects. Decreased time spent in the drug-paired context indicates conditioned aversive effects of a drug. When evaluating the effects of an antagonist on drug-induced CPP, the antagonist can be administered either before each conditioning session or before tests of conditioning. The former assesses development of drug-induced CPP while the latter assesses CPP expression.

CPP studies use an unbiased or biased design. In the unbiased design, animals exhibit no innate preference for either set of place cues and pairing of drug with each environmental context is counterbalanced. In a biased design, animals exhibit a preference for one of the environments and drug administration is typically paired with the least-preferred environment. When interpreting data from CPP studies, it is important to note that drug-induced increases in preference observed in biased procedures may reflect anxiolytic (e.g, decrease in aversion) or rewarding effects of a drug whereas the unbiased design does not suffer from this potential confound (26). Self-administration and CPP measure distinct reward processes (26) and clear evidence of a dissociation between the results of the two procedures has been obtained (27).

15.4.4 Intracranial Self-Stimulation

Since the discovery by olds that animals will voluntarily work to obtain electrical stimulation of the brain (28, 29), intracranial self-stimulation (ICSS) has been used to identify the neural substrates mediating the rewarding effects of various stimuli (21, 30, 31). In ICSS, animals are trained to emit an operant response to receive rewarding electrical stimulation of the medial forebrain bundle or to brain regions such as the prefrontal cortex, ventral tegmental area (VTA), dorsal striatum, and Nacc. Work by various investigators has shown that stimulants and other abused drugs enhance ICSS. Response rates increase and the minimum stimulus current (threshold) that maintains operant responding decreases (30).

15.5 Nonselective Opioid Receptor Antagonists

Naloxone and naltrexone are nonselective opioid receptor antagonists. Although they bind with highest affinity to MOPr, they also bind with high affinity to DOPr and KOPr (32, 33). Studies using these antagonists have provided important information about opioid/stimulant interactions. Importantly, however, the role of specific opioid receptor types in mediating their effects cannot be determined.

15.5.1 Drug Self-Administration

Both naloxone and naltrexone decrease the acquisition of cocaine self-administration in rodents. Using a single session i.v. self-administration paradigm in mice, Kuzmin et al. (34) showed that naloxone (1.0 mg/kg; subcutaneous, s.c.) decreased cocaine (0.4 μg/infusion) self-administration. A rightward shift in the cocaine dose-response curve was seen, indicating decreased sensitivity to the acute rewarding effects of cocaine. Decreased acquisition of cocaine self-administration is also observed in response to naltrexone (35–37). In rats that were food deprived to increase the rate of acquisition of operant responding, once daily administration of naltrexone (0.1–1.0 mg/kg/day × 5 days; s.c) dose-dependently decreased acquisition of cocaine (0.12 mg/kg/infusion; i.v.) self-administration. Interestingly, acquisition of cocaine self-administration (0.06 or 0.25 mg/kg/infusion) was unaltered and a trend toward a naltrexone-induced increase in drug infusions in response to the higher dose of cocaine was seen (35). The finding that naltrexone suppresses self-administration of a moderate dose of cocaine is consistent with a decrease in the rewarding effects of cocaine. Similarly, the increased responding for the higher cocaine dose may indicate a rightward shift in the cocaine-effect curve. Since, however, other doses on the descending limb of the dose-effect curve were not evaluated, questions exist as to whether the effects observed reflect attenuation or potentiation of the rewarding effects of high doses of cocaine. Whether similar effects would occur in food-satiated animals is unknown.

The brain regions where naltrexone acts to modulate acquisition of cocaine self-administration have been examined. Intracerebroventricular infusion of naltrexone (5.0 μg) decreased acquisition of self-administration in rats. The effective dose was substantially lower than that effective systemically, confirming a central nervous system (CNS) mechanism (36). Infusion of naltrexone (0.1 or 1.0 μg) into the VTA produced a similar effect, whereas its infusion into either the caudate nucleus, central nucleus of the amygdala, Nacc, or medial prefrontal cortex failed to modify behavior (37). These findings suggest that blockade of VTA opioid receptors is sufficient to reduce acquisition of cocaine self-administration.

In contrast to the above studies, chronic pretreatment of a high dose of naltrexone (10 mg/kg/day × 12 days) preceding the start of cocaine self-administration increased the acquisition of cocaine (0.16 mg/kg/infusion) self-administration in rats (38). The opposite effect observed in this as compared to other studies may result from the use of a high dose of antagonist. Alternatively, it may reflect differences in the antagonist treatment schedule employed (e.g., chronic vs subacute). Chronic naltrexone treatment upregulates multiple opioid receptor types and the receptor types affected varies as a function of dose (39, 40). Prolonged treatment with naltrexone and resultant opioid receptor upregulation may, thus, enhance rather than decrease the effects of psychostimulants.

Data regarding the effects of these antagonists on the maintenance of cocaine self-administration are conflicting (41, 42) versus (43–45). Acute pretreatment with either naltrexone or naloxone (0.1–10 mg/kg; s.c.) dose-dependently decreased cocaine self-administration in rats trained to self-administer a low (0.1 and 0.3 mg/kg/infusion) but not a high dose of cocaine (41). Self-administration of nicotine (0.03 mg/kg/infusion) was unaltered, indicating a specific interaction of antagonists with cocaine (41). These findings contrast with those showing no effect of a similar dose range of naltrexone (0.01–10 mg/kg; intraperitoneally, i.p.) (44) and with those showing that naltrexone (0.5–2.0 mg/kg; i.v.) increases responding for cocaine (0.1 mg/kg) in food-satiated but not food-deprived rats (45). Methodological differences may account for the contrasting results. An enhancement of self-administration was seen when a continuous cocaine access procedure (24-h session) was used, whereas a decrease was observed when self-administration sessions were 60 min in duration (41). As will become apparent, methodological differences abound in the literature and should be considered when interpreting studies examining opioid/psychostimulant interactions.

Studies in nonhuman primates indicate either no or nonspecific effects of these antagonists. Treatment with naloxone (0.01–4.0 mg/kg; i.m.) for 7–10 days did not alter cocaine self-administration in rhesus monkeys (46). Although daily treatment with naltrexone (0.32 or 3.20 mg/kg over 60 min) decreased cocaine self-administration, food self-administration was reduced (42), indicating a generalized disruption of behavior. A later study by the same laboratory showed no effect of naltrexone (0.4 mg/kg/day) on cocaine self-administration (43). These findings contrast with those in the rodent and may indicate important species differences. However, it is noteworthy that in primate studies, animals were receiving buprenorphine, a long-acting mixed opioid receptor antagonist. Therefore, drug history may contribute to the lack of observed effects (43). Furthermore, in contrast to rodent studies, naltrexone was administered repeatedly for 10–15 days via slow, i.v. infusion. Distinct neuroadaptations may occur in response to continuous versus repeated, intermittent administration of antagonists.

Three studies have investigated the effects of naltrexone on reinstatement of cocaine seeking in response to a priming injection of cocaine (23, 47, 48). Using a within-session reinstatement procedure in rats, no effect of acute naltrexone (1.6 and 3.2 mg/kg; i.v.) on reinstatement produced by a priming injection of cocaine (3.2 mg/kg; i.v.) was observed (23). Another study reported no effect of acute naltrexone (3.0 mg/kg) when the antagonist was administered before the first test session. However, a significant decrease was observed when naltrexone was administered before the second and third reinstatement sessions (48). Therefore, while acute opioid receptor blockade may be ineffective in attenuating cocaine-primed reinstatement of cocaine responding, repeated receptor blockade may have marked effects.

Pretreatment of rats with naltrexone (1.0 mg/kg; i.p.) decreased cue-induced reinstatement of methamphetamine-associated responding. Interestingly, however, a higher dose of naltrexone (3.2 mg/kg; i.p.) did not affect reinstatement produced by a priming injection (1 mg/kg; i.p.) of this psychostimulant (47). Although additional studies are necessary, these results (Table 15.1) suggest that acute opioid receptor blockade may be effective in attenuating acquisition of stimulant self-administration and in decreasing compulsive drug seeking evoked by cues that have signaled stimulant exposure.

15.5.2 Conditioned Place Preference

Naloxone attenuates the development of stimulant-induced CPP in rodents (34, 49, 50). Pretreatment of rats with a dose of naloxone (0.02 mg/kg; s.c.) that was ineffective, by itself, in producing a conditioned response, attenuated CPP produced by a low dose of amphetamine (1.0 mg/kg; s.c.) (49). Similar results have been reported in mice for

Table 15.1 Self-administration: acquisition, maintenance, and reinstatement

Opioid receptor antagonist type	Acquisition of self-administration	Maintenance of self-administration	Reinstatement
Nonselective: naloxone	*Cocaine*: -mice: ↓	*Cocaine*: -rats: ↓ -nonhuman primates: NE	
Naltrexone	*Cocaine*: -rats: ↓; ↑ w/chronic pretreatment	*Cocaine*: -rats: ↓, ↑, NE -nonhuman primates: ↓, NE *Nicotine*: -rats: NE	*Cocaine responding*: -rats: NE on cocaine-primed, ↓ w/repeated testing *Methamphetamine responding*: -rats: NE on methamphetamine-primed, ↓ cue-induced
MOPr	–	*Cocaine*: -β-FNA (rats): (intra-VTA and Nacc admin) ↓ for PR schedule, NE for FR1 schedule; NE for intradorsal Str admin	*Cocaine responding*: -CTAP (rats): (intraventral pallidum admin) ↓ cocaine-primed
DOPr	–	*Cocaine*: -naltrindole: (rats) NE, ↓; (nonhuman primates) NE, ↓ -chronic naltrindole (rats): NE	–
KOPr	–	*Cocaine*: -nor-BNI: (rats) ↓; (nonhuman primates) NE *Concurrent choice food/ cocaine task*: -nor-BNI (nonhuman primates): NE	*Cocaine responding*: -nor-BNI (rats): (ICV admin) NE on cocaine-primed -JDTic (rats): NE on cocaine-primed, ↓ in footshock-induced

↓ indicates a decrease or blockade, ↑ indicates an increase, and NE indicates no effect by the antagonist

cocaine-induced CPP (34). Evidence that blockade of opioid receptors in the ventral pallidum, a brain region implicated in mediating the rewarding effects of cocaine (51, 52), is sufficient to produce these effects has been obtained. Intrapallidal infusion of naloxone (0.01 μg), at a dose that does not produce an aversion by itself, blocks cocaine-induced (10 mg/kg) CPP (50).

To date, only one study has evaluated the effect of antagonists on the expression of stimulant-evoked CPP (53). Acute injection of naloxone (1.0 mg/kg; s.c.) before testing was ineffective in blocking the expression of cocaine-induced (10.0 mg/kg) CPP in mice. However, this same treatment attenuated the expression of nicotine-evoked CPP (1.0 mg/kg). Antagonist pretreatment prevented the increase in CREB phosphorylation associated with the expression of nicotine CPP, suggesting a more global role of endogenous opioid systems in modulating the conditioned response to this drug of abuse (53).

15.5.3 Intracranial Self-Stimulation

The influence of naloxone on the enhancement of ICSS produced by amphetamine (31, 54, 55), cocaine (56, 57), and nicotine (58) has been investigated (Table 15.2). Amphetamine decreases the threshold to maintain ICSS of the median forebrain bundle, prefrontal cortex, and dorsal tegmentum. Doses of naloxone

Table 15.2 Conditioned place preference (CPP) and intracranial self-stimulation (ICSS)

Opioid receptor antagonist type	CPP	ICSS
Nonselective: naloxone	*Cocaine-induced*: -rats: ↓ development -mice: ↓ development, NE on expression *Amphetamine-induced*: -rats: ↓ development *Nicotine-induced*: -mice: ↓ expression	*ICSS alone*: -rats: ↓ responding (MFB, PFC, DT) *Amphetamine ICSS*: -rats: NE (PFC) or ↓ (MFB, DT) effect of amphetamine *Cocaine ICSS*: -rats: NE (PFC) or ↓ (MFB, VTA) effect of cocaine *Nicotine ICSS*: -rats: NE (MFB) on effect of nicotine
MOPr	–	–
DOPr	*Cocaine- and methamphetamine-induced*: -naltrindole (rats): NE w/low doses, NE and ↓ w/higher doses -naltriben (rats): NE w/low doses, ↓ w/higher doses Sensitization of cocaine-induced CPP: -naltrindole (rats): ↓	*Cocaine ICSS*: -naltrindole (rats): ↓ (MFB) effect of cocaine *MDMA ICSS*: -naltrindole (rats): ↓ (MFB) effect of MDMA
KOPr	*Stress-induced potentiation of cocaine-induced CPP*: -nor-BNI (mice): ↓	*ICSS alone*: -ANTI (rats): NE (MFB) -nor-BNI (rats): NE (LH)

↓ indicates a decrease or blockade, ↑ indicates an increase, and NE indicates no effect by the antagonist

For ICSS, the brain region in ( ) refers to the brain region where ICSS was administered: *MFB* medial forebrain bundle, *PFC* prefrontal cortex, *DT* dorsal tegmentum, *VTA* ventral tegmental area, *LH* lateral hypothalamus

(2.0 or 4.0 mg/kg; i.p.) that were ineffective in altering median forebrain bundle ICSS blocked the decrease in ICSS thresholds produced by systemically administered amphetamine (54). A subsequent study showed that naloxone (0.1–10.0 mg/kg; i.p.) alone dose-dependently decreased responding for ICSS of the forebrain bundle, prefrontal cortex, and dorsal tegmentum. Naloxone (10 mg/kg; i.p.) attenuated the amphetamine-evoked facilitation of dorsal tegmental ICSS whereas no alteration in prefrontal cortical ICSS was seen (55). An attenuated response to amphetamine (0.1–1.0 mg/kg; s.c.) is observed when lower doses of naloxone (≥1.0 mg/kg) and an FI reinforcement schedule were used (31).

Cocaine enhances ICSS of the medial forebrain bundle, VTA, medial prefrontal cortex, and sulcal prefrontal cortex as evidenced by a lowering of the thresholds needed to produce self-stimulation (56, 57). Response rates for stimulation of the medial prefrontal cortex and the sulcal prefrontal cortex are increased (57). Naloxone pretreatment (4 mg/kg; i.p.) attenuated the cocaine-evoked (10.0 or 15.0 mg/kg) decrease in thresholds for ICSS of the medial forebrain bundle and the VTA (56). Only one study has evaluated the effects of naloxone on stimulation of the medial prefrontal and sulcal prefrontal cortex. No effect of a low dose of naloxone (0.5 mg/kg) on cocaine (15 mg/kg) – evoked alterations of response rates and thresholds was seen (57). The dose used, however, was substantially lower than those shown to affect stimulation in other areas. Therefore, effects may be seen if doses greater than or equal to 1.0 mg/kg were tested (31, 54). Taken together, these data indicate that moderate doses of naloxone attenuate the enhancement of reward produced by stimulants. Differences in the effects of low versus moderate high doses of naloxone may reflect differential blockade of one or more opioid receptor types and highlight the need for testing multiple doses of antagonists.

Only one study has investigated the effects of nicotine on ICSS. Acute nicotine (0.125–0.75 mg/kg; s.c.) administration lowered the threshold required for ICSS in the medial forebrain bundle. However, naloxone (0.5–16 mg/kg) (58) did not alter this effect. As shown in Table 15.2, these data contrast with those obtained for cocaine and amphetamine and with CPP data demonstrating a naloxone-induced reduction in the expression of nicotine-induced CPP (53). Together, these data suggest a critical role of endogenous opioid systems in mediating the rewarding effects of amphetamine and cocaine. Furthermore, although opioid systems may contribute to the conditioned rewarding effects of nicotine, they are not necessary for the interaction of nicotine with brain reward pathways.

15.5.4 Neurochemistry

Acute administration of stimulants increases extracellular DA concentrations in the Nacc and dorsal striatum (59). Increased mesoaccumbal DA transmission is thought to mediate the locomotor-activating and rewarding effects of stimulants (60), whereas increased mesostriatal DA transmission is implicated in mediating stimulant-evoked stereotypy and the habit-like behavior that characterizes addiction (61–63). Alterations in mesoaccumbal DA neurotransmission have also been implicated in the expression of behavioral sensitization, a process whereby the repeated intermittent administration of stimulants results in a persistent enhancement of their locomotor-activating and rewarding effects (64–66).

The technique of in vivo microdialysis has been used in conjunction with locomotor activity measures to examine the involvement of opioid receptors in modulating the behavioral and neurochemical effects of stimulants (67, 68). Pretreatment with naloxone (5.0 mg/kg; s.c.) attenuated amphetamine-induced increases in locomotor activity and decreased the striatal DA response to amphetamine (67). These findings were replicated and extended in a subsequent study using naloxone (5.0 mg/kg; s.c.). Amphetamine-induced increases in extracellular DA in both the striatum and the Nacc were attenuated by naloxone, as was amphetamine-induced increases in locomotion. Interestingly, the same dose of naloxone was ineffective in altering cocaine-induced increases in extracellular DA or locomotor activity (68), suggesting a distinct role of opioid receptors in mediating the neurochemical and behavioral-activating effects of amphetamine, but not cocaine.

VTA perfusion of morphine increases extracellular DA and decreases extracellular gamma-aminobutyric acid (GABA) concentrations in this same region; effects that are blocked by a moderate dose of naloxone (2 mg/kg) (69). GABAB receptor stimulation decreases amphetamine-induced locomotor behavior and the peak level of amphetamine-evoked striatal DA release (70), suggesting that inhibition of GABAB receptors may contribute to the increase in extracellular DA induced by amphetamine. Given that acute amphetamine administration increases PENK expression, amphetamine-induced increases in extracellular DA may reflect direct and indirect effects on DA neurotransmission that occur as a consequence of amphetamine-evoked increases in the release of endogenous opioid peptides (e.g., enkephalin) (68).

Mesoaccumbal and mesostriatal DA neurons express opioid peptides and receptors (71, 72). Microdialysis studies have shown that the basal activity of VTA DA neurons projecting to the Nacc is regulated by endogenous opioid peptide systems (2). In view of the role of mesoaccumbal DA neurons in mediating the behavioral effects of drugs of abuse, Holtzman and colleagues (73) examined whether opioid receptor blockade at the level of the DA cell body or terminals attenuates amphetamine-evoked increases in DA. Infusion of naloxone methiodide, which does not cross the blood-brain barrier, into the VTA attenuated amphetamine-induced increase in extracellular DA in the Nacc (73). In contrast, infusion into the Nacc was without effect. Similarly, its administration into the substantia nigra but not the striatum attenuated amphetamine-induced increases in striatal DA concentrations. These results indicate that amphetamine-evoked increases in accumbal and striatal DA levels are mediated, at least in part, via the release of endogenous opioid peptides and the resultant activation of opioid receptors at the level of the DA cell body. Further, they suggest that although opioid receptors are located in DA terminal regions and can regulate basal DA release, they do not mediate the interaction of opioid receptor antagonists with this stimulant.

15.6 Selective MOPr Antagonists

MOPr, endorphins, endomorphins, and enkephalins are present in the mesocorticolimbic and mesostriatal DA systems. β-Endorphin (74) and enkephalins (75) bind with high affinity to MOPr and DOPr, while endormophin-1 and -2 bind with high affinity and selectivity to MOPr (74). MOPr mRNA and binding sites are enriched in the striatum, Nacc, and ventral pallidum (76); areas implicated in mediating the effects of psychostimulants. Although opioid receptor density is low in the VTA, MOPr protein and mRNA are present (77). MOPr is preferentially located on non-DA dendrites and axon terminals, but some scattered DA cells expressing MOPr are seen (78). Although non-DA cells are the primary sites of MOPr action in the VTA, MOPr agonists and antagonists can influence DA release at the level of the DA terminal (79). MOPr immunoreactivity is observed in the Nacc, and in the shell, MOPr are localized on the plasma membrane and axon terminals of GABA neurons (80). Despite anatomical evidence that MOPr is strategically positioned to modulate reward circuitry, few studies have investigated the influence of selective MOPr antagonists in animal models of reward. Such studies are essential since, as noted above, naloxone and naltrexone bind to MOPr, DOPr, and KOPr.

15.6.1 Drug Self-Administration

Infusion of the irreversible MOPr antagonist beta-funaltrexamine (β-FNA) into either the VTA or Nacc significantly decreased cocaine self-administration in rats maintained on a PR schedule of reinforcement (Table 15.1). This effect was apparent for 5 days after antagonist infusion indicating its relative persistence. In contrast, responding of animals performing cocaine self-administration on an FR1 schedule was unaltered. Antagonist administration into the dorsal striatum had no effect on self-administration maintained on either schedule indicating regional specificity (81). The attenuation of self-administration under one reinforcement schedule but not another highlights the importance of this variable in evaluating and detecting opioid/stimulant interactions. Indeed as discussed above, differences in the effects of naloxone and naltrexone were observed in ICSS studies that used FR vs FI schedules, and in self-administration studies which differed in FR response requirements. As discussed by Roberts et al. (82), FR schedules provide a sensitive assay for evaluating the rate of drug intake, while PR schedule measures motivational aspects of drug reinforcement (22). The marked effect of β-FNA on cocaine under a PR schedule suggests that blockade of mesoaccumbal MOPr may selectively decrease motivation to self-administer cocaine.

The selective MOPr antagonist, Cys-Tyr-D-Trp-Arg-Thr-Pen-Thr-NH2 (CTAP), has been used to evaluate the effects of MOPr blockade on the reinstatement of cocaine self-administration produced by a priming injection of cocaine or morphine (83). Intraventral pallidal administration of CTAP (0.03–3.0 μg) dose-dependently decreased reinstatement produced by either drug. Although intra-accumbal administration of

CTAP reduced cocaine-primed reinstatement, this effect was not statistically significant, indicating that diffusion of the antagonist cannot account for efficacy of the ventral pallidal injection site. These data suggest that reinstatement of cocaine-seeking behavior produced by drug priming is dependent on ventral pallidal MOPr.

15.6.2 Neurochemistry

Studies examining the influence of MOPr antagonists on the neurochemical effects of stimulants are limited. Selective blockade of CNS MOPr receptors by intracisternal infusion of β-FNA (10 μg) attenuated amphetamine-induced (s.c.) increases in extracellular DA concentrations that occur in the Nacc. This effect was pathway specific since no alteration in the striatal DA response was seen (84). The results in the striatum contrast with those observed with nonselective opioid receptor antagonists (see above) and may indicate an involvement of multiple opioid receptor types in mediating the effects of naloxone and naltrexone in striatum. The efficacy of MOPr blockade in attenuating amphetamine-evoked DA increased in the Nacc, however, clearly demonstrates that the blockade of centrally located MOPr is sufficient to inhibit the response of accumbal DA neurons to acute amphetamine.

The mechanisms by which MOPr antagonists interact with amphetamine is unclear. MOPR agonists increase extracellular DA concentrations in the Nacc, an effect that has been attributed to hyperpolarization of GABAergic neurons in the VTA and disinhibition of DA neurons projecting to the nucleus accumbens (85). Consistent with this hypothesis, infusion of morphine or selective MOPr agonists into the VTA inhibit GABA release in this region (69, 86). Studies with selective MOPr antagonists have also revealed tonically active VTA MOPr that regulate basal GABA release in the VTA and DA release in the Nacc (2, 86, 87). Therefore, MOPr blockade in the VTA, by preventing GABA inhibition of DA neuronal activity may underlie the reduction in amphetamine-evoked DA levels. Amphetamine-evoked release of opioid peptides in the VTA has not been examined. However, microdialysis studies have shown that acute administration of amphetamine as well as cocaine increase β-endorphin release in the Nacc (88).

Kalivas and colleagues have begun to examine the influence of MOPr blockade on neurochemical alterations that occur during compulsive drug seeking (83). Using microdialysis in combination with a reinstatement procedure, these investigators focused on the ventral pallidum. This region is innervated by spiny neurons originating in the Nacc that release GABA and enkephalin (89) and is implicated in mediating the rewarding effects of cocaine. Furthermore, blockade of pallidal MOPr attenuates the conditioned rewarding effects of cocaine (50–52). In animals in which cocaine self-administration was extinguished, a priming injection of cocaine reinstated compulsive cocaine seeking, an effect that was attenuated by intrapallidal infusion of the MOPr antagonist, CTAP. In contrast to MOPr blockade, administration of morphine reinstated lever pressing for cocaine. Microdialysis studies revealed a marked reduction in GABA levels in response to the priming injection of cocaine (83). This decrease was attenuated by CTAP, suggesting the possibility that the MOPr antagonist-induced attenuation of reinstatement may be linked to a normalization of GABA levels. However, the cocaine-evoked reduction in GABA levels was observed in animals that reinstated lever pressing and in those that did not. Therefore, although MOPr blockade attenuates reinstatement, the role of GABA in reinstatement and the effects of CTAP remain ill defined. A cocaine-induced, MOPR-dependent reduction in ventral pallidal GABA levels may be a necessary, but not sufficient for reinstatement of compulsive cocaine seeking. A role of ventral pallidal GABA in behavioral activation and sensitization has been suggested and the effects observed may reflect these processes or adaptations that occur as a consequence of repeated cocaine exposure. Interestingly, withdrawal from contingent or noncontingent cocaine administration increases PENK in the Nacc and neurons expressing this opioid peptide project to the ventral tegmentum (90).

15.7 Selective DOPr Antagonists

DOPr are enriched in the mesoaccumbal and mesostriatal systems. Expression of DOPr mRNA and binding sites is higher in the Nacc shell as compared to the core. In the shell, DOPr are localized primarily on non-DA terminals and dendritic spines that contain GABA and other neuropeptides (91). Enkephalins bind to both MOPr and DOPr but bind with higher affinity to DOPr (74, 79). PENK mRNA is high in both accumbal subregions (92).

15.7.1 Drug Self-Administration

The effects of selective DOPr antagonists on the maintenance of cocaine self-administration have been investigated in rats (93, 94) and rhesus monkeys (Table 15.1) (95). Using a FR schedule in rats, De Vries et al. (94) reported no effect of acute naltrindole (0.3–3.0 mg/kg; i.p.) administration on cocaine (0.25 and 1.0 mg/kg/infusion) self-administration. The antagonist doses employed were those previously shown to be DOPr selective in other assays and to attenuate the development of behavioral sensitization to cocaine (96, 97). Therefore, the lack of effect cannot be attributed to an ineffective dose range. A higher dose of naltrindole (10 mg/kg) resulted in a slight, but nonsignificant attenuation of low-dose cocaine self-administration. However, locomotor activity was reduced, indicating a generalized depression of behavior. In a separate series of experiments, rats self-administering cocaine were pretreated once daily with naltrindole (1.0 mg/kg) for 3 consecutive days. Cocaine self-administration was assessed 24 h following treatment cessation. Again, no alteration in responding for cocaine was seen. These findings contrast with those showing a marked reduction in cocaine responding in response to higher doses of naltrindole (93). An explanation for the discrepant results is not readily apparent since the rat strain did not differ and both the cocaine dose and the FR schedule employed were similar. Although the latter study used female rats, gender differences in DOPr-mediated responses have not been reported. However, a dose of 3.0 mg/kg (s.c.) exhibits KOPr-like activity and receptor selectivity may be an issue (98).

Only one study has examined the influence of DOPr antagonists on cocaine self-administration in nonhuman primates. As with the rat, variable effects were observed. Naltrindole decreased self-administration in three of four animals. As discussed by Negus (95), the profile of antagonism differed from that seen against DOPr agonists. In studies of cocaine, the dose-response curve for naltrindole was biphasic rather than linear, and not all animals exhibited a similar response. Furthermore, in contrast to DOPr agonists, when effective doses of antagonist were retested, a decrease or no antagonism was seen (95). Together the findings in rodents and nonhuman primates indicate inconsistent effects of DOPr antagonists on cocaine self-administration. Whether these inconsistencies reflect individual differences in DOPr modulation that could be exploited therapeutically is unclear. Given, however, the narrow dose-effect curve observed in both rodent and primate studies, this possibility appears unlikely.

15.7.2 Conditioned Place Preference

Low doses of naltrindole or naltriben (0.03–0.3 mg/kg) are ineffective in attenuating CPP produced by cocaine or methamphetamine in rodents (99). However, higher doses (1.0–3.0 mg/kg) attenuated the conditioned rewarding effects of these agents in all but one study (94, 99, 100). Although these studies suggest an involvement of DOPr in the conditioning of psychostimulant reward, this interpretation should be viewed with some caution. First, it is based on the assumption that the effective doses are DOPr selective. Consistent with this assumption, in vitro findings have demonstrated a markedly higher affinity of naltrindole and naltriben for DOPr than other opioid receptor subtypes. However, evidence that naltrindole exerts KOPr-mediated effects at doses exceeding 1.0 mg/kg has been obtained (98).

Prior, intermittent administration of stimulants and other drugs of abuse results in a long-lasting augmentation of their behavioral effects. This phenomenon referred to as sensitization has been hypothesized to lead to an incentive-salience state described as "wanting" and to contribute to the wanting or craving that characterizes addiction (65, 66). Sensitization to the conditioned rewarding effects of cocaine has been demonstrated (97, 101, 102). In animals with a prior history of cocaine or amphetamine administration, the minimum dose of drug that produces CPP is decreased and the magnitude of conditioning is increased, consistent with the development of sensitization. This sensitized response is evident when conditioning commences weeks after the cessation of repeated drug treatment, indicating it is long-lasting. Studies in rats have shown that low doses of naltrindole or naltriben (0.03–0.3 mg/kg) administered in combination with repeated injections of cocaine prevent the development of the enhanced conditioned response to cocaine. When the same doses of antagonists were administered during conditioning, no attenuation of CPP was seen (97).

15.7.3 Intracranial Self-Stimulation

The influence of naltrindole on cocaine- (103) and methylenedioxymethamphetamine (MDMA)- (104) evoked alterations in medial forebrain bundle self-stimulation has been evaluated in rats (Table 15.2). Naltrindole (3.0 mg/kg) did not alter response rates, but blocked cocaine-induced (5 mg/kg) increases in responding for lower intensities of brain stimulation (103). A higher dose of naltrindole (10.0 mg/kg) blocked the MDMA-induced (2 mg/kg; s.c.) increase in ICSS (104).

15.7.4 Neurochemistry

Selective DOPr antagonists attenuate amphetamine-evoked increases in extracellular DA levels in a region-specific manner. In vivo microdialysis revealed a reduction in amphetamine-evoked striatal DA levels in response to intracisternal infusion of naltrindole (3.0–30.0 μg). In contrast, the increase in accumbal DA levels produced by the same doses of amphetamine was unaffected by antagonist treatment (84). These results are opposite to those observed with a selective MOPr antagonist, suggesting that MOPr and DOPr antagonists differentially affect amphetamine-induced release of DA in the striatum and Nacc.

The effect of intrastriatal perfusion of naltrindole on amphetamine-evoked striatal glutamate levels has been investigated (105). As with DA, naltrindole (10–100 μM) decreased amphetamine-evoked glutamate levels in a concentration-dependent manner. A selective DOPr agonist reversed the effect of naltrindole, confirming DOPr mediation.

15.8 Selective KOPr Antagonists

DYN immunoreactivity is found in the mesoaccumbal and mesostriatal systems, as well as in their afferent and efferent projection sites (106). KOPr protein is enriched in regions comprising these systems (107). In the Nacc, the majority of KOPr immunoreactivity is found in axons (108) and terminals having the morphological features of DA containing neurons (109). This localization of KOPr is consistent with neurochemical studies indicating that KOPr in the Nacc regulates the activity of mesoaccumbal DA neurons. Colocalization of KOPr with the DA transporter in axons of accumbal DA neurons has been described (110). Such findings are important in view of evidence that synthetic KOPr agonists regulate DA transporter function in the Nacc (111) and the involvement of this transporter in the action of stimulants.

15.8.1 Drug Self-Administration

The effects of selective KOPr antagonists on cocaine self-administration have been studied in rats (112) and nonhuman primates (Table 15.1) (113, 114). In rats, treatment with the long-acting selective KOPr antagonist norbinaltorphimine 48 h before initiation of daily cocaine self-administration sessions suppressed responding for a low dose of cocaine (0.03 mg/infusion). Self-administration of a higher dose (0.06 mg/infusion) (112) was unaffected. Although the low-dose response suppression is consistent with an attenuation of reward, testing of additional cocaine doses is needed to verify this hypothesis. In rhesus monkeys reliably self-administering cocaine, norbinaltorphimine (0.064 mg/kg/min × 50 min; i.v.) failed to alter cocaine or food self-administration, but blocked the decrease in cocaine (0.01 and 0.032 mg/kg/injection) self-administration produced by KOPr agonists (113). The same treatment did not affect responding for cocaine in a concurrent choice procedure for food and cocaine (114).

Two studies have examined the involvement of KOPr in reinstatement of cocaine responding produced by footshock or a priming injections of cocaine. In contrast to selective KOPr agonists that attenuate reinstatement produced by a priming injection of cocaine, intracerebroventricular infusion of norbinaltorphimine was ineffective in modulating compulsive cocaine seeking (115). Similarly, a novel KOPr antagonist, (3*R*)-7-hydroxy-*N*-{(1*S*)-1-{[(3*R*,4*R*)-4-(3-hydroxyphenyl)-3,4-dimethyl-1-piperidinyl]methyl}-2-methylpropyl}-1,2,3,4-tetrahydro-3-isoquinoline-carboxamide (JDTic) administered 24 h before testing failed to modify cocaine-evoked reinstatement of responding. However, footshock-induced reinstatement of cocaine seeking produced was attenuated, indicating that KOPr blockade may affect stress-induced reinstatement of compulsive cocaine seeking (116).

15.8.2 Conditioned Place Preference

KOPr agonists attenuate the enhancement of cocaine-induced CPP produced by prior repeated administration of cocaine, suggesting that an increase in the activity of KOPr systems attenuates the development of sensitization to the conditioned rewarding effects of cocaine (117). Although norbinaltorphimine prevented agonist-induced attenuation of sensitization, administration of the antagonist alone did not affect the development of the sensitization, suggesting that endogenous KOPr systems do not modulate this response.

Stress increases DYN levels (118). In view of the link between stress and vulnerability to addiction, attention has focused on the role of KOPr systems in modulating stress-induced alterations in the rewarding effects of cocaine. In contrast to its lack of effect on the development of sensitization to the conditioned rewarding effects of cocaine, pretreatment with norbinaltorphimine prevents stress-induced potentiation of cocaine-evoked CPP in mice (119–121). These findings parallel those of reinstatement studies and suggest that blockade of KOPr may be effective in the treatment of stress-induced relapse to cocaine addiction.

15.8.3 Intracranial Self-Stimulation

Withdrawal from various drugs of abuse increases the threshold amount of stimulation required to sustain ICSS. This finding has been interpreted as reflecting anhedonia (122, 123). Consistent with this interpretation, antidepressants attenuate withdrawal-induced elevations in thresholds. Synthetic KOPr agonists increase ICSS thresholds, suggesting that KOPr activation produces depressant-like behavior in experimental animals (124). Although KOPr antagonists can decrease this effect, there is no effect of KOPr antagonists norbinaltorphimine (125) or 5′-acetamidinoethylnaltrindole (ANTI) (124, 126) on ICSS alone. Other approaches have been used to demonstrate antidepressant-like effects of KOPr antagonists. Decreasing activity of CREB, a transcription factor that regulates PDYN expression activity, in the Nacc produces an antidepressant-like effect in rodent models. Intra-accumbal infusion of norbinaltorphimine produced a similar behavioral phenotype indicating that KOPr blockade in this region is sufficient to produce an antidepressant-like effect. Antidepressant-like effects of other KOPr antagonists, including ANTI, have been observed in the forced swim test (126).

15.8.4 Neurochemistry

Both pharmacological and gene-targeting techniques have shown that endogenous KOPr systems regulate the basal activity of mesoaccumbal DA neurons. In contrast to KOPr agonists, which decrease mesoaccumbal DA transmission, infusion of norbinaltorphimine into the Nacc increases DA levels in this brain region. No alteration in accumbal DA levels is observed following antagonist infusion into the VTA, indicating that a tonically active KOPr system located at the level of the DA nerve terminal inhibits DA release (2). Studies in mice lacking the KOPr gene have provided additional data consistent with this hypothesis (127). Striatal DA levels are increased following intra-striatal infusion of norbinaltorphimine, indicating tonic KOPr inhibition of mesostriatal DA transmission (128). KOPr antagonist infusion into the substantia nigra reticulata increases extracellular DA concentrations in this region as well as the striatum, suggesting a critical role of KOPr in regulating dendritic and terminal DA release in the mesostriatal system.

The repeated administration of stimulants increases PDYN expression in the striatum (3, 129, 130). Decreases in Nacc expression have been reported. Similar effects are observed in response to other manipulations that enhance DA transmission (131). In view of the inhibitory effects of KOPr agonists on DA transmission, it has been hypothesized that the activity of KOPr systems is increased in response to stimulant use and that this increase is a homeostatic mechanism that opposes DA neuronal dysregulation. Consistent with this hypothesis coadministration of KOPr agonists with cocaine prevents alterations in basal and cocaine-evoked DA dynamics that occur in the Nacc as a consequence of repeated cocaine administration (111). Although the ability of KOPr antagonists to normalize these alterations has not been examined, a recent microdialysis study showed that prior administration of norbinaltorphimine results in a marked increase in cocaine-evoked DA levels in the Nacc (127). A similar effect is observed in mice lacking the KOPr gene, suggesting that hypofunction of KOPr systems may lead to enhanced vulnerability to cocaine. Both manipulations led to an enhancement of the locomotor-activating effects of cocaine. The magnitude of the response was analogous to animals that had received a repeated cocaine treatment regimen that produces behavioral sensitization, suggesting that lack of KOPr may result in a sensitized phenotype.

15.9 Conclusions

Consistent with the postulated role of endogenous opioid systems in the regulation of mood and incentive motivation, pretreatment with naloxone attenuates the rewarding effects of ICSS. In contrast to nonselective antagonists, DOPr and KOPr antagonists alone do not alter ICSS. Studies, however, examining the influence of selective MOPr antagonists are lacking. Therefore, although it is apparent that endogenous opioid systems regulate the setpoint for reward, whether MOPr or multiple opioid receptor systems subserve this function awaits clarification. Given the documented role of MOPr in the regulation of mesoaccumbal DA transmission, studies evaluating the role of this opioid receptor type are warranted.

Data from both humans and experimental animals are consistent with the hypothesis that stimulant use modulates the activity of endogenous opioid systems. Studies assessing the effects of naloxone and naltrexone clearly indicate that the activity of opioid systems is critical for the conditioning of psychostimulant reward and the facilitation of ICSS produced by amphetamine and cocaine. Most studies have shown that these antagonists attenuate cocaine self-administration and the reinstatement of compulsive cocaine seeking. However, as discussed, these findings have not been universal and may reflect differences in the reinforcement schedules employed, degree of food deprivation, as well as the species tested. Taken together, published data provide strong evidence that endogenous opioid peptide systems are a critical component of brain circuits that are engaged by stimulants and which mediate their rewarding effects. A far less consistent picture has emerged from studies examining the effects of selective opioid receptor antagonists. Such inconsistencies may reflect the limited data set available as well as differences in the procedures used. Alternatively, they may indicate that the function of one opioid receptor system (e.g., MOPr) is readily subserved by another (e.g., DOPr). If such is the case, then effective treatments that target opioid systems will require the blockade of multiple opioid receptor types.

As is apparent from this chapter, many questions remain as to the mechanisms mediating the interactions of opioid receptor antagonists with psychostimulants. In view of recent data indicating an association between vulnerability to drug abuse and polymorphisms of genes encoding opioid receptors and their endogenous ligands (132, 133), preclinical studies addressing this issue are essential.

Acknowledgments This work was supported by the Intramural Research Program of the National Institutes of Health, National Institute on Drug Abuse. A special thank to Teyana Joseph for her administrative assistance.

References

1. Substance Abuse and Mental Health Services Administration. Results from the 2004 National Survey on Drug Use and Health: National Findings (Office of Applied Studies, NSDUH Series H-28, DHHS Publication No. SMA 05-4062). 2005. Rockville, MD.
2. Spanagel R, Herz A, Shippenberg T. Opposing tonically active endogenous opioid systems modulate the mesolimbic dopaminergic pathway. PNAS 1992; 89(6):2046–2050.
3. Daunais JB, Roberts DC, McGinty JF. Cocaine self-administration increases preprodynorphin, but not c-fos, mRNA in rat striatum. Neuroreport 1993; 4(5):543–546.
4. Hurd YL. Cocaine effects on dopamine and opioid peptide neural systems: implications for human cocaine abuse. NIDA Res Monogr 1996; 163:94–116.
5. Hurd YL, Svensson P, Ponten M. The role of dopamine, dynorphin, and CART systems in the ventral striatum and amygdala in cocaine abuse. Ann N Y Acad Sci 1999; 877:499–506.
6. Simpson JN, Wang JQ, McGinty JF. Repeated amphetamine administration induces a prolonged augmentation of phosphorylated cyclase response element-binding protein and Fos-related antigen immunoreactivity in rat striatum. Neuroscience 1995; 69(2):441–457.
7. Unterwald EM, Cox BM, Kreek MJ, Cote TE, Izenwasser S. Chronic repeated cocaine administration alters basal and opioid-regulated adenylyl cyclase activity. Synapse 1993; 15(1):33–38.
8. Unterwald EM, Fillmore J, Kreek MJ. Chronic repeated cocaine administration increases dopamine D1 receptor-mediated signal transduction. Eur J Pharmacol 1996; 318(1): 31–35.
9. Beninger RJ, Hahn BL. Pimozide blocks establishment but not expression of amphetamine-produced environment-specific conditioning. Science 1983; 220(4603):1304–1306.
10. Beninger RJ, Herz RS. Pimozide blocks establishment but not expression of cocaine-produced environment-specific conditioning. Life Sci 1986; 38(15):1425–1431.
11. Morency MA, Beninger RJ. Dopaminergic substrates of cocaine-induced place conditioning. Brain Res 1986; 399(1):33–41.
12. Yokel RA, Wise RA. Increased lever pressing for amphetamine after pimozide in rats: implications for a dopamine theory of reward. Science 1975; 187(4176):547–549.
13. Crespo JA, Manzanares J, Oliva JM, Corchero J, Palomo T, Ambrosio E. Extinction of cocaine self-administration produces a differential time-related regulation of proenkephalin gene expression in rat brain. Neuropsychopharmacology 2001; 25(2):185–194.
14. Kelley AE. Ventral striatal control of appetitive motivation: role in ingestive behavior and reward-related learning. Neurosci Biobehav Rev 2004; 27(8):765–776.

15. Spangler R, Ho A, Zhou Y, Maggos CE, Yuferov V, Kreek MJ. Regulation of kappa opioid receptor mRNA in the rat brain by "binge" pattern cocaine administration and correlation with preprodynorphin mRNA. Brain Res Mol Brain Res 1996; 38(1):71–76.
16. Przewlocka B, Lason W. Adaptive changes in the proenkephalin and D2 dopamine receptor mRNA expression after chronic cocaine in the nucleus accumbens and striatum of the rat. Eur Neuropsychopharmacol 1995; 5(4):465–469.
17. Wang JQ, McGinty JF. Muscarinic receptors regulate striatal neuropeptide gene expression in normal and amphetamine-treated rats. Neuroscience 1996; 75(1):43–56.
18. Gonzalez-Nicolini MV, Berglind W, Cole KS, Keogh CL, McGinty JF. Local mu and delta opioid receptors regulate amphetamine-induced behavior and neuropeptide mRNA in the striatum. Neuroscience 2003; 121(2):387–398.
19. Hurd YL, Herkenham M. Molecular alterations in the neostriatum of human cocaine addicts. Synapse 1993; 13(4):357–369.
20. Arnold JM, Roberts DC. A critique of fixed and progressive ratio schedules used to examine the neural substrates of drug reinforcement. Pharmacol Biochem Behav 1997; 57(3): 441–447.
21. Sanchis-Segura C, Spanagel R. Behavioural assessment of drug reinforcement and addictive features in rodents: an overview. Addict Biol 2006; 11(1):2–38.
22. Richardson NR, Roberts DC. Progressive ratio schedules in drug self-administration studies in rats: a method to evaluate reinforcing efficacy. J Neurosci Methods 1996; 66(1):1–11.
23. Comer SD, Lac ST, Curtis LK, Carroll ME. Effects of buprenorphine and naltrexone on reinstatement of cocaine-reinforced responding in rats. J Pharmacol Exp Ther 1993; 267(3):1470–1477.
24. Childress AR, Ehrman R, Roohsenow DJ, Robbins SJ, O'Brien CP. Classically conditioned factors in drug dependence. In: Lowinson W, Luiz P, Millman RB, Langard JG, editors. Substance abuse: a comprehansive text book. Baltimore: Williams & Wilkins, 1992: 56–69.
25. O'Brien CP, McLellan AT. Myths about the treatment of addiction. Lancet 1996; 347(8996): 237–240.
26. Bardo MT, Bevins RA. Conditioned place preference: what does it add to our preclinical understanding of drug reward? Psychopharmacology (Berl) 2000; 153(1):31–43.
27. Bardo MT, Valone JM, Bevins RA. Locomotion and conditioned place preference produced by acute intravenous amphetamine: role of dopamine receptors and individual differences in amphetamine self-administration. Psychopharmacology (Berl) 1999; 143(1):39–46.
28. Olds J. Self-stimulation of the brain; its use to study local effects of hunger, sex, and drugs. Science 1958; 127(3294):315–324.
29. Olds J, Milner P. Positive reinforcement produced by electrical stimulation of septal area and other regions of rat brain. J Comp Physiol Psychol 1954; 47(6):419–427.
30. Schaefer GJ. Opiate antagonists and rewarding brain stimulation. Neurosci Biobehav Rev 1988; 12(1):1–17.
31. Schaefer GJ, Michael RP. Interactions of naloxone with morphine, amphetamine and phencyclidine on fixed interval responding for intracranial self-stimulation in rats. Psychopharmacology (Berl) 1990; 102(2):263–268.
32. Magnan J, Paterson SJ, Tavani A, Kosterlitz HW. The binding spectrum of narcotic analgesic drugs with different agonist and antagonist properties. Naunyn Schmiedebergs Arch Pharmacol 1982; 319(3):197–205.
33. Emmerson PJ, Liu MR, Woods JH, Medzihradsky F. Binding affinity and selectivity of opioids at mu, delta and kappa receptors in monkey brain membranes. J Pharmacol Exp Ther 1994; 271(3):1630–1637.
34. Kuzmin AV, Gerrits MA, Van Ree JM, Zvartau EE. Naloxone inhibits the reinforcing and motivational aspects of cocaine addiction in mice. Life Sci 1997; 60(18):L-64.
35. De Vry J, Donselaar I, Van Ree JM. Food deprivation and acquisition of intravenous cocaine self-administration in rats: effect of naltrexone and haloperidol. J Pharmacol Exp Ther 1989; 251(2):735–740.

36. Ramsey NF, Van Ree JM. Intracerebroventricular naltrexone treatment attenuates acquisition of intravenous cocaine self-administration in rats. Pharmacol Biochem Behav 1991; 40(4): 807–810.
37. Ramsey NF, Gerrits MA, Van Ree JM. Naltrexone affects cocaine self-administration in naive rats through the ventral tegmental area rather than dopaminergic target regions. Eur Neuropsychopharmacol 1999; 9(1–2):93–99.
38. Ramsey NF, Van Ree JM. Chronic pretreatment with naltrexone facilitates acquisition of intravenous cocaine self-administration in rats. Eur Neuropsychopharmacol 1990; 1(1): 55–61.
39. Tempel A, Gardner EL, Zukin RS. Neurochemical and functional correlates of naltrexone-induced opiate receptor up-regulation. J Pharmacol Exp Ther 1985; 232(2):439–444.
40. Lesscher H, Bailey A, Burbach J, Van Ree J, Kitchen I, Gerrits M. Receptor-selective changes in μ-, Δ- and κ-opioid receptors after chronic naltrexone treatment in mice. Eur J Neurosci 2003; 17(5):1006–1012.
41. Corrigall WA, Coen KM. Opiate antagonists reduce cocaine but not nicotine self-administration. Psychopharmacology (Berl) 1991; 104(2):167–170.
42. Mello NK, Mendelson JH, Bree MP, Lukas SE. Buprenorphine and naltrexone effects on cocaine self-administration by rhesus monkeys. J Pharmacol Exp Ther 1990; 254(3):926–939.
43. Mello NK, Lukas SE, Mendelson JH, Drieze J. Naltrexone-buprenorphine interactions: effects on cocaine self-administration. Neuropsychopharmacology 1993; 9(3):211–224.
44. Ettenberg A, Pettit HO, Bloom FE, Koob GF. Heroin and cocaine intravenous self-administration in rats: mediation by separate neural systems. Psychopharmacology (Berl) 1982; 78(3):204–209.
45. Carroll ME, Lac ST, Walker MJ, Kragh R, Newman T. Effects of naltrexone on intravenous cocaine self-administration in rats during food satiation and deprivation. J Pharmacol Exp Ther 1986; 238(1):1–7.
46. Killian AK, Bonese K, Schuster CR. The effects of naloxone on behavior maintained by cocaine and heroin injections in the rhesus monkey. Drug Alcohol Depend 1978; 3(4):243–251.
47. Anggadiredja K, Sakimura K, Hiranita T, Yamamoto T. Naltrexone attenuates cue- but not drug-induced methamphetamine seeking: a possible mechanism for the dissociation of primary and secondary reward. Brain Res 2004; 1021(2):272–276.
48. Gerrits MA, Kuzmin AV, Van Ree JM. Reinstatement of cocaine-seeking behavior in rats is attenuated following repeated treatment with the opioid receptor antagonist naltrexone. Eur Neuropsychopharmacol 2005; 15(3):297–303.
49. Trujillo KA, Belluzzi JD, Stein L. Naloxone blockade of amphetamine place preference conditioning. Psychopharmacology (Berl) 1991; 104(2):265–274.
50. Skoubis PD, Maidment NT. Blockade of ventral pallidal opioid receptors induces a conditioned place aversion and attenuates acquisition of cocaine place preference in the rat. Neuroscience 2003; 119(1):241–249.
51. Hubner CB, Koob GF. The ventral pallidum plays a role in mediating cocaine and heroin self-administration in the rat. Brain Res 1990; 508(1):20–29.
52. Gong W, Neill D, Justice JB, Jr. Conditioned place preference and locomotor activation produced by injection of psychostimulants into ventral pallidum. Brain Res 1996; 707(1):64–74.
53. Walters CL, Cleck JN, Kuo YC, Blendy JA. Mu-opioid receptor and CREB activation are required for nicotine reward. Neuron 2005; 46(6):933–943.
54. Esposito RU, Perry W, Kornetsky C. Effects of d-amphetamine and naloxone on brain stimulation reward. Psychopharmacology (Berl) 1980; 69(2):187–191.
55. Franklin KB, Robertson A. Effects and interactions of naloxone and amphetamine on self-stimulation of the prefrontal cortex and dorsal tegmentum. Pharmacol Biochem Behav 1982; 16(3):433–436.
56. Bain GT, Kornetsky C. Naloxone attenuation of the effect of cocaine on rewarding brain stimulation. Life Sci 1987; 40(11):1119–1125.

57. McGregor IS, Atrens DM, Jackson DM. Cocaine facilitation of prefrontal cortex self-stimulation: a microstructural and pharmacological analysis. Psychopharmacology (Berl) 1992; 106(2):239–247.
58. Huston-Lyons D, Kornetsky C. Effects of nicotine on the threshold for rewarding brain stimulation in rats. Pharmacol Biochem Behav 1992; 41(4):755–759.
59. Di Chiara G, Imperato A. Drugs abused by humans preferentially increase synaptic dopamine concentrations in the mesolimbic system of freely moving rats. Proc Natl Acad Sci USA 1988; 85(14 – July 15, 1988):5274–5278.
60. Wise RA, Bozarth MA. A psychomotor stimulant theory of addiction. Psychol Rev 1987; 94(4):469–492.
61. Iversen SD, Kelly PH, Miller RJ, Seviour P. Proceedings: amphetamine and apomorphine responses in the rat after lesion of mesolimbic or striatal dopamine neurones. Br J Pharmacol 1975; 54(2):244p.
62. Kelly PH, Seviour PW, Iversen SD. Amphetamine and apomorphine responses in the rat following 6-OHDA lesions of the nucleus accumbens septi and corpus striatum. Brain Res 1975; 94(3):507–522.
63. Ito R, Dalley JW, Robbins TW, Everitt BJ. Dopamine release in the dorsal striatum during cocaine-seeking behavior under the control of a drug-associated cue. J Neurosci 2002; 22(14):6247–6253.
64. Kalivas PW, Sorg BA, Hooks MS. The pharmacology and neural circuitry of sensitization to psychostimulants. Behav Pharmacol 1993; 4(4):315–334.
65. Robinson TE, Berridge KC. The neural basis of drug craving: an incentive-sensitization theory of addiction. Brain Res Rev 1993; 18(3):247–291.
66. Robinson TE, Berridge KC. Incentive-sensitization and addiction. Addiction 2001; 96(1):103–114.
67. Hooks MS, Jones DN, Justice JB, Jr., Holtzman SG. Naloxone reduces amphetamine-induced stimulation of locomotor activity and in vivo dopamine release in the striatum and nucleus accumbens. Pharmacol Biochem Behav 1992; 42(4):765–770.
68. Schad CA, Justice JB, Jr., Holtzman SG. Naloxone reduces the neurochemical and behavioral effects of amphetamine but not those of cocaine. Eur J Pharmacol 1995; 275(1):9–16.
69. Klitenick MA, DeWitte P, Kalivas PW. Regulation of somatodendritic dopamine release in the ventral tegmental area by opioids and GABA: an in vivo microdialysis study. J Neurosci 1992; 12(7):2623–2632.
70. Zhou W, Mailloux AW, Jung BJ, Edmunds HS, Jr., McGinty JF. GABAB receptor stimulation decreases amphetamine-induced behavior and neuropeptide gene expression in the striatum. Brain Res 2004; 1004(1–2):18–28.
71. Moore RY, Bloom FE. Central catecholamine neuron systems: anatomy and physiology of the dopamine systems. Annu Rev Neurosci 1978; 1:129–169.
72. Pollard H, Llorens-Cortes C, Schwartz JC. Enkephalin receptors on dopaminergic neurones in rat striatum. Nature 1977; 268(5622):745–747.
73. Schad CA, Justice JB, Jr., Holtzman SG. Endogenous opioids in dopaminergic cell body regions modulate amphetamine-induced increases in extracellular dopamine levels in the terminal regions. J Pharmacol Exp Ther 2002; 300(3):932–938.
74. Zadina JE, Hackler L, Ge LJ, Kastin AJ. A potent and selective endogenous agonist for the mu-opiate receptor. Nature 1997; 386(6624):499–502.
75. Garzon M, Pickel VM. Ultrastructural localization of enkephalin and mu-opioid receptors in the rat ventral tegmental area. Neuroscience 2002; 114(2):461–474.
76. Mansour A, Fox CA, Thompson RC, Akil H, Watson SJ. mu-Opioid receptor mRNA expression in the rat CNS: comparison to mu-receptor binding. Brain Res 1994; 643(1–2): 245–265.
77. Mansour A, Fox CA, Burke S, Akil H, Watson SJ. Immunohistochemical localization of the cloned mu opioid receptor in the rat CNS7. J Chem Neuroanat 1995; 8(4):283–305.
78. Garzon M, Pickel VM. Plasmalemmal mu-opioid receptor distribution mainly in nondopaminergic neurons in the rat ventral tegmental area. Synapse 2001; 41(4):311–328.

79. Shippenberg TS, Chefer VI. Opioid modulation of psychomotor stimulant effects. In: Maldonado R, editor. Molecular biology of drug addiction. Totowa, NJ: Humana Press, 2003: 107–132.
80. Svingos AL, Moriwaki A, Wang JB, Uhl GR, Pickel VM. mu-Opioid receptors are localized to extrasynaptic plasma membranes of GABAergic neurons and their targets in the rat nucleus accumbens. J Neurosci 1997; 17(7):2585–2594.
81. Ward SJ, Martin TJ, Roberts DC. Beta-funaltrexamine affects cocaine self-administration in rats responding on a progressive ratio schedule of reinforcement. Pharmacol Biochem Behav 2003; 75(2):301–307.
82. Roberts DC, Bennett SA, Vickers GJ. The estrous cycle affects cocaine self-administration on a progressive ratio schedule in rats. Psychopharmacology (Berl) 1989; 98(3):408–411.
83. Tang XC, McFarland K, Cagle S, Kalivas PW. Cocaine-induced reinstatement requires endogenous stimulation of mu-opioid receptors in the ventral pallidum. J Neurosci 2005; 25(18):4512–4520.
84. Schad CA, Justice JB, Jr., Holtzman SG. Differential effects of delta- and mu-opioid receptor antagonists on the amphetamine-induced increase in extracellular dopamine in striatum and nucleus accumbens. J Neurochem 1996; 67(6):2292–2299.
85. Johnson SW, North RA. Opioids excite dopamine neurons by hyperpolarization of local interneurons. J Neurosci 1992; 12(2):483–488.
86. Chefer VI, Zapata A., Shippenberg T.S., Denoroy L. delta-Opioid receptor regulation of somatodendritic dopamine, glutamate, and GABA in the ventral tegmental area of the freely moving rat. Society for Neuroscience Abstracts. 2006.
87. Zhou W, Mailloux A, McGinty J. Intracerebral baclofen administration decreases amphetamine-induced behavior and neuropeptide gene expression in the striatum. Neuropsychopharmacology 2005; 30(5):880–890.
88. Olive MF, Koenig HN, Nannini MA, Hodge CW. Stimulation of endorphin neurotransmission in the nucleus accumbens by ethanol, cocaine, and amphetamine. J Neuroscience 2001; 21(RC184):1–5.
89. Zahm DS, Zaborszky L, Alones VE, Heimer L. Evidence for the coexistence of glutamate decarboxylase and Met-enkephalin immunoreactivities in axon terminals of rat ventral pallidum. Brain Res 1985; 325(1–2):317–321.
90. Lu XY, Ghasemzadeh MB, Kalivas PW. Expression of D1 receptor, D2 receptor, substance P and enkephalin messenger RNAs in the neurons projecting from the nucleus accumbens. Neuroscience 1998; 82(3):767–780.
91. Svingos AL, Clarke CL, Pickel VM. Localization of the delta-opioid receptor and dopamine transporter in the nucleus accumbens shell: implications for opiate and psychostimulant cross-sensitization. Synapse 1999; 34(1):1–10.
92. Mansour A, Thompson RC, Akil H, Watson SJ. Delta opioid receptor mRNA distribution in the brain: comparison to delta receptor binding and proenkephalin mRNA. J Chem Neuroanat 1993; 6(6):351–362.
93. Reid LD, Glick SD, Menkens KA, French ED, Bilsky EJ, Porreca F. Cocaine self-administration and naltrindole, a delta-selective opioid antagonist. Neuroreport 1995; 6(10):1409–1412.
94. De Vries TJ, Babovic-Vuksanovic D, Elmer G, Shippenberg TS. Lack of involvement of delta-opioid receptors in mediating the rewarding effects of cocaine. Psychopharmacology (Berl) 1995; 120(4):442–448.
95. Negus SS, Mello NK, Portoghese PS, Lukas SE, Mendelson JH. Role of delta opioid receptors in the reinforcing and discriminative stimulus effects of cocaine in rhesus monkeys. J Pharmacol Exp Ther 1995; 273(3):1245–1256.
96. Heidbreder C, Goldberg SR, Shippenberg TS. Inhibition of cocaine-induced sensitization by the delta-opioid receptor antagonist naltrindole. Eur J Pharmacol 1993; 243(2):123–127.
97. Shippenberg TS, Heidbreder C. The delta-opioid receptor antagonist naltrindole prevents sensitization to the conditioned rewarding effects of cocaine. Eur J Pharmacol 1995; 280(1): 55–61.

98. Stewart PE, Holper EM, Hammond DL. Delta antagonist and kappa agonist activity of naltriben: evidence for differential kappa interaction with the delta 1 and delta 2 opioid receptor subtypes. Life Sci 1994; 55(4):L79–L84.
99. Suzuki T, Mori T, Tsuji M, Misawa M, Nagase H. The role of delta-opioid receptor subtypes in cocaine- and methamphetamine-induced place preferences. Life Sci 1994; 55(17):L339–L344.
100. Menkens K, Bilsky EJ, Wild KD, Portoghese PS, Reid LD, Porreca F. Cocaine place preference is blocked by the delta-opioid receptor antagonist, naltrindole. Eur J Pharmacol 1992; 219(2):345–346.
101. Lett BT. Repeated exposures intensify rather than diminish the rewarding effects of amphetamine, morphine, and cocaine. Psychopharmacology (Berl) 1989; 98(3):357–362.
102. Sala M, Braida D, Colombo M, Groppetti A, Sacco S, Gori E, et al. Behavioral and biochemical evidence of opioidergic involvement in cocaine sensitization. J Pharmacol Exp Ther 1995; 274(1):450–457.
103. Reid LD, Hubbell CL, Glaccum MB, Bilsky EJ, Portoghese PS, Porreca F. Naltrindole, an opioid delta receptor antagonist, blocks cocaine-induced facilitation of responding for rewarding brain stimulation. Life Sci 1993; 52(9):L67–L71.
104. Reid LD, Hubbell CL, Tsai J, Fishkin MD, Amendola CA. Naltrindole, a delta-opioid antagonist, blocks MDMA's ability to enhance pressing for rewarding brain stimulation. Pharmacol Biochem Behav 1996; 53(2):477–480.
105. Rawls SM, McGinty JF. Delta opioid receptors regulate calcium-dependent, amphetamine-evoked glutamate levels in the rat striatum: an in vivo microdialysis study. Brain Res 2000; 861(2):296–304.
106. Van Bockstaele EJ, Gracy KN, Pickel VM. Dynorphin-immunoreactive neurons in the rat nucleus accumbens: ultrastructure and synaptic input from terminals containing substance P and/or dynorphin. J Comp Neurol 1995; 351(1):117–133.
107. Mansour A, Burke S, Pavlic RJ, Akil H, Watson SJ. Immunohistochemical localization of the cloned [kappa]1 receptor in the rat CNS and pituitary. Neuroscience 1996; 71(3):671–690.
108. Meshul CK, McGinty JF. Kappa opioid receptor immunoreactivity in the nucleus accumbens and caudate-putamen is primarily associated with synaptic vesicles in axons. Neuroscience 2000; 96(1):91–99.
109. Svingos AL, Colago EE, Pickel VM. Cellular sites for dynorphin activation of kappa-opioid receptors in the rat nucleus accumbens shell. J Neurosci 1999; 19(5):1804–1813.
110. Svingos AL, Chavkin C, Colago EE, Pickel VM. Major coexpression of kappa-opioid receptors and the dopamine transporter in nucleus accumbens axonal profiles. Synapse 2001; 42(3):185–192.
111. Thompson AC, Zapata A, Justice JB, Jr., Vaughan RA, Sharpe LG, Shippenberg TS. Kappa-opioid receptor activation modifies dopamine uptake in the nucleus accumbens and opposes the effects of cocaine. J Neurosci 2000; 20(24):9333–9340.
112. Kuzmin AV, Gerrits MAFM, Van Ree JM. [kappa]-Opioid receptor blockade with nor-binaltorphimine modulates cocaine self-administration in drug-naive rats. Eur J Pharmacol 1998; 358(3):197–202.
113. Negus SS, Mello NK, Portoghese PS, Lin CE. Effects of kappa opioids on cocaine self-administration by rhesus monkeys. J Pharmacol Exp Ther 1997; 282(1):44–55.
114. Negus SS. Effects of the kappa opioid agonist U50,488 and the kappa opioid antagonist nor-binaltorphimine on choice between cocaine and food in rhesus monkeys. Psychopharmacology 2004; 176(2):204–213.
115. Schenk S, Partridge B, Shippenberg TS. Reinstatement of extinguished drug-taking behavior in rats: effect of the kappa-opioid receptor agonist, U69593. Psychopharmacology (Berl) 2000; 151(1):85–90.
116. Beardsley P, Howard J, Shelton K, Carroll F. Differential effects of the novel kappa opioid receptor antagonist, JDTic, on reinstatement of cocaine-seeking induced by footshock stressors vs cocaine primes and its antidepressant-like effects in rats. Psychopharmacology 2005; 183(1):118–126.

117. Shippenberg TS, LeFevour A, Heidbreder C. kappa-Opioid receptor agonists prevent sensitization to the conditioned rewarding effects of cocaine. J Pharmacol Exp Ther 1996; 276(2):545–554.
118. Przewlocki R, Lason W, Hollt V, Silberring J, Herz A. The influence of chronic stress on multiple opioid peptide systems in the rat: pronounced effects upon dynorphin in spinal cord. Brain Res 1987; 413(2):213–219.
119. McLaughlin JP, Marton-Popovici M, Chavkin C. Kappa opioid receptor antagonism and prodynorphin gene disruption block stress-induced behavioral responses. J Neurosci 2003; 23(13):5674–5683.
120. McLaughlin JP, Li S, Valdez J, Chavkin TA, Chavkin C. Social defeat stress-induced behavioral responses are mediated by the endogenous kappa opioid system. Neuropsychopharmacology 2006; 31(6):1241–1248.
121. McLaughlin J, Land B, Li S, Pintar J, Chavkin C. Prior activation of kappa opioid receptors by U50, 488 mimics repeated forced swim stress to potentiate cocaine place preference conditioning. Neuropsychopharmacology 2006; 31(4):787–94.
122. Markou A, Hauger RL, Koob GF. Desmethylimipramine attenuates cocaine withdrawal in rats. Psychopharmacology (Berl) 1992; 109(3):305–314.
123. Wise RA, Munn E. Withdrawal from chronic amphetamine elevates baseline intracranial self-stimulation thresholds. Psychopharmacology (Berl) 1995; 117(2):130–136.
124. Todtenkopf MS, Marcus JF, Portoghese PS, Carlezon WA, Jr. Effects of kappa-opioid receptor ligands on intracranial self-stimulation in rats. Psychopharmacology (Berl) 2004; 172(4):463–470.
125. Carr KD, Papadouka V, Wolinsky TD. Norbinaltorphimine blocks the feeding but not the reinforcing effect of lateral hypothalamic electrical stimulation. Psychopharmacology (Berl) 1993; 111(3):345–350.
126. Mague SD, Pliakas AM, Todtenkopf MS, Tomasiewicz HC, Zhang Y, Stevens WC, Jr., et al. Antidepressant-like effects of kappa-opioid receptor antagonists in the forced swim test in rats. J Pharmacol Exp Ther 2003; 305(1):323–330.
127. Chefer VI, Czyzyk T, Bolan EA, Moron J, Pintar JE, Shippenberg TS. Endogenous kappa-opioid receptor systems regulate mesoaccumbal dopamine dynamics and vulnerability to cocaine. J Neurosci 2005; 25(20):5029–5037.
128. You ZB, Herrera-Marschitz M, Terenius L. Modulation of neurotransmitter release in the basal ganglia of the rat brain by dynorphin peptides. J Pharmacol Exp Ther 1999; 290(3):1307–1315.
129. Mathieu-Kia AM, Besson MJ. Repeated administration of cocaine, nicotine and ethanol: effects on preprodynorphin, preprotachykinin A and preproenkephalin mRNA expression in the dorsal and the ventral striatum of the rat. Mol Brain Res 1998; 54(1):141–151.
130. Brandon CL, Steiner H. Repeated methylphenidate treatment in adolescent rats alters gene regulation in the striatum. Eur J Neurosci 2003; 18(6):1584–1592.
131. Gerfen CR, McGinty JF, Young WS, III. Dopamine differentially regulates dynorphin, substance P, and enkephalin expression in striatal neurons: in situ hybridization histochemical analysis. J Neurosci 1991; 11(4):1016–1031.
132. Dahl JP, Weller AE, Kampman KM, Oslin DW, Lohoff FW, Ferraro TN, et al. Confirmation of the association between a polymorphism in the promoter region of the prodynorphin gene and cocaine dependence. Am J Med Genet B Neuropsychiatr Genet 2005; 139(1):106–108.
133. Luo X, Kranzler HR, Zhao H, Gelernter J. Haplotypes at the OPRM1 locus are associated with susceptibility to substance dependence in European-Americans. Am J Med Genet B Neuropsychiatr Genet 2003; 120(1):97–108.

Chapter 16
Potential Use of Opioid Antagonists in the Treatment of Marijuana Abuse and Dependence

B. Le Foll, Zuzana Justinova, G. Tanda, Marcello Solinas, Peter Selby, and Steven R. Goldberg

Abstract Cannabinoids are usually abused by humans in the form of marijuana. They are the most frequently abused illicit class of drugs in the United States, but no pharmacological treatment is currently available to help in reducing marijuana abuse and dependence. Although the dopaminergic system plays a critical role in the reinforcing effects of drugs of abuse, other neurotransmitter systems are implicated. Notably, opioid systems appear to be critically involved in various behavioral and neurochemical effects of various abused drugs, including delta 9-tetrahydrocannabinol (Δ^9-THC), the main psychoactive ingredient in marijuana, and clinical trials have demonstrated the utility of opioid antagonists in the treatment of alcohol dependence. Opioid antagonists reduce the dopamine-releasing effects of Δ^9-THC in rats and attenuate various behavioral effects of Δ^9-THC and synthetic cannabinoid CB_1 receptor agonists in mice, rats, and monkeys. These opioid–cannabinoid interactions are bidirectional, since the CB_1 receptor antagonist SR141716A reduces, but does not completely block, some reinforcing effects of opioids. Moreover, Δ^9-THC is actively self-administered by squirrel monkeys and this behavior is markedly reduced by naltrexone treatment. Although naltrexone does not appear to significantly alter subjective responses to smoked marijuana or oral Δ^9-THC in the few acute studies conducted in humans, the strong preclinical evidence from animal studies for reductions in the reinforcing and other abuse-related behavioral and neurochemical effects of Δ^9-THC by opioid antagonists suggests that they remain promising candidates for treatment of marijuana abuse and dependence in humans. This hypothesis should be validated in clinical trials involving chronic treatment with opioid antagonists such as naltrexone.

Keywords: Δ^9-THC; Marijuana; Opioid receptors; Cannabinoid receptors; Clinical trials; Drug dependence

B. Le Foll (✉), Z. Justinova, G. Tanda, M. Solinas, P. Selby, and S.R. Goldberg
Translational Addiction Research Laboratory,
Centre for Addiction and Mental Health (CAMH), University of Toronto,
33 Russell Street, Toronto, Canada M5S 2S1
e-mail: bernard_lefoll@camh.net

R. Dean et al. (eds.), *Opiate Receptors and Antagonists*,

16.1 Introduction

Opioid receptor antagonists are currently used for the treatment of opiate and alcohol dependence, but their use has not yet been validated for the treatment of other types of drug dependence, such as marijuana dependence. This chapter focuses on recent experimental evidence that supports the use of opioid antagonists as medications for the treatment of marijuana dependence. Although a large amount of preclinical evidence suggests that an opioid antagonist approach could be efficacious in reducing marijuana's physiological and behavioral effects, including its rewarding/reinforcing effects, adequate animal models for validating this hypothesis were lacking until recently and this has hampered the development of clinical trials in this area.

Here, we will first summarize the main preclinical experimental findings in animals indicating potential utility of opioid antagonists in the treatment of marijuana dependence, findings primarily related to the effects of opioid receptor blockade on the neurochemical and behavioral effects of delta 9-tetrahydrocannabinol (Δ^9-THC), the main psychoactive ingredient in marijuana. Special emphasis will be given to recent studies in rodents and monkeys of the effects of opioid antagonists on Δ^9-THC-induced dopamine release in the nucleus accumbens, Δ^9-THC-induced subjective effects assessed by two-lever choice drug-discrimination procedures, and rewarding/reinforcing effects of Δ^9-THC assessed by conditioned place preference (CPP) and intravenous drug self-administration procedures. The current status of experimental research in human subjects will also be summarized and possible future directions for clinical research will be discussed.

16.2 Historical Evolution of Research on Cannabinoids

Marijuana is the most widely used illicit drug in the United States. Although marijuana extracts usually contain a large number of different psychotropic substances, only a few of them are present in concentrations sufficient to induce psychotropic effects in humans and Δ^9-THC is believed to be responsible for most psychotropic effects of marijuana. Two forms of cannabinoid receptors, CB_1 and CB_2, have been cloned (1–3). The CB_1 receptor, and its splice variant the CB_{1A} receptor, are predominantly found in the brain, with the highest density in the hippocampus, cerebellum, cortex, and striatum, whereas CB_2 receptors are primarily located peripherally, principally associated with the immune system (4), but are also located in the brain (5). New data indicate that additional forms of cannabinoid receptors (non-CB_1/non-CB_2) may exist [see Wilson and Nicoll (6)]. Δ^9-THC appears to produce its effects by duplicating the effects of natural endogenous ligands for CB_1 receptors (anandamide, 2-arachidonylglycerol and, perhaps, noladin ether), which have a shorter duration of action than synthetic or plant-derived cannabinoids. Endogenous cannabinoids are also implicated in a variety of central nervous system functions, including reward/reinforcement, cognitive processes, including memory and pain (6). Central nervous system effects produced by Δ^9-THC have been linked to cannabinoid CB_1 receptors. As with other drugs of abuse, Δ^9-THC administration produces elevations in dopamine levels in the shell of the nucleus accumbens of rats (7), which are blocked by cannabinoid CB_1 receptor antagonists such as Rimonabant (SR141716) (8). The discovery that an opioid antagonist could also block the dopamine-releasing effects of THC in the nucleus accumbens shell suggested opioid system involvement in the abuse-related effects of marijuana and cannabinoids. There is increasing experimental evidence from animal studies for reciprocal functional interactions between endogenous brain cannabinoid and opioid systems (9). Endogenous cannabinoid and opioid neurotransmitter systems are both involved in the regulation of physiological processes such as thermoregulation, blood pressure, and antinociception, and in the control of behaviors such as locomotion and eating and various types of drug dependence. We will focus here on the neurochemical and behavioral findings in relation to marijuana abuse and dependence.

16.3 Effects of Opioid Antagonists in Animal Models of Δ^9-THC Abuse and Dependence

A variety of animal models are currently available to study the cardinal features of drug abuse and dependence (10–21). We will present the effects of opiate receptor blockade on neurochemical effects of cannabinoids (Δ^9-THC-induced dopamine release); on the withdrawal states associated with abrupt termination of cannabinoid action (administration of selective CB_1 receptor antagonists after chronic Δ^9-THC exposure); on animals models for the subjective effects of administered Δ^9-THC (drug discrimination); on the rewarding/reinforcing properties of Δ^9-THC and other synthetic CB_1 receptor agonists (intravenous drug self-administration, CPP, and intracranial self-stimulation procedures); and on the influence of environmental stimuli on drug-seeking and drug-taking behavior (CPP, second-order schedules of drug self-administration, reinstatement of extinguished drug-seeking behavior, and other relapse models). The difficulties involved in obtaining reliable models of Δ^9-THC-induced CPP and Δ^9-THC self-administration in rodents have been previously reviewed and will not be presented here in detail [see Justinova et al. (22)].

16.3.1 Effects of Opioid Antagonists on Δ^9-THC-Induced Changes in Dopamine Neurotransmission

Despite contrasting results obtained in early in vitro (23–25) and in vivo (26–28) rodent studies about the ability of Δ^9-THC to increase brain levels of dopamine in striatal areas, evidence collected in the last decade using more sophisticated electrophysiology (29, 30) and microdialysis (7, 31–33) techniques clearly show that Δ^9-THC administration significantly increases dopamine neurotransmission by increasing the firing rate of dopaminergic neurons projecting to the nucleus accumbens (29, 30), an effect that is blocked by Rimonabant (30). The increases in dopamine levels in the shell of the accumbens induced by Δ^9-THC or the synthetic CB_1 agonist WIN 55,212-2 are blocked by Rimonabant, indicating an involvement of CB_1 receptors (32). Although some effects of Δ^9-THC are not blocked by opioid antagonists such as naloxone (29), several investigators have shown that various antagonists of mu-opioid receptors can effectively block or markedly reduce Δ^9-THC-induced dopamine release in the shell of nucleus accumbens (7, 32) (Fig. 16.1).

Similar effects have been obtained by selectively administrating the mu-opioid antagonist naloxonazine into the ventral tegmental area (VTA) of rats (32), suggesting that THC can increase endogenous opioid tone in the VTA and that mu-opioid receptors in the VTA mediate the effects of THC on dopamine release in the nucleus accumbens shell (34). In support of this hypothesis, it has recently been shown that THC administration increases levels of the endogenous opioid β-endorphin in the VTA and that that elevated β-endorphin levels in the VTA facilitate the discrimination of THC's effects (35). Because the VTA and the mesolimbic dopamine

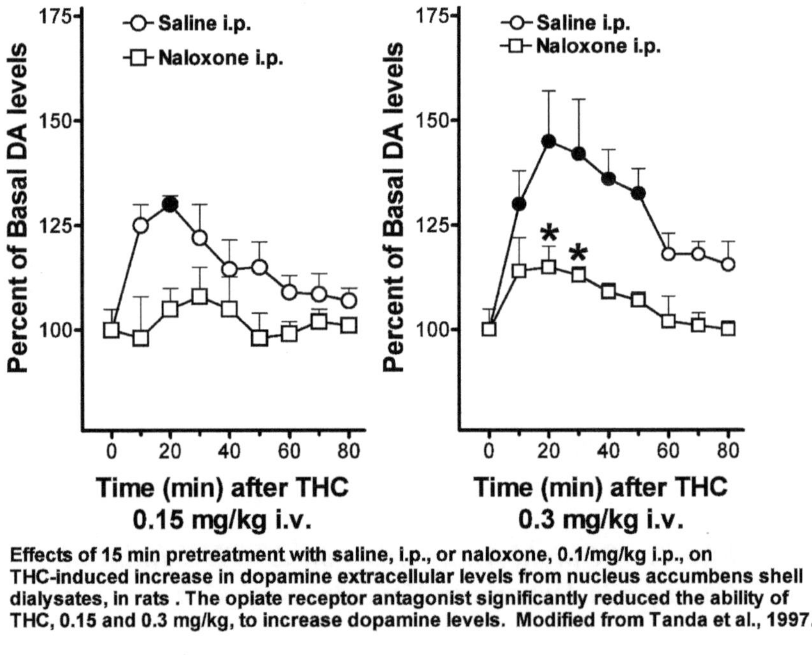

Fig. 16.1 Effects of opioid antagonists on tetrahydrocannabinol (*THC*)-induced dopamine release in the shell of the nucleus accumbens

terminal fields in the accumbens shell are believed to be fundamental substrates for the motivational rewarding/reinforcing effects of drugs abused by humans (36), the ability of opioid antagonists to influence the actions of Δ^9-THC on dopaminergic neurotransmission in the mesolimbic dopamine reward system suggests their therapeutic potential as medications for marijuana abuse and dependence.

16.3.2 Effects of Opioid Antagonists on THC Discrimination

Humans abusing psychoactive drugs report characteristic subjective effects and drug discrimination procedures in rats and monkeys are extensively used as animal models for subjective reports of drug effects in humans (37–40). These interoceptive subjective effects of drugs are most frequently assessed in humans through the use of performance assessment tasks and subject-rating scales. In animals, the interoceptive effects of drugs can serve as discriminative stimuli to indicate how to obtain a reinforcer such as a food pellet or how to avoid an electric shock. For this purpose, animals are trained under a discrete-trial schedule of food-pellet delivery or stimulus-shock termination to respond on one lever after an injection of a training dose of a drug and on the other lever after an injection of vehicle. Once animals learn to reliably make this discrimination, the subjective effects of different drugs can be compared and the modulation of subjective effects of drugs of abuse by various pharmacological ligands can be measured.

The discriminative-stimulus effects of THC show a high degree of pharmacological specificity. Only drugs that activate cannabinoid CB_1 receptors have been found to fully generalize to the discriminative-stimulus effects of THC and, until recently, only drugs that block CB_1 receptors have been found to antagonize the discriminative-stimulus effects of THC (41–44). Investigating the role played by different opioid receptor subtypes in the discriminative-stimulus effects of THC helps to reveal the general neurobiological mechanisms involved in the behavioral effects of THC but also to elucidate similarities or differences between opioid system modulation of the discriminative-stimulus and rewarding effects of THC.

Rodent studies showed that discriminative-stimulus effects of THC can be potentiated by the opioid agonist morphine and reduced by the opioid antagonists naloxone and naltrexone, and that this modulation of THC's discriminative effects is related to its ability to increase the extracellular levels of β-endorphin in the VTA (35, 45). Moreover, selective agonists or antagonists at delta-opioid and kappa-opioid receptors do not alter the discriminative-stimulus effects of THC and do not block heroin-induced potentiation of THC discrimination. Thus, the discriminative effects of THC appear to be modulated by mu-opioid receptor activation (45). In these and previous experiments, heroin did not produce THC-like effects when administered alone (35, 41, 43, 46), and naltrexone did not completely block the effects of the training dose of THC (35, 41, 47). These results suggest that the endogenous opioid system does not mediate, but instead facilitates the discriminative-stimulus effects of THC in rodents.

16.3.3 Effects of Opioid Antagonists on the Cannabinoid Withdrawal Syndrome

The withdrawal syndrome that results from abrupt interruption of cannabis use has recently become a main area of research (48). Physical withdrawal signs are usually hard to detect in humans, a fact that could be related to the high lipophilicity of THC, which allows it to be stored in fat tissue, from which it is slowly released over long periods of time, thus supplying the body with a “THC reservoir” during periods of abstinence. In recent years, a growing number of people have been seeking treatment for cannabis withdrawal and this has reached the attention of researchers and clinicians, resulting in publications about this topic being made available [see Budney and Hughes (48) and references herein]. The cannabinoid withdrawal syndrome can be demonstrated in laboratory animals by spontaneous withdrawal (49–51), and by precipitated withdrawal with a selective cannabinoid CB_1 receptor antagonist (52, 53). A cannabinoid withdrawal syndrome can also be precipitated by opioid antagonists in animals made dependent on THC and this was first described by two different research groups in the 1970; Hirschhorn and Rosecrans (54) and Kaymakcalan et al. (49) described “narcotic-like” withdrawal signs precipitated by naloxone in rats chronically treated with THC. Since THC induces release of endogenous opioids in the brain (35, 55), these signs may be partly due to adaptive changes in the endogenous opioid system. Moreover, it has been reported that somatic expression of the cannabinoid withdrawal syndrome is significantly reduced in pre-proenkephalin knockout mice (56) and in mu-opioid receptor knockout mice (57), suggesting, again, that the endogenous opioid system is involved in the development and expression of cannabinoid dependence. However, at variance with these results, there are reports that significant signs of withdrawal from THC do not occur after opioid antagonist administration in mice (57), and that there are no significant differences in signs of withdrawal from THC in mu-opioid receptor knockout mice and their littermate controls (58). Also, in THC-dependent rhesus monkeys, opioid antagonists do not appear to precipitate withdrawal signs (59).

16.3.4 Effects of Opioid Antagonists on THC-Induced CPPs

With CPP procedures, a distinctive environment is repeatedly associated with the effects of an administered dose of a psychoactive drug and a distinctively different environment is repeatedly associated with administration of its vehicle. A CPP is demonstrated when a test trial is conducted with no drug or vehicle administration and, during the test trial, the environment repeatedly associated with the drug elicits approach behavior and increased time is spent in the drug-associated environment compared to the vehicle-associated environment (a place preference).

Compared to other drugs of abuse, very limited work has been done with THC or synthetic CB_1 agonists in rats or mice and experimental parameters such as dose of cannabinoid and pretreatment time, preexposure to cannabinoid before conditioning trials, and enriched housing conditions appear critical for the demonstration of significant cannabinoid-induced CPPs (60–62). THC and other synthetic CB_1 agonists may also induce conditioned place aversions (CPA) (58). In mice and rats, THC has been reported to produce either CPP or CPA in different studies. Although cannabinoids tend to produce CPA (60, 63–65) in most reported studies with rodents, there have been some reports of THC-induced CPP (60, 66, 67) and administration of the opioid antagonist naloxone appears able to block the acquisition of THC-induced CPP when they occur (66). The influence of the different opioid receptor subtypes in THC-induced CPP has been explored with experiments using genetic ablation of receptors in mice.

The deletion of mu-opioid receptors abolished the ability of THC to induce CPP, whereas deletion of kappa-opioid receptors abolished the acquisition of THC-induced CPA and unmasked THC-induced CPP (58) (Fig. 16.2). These experiments

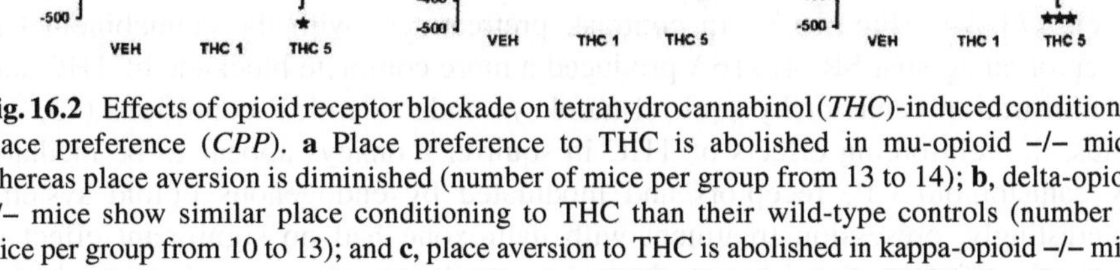

Fig. 16.2 Effects of opioid receptor blockade on tetrahydrocannabinol (*THC*)-induced conditioned place preference (*CPP*). **a** Place preference to THC is abolished in mu-opioid –/– mice, whereas place aversion is diminished (number of mice per group from 13 to 14); **b**, delta-opioid –/– mice show similar place conditioning to THC than their wild-type controls (number of mice per group from 10 to 13); and **c**, place aversion to THC is abolished in kappa-opioid –/– mice (number of mice per group from 11 to 12) mice. THC1 (1 mg/kg, i.p.); THC5 (5 mg/kg, i.p.). Mice conditioned to the dose of 1 mg/kg THC received a previous THC injection (1 mg/kg, i.p.) in their home cage, 24 h before the start of the conditioning phase. In wild-type mice, THC1 conditions reveal THC place preference, whereas THC5 conditions show THC place aversion. Values are expressed as mean ± standard error of the mean (*SEM*). Scores were calculated as the difference between test and preconditioning time spent in the drug-paired compartment. $^{*}p < 0.05$, ★★ $p < 0.01$, comparison between treatments; $^{**}p < 0.01$, comparison between genotypes (one-way ANOVAs). Reprinted from Ghozland (58) with permission

suggest an involvement of mu- and kappa-opioid receptors in the motivational effects of cannabinoids studied with CPP procedures.

16.3.5 Effects of Opiates Antagonists on Intravenous Drug Self-Administration

With intravenous drug self-administration procedures, a catheter implanted in a jugular vein allows the animal to intravenously self-administer a small amount of drug by pressing a lever. The administration of drug constitutes the event that positively reinforces the lever-pressing behavior and reward is inferred if the frequency of responding subsequently increases (defining reinforcement). Under a fixed-ratio schedule of intravenous drug injection, a fixed number of lever-presses is required to obtain each injection of drug (e.g., 1 lever press for a fixed-ratio 1, i.e., fixed-ratio 1, schedule). Once an animal has been learned to self-administer the drug, the influences of drug priming, stressors or presentation of drug-associated cues on drug self-administration behavior, or relapse to extinguished drug-seeking behavior can be studied and this provides useful measures of variables controlling drug-taking behaviour or relapse to drug-seeking behavior (68, 69).

Evidence for a role of opioid neurotransmitter systems in the modulation of the reinforcing effects of cannabinoids comes from rodent drug self-administration studies in which naloxone pretreatment reduced self-administration behavior maintained by the synthetic cannabinoid CB_1 receptor agonists WIN55,212-2, HU-210 (70) and CP55,940 (71, 72).

Recent demonstrations in squirrel monkeys of strong and persistent intravenous self-administration of the natural cannabinoid in marijuana, THC (73, 74), provide an opportunity to explore whether the reinforcing effects of THC in nonhuman primates would be similarly reduced by opioid receptor blockade.

In results reproduced in Fig. 16.3, naltrexone produced a significant downward shift and a flattening of the THC dose-response curve for self-administration, but THC self-administration behavior remained well above vehicle substitution levels (73, 74) (Fig. 16.3). In contrast, pretreatment with the cannabinoid CB_1 receptor antagonist SR141716A produced a more complete blockade of THC self-administration behavior by squirrel monkeys under identical conditions (73, 74). Thus, the reinforcing effects of THC in squirrel monkeys appear to be mediated by cannabinoid CB_1 receptors and modulated by endogenous opioid systems. Interestingly, presession treatment with naltrexone had no significant effect on responding for cocaine in control monkeys under the same fixed-ratio schedule of intravenous drug injection, suggesting little, if any, involvement of opioid systems in the reinforcing effects of cocaine in squirrel monkeys (75). This result is in accordance with previous reports that opioid antagonists do not alter cocaine self-administration in primates (76, 77). However, there is a growing literature that indicates that opioid systems may be involved in some aspects of drug-taking and drug-seeking behavior (78–81).

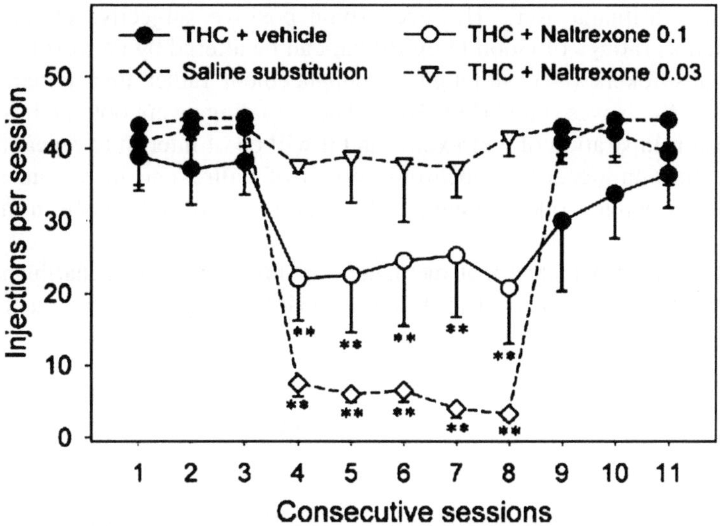

Fig. 16.3 Effects of opioid receptor blockade on tetrahydrocannabinol (*THC*)-self administration by squirrel monkeys. Effects of presession treatment with 0.03 and 0.1 mg/kg naltrexone on self-administration responding maintained by intravenous THC injections over consecutive sessions. Number of injections per session during THC (4 μg/kg/injection) self-administration sessions after pretreatment with vehicle (sessions 1–3 and 9–11) or naltrexone (sessions 4–8), and number of injections per session during self-administration sessions when saline was substituted for THC (sessions 4–8) are shown. Symbols represent the means (± SEM) of injections per session from four monkeys. $^{**}p < 0.01$, post hoc comparisons with the last THC session before naltrexone pretreatment or saline substitution (session 3) after significant one-way ANOVA for repeated measures main effect, Dunnett's test. Reprinted from Justinova (75) with permission

16.4 Research in Human Subjects

To determine if these preclinical findings can be applied to clinical situations, it is important to review the clinical studies that have evaluated the effects of opioid antagonist on effects of cannabinoids in humans.

16.4.1 Current Clinical Research with Humans

Although there is a large body of preclinical findings in experimental animals suggesting that opioid receptor antagonists may be a useful pharmacological tool for the treatment of marijuana dependence, only a few clinical studies have evaluated the effects of naltrexone on physiological or subjective effects of cannabinoid in humans. Interestingly, acute naltrexone pretreatments did not alter the antinociceptive or subjective effects of smoked marijuana (82) or oral THC (83) in current marijuana users. However, some positive subjective effects of oral THC, such as ratings of Good Drug Effect, can be altered by naltrexone in heavy marijuana smokers (84), although an enhancement rather than a reduction in subjective effects was found (Fig. 16.4). These findings were obtained using only an acute administration of naltrexone, and it will be of interest to repeat the same experiments administering subchronic doses of naltrexone in human subjects, which might better model a potential therapeutic use of naltrexone in marijuana smokers.

There is some evidence that methadone treatment increases marijuana use in males (85). However, it is unclear if this is a pharmacological effect or a behavioral

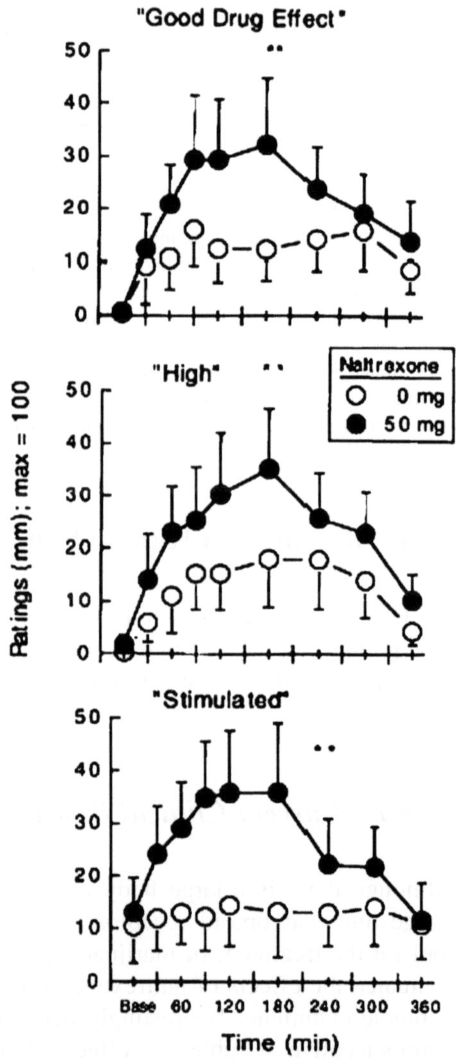

Fig. 16.4 Effects of opioid receptor blockade by naltrexone on subjective effects of smoked marijuana in humans. Time course for selected subjective-effects ratings portrayed as a function of tetrahydrocannabinol (*THC*) (30 mg) and naltrexone (oral, 50 mg) dose condition. *Asterisks* denote a significant difference between active and placebo naltrexone on data averaged over the 60–300 min following THC administration ($^{*}p < 0.01$; $^{**}p < 0.005$). *Error bars* represent standard error of the mean (*SEM*). Reprinted from Haney (84) with permission

effect resulting from reduced illicit opiate use and the policies of methadone clinics toward THC use. Moreover, the use of THC in methadone-maintained patients does not appear to affect clinical outcomes (86–88). Although in one study, regular users of THC in a methadone program were less likely to use other drugs (89), in another pooled analysis of methadone patients in contingency management programs, THC use did not increase the use of heroin over nonusers of THC (87). The authors also noted that being maintained on methadone did not increase the use of THC (87). In contrast to the many preclinical findings suggesting a clear modulatory role of the opioid system on the behavioral and neurochemical effects of cannabinoids in animals, clinical findings do not yet provide clear indications of opioid system modulation of cannabinoid effects in humans.

16.4.2 Future Directions for Clinical Research

The limitations of the studies done in humans include the use of single doses and measurements of acute effects in a few subjects (57, 58). If these experiments were applied to naltrexone use in the treatment of alcohol dependence in humans, the drug would never have been introduced into clinical practice for this indication (90). More extensive dose-ranging studies with doses given chronically over time in larger numbers of subjects are needed. In addition, since naltrexone plasma levels and beta hydroxyl naltrexone are subject to interindividual differences, dose titration-to-effect studies may be necessary to observe consistent effects. Alternatively, newer depot formulations of naltrexone and nalmaphene, given once per month, hold promise to increase adherence to treatment and may mitigate potential kinetic problems associated with these opioid antagonists (91–94). Finally, the role of opioid antagonists in relapse prevention, that is, in users who have been "detoxified" from THC, is also not clear and needs further study.

16.5 Conclusions

It appears at first view that the findings in humans are not consistent with findings obtained in rodents and primate studies, where decreases in various behavioral effects of THC after naloxone or naltrexone treatment were generally found. That may be due to species differences between rodents and human or nonhuman primates in functional interactions between opioid and cannabinoid systems or to the use of relatively high doses of naltrexone (e.g., 50 mg, oral) in long-term, heavy marijuana smokers tolerant to many of THC's effects (84). The strong body of evidence that indicates that opioid receptor blockade can reduce the reinforcing and motivational effects of cannabinoids strongly support the implementation of further clinical trials in this area.

Acknowledgments Preparation of this paper was supported in part by the Intramural Research Program of the National Institute on Drug Abuse, National Institutes of Health, and Department of Health and Human Services.

References

1. Matsuda LA, Lolait SJ, Brownstein MJ, Young AC, Bonner TI. Structure of a cannabinoid receptor and functional expression of the cloned cDNA. Nature 1990;346:561–4.
2. Gerard CM, Mollereau C, Vassart G, Parmentier M. Molecular cloning of a human cannabinoid receptor which is also expressed in testis. Biochem J 1991;279 (Pt 1):129–34.
3. Munro S, Thomas KL, Abu-Shaar M. Molecular characterization of a peripheral receptor for cannabinoids. Nature 1993;365:61–5.
4. Howlett AC, Barth F, Bonner TI, Cabral G, Casellas P, Devane WA, Felder CC, Herkenham M, Mackie K, Martin BR, Mechoulam R, Pertwee RG. International union of pharmacology. XXVII. Classification of cannabinoid receptors. Pharmacol Rev 2002;54:161–202.
5. Van Sickle MD, Duncan M, Kingsley PJ, Mouihate A, Urbani P, Mackie K, Stella N, Makriyannis A, Piomelli D, Davison JS, Marnett LJ, Di Marzo V, Pittman QJ, Patel KD, Sharkey KA. Identification and functional characterization of brainstem cannabinoid CB_2 receptors. Science 2005;310:329–32.
6. Wilson RI, Nicoll RA. Endocannabinoid signaling in the brain. Science 2002;296:678–82.
7. Chen JP, Paredes W, Li J, Smith D, Lowinson J, Gardner EL. Delta 9-tetrahydrocannabinol produces naloxone-blockable enhancement of presynaptic basal dopamine efflux in nucleus accumbens of conscious, freely-moving rats as measured by intracerebral microdialysis. Psychopharmacology (Berl) 1990;102:156–62.
8. Tanda G, Di Chiara G. Cannabinoid and heroin activation of mesolimbic dopamine transmission by a common m1 opioid receptor mecanism. Science 1997;276:2048–50.
9. Manzanares J, Corchero J, Fuentes JA. Opioid and cannabinoid receptor-mediated regulation of the increase in adrenocorticotropin hormone and corticosterone plasma concentrations induced by central administration of delta(9)-tetrahydrocannabinol in rats. Brain Res 1999;839:173–9.
10. Schuster CR, Woods JH. The conditioned reinforcing effects of stimuli associated with morphine reinforcement. Int J Addict 1968;3:223–30.
11. Goldberg SR. Stimuli associated with drug injections as events that control behavior. Pharmacol Rev 1975;27:325–40.
12. Goldberg SR, Kelleher RT, Morse WH. Second-order schedules of drug injection. Fed. Proc. 1975;34:1771–6.
13. Spealman RD, Goldberg SR. Drug self-administration by laboratory animals: control by schedules of reinforcement. Annu Rev Pharmacol Toxicol 1978;18:313–39.
14. Goldberg SR, Spealman RD, Kelleher RT. Enhancement of drug-seeking behavior by environmental stimuli associated with cocaine or morphine injections. Neuropharmacology 1979;18:1015–7.
15. Goldberg SR, Kelleher RT, Goldberg DM. Fixed-ratio responding under second-order schedules of food presentation or cocaine injection. J Pharmacol Exp Ther 1981;218:271–81.
16. Katz JL, Goldberg SR. Preclinical assessment of abuse liability of drugs. Agents Actions 1988;23:18–26.
17. Markou A, Weiss F, Gold LH, Caine B, Schulteis G, Koob GF. Animal models of drug craving. Psychopharmacology 1993;112:163–82.
18. Everitt BJ, Robbins TW. Second-order schedules of drug reinforcement in rats and monkeys: measurement of reinforcing efficacy and drug-seeking behaviour. Psychopharmacology (Berl) 2000;153:17–30.

19. Schindler CW, Panlilio LV, Goldberg SR. Second-order schedules of drug self-administration in animals. Psychopharmacology(Berl) 2002;163:327–44.
20. Deroche-Gamonet V, Belin D, Piazza PV. Evidence for addiction-like behavior in the rat. Science 2004;305:1014–7.
21. Vanderschuren LJ, Everitt BJ. Drug seeking becomes compulsive after prolonged cocaine self-administration. Science 2004;305:1017–9.
22. Justinova Z, Goldberg SR, Heishman SJ, Tanda G. Self-administration of cannabinoids by experimental animals and human marijuana smokers. Pharmacol Biochem Behav 2005;81: 285–99.
23. Bloom AS, Dewey WL. A comparison of some pharmacological actions of morphine and delta 9-tetrahydrocannabinol in the mouse. Psychopharmacology (Berl) 1978;57:243–8.
24. Rodriguez de Fonseca F, Carrera MR, Navarro M, Koob GF, Weiss F. Activation of corticotropin-releasing factor in the limbic system during cannabinoid withdrawal. Science 1997; 276:2050–4.
25. Navarro M, Fernandez-Ruiz JJ, de Miguel R, Hernandez ML, Cebeira M, Ramos JA. An acute dose of delta 9-tetrahydrocannabinol affects behavioral and neurochemical indices of mesolimbic dopaminergic activity. Behav Brain Res 1993;57:37–46.
26. Ng Cheong Ton JM, Gerhardt GA, Friedemann M, Etgen AM, Rose GM, Sharpless NS, Gardner EL. The effects of delta 9-tetrahydrocannabinol on potassium-evoked release of dopamine in the rat caudate nucleus: an in vivo electrochemical and in vivo microdialysis study. Brain Res 1988;451:59–68.
27. Sakurai-Yamashita Y, Kataoka Y, Fujiwara M, Mine K, Ueki S. Delta 9-tetrahydrocannabinol facilitates striatal dopaminergic transmission. Pharmacol Biochem Behav 1989;33: 397–400.
28. Castaneda E, Moss DE, Oddie SD, Whishaw IQ. THC does not affect striatal dopamine release: microdialysis in freely moving rats. Pharmacol Biochem Behav 1991;40:587–91.
29. French ED, Dillon K, Wu X. Cannabinoids excite dopamine neurons in the ventral tegmentum and substantia nigra. Neuroreport 1997;8:649–52.
30. Gessa GL, Melis M, Muntoni AL, Diana M. Cannabinoids activate mesolimbic dopamine neurons by an action on cannabinoid CB_1 receptors. Eur J Pharmacol 1998;341:39–44.
31. Chen JP, Paredes W, Lowinson JH, Gardner EL. Strain-specific facilitation of dopamine efflux by delta 9-tetrahydrocannabinol in the nucleus accumbens of rat: an in vivo microdialysis study. Neurosci Lett 1991;129:136–80.
32. Tanda G, Pontieri FE, Di Chiara G. Cannabinoid and heroin activation of mesolimbic dopamine transmission by a common mu1 opioid receptor mechanism. Science 1997;276:2048–50.
33. Malone DT, Taylor DA. Modulation by fluoxetine of striatal dopamine release following Delta 9-tetrahydrocannabinol: a microdialysis study in conscious rats. Br J Pharmacol 1999;128:21–6.
34. Di Chiara G, North RA. Neurobiology of opiate abuse. Trends Pharmacol Sci 1992;13: 185–93.
35. Solinas M, Zangen A, Thiriet N, Goldberg SR. Beta-endorphin elevations in the ventral tegmental area regulate the discriminative effects of Delta-9-tetrahydrocannabinol. Eur J Neurosci 2004;19:3183–92.
36. Wise RA. Forebrain substrates of reward and motivation. J Comp Neurol 2005;493:115–21.
37. Holtzman SG. Drug discrimination studies. Drug Alcohol Depend 1985;14:263–82.
38. Stolerman IP, Samele C, Kamien JB, Mariathasan EA, Hague DS. A bibliography of drug discrimination research, 1992–1994. Behav Pharmacol 1995;6:643–68.
39. Colpaert FC. Drug discrimination in neurobiology. Pharmacol Biochem Behav 1999;64:337–45.
40. Le Foll B, Goldberg SR. Cannabinoid CB_1 receptor antagonists as promising new medications for drug dependence. J Pharmacol Exp Ther 2005;312:875–83.
41. Browne RG, Weissman A. Discriminative stimulus properties of delta 9-tetrahydrocannabinol: mechanistic studies. J Clin Pharmacol 1981;21:227S–234S.

42. Barrett RL, Wiley JL, Balster RL, Martin BR. Pharmacological specificity of delta 9-tetrahydrocannabinol discrimination in rats. Psychopharmacology (Berl) 1995;118:419–24.
43. Wiley JL, Lowe JA, Balster RL, Martin BR. Antagonism of the discriminative stimulus effects of delta 9-tetrahydrocannabinol in rats and rhesus monkeys. J Pharmacol Exp Ther 1995;275:1–6.
44. Solinas M, Panlilio LV, Antoniou K, Pappas LA, Goldberg SR. The cannabinoid CB_1 antagonist N-piperidinyl-5-(4-chlorophenyl)-1-(2,4-dichlorophenyl) -4-methylpyrazole-3-carboxamide (SR-141716A) differentially alters the reinforcing effects of heroin under continuous reinforcement, fixed ratio, and progressive ratio schedules of drug self-administration in rats. J Pharmacol Exp Ther 2003;306:93–102.
45. Solinas M, Goldberg SR. Involvement of mu-, delta- and kappa-opioid receptor subtypes in the discriminative-stimulus effects of delta-9-tetrahydrocannabinol (THC) in rats. Psychopharmacology (Berl) 2005;179:804–12.
46. Jarbe TU, Henriksson BG. Discriminative response control produced with hashish, tetrahydrocannabinols (delta 8-THC and delta 9-THC), and other drugs. Psychopharmacologia 1974; 40:1–16.
47. Jarbe TU, Ohlin GC. Stimulus effects of delta(9)-THC and its interaction with naltrexone and catecholamine blockers in rats. Psychopharmacology (Berl) 1977;54:193–5.
48. Budney AJ, Hughes JR. The cannabis withdrawal syndrome. Curr Opin Psychiatry 2006; 19:233–8.
49. Kaymakcalan S, Ayhan IH, Tulunay FC. Naloxone-induced or postwithdrawal abstinence signs in delta 9-tetrahydrocannabinol-tolerant rats. Psychopharmacology (Berl) 1977;55: 243–9.
50. Costa B, Giagnoni G, Colleoni M. Precipitated and spontaneous withdrawal in rats tolerant to anandamide. Psychopharmacology (Berl) 2000;149:121–8.
51. Aceto MD, Scates SM, Martin BB. Spontaneous and precipitated withdrawal with a synthetic cannabinoid, WIN 55212-2. Eur J Pharmacol 2001;416:75–81.
52. Aceto MD, Scates SM, Lowe JA, Martin BR. Cannabinoid precipitated withdrawal by the selective cannabinoid receptor antagonist, SR 141716A. Eur J Pharmacol 1995;282:R1–2.
53. Tanda G, Loddo P, Di Chiara G. Dependence of mesolimbic dopamine transmission on delta 9-tetrahydrocannabinol. Eur J Pharmacol 1999;376:23–6.
54. Hirschhorn ID, Rosecrans JA. Morphine and delta 9-tetrahydrocannabinol: tolerance to the stimulus effects. Psychopharmacologia 1974;36:243–53.
55. Valverde O, Noble F, Beslot F, Dauge V, Fournie-Zaluski MC, Roques BP. Delta 9-tetrahydrocannabinol releases and facilitates the effects of endogenous enkephalins: reduction in morphine withdrawal syndrome without change in rewarding effect. Eur J Neurosci 2001;13:1816–24.
56. Valverde O, Maldonado R, Valjent E, Zimmer AM, Zimmer A. Cannabinoid withdrawal syndrome is reduced in pre-proenkephalin knock-out mice. J Neurosci 2000;20:9284–9.
57. Lichtman AH, Fisher J, Martin BR. Precipitated cannabinoid withdrawal is reversed by Delta (9)-tetrahydrocannabinol or clonidine. Pharmacol Biochem Behav 2001;69:181–8.
58. Ghozland S, Matthes HW, Simonin F, Filliol D, Kieffer BL, Maldonado R. Motivational effects of cannabinoids are mediated by mu-opioid and kappa-opioid receptors. J Neurosci 2002;22:1146–54.
59. Beardsley PM, Balster RL, Harris LS. Dependence on tetrahydrocannabinol in rhesus monkeys. J Pharmacol Exp Ther 1986;239:311–9.
60. Lepore M, Vorel SR, Lowinson J, Gardner EL. Conditioned place preference induced by delta 9-tetrahydrocannabinol: comparison with cocaine, morphine, and food reward. Life Sci 1995;56:2073–80.
61. Valjent E, Maldonado R. A behavioural model to reveal place preference to delta 9-tetrahydrocannabinol in mice. Psychopharmacology (Berl) 2000;147:436–8.
62. Gobbi G, Bambico FR, Mangieri R, Bortolato M, Campolongo P, Solinas M, Cassano T, Morgese MG, Debonnel G, Duranti A, Tontini A, Tarzia G, Mor M, Trezza V, Goldberg SR, Cuomo V, Piomelli D. Antidepressant-like activity and modulation of brain

monoaminergic transmission by blockade of anandamide hydrolysis. Proc Natl Acad Sci USA 2005;102:18620–5.
63. Parker LA, Gillies T. THC-induced place and taste aversions in Lewis and Sprague-Dawley rats. Behav Neurosci 1995;109:71–8.
64. Mallet PE, Beninger RJ. Delta 9-tetrahydrocannabinol, but not the endogenous cannabinoid receptor ligand anandamide, produces conditioned place avoidance. Life Sci 1998;62:2431–9.
65. Cheer JF, Kendall DA, Marsden CA. Cannabinoid receptors and reward in the rat: a conditioned place preference study. Psychopharmacology (Berl) 2000;151:25–30.
66. Braida D, Iosue S, Pegorini S, Sala M. Delta 9-tetrahydrocannabinol-induced conditioned place preference and intracerebroventricular self-administration in rats. Eur J Pharmacol 2004;506:63–9.
67. Le Foll B, Wiggins M, Goldberg SR. Nicotine pre-exposure does not potentiate the locomotor or rewarding effects of Delta-9-tetrahydrocannabinol in rats. Behav Pharmacol 2006; 17:195–9.
68. Shalev U, Grimm JW, Shaham Y. Neurobiology of relapse to heroin and cocaine seeking: a review. Pharmacol Rev 2002;54:1–42.
69. Le Foll B, Goldberg SR. Control of the reinforcing effects of nicotine by associated environmental stimuli in animals and humans. Trends Pharmacol Sci 2005;26:287–93.
70. Navarro M, Carrera MR, Fratta W, Valverde O, Cossu G, Fattore L, Chowen JA, Gomez R, del Arco I, Villanua MA, Maldonado R, Koob GF, Rodriguez de Fonseca F. Functional interaction between opioid and cannabinoid receptors in drug self-administration. J Neurosci 2001;21:5344–50.
71. Braida D, Pozzi M, Parolaro D, Sala M. Intracerebral self-administration of the cannabinoid receptor agonist CP 55,940 in the rat: interaction with the opioid system. Eur J Pharmacol 2001;413:227–34.
72. Braida D, Pozzi M, Cavallini R, Sala M. Conditioned place preference induced by the cannabinoid agonist CP 55,940: interaction with the opioid system. Neuroscience 2001;104:923–6.
73. Tanda G, Munzar P, Goldberg SR. Self-administration behavior is maintained by the psychoactive ingredient of marijuana in squirrel monkeys. Nat Neurosci 2000;3:1073–4.
74. Justinova Z, Tanda G, Redhi GH, Goldberg SR. Self-administration of delta 9-tetrahydrocannabinol (THC) by drug naive squirrel monkeys. Psychopharmacology (Berl) 2003;169: 135–40.
75. Justinova Z, Tanda G, Munzar P, Goldberg SR. The opioid antagonist naltrexone reduces the reinforcing effects of Delta 9 tetrahydrocannabinol (THC) in squirrel monkeys. Psychopharmacology (Berl) 2004;173:186–94.
76. Killian AK, Bonese K, Schuster CR. The effects of naloxone on behavior maintained by cocaine and heroin injections in the rhesus monkey. Drug Alcohol Depend 1978;3:243–51.
77. Winger G, Skjoldager P, Woods JH. Effects of buprenorphine and other opioid agonists and antagonists on alfentanil- and cocaine-reinforced responding in rhesus monkeys. J Pharmacol Exp Ther 1992;261:311–7.
78. Mello NK, Kamien JB, Mendelson JH, Lukas SE. Effects of naltrexone on cocaine self-administration by rhesus monkey. NIDA Res Monogr 1990;105:617–8.
79. Kiyatkin EA, Brown PL. Naloxone depresses cocaine self-administration and delays its initiation on the following day. Neuroreport 2003;14:251–5.
80. Bain GT, Kornetsky C. Naloxone attenuation of the effect of cocaine on rewarding brain stimulation. Life Sci 1987;40:1119–25.
81. Spano MS, Fattore L, Cossu G, Deiana S, Fadda P, Fratta W. CB_1 receptor agonist and heroin, but not cocaine, reinstate cannabinoid-seeking behaviour in the rat. Br J Pharmacol 2004;143:343–50.
82. Greenwald MK, Stitzer ML. Antinociceptive, subjective and behavioral effects of smoked marijuana in humans. Drug Alcohol Depend 2000;59:261–75.
83. Wachtel SR, de Wit H. Naltrexone does not block the subjective effects of oral Delta (9)-tetrahydrocannabinol in humans. Drug Alcohol Depend 2000;59:251–60.

84. Haney M, Bisaga A, Foltin RW. Interaction between naltrexone and oral THC in heavy marijuana smokers. Psychopharmacology (Berl) 2003;166:77–85.
85. Lollis CM, Strothers HS, Chitwood DD, McGhee M. Sex, drugs, and HIV: does methadone maintenance reduce drug use and risky sexual behavior? J Behav Med 2000;23:545–57.
86. Nixon LN. Cannabis use and treatment outcome in methadone maintenance. Addiction 2003;98:1321–2; author reply 1322–3.
87. Epstein DH, Preston KL. Does cannabis use predict poor outcome for heroin-dependent patients on maintenance treatment? Past findings and more evidence against. Addiction 2003;98:269–79.
88. Seivewright N. Methadone treatment outcomes appear mainly unaffected by cannabis use. Addiction 2003;98:251–2.
89. Saxon AJ, Calsyn DA, Blaes PA, Haver VM, Greenberg DM. Marijuana use by methadone maintenance patients. NIDA Res Monogr 1990;105:306–7.
90. Rush CR, Ali JA. Naltrexone does not attenuate the acute behavioral effects of ethanol or pentobarbital in humans. Behav Pharmacol 1999;10:401–13.
91. Paudel KS, Nalluri BN, Hammell DC, Valiveti S, Kiptoo P, Hamad MO, Crooks PA, Stinchcomb AL. Transdermal delivery of naltrexone and its active metabolite 6-beta-naltrexol in human skin in vitro and guinea pigs in vivo. J Pharm Sci 2005;94:1965–75.
92. Dean RL. The preclinical development of Medisorb Naltrexone, a once a month long acting injection, for the treatment of alcohol dependence. Front Biosci 2005;10:643–55.
93. Costantini LC, Kleppner SR, McDonough J, Azar MR, Patel R. Implantable technology for long-term delivery of nalmefene for treatment of alcoholism. Int J Pharm 2004;283:35–44.
94. Comer SD, Sullivan MA, Yu E, Rothenberg JL, Kleber HD, Kampman K, Dackis C, O'Brien CP. Injectable, sustained-release naltrexone for the treatment of opioid dependence: a randomized, placebo-controlled trial. Arch Gen Psychiatry 2006;63:210–8.

Chapter 17
Naltrexone in Smoking Cessation: A Review of the Literature and Future Directions

Andrea King, Rachel Torello, Suchitra Krishnan-Sarin, and Stephanie O'Malley

Abstract There are a number of efficacious pharmacotherapies currently available for smoking cessation, including nicotine replacement, buproprion, and varenicline. Each of these FDA-approved treatment options operates by a different mechanism of action to increase smoking quit rates. This chapter reviews the existing literature that addresses the role of the endogenous opioid system in nicotine dependence and smoking cessation. Human laboratory studies have shown mixed support for the opioid antagonist naltrexone altering cigarette craving, withdrawal, and smoking behavior. There are few published placebo-controlled randomized clinical trials of naltrexone in smoking cessation. While several of these clinical trials have indicated that naltrexone, particularly in combination with nicotine patch, may improve quit rates, other studies have not shown this effect. This inconsistency may, in part, be due to individual differences, such as sex, history of depression, weight gain, alcohol use, and genetic variables.

Keywords: Naltrexone; Opioid antagonist; Smoking cessation; Nicotine dependence

17.1 Introduction

In 2006, the centers for disease control (CDC) reported that ~21% of all adults (45.1 million people) in the United States smoke cigarettes, and that smoking remains the leading preventable cause of death in the United States (1). Tobacco use exacts a devastating toll

A. King (✉)
Department of Psychiatry, University of Chicago,
5841 S. Maryland Avenue, Chicago, IL 60637
e-mail: aking@bsd.uchicago.edu

R. Torello
The Chicago School of Professional Psychology,
Chicago, IL 60610

S. Krishnan-Sarin and S. O'Malley
Department of Psychiatry, Yale University School of Medicine,
New Haven, CT 06519

R. Dean et al. (eds.), *Opiate Receptors and Antagonists*,

on death and disease, particularly in terms of cancer, and cardiovascular and pulmonary disease. While long-term quit rates are generally low in unaided cessation attempts (~6%) (2), the use of FDA-approved pharmacotherapies, such as nicotine replacement, bupropion, and/or varenicline can double or triple smoking abstinence rates (3–7). However, because some patients either do not respond to these treatments or have contraindications for their use, additional medication adjuncts are needed for smoking cessation.

One possible pharmacotherapeutic agent for smoking cessation may be naltrexone, a primary mu opioid receptor (MOR) antagonist that is currently FDA-approved for the treatment of opioid and alcohol dependence. There is mixed evidence for the efficacy of naltrexone for the treatment of nicotine dependence. In this chapter, we review peer-reviewed investigations on naltrexone and smoking behavior, including both human laboratory and clinical treatment trials. Finally, we discuss potential individual difference factors which may play an important role in response to opioid antagonist treatment for smoking cessation.

17.1.1 Opioid Mediation of Smoking Behavior

Nicotine, the active ingredient in tobacco, affects various neuroregulatory systems, including the endogenous opioid system (8). Basic science research has demonstrated an association between opioids and nicotine (9–17). In addition, translational animal and human research studies have shown the similarities in mild opiate and nicotine withdrawal (18, 19). These withdrawal-like symptoms are precipitated by infusion of naloxone in both nicotine-dependent rats and humans (19, 20) and can be reversed with infusion of an opioid agonist, such as morphine (21). Hence, there is a preponderance of evidence from basic science and animal-based studies that nicotine may act at least in part through opioid mechanisms.

The opioid system may be involved in nicotine reinforcement through the dopaminergic brain reward pathway (22, 23). Evidence for a stimulatory effect of opiates on dopamine function comes from electrophysiological (24, 25) and behavioral animal studies (26). Also, endogenous opioids may also affect nicotine reward through interactions with nicotinic receptors (9, 10). Mu opiate receptors have also been demonstrated to be involved in the development of tolerance and dependence on nicotine (27–29). A greater understanding of neurobiological as well as behavioral and subjective pathways underlying opioid–nicotine interactions is crucial for developing and testing opioid antagonist treatment strategies in smoking cessation.

17.2 Human Laboratory Studies of Naltrexone and Acute Smoking

Human behavioral studies can provide a model to examine the mechanisms of action of a drug on indices of the target behavior and may inform design and methods for treatment studies. Preclinical human research investigations of naltrexone's effects on cigarette smoking have focused on specific subcomponents of tobacco addiction such as self-report subjective states and mood, withdrawal symptoms, smoking urges, and behavioral responses (i.e., after a single cigarette, choice or ad libitum smoking, and reinforcing value of nicotine). Significant effects of naltrexone altering one or more of these components may elucidate appropriate dosing, timing and length of medication delivery, adjunctive treatments, and potential smoker subgroups to target treatment toward.

The first comprehensive human laboratory study of oral naltrexone on smoking indices resulted in mixed findings (30). The study used a within-subjects design and participants were randomized to naltrexone or placebo blocks separated by a 10-day washout period in between blocks. Twelve heavy cigarette smokers (average 28.6 cigarettes daily) were tested in this study. Subjects took part in a 1-h baseline afternoon laboratory session where they completed self-report measures before and after smoking one cigarette of their normal brand. Subjects were then given 50 mg naltrexone or placebo at the end of the session and instructed to abstain from cigarette smoking for the next 24 h. At that time, they returned to the laboratory for an identical laboratory session. This second laboratory session was followed by administration of 100 mg naltrexone (or identical placebo), and subjects were instructed to record their ad libitum cigarette consumption over the next 48 h in the natural environment. The results of this study showed that naltrexone reduced the perceived difficulty in abstaining over the first 24 h of abstinence. The 50 mg naltrexone dose did not affect withdrawal symptoms during the 24-h interval, but the 100 mg dose did increase withdrawal-like mood states during the 48 h of ad libitum smoking. Naltrexone also did not alter reported subjective rewarding effects of smoking or amount smoked during the 48 h of ad libitum smoking. Taking the results together, the authors concluded that they could not find evidence for naltrexone altering the reinforcing properties of smoking under normal conditions.

Another well-controlled laboratory paradigm examining naltrexone's effects on acute smoking behavior was conducted a few years later; however, this study showed a different pattern of results (31). Subjects were 43 young adult smokers (average age = 24 years, 50% females), who smoked on average 19 cigarettes daily for 7 years. The study was conducted entirely in a controlled General Clinical Research Center (GCRC) environment. Ad libitum smoking behaviors were measured for 3 days during which subjects were administered either 50 mg naltrexone twice daily (100 mg daily dose) versus placebo. Results indicated that, compared to placebo, naltrexone significantly reduced smoking behaviors, in terms of numbers of cigarettes smoked and plasma nicotine levels, as well as lowered self-reported ratings of smoking satisfaction. However, naltrexone did not reduce overall expired air carbon monoxide (CO) levels, or subjective variables such as self-reported mood states and withdrawal symptoms. The results indicated some support for naltrexone in diminishing select aspects of smoking reward and behavior, but the findings were mixed, as CO and other subjective measures were not altered by naltrexone.

Given evidence that opioid antagonism might precipitate a mild withdrawal-like state and result in unpleasant subjective mood (19, 20), which would likely bode poorly for treatment, several human laboratory studies have examined the mechanisms of naltrexone combined with a nicotine agonist treatment on smoking responses. Hutchison et al. (32) conducted a between-subjects study and randomized ten smokers (5 female) to 50 mg naltrexone and ten smokers (5 female) to identical placebo (32). This sample was older than in prior laboratory studies of naltrexone (average age = 39.5 years) and subjects averaged 26.1 cigarettes smoked daily for a duration of 23 years. Subjects were given a 21 mg nicotine patch and were instructed to abstain from smoking for ~9 h. In the laboratory the next morning, they were given either 50 mg naltrexone or placebo pill, and several hours later took part in a smoking cue paradigm. Subjective measures were obtained before and after the cue, which was, holding a lit cigarette for 1 min. Naltrexone compared with placebo significantly decreased ratings of urge to smoke, negative affect, and withdrawal. The results indicated that naltrexone, in the context of treatment with nicotine replacement, attenuated smoking urges and negative mood states produced by a smoking cue. However, the preliminary nature of the study, with a relatively small sample size and lack of measurement of other effects, such as smoking levels, limited the generalizability of the findings.

Naltrexone alone, and in combination with nicotine patch, was also studied in a double-blind, within-subjects laboratory study (33). Subjects (n = 19, 11 women; average age 38.3 years) were adult moderate-to-heavy smokers who smoked on average 23.4 cigarettes daily for 19.6 years. They participated for 1 month and received 1 week of each of four different 50 mg naltrexone/placebo pill and 21 mg patch/placebo patch combinations in random order. Subjects were not given any specific instructions to alter smoking behaviors even though at some intervals in the study they were taking 21 mg patch daily. They rated their ad libitum responses to smoking as well as mood and withdrawal states in their natural environment during the first 6 days of each trial and then rated responses to nicotinized and denicotinized cigarettes in a controlled laboratory session on the last day of each week. Unlike prior laboratory studies, this study examined smoking behaviors via a controlled smoking device and measures were obtained in the laboratory ~1 h rather than several hours after pill administration. Results from the ad libitum smoking period in the natural environment showed that naltrexone attenuated ratings of the wakefulness of cigarettes and increased negative mood states. Naltrexone with patch increased the aversiveness of the first cigarette of the day but no other interactions on mood or withdrawal symptoms were observed. In the laboratory sessions, naltrexone appeared to reverse some of the effects of patch, including aversiveness, craving reduction, negative affect, wakefulness, and amount of ad libitum smoking. The findings were interpreted as showing evidence for the interaction between the opioid system and aspects of smoking behavior, but potential clinical applications for naltrexone in treatment were not supported given that naltrexone did not alter behavior or subjective responses in a manner that may be deemed helpful for clinical indications.

While many of these laboratory studies indicated mixed support for naltrexone altering human smoking behaviors and subjective response, in some cases the sample characteristics (young smokers in their 20s, which is younger than the median age for cessation treatment) or the laboratory paradigm (smoking during the 21 mg patch) may not translate directly to the clinical setting. A study by King and Meyer was designed to examine naltrexone on aspects of smoking behavior that may occur in early treatment, such as early abstinence, smoking a single cigarette (i.e., a "slip") and/or continuing with smoking behavior (i.e., a "relapse") (34). Subjects ingested either 50 mg naltrexone or identical placebo (in random order) the morning after overnight observed abstinence from smoking at the GCRC. They completed subjective measures 2 h after pill ingestion, followed immediately by smoking a single cigarette of their preferred brand, a 1-h rest period, and then a 2-h choice smoking paradigm. Twenty-two adult nicotine-dependent smokers (10 female), of an average age of 32.5 years, who smoked 25.3 cigarettes daily for 13.9 years, were examined in this within-subjects study. Results showed that naltrexone did not affect subjective measures of craving or mood 2 h after ingestion (i.e., during the first few hours of abstinence). Naltrexone compared with placebo significantly attenuated self-report ratings of smoking pleasure and craving after the first cigarette. Naltrexone also decreased the number of cigarettes chosen in the choice phase, which was confirmed by objective measures including expired air CO and plasma nicotine levels. This study demonstrated that naltrexone may significantly interact with nicotine response during an initial smoking exposure and attenuate smoking behaviors upon subsequent choice to continue to smoke.

To further examine effects of naltrexone on smoking, a second study in the same laboratory was conducted to examine naltrexone compared with placebo on response to a smoking cue, subjective effects before and after smoking, and behavioral choice for smoking (35). The sample included the largest within-subject sample size to date (n = 44 smokers, 21 female). Subjects' average age was 37 years and cigarette smoking averaged 20.7 cigarettes daily for 18.7 years. They participated in a similar study paradigm at the GCRC as in the first study (34). The difference was that this study also included a smoking cue (holding a lit cigarette for 1 min) 2 h after study drug, followed 1 h later by a single cigarette and then choice smoking for 2 h. The results showed that, similar to the first study, naltrexone compared with placebo decreased choice smoking behavior, which was confirmed by expired air CO readings and plasma nicotine levels. Naltrexone also increased negative affect and subjective side effects, such as sedation, and decreased positive affect after the first cigarette. However, unlike prior studies (32, 34), compared with placebo treatment, naltrexone did not alter ratings of craving or pleasure to the single cigarette or responses to the cue. The authors suggested that response to the cue may have been masked by high baseline smoking urge ratings as the subjects were moderately heavy smokers deprived of smoking for 14 h. Moreover, the addition of the cue may have altered subsequent response to smoking, as desire to smoke ratings in the placebo condition did not return to baseline levels 1 h after the cigarette as they did in the first study. Taken together, both studies suggested a main effect of naltrexone in decreasing smoking behavior, corroborated by lower expired air CO and plasma nicotine levels, but the precise mechanism underlying naltrexone's effects on smoking behavior remains to be determined.

The two most recent laboratory-based studies examining naltrexone on cigarette smoking have employed somewhat different methodologies than used in the prior laboratory studies. In one study, 26 nicotine-dependent smokers (11 female) with an average age of 44 years and who smoked 17.9 cigarettes daily were examined in a within-subjects study of naltrexone's effects on the relative reinforcing value of nicotine as measured a smoking topography machine (36). Smoking choice behavior for nicotine versus nonnicotine factors (i.e., more smoking for nicotine would indicate greater reinforcing value) was the primary dependent measure. Puff choices out of 16 required puff for cigarettes containing 0.6 mg versus 0.05 mg nicotine were examined. Naltrexone (50 mg) or identical placebo was given in random order and smoking choices were examined 2–3 h later. Naltrexone significantly increased nausea and dizziness ratings in the first few hours of smoking abstinence compared with placebo, and decreased the reinforcing value of nicotine, as the ratio of choice puffing for the nicotinized versus denicotinized cigarettes was lower compared with the placebo session. However, naltrexone did not significantly affect self-reported smoking satisfaction or liking. Since behavior outcome (smoking choices for nicotinized vs denicotinized cigarettes) differed between the naltrexone and placebo conditions, interpretation of subjective responses may be difficult. The findings of naltrexone altering the reinforcing value of nicotine, that is, apart from general smoking behavior, support an opioid–nicotine interaction and may identify an underlying mechanism for results from prior laboratory studies.

The only laboratory-based study of naltrexone and smoking that specifically employed participants who desired to quit smoking also showed mixed results (37). The preponderance of evidence of naltrexone's effects on acute smoking from laboratory studies thus far has focused on smokers who do not desire to quit, which may limit applicability to clinical settings (38). In this between-subjects study by Lee and colleagues (37), 25 male smokers were randomized to either 2 weeks of naltrexone (n = 13) or placebo (n = 12). Subjects' average age was 31.4 years and they smoked on average 20.3 cigarettes daily for 12.7 years. Because the study was designed to observe natural effects of the study drug on smoking behaviors, subjects were encouraged to but not required to quit smoking. No adjunct counseling or self-help materials were included. At the end of the first and second weeks, subjects were examined in the laboratory on their responses to sham smoking (putting an unlit cigarette to the lips) as well as regular smoking of a cigarette of their preferred brand. Unlike most other studies, the study drug was taken in the evening with variable dosing and while the goal was 25 mg daily for the first week and 50 mg daily for the second week, the average dose was 23.5 mg daily in the first week and 37.1 mg daily in the second week.

Over the 2-week period, naltrexone significantly reduced ad libitum smoking levels and this was verified by expired air CO levels. In the laboratory session, naltrexone reduced self-reported craving after the sham smoking compared with placebo. While naltrexone did decrease smoking and craving, the authors concluded that since only one of the thirteen naltrexone-treated subjects had completely quit smoking, it may have limited utility in smoking cessation. However, the paradigm may not have provided an adequate test of naltrexone effects on cessation, as the between-subjects study had a small sample size and limited statistical power, and contained potential mixed messages about quitting smoking, with no specific cessation goals or behavioral self-help adjuncts offered. Also, inclusion of sham smoking in the experimental sessions conducted during the treatment period might have confounded measurement of smoking urges and encouraged smoking exposure.

Taking results of these laboratory-based studies of naltrexone on smoking response together, a majority of the studies (5 of 7 studies) examining smoking behaviors have shown that naltrexone, compared with placebo, attenuates ad libitum smoking levels and/or choice smoking behaviors for cigarettes or nicotine. Results on the subjective effects are more variable, with some studies showing naltrexone reduction in ratings of smoking pleasure and satisfaction (31, 34), cigarette urges (32, 37), and perceived difficulty in abstaining (30), while others have found naltrexone to augment withdrawal-like effects or negative mood (30, 33, 35, 36).

The discrepancy in findings across laboratory studies may be due to differences in study paradigms in the timing of measures, types of measures employed, and the characteristics of the subject samples. First, some studies did not report pertinent subject-related factors, such as the sex ratio, or only employed male subjects without stating a rationale for the exclusion of female. Other studies did not state specific frequencies or incidence of side effects or rationale behind study parameters, such as requiring success in a baseline period of abstinence after naltrexone or placebo initial dosing for study inclusion. Second, given the extensive first-pass metabolism of oral naltrexone and rapid transformation to the metabolite 6-β-naltrexol, differences in time course, dosing, and acute versus repeated administration may play a role in the different results across studies. Third, translating human preclinical studies to clinical treatment trials can be difficult for various reasons and the effects of naltrexone on subjective and objective smoking responses may be complex. Differences across studies in sample characteristics and subjects' motivation to participate (i.e., nontreatment seeking), short-term versus long-term dosing, and paradigm focus (abstinence, response to cues, demand characteristics, and use of nicotine replacement) and may all play a large role in identifying or failing to identify significant drug effects. Finally, these laboratory studies were largely conducted with small sample sizes, low statistical power, and none have extensively examined potential individual difference factors in response to naltrexone.

17.3 Clinical Trials

The use of naltrexone for smoking cessation has emerged out of the biochemical and behavioral data obtained from several of the aforementioned laboratory studies. To apply these findings clinically, additional studies began to use a variety of designs that involve both naltrexone alone (39, 40), as well as in combination with nicotine replacement (41–43). Several published reports of naltrexone in smoking cessation have reported only preliminary or descriptive data (44, 45) or were open-label trials (46). Other studies have some methodological limitations such as not employing a placebo control (47) or analyzing only treatment completer data (48). For the purposes of this chapter, only those investigations employing intent-to-treat analyses, adequate follow-up (6 months or longer) with biochemical verification and appropriate placebo-controlled randomized designs were reviewed.

Wong and colleagues (39) conducted a double-blind, placebo-controlled trial of naltrexone versus placebo in smoking cessation. The study was one site of a larger multisite trial, but the results from the other study sites were not reported. The main dependent measure was abstinence rates, with secondary measures including completion rates and self-report side effects, and craving. Subjects were 100 male and female heavy smokers with an average of 27.8 cigarettes smoked per day at baseline. They were randomized according to a 2 × 2 design using 50 mg daily naltrexone versus placebo, and nicotine patch versus no patch (i.e., a placebo patch condition was not employed). Both study drugs were initiated beginning upon each participant's quit day and continued for 12 weeks: nicotine patch dose was 21 mg daily for the first 8 weeks followed by 14 mg daily for the remaining 4 weeks, and naltrexone (or placebo) was taken at 50 mg daily for the entire 12 weeks. At each of the eight study appointments, participants were provided with brief 15–20 min counseling [using the American Lung Association (ALA) *Freedom from Smoking* materials] conducted by research assistant.

Overall, 68% of subjects completed participation through to the end of treatment at 12 weeks. These rates were lower with naltrexone, particularly in those taking naltrexone alone (i.e., 39% completion in naltrexone only vs 69% placebo only, 88% placebo and patch, and 73% naltrexone and patch). Naltrexone produced greater side effects than placebo in terms of headache (57% naltrexone only vs 23% placebo only) and sleep disturbance (22% naltrexone only, vs 0% placebo only). Severe side effects were rare, and only three participants were discontinued from treatment due to adverse effects, all of whom were randomized to naltrexone, alone or with patch.

Smoking quit rates were determined by continuous abstinence (i.e., no smoking at any point in the study) and 7-day point prevalence at 12 and 24 weeks, both confirmed by expired air CO levels. Naltrexone, either with or without the patch, was found to have no effect on smoking quit rates at any point in the trial. However, strong effects for the patch versus no patch were observed, with 12-week continuous abstinence rates of 31% and 36% for patch either with or without naltrexone, compared with 9% and 12% for no patch either with or without naltrexone. Similar findings were observed for self-reported craving, with no effects of naltrexone but significant effects of patch versus no patch in reducing craving (i.e., intention and desire to smoke with smoking anticipated as pleasurable). The conclusion of the study was that there was no evidence for the efficacy of naltrexone in smoking cessation, despite prior laboratory and short-term studies suggesting that naltrexone may decrease smoking levels in controlled settings.

In contrast, another early placebo-controlled investigation of naltrexone in smoking cessation showed positive effects of naltrexone on outcome (40). In this study, 80 participants smoking an average of 34.3 cigarettes per day at baseline were randomly assigned to receive either placebo or naltrexone monotherapy for 4 weeks in addition to brief individual counseling employing the ALA program. The naltrexone dose began at 25 mg per day ~3 days before quit day. Depending on each participant's ability to tolerate the medication, the dose was increased to 50 mg on quit day and potentially increased to up to 75 mg.

Dosing schedules were not standardized, and occurred at the discretion of the research staff.

In this study, dropout during the 3-day prequit interval occurred in 25% of those assigned to naltrexone and 5% of those in placebo. Reasons for dropout were variable, but often included reported negative side effects such as nausea, dizziness, sleeplessness, and concentration difficulty. Outcome was only assessed in those who remained in the trial upon the quit date (n = 68). At the end of the treatment phase at 4 weeks, naltrexone directionally increased quit rates compared with placebo (46.7% naltrexone vs 26.3% placebo). Quit rates remained proportionally higher in the naltrexone compared with placebo group at 6 months, although not statistically significant (26.7% naltrexone vs 15.2% placebo). Posthoc stratifications by sex and history of major depression showed that both variables related to better outcomes with naltrexone treatment. However, caution should be taken in interpreting these results given the small sample size and the fact that a strict intent-to-treat analysis was not conducted.

On the basis of evidence of nicotine withdrawal in the presence of naltrexone, a growing body of literature has looked at the efficacy of combined naltrexone with concomitant nicotine replacement therapy. Such combination pharmacotherapy may aid cessation rates by reducing withdrawal effects by nicotine agonist therapy and reducing aspects of nicotine reward or craving, putatively with naltrexone. Indeed, the prevalence and nature of the side effects and dropout rates in the naltrexone treated groups in the two studies reviewed add support to animal and human laboratory data demonstrating opioid blockade may produce nicotine and mild opiate withdrawal-like states (19, 21). The most recent comprehensive studies of naltrexone in smoking treatment have both employed nicotine patch therapy as a standard platform treatment with which to examine the efficacy of naltrexone on quit rates.

The largest oral naltrexone and transdermal nicotine patch combined treatment study included 400 male and female participants in a 6-week, dose ranging clinical trial (42). Participants were treatment-seeking and recruited from the community and smoked on average 27.4 cigarettes daily. All subjects received the nicotine patch and brief behavioral counseling (45 min with a nurse at the first visit and 15 min sessions with a research assistant at subsequent visits). The nicotine patch dose was 21 mg and patch use began on the quit date and continued for 6 weeks. Participants were randomly assigned to either the placebo group or one of three naltrexone dose groups (25, 50, 100 mg/day). The study drug was initiated on the day after the quit date (the second day of nicotine patch use) and the dose was titrated on an escalating scale, depending on the dose group (i.e., 12.5 mg for 1 day, 25 mg for 1 day, 50 mg for 2 days, and 100 mg thereafter for 6 weeks). The two primary dependent measures were prolonged abstinence quit rates at 6 weeks (not smoking at all allowing for a 2-week grace period after the quit date) and weight gain in abstainers at the same interval. In the intent-to-treat sample, the naltrexone effect was not statistically significant for prolonged abstinence, although there was a marginally significant increase in quit rates for 100 mg maltrexone compared with placebo based on continuous abstinence (i.e., no grace period allowed, 51.5% vs 38.7%, respectively). However, among the ~74% of the sample who completed the 6 weeks of treatment, naltrexone (100 mg) produced significantly higher continuous abstinence quit rates compared with placebo (71.6% vs 48%).

For secondary outcome measures, while the 25 mg and 50 mg doses did not improve quit rates beyond that of placebo, both doses resulted in less weight gain over the first 6 weeks of cessation in abstainers compared with placebo (1.5 and 2.4 pound in the 25 and 50 mg groups, respectively, vs 4.2 pound in placebo). In contrast, while the 100 mg dose resulted in a greater number of participants having dose reductions or discontinuation during the trial (17.5% vs 3.2% in placebo), this dose produced more rapid and greater reductions in withdrawal symptoms and smoking urges over time. In summary, the results of this trial were mixed in terms of support for naltrexone: while robust intent-to-treat analyses did not show statistically significant increases in quit rates with naltrexone, the treatment completer analyses showed efficacy for the 100 mg dose, which was supported by results showing greater reduction in withdrawal and smoking urges over time with that dose. On the contrary, in those who successfully quit, the weight gain was not significantly reduced with the 100 mg dose but rather the 25 and 50 mg doses. Although effects were noted during treatment, at 3-, 6-, and 12-month follow-up, the advantage of naltrexone was no longer apparent. The authors suggested that dosing choices may eventually be determined based on patient matching of goals and characteristics. Also, since treatment effects did not extend to follow-up, treatment with naltrexone for more extended periods of time may be indicated.

The second study examining naltrexone in combination with nicotine patch and standard individual counseling was conducted in 110 (56 female) treatment-seeking smokers (41). These participants smoked an average of 21.1 cigarettes per day at baseline, which is ~22% less than participants in the O'Malley study (42). Participants in this trial were randomly assigned to receive either naltrexone (50 mg/day) or placebo for 8 weeks, but unlike O'Malley, medication was initiated 3 days before quit day, at 25 mg per day. Beginning on quit day, all subjects received the nicotine patch for 4 weeks (21 mg for the first 2 weeks, 14 mg the third week, and 7 mg the fourth week) and increased dose of naltrexone to 50 mg daily, and continued at that dose (or placebo) for the remaining 8 weeks. In addition, all participants received six 45-min individual behavioral therapy sessions delivered by a master's or doctoral level therapist. Counseling began 2 weeks before quit day and ended 4 weeks after the quit date.

As in the O'Malley study (42), there were few adverse effects with naltrexone combined with nicotine patch. The main side effects associated with naltrexone in the first week of treatment were nausea, sedation, lightheadedness, and feeling flushed/warm; at 4 weeks, only lightheadedness remained significantly elevated in the naltrexone versus placebo group. Dropout rates between the groups were also similar (15% naltrexone vs 22% placebo discontinued before end of treatment at 8 weeks).

For the overall sample, naltrexone directionally improved prolonged abstinence quit rates (no smoking after allowing a 1-week grace period) compared with placebo, but this was not statistically significant at either end of treatment or follow-up (48% vs 41% at 8 weeks; 27% vs 19% at 24 weeks). However, when stratifying the sample by sex, differences in treatment response between the sexes emerged. Among placebo-treated participants, women had significantly lower quit rates than men (39% vs 67%, respectively), similar to the "gender gap" in outcome demonstrated in other studies (49–54). In contrast, among naltrexone-treated participants, women's quit rates were similar to those of men (58% vs 62%, respectively). Further, naltrexone significantly reduced men's and women's cessation-related weight gain, and also selectively reduced women's urge to smoke to relieve negative affect and withdrawal. The results suggest continued examination of naltrexone as an adjunct in smoking cessation, particularly in female smokers, who have historically shown worse outcomes with traditional treatment methods.

17.4 Sources of Individual Differences in Response to Naltrexone

Compared with laboratory studies, there are very few clinical studies examining naltrexone in smoking cessation, and of these studies, only very few of them have employed robust research methodology including random assignment, double-blinding, standardizing dose levels, and intent-to-treat analyses. The 2006 Cochrane Review (55) indicated that while no trials in their meta-analysis detected a significant difference in quit rates between naltrexone and placebo, collectively the confidence intervals are compatible with both clinically significant benefit and possible negative effects of naltrexone in promoting smoking abstinence. The review concluded that data from larger trials is necessary to determine whether naltrexone may be efficacious in smoking cessation. In addition, analyses of secondary variables of interest, such as weight gain, or post-hoc sample stratifications on sex, have revealed potentially important individual difference factors that may be relevant in terms of identifying patients most likely to benefit from adjunct treatment with naltrexone. In this final section of this chapter, we review five potential individual difference factors which may mediate or moderate response to naltrexone in smoking cessation, including sex differences, depression, weight gain concerns, alcohol drinking patterns, and genetic variants.

17.4.1 Sex Differences

There is increasing evidence that female smokers show poorer outcome in smoking cessation compared to their male counterparts, although there is still some debate, especially in interpreting trials that do not a priori stratify for gender (56). Several theories have emerged to explicate reasons for women having lower success than men in smoking treatment, including females' increased affective symptoms and higher prevalence of depression, greater withdrawal complications during cessation, concerns about weight gain, and lack of social support (57). Also, lower dependency on nicotine relative to the nonassociative aspects of smoking has been demonstrated in female smokers (58). The implication of female smokers' differential nicotine-dependence profile is relevant in terms of optimizing and targeting cessation options since several pharmacotherapy studies with nicotine replacement therapy shown lower quit rates in women versus men (49, 51, 53, 54).

King's (41) findings are similar to those demonstrated by Covey et al. (40), who observed that 50–75 mg doses of naltrexone were associated with improved quit rates for female smokers at 4 weeks (39% naltrexone vs 15% placebo), but this was not the case for males. These findings suggest potential sex differences with regard to quitting smoking via naltrexone augmentation of the nicotine patch, such that women may benefit more than men from this type of combined pharmacotherapy (40, 41, 59).

17.4.2 Depression History and Symptoms

Another clinical observation associated with outcome pertains to smokers with a history of Major Depressive Disorder (MDD). Covey et al. (40) found that, at the end of the 4-week treatment, quit rates for participants with a history of MDD were 57.1% for those on naltrexone and 13.6% for those taking placebo. At 6-month follow-up, those participants with a history of MDD taking naltrexone had a significantly higher quit rate (28.6%; n = 14) at 6 months than those on placebo (9.1%; n = 22). Similarly, post-hoc analyses of data in the King et al. study have indicated that even in a nondepressed sample, subclinical depressive symptoms may affect outcome with naltrexone: smokers with higher scores on the Beck Depression Inventory had worse quit rates in the placebo group, but not in the naltrexone group (60). In contrast, studies that have excluded participants who have a history of depression have not found positive effects of naltrexone on quit rates (39) and this individual difference factor may be one potential explanation for discrepancy across studies.

17.4.3 Cessation-Related Weight Gain

The average weight gain for individuals who are continuously abstinent from smoking is ~10–13 pounds in the first year, with most of the weight gain occurring within the first 6 months postcessation (61, 62). This may be due to decreases in metabolism, increased appetite, and/or behavioral changes (i.e., substituting eating for smoking) following smoking cessation. Clinically, weight gain during cessation may bode poorly for outcome and even anticipation of weight gain may deter some smokers from even attempting to quit, particularly for female smokers (63–66). There is evidence that naltrexone at 25 mg and 50 mg doses may significantly decrease the weight gain associated with cessation (41, 42). While naltrexone-treated patients still gained some weight during early smoking abstinence, the amount was significantly reduced compared to placebo (i.e., ~3 pounds less weight gain in the first 4–6 weeks). Pending the outcome of ongoing and future research, naltrexone may show efficacy particularly for weight-concerned and/or female smokers who tend to be more sensitive to weight-related changes than many of their male counterparts.

17.4.4 *Alcohol Drinking Patterns*

Given that naltrexone is approved for the treatment of alcohol dependence, smokers who drink alcohol excessively represent a sizeable subgroup in which combined use of naltrexone and other approved smoking cessation therapies may be helpful. Daily smokers are more than four times as likely to drink hazardously compared to nonsmokers (67) and over 22% of individuals with nicotine dependence also meet criteria for an alcohol use disorder (68). Moreover, alcohol consumption has been shown to increase smoking behavior (69–73). Given this, clinical practice guidelines for treating tobacco dependence (74) suggest that smokers be advised to reduce or avoid alcohol consumption during a quit attempt. With this background in mind, naltrexone could be useful to smokers who drink heavily by reducing the frequency of hazardous drinking which is otherwise harmful and which may also promote smoking relapse. Preliminary results from the trials by O'Malley et al. (42) and King et al. (41) suggest that naltrexone, compared to placebo, results in reductions in alcohol consumption in the absence of specific counseling to alter drinking patterns during a smoking cessation attempt (75, 76).

17.4.5 *Genetic Variants*

The MOR gene, OPRM1, is emerging as a key factor related to addictions to a number of substances. For example, the presence of the G allele of the OPRM1 gene has been associated with greater response to alcohol (77) and opiate antagonists (78). In the tobacco area, recent evidence suggests that the presence of polymorphisms in the OPRM1 gene may result in increased susceptibility of smoking initiation and nicotine dependence (79). The presence of a functional A118G variant of the OPRM1 gene, which is associated with reduced MOR expression (80) and partial loss of function (81), has been associated with improved treatment response to nicotine replacement therapy (82, 83), as well as reduced nicotine reinforcement in women (84). With respect to naltrexone treatment, one would predict that since the primary site of action of naltrexone is the MOR that polymorphisms in the OPRM1 gene should alter response. Indeed, in clinical trials examining the efficacy of naltrexone in the treatment of alcohol dependence, the presence of at least one copy of the G allele of OPRM1 was associated with better treatment outcomes (85). It has yet to be established whether such genetic treatment outcome linkages may be present with opioid polymorphisms and response to opioid antagonist treatment for nicotine dependence.

17.5 Future Directions and Ongoing Research

Evidence from both preclinical and clinical trials demonstrates that naltrexone alters some aspects of cigarette smoking behavior and may potentially improve treatment outcome for some smokers. However, comprehensive and large-scale research is currently lacking. There are ongoing research studies examining the role of sex differences, depression and affective symptomology, weight concerns, alcohol drinking levels, and genetic variants as potential individual difference factors that may relate to response to naltrexone in smoking cessation. While the exact therapeutic role for opioid antagonist treatment in nicotine dependence has not yet been established, continued large-scale and comprehensive clinical trials, as well as further preclinical research, will help elucidate if naltrexone may be effective in augmenting smoking cessation outcomes.

Acknowledgments This work was supported by # R01-DA016834, R01-AA013746, and CCSG P30-CA14599. Appreciation is expressed to Megan Conrad for technical assistance

References

1. Tobacco use among adults – United States, 2005. MMWR Morb Mortal Wkly Rep 2006; 55:1145–1148.
2. Smoking cessation during previous year among adults – United States, 1990 and 1991. MMWR Morb Mortal Wkly Rep 1993;42:504–507.
3. Fiore MC, Bailey WC, Cohen SJ, Dorfman SF, Goldstein MG, Gritz ER, Heyman RB, Jaen CR. Treating tobacco use and dependence: Clinical practice guidelines. AHRQ Pub. No. 00-0032. Washington, DC: US Department of Health and Human Services, Public Health Service, 2000.
4. Gonzales D, Rennard SI, Nides M, Oncken C, Azoulay S, Billing CB, Watsky EJ, Gong J, Williams KE, Reeves KR. Varenicline, an $\alpha4\beta2$ nicotinic acetylcholine receptor partial agonist, vs. sustained-release bupropion and placebo for smoking cessation: A randomized controlled trial. JAMA 2006;296:47–55.
5. Jorenby DE, Leischow SJ, Rennard SI, Johnston AJ, Hughes AR, Smith SS, Muramotot ML, Daughton DM, Doan K, Fiore MC, Baker TB. A controlled trial of sustained-release bupropion, a nicotine patch, or both for smoking cessation. N Eng J Med 1999;340:685–691.
6. Jorenby DE, Hays JT, Rigotti NA, Azoulay S, Watsky EJ, Williams KE, Billing CB, Gong J, Reeves KR. Efficacy of Varenicline, an $\alpha4\beta2$ nicotinic acetylcholine receptor partial agonist vs placebo or sustained-release bupropion for smoking cessation: A randomized controlled trial. JAMA 2006;296:56–63.
7. Tonstad S, Tønnesen P, Hajek P, Williams KE, Billing CB, Reeves KR; for the Varenicline Phase 3 Study Group. Effect of maintenance therapy with Varenicline on smoking cessation: A randomized controlled trial. JAMA 2006;296:64–71.
8. Pomerleau OF, Rosencrans J. Neuroregulatory effects of nicotine (Rev). Psychoneuroendocrinology 1989;14:407–423.
9. Almeida LEF, Pereira EFR, Alkondon M, Fawcett WP, Randall WR, Albuquerque EX. The opioid antagonist naltrexone inhibits activity and alters expression of α and $\alpha4\beta2$ nicotinic receptors in hippocampal neurons: Implications for smoking cessation programs. Neuropharmacology 2000;39:2740–2755.

10. Almeida LE, Pereira EF, Camara A, Maelicke A, Albuquerque E. Sensitivity of neuronal nicotinic acetylcholine receptors to the opiate antagonists naltrexone and naloxone: Receptor blockade and up-regulation. Bioorg Med Chem Lett 2004;14:1879–1887.
11. Boyadjieva NI, Sarkar DK. The secretory response of hypothalamic β-endorphin neurons to acute and chronic treatments and following nicotine withdrawal. Life Sci 1997;61:59–66.
12. Davenport KE, Houdi AA, Van Loon GR. Nicotine protects against μ-opioid receptor antagonism by β-funaltrexamine: Evidence for nicotine-induced release of endogenous opioids in brain. Neurosci Lett 1990;113:40–46.
13. Opitz K, Weischer ML. Volitional oral intake of nicotine in tupaias: Drug-induced alterations. Drug Alcohol Depend 1988;21:99–104.
14. Sahley TL, Berntson GG. Antinociceptive effects of central and systemic administrations of nicotine in the rat. Psychopharmacology (Berl) 1979;65(3):279–283.
15. Tomé AR, Izaguirre V, Rosário LM, Ceña V, González-García C. Naloxone inhibits nicotine-induced receptor current and catecholamine secretion in bovine chromaffin cells. Brain Res 2001;903:63–65.
16. Tripathi HL, Martin BR, Aceto MD. Nicotine-induced antinociception in rats and mice: Correlation with nicotine brain levels. J Pharmacol Exp Ther 1982;221:91–96.
17. Wewers ME, Dhatt RK, Snively TA, Tejwani GA. The effect of chronic administration of nicotine on antinociception, opioid receptor binding and met-enkephalin levels in rats. Brain Res 1999;822:107–113.
18. Gianutsos G, Drawbaugh R, Hynes M, Lal H. The narcotic withdrawal syndrome in the rat. In: Ehrenpreis S, Neidle A, eds. Methods in Narcotics Research. New York: Dekker 1975:293–309.
19. Krishnan-Sarin S, Rosen MI, O'Malley SS. Naloxone challenge in smokers: Preliminary evidence of an opiod component in nicotine dependence. Arch Gen Psychiatry 1999;56:663–668.
20. Malin D, Lake J, Carter V, Cunningham J, Wilson O. Naloxone precipitates nicotine abstinence syndrome. Psychopharm 1993;112:339–342.
21. Malin D, Lake J, Payne M, Short P, Carter V, Cunningham J, Wilson O. Nicotine alleviation of nicotine abstinence syndrome is naloxone-reversible. Pharmacol Biochem Behav 1996;53:81–85.
22. Pomerleau OF. Endogenous opioids and smoking: A review of progress and problems. Psychoneuroendocrinology 1998;23:115–130.
23. Watkins SS, Koob GF, Markou A. Neural mechanisms underlying nicotine addiction: Acute positive reinforcement and withdrawal. Nicotine Tob Res 2000;2:19–37.
24. Gysling K, Wang RY. Morphine-induced activation of A 10 dopamine neurons in the rat. Brain Res 1983;277:119–127.
25. Matthews RT, German DC. Electrophysiological evidence for excitation of rat ventral tegmental area dopamine neurons by morphine. Neuroscience 1984;11:129–152.
26. David V, Durkin TP, Cazala P. Differential effects of the dopamine D_2/D_3 receptor antagonist sulpiride on self-administration of morphine into the ventral tegmental area or the nucleus accumbens. Psychopharmacology (Berl) 2002;160:307–317.
27. Berrendero F, Kieffer BL, Maldonado R. Attenuation of nicotine-induced antinociception, rewarding effects, and dependence in mu-opiod receptor knock-out mice. J Neurosci 2002;22:10935–10940.
28. Berrendero F. Mendizabal V. Robledo P. Galeote L. Bilkei-Gorzo A. Zimmer A. Maldonado R. Nicotine-induced antinociception, rewarding effects, and physical dependence are decreased in mice lacking the preproenkephalin gene. J Neurosci 2005;25:1103–1112.
29. Galeote L, Kieffer BL, Maldonado R, Berrendero F. Mu-opioid receptors are involved in the tolerance to nicotine antinociception. J Neurochem 2006;97(2):416–423.
30. Sutherland G, Stapleton JA, Russell MA, Feyerabend C. Naltrexone, smoking behaviour and cigarette withdrawal. Psychopharmacology (Berl) 1995;120:418–425.
31. Wewers ME, Dhatt R, Tejwani GA. Naltrexone administration affects ad libitum smoking behavior. Psychopharmacology (Berl) 1998;140:185–190.

32. Hutchison KE, Monti PM, Rohsenow DJ, Swift RM, Colby SM, Gnys M, Niaura RS, Sirota AD. Effects of naltrexone with nicotine replacement on smoking cue reactivity: Preliminary results. Psychopharmacology (Berl) 1999;142:139–143.
33. Brauer LH, Behm FM, Westman EC, Patel P, Rose JE. Naltrexone blockade of nicotine effects in cigarette smokers. Psychopharmacology 1999;143:339–346.
34. King AC, Meyer PJ. Naltrexone alteration of acute smoking response in nicotine-dependent subjects. Pharmacol Biochem Behav 2000;66:563–572.
35. Epstein AM, King AC. Naltrexone attenuates acute cigarette smoking behavior. Pharmacol Biochem Behav 2004;77:29–37.
36. Rukstalis M, Jepson C, Strasser A, Lynch KG, Perkins K, Patterson F, Lerman C. Naltrexone reduces the relative reinforcing value of nicotine in a cigarette smoking choice paradigm. Psychopharmacology (Berl) 2005;180:41–48.
37. Lee YS, Joe KH, Sohn IK, Na C, Kee BS, Chae SL. Changes of smoking behavior and serum adrenocorticotropic hormone, cortisol, prolactin, and endogenous opioid levels in nicotine dependence after naltrexone treatment. Prog Neuropsychopharmacol Biol Psychiatry 2005;29:639–647.
38. Perkins KA, Stitzer M, Lerman C. Medication screening for smoking cessation: A proposal for new methodologies. Psychopharmacology (Berl) 2006;184:628–636.
39. Wong GY, Wolter TD, Croghan GA, Croshan IT, Offord EP, Hurt RD. A randomized trial of naltrexone for smoking cessation. Addiction 1999;94:1227–1237.
40. Covey LS, Glassman AH, Stetner F. Naltrexone effects on short-term and long-term smoking cessation. J Addict Dis 1999;18:31–40.
41. King AC, de Wit H, Riley RC, Cao D, Niaura R, Hatsukami D. Efficacy of naltrexone in smoking cessation: A preliminary study and an examination of sex differences. Nicotine Tob Res 2006;5:1–12.
42. O'Malley SS, Cooney JL, Krishnan-Sarin S, Dubin JA, McKee SA, Cooney NL, Blakeslee A, Meandzija B, Romano-Dahlgard D, Wu R, Makuch R, Jatlow P. A controlled trial of naltrexone augmentation of nicotine replacement for smoking cessation. Arch Intern Med 2006;166:667–674.
43. O'Malley SS, Krishnan-Sarin S, Meandzija B. Naltrexone treatment of nicotine dependence: A preliminary study. Poster presented at third annual scientific conference of the Society for Research on Nicotine and Tobacco, Nashville, TN, 1997.
44. King AC. Role of naltrexone in initial smoking cessation: Preliminary findings. Alcohol Clin Exp Res 2002;26:1942–1944.
45. Krishnan-Sarin S, Meandzija B, O'Malley S. Naltrexone and nicotine patch in smoking cessation: A preliminary study. Nicotine Tob Res 2003;5:851–857.
46. Roozen HG, van Beers S, Weevers HJ, Breteler M, Willemsen M, Postmus P, Kerkhof A. Effects on smoking cessation: Naltrexone combined with a cognitive behavioral treatment based on the community reinforcement approach. Subst Use Misuse 2006;41:45–60.
47. Ahmadi J, Ashkani H, Ahmadi M, Ahmadi N. Twenty-four week maintenance treatment of cigarette smoking with nicotine gum, clonidine and naltrexone. J Subst Abuse Treat 2003;24:251–255.
48. Byars JA, Frost-Pineda K, Jacobs WS, Gold MS. Naltrexone augments the effects of nicotine replacement therapy in female smokers. J Addict Dis 2005;24:49–60.
49. Bjornson W, Rand C, Connett JE, Lindgren P, Nides M, Pope F, Buist AS, Hoppe-Ryan C, O'Hara P. Gender differences in smoking cessation after 3 years in the lung health study. Am J Public Health 1995;85:223–230.
50. Cepeda-Benito A, Reynoso JT, Erath S. Meta-analysis of the efficacy of nicotine replacement therapy for smoking cessation: Differences between men and women. J Consult Clin Psychol 2004;72:712–722.
51. Royce JM, Corbett K, Sorensen G, Ockene J. Gender, social pressure, and smoking cessations: The Community Intervention Trial for Smoking Cessation (COMMIT) at baseline. Soc Sci Med 1997;44:359–370.

52. Scharf D, Shiffman S. Are there gender differences in smoking cessation, with and without bupropion? Pooled-and-meta-analyses of clinical trials of bupropion SR. Soc for the Study of Addiction 2004;99:1462–1469.
53. Senore C, Battista RN, Shapiro SH, Segnan N, Ponti A, Rosso S, Aimar D. Predictors of smoking cessation following physicians' counseling. Prev Med 1998;27:412–421.
54. Wetter DW, Kenford SL, Smith SS, Fiore MC, Jorneby DE, Baker TB. Gender differences in smoking cessation. J Consult Clin Psychol 1999;67:555–562.
55. David S, Lancaster T, Stead LF, Evins AE. Opioid antagonists for smoking cessation. Cochrane Database of Systematic Reviews 2006;4. Art. No.: CD003086. DOI: 10.1002/14651858.CD003086.pub2.
56. Killen JD, Fortmann SP, Varady A, Kraemer HC. Do men outperform women in smoking cessation trials? Maybe, but not by much. Exp Clin Psychopharmacol 2002;3:295–301.
57. Perkins KA. Smoking cessation in women: Special considerations. CNS Drugs 2001;15:391–411.
58. Perkins KA. Sex differences in nicotine vs. non-nicotine reinforcement as determinants of tobacco smoking. Exp Clin Psychopharmacol 1996;4:166–177.
59. O'Malley S, Cooney J, Krishnan-Sarin S, McKee S, Meandzija B, Dubin J, Cooney N, Makuch R, Wu R, Romano-Dahlgard D, Blakeslee A, LaVelle E. Do sex differences influence response to naltrexone for smoking cessation? Poster presented at the annual meeting of the society for research on nicotine and tobacco, Prague, Czech Republic, March 21, 2007.
60. Walsh Z, Epstein A, Munisamy G, King A. The impact of depressive symptoms on the efficacy of naltrexone in smoking cessation. J Addict Dis 2008;27:65–72.
61. Klesges RC, Winders SE, Meyers AW, Eck LH, Ward KD, Hultquist CM, Ray JW, Sadish WR. How much weight gain occurs following smoking cessation? A comparison of weight gain using both continuous and point prevalence abstinence. J Consult Clin Psychol 1997;65:286–291.
62. Hudmon KS, Gritz ER, Clayton S, Nisenbaum R. Eating orientation, postcessation weight gain, and continued abstinence among female smokers receiving an unsolicited smoking cessation intervention. Health Psychol 1999;18:29–36.
63. Meyers AW, Klesges RC, Winders SE, Ward KD, Peterson BA, Eck LH. Are weight concerns predictive of smoking cessation? A prospective analysis. [Journal Article. Research Support, Non-U.S. Govt. Research Support, U.S. Govt, P.H.S.] J Consult Clin Psychol 1997;65:448–452.
64. Nides M, Rand C, Dolce J, Murray R, O'Hara P, Voelker H, Connett J. Weight gain as a function of smoking cessation and 2-mg nicotine gum use among middle-aged smokers with mild lung impairment in the first 2 years of the Lung Health Study. J Health Psychol 1994;13:354–361.
65. Pirie PL, Murray DM, Leupker RV. Gender differences in cigarette smoking and quitting in a cohort of young adults. Am J Public Health 1991;81:324–327.
66. Swan GE, Ward MN, Carmelli D, Jack LM. Differential rates of relapse in subgroups of male and female smokers. J Clin Epidemiol 1993;46:1041–1053.
67. McKee SA, Falba T, O'Malley SS, Sindelar J, O'Connor PG. Smoking status as a clinical indicator for alcohol misuse in US adults. Arch Int Med 2007;167:716–721.
68. Grant BF, Hasin DS, Chou PS, Stinson FS, Dawson DA. Nicotine dependence and psychiatric disorders in the United States. Arch Gen Psychiatry 2004;61:1107–1115.
69. Baer JS, Lichenstein E. Classification and prediction of smoking relapse episodes: An exploration of individual differences, J Consult Clin Psychol 1988; 6:104–110.
70. McKee SA, Krishnan-Sarin S, Shi J, Mase T, O'Malley SS. Modeling the effect of alcohol on smoking lapse behavior. Psychopharmacology (Berl) 2006;189:201–210.
71. Shiffman SM, Fischer LA, Paty J, Gnys M, Hickcox M, Kassel JD. Drinking and smoking: A field study of their association. Ann Behav Med 1994;16:203–209.
72. Shiffman S, Paty JA, Gnys M, Kassel JA, Hickcox M. First lapses to smoking: Within-subjects analysis of real-time reports. J Consult Clin Psychol 1996;64:366–379.

73. Zimmerman RS, Warheit GJ, Ulbrich PM, Auth JB. The relationship between alcohol use and attempts and success at smoking cessation. Addict Behav 1990;15:197–207.
74. Fiore MC, Bailey WC, Cohen SJ, et al. Treating Tobacco Use and Dependence. Clinical Practice Guideline. Rockville, MD: U.S. Department of Health and Human Services. Public Health Service. June 2000.
75. O'Malley SS, Krishnan-Sarin J, Cooney J, Dubin N, Cooley S, McKee S, Meandzija B, Wu R, Blakeslee A, Makuch R, Jatlow P. Dose dependent effects on naltrexone on hazardous drinking in prospective randomized study for naltrexone for smoking cessation. Alcohol Clin Exp Res 2005;29:78A. Suppl.S.
76. King AC, Vanier C, Cao D, Wilcox T. Naltaxone decreases alcohol drinking levels in smoking cessation. Poster presented at the Research Society on Alcholism 30th Annual Meeting, Washington, D.C. 2008.
77. Ray LA, Hutchison KE. A polymorphism of the μ-opioid receptor gene (OPRM1) and sensitivity to the effects of alcohol in humans. Alcohol Clin Exp Res 2004;28:1789–1795.
78. Wand GS, McCaul M, Yang X, Reynolds J, Gotjen D, Lee S, Ali A. The μ-opioid receptor gene polymorphism (A118G) alters HPA axis activation induced by opioid receptor blockade. Neuropsychopharmacology 2002;26:106–114.
79. Zhang L, Kendler KS, Chen X. The μ-opioid receptor gene and smoking initiation and nicotine dependence. Behav Brain Funct 2006 Aug 4;2:28.
80. Beyer A, Koch T, Schroder H, Schulz S, Hollt V. Effect of the A118G polymorphism on binding affinity, potency and agonist-mediated endocytosis, desensitization, and resensitization of the human mu-opioid receptor. J Neurochem 2004;89:553–560.
81. Zhang Y, Wang D, Johnson AD, Papp AC, Sadee W. Allelic expression imbalance of human opioid receptor (OPRM1) caused by variant A118G. J Biol Chem 2005;280:32618–32624.
82. Lerman C, Wileyto EP, Patterson F, Rukstalis M, Audrain-McGovern J, Restine S, Shields PG, Kaufmann V, Redden D, Benowitz N, Berrettini WH. The functional μ-opioid receptor (OPRM1) Asn40Asp variant predicts short-term response to nicotine replacement therapy in a clinical trial. Pharmacogenomics J 2004;4:184–192.
83. Munafò MR, Elliot KM, Murphy MFG, Walton RT, Johnstone EC. Association of the mu-opiod receptor gene with smoking cessation. Pharmacogenomics J 2007:1–9.
84. Ray R, Jepson C, Patterson F, Strasser A, Rukstalis M, Perkins K, Lynch KG, O'Malley S, Berrettini WH, Lerman C. Association of OPRM1 A118G variant with the relative reinforcing value of nicotine. Psychopharmacology (Berl) 2006;188:355–363.
85. Oslin DW, Berrettini W, Kranzler HR, Pettinati H, Gelernter J, Volpicelli JR, O'Brien CP. A functional polymorphism of the μ-opioid receptor gene is associated with naltrexone response in alcohol dependent patients. Neuropsychopharmacology 2003;28:1546–1552.

Part IV
Alcohol and Ingestive Behaviors

Chapter 18
Opioid Antagonists and Ethanol's Ability to Reinforce Intake of Alcoholic Beverages: Preclinical Studies

Larry D. Reid

Abstract A review of preclinical research leading to the use of opioid antagonists as medicines for alcohol abuse and alcohol dependence is presented. There is also a discussion of the how studies using laboratory animals can address many of the remaining issues associated with using drugs to treat alcohol use disorders. The case is made that recent findings associated with the development of opioid antagonists as medicines for alcoholism provides a revolutionary approach to treating alcoholism (and drug addiction, in general). The actualization of the prospects provided by the revolutionary approach is apt to yield the first truly effective treatments for alcoholism.

Keywords: Alcohol abuse; Alcohol dependence; Alcoholism; Opioids; Morphine; Naloxone; Naltrexone; Endorphins

18.1 Introduction: Alcoholism is a Problem with a Long History

Some people drink alcoholic beverages too much, too often. This is a problem because ethanol, the salient ingredient of alcoholic beverages, is toxic. For thousands of years, there has been rancorous debate concerning religious and political decisions about what exactly is too much, too often and the debate continues. Over the years, some consensus has emerged. Everyone agrees, for example, that drinking alcoholic beverages is not a good idea for pregnant women (increases the risk of birth defects including fetal alcohol syndrome). Nearly everyone agrees, for another example, that *other* people should not drive a car when intoxicated. In terms of drinking and driving, we have even been able to codify, in many jurisdictions, the blood ethanol level that produces impairments in judgment and motor coordination.

L.D. Reid
Department of Cognitive Science, Carnegie Hall,
Rensselaer Polytechnic Institute, RPI Campus, Troy, NY 12180
e-mail: reidl@rpi.edu

R. Dean et al. (eds.), *Opiate Receptors and Antagonists*,

In societies where the sale of alcoholic beverages is sanctioned, alcoholic beverages are popular and can be sold at premium prices. In those societies, some people drink excessively as defined by the emergent toxic consequences (a host of health and social problems). In some societies, the incidence of problematic drinking occurs with a significant proportion of the population and that, in turn, has profound unhealthy consequences for that society.

When there is significant incidence of problematic drinking, both formal and informal sanctions are usually applied. During certain periods in Western democracies, complete prohibition of the distribution of alcoholic beverages has been tried. In some societies dominated by religions prohibiting the use of alcoholic beverages, for example, many Muslim countries, prohibition is part of the societies' code. Among societies permitting sales, it is common to restrict sales (e.g., no sales to minors) and to restrict sales by heavy taxation. Drunkenness is often met with considerable social scorn and drunkards are often socially ostracized.

Despite sanctions, some people habitually drink to intoxication. When that happens, remedies are proposed. Remedies have varied from extremely harsh punishment for violators of sanctions to mild social distancing. Remarkably, even harsh sanctions and the accumulation of serious toxic effects are often not sufficient to curb some people's habitual use of alcoholic beverages. Despite a host of negative consequences, some people drink inordinate amounts of alcoholic beverages taking large amounts of ethanol on nearly a daily basis.

Alcoholic is a common label for persons who apparently cannot control their drinking. The germane condition of the alcoholic has been labeled alcoholism (there are more formal labels, but they do not add much to the discussion). Alcoholism is a moral problem involving temptation, choices, and serious consequences; however, labeling the alcoholic a sinner may mute but has not curbed alcoholism. Alcoholism remains a problem, although sanctions for habitual drunkenness and related behavioral problems have been refined, and then refined again and again, and the so-called refinements exercised across thousands of years.

The fact that even rational argument and harsh sanctions are not sufficient to curb an alcoholic's drinking has been perplexing. The common resolution is to come to the conclusion that the alcoholic suffers from an affliction and is somehow different from the non alcoholic. This has been codified in theories of alcoholism. During the thousands of years alcoholism has been a problem, many theories of alcoholism have been generated.

Progress toward understanding alcoholism was static for thousands of years mired in arguments about moral, theoretical, and commercial issues. A major change occurred with the modern development of the biological and social sciences. Alcoholism became a topic of scientific investigation; various theories of alcoholism began to be tested systematically. Accompanying that change was a conceptualization that put alcoholism in the category of a disease (a change that began in America with the writings of Benjamin Rush, a physician and signer of the Declaration of Independence, a revolutionary in more than one sense). The alcoholic was seen as an unfortunate victim rather than, or as well as, a sinner. Eventually, and importantly, money was allocated from the public coffer to scientifically investigate alcoholism.

Accompanying the idea that science might be successfully applied to social, even moral, problems (if redefined as a disease) were the developments in the theory of evolution. This, in turn, indicated that problems germane to alcoholism might be investigated in the laboratory using animals. The idea that moral problems such as alcoholism can be addressed in the animal laboratory is controversial, especially in societies where moral issues are thought to be the exclusive purview of religious authorities and surely not subject to assessment by results from a study done on rats!

Even within the framework of modern science, seldom, if ever, does a single research result from the animal laboratory have direct applicability to a human problem. What does have applicability is rational theory. In the animal laboratory, theories and their derived predictions can be assessed; theories refined; and, new approaches discovered. Theory is also refined in the laboratory using humans as subjects and in the systematic feedback of science-based clinical trials. The ultimate test of theory is, of course, applicability in resolving problems.

The new science of alcohol abuse and alcoholism (AAA) made progress. Some ideas did not find support, others did. Despite progress on some issues, until recently, the success rates for treating alcoholics remained much the same as before. Relapse rates were high. It is relatively easy to get alcoholics, on occasion, to stop drinking briefly, but within 3 months or so, about 70–80% return to drinking at pretreatment amounts or more. Further, and most disappointing, it did not appear to make much difference what kind of treatment was applied, whether the treatment involved professionals or lay persons, or which theoretical orientation (including some theories derived from scientific research) was guiding treatment. There were variable outcomes from treatments, but the relevant variables had to do with the quality of the patient rather than variables of treatment. If patients were employed, supported by significant others (e.g., family or employer), and were in treatment for the first time, the expected success rates (measured in terms of abstinence or near abstinence for a year) were about 50%. Among patients who were periodically unemployed, with no significant other looking after them and had been in treatment many times, the expected success rates dropped to less than 10% (1, 2). An implication of these kinds of outcomes is that extant theories were not sufficiently well developed to guide treatment and more research was needed. Also, any emergent treatment would have to get a better success rate, on average, than 20–30% abstinence (or near abstinence or drinking with no problems) at the 1- or 2-year benchmark to be considered effective and a higher rate with patients entering treatment for the first time.

Dole [(3), p. 361] summarized the situation in 1986 by saying: "Alcoholics relapse. Despite medical care, counseling, and good intensions, alcoholics find it difficult to remain abstinent. The typical course of this disease is a series of treatments and relapses, progressive deterioration, and premature death." He said that the extant data indicated available treatments were not particularly effective: "The medical benefits of detoxification, rest, and good diet are undeniable, but a few weeks of intensive treatment do not ensure continued abstinence and may in fact have little influence on the long term course of the disease" [(3), p. 361].

I believe that a serious change, indeed, a scientific revolution occurred during the 1980s and early 1990s that has had and will continue to have profound influence on how we think about alcoholism. Previously, the prevailing remedies for alcoholism were to restrict the use of alcoholic beverages, punish excessive use of alcoholic beverages, treat the mental disorders that supposedly led to excessive drinking, or develop sufficient will-power to overcome the temptation presented by the availability of alcoholic beverages. When the ordinary developmental processes (involving parental training, secular and religious education) failed to develop sufficient character to overcome temptation, psychotherapy of various kinds was invoked to remedy the situation. The myriad psychotherapies, group therapies, and support groups were occasionally shown to be successful, but the problems of AAA were extant despite applications of various kinds of medical and psychological therapy (cure rates never being consistently better than cure rates from no treatment). Alcoholism remained one of the most serious health and social problems of Western democracies despite wide-spread availability of expensive treatments.

Before the revolutionary thinking about alcoholism, the prevailing scientific theories of AAA were based in the general idea that ethanol was a negative reinforcer, that is, it provided relief, in one form or another. The alcoholic was afflicted by a disease or by the "slings and arrows of outrageous fortune" and ethanol provided relief from such aversive conditions. The relief reinforced the act of drinking. Drinking, in turn, might produce aversive states (e.g., withdrawal symptoms or conditioned withdrawal symptoms) that set the circumstances for ethanol to again reinforce the act of drinking. We have gone from tension reduction, to anxiety reduction, to stress reduction, to stress response dampening hypotheses across the last few years (4). There were similar deficiencies theories: The alcoholic lacked something that ethanol somehow provided, thereby providing relief from an unpleasant condition. When, for example, the idea was extant that ethanol's metabolism provided an opioid-like compound and the endogenous opioids had been discovered, the idea was that ethanol provided missing endogenous opioidergic stimulation thereby restoring some sort of normality that was reinforcing (5, 6).

These negative reinforcement theories had facts that fit the theory. There was available an extensive literature studying negative reinforcement in the laboratory (e.g., fear being established by footshock in rats and then studying fear-reduction as reinforcement). Ethanol withdrawal symptoms are aversive and ethanol does relieve them. Anxiety and depression are often correlates of alcoholism. Alcoholism and addiction to opioids have features in common. These theories guided both the practice of treating alcoholism and the laboratory science directed toward studying potentially relevant variables (e.g., there was extensive study of withdrawal symptoms). It followed from such theory that the cure for AAA was to treat the anxiety (tension, stress) thereby eliminating the need to drink.

When the benzodiazepine antianxiety agents Librium and Valium were popular, the idea was that their effects would be effective treatments because they reduced anxiety and anxiety sustained alcohol use. This idea supported extensive prescription of these agents to persons presenting with AAA. As detailed next, this approach was not only ineffective, but probably dangerous.

The research program developed by Jane Stewart and Harriet de Wit (7), studying the reinstatement of extinguished responding previously sustained by addictive drugs, supports the idea that agents producing similar effects to the originally worked-for-drug have the effect of reinstating vigorous responding. This is an interesting conclusion derived from the animal laboratory. The implication is that a drug producing similar effects to ethanol is apt to evoke behavior previously maintained by ethanol, that is, its prescription being contrary to maintaining abstinence. Benzodiazepines used as antianxiety agents produce similar effects to ethanol, both modifying the GABA receptor. The prescription of benzodiazepines to treat the anxiety of recovering alcoholics is, therefore, problematic. The widespread prescription of benzodiazepines and their failure to be helpful (and perhaps harmful) had many consequences. One consequence salient to our topic is that people attempting to treat AAA became very suspicious of the use of any drug to help the recovering alcoholic.

Even though benzodiazepines are not helpful in sustaining abstinence, they are effective in preventing alcohol withdrawal symptoms from reaching problematic levels. Using drugs to prevent the serious effects of alcohol withdrawal, such as risk of seizures, is not controversial. The common site of action of benzodiazepines and alcoholic beverages also accounts for their cumulative effects with respect to driving a car, etc.

18.2 A Scientific Revolution in Theory of Addictions

The ground work for a revolution in thinking about AAA came from the laboratory study of other addictive agents, for example, morphine and cocaine. The fact that laboratory animals such as rats and monkeys would work for small doses of these agents without being stressed, made anxious, or made previously dependent upon them presented serious problems for negative reinforcement theories of addiction (no apparent negative reinforcement, yet sustained intake). Some theories of addiction to opioids, for example, might feature existential angst as the reason that persons used opioids. However, that theory was difficult to reconcile with rats pressing for injections of morphine. Rats are smart, but they probably are not extensively worried about the meaning of life.

The work showing that laboratory animals readily self-administered most drugs abused by people was followed by studies showing that those same agents enhanced pressing for direct electrical stimulation of the medial forebrain bundle as it coursed through the hypothalamus. Those same agents also established conditioned place preferences (CPP). New theories of drug abuse emerged from these studies which were presented in a 1983 edited book (8). There was the recognition that drugs of abuse were euphorigens and that they achieved their ability to be euphorigenic by acting on the very substrates that are active when ordinary stimuli induce positive effect. This positive effect could be conditioned to the circumstances of the drug-induced effect to produce secondary reinforcers having powerful motivational effects. Elaborations of these ideas are our modern theories of drug addiction.

Another line of research provides background for the revolution in thinking about alcoholism. Soon after the discovery of the endogenous opioid system, it became apparent that the system was extensive and involved brain areas not usually associated with pain (the most likely behavior given morphine's well-known analgesic effects). The prevailing notion was that naloxone, the classic opioid antagonist, was inert except in morphine-dependent animals. When naloxone is injected into rats and one just watches them, nothing appears to happen. When, however, they are subjected to testing for their effects on motivations, a different picture emerges. Naloxone reduces intakes of water and food [e.g., (9, 10)]. Naloxone enhances some sexual behaviors [e.g. (11)]. Naloxone modifies social behaviors in young animals (12). It became apparent that the endogenous opioid system was part of the system involved in motivation and emotion.

18.3 The Revolution and Alcoholism

The experiment that should have clearly started a revolution in thinking about alcoholism was a 1980-study using monkeys by Altshuler, Phillips, and Feinhandler (13). They demonstrated that naltrexone (NTX), the long acting opioid antagonist, at doses of 1, 3, and 5 mg/kg, dose-relatedly decreased intravenous self-administration of dilute solutions of ethanol. The results, however, did not fit nicely with the conclusions drawn from other studies. Consequently, it took further study before the results of the study had its full impact.

At the time of the Altshuler et al. study, the research with the morphine on intake of alcoholic beverages showed that doses of 7.5–60 mg/kg reduced intakes among rats, mice and hamsters (14–19). Further, there was evidence of stereospecificity of agonist's effects since levorphanol, but not dextrorphan, reduced intakes of alcohol (14, 16, 17). Similar reductions in intake were seen with methadone (a long acting agonist) at doses of 15 and 30 mg/kg (14, 16) and with LAAM (an even longer acting agonist) at doses of 5 and 10 mg/kg (14). Using rats, 200 μg of Met-enkephalin administered intracerebroventricularly reduced intake of an ethanol solution on the day of and the day after its administration (15).

Naloxone, at doses of 1–2.5 mg/kg reduced rats' intakes of alcoholic beverage in drinking sessions of 0.5- to 8-h long (20, 21), but similar doses (0.1–5 mg/kg) did not reduce intakes in sessions 24-h long (14). Among hamsters with 24-h access to a 15% ethanol solution, 2 mg/kg of naloxone given every 6 h had no reliable effect on intakes (22). NTX in doses of 0.1–5 mg/kg had no reliable effect on rats' intakes when they had an opportunity to drink for 24 h (14). NTX, 2 mg/kg, apparently increased hamsters' 18-h intake of an alcoholic beverage (17). NTX, 10 mg/kg, blocked the decrease in intake of alcoholic beverage among rats produced by 60 mg/kg of morphine (15).

Both agonists and antagonists at opioid receptors reduced intake of alcoholic beverage, in contrast to what might be predicted based on the known pharmacodynamics of these agents (one would expect bipolar, opposite results from administration of known agonists and antagonists). There were mixed results from assessments of opioid antagonists. Although the extent of the laboratory data was small [we (23) found only 13 reports published before 1983 on opioids' effects on intake of alcoholic beverage, none before 1973], there was considerable discussion of the relationship between opioids and alcoholism. We (23) found 7 reviews citing the small laboratory literature. Most reviews touted ideas centered about deficiency (negative reinforcement) hypotheses of alcoholism, that is, somehow morphine, by fulfilling some sort of need, reduced the motivation that sustained alcohol intake (5). It was into this confusing picture that Altshuler et al.'s extraordinary experiment (13) was reported and it did not have inordinate impact upon the extant thinking about AAA.

On the basis of our experience studying morphine's effects on pressing for rewarding intracranial stimulation [(24, 25), and for a review of the early work (26)] and our experience studying both agonists' and antagonists' effects on ingestion of food and water [(27, 28), for a review of the early work (28, 29)], we realized that the early studies of agonists and antagonists on the consumption of alcoholic beverage often did not take into account the pharmacokinetics of these agents. The doses of naloxone and NTX used with the rodents were not sufficiently large to provide antagonism for the duration of the testing, so the measurements were of antagonist and post antagonists' effects. The doses of morphine used were inordinately large. In the first study (18), the dose was 60 mg/kg, a dose sufficient to produce catatonia and conditioned taste aversions (24). Smaller doses of agonists are all that is necessary to mimic any actions of the endogenous opioids and it was small doses of morphine that enhanced pressing for rewarding brain stimulation (26, 30), produced CPPs (31), and increased intakes of palatable substances such as sweetened water (26).

The issue became how to test the effects of opioids on alcohol's effects, that is, how to get laboratory subjects to voluntarily take sufficient alcoholic beverage during a short period (1- or 2-h a day) to have high blood ethanol levels so that the effects of small doses of morphine and naloxone could be tested. We did this by arranging for rats to take a palatable alcoholic beverage for 2 h/day for many days. We deprived them of water before hand, and presented them with a choice to drink water, the alcoholic beverage, or both. Under such circumstance, rats gradually increase their intake of alcoholic beverage until they are taking over 2 g/kg of pure ethanol during a 2-h period, sufficient ethanol to produce overt signs of drunkenness. They also take sufficient water to maintain a healthy rate of growth. After about 3 weeks on such a daily regimen, intakes of ethanol remain rather stable for many days thereafter. Figure 18.1 is a summary of many studies using this general procedure.

We [summarized in (23)] found that doses of morphine ranging from 0.5 mg/kg to about 7.5 mg/kg given 10–30 min before a 1- or 2-h drinking session increased intakes of alcoholic beverage (smaller doses need to be given closer to the time of testing and the testing session needs to be shorter in order to have morphine in circulation during the time of testing). Doses of 1–2 mg/kg given 20 min before a 2-h drinking session produce near maximal increases in intakes achievable by single injections of morphine. Doses larger than 7.5 mg/kg decreased intakes. Larger doses

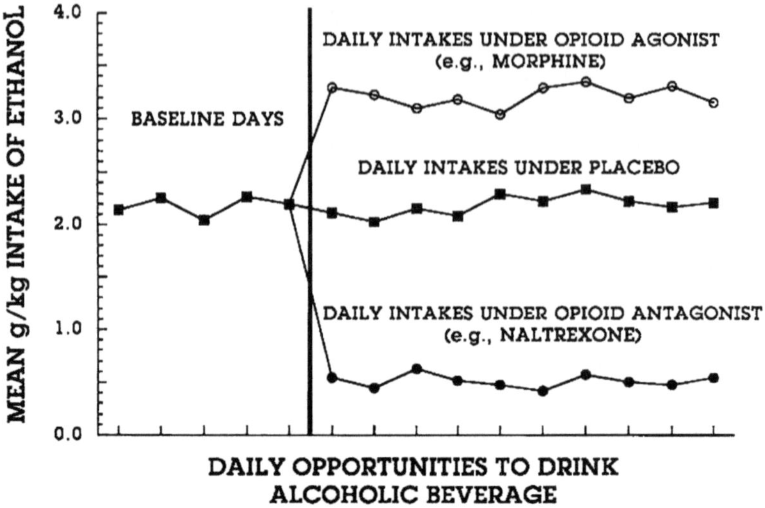

Fig. 18.1 This figure depicts a summary of a number of experiments, with data-points being the average across those experiments. The rats had 2 h a day to drink alcoholic beverage having a high concentration of ethanol (12%). Under a regimen involving a number of setting conditions fostering the intake of the beverage, the amount of ethanol drunk gradually increases so that, in about 3 weeks, the rats are taking over 2 g/kg a day. The data-points designated baseline days depicts the rather stable average intake of a group of rats after intakes have become stable. After baseline, before daily opportunity to drink, subjects are injected with either small doses of morphine, doses of an opioid antagonist, or the carrier of those drugs (placebo). Morphine reliably increases intakes. Opioid antagonists reliably decrease ethanol-intake (but do not decrease intakes to zero)

can increase intakes, if there has been some tolerance to morphine's effects. Doses of morphine given intraventricularly ranging from 0.03 to 10.0 μg/rat produced significant increases in intakes. Agonists that do not cross the blood brain barrier do not enhance intakes at any dose tested (32).

The initial studies [e.g., (33–35)] showing that small doses of morphine enhanced intakes of ethanol used male rats, sweetened alcoholic beverage, and rats motivated to be alert and ready to drink by mild water deprivation (mild in that it did not reduce ordinary rate of body weight gain) and provisioning of both water and beverage on a 2-h a day schedule, food always available. Because the procedures ensured a baseline level of ethanol intake that was large, the enhanced intakes were clearly significant from the view of "does a manipulation induce sufficient intake to have clinical relevance?" We then engaged a prolonged series of experiments to determine if the small-dose-morphine effect, exemplified by doses of 1 or 2 mg/kg enhancing intake of ethanol, was peculiar to variables of the initial studies [summarized in (23)].

Small doses of morphine enhance intakes of alcoholic beverages:

- When the alcoholic beverage is flavored with sweeteners or not (just ethanol and water),
- When the ethanol and water solution is flavored with the taste of beer,

- When the testing sessions occur during the night or the day,
- When testing is under the conditions of individual or group housing,
- When rats were mildly deprived of water or food or not deprived,
- Among male and female rats,
- Among rats of various ages,
- When baseline intakes are small, but not zero, and baseline intakes are large,
- When testing is during the initial days of presentation of alcoholic beverage, but not the first days, and when it is after many days of presentation of beverage,
- Regardless of whether the rats are made dependent upon morphine or not, and
- Among rats of different strains.

In brief, the small-dose-morphine effect is a highly reliable effect that is not dependent upon the rather arbitrary selection of variables that are inherent to any one experiment. Further, small doses of other agonists, for example, methadone (36) and fentanyl (37) enhance intakes of alcoholic beverage.

Very small doses of morphine can enhance intakes of alcoholic beverage when applied intraventricularly, for example, 1 μg/rat. This dose is about 120 times smaller, on a molar basis, than the dose of Met-enkephalin that was shown to reduce intakes (15, 23).

We (38) asked the critical question of whether the small-dose-morphine effect waned with repeated administration of morphine: if endogenous opioidergic systems were to be considered salient to excessive intake of alcoholic beverages (which among alcoholics is sustained for prolonged periods), then the effect should not disappear after several administrations of morphine. Small doses of morphine increased intake of alcoholic beverage for 100 days with no indication that the effect would wane with continuation of testing.

With nearly every study of the small-dose-morphine effect, doses of naloxone or NTX were also administered. Doses of naloxone and NTX reliably reduced intakes of alcoholic beverages when intakes of ethanol were both large and small. Given the results of these experiments, the issue of a lack of a bipolar effect of agonists and antagonists is no longer an issue. Small doses of agonists enhance intakes, antagonists reduce intakes. Large doses of morphine, which induces behaviors incompatible with drinking (such as catatonia), reduces intakes, but the effects of large doses are probably irrelevant to building theory of opioidergic effects on alcoholic beverages. The results of the study by Altshuler et al. (13), showing NTX reduced monkey's self-administration of injections of ethanol, with similar results by Myers et al. (39), now appear to be more definitive in the context of findings of the small-dose-morphine effect and further recognition of the pharmacokinetics of opioid antagonists when given to rodents.

Figure 18.2 is a summary of another group of experiments. Rats were fixed with osmotic pumps for the constant delivery of small amounts of morphine. The opioid manipulations began with the first presentations (2 h daily) of a palatable, concentrated (12% ethanol) alcoholic beverage. Notice the intakes of the placebo controls: they gradually increase intakes across days of presentation; the ethanol solution is probably becoming more palatable as the postingestive effects of ethanol are paired with the taste of the beverage (40) and there is tolerance to some of ethanol's effects.

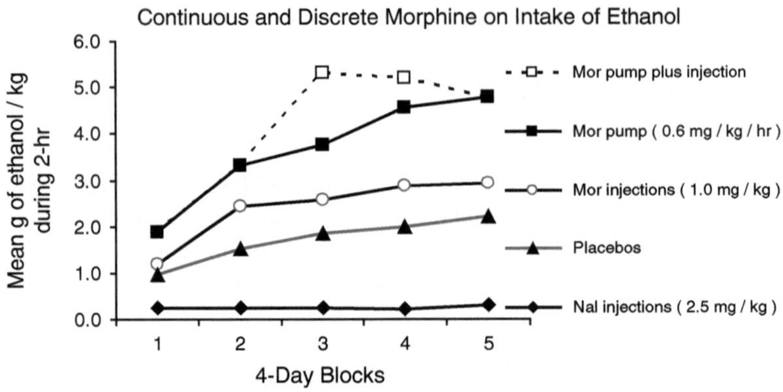

Fig. 18.2 The average intake of ethanol by male rats with a daily regimen of opportunity to take a palatable alcoholic beverage daily, 2h a day, for 20 days while various opioidergic manipulations were programmed. The first chance to take beverage was Day 1 of the 20 days. There were two groups fitted with osmotic pumps for the continuous delivery of morphine (Mor pump). They had the same treatment for the first 8 days, and then one group continued to receive the morphine of the pump, but also received a small injection of morphine daily across the next 8 days (*open squares*)

Morphine, 1.0mg/kg, given daily before the chance to drink enhances intakes as soon as the rats are taking enough ethanol to have clear central neural effects, but not before that. Naloxone when presented before the initial opportunities to drink prevents the development of gain in intake of alcoholic beverage usually seen with daily presentation of alcoholic beverages, a finding recently confirmed with alcohol preferring rats (41).

Two groups of rats were fitted with osmotic pumps for the continuous delivery of small amounts of morphine. Morphine delivered by way of pumps enhanced intakes much the same way as when small doses of morphine were injected daily (any apparent difference between the pump group and injected group could easily be a function of slight differences in doses; one should not come to the conclusion, from Fig. 18.2, that morphine by way of pumps is more effective than morphine by way of injections). After 8 days, one group receiving morphine by way of pumps was also given an injection of morphine just before the 2-h chance to drink. Notice that the addition of the injection further enhanced intakes.

I believe that these data support the conclusion that a surfeit of opioidergic activity (a high basal rate of endogenous opioid activity), a surge in opioidergic activity or both could enhance intakes of alcoholic beverage. The surge in activity could be from a low basal level or from a high basal level. Persons at risk for AAA due to family history have a low basal level of β-endorphin, but ethanol produces more release among them than their low risk counterparts (42).

We (43) tested predictions from the supposition that either a surfeit of opioidergic activity or a deficit was a controlling condition for enhanced intakes. There was strong support for the conclusion that a surfeit of opioid activity enhanced intakes and that a deficit decreased activity. The conclusion is both a high basal opioidergic tone and a surge in opioid activity are conditions for extraordinarily large amounts of voluntary intakes of alcoholic beverages. Both conditions can be blocked by a long acting opioid antagonist, NTX.

By 1985, there was sufficient information from the experimental laboratory to support the conclusion that NTX would be an effective medicine for treating excessive intake of alcoholic beverage, the defining problem of alcoholism. The patent on NTX was held by DuPont. With the introduction of William Schmidt, who was then working at DuPont, I presented the findings to an assembly of DuPont's scientists and administrators with the idea that there was sufficient information for a clinical trial of NTX as a medicine for alcoholism. Subsequently, Joseph Volpicelli working with Charles O'Brien also presented data and their rationale for why NTX would be an effective medicine for alcoholism. The result, in both instances, was that although the data and the ideas were interesting, DuPont was not inclined to fund further research. To the great credit of Volpicelli and O'Brien, they arranged a clinical trial of NTX despite little support from industry or governmental sources. Their first written report, involving their first wave of patients, appeared in 1990 (44) in an edited book emerging from a 1989 symposium. With knowledge of Volpicelli and O'Brien's favorable results, a group at Yale University, led by Stephanie O'Malley, began a clinical trial. O'Malley et al.'s preliminary results were presented at a 1990 symposium (45). Full reports of both trials appeared in 1992 (46, 47), considerably after Altshuler et al.'s preclinical results (13) were published.

Volpicelli et al. (46) and O'Malley et al.'s (47) results provided strong support for the conclusion that NTX was an effective adjunct to psychotherapy with the aim of reducing the excessive drinking of persons with a history of alcoholism. In fact, these two studies are the first double-blind, placebo-controlled, multicenter trial to confirm that any variable arranged by clinicians was effective in stemming uncontrolled drinking by alcoholics. The results were sufficiently convincing that DuPont fostered further research and the work necessary to get the Food and Drug Administration (FDA) to approve NTX as a medicine for alcohol dependence and to begin marketing NTX.

It is significant that nearly 50 years earlier, the FDA approved Antabuse, an agent that causes sickness upon drinking alcoholic beverages, as a medicine for treating alcoholism. Between the approval of Antabuse and NTX, no other medicines were approved. Antabuse punishes drinking, in line with the then extant view of alcoholism. NTX works differently and therein lays a foundation for a different way, a revolutionary way, of thinking about alcoholism. What is revolutionary about the preclinical and clinical research involved with opioids and the voluntary intake of alcoholic beverages is the idea that the alcoholics' appetite for alcoholic beverages was modifiable by way of a drug. Previous thinking seem to presume that the alcoholic had a fixed (almost not modifiable), high motivation to drink alcoholic beverages. This idea is strengthened by the demonstration of genetic correlates to drinking and the idea that alcoholism is a disease. Treatments were designed to punish the manifestation of that appetite (e.g., giving Antabuse), designed to strengthen character sufficiently to overcome the gnawing temptation to drink that was characteristic of alcoholism, or designed to treat the mental illness, or deficiency, that made it difficult to control drinking. The idea that a drug, for example, an opioid antagonist, might modify the motivation to drink or modify the motivation to drink once drinking had begun was novel. It was like building character by taking a drug – it just did not make sense to many people.

Despite the favorable results from the clinic and a growing body of convincing laboratory data, NTX was and is not (48, 49) widely accepted as an effective intervention in treating alcoholism. In part, this was due to the poor experiences with other psychotropic drugs such as benzodiazepines leading to the general conclusion, among those treating alcoholics, that using drugs to treat alcoholism was a poor idea. There were extant theories of alcoholism that were not compatible with the idea that any medicine could deal with the moral problem of habitual drinking even though, paradoxically, many agreed that alcoholism was a disease. The first clinical studies used a single dose of NTX, did not deal with the issue of long-term compliance, and involved only 12 weeks of dosing. A number of issues remained for both preclinical and clinical research.

18.4 Tolerance to Naltrexone's Effects

With respect to using opioid antagonists as adjuncts to psychotherapy for AAA, a significant issue is whether there is tolerance to the antagonists' initially beneficial effects, that is, do antagonists' effects wane with continuous use? The issue can and has been addressed in the laboratory where one can continuously provide the temptation to drink.

If a salient effect of NTX is to reduce consumption once begun, NTX might reduce each bout of drinking, but the number of drinking bouts may increase with continuous opportunity to drink. This circumstance seems to have limited NTX's ability to be an antiobesity drug; NTX reduced meal size but increased number of snacks (29). NTX retains its ability to be an effective medicine for binge eating disorders (decreased binge durations which are more discrete) (29, 50–52).

Figure 18.1 shows the effects of ten repeated injections of naloxone and no apparent waning of effect. Using rats, we (53) gave 10.0 mg/kg of NTX for 30 days before 2-h daily access to sweetened alcoholic beverage and found similar reductions of intakes on the first and the last days of administration. Stromberg et al. (54) gave 1.0 mg/kg for 60 days before limited daily access to an alcoholic beverage of only water and ethanol. They found that NTX did not loose its effectiveness. We (55) gave NTX, again, but in doses of 5.0 and 3.0 mg/kg and observed a decrement in effectiveness. Across these studies there is an apparent lack of dose-orderly effects 1 and 10 mg/kg showing persistent effects, 3 and 5 mg/kg showing signs of tolerance. However, as detailed in the discussion of Reid et al. (56), the apparent inconsistency of effects is understandable when you take into account the amount of alcohol taken during baselines. The daily intakes of the Stromberg et al. study (54) were small and a small dose of NTX was sufficient to persistently reduce intakes. Our studies arranged for rats to take considerably larger amounts of alcohol during 2-h daily sessions. Under those circumstances, the dose of 10.0 mg/kg was sufficient to sustain suppressed intakes, whereas doses of 3.0 and 5.0 mg/kg were not. As shown by studies of opioid antagonists and intake of palatable non-alcoholic beverages (57), a dose of an antagonist sufficient to reduce intake of a less palatable solution may not be sufficient to reduce intake of a more palatable one, that is, the dose–response curve for highly reinforcing beverages is shifted to the right compared to curves for less reinforcing beverages. In other words, there are probably orderly dose–response curves for each level of intake of alcoholic beverage. Stated differently, large doses of NTX will be necessary to persistently mute alcoholic beverage intake when that intake is highly motivated as indexed by the amount of intake. Multiple injections of NTX or continuous NTX by way of osmotic pumps increase the number of opioid receptors [for an early review of the literature see (58), for a later review see Unterwald, this book, also (59–61)]. Overstreet et al. (59) measured alcohol intake in alcohol preferring rats in both limited and continuous access situations. They also developed dose–response effects for naloxone injections during initial days of its application (ED50 = 2.1 mg/kg). Naloxone retained its ability to suppress intakes when the opportunity to drink was limited (14 daily opportunities of short duration). However, naloxone's effects waned, when naloxone was given continuously by way of osmotic pumps and the opportunity to drink was extended to 24 h daily. Autoradiographic measurement using the ligand (3H)(D-Ala2,N-Me-Phe4,Gly-ol5)(tyrosyl-3,5–3H)-enkephalin, specific for the μ receptor, showed that rats chronically exposed to naloxone and showing tolerance to naloxone's suppression of drinking exhibited 17–250% increases in the binding.

Similar results to those of Overstreet et al. (59) were found by Cowen et al. (60) using NTX as the opioid antagonist and the autoradiographic examination of another ligand for the μ receptor. Hyytia et al. (61) provided continuous naloxone by way of osmotic pumps while measuring intakes during limited daily access in alcohol preferring rats and measured opioid density with respect to μ, δ, and κ receptors. Naloxone decreased intakes. Naloxone increased receptor density with respect to all three kinds of receptors. Tests for functionality of this upregulation (e.g., dose–response curves for agonist analgesia) also showed that the upregulation was meaningful in terms of expected effects from agonists.

Measures of opioid receptor density in many situations (58) including situations where ethanol intake is of interest (58, 60, 61) indicate that the effects of chronic opioid antagonism sets in motion events that attempt to counter the effect of opioid antagonism as indexed by opioid receptor upregulation. This circumstance may limit the effectiveness of NTX-treatment for AAA. Recently, there has been a germane test (62). Wistar, male rats were given NTX or placebo between opportunities to drink alcoholic beverage (10% ethanol in water). Post NTX, the NTX-treated rats drank more ethanol than the placebo-treated. The implication for treatment of alcoholism is obvious: there needs to be special attention to the end of NTX-treatment (see comments given below).

Generalizing: opioid antagonism is more likely to be effective when the alcoholic beverage (or meals) are made available for a limited time, because the antagonists limit the length of bouts of ingestion (57). On the surface, NTX-treatment might reduce excessive drinking and thereby allow the alcoholic to drink socially; however, if NTX-treatment reduced each bout of drinking but increased the number of instances of drinking, the toxic effects of ethanol would continue to accrue. An extrapolation from the generalization is that treatments for alcoholism should strive for abstinence, thereby making it more likely that relapses will be discrete events for which NTX can be helpful. This approach is also much more acceptable to the alcoholism treatment community who thoroughly believe that an alcoholic cannot return to moderate levels of drinking without returning to alcoholism.

Recall that continuous morphine, by way of minipumps, induced considerable intake of alcoholic beverage and that an injection of a small dose of morphine, in addition to the morphine provided by the minipumps, induced even more intake (23, 63) (Fig. 18.2). The opposite of that might be an effective therapy for AAA. The long acting NTX provided by injection (64) would be the opposite of morphine by way of minipumps. Recently, Hernandez-Avila et al. found that targeted oral dosing with NTX was moderately effective in men being treated for AAA [also see (65)]. Targeted dosing refers to instructions to take NTX before being in a situation that is apt to elicit the motivation to drink alcoholic beverages. The targeted dosing could be the opposite of the injection of a small dose of morphine. The patient would be instructed to take the monthly injection and to take NTX orally before any situation that in the past has elicited uncontrolled drinking. This dosing regimen, of course, should be accompanied by counseling providing rationale for such a regimen and the learning of skills for abstinence without NTX's help.

The regimen of continuous, relatively large doses NTX by way of monthly injections and targeted oral dosing will likely override the effects of upregulation of receptors and mute opioid mediated incentive motivation (see below). The continuous NTX should be large enough to help prevent relapse (64), without inordinate side effects. The targeted dosing is designed to provide sufficiently more NTX to overcome tolerance induced by continuous NTX and to meet the demand characteristics of a high motivation to drink and to ensure effectiveness in curbing excessive drinking on the occasional slip. Also, such a regimen is apt to help establish routines that might be useful when injections of NTX are discontinued. Monthly injections of NTX will probably have side effects similar to daily oral doses [likely muting some capacity for pleasure, (66)] that will probably limit its use to a couple of years. The discontinuance of injections of NTX will be a particularly dangerous time for the alcoholic: perception of help no longer being available and probably increased opioidergic tone (rebound from antagonism) which is apt to encourage excessive drinking. With a regimen of targeted NTX administration being established, the transition from continuous NTX to no NTX is apt to be made easier. Fortunately, a year or two and surely 5 years of abstinence or no problematic drinking are usually sufficient for male alcoholics to remain abstinent for the balance of their lives (67).

As we studied the enduring effects of naloxone or NTX, two features of their effects were seen again and again. First, the antagonists did not reduce intakes to zero (the rats always took some of the presented beverage). Second, upon termination of antagonist administration, intakes promptly returned to pre-NTX levels.

The administration of small doses of morphine and administration of large doses of antagonists worked like turning on and off switches for an electrical device: with morphine, more drinking, with antagonists less drinking (Fig. 18.1 for initial effects). The only time antagonists were effective in reducing intakes to zero, or close to zero, were when the antagonists were given before the habit of drinking was established, that is, from the first presentation of an alcoholic beverage, even an ostensibly palatable beverage (Fig. 18.2). These features of NTX's effects have important implications for developing effective treatments with both advantages and disadvantages.

The disadvantage of the prompt return to high levels of drinking with the termination of NTX-treatment is obvious. It would be nice if NTX's effects were not only enduring when it was applied and if NTX's effects carried over to a period following NTX-treatment; but based on results from the animal laboratory, the carryover effect, if any, is surely limited. The advantages are not so obvious. The advantage of the limitation of NTX to not completely suppress drinking is that NTX mutes the motivation to drink, but does not completely reduce it, thereby providing the circumstances for counter conditioning the cues that are inherent to the motivation for habitual drinking (if no motivation is present there is no opportunity for training to counter the motivation). NTX provides the opportunity to learn new habits that will replace, counter, the habit of drinking. The next section is related to this possibility.

A regimen of NTX-treatment provides the opportunity to unlearn, extinguish, features of the habit of drinking by providing temptation without the danger of complete relapse. How do you train abstinence? By counter conditioning the cues that evoke the habit of drinking, but that cannot be done when there is high motivation to drink and the accompanying relapse to extensive drinking which is antithetical to treatment.

18.5 Secondary Reinforcers That Strengthen the Habit to Drink and Their Opioid Involvement

There is recognition that to reduce relapse rates among treated alcoholics, it will be necessary to reduce the salience of learned motivations that develop with pairing of ethanol's CNS effects with salient events surrounding the drinking. The issue is not whether motivation to drink alcoholic beverages is strengthened by the association between the post ingestive effects of ethanol and other events incrementing positive effect (e.g., fun at parties, good food, attending sporting events, etc.). The issue is not whether environmental events paired with ethanol-induced increments in positive effect can come to have motivational relevance as a result of that pairing. No one doubts these possibilities. Theories of alcoholism that merely restate the possibilities for incentive salience are vacuous in that they state the obvious. The issue is how to undo all of the learning associated with drinking alcoholic beverages that makes it difficult to stop the habit of drinking them.

The prime purpose, it seems to me, in developing a procedure that allows the easy measurement of ethanol-induced incentive motivation is to find out how to increase and decrease it. When you can control events in the laboratory, then it is likely that a useful concept can be derived. Procedures have been developed to index the potential of ethanol to establish conditioned responses having motivational salience as indexed by easy to quantify, reliable responses of rodents. Among those procedures are (a) strength of extinction, (b) strength of reinstatement of extinguished responding after apparent extinction by presentation of potentially salient stimuli, and (c) the CPP test.

Pavlov and Skinner were leaders in the study of how the judicious presentation of food and beverages could be used to develop habits. From the research traditions of Pavlov and Skinner, the lessons learned concerning the persistence of habits seem particularly applicable. The treatment of alcoholism is, in essence, an attempt to extinguish the habit of drinking alcoholic beverages.

When behavior (for example, a rat pressing bar for the opportunity to eat a small amount of food) is well-established by presentation of a rewarding ingestible (positive reinforcers) and the presentation of the reward is no longer presented, the habits (e.g., bar pressing) that were developed do not stop abruptly, but gradually decrease, a process called extinction. The persistence of responding under the contingency of extinction can be thought of as an index of the strength of the habit. Variables can be manipulated to see how they might affect that persistence of responding.

Strength of habit can be indexed by making the response requirements more stringent and seeing how much work will be expended for a unit of reward. In a Skinner box, rats can be asked, for example, to press a bar (a lever, but using the term "bar" seems more appropriate in this context) for a sip of alcoholic beverage. When they do that regularly, the cost of the sip can be changed by requiring more presses before the opportunity to drink is presented. One of the first lessons taught by Skinner and his colleagues was that positive reinforcers need not be large and did not have to occur with every bar press for the habit of bar pressing to be sustained. An alcoholic need not get an increment in positive effect from every instance of drinking for habitual drinking to be sustained. In fact, periodic reinforcement induces more resistance to extinction than continuous reinforcement.

Another lesson learned is that stimuli paired with the presentation of a positive reinforcer (an instance of positive effect) can become a reinforcer by virtue of that pairing. The paired stimulus when it has achieved reinforcing strength is called a secondary reinforcer. The stimuli surrounding and the act of bar pressing themselves become secondary reinforcers to the primary reinforcer of consummation (in our case the drinking of an alcoholic beverage which, in turn, induces an increment in positive effect or relieves an aversive state). The change in effect is the primary event that in turn is associated with the act of drinking. In the case of alcohol related habits, the change in effect is ethanol-induced and is paired with the act of drinking which includes the taste of the alcoholic beverage and the circumstances of that drinking.

Secondary reinforcers have motivational relevance, that is, induce movement toward the primary reinforcer. When they do that, the circumstance is called an incidence of incentive motivation. By virtue of ethanol's ability to induce an increment in positive effect being paired with many circumstances (but usually always with the act of drinking alcoholic beverage), the habit of drinking not only becomes persistent but is motivated by pervasive instances of incentive motivations. The conscious manifestation of the incentive motivations is craving. The issue is how to reduce the incentives to drink and to extinguish the habit of drinking, that is, how to prevent relapse.

To study variables that might change the events of the habit of drinking, one can establish those habits in the laboratory and then manipulate various events to see which are salient. One procedure that seems relevant is called reinstatement. A rat can be taught to press a bar for a sip of alcoholic beverage. Once the habit is established, the bar press can be made to no longer yield a sip and the bar pressing gradually stops, that is, extinction occurs. Then, events can be programmed to see which of them will reinstate the apparently extinguished habit of bar pressing. When responding is reinstated, it has been called spontaneous recovery (by Pavlov no less); but the better name is reinstatement, since the term spontaneous gives the idea that the behavior occurs without being elicited by salient variables and recovery means something else in the alcohol treatment literature (68).

What events reinstate extinguished responding for alcoholic beverage or more generally for any extinguished behavior? Events such as tones, lights, and certain smells that have been previously paired with drinking reinstate bar pressing [for a review (69)]. A small amount of ethanol will reinstate responding (70, 71). As mentioned previously, drugs producing some of the same central neural events as ethanol reinstate extinguished responding (7).

Here is what is salient: nonspecific opioid antagonists reduce the effectiveness of events that usually reinstate responding (72–74). Opioid antagonists weaken the incentive motivations that usually sustain the habit of drinking as indexed by studies using bar pressing, or other operants, as an index of habit strength (75–78).

One laboratory procedure, using rodents, useful in indexing the potential for the positive effect of drugs to induce a preference for the place where that drug was experienced is the CCP test. The CPP test can be an index of incentive motivation. The particular procedures were first described in Rossi and Reid (31) as they assessed whether morphine's enhancement of pressing for rewarding brain stimulation was related to morphine's ability to induce positive effect or reduced positive effect thereby eliciting more pressing (an issue of some controversy at the time of the experiment). The fact that small doses of morphine established a preference for the place of morphine's experience seems to have settled the issue. The procedure was first used to assess the potential of an agent's ability to elicit positive effect shortly thereafter (79). The name for the test, that is, the CPP test, was chosen by Mike Bozarth, Ron Mucha, and me at a meeting at RPI (with input from Derek van der Kooy) who were the first investigators to recognize the potential of the test and, thereby, begin using it extensively. As we anticipated, this consensus on a name facilitated literature searches (80, 81).

The fact that drugs such as morphine and cocaine had the potential to get individuals, either people or laboratory animals, to spend time in the place where they had previously experienced the drugs' effects was not a new finding; and if that common observation was all the experiments using the CPP confirmed, the results are trivial. Using the procedures to assess ideas germane to addictions is not trivial.

With rats, establishing a CPP using morphine, heroin, cocaine, and other drugs frequently abused by people is relatively easy and can be accomplished rather quickly. Establishing a CPP following injections of ethanol proved to be more difficult. The first attempts at establishing a CPP with rats and using ethanol injections were not successful (e.g., Borman and Cunningham (82) cite 16 papers showing that ethanol was not effective in establishing a CPP using rats as subjects).

When rats are presented with even a very palatable alcoholic beverage, they do not begin taking large amounts of it for days. With rats, it takes a number of opportunities to drink before they drink large amounts of ethanol. The first demonstration (83) of a CPP following injections of small doses of ethanol [doses sufficiently large to produce noticeable effects on behavior, but not much larger (84)] used rats that had considerable experience drinking alcoholic beverages. That study also separated by a few minutes (4 min) the immediate effects of the necessarily large volume injection, which are likely to be unpleasant, from the putative place of the experience of ethanol. Also, the time in the place of ethanol's effects was short (4 min) thereby capturing the first effects of ethanol on brain without the direct experience of the injection. Under these conditions, a CPP was established. Given the procedural variables of previous experiments and the variables of this experiment, we hypothesized that "it was getting drunk that was fun, not being drunk" (p. 487). Other studies (85–88), using rats, demonstrated that a CPP was established when many injections of ethanol were programmed.

Cunningham et al. (89) confirmed what was observed earlier that using mice to study ethanol-induced CPPs was easier than using rats (initial applications of ethanol in mice have greater positive effect than in rats who need some experience with ethanol before ethanol's positive effective potential is manifest in laboratory tests). Therefore, he cleverly chose to study mice. Cunningham and his colleagues and others [e.g., (90–93)] have identified many procedural details useful in designing experiments to study ethanol's ability to establish a CPP. He and his colleagues (91) confirmed, for example, that the immediate effects of handling, injections or oral gavage (92) might have aversive qualities that would obscure ethanol's ability to elicit positive effect and confirmed that it was the rise in blood ethanol levels and its early effects in brain that were salient to establishing a CPP. Ethanol itself, of course, can have aversive properties associated with overdosing (i.e., effects that emerge subsequent to drinking that include confusion and nausea) and withdrawal effects (94).

With knowledge of procedural details that allow the measurement of ethanol's capacity to induce positive effect, Cunningham and his colleagues have made important observations. They (95) showed, for example, that once an ethanol-CPP was established that it was extraordinarily resistant to extinction. Importantly, they showed that an opioid antagonist facilitated extinction of a CPP. They confirmed our observation (96, 97) that in the circumstances under which ethanol established a conditioned place aversion, that naloxone accentuates that aversion (82) and prolongs extinction of that aversion (95). As Cunningham et al. (95) pointed out, the ability of an opioid antagonist to accentuate any conditioned aversive effects of ethanol and suppress conditioned rewarding effect "would presumably lead to a more rapid weakening of behaviors instrumental in obtaining alcohol" (p. 69) [also see (98) for a similar finding].

Just as naloxone might not blunt initial intake of ethanol but decreases overall intake, naloxone does not readily appear to prevent the establishment of a CPP, but does blunt a CPP when measurements are taken subsequently (95, 99). When naloxone is given before a test for conditioning, the putative CPP is manifest during the first minutes of testing but suppressed by naloxone during subsequent minutes of testing (95, 100). Interestingly, it was also shown that a priming dose of ethanol that was sufficient to reinstate a CPP was not effective when the mice where under the influence of naloxone (101). The endogenous opioid system seems particularly salient to the effects of ethanol in terms of events that sustain an interest in the effect induced by ethanol. Middaugh and Bandy (102) found that NTX reduced an ethanol-CPP compared to controls.

Matsuzawa et al. (103) also found that opioid antagonists reduced a CPP established in rats that had been subjected to 10 min of 1 s of footshock every 4 s just before being injected during a procedure for induction of an ethanol-CPP. Results from similar studies (7, 104) have been cited as support for the idea that somehow ethanol relieves stress. Note, however, that being placed in a safe place after being shocked for 10 min is probably a pleasurable event. We (96, 97) found that small doses of morphine given before procedures for an induction of an ethanol-CPP enhanced the CPP, a finding confirmed by Matsuzawa et al. (105). The stress enhanced ethanol-CPP was blocked by naloxone (105).

There are two different situations exemplified by the Matsuzawa et al.'s (103) study, the clear stress (distress) of the 10 min of shock and the emotions associated with the end of that stress (I guess the rats were happy it ended). Note the rats did nothing to end the shock; there was no negative reinforcement in the traditional sense of the word.

There is a germane study with people. Helzer et al. (4) have 2 years of daily data on emotional status and incidence of drinking alcoholic beverages. Stress was related to drinking, but in a way just the opposite of what might be proposed by some theorists: There was little support for the idea that people "drink to cope." Drinking seemed to set the circumstances for stress, rather than the opposite. Drinking occurred most often with celebrations.

Using ethanol-induced CPP-test with mice, Bechtholt and Cunningham made an important finding: opioid antagonists were effective in reducing the expression of a CPP when applied to the ventral tegmental area, but not when applied to the accumbens n. There are other studies [e.g., (106)] attempting to locate the circuitry of opioid modulation of drinking by applying antagonists to sites within the brain. The limited numbers of sites assessed generally confirm that relevant sites are associated with the medial forebrain bundle system, but that topic is not the focus here.

From the studies of indices of incentive motivation established using ethanol's effects as the unconditioned stimulus, an important generalization is derived: the circuits of that incentive motivation have important elements that are opioidergic and that opioid antagonists can be used to mute incentive motivation germane to the habit of drinking alcoholic beverages. A regimen of NTX-treatment provides the opportunity to unlearn, extinguish, features of the habit of drinking by providing temptation without the danger of complete relapse. How do you do that? By counterconditioning the cues that evoke the habit of drinking; but that cannot be done when there is high motivation to drink and high risk for relapse to extensive drinking which is antithetical to treatment. The counterconditioning of the incentive motivations to drink can be modeled after the counterconditioning methods of fear-extinction as exemplified in systematic desensitization therapy of Wolpe (107, 108) which are compatible with other features of cognitive behavioral therapy, an efficient therapy when combined with NTX (109).

It would be undesirable to have a medicine that completely blocked the propensity to drink alcoholic beverages. Such a circumstance would not provide the circumstance to extinguish the habit of drinking. Complete blockage would also induce severe side effects, because of the overlap between circuits sustaining consumption of alcoholic beverages with the circuits of nutrition, the topic of the next section.

18.6 Specificity of Naltrexone

Naloxone and NTX bind to μ, δ, and κ receptors. Circuits having endogenous opioid components are scattered throughout the brain. The issue is which of these opioid systems are critical to NTX's ability to modulate intake of alcoholic beverages.

18.6.1 Overlap with Eating Disorders

On the basis of our general knowledge of brain, the conclusion is: There is no neural circuit specific for drinking alcoholic beverages. There are circuits related to the learning associated with experiencing the effects of ethanol, but those circuits are established secondarily to the initial effects of ethanol. There is, however, specific circuitry associated with ingestion and an endogenous opioid system modulates ingestion [for early reviews see (26, 29, 110–112) for up-to-date review see Bodnar, this book]. Since intake of alcoholic beverage is an ingestive behavior and alcoholic beverages have ready calories and variable tastes (which, in turn, regulate intakes), it is reasonable to suppose that there is considerable communality between the circuitry associated with ingestion in general and that associated with the specific ingestion of alcoholic beverages (29).

The incidence of eating disorders is high among alcoholics and the incidence of alcoholism is high among those with eating disorders. For example, bulimia, an eating disorder associated with binge eating and more common among women, covaries with alcoholism (113–115). According to one sample, a substantial number, more than 25%, of women with eating disorder develop their eating disorder before developing their alcohol use disorders (116). The incidence of AAA and bulimia is, in turn, associated with depression and anxiety (114) and, in one study, associated with anxiety about over indulgence (117).

Strangely, from my perspective and given the relationship between binge eating and AAA, both men and women alcoholics are generally lean and the association between extent of drinking alcoholic beverages and obesity is negative (118–121). Alcoholics may have "beer bellies," as indexed by waist to hip ratios (122, 123), but generally, otherwise, they tend to be lean. The leaner body reduces the risk of type 2 diabetes (124).

One factor that might contribute to alcoholics being leaner than their counterparts is that alcohol induces a higher metabolic rate. Also, there is the finding that intake of carbohydrates, particularly sugar, is smaller among women who drank: The intake of a candy bars is inversely related to intake of alcoholic beverages (120). The very obese are seldom alcoholic.

Among rats, the finding is that there is an association between extent of intake among sweet beverages and alcoholic beverages (125), but the measures of intake are often not done simultaneously (e.g., a strain of rats that takes a lot of alcohol is tested to see if it takes a lot of saccharin solution in a different situation). One can sweeten alcoholic beverages and get more intake of ethanol. Providing a sweet alternative to even palatable alcoholic beverages reduces intake of ethanol. And strangely, providing an opportunity to take saccharin for a number of days without the opportunity to take an alcoholic beverage has carryover effects of reducing intake of ethanol (126).

Kleiner et al. (121) summarize a theory by saying "overeating may compete with alcohol for brain reward sites, making alcohol ingestion less reinforcing" (p. 105). Alternatively, I suggest that both bulimics and alcoholics share a vulnerability: they both get considerable opioid-related pleasure from certain ingesta, specifically calorie-dense sweets and alcoholic beverages after there is a history of intake of the beverages, and have a difficult time stopping ingestion once begun. The social circumstances determine whether sugary food or alcoholic beverages is easily obtainable. For young women, eating chocolate candy is clearly more socially acceptable than drinking alcoholic beverages in either a tavern or alone, hence they are more at risk for eating disorders than alcoholism. Although satiation is delayed for both overeaters and drinkers, it is not totally disabled so that if one fills up with beer, there is satiation for carbohydrates. And if one fills up with cake and candy, there is not a carbohydrate appetite for alcoholic beverage. Also, the habits tend to be mutually exclusive by virtue of having different cues eliciting the initiation of their respective overindulgences. Regardless of how one thinks about it, the findings are concordant with the observation that taverns typically do not sell cake and candy bars.

In summary and as Froehlich et al. (127) put it, although opioid antagonists attenuate the reinforcing properties of food and water, "ethanol drinking is a subset of consummatory behaviors that is particularly sensitive to opioid receptor blockade" (p. 385). That subset probably includes saccharin-sweetened water and some sweets (76, 125, 128). I have used the term alcoholic beverage throughout this discussion because the taste and nutritional features of alcoholic beverages are salient to the habitual use of alcoholic beverages. Hoebel and his colleagues [e.g., (129)] are actively assessing the relationship between neuromodulators salient to ingestion in general and those more particular to ingestion of alcoholic beverages. Along these lines, there are indications of a relationship between circulating levels of leptin (a neuromodulator of eating) and craving for and relapse to drinking among persons being treated for alcoholism (130).

Hoebel, Leibowitz, and their colleagues (131) have recently published the results from a series of experiments (including a nice review of the relationship of the relatedness of eating disorders to alcoholism in terms of their neurochemical communality) that have considerable bearing on opioids and alcoholism. They have shown that ethanol, whether injected or taken orally, induces a significant increase in galanin, enkephalin, and dynorphin in the paraventricular nucleus of the hypothalamus. They also showed that ethanol increased circulating levels of triglycerides and point out there is literature supporting a relationship between eating fat and drinking ethanol. They conclude that galanin and the endogenous opioids are part of a positive feedback loop that "may work closely together in stimulating consumption of ethanol as well as increasing intake of a fat-rich diet" (p. 257). Their findings have important implications for the use of opioid antagonists in the control of ingestive disorders, including alcoholism.

18.6.2 Overlap with Analgesia

There is evidence indicating that the system of opioid analgesia and the system of regulating ingestion of alcoholic beverages do not overlap. There is tolerance to opioid analgesia and no apparent tolerance to the effects of small doses of morphine to increase intake of alcoholic beverage (132). Not all opioid analgesics enhance rats' intake of alcoholic beverages. The more compelling data is that associated with the injections of small doses (25–100 μg/kg) of diprenorphine.

Diprenorphine is an antagonist to morphine's analgesia, but increases intakes of alcoholic beverages (133). Small doses of morphine plus small doses of diprenorphine increase drinking. Diprenorphine will also block the suppressive effects of large doses of morphine on voluntary intake of alcoholic beverages (134).

Although there is no apparent relationship between the opioidergic system salient to ingestion and the system salient to analgesia that does not mean that the two systems have different types of opioid receptors as part of the system. The two systems (one for positive effect from ingestion and one for pain) could be separated anatomically and use the same kind of receptors. The kind of opioid receptor involved in NTX's beneficial effects on alcohol consumption is the next topic.

18.6.3 Kind of Opioid Receptors

Almost by definition the μ receptor is probably involved in morphine and naloxone's bipolar effects on intake of alcoholic beverages. Studies in which antagonists specific for the μ and δ receptor have been tested on ethanol's salient characteristics have shown that these agents, generally, reduce intakes of alcoholic beverages and block conditioned effects of ethanol similarly to NTX (103, 105, 135–139). The circumstance is different for the κ receptor. Agonists at the κ receptor reduce drinking (140) and antagonists enhance drinking (140).

Mice genetically modified to be without μ receptors respond in behavioral tests as if they were under the effects of large doses of NTX (141–144). Genetically altered mice without the ability to produce preproenkephalin (145) and other mice that are deficient in β-endorphin react to ethanol in much the same way as their wild counterparts. Actually, and germane to speculations focusing on β-endorphin (42, 146, 147), β-endorphin deficient mice, under some circumstances, take more alcoholic beverage than their unaltered counterparts and show more signs of an ethanol-CPP than their counterparts (148–150).

Hayward et al. (151) observed ordinary intake of alcoholic beverage among mice lacking both enkephalins and β-endorphin. If both enkephalins and endorphin are missing in the genetically engineered mice and ethanol is still reinforcing, the question becomes: what is the ligand for the μ receptor? Hayward et al. (151) inferred that another μ-ligand might be salient and suggested endomorphin. I could find no studies manipulating levels of endomorphin while measuring intake of alcoholic beverages.

Banks and his colleagues (152) first did exceptional research showing that preproenkephalin targeted antisenses (they used three of them with slightly different strands of DNA) crossed the blood brain barrier. They then used the antisenses to reduce the production of preproenkephalin in mice provided an opportunity to drink alcoholic beverage. With some antisenses preparations muting the production of enkephalins, intake of alcoholic beverage was increased. The results are concordant with those of Hayward et al. (151).

Mice without δ receptors show increased intakes of alcoholic beverage (153), not the same as when δ antagonists are administered. Mice without κ receptors show decreased intakes of alcoholic beverages (154), not the same as when κ antagonists are administered. There is clearly something systematic happening, and it does not fit with the idea that the administration of a specific antagonist and the knock-out of a specific receptor for which that specific antagonist is supposed to act produce the same kind of effect. In addition, mice without enkephalins and β-endorphin do not behave as mice given naloxone or NTX.

In summary, there are data to support the theory that the μ receptor is salient to ethanol's ability to sustain its own intake. With respect to ethanol's ability to reinforce its own intake, it has yet to be determined which endogenous ligand or ligands for that receptor are salient.

The results of the research to find the kind of receptor and the endogenous ligand for the receptors of naloxone and NTX's salient effects for alcoholism do not fit nicely with one another. Some resolution to the discord is to presume that as endogenous circuits that are critical to sustaining intake do that, they also provide signal for satiety. A bout of drinking has events that initiate drinking, sustain that drinking once begun and events that terminate the bout. These events are chained together to guide behavior to ingestion, when that is appropriate, and to stop ingestion. Ingestion needs to stop to allow other behavior to emerge, but satiation also is adaptive in many circumstances because it prevents poisoning due to overindulgence. Reducing the signal for satiety could increase intakes. There could be separate opioidergic components to the various segments of a bout of drinking, some having one kind of receptor and others having another kind of receptor. A circuit involving μ receptors is apparently part of a circuit involved with the early stages of a bout of drinking and when that circuit is activated for a sufficiently long time begins to provide a signal for negative feedback to reduce the bout. Given this framework, one can imagine how the disturbance of anyone of the parts of the system can produce behavior that is different than what would be predicted if one merely assumes that all of the parts work as if they were one and gross measures of intake were sufficient to index all parts of a bout or bouts of drinking. The work manipulating separately the μ and κ receptors certainly indicates that they are components of separate systems. Some years ago, I guessed that much of the endogenous opioid circuitry was part of a system whose function was foraging (26). Opioids provided the feedback (in terms of increments in positive effect) to guide approach behavior (which is a manifestation of positive effect) toward food and drink while at the same time suppressing some signals of danger that would inhibit approach and having circuitry to suppress other motivations (e.g., sex) when nutritional needs were not being met. Satiety reduces foraging for food. There are enough dynamic parts of such a system that one can build models using the data of research manipulating any one or two of the opioidergic systems that can account for just about any set of outcomes.

18.7 Opioids and Sex of the Drinker

NTX may not be effective (or considerably less effective) in women compared to men [e.g., (64, 155)]. The work of Phillips et al. (156) with mice indicates that females react differently than males to large doses of NTX.

As the social barriers designed to curb women's drinking become less salient, the incidence of alcoholism among women is increasing [e.g., (157)]. Studies with various strains of rats and mice frequently indicate that females voluntarily drink more alcoholic beverages than males. Female mice were more likely to establish an ethanol-induced CPP than males (142). Any previously observed reduced incidence of alcoholism in women compared to men is, therefore, probably not a consequence of being female itself, but rather due to extant social constraints on women's drinking. Given these circumstances, it is reasonable to predict that the incidence of female alcoholism and the concomitant problems will increase dramatically.

The question of why NTX may be less effective in females is the kind of question that further research in the animal laboratory might contribute an answer. Recently, we (158, 159) have studied the effects of estradiol valerate on female rats' intakes of alcoholic beverages.

Continuous dosing with estradiol initially reduces intake and subsequently enhances intakes of alcoholic beverages. The enhancement can be substantial and surprisingly long lasting (159, 160). Juarez et al. (161), citing studies demonstrating that estrogen treatments modulate opioid receptors, theorized that estradiol's initial effects (reduced intakes) were due to an initial down regulation of opioid receptors (an effect similar to opioid antagonism), but subsequently, there was up regulation of opioid receptors (an effect similar to that of an opioid agonist). Such a sequence of events would account for estradiol's initial reduction in intake of alcoholic beverages and the subsequently enhanced intakes.

There are implications that can be drawn from the initial studies of estradiol and intake of alcoholic beverages. First, the conclusion that estradiol reduces intakes of alcohol (162–164) is an overgeneralization, because there are clear instances where that is not the case. Second, a question is raised about the safety of prescribing estrogenic medicines. Third, for NTX to be effective in women, it may take larger doses.

18.8 Combining Drugs to Achieve Better Outcomes of Treatments

Rezvani (165) has been an advocate for combining drugs to achieve a more favorable outcome from treatments. The general idea is that alcoholism is a multifaceted problem needing multiple approaches. Relatedly, AAA is accompanied by other disorders, particularly mood and anxiety disorders and those disorders are often addressed by the prescription of drugs. There is a high incidence of alcoholism among schizophrenics and their medications should be compatible with any medicines for alcoholism (see the chapter in this book by Petrakis). There are also other issues associated with the use of a combination of drugs including the possibility that some drugs might enhance the motivation to drink (as mentioned, agonists at opioid and benzodiazepine receptors). There is a general rule that the more drugs a person is taking the greater the risk of adverse drug reactions and the incidence of adverse drug reactions is alarmingly high (166). There are also issues associated with the fact that many of those currently presenting with AAA are also frequent users of other recreational drugs, in particular marijuana and cocaine (167).

We can not summarize here all of the studies in which a combination of drugs have been assessed for their ability to modulate intake of alcoholic beverages. There are, however, some clear guidelines for combining drugs. As mentioned, benzodiazepine agonists are clearly not a reasonable medicine to treat anxiety that might accompany alcoholism. Opioid agonists and any other agent that would increase rats' intake of alcoholic beverages should probably be shunned in favor of similar agents that do not. Agents that might reduce cognitive functioning (e.g., acetylcholine antagonists or agents with significant cholinergic binding) should be avoided on general grounds, but also on the grounds that the recovering alcoholic has important, difficult learning to do.

Isradipine and other calcium channel antagonists can be used with NTX to treat hypertension that often accompanies AAA, because they are safe to use and may also decrease propensity to take alcoholic beverages (55, 56, 168–171).

There is no basis in the claim that marijuana may be a suitable drug to substitute for propensity to take alcoholic beverages or would help relieve the events of alcohol withdrawal. In fact, preclinical research suggests just the opposite, agonists increase rats' intakes of alcoholic beverages and cannabinoid antagonists decrease intakes (172–174). An antagonist at the cannabinoid receptor and naloxone together reduced work for beer more than either alone, opening the possibility of having a treatment that might be particularly useful for patients presenting with both AAA and marijuana use disorder (174).

Given the distinct possibility that the stress and anxiety which are correlated with alcoholism is a product of the alcoholism, rather than the cause of alcoholism (175–177), it is reasonable to presume that an effective medicine for the comorbid anxiety will be a medicine that helps reduce alcoholism.

18.9 Theory Incorporating the Lessons of the Revolution

An excellent framework for building theory of AAA is Mowrer's two-factor learning theory (178). Mowrer's theory differs from the usual discussions of two-factor learning theory which emphasize fear and its reduction. Mowrer also spoke of positive emotions and the conditioning that occurs with positive events. Mowrer called the opposite of fear "hope." In more modern parlance, it might be called incentive motivation (179). What can be added to Mowrer's framework is the understanding that ethanol can induce an increment in positive effect in some people more so than others. The positive effect is easily conditionable to the place and events of that effect, thereby setting the circumstances for secondary reinforcement and incentive motivations (manifest on occasions as craving) to strengthen the habit of drinking.

An important elaboration is that the positive effect induced by ethanol is a product of activity in a circuit that has neurochemical coding involving the endogenous opioids. That circuit is also involved in the elaborations we call secondary reinforcement, incentive motivation. A further extension is the understanding that ethanol is clearly toxic to brain long before it is obvious to casual observation and that is manifest as reduced cognitive ability to cope, to change habitual behavior, and to learn alternatives to drinking.

An application of this theory is using opioid antagonists as adjuncts to psychotherapy. The psychotherapies most likely to succeed are those that explicitly attempt to countercondition the incentive motivations that sustain the habit of drinking and to develop alternative habits (180, 181). Such counterconditioning may be facilitated by NTX-treatment. Another application is to start the treatment regimen using NTX much earlier than is usually practiced, before cognitive impairment makes learning new habits difficult. Both preclinical research (41) and initial results of using NTX in the clinic with adolescents indicate both efficacy and safety (182).

The revolutionary idea that we can use drugs to modify the motivation to drink is extant. With continued scientific research, we can expect more successful treatments will be developed using new, better drugs than single oral doses of NTX and better combinations of drugs. Psychotherapies can be enhanced as they focus on the opportunities presented by pharmacotherapy. The thousands-year-old problem of alcoholism will yield to further research and development. Now, we have new perspectives, largely developed from preclinical research, and new applications that can make a difference to the millions who can not seem to control their drinking and drink too much, too often.

Acknowledgment I publicly acknowledge Meta Reid's help and hope I have made my appreciation clearly apparent to her.

References

1. Hunt WA, Barnett LW, Branch LG. Relapse rates in addiction programs. J Clin Psychol 1971; 27:455–456.
2. Miller WR, Walters ST, Bennett ME. How effective is alcoholism treatment in the United States? J Stud Alcohol 2001;62:211–220.
3. Dole VP. On the relevance of animal models to alcoholism in humans. Alcohol Clin Exp Res 1986;10:361–363.
4. Helzer JE, Badger GJ, Searles JS, Rose GL, Mongeon JA. Stress and alcohol consumption in heavily drinking men: 2 years of daily data using interactive voice response. Alcohol Clin Exp Res 2006;30:802–811.
5. Blum K, Hamilton MG, Wallace JE. Alcohol and opiates: A review of common neurochemical and behavioral mechanisms. In: Blum K, ed. Alcohol and Opiates: Neurochemical and Behavioral Mechanisms. New York: Academic Press, 1977:203–236.
6. Blum K, Briggs AH, Elston SFA, Hirst M, Hamilton MG, Verebey K. A common denominator theory of alcohol and opiate dependence: Review of similarities and differences. In: Rigter H, Crabbe JC, eds. Alcohol Tolerance and Dependence. New York: Elsevier Biomedical Press, 1980:339–370.
7. Stewart J. Pathways to relapse: The neurobiology of drug- and stress-induced relapse to drug taking. J Psychiatry Neurosci 2000;25:125–136.
8. Smith JE, Lane JD, eds. The Neurobiology of Opiate Reward Processes. New York: Elsevier Biomedical Press, 1983.
9. Rockwood GA, Reid LD. Naloxone modifies sugar-water intake in rats drinking with open gastric fistulas. Physiol Behav 1982;29:1175–1178.
10. Ostrowski NL, Foley TL, Lind MD, Reid LD. Naloxone reduces fluid intake: Effects of water and food deprivation. Pharm Biochem Behav 1980;12:431–435.
11. Ostrowski NL, Stapleton JM, Noble RG, Reid LD. Morphine and naloxone's effect on sexual behavior of the female golden hamster. Pharm Biochem Behav 1979;11:673–681.
12. Herman BH, Panksepp J. Effects of morphine and naloxone on separation distress and approach attachment: Evidence for opiate mediation of social affect. Pharm Biochem Behav 1978;9:213–220.
13. Altshuler HL, Philips PE, Feinhandler DA. Alteration of ethanol self-administration by naltrexone. Life Sci 1980;26:679–688.
14. Ho AKS, Chen RCA, Morrison JM. Interactions of narcotics, narcotic-antagonists, and ethanol during acute, chronic, and withdrawal states. Ann N Y Acad Sci 1976;281:297–310.
15. Ho AKS, Rossi N. Suppression of ethanol consumption by MET-enkephalin in rats. J Pharmac Pharmacol 1982;34:118–119.
16. Ho AKS, Tsai CS, Chen RCA, Braude MC. Drug interaction between alcohol and narcotic agents in rats and mice. The Pharmacologist 1975;17:197.

17. Ross D, Hartmann RJ, Geller I. Ethanol preference in the hamster: Effects of morphine sulfate and naltrexone, a long-acting morphine antagonist. Proc West Pharmacol Soc 1976; 19:326–330.
18. Sinclair JD, Adkins J, Walker S. Morphine-induced suppression of voluntary alcohol drinking in rats. Nature 1973;246:425–427.
19. Sinclair J, Rusi M, Airaksinen MM, Altshuler HL. Relating TIQ's, Opiates and Ethanol. β-carbolines and Tetrahydroquinolines: Progress in Clinical and Biological Research. New York: Alan R. Liss, Inc., 1982:365–376.
20. Marfaing-Jallat P, Miceli D, LeMagnen J. Decrease in ethanol consumption by naloxone in naive and dependent rats. Pharm Biochem Behav 1983;18(suppl. 1):537–539.
21. Sinden JD, Marfaing-Jallat P, LeMagnen J. The effect of naloxone on intragastric ethanol self-administration. Pharm Biochem Behav 1983;19:1045–1048.
22. Blum K, Wallace JE, Eubanks JD, Schwertner HA. Effects of naltrexone on ethanol withdrawal, preference and narcosis. Pharmacologist 1975;17:197.
23. Hubbell CL, Reid LD. Opioids modulate rats' intakes of alcoholic beverages. In: Reid LD, ed. Opioids, Bulimia, Alcohol Abuse & Alcoholism. New York: Springer-Verlag, 1990:145–174.
24. Bush HD, Bush MF, Miller MA, Reid LD. Addictive agents and intracranial stimulation: Daily morphine and lateral hypothalamic self-stimulation. Physiol Psychol 1976;4:79–85.
25. Collaer ML, Magnuson DJ, Reid LD. Addictive agents and intracranial stimulation (ICS): Pressing for ICS before and after self-administration of sweetened morphine solutions. Physiol Psychol 1977;5:425–428.
26. Reid LD, Siviy SM. Administration of opiate antagonists reveal endorphinergic involvement in reinforcement processes. In: Smith JE, Lane JD, eds. The Neurobiology of Opiate Reward Processes. New York: Elsevier Biomedical Press, 1983:257–279.
27. Wu M-F, Lind MD, Stapleton JM, Reid LD. Dose-response relationship between naloxone injections and intake of sucrose solution. Bull Psychon Soc 1981;17:101–103.
28. Stapleton JM, Ostrowski NL, Merriman VJ, Lind MD, Reid LD. Naloxone reduces fluid consumption in water deprived and nondeprived rats. Bull Psychon Soc 1979;13:237–239.
29. Reid LD. Endogenous opioid peptides and regulation of drinking and feeding. Am J Clin Nutr 1985;42:1099–1132.
30. Reid LD, Bozarth MA. Addictive agents and intracranial stimulation (ICS): The effect of various opioids on pressing for ICS. Proceedings of the Fortieth Annual Scientific Meeting of the Committee on Problems on Drug Dependence, 1978:729–741.
31. Rossi NA, Reid LD. Affective states associated with morphine injections. Physiol Psychol 1976; 4:269–274.
32. Linseman MA. Central vs. peripheral mediation of opioid effects on alcohol consumption in free-feeding rats. Pharm Biochem Behav 1989;33:407–413.
33. Reid LD, Hunter GA. Morphine and naloxone modulate intake of ethanol. Alcohol 1984;1:33–37.
34. Beaman CM, Hunter GA, Dunn LL, Reid LD. Opioids, benzodiazepines and intake of ethanol. Alcohol 1984;1:39–42.
35. Hunter GA, Beaman C, Dunn LL, Reid LD. Selected opioids, ethanol and intake of ethanol. Alcohol 1984;1:43–46.
36. Mudar PJ, LeCann NC, Czirr SA, Hubbell CL, Reid LD. Methadone, pentobarbital, pimozide and ethanol-intake. Alcohol 1986;3:303–308.
37. Czirr SA, Hubbell CL, Milano WC, Frank JM, Reid LD. Selected opioids modify intake of sweetened ethanol solution among female rats. Alcohol 1987;4:157–160.
38. Hubbell CL, Abelson ML, Burkhardt CA, Herlands SE, Reid LD. Constant infusions of morphine and intakes of sweetened ethanol solution among rats. Alcohol 1988;5:409–415.
39. Myers RD, Borg S, Mossberg R. Antagonism by naltrexone of voluntary alcohol selection in the chronically drinking macaque monkey. Alcohol 1986;3:383–388.
40. Kiefer SW, Bice PJ, Badia-Elder N. Alterations in taste reactivity to alcohol in rats given continuous alcohol access followed by abstinence. Alcohol Clin Exp Res 1994;18:555–559.
41. Sable HJ, Bell RL, Rodd ZA, McBride WJ. Effects of naltrexone on the acquisition of alcohol intake in male and female periadolescent and adult alcohol-preferring (P) rats. Int J Adolesc Med Health 2006;18:139–149.

42. Gianoulakis C, Angelogianni P, Meaney M, Thavundayil J, Tawar V. Endorphins in individuals with high and low risk for development of alcoholism. In: Reid LD, ed. Opioids, Bulimia, Alcohol Abuse & Alcoholism. New York: Springer-Verlag, 1990:229–246.
43. Reid LD, Hubbell CL. Opioids modulate rats' propensities to take alcoholic beverages. In: Naranjo CA, Sellers EM, eds. Novel Pharmacological Interventions for Alcoholism. New York: Springer-Verlag, 1992:121–134.
44. Reid LD, ed. Opioids, Bulimia, and Alcohol Abuse & Alcoholism. New York: Springer-Verlag, 1990.
45. O'Malley SS, Jaffe AJ, Chang G, Witte RS, Schottenfeld RS, Rounsaville B. Naltrexone in the treatment of alcohol dependence: Preliminary findings. In: Naranjo CA, Sellers EM, eds. Novel Pharmacological Interventions for Alcoholism. New York: Springer-Verlag, 1992:148–157.
46. Volpicelli JR, Alterman AI, Hayashida M, O'Brien CP. Naltrexone in the treatment of alcohol dependence. Arch Gen Psychiatry 1992;49:876–880.
47. O'Malley SS, Jaffe AJ, Chang G, Schottenfeld RS, Meyer RE, Rounsaville B. Naltrexone and coping skills therapy for alcohol dependence. A controlled study. Arch Gen Psychiatry 1992; 49:881–887.
48. Mark T. What will it take for physicians to embrace alcoholism medications? Alcohol Clin Exp Res 2006;30:257A.
49. Hilton M. Barriers to wider use of pharmacotherapy in clinical practice. Alcohol Clin Exp Res 2006;30:257A.
50. Alger SA, Schwalberg MJ, Bigaouette JM, Howard LJ, Reid LD. Using drugs to manage binge-eating among obese and normal weight patients. In: Reid LD, ed. Opioids, Bulimia, Alcohol Abuse & Alcoholism. New York: Springer-Verlag, 1990:131–142.
51. Jonas JM. Naltrexone and bulimia: Initial observations. In: Reid LD, ed. Opioids, Bulimia, Alcohol Abuse & Alcoholism. New York: Springer-Verlag, 1990:123–130.
52. Atkinson RL, Berke LK, Drake CR, Bibbs ML, Williams FL, Kaiser DL. Effects of long-term therapy with naltrexone on body weight in obesity. Clin Pharm Ther 1985;36:419–422.
53. Gardell LC, Hubbell CL, Reid LD. Naltrexone persistently reduces rats intake of a palatable alcoholic beverage. Alcohol Clin Exp Res 1996;20:584–588.
54. Stromberg M, Volpicelli J, O'Brien C. Effects of naltrexone administered repeatedly across 30 or 60 days on ethanol consumption using a limited access procedure in the rat. Alcohol Clin Exp Res 1998;22:2186–2191.
55. Gardell LC, Reid LD, Boedeker KL, Liakos TM, Hubbell CL. Isradipine and naltrexone in combination with isradipine interact with a period of abstinence to reduce rats' intakes of an alcoholic beverage. Alcohol Clin Exp Res 1997;21:1592–1598.
56. Reid ML, Hubbell CL, Douglass AV, Boedeker KL, Reid LD. Research with rats germane to medication for alcoholism: Consequences of noncompliance. Alcohol 2001;24:169–177.
57. Cooper SJ, Kirkham TC. Basic mechanisms of opioids' effects on eating and drinking. In: Reid LD, ed. Opioids, Bulimia, Alcohol Abuse & Alcoholism. New York: Springer-Verlag, 1990: 91–110.
58. Unterwald EM, Zukin RS. The endogenous opioidergic systems. In: Reid LD, ed. Opioids, Bulimia, and Alcohol Abuse & Alcoholism. New York: Springer-Verlag, 1990:49–72.
59. Overstreet DH, Kampov-Polevoy AB, Rezvani AH, Braun C, Bartus RT, Crews FT. Suppression of alcohol intake by chronic naloxone treatment in P rats: Tolerance development and elevation of opiate receptor binding. Alcohol Clin Exp Res 1999;23:1761–1771.
60. Cowen MS, Rezvani AH, Jarrott B, Lawrence AJ. Ethanol consumption by Fawn-Hooded rats following abstinence: Effect of naltrexone and changes in mu-opioid receptor density. Alcohol Clin Exp Res 1999;23:1008–1014.
61. Hyytia P, Ingman K, Soini SL, Laitinen JT, Korpi ER. Effects of continuous opioid receptor blockade on alcohol intake and up-regulation of opioid receptor subtype signaling in a genetic model of high alcohol drinking. Naunyn Schmiedebergs Arch Pharmacol 1999;360:391–401.
62. Juarez J, de Tomasi Eliana B. Alcohol consumption is enhanced after naltrexone treatment. Alcohol Clin. Exp. Res. 2007;31:260–264.
63. Hubbell CL, Abelson ML, Burkhardt CA, Herlands SE, Reid LD. Constant infusions of morphine and intakes of sweetened ethanol solutions among rats. Alcohol 1988;5:409–415.

64. Garbutt JC, Kranzler HR, O'Malley SS, et al. Efficacy and tolerability of long-acting injectable naltrexone for alcohol dependence: A randomized controlled trial. JAMA 2005; 293:1617–1625.
65. Heinala P, Alho H, Kiianmaa K, Lonnqvist J, Kuoppasalmi K, Sinclair J. Targeted use of naltrexone without prior detoxification in the treatment of alcohol dependence: A factorial double-blind, placebo-controlled trial. J Clin Psychopharmacol 2001;21:287–292.
66. Morgan CJ, Kosten TR. Potential toxicities of high doses of naltrexone in patients with appetitive disorders. In: Reid LD, ed. Opioids, Bulimia, Alcohol Abuse & Alcoholism. New York: Springer-Verlag, 1990:261–273.
67. Valliant GE. The Natural History of Alcoholism Revisited. Cambridge, MA: Harvard University Press, 1995.
68. Rodd ZA, Bell RL, Sable HJK, Murphy JM, McBride WJ. Recent advances in animal models of alcohol craving and relapse. Pharm Biochem Behav 2004;79:439–450.
69. Le A, Shaham Y. Neurobiology of relapse to alcohol in rats. Pharmacol Ther 2002;94:137–156.
70. Le AD, Quan B, Juzytch W, Fletcher PJ, Joharchi N, Shaham Y. Reinstatement of alcohol-seeking by priming injections of alcohol and exposure to stress in rats. Psychopharmacology 1998;135:169–174.
71. Le AD, Poulus CX, Harding S, Watchus J, Joharchi N, Shaham Y. Effects of naltrexone and fluoxetine on alcohol self-administration and reinstatement of alcohol seeking induced by priming injections of alcohol and exposure to stress. Neuropsychopharmacology 1999; 21:435–444.
72. Burattini C, Gill TM, Aicardi G, Janak PH. The ethanol self-administration context as a reinstatement cue: Acute effects of naltrexone. Neuroscience 2006;139:877–887.
73. Ciccocioppi R, Martin-Fardon R, Weiss F. Effect of selective blockade of μ_1 or δ opioid receptors on reinstatement of alcohol-seeking behavior by drug-associated stimuli in rats. Neuropsychopharmacology 2002;27:391–399.
74. Katner SN, Magalong JG, Weiss F. Reinstatement of alcohol-seeking behavior by drug-associated discriminative stimuli after prolonged extinction in the rat. Neuropsychopharmacology 1999; 20:471–479.
75. Bienkowski B, Kostowski W, Koros E. Ethanol-reinforced behavior in the rat: Effects of naltrexone. Eur J Pharmacol 1999;374:321–327.
76. Eiler WJ, 2nd, Woods JE, 2nd, Masters J, et al. Brain stimulation reward performance and sucrose maintained behaviors in alcohol-preferring and -nonpreferring rats. Alcohol Clin Exp Res 2005;29:571–583.
77. McGregor IS, Gallate JE. Rats on the grog: Novel pharmacotherapies for alcohol craving. Addictive Behav 2004;29:1341–1357.
78. Chow BL, Sellers EM, Tomkins DM. Effect of naltrexone and its derivatives, nalmefene and naltrindole, on conditioned anticipatory behaviour and saccharin intake in rats. Behav Pharmacol 1997;8:725–735.
79. Stapleton JM, Lind MD, Merriman VJ, Bozarth MA, Reid LD. Affective consequences and subsequent effects on morphine self-administration of d-ala^2-methionine enkephalin. Physiol Psychol 1979;7:146–152.
80. Schechter MD, Calcagnetti DJ. Trends in place preference conditioning with a cross-indexed bibliography; 1957–1991. Neurosci Biobehav Rev 1993;17:21–41.
81. Schechter MD, Calcagnetti DJ. Continued trends in the conditioned place preference literature from 1992 to 1996, inclusive, with a cross-indexed bibliography. Neurosci Biobehav Rev 1998;22:827–846.
82. Bormann NM, Cunningham CL. The effects on naloxone on expression and acquisition of ethanol place conditioning in rats. Pharm Biochem Behav 1997;58:975–982.
83. Reid LD, Hunter GA, Beaman CM, Hubbell CL. Toward understanding ethanol's capacity to be reinforcing: A conditioned place preference following injections of ethanol. Pharm Biochem Behav 1985;22:483–487.
84. Shippenberg TS, Altshuler HL. A drug discrimination analysis of ethanol-induced behavioral excitation and sedation: The role of endogenous opiate pathways. Alcohol 1985;2:197–201.

85. Bienkowsky P, Kuca P, Kostowski W. Conditioned place preference after prolonged pre-exposure to ethanol. Pol J Pharmacol 1995;47:189–191.
86. Bozarth MA. Evidence for the rewarding effects of ethanol using the conditioned place preference method. Pharm Biochem Behav 1990;35:485–487.
87. Gauvin DV, Holloway FA. Historical factors in the development of ETOH-conditioned place preference. Alcohol 1992;9:1–7.
88. Bienkowsky P, Kuca P, Piasecki J, Kostowski W. Low dose of ethanol induces conditioned place preference in rats after repeated exposures to ethanol or saline injections. Alcohol Alcohol 1996;31:547–553.
89. Cunningham C, Niehus J, Noble D. Species difference insensitivity to ethanol's hedonic effects. Alcohol 1993;10:97–102.
90. Cunningham C, Ferree NH, Howard MA. Apparatus bias and place conditioning with ethanol in mice. Psychopharmacology 2003;170:409–422.
91. Bechtholt AJ, Gremel CM, Cunningham CL. Handling blocks expression of conditioned place aversion but not conditioned place preference produced by ethanol in mice. Pharm Biochem Behav 2004;79:739–744.
92. Cunningham CL, Clemans JM, Fidler TL. Injection timing determines whether intragastric ethanol produces conditioned place preference or aversion in mice. Pharm Biochem Behav 2002;72:659–668.
93. Kelley BM, Bandy AL, Middaugh LD. A study examining ethanol-conditioned place preference in C57BL/6J mice. Alcohol Clin Exp Res 1997;21:1661–1166.
94. Morse AC, Schulteis G, Holloway FA, Koob GF. Conditioned place aversion to the "hangover" phase of acute ethanol administration in the rat. Alcohol 2000;22:19–24.
95. Cunningham CL, Henderson CM, Bormann NM. Extinction of ethanol-induced conditioned place preference and conditioned taste aversion: Effects of naloxone. Psychopharmacology 1998;139:62–70.
96. Marglin SH, Reid LD. Opioids modulate rats' reactivities to alcohol. In: Reid LD, ed. Opioids, Bulimia, Alcohol Abuse & Alcoholism. New York: Springer-Verlag, 1990:175–191.
97. Marglin SH, MacKechnie DK, Mattie ME, Hui Y, Reid LD. Ethanol with small doses of morphine establishes a conditioned place preference. Alcohol 1988;5:309–313.
98. Froehlich JC, Badia-Elder NE, Zink RW, McCullough DE, Portoghese PS. Contribution of the opioid system to alcohol aversion and alcohol drinking behavior. J Pharmacol Exp Ther 1998;287:284–292.
99. Monti PM, Tidey J, Czachowski CL, et al. Building bridges: The transdisciplinary study of craving from the animal laboratory to the lamppost. Alcohol Clin Exp Res 2004;28:279–287.
100. Cunningham C, Dickinson S, Okorn D. Naloxone facilitates extinction but does not affect acquisition or expression of ethanol-induced conditioned place preference. Exp Clin Pscyhopharmacol 1995;3:330–343.
101. Kuzman A, Sandin J, Terenius L, Ogren SO. Acquisition, expression, and reinstatement of ethanol-induced conditioned place preference in mice: Effects of opioid receptor-like 1 receptor agonists and naloxone. J Phamacol Exp Ther 2003;304:310–318.
102. Middaugh LD, Bandy AL. Naltrexone effects on ethanol consumption and response to ethanol conditioned cues in C57BL/6 mice. Psychopharmacology 2000;151:321–327.
103. Matsuzawa S, Suzuki T, Misawa M, Nagase H. Involvement of μ– and δ–opioid receptors in the ethanol-associated place preference in rats exposed to foot shock stress. Brain Res 1998; 803:169–177.
104. Stewart J. Stress and relapse to drug seeking: Studies in laboratory animal shed light on mechanisms and sources of long-term vulnerability. Am J Addict 2003;12:1–17.
105. Matsuzawa S, Suzuki T, Misawa M, Nagase H. Different roles of μ–, δ, and κ–opioid receptors in ethanol-associated place preference in rats exposed to conditioned fear stress. Eur J Pharmacol 1999;368:9–16.
106. Heyser CJ, Roberts AJ, Schulteis G, Koob GF. Central administration of an opiate antagonist decreases oral ethanol self-administration in rats. Alcohol Clin Exp Res 1999;23: 1468–1476.

107. Wolpe J. Conditioned inhibition of craving in drug addiction: A pilot experiment. Behav Res Ther 1965;18:285–288.
108. Wolpe J, Salter A, Reyna LJ, eds. The Conditioning Therapies. The Challenge in Psychotherapy. New York: Holt, Rinehart and Winston, 1965.
109. Anton RF, Moak DH, Latham P, et al. Naltrexone combined with either cognitive behavioral or motivational enhancement therapy for alcohol dependence. J Clin Psychopharmacol 2005;25:349–357.
110. Morley JE, Levine AS. The role of the endogenous opiates as regulators of appetite. Am J Clin Nutr 1982;35:757–761.
111. Sanger DJ. Endorphinergic mechanisms in the control of food and water intake. Appetite 1981;2:193–208.
112. Morley JE, Levine AS, Yim GK, Lowry MT. Opioid modulation of appetite. Neurosci Biobehav Rev 1983;7:281–305.
113. Jonas JM. Do substance-abuse, including alcoholism, and bulimia covary? In: Reid LD, ed. Opioids, Bulimia, Alcohol Abuse & Alcoholism. New York: Springer-Verlag, 1990:247–258.
114. Dansky BS, Brewerton TD, Kilpatrick DG. Comorbidity of bulimia nervosa and alcohol use disorders: Results from the National Women's Study. Int J Eat Disord 2000;27:180–190.
115. Timmerman MG, Wells LA, Chen SP. Bulimia nervosa and associated alcohol abuse among secondary school students. J Am Acad Child Adolesc Psychiatry 1990;29:118–122.
116. Franko DL, Dorer DJ, Keel PK, Jackson S, Manzo MP, Herzog DB. How do eating disorders and alcohol use disorders influence each other? Int J Eat Disord 2005;38:200–207.
117. Sinha R, Robinson J, Merikangas K, Wilson GT, Rodin J, O'Malley SS. Eating pathology among women with alcoholism and/or anxiety disorders. Alcohol Clin Exp Res 1996; 20:1184–1191.
118. Addolorato G, Capristo E, Greco AV, Caputo F, Stefanini GF, Gasbarrini G. Three months of abstinence from alcohol normalizes energy expenditure and substrate oxidation in alcoholics: A longitudinal study. Am J Gastroenterol 1998;93:2476–2481.
119. Leibel RL, Dufour M, Hubbard VS, Lands WE. Alcohol and calories: A matter of balance. Alcohol 1993;10:427–434.
120. Colditz GA, Giovannucci E, Rimm EB, et al. Alcohol intake in relation to diet and obesity in women and men. Am J Clin Nutr 1991;54:49–55.
121. Kleiner KD, Gold MS, Frost-Pineda K, Lenz-Brunsman B, Perri MG, Jacobs WS. Body mass index and alcohol use. J Addict Dis 2004;23:105–118.
122. Addolorato G, Capristo E, Marini M, et al. Body composition changes induced by chronic ethanol abuse: Evaluation by dual energy X-ray absorptiometry. Am J Gastroenterol 2000; 95:2323–2327.
123. Koppes LL, Twisk JW, Van Mechelen W, Snel J, Kemper HC. Cross-sectional and longitudinal relationships between alcohol consumption and lipids, blood pressure and body weight indices. J Stud Alcohol 2005;66:713–721.
124. Carlsson S, Hammar N, Grill V, Kaprio J. Alcohol consumption and the incidence of type 2 diabetes: A 20-year follow-up of the Finnish twin cohort study. Diabetes Care 2003; 26:2785–2790.
125. Kampov-Polevoy AB, Garbutt JC, Janowsky DS. Association between preference for sweets and excessive alcohol intake: A review of animal and human studies. Alcohol Alcohol 1999; 34:386–395.
126. Kampov-Polevoy AB, Overstreet DH, Rezvani AH, Janowsky DS. Suppression of ethanol intake in alcohol-preferring rats by prior voluntary saccharin consumption. Pharm Biochem Behav 1995;52:59–64.
127. Froehlich JC, Harts J, Lumeng L, Li T-K. Naloxone attenuates voluntary ethanol intake in rats selectively bred for high ethanol preference. Pharm Biochem Behav 1990;35:385–290.
128. Phillips TJ, Broadbent J, Burkhart-Kasch S, et al. Genetic correlational analyses of ethanol reward and aversion phenotypes in short-term selected mouse lines bred for ethanol drinking or ethanol-induced conditioned taste aversion. Behav Neurosci 2005;119:892–910.

129. Schneider ES, Rada P, Darby R, Leibowitz SF, Hoebel BG. Hypothalamic orexin preferentially stimulates alcohol intake over food and water in rats. Alcohol Clin Exp Res 2006;30: 129A.
130. Kiefer F, Jahn H, Otte C, Demiralay C, Wolf K, Weidemann K. Increasing leptin precedes craving and relapse during pharmacological abstinence maintenance treatment of alcoholism. J Psychiatr Res 2005;39:545–551.
131. Chang G-Q, Karatayev O, Ahsan R, et al. Effect of ethanol on hypothalamic opioid peptides, enkephalin, and dynorphin: Relationship with circulating triglycerides. Alcohol Clin Exp Res 2007;31:249–259.
132. Hubbell CL, Czirr SA, Hunter GA, Beaman CM, LeCann NC, Reid LD. Consumption of ethanol solution is potentiated by morphine and attenuated by naloxone persistently across repeated daily administrations. Alcohol 1986;3:39–54.
133. Reid LD, Czirr SA, Bensinger CC, Hubbell CL, Volanth AJ. Morphine and diprenorphine together potentiate intake of alcoholic beverages. Alcohol 1987;4:161–168.
134. Reid LD. Prospects for developing more specific antagonists, I. In: Reid LD, ed. Opioids, Bulimia, Alcohol Abuse & Alcoholism. New York: Springer-Verlag, 1990:275–280.
135. Hyytia P. Involvement of mu-opioid receptors in alcohol drinking by alcohol-preferring AA rats. Pharmacol Biochem Behav 1993;45:697–701.
136. June HL, McCane SR, Zink RW, Portoghese PS, Li T-K, Froehlich JC. The δ_2-opioid receptor antagonist naltriben reduces motivated responding for ethanol. Psychopharmacology 1999;147:81–89.
137. Stromberg MF, Casale M, Volpicelli L, Volpicelli JR, O'Brien CP. A comparison of the effects of the opioid antagonists naltrexone, naltrindole, and beta-funaltrexamine on ethanol consumption in the rat. Alcohol 1998;15:281–289.
138. Le AD, Poulos CX, Quan B, Chow S. The effects of selective blockade of delta and mu opiate receptors on ethanol consumption by C57BL/6 mice in a restricted access paradigm. Brain Res Bull 1993;630:330–332.
139. Franck J, Lindholm S, Raaschou P. Modulation of volitional ethanol intake in the rat by central delta-opioid receptors. Alcohol Clin Exp Res 1998;22:1185–1189.
140. Sandi C, Borrell J, Guaza C. Involvement of kappa type opioids on ethanol drinking. Life Sci 1988;42:1067–1075.
141. Roberts AJ, McDonald JS, Heyser CJ, et al. mu-Opioid receptor knockout mice do not self-administer alcohol. J Pharmacol Exp Ther 2000;293:1002–1008.
142. Hall FS, Sora I, Uhl GR. Ethanol consumption and reward are decreased in μ-opiate receptor knockout mice. Psychopharmacology 2001;154:43–49.
143. Becker A, Grecksch G, Kraus J, Loh HH, Schroeder H, Hollt V. Rewarding effects of ethanol and cocaine in mu opioid receptor-deficient mice. Nauyn Schmiedebergs Arch Pharmacol 2002;365:296–302.
144. Ghozland S, Kathleen C, Kieffer BL, Roberts AJ. Lack of stimulant and anxiolytic-like effects of ethanol and accelerated development of ethanol dependence in mu-opioid receptor knockout mice. Neuropsychopharmacology 2005;49:493–501.
145. Koenig HN, Olive MF. Ethanol consumption patterns and conditioned place preference in mice lacking preproenkephalin. Neurosci Lett 2002;325:75–78.
146. Zalewska-Kaszubska J, Czarnecka E. Deficit in beta-endorphin peptide and tendency to alcohol abuse. Peptides 2005;26:701–705.
147. Oswald LM, Wand GS. Opioids and alcoholism. Physiol Behav 2004;81:339–358.
148. Grahame NJ, Low MJ, Cunningham CL. Intravenous self-administration of ethanol in beta-endorphin-deficient mice. Alcohol Clin Exp Res 1998;22:1093–1098.
149. Grahame NJ, Mosemiller AK, Low MJ, Froehlich JC. Naltrexone and alcohol drinking in mice lacking β-endorphin by site-directed mutagenesis. Pharm Biochem Behav 2000; 67:729–766.
150. Grisel JE, Mogil JS, Grahame NJ, et al. Ethanol oral self-administration is increased in mutant mice with decreased β–endorphin expression. Brain Res 1999;835:62–67.

151. Hayward MD, Hansen ST, Pintar JE, Low MJ. Operant self-administration of ethanol in C57BL/6 mice lacking β-endorphin and enkephalin. Pharm Biochem Behav 2004; 79:171–181.
152. Banks WA, Jaeger LB, Urayama A, et al. Preproenkephalin targeted antisenses cross the blood-brain barrier to reduce brain methionine enkephalin levels and increase voluntary ethanol drinking. Peptides 2006;27:784–796.
153. Roberts AJ, Gold LH, Polis I, et al. Increased ethanol self-administration in delta-opioid receptor knockout mice. Alcohol Clin Exp Res 2001;25:1249–1256.
154. Kovacs KM, Szakall I, O'Brien D, et al. Decreased oral self-administration of alcohol in kappa-opioid receptor knock-out mice. Alcohol Clin Exp Res 2005;29:730–738.
155. Hernandez-Avila CA, Song C, Kuo L, Tennen H, Armeli S, Kranzler HR. Targeted versus daily naltrexone: Secondary analysis of effects on average daily drinking. Alcohol Clin Exp Res 2006;30:860–865.
156. Phillips TJ, Wenger CD, Dorow JD. Naltrexone effects on ethanol drinking acquisition and on established ethanol consumption in C57BL/6J mice. Alcohol Clin Exp Res 1997;21: 691–702.
157. Holdcraft LC, Iacono WG. Cohort effects on gender differences in alcohol dependence. Addiction 2002;97:1025–1036.
158. Reid LD, Marinelli PW, Bennett SM, et al. One injection of estradiol valerate induces dramatic changes in rats' intake of alcoholic beverages. Pharm Biochem Behav 2002;72: 601–616.
159. Reid ML, Hubbell CL, Reid LD. A pharmacological dose of estradiol can enhance appetites for alcoholic beverages. Pharm Biochem Behav 2003;74:381–388.
160. Marinelli PW, Quirion R, Gianoulakis C. Estradiol valerate and alcohol intake: A comparison between Wistar and Lewis rats and the putative role of endorphins. Behav Brain Res 2003;139:59–67.
161. Juarez J, Barrios de Tomasi E, Virgen M. Effects of estradiol treatment on voluntary and forced alcohol consumption in male rats. Pharm Biochem Behav 2002;71:259–268.
162. Sandberg D, Stewart J. Effects of estradiol benzoate and MER-25 on ethanol consumption in the ovariectomized rat. J Comp Physiol Psychol 1982;96:635–648.
163. Sandberg D, David S, Stewart J. Effects of estradiol benzoate on the pattern of eating and ethanol consumption. Physiol Behav 1982;29:61–65.
164. Eckel LA. Estradiol: A rhythmic, inhibitory, indirect control of meal size. Physiol Behav 2004;82:35–41.
165. Rezvani AH, Overstreet DH, Mason GA, et al. Combination pharmacotherapy: A mixture of small doses of naltrexone, fluoxetine, and a thyrotropin-releasing hormone analogue reduces alcohol intake in three strains of alcohol-preferring rats. Alcohol Alcohol 2000;35:76–83.
166. Lazarou J, Pmeranz BH, Corey PN. Incidence of adverse drug reactions in hospitalized patients: A meta-analysis of prospective studies. JAMA 1998;279:1200–1205.
167. Sable HJK, White SL, Steinpreis RE. Effects of chronic naltrexone treatment in rats on place preference and locomotor activation after acute administration of cocaethylene or ethanol plus cocaine. Alcohol 2004;33:51–61.
168. Croog SH, Elias MF, Colton T, et al. Effects of antihypertensive medications on quality of life in elderly hypertensive women. Am J Hypertens 1994;7:329–339.
169. Perry HM, Jr, Hall W, Ryder Benz J, et al. Efficacy and safety of atenolol, enalapril, and isradipine in elderly hypertensive women. Am J Med 1994;96:77–86.
170. Cramer CM, Gardell LC, Boedeker KL, Harris JR, Hubbell CL, Reid LD. Isradipine combined with naltrexone persistently reduces the reward-relevant effects of cocaine and alcohol. Pharm Biochem Behav 1998;60:345–356.
171. De Beun R, Schneider R, Klein A, Lohmann A, De Vry J. Effects of nimodipine and other calcium channel antagonists in alcohol-preferring AA rats. Alcohol 1996;13:263–271.
172. McGregor IS, Dam KD, Mallet PE, Gallate JE. Delta9-THC reinstates beer- and sucrose-seeking behaviour in abstinence rats: Comparison with midazolam, food deprivation and predator odour. Alcohol Alcohol 2005;40:35–45.

173. Gessa GL, Serra S, Vacca G, Carai MA, Colombo G. Suppressing effect of the cannabinoid CB1 receptor antagonist, SR147778, on alcohol intake and motivational properties of alcohol in alcohol-preferring sP rats. Alcohol Alcohol 2005;40:46–53.
174. Gallate JE, Mallet PE, McGregor IS. Combined low dose treatment with opioid and cannabinoid receptor antagonist synergistically reduces the motivation to consume alcohol in rats. Psychopharmacology 2004;173:210–216.
175. Da Silva GE, Ramos A, Takahashi RN. Comparison of voluntary ethanol intake by two pairs of rat lines used as genetic models of anxiety. Braz J Med Biol Res 2004;37:1511–1517.
176. Langen B, Fink H. Anxiety as a predictor of alcohol preference in rats? Prog Neuropsychopharmacol Biol Psychiatry 2004;28:961–968.
177. Henniger MS, Spanagel R, Wigger A, Landgraf R, Holter SM. Alcohol self-administration in two rat lines selectively bred for extremes in anxiety-related behavior. Neuropsychopharmacology 2002;26:729–736.
178. Mowrer OH. Learning Theory and Behavior. New York: John Wiley & Sons, Inc., 1960.
179. Krank MD. Pavlovian conditioning with ethanol: Sign-tracking (autoshaping), conditioned incentive, and ethanol self-administration. Alcohol Clin Exp Res 2003;27:1592–1598.
180. Hunt GM, Azrin NH. A community-reinforcement approach to alcoholism. Behav Res Ther 1973;11:91–104.
181. Azrin NH. Improvements in the community-reinforcement approach to alcoholism. Behav Res Ther 1976;14:339–348.
182. Deas D, May MP, Randall C, Johnson N, Anton R. Naltrexone treatment of adolescent alcoholics: An open-label pilot study. J Child Adolesc Psychopharmacol 2005;15:723–728.

Chapter 19
Clinical Use of Opioid Antagonists in the Treatment of Alcohol Dependence

Raymond F. Anton

Abstract The opiate system is one of a few brain neurotransmitter systems implicated in alcohol reward and reinforcement. Alterations in this system might underlie risk for the development of alcoholism. However, most germane to this chapter is the use of opiate receptor antagonist drugs as medications to treat alcohol dependence. Accumulating evidence from both basic and clinical studies points to the efficacious use of drugs such as naltrexone and nalmefene in both reducing heavy drinking and preventing relapse. Studies in mice, rats, nonhuman primates, and man all provide support for the ability of these agents to reduce alcohol consumption.

Human laboratory studies have shown that opiate antagonists will reduce alcohol consumption, reduce initial cognitive stimulation caused by alcohol, and reduce craving along with normalizing its neuroanatomical correlates. Clinical trials have generally found naltrexone to be more efficacious than placebo as ellucidated in several meta-analyses. It is becoming increasingly evident that compliance with naltrexone is extremely important for its effects to be fully recognized. Limitations to compliance include adverse effects, patient motivation to cut-down or cease alcohol consumption, costs, and belief in potential benefit of treatment. Several large clinical trials in the United States, the extended release naltrexone trial (Vivatrol™ Study) and the NIH funded COMBINE Study have both shown naltrexone to be more efficacious than placebo. Both trials employed compliance enhancing strategies. For the Vivatrol™ Study it was once monthly extended-release naltrexone injections, and for the COMBINE Study it was the use of medical management counseling that specifically supported compliance. In general, naltrexone seems to work best in the context of a structured psychosocial or compliance enhancing counseling context. Adverse effect management, liver toxicities, and pain management are all limitations that need to be addressed during treatment.

R.F. Anton
Center for Drug and Alcohol Programs, Institute of Psychiatry, Charleston, SC 29425
e-mail: antonr@musc.edu

R. Dean et al. (eds.), *Opiate Receptors and Antagonists*,

It is clear that opiate antagonist medications do not work for everyone. It has been suggested that higher levels of craving, family history of alcohol dependence, high motivation for treatment, and genetic disposition all contribute to success. Of particular interest is the recent suggestion that those alcoholics with a genetic difference at one nucleotide (single nucleotide polymorphism or SNP A118G) in the mu opiate receptor coding gene will be more sensitive to naltrexone effects and show greater efficacy during treatment.

Keywords: Alcohol dependence; Opiate antagonists; Naltrexone; Clinical studies

19.1 Introduction

It has been known for almost 30 years that the brain opiate system played some role in alcohol effects. Early studies in animals showed that opiate receptor antagonists, particularly those that blocked the mu type receptor, could alter some of alcohol's effects in animals. It took about 15 years to recognize the potential of drugs like naltrexone for the treatment of alcohol dependence. Landmark studies done at the University of Pennsylvania and Yale University School of Medicine and published in 1992 (1, 2) led to subsequent Food and Drug Administration (FDA) approval of naltrexone for the treatment of alcohol dependence in 1994. Over the ensuing years considerable data have accumulated at the basic science level to confirm the definitive effect of opiate antagonists in reducing the reinforcing and cue induced motivational aspects of alcohol consumption. Clinical trials have been conducted in many countries, a needed effort considering that the initial FDA approval of naltrexone's use in alcohol dependence was based on just two single-site academic studies. In addition, clinical laboratory paradigms have been developed to examine the mechanisms of naltrexone's effects in alcoholics as well as to bridge the gap between basic and clinical science in the development of new compounds to treat alcoholism. In many ways, naltrexone has "broken the log jam" in drug development for alcoholism. A few large well-conducted clinical trials have recently confirmed naltrexone's utility with less intensive psychosocial interventions. Naltrexone, along with another opiate antagonist, nalmefene, has captured the interest of alcohol researchers, clinicians, patients, and now an increasing number of pharmaceutical companies. In fact, an extended-release injectable formulation of naltrexone has been approved and is being currently marketed.

This chapter will review what is known about opiate antagonists in the treatment of alcohol dependence in humans. In order to do this adequately, it will first develop the bridge between basic and clinical science, and then discuss clinical studies and trials. Given the limitations of space, this chapter does not attempt to be a "comprehensive review" but does abstract and present important data to illustrate overriding points and ideas.

19.2 Evidence for the Clinical Use of Opioid Antagonists in the Treatment of Alcohol Dependence

19.2.1 Translation from Basic Science to Clinical Utility

Opiate antagonist medications, such as naltrexone and nalmefene, reduce free choice drinking (3, 4) and reinforced responding (5) in animals. This reduction in free choice drinking and reinforced responding has been related to a naltrexone-induced decrease in dopamine release, as measured by microdialysis, in the nucleus accumbens (6, 7), the purported brain reward center for substances of abuse (8). It has been shown that rodents, when placed in an environment in which they had previously consumed alcohol, increase dopamine in the nucleus accumbens even before they were able to taste or drink it. This animal equivalent to a human expectancy or "craving" effect was also reduced by naltrexone (7, 9). Whether the effect of naltrexone is directly on nucleus accumbens cells or, more likely, an indirect decrease in output of dopamine from the ventral tegmental area is open to question. Suffice it to say that the mu opiate receptor blockade by naltrexone will reduce dopamine elevation in an important brain area which subserves reinforcement and which transmits signals to higher association areas (e.g., cingluate gyrus and prefrontal areas) that subserve memory for reinforced behaviors and substances of abuse. Recent data from our lab at the Medical University of South Carolina Center for Drug and Alcohol Programs suggest that naltrexone reduces activation in the above areas when alcoholics are viewing pictures in a functional imaging paradigm (10). Taken together, data from animals and man suggest that naltrexone can disrupt the normal brain circuitry underlying addiction, forming the basis for its efficacy as a therapeutic agent for the treatment of alcohol dependence.

19.2.2 Human Laboratory Models of Heavy Drinking

A crucial bridge between animal observations and clinical efficacy is the determination of the effect of opiate antagonists under controlled alcohol consumption paradigms. While work with cue-induced neuroimaging techniques holds considerable promise, ultimately how a medication affects drinking behavior is crucial in determining its clinical efficacy. Our group at Medical University of South Carolina (MUSC) and others have examined both naltrexone and nalmefene (another clinically safe opiate antagonist) in clinical lab settings (11–14). In our initial study, nontreatment seeking alcoholics were placed on naltrexone, nalmefene, or placebo for 7 days under double blind natural conditions, prior to being given a priming drink of their preferred beverage in a bar lab setting. After 45 min they were allowed to consume a limited amount of drinks (4 total) in a free choice paradigm where they chose between alcohol or money (14). We evaluated whether they had

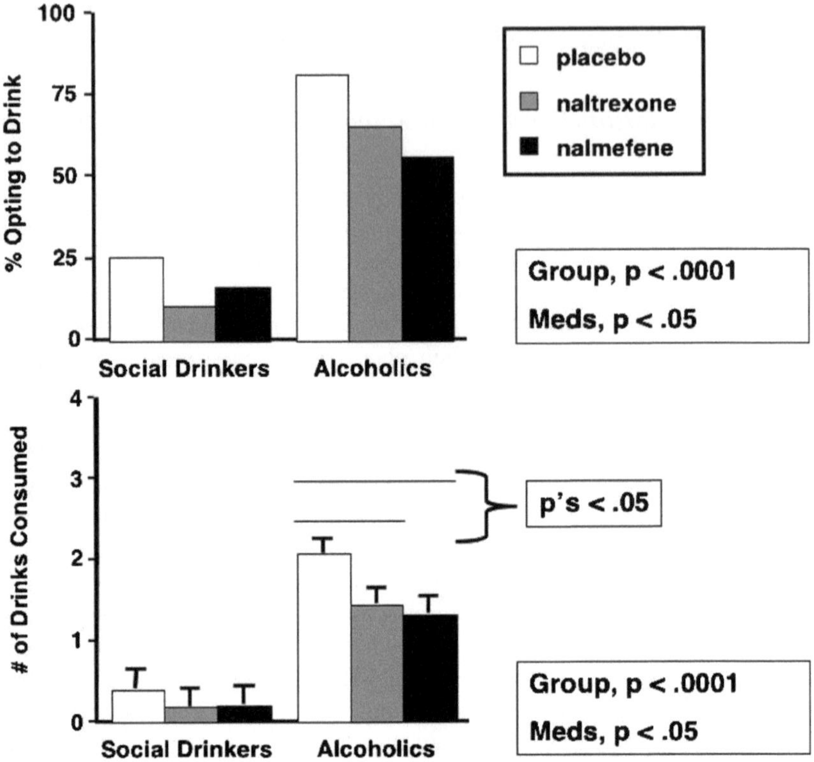

Fig. 19.1 Free choice drinking in a bar lab setting by social drinkers and nontreatment seeking alcoholics after a priming drink depending on medication treatment during the 7 days previous. Source: Drobes et al. (14)

any additional drinks, and how many, after the priming drink. As can be seen in Fig. 19.1, fewer alcoholics pretreated with naltrexone and nalmefene opted to drink more alcohol than those pretreated with placebo. Those on the medications also consumed less drinks if they did choose to drink.

In a follow-up study (13) a similar paradigm was used but in this follow-up study, less alcohol was given as a priming drink and more drinks (8 total) could be chosen afterwards. One group was allowed to drink immediately (short delay) after the priming drink and the other group was subject to a 45 min long delay before opting to drink. This time, naltrexone reduced drinking and delayed the progression of drinking *only* in the group that was forced to wait for 45 min (Fig. 19.2). Interestingly, our group discovered that the positive relationship between the priming drink induced stimulation (cognitive and motoric) and further drinking was reversed by naltrexone (Fig. 19.3).

These series of experiments done by the MUSC lab and others have shown that the pharmacological effects of naltrexone can be measured directly. Since the people recruited for these studies had no motivation to reduce or quit drinking, it

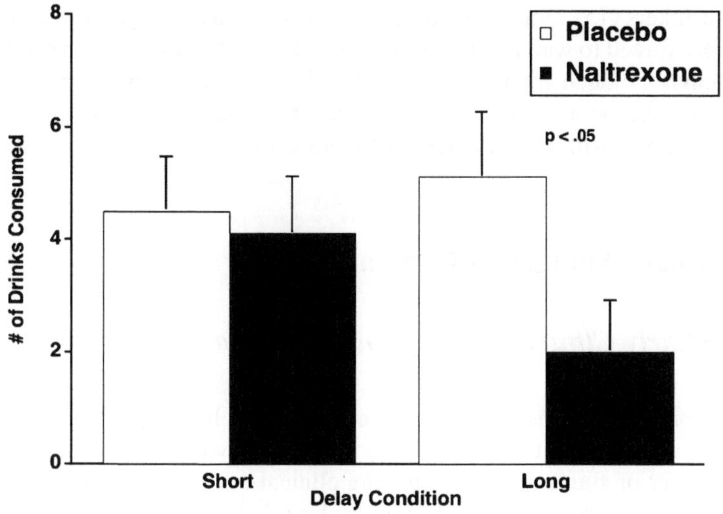

Fig. 19.2 Medication x delay condition. Source: Anton et al. (13)

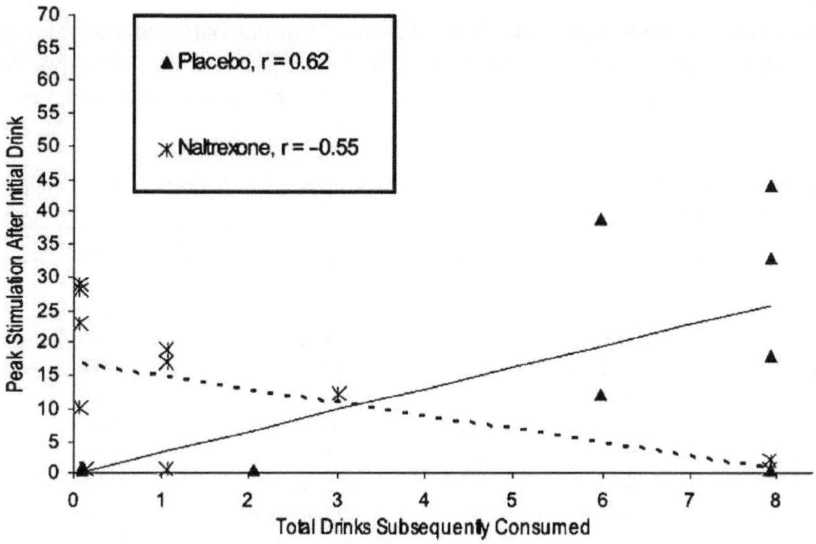

Fig. 19.3 Relationship of stimulation after a priming drink of alcohol to subsequent free choice drinking in nontreatment seeking alcoholics in a bar lab setting. Source: Anton et al. (13)

was intriguing to see that the opiate antagonists caused a reduction of alcohol intake under controlled drinking (bar lab) conditions. This may be seen as a pure pharmacological effect since motivation to alter drinking behavior was lacking. Also, there was an indication that naltrexone might interfere with the initial stimulatory effect of alcohol, an effect that might be more pronounced in heavy drinkers as compared to social drinkers (15). Finally, naltrexone only reduced and/or slowed drinking if a person were forced to wait awhile prior to consuming the next drink. This important drug by environmental interaction might explain why cognitive behavioral therapies or other techniques which boost motivation to control drinking (16, 17) might interact positively with opiate antagonist medications.

19.3 Opiate Antagonist Clinical Trials

19.3.1 Early Clinical Trials – Initial Efficacy and Questions

The two opiate antagonists that have been studied clinically are naltrexone and nalmefene, with the vast majority being conducted with naltrexone. There have been a number of single-site and multisite clinical trials that support the utility of naltrexone in reducing relapse to heavy drinking in alcoholics. A number of these trials are summarized in Table 19.1. The FDA approved naltrexone in 1994 for the prevention of relapse in alcohol-dependent individuals based on two single-site studies (1, 2).

Although the published controlled trials used similar outcome variables, such as percent of days abstinent (PDA) and time to relapse to a day of heavy drinking, they generally excluded patients with other substance abuse or psychiatric

Table 19.1 Summary of trials of naltrexone/nalmefene in the context of either CBT or supportive/12-step counseling

CBT/similar techniques (n = 947)			Supportive/12-step therapy (n = 1,543)		
O'Malley	1992	+	O'Malley	1992	+
Heinälä	2001	+	Heinälä	2001	0
Balldin	2003	+	Balldin	2003	0
Volpicelli	1992	+	Chick	2000	0
Volpicelli	1997	(+)	Krystal	2001	0
Anton	1999	+	Morris	2001	+
Mason	1999	+	Latt	2002	+
Kranzler	2000	0	Gastpar	2002	0
Monti	2001	(+)	Rybakowski[a]	1997	0
Monterosso	2001	+	Auriacombe[b]	2000	0

There was a significant difference ($p < 0.05$) between drug and placebo

A + sign indicated significant difference of naltrexone over placebo

+, ITT; (+), completers

[a] Rybakowski JK, Ziółkowski M, Volpicelli JR. A study of lithium, carbamazepine and naltrexone in male patients with alcohol dependence – results of four months of treatment. Abstract ESBRA, 1997

[b] Auriacombe M, Robinson M, Grabot D, Tignol J. Naltrexone is ineffective to prevent relapse to alcohol in a realistic out-patient setting. A double blind one-year controlled study. Abstract CPDD, 2000

CBT cognitive behavioral therapy

comorbidity. Most alcoholics were of moderate or greater severity and were generally motivated to seek treatment and participate in a clinical trial. Overall, three meta-analyses (18–20) including many of the trials in Table 19.1, have supported the utility of naltrexone over placebo. For the common variable "relapse to heavy drinking (four or more drinks for women and five or more for men in a given day)," naltrexone appears to produce about a 15–25% reduction of risk over placebo. In two studies (16, 17) done by our MUSC group utilizing cognitive behavioral therapy (CBT), the risk reduction for relapse during naltrexone compared to placebo treatment was exactly 22%. However, one meta-analysis reported a significant 19% increase in percent days abstinent of naltrexone over placebo (19) while another reported a nonsignificant 3% increase (18). Moreover, there is some suggestion that naltrexone may increase the number of people completely abstinent during the trial since all three meta-analyses show a trend (about a 10–15% increase in complete abstinence rates of naltrexone over placebo) in that direction. Overall, there seems to be some consensus in the literature that naltrexone helps more with a reduction in heavy drinking and less in the maintenance of total abstinence. However, the treatment outcome differences might to some degree be related to the goals of the individual patient at the start of treatment. This will be discussed later in this chapter. In our work at MUSC, we have found that subjects entering clinical trials have varying goals and motivations toward alcohol treatment. Some desire complete abstinence while others initially choose a goal of moderation or reduction in intake, which makes a standard outcome variable somewhat difficult.

In the Unites States, a large Veterans Administration multisite naltrexone trial (21) failed to show statistical benefit of naltrexone over placebo. This trial had several differences compared to other positive naltrexone studies. The most salient of these differences were (1) subjects were older and more severely alcohol affected; (2) the background psychosocial intervention (12-step facilitation) may have been more varied; (3) the drop out rate was slightly higher; and (4) there is more variability inherent in multisite, compared to single-site studies. In fact, a number of studies have indicated that naltrexone works best when combined with a relapse prevention (coping skills, CBT) approach. In general, when naltrexone and/or nalmefene were studied, without concomitant use of defined relapse prevention interventions, its efficacy has been less robust (22). At the time of that review, six out of seven studies showed a significant reduction in relapse when relapse prevention or CBT was utilized along with naltrexone or nalmefene, while only two out of seven studies showed such an effect when only supportive/12-step therapy was utilized (Table 19.1). Furthermore, a 28% reduction in relapse was observed when opiate antagonists were utilized with relapse prevention/CBT interventions.

In this context, it was interesting to see that a clinical trial of nalmefene in the United States utilizing Motivational Enhancement Therapy (MET) did not show efficacy on relapse to heavy drinking or heavy drinking days (17). This was consistent with a trial published from our MUSC group that found naltrexone to work better with CBT rather than MET in the prevention of relapses (23). These experiences lead to questions in the field as to how naltrexone should be utilized in clinical practice. At the same time, questions were being asked regarding the utility of combining naltrexone with another reportedly efficacious medication, acamprosate, for the treatment of alcohol dependencies.

19.3.2 The COMBINE Study in the US

Given the above data the National Institute of Alcohol Abuse and Alcoholism (NIAAA) convened a group of the top alcohol clinical trial experts to design a study that would address some of the questions regarding the use of naltrexone. The study was designed to address the following two key questions on the efficacy of naltrexone: (1) Does naltrexone work only in the context of specialized alcohol counseling versus a more supportive medical management (MM) approach? and (2) Does the combination of naltrexone and acamprosate work better than naltrexone alone? The 16-week study with one year follow-up, addressed these and other questions (24, 25).

Patients (n = 1,383) were assigned to one of eight groups and treated with one of the following four study drug regimens: (1) naltrexone (100 mg/day); (2) acamprosate (3,000 mg/day); (3) both; or (4) their matching placebos. Patients were also assigned to either receive MM alone or MM with Combined Behavioral Intervention (CBI). MM was designed to be a nine-session intervention which could be delivered by health care professionals (physicians, nurses, and physician assistants) and consisted of education of alcohol effects, motivation to maintain abstinence, encouragement to attend Alcoholics Anonymous meetings, and a continual review and reinforcement of medication adherence (26, 27). CBI (28, 29) developed for the COMBINE Study included elements of three approaches: (1) MET; (2) Cognitive Behavioral Therapy; and (3) 12-step facilitation as used in Project MATCH (30). It allowed for client-based modules to be utilized in a flexible fashion over a 20-session maximum (in reality, patients only utilized a median of nine sessions). Subjects were assessed over 16 weeks of treatment and again at week 26, 52, and 68 after randomization (up to 1 year after treatment).

The study collected 94% of the drinking data during the 16 weeks of treatment and 82% of the drinking data up to 1-year follow-up. The results were intriguing and somewhat unexpected. There was a statistically significant interaction between the type of counseling and naltrexone. There was more percent days absent (PDA), less relapse to the first heavy drinking day, and a better clinical global outcome in those receiving MM with either naltrexone or CBI therapy as compared to those who only received placebo. There was no additive effect of naltrexone and acamprosate or naltrexone and CBI. The interaction of naltrexone and counseling on good clinical outcome (being abstinent or having moderate drinking without problems during the last 8 weeks of treatment) is given in Fig. 19.4.

The odds ratio (95% CI) of having a good clinical outcome compared to MM + placebo was 1.82 (1.26–2.65) if treated with MM + CBI without naltrexone, 1.93 (1.33–2.80) if treated with MM + CBI with naltrexone, and 2.16 (1.46–3.20) if

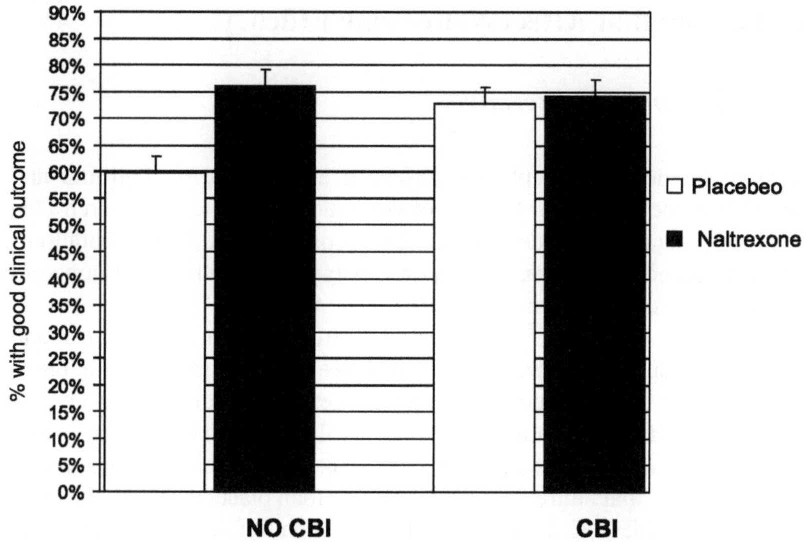

Fig. 19.4 Those acheiving a good clinical outcome (GCO) in the COMBINE Study. Naltrexone was better than placebo in the context of medical management but not when given simultaneously with Combined Behavioral Intervention (see text). Naltrexone by CBI interaction, $p = 0.02$. GCO defined as No more than 2-day heavy drinking over 8 weeks and no more than 11 drinks (women) or 14 drinks (men) per week and no alcohol problems. Source: Anton et al. (25)

treated with MM + naltrexone without CBI. Putting it another way, the odds of having a good clinical outcome were almost twice as great if a person received naltrexone in the context of MM. Adding specialized counseling to naltrexone did not add much to the naltrexone by itself.

These findings have wide ranging implications. First of all, they imply that naltrexone can be given without specialized alcohol counseling as long as good MM techniques, similar to those used in the study, are employed. Although the MM was conducted primarily by physicians and nurses (who were responsible for the majority of the counseling) in a clinical trial setting with substance abuse investigators, the techniques are not dissimilar to those employed in the management of other chronic diseases where education, support, and treatment adherence are considered the primary agenda. Why naltrexone and CBI were not additive remains a question for further exploration. It is possible that CBI maximized treatment gains in a way that CBT in prior studies was not able to do, thereby not allowing naltrexone room for enhancement. Alternatively, CBI and naltrexone might work better for certain individuals, a distinction that could have been lost in a large multisite trial of heterogeneous individuals and therapists. It was disappointing that acamprosate did not enhance naltrexone's efficacy, an effect that was hypothesized at the initiation of the trial and subsequently suggested by a previously reported small study (31).

19.4 Factors that Affect Naltrexone Efficacy

19.4.1 Treatment Adherence

The role of medication compliance has been emphasized by Pettinati and colleagues (32) at the Center for Studies of Addiction, Treatment Research Division. In reanalyzing data from several clinical trials completed at their Philadelphia site, a marked difference in naltrexone response between compliant and noncompliant individuals emerged as shown in Fig. 19.5.

As can be seen in Fig. 19.5, the effect of naltrexone is much greater in adherent patients. Our group at MUSC has recently reevaluated data from a previously published clinical trial in which we used two measures of medication compliance, microchip embedded medication bottle caps (MEMS caps) and urinary riboflavin measurements of riboflavin-enhanced study capsules. In the intent-to-treat analysis (17) we showed that naltrexone worked better than placebo only in the context of CBT and not with MET. Evaluating the efficacy of naltrexone in the most compliant subjects (those with greater than 80% pill bottle opening and 75% positive urine riboflavins), the effect size of the naltrexone by CBT interaction increased from 0.2 to 0.5, indicating more than a doubling of efficacy (33) in those with maximal compliance. These data taken together with that of Pettinati and colleagues indicate the important role of medication compliance in the effectiveness of naltrexone.

Others have written about the importance of adherence in the treatment of alcoholism (34). It is clear that a number of factors affect adherence: (1) patient motivation for treatment and acceptance of goals of treatment; (2) simplicity of medication regimen, that is, how many times a day medication must be taken or the need for ancillary lab tests; (3) adverse symptoms of the medication; (4) monitoring visits to support compliance; (5) support from important others; and (6) negative

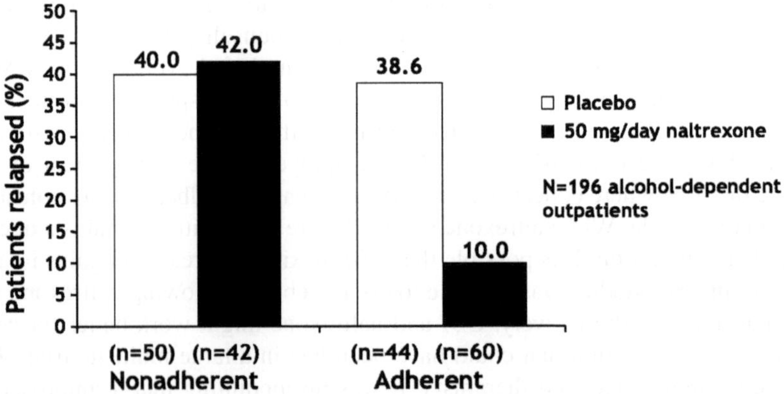

Fig. 19.5 Rates of relapse in alcohol-dependent patients by treatment adherence and medication group. Adherent = took naltrexone as prescribed and attended at least 80% of clinical visits. Source: Pettinati et al. (32)

consequences of not adhering to treatment, for example, job or marital loss. Several authors (35, 36) have suggested that high levels of side effects during the first several weeks of treatment will reduce compliance and that higher craving at study entry, as well as a greater belief in the medication's efficacy, may predict better medication compliance. Fortunately, the oral form of naltrexone needs to be taken only once a day which should enhance adherence. Naltrexone does, however, have some uncomfortable side effects (headaches, GI distress, and fatigue) that could be limiting, especially in subjects with lower motivation for treatment. These side effects moderate considerably after the first several weeks of treatment and might be dose, or blood level, related (37). Nevertheless, the side effects of the medication coincide with the highest risk period for relapse, which is the first month of treatment. This is why everything possible should be done to support treatment adherence during this period, including frequent patient visits and monitoring. Titration of oral naltrexone, especially in women, over the first several weeks of treatment seems to be important. Therefore, doses starting at 25 mg and going to up to 50 or 100 mg appears to be a reasonable plan.

19.4.2 Long Acting Injectable Naltrexone

In mid-2006, the FDA approved a long acting intramuscular injectable (extended release – XL) formulation of naltrexone (Vivatrol™). This approval was based on a US multisite trial in which XL naltrexone was given once a month over 6 months along with 12 sessions of health care professional supportive/educative counseling (38). The 627 alcohol dependent participants were randomly assigned to receive one of two doses of XL naltrexone (190 mg, 380 mg) or inactive placebo injections. The 380 mg XL dose was formulated to be roughly bioequivalent to 50 mg of naltrexone daily. After an initial peak, release serum levels are maintained at about 2 ng/ml without the daily peaks and troughs of oral naltrexone (39). The compliance with the injections was reasonably high, and equal to or better than oral naltrexone compliance, with 64% of participants receiving all 6-monthly injections and 74% receiving 4-monthly injections. However, participants in the high dose XL group dropped out twice as often as the placebo group (14.1% vs 6.7%) secondary to adverse effects. Theoretically, the XL formulation with lower overall accumulated naltrexone levels should lead to less adverse effects than oral naltrexone and to better overall adherence; but, since there was no oral dose naltrexone comparison group in this study, this question remains unaddressed. Nevertheless, the high dose XL naltrexone (approved by the FDA) reduced the risk of heavy drinking by 25%, which is very consistent with the oral naltrexone studies combined with behavioral counseling. Of interest, the efficacy of XL naltrexone seems to be more significant in men compared to women and also in those who had some abstinence at the beginning of the trial. This trial is significant in that it supports the pharmacological action of naltrexone in the context of high compliance and non-intensive counseling. Taken together with the results of the COMBINE Study and other data (40), these data suggest that expanded use of naltrexone in various heath care settings is possible, thereby broadening access to treatment for many individuals not being served at this time.

19.5 Longer-Term Follow-up of Individuals Treated with Naltrexone

Most studies with naltrexone have been designed for 12–16 weeks. The question remains as to how long alcohol-dependent patients should be treated with naltrexone. Data do exist, however, on what happens to individuals after treatment with naltrexone ends. Several studies have shown that relapse to heavy drinking is high after termination of naltrexone, even if individuals had received concomitant relapse prevention or CBT (25, 41, 42). For instance, in the COMBINE Study, while the effects observed during treatment were still evident, the results were no longer significant 1 year after treatment. Our MUSC group previously showed (42) that over the first several months after naltrexone and CBT ended that individuals had a gradual return to heavier drinking such that, by the end of follow-up, average drinking levels looked similar to those previously treated with placebo. Taken together, these data suggest that, at least for some individuals (most likely those that did not attain complete abstinence by the end of the trial) more treatment is indicated. O'Malley et al. (40) showed that patients who do well on naltrexone during 10 weeks in the context of MM, continue to maintain reduced drinking levels if maintained on naltrexone for up to 6 months. Future investigation will have to determine which individuals need continued or intermittent treatment over the long run. Clinical observation suggests that those without complete abstinence and those with a high level of craving at the end of an initial 12–16-week course of treatment are in the greatest need of maintenance medication or booster counseling sessions.

19.6 Patient Variables Affecting Response

Reports of naltrexone use in alcoholics with comorbid cocaine dependence have generally been negative (43, 44). Other studies have suggested some utility of naltrexone coupled with brief intervention (45) or when used in an intermittent "targeted" fashion to reduce drinking in high-risk situations (46) in heavy/early problem drinkers. One study reported that naltrexone was well-tolerated in older alcoholics (47) and appeared to reduce drinking in those that could not remain abstinent.

One of the most exciting developments of recent years has been the ability to genotype individuals to predict treatment response (pharmacogenomics). Oslin and colleagues (48) reported that alcoholics with a single nucleotide polymorphism (SNP) in the gene coding for the mu opiate receptor (OPRM1) leads to a functional amino acid substitution (asn40asp) in the mu opiate receptor protein. Those with the asn40asp substitution have a greater rate of responding to naltrexone than those (asn40asn) who do not. This SNP occurs in about 20% of the population. Others (49) have reported that those with this mutation also respond more strongly to alcohol. Data from the COMBINE Study will support this initial observation.

19.7 Side Effects and Clinical Use

Naltrexone side effects have generally been moderate at the 50-mg dose, the dosage used in most studies. They include gastrointestinal problems (nausea, vomiting, and abdominal pain) and central nervous system-related symptoms (headache, fatigue). The US Product Label (as described in the Physicians Desk Reference) warns that significant hepatotoxicity may occur with naltrexone; however, this label has remained for the XL naltrexone although there are little data presently to support or refute its applicability. Historically, heptotoxicity has been mostly observed in morbidly obese subjects receiving higher doses of the medication, while many clinical trials, including a safety study conducted for FDA review (50), did not observe significant hepatoxicity. However, a report (51) of an interaction between nonsteroidal antiinflammatory drugs (NSAIDs) and high dose naltrexone (>100 mg/day) leading to hepatoxicity should be noted. While the exact risk of this interaction is unknown, clinicians should be careful at using high doses of naltrexone and warn their patients of this potentially dangerous drug effect.

In the COMBINE Study (25), 12 individuals had treatment emergent increases in AST or ALT to five times greater than normal. Of these 12 cases, 11 subjects were taking 100 mg of naltrexone. While most of these individuals were drinking heavily, other causes of this elevation could not be determined. Most of these resolved when the medication was discontinued.

Another caution should be noted in the use of naltrexone. Since naltrexone is an opiate antagonist, individuals abusing opiates may experience opiate withdrawal, while those receiving opiates for analgesia will find them ineffective during naltrexone treatment. Therefore, a complete medication history and a urine drug screen may be indicated prior to initiating naltrexone therapy. In addition, if acute opiate analgesia is required during the course of treatment, caution should be taken. Higher doses of opiates may be required and signs of respiratory distress should be monitored. The patient should carry a card explaining these issues and provide it to health care personnel in an emergency situation.

19.8 Summary

Considerable data are now available from both basic and clinical laboratories, as well as from well-conducted clinical trials, supporting the role of opiate antagonists in the treatment of alcohol dependence. There are two FDA approved naltrexone formulations (oral and injectable extended release) now on the market in the United States. Meta-analysis and recently published large trials (25, 38) all suggest its utility with effect sizes in the 0.2 range. Maximizing compliance and motivation is likely to increase the effectiveness of naltrexone. It is also clear that many patients need extended treatment past an initial 3–4 months.

The primary challenge for the future is to identify individual patient factors that might predict increased rate of response to naltrexone since it is clear that not everyone (perhaps only 1 in 6) respond well to the medication. Perhaps genetic subtyping, as mentioned above, will lead to greater prediction of response as we go forward into the new age of "personalized medicine." New formulations of opiate antagonists that bind more specifically to brain mu or delta opiate receptors, perhaps in different regions of the brain, might allow for greater efficacy with less adverse effects. The combination of naltrexone with other medications to treat alcohol dependence might also be a fruitful area of investigation leading to enhanced clinical utility.

References

1. Volpicelli JR, Alterman AI, Hayashida M, O'Brien CP. Naltrexone in the treatment of alcohol dependence. Arch Gen Psychiatry 1992;49:876–80.
2. O'Malley SS, Jaffe AJ, Chang G, Schottenfeld RS, Meyer RE, Rounsaville B. Naltrexone and coping skills therapy for alcohol dependence. Arch Gen Psychiatry 1992;49:881–7.
3. Sinclair JD. Laboratory animal research in the discovery and development of the new alcoholism treatment using opioid antagonists. Scand J Lab Anim Sci 1996;23:379–90.
4. Kornet M, Goosen C, Van Ree JM. Effect of naltrexone on alcohol consumption during chronic alcohol drinking and after a period of imposed abstinence in free-choice drinking rhesus monkeys. Psychopharmacology (Berl) 1991;104:367–76.
5. Williams KL, Woods JH. Conditioned effects produced by naltrexone doses that reduce ethanol-reinforced responding in rhesus monkeys. Alcohol Clin Exp Res 1999;23(4):708–15.
6. Benjamin D, Grant ER, Pohorecky LA. Naltrexone reverses ethanol-induced dopamine release in the nucleus accumbens in awake, freely moving rats. Brain Res 1993;621:137–40.
7. Gonzales RA, Weiss F. Suppression of ethanol-reinforced behavior by naltrexone is associated with attenuation of the ethanol-induced increase in dialysate dopamine levels in the nucleus accumbens. J Neurosci 1998;18(24):10663–71.
8. Koob GF, Roberts AJ, Schulteis G, et al. Neurocircuitry targets in ethanol reward and dependence. Alcohol Clin Exp Res 1998;22(1):3–9.
9. Middaugh LD, Szumlinski KK, Patten YV, Marlowe A-LB, Kalivas PW. Chronic ethanol consumption by C57BL/6 mice promotes tolerance to its interoceptive cues and increases extracellular dopamine, an effect blocked by naltrexone. Alcohol Clin Exp Res 2003;27(12): 1892–900.
10. Myrick H, Anton RF, Li X, Henderson S, Randall PK, Voronin K. Effect of naltrexone and ondansetron on alcohol cue-induced activation of the ventral striatum in alcohol-dependent people. Arch Gen Psych 2008;65(4):466–475.
11. O'Malley SS, Krishnan-Saria S, Farren C, Sinha R, Kreek MJ. Naltrexone decreases craving and alcohol self-administration in alcohol-dependent subjects and activates the hypothalamo-pituitary-adrenocortical axis. Psychopharmacology (Berl) 2002; 160:19–29.
12. Drobes DJ, Anton RF, Thomas SE, Voronin K. Effects of naltrexone and nalmefene on subjective response to alcohol among non-treatment seeking alcoholics and social drinkers. Alcohol Clin Exp Res 2004;28(9):1362–70.

13. Anton RF, Drobes DJ, Voronin K, Durazo-Avizu R, Moak D. Naltrexone effects on alcohol consumption in a clinical laboratory paradigm: temporal effects of drinking. Psychopharmacology (Berl) 2004;173:32–40.
14. Drobes DJ, Anton RF, Thomas SE, Voronin K. A clinical laboratory paradigm for evaluating medication effects on alcohol consumption: naltrexone and nalmefene. Neuropsychopharmacology 2003;28:755–64.
15. Thomas SE, Drobes DJ, Voronin K, Anton RF. Following alcohol consumption, nontreatment-seeking alcoholics report greater stimulation but similar sedation compared with social drinkers. J Stud Alcohol 2004;65(3):330–5.
16. Anton RF, Moak DH, Waid LR, Latham PK, Malcolm RJ, Dias JK. Naltrexone and cognitive behavioral therapy for the treatment of outpatient alcoholics. Am J Psychiatry 1999;156(11): 1758–64.
17. Anton RF, Moak DH, Latham PK, et al. Naltrexone combined with either cognitive behavioral or motivational enhancement therapy for alcohol dependence. J Clin Psychopharmacol 2005;25(4):1–9.
18. Streeton C, Whelan G. Naltrexone, a relapse prevention maintenance treatment of alcohol dependence: a meta-analysis of randomized controlled trials. Alcohol Alcohol 2001;36(6): 544–52.
19. Kranzler HR, Van Kirk J. Efficacy of naltrexone and acamprosate for alcoholism treatment: a meta-analysis. Alcohol Clin Exp Res 2001;25(9):1335–41.
20. Bouza C, Magro A, Munoz A, Amate J. Efficacy and safety of naltrexone and acamprosate in the treatment of alcohol dependence: a systematic review. Addiction 2004;99:811–28.
21. Krystal JH, Cramer JA, Krol WF, Kirk GF, Rosenheck RA, the Veterans Affairs Naltrexone Cooperative Study Group. Naltrexone in the treatment of alcohol dependence. N Engl J Med 2001;345(24):1734–9.
22. Berglund M, Thelander S, Salaspuro M, Franck J, Andreasson S, Ojehagen A. Treatment of alcohol abuse: an evidence-based review. Alcohol Clin Exp Res 2003;27(10):1645–56.
23. Anton RF, Pettinati H, Zweben A, et al. A multisite dose ranging study of nalmefene in the treatment of alcohol dependence. J Clin Pharmacol 2004;24:421–8.
24. The COMBINE Study Group. Testing combined pharmacotherapies and behavioral interventions in alcohol dependence: rationale and methods. Alcohol Clin Exp Res 2003;27:1107–22.
25. Anton RF, O'Malley SS, Ciraulo DA, et al. Combined pharmacotherapies and behavioral interventions for alcohol dependence: the COMBINE study: a randomized controlled trial. JAMA 2006;295(17):2003–17.
26. Pettinati HM, Weiss RD, Miller WR, Donovan D, Ernst DB, Rounsaville BJ. Medical Management (MM) treatment manual. COMBINE monograph series. In: DHHS Pub. No (NIH) 04-5289; 2004.
27. Pettinati HM, Weiss RD, Dundon W, et al. A structured approach to medical management: a psychosocial intervention to support pharmacotherapy in the treatment of alcohol dependence. J Stud Alcohol 2005;66(4):S170(9).
28. Miller WR. Combined behavioral intervention manual.In: DHHS Pub. No. (NIH) 04-5288; 2004.
29. Longabaugh R, Zweben A, Locastro JS, Miller WR. Origins, issues and options in the development of the combined behavioral intervention. J Stud Alcohol 2005;66(4):S179(9).
30. Project MATCH Research Group. Matching alcohol treatments to client heterogeneity: project MATCH posttreatment drinking outcomes. J Stud Alcohol 1997;58:7–29.
31. Kiefer F, Jahn H, Tarnaske T, et al. Comparing and combining naltrexone and acamprosate in relapse prevention of alcoholism. Arch Gen Psychiatry 2003;60(1):92–9.
32. Pettinati HM, Volpicelli JR, Pierce JD, Jr., O'Brien CP. Improving naltrexone response: an intervention for medical practitioners to enhance medication compliance in alcohol dependent patients. J Addict Dis 2000;19(1):71–83.
33. Crissman AM, Latham PK, Moak D, Voronin K, Anton R. Comparison of microchip embedded medication bottle caps and urine riboflavin as indicators of medication compliance in an alcohol pharmacotherapy trial. Alcohol Clin Exp Res 2005;29(5):162A.

34. Weiss RD. Adherence to pharmacotherapy in patients with alcohol and opioid dependence. Addiction 2004;99(11):1382–92.
35. Rohsenow DJ, Colby SM, Monti PM, et al. Predictors of compliance with naltrexone among alcoholics. Alcohol Clin Exp Res 2000;24(10):1542–9.
36. Oncken C, Van Kirk J, Kranzler HR. Adverse effects of oral naltrexone: analyais of data from two clinical trials. Psychopharmacology (Berl) 2001;154(4):397–402.
37. King AC, Volpicelli JR, Gunduz M, O'Brien CP, Kreek MJ. Naltrexone biotransformation and incidence of subjective side effects: a preliminary study. Alcohol Clin Exp Res 1997;21(5): 906–9.
38. Garbutt J, Kranzler H, O'Malley S, et al. Efficacy and tolerability of long-acting injectable naltrexone for alcohol dependence. JAMA 2005;293(13):1617–25.
39. Dunbar JL, Turncliff RZ, Dong Q, Silverman BL, Ehrich EW, Lasseter KC. Single- and multiple-dose pharmacokinetics of long-acting injectable naltrexone. Alcohol Clin Exp Res 2006;30(3):480–90.
40. O'Malley SS, Rounsaville BJ, Farren C, et al. Initial and maintenance naltrexone treatment for alcohol dependence using primary care vs speciality care: a nested sequence of 3 randomized trials. Arch Intern Med 2003;163:1695–704.
41. O'Malley SS, Jaffe AJ, Chang G, et al. Six-month follow-up of naltrexone and psychotherapy for alcohol dependence. Arch Gen Psychaitry 1996;53:217–24.
42. Anton RF, Moak DH, Latham PK, et al. Posttreatment results of combining naltrexone with cognitive-behavior therapy for the treatment of outpatient alcoholics. J Clin Psychopharmacol 2001;21(1):72–7.
43. Hersh D, Van Kirk JR, Kranzler HR. Naltrexone treatment of comorbid alcohol and cocaine use disorders. Psychopharmacology (Berl) 1998;139:44–52.
44. McCaul B, Wand GS, Sullivan J, Mumford G, Quigley J. Beta-naltrexol level predicts alcohol relapse. Alcohol Clin Exp Res 1997;21(3):32A.
45. Bohn MJ, Kranzler HR, Beazoglou D, Staehler BA. Naltrexone and brief counseling to reduce heavy drinking. Results of a small clinical trial. Am J Addict 1994;3(2):91–9.
46. Kranzler HR, Tennen H, Penta C, Bohn MJ. Targeted naltrexone treatment of early problem drinkers. Addict Behav 1997;22(3):431–6.
47. Oslin D, Liberto JG, O'Brien J, Krois S. Tolerability of naltrexone in treating older alcohol-dependent patients. Am J Addict 1997;6(3):266–70.
48. Oslin DW, Berrettini W, Kranzler HR, et al. A functional polymorphism on the μ-opioid receptor gene is associated with naltrexone response in alcohol-dependent patients. Neuropsychopharmacology 2003;28:1546–52.
49. Ray LA, Hutchinson KE. A polymorphism of the μ-opioid receptor gene *(oprm1)* and sensitivity to the effects of alcohol in humans. Alcohol Clin Exp Res 2004;28(12):1789–95.
50. Croop RS, Faulkner EB, Labriola DF, Group tNUS. The safety profile of naltrexone in the treatment of alcoholism. Results from a multicenter usage study. Arch Gen Psychiatry 1997;54: 1130–5.
51. Kim SW, Grant JE, Adson DE, Remmel RP. A preliminary report on possible naltrexone and nonsteroidal analgesic interactions. J Clin Psychopharmacol 2001;21(6):632–4.
52. Anton RF, Oroszi G, O'Malley SS, Couper DJ, Swift R, Pettinati HM, Goldman D. An evaluation of mu-opioid receptor (OPRM1) as a predictor of naltrexone response in the treatment of alcohol dependence: Results from the combined pharmacotherapies and behavioral interventions for alcohol dependence (COMBINE) Study. Arch Gen Psych 2008;65(2):135–144.

Chapter 20
Preclinical Effects of Opioid Antagonists on Feeding and Appetite

Richard J. Bodnar

Abstract A large component of the evidence linking the endogenous opioid system to the control of food intake and body weight has been derived from the ability of general and selective opioid antagonists to block food intake under a number of homeostatically mediated and reward-mediated conditions. This chapter will examine the role of general and specific opioid receptor subtype antagonist involvement in the mediation of (1) the palatable and hedonic aspects of food intake and food choice, including ingestion of simple sugars and fats; (2) the ingestive response to homeostatic regulatory challenges including food deprivation, glucoprivation, and lipoprivation; (3) body weight regulation in normophagic, genetically-obese, diet-obese and stressed animals; and (4) pharmacologically-induced feeding. Detailed description of the central sites of antagonist will be provided, as well as comparing opioid antagonist effects with those derived from molecular gene expression and knockout and knockdown (antisense) approaches. The pervasive effects of opioid antagonists on the different aspects of feeding behavior make the development of more selective antagonist peptide analogues and drugs attractive target systems for the treatment of obesity and diabetes and intake of macronutrients associated with these important dysfunctions.

Keywords: Body weight regulation; Feeding behavior; Food deprivation; Gene expression; Homeostatic challenges; Palatability; Pharmacologically induced feeding

20.1 Introduction

Within 1 year of the discovery of the opiate receptor in 1973 (1–3), Steven Holtzman (4) made the seminal observation that the general opiate antagonist, naloxone reduced food intake elicited by food deprivation to the same degree as the well-known anorectic,

R.J. Bodnar
Department of Psychology and Neuropsychology, Queens College, City University of New York, Flushing, NY 11367
e-mail: richard.bodnar@qc.cuny.edu

R. Dean et al. (eds.), *Opiate Receptors and Antagonists*,

D-amphetamine, and that combined treatment with naloxone and D-amphetamine produced synergitic degrees of inhibition. That finding, together with the initial discoveries that endogenous opioid peptides such as beta-endorphin (5), enkephalin (6, 7), and dynorphin (8, 9) elicited potent feeding responses, indicated that the endogenous opioid system was involved in the modulation of feeding and appetite. Indeed, the endogenous opioid system has subsequently been implicated in virtually all aspects of food intake and body weight regulation, with a number of classic reviews focusing on the opioid integration of sensory, emotional and energy state ingestive information (e.g., 10, 11), or more specifically on the modulation of the hedonic or palatable aspects of food (e.g., 12–15). Given the widespread effects of the endogenous opioid system upon different mechanisms regulating the appetitive and consummatory aspects of food intake and body weight regulation, the present chapter will systematically evaluate opioid antagonist involvement in the mediation of (1) the palatable and hedonic aspects of food intake and food choice including ingestion of simple sugars and fats; (2) the ingestive response to homeostatic regulatory challenges including food deprivation, glucoprivation, and lipoprivation; (3) body weight regulation in normophagic, genetically-obese, diet-obese, and stressed animals; and (4) pharmacologically-induced feeding. In each of these particular sections, empirical evidence will be presented for opioid receptor involvement through the analysis of (a) general opioid antagonists, (b) specific opioid receptor subtype antagonists, (c) central sites of action, and where applicable, and (d) molecular gene expression and knockout and knockdown (antisense, AS) approaches.

20.2 Opioid Antagonist Effects upon Palatable and Hedonic Aspects of Food Intake

20.2.1 Behavioral Role of General and Specific Opioid Antagonists

20.2.1.1 General Opioid Antagonist Effects

Both naloxone and naltrexone antagonists decrease intake of sucrose and saccharin solutions as well as high-fat or high-sugar diets (16–18) to a greater degree than normal diets (19) with its effects apparent as early as 6 days of age (20), and persisting whether the animals were fed on a restricted or an ad libitum regimen (21). Naloxone reduces sucrose intake without affecting eating latency or rate, suggesting effects upon the maintenance, rather than the initiation of intake (e.g., 22, 23), and affects the hedonic and orosensory characteristics because it continued to inhibit sucrose intake in vagotomized rats (24), shifted the sucrose concentration threshold to the right in sham-fed rats (25, 26), altered taste reactivity (27, 28), and more potently reduced intake of preferred relative to nonpreferred diets (29, 30). Recent analyses of eight inbred and one outbred mouse strains revealed up to a 35-fold difference in the potency of systemic naltrexone to inhibit sucrose intake in highly-sensitive (e.g., C57BL/10J) relative to less-sensitive (e.g., SWR/J, 129P3/J) strains, suggesting profound genetic variance (31). Conditioned flavor preferences in animals are observed for novel flavors paired with simple sugars relative to novel flavors paired with saccharin (flavor–flavor conditioning), but naltrexone failed to alter either the acquisition or expression of sucrose flavor–flavor conditioning in sham-feeding rats (32) or of fructose flavor–flavor conditioning in real-feeding rats (33). Naltrexone also failed to alter either the acquisition or expression of flavor preferences conditioned by intragastric sucrose (34), but dose-dependently reduced the expression, but not the acquisition of a sucrose-conditioned place preference (35). Sucrose-preferring rats that have sucrose restricted display reductions in the total amount of energy generated by sucrose relative to starch following naltrexone infusions. In contrast, sucrose-preferring rats without subsequent sucrose restrictions failed to show reductions in sucrose preference (36). A suggestion that naloxone acts to modify nutrient selection by selectively reducing fat intake (37, 38) was supported by dose-dependent decreases in the licks for intralipid solutions (39).

20.2.1.2 Opioid Receptor Subtype Antagonist Effects

Ventricular administration of selective mu and kappa, but not delta-1 opioid antagonists reduces intake of palatable fat or sucrose diets (40–43). Like general opioid antagonism, ventricular administration of general, mu and kappa, but not mu-1 or delta opioid antagonists reduces sucrose intake in sham-feeding rats by shifting effective sucrose concentrations to the right and producing delayed effects (44). In contrast, maltose dextrin intake was reduced by only mu antagonists in real-feeding rats and by kappa and delta-1 antagonists in sham-feeding rats, whereas only delta antagonists reduced saccharin intake in real-feeding rats (45, 46).

20.2.1.3 Central Sites of Action of General and Specific Opioid Antagonists

Naltrexone reduces intake of both preferred and nonpreferred diets following administration into the hypothalamic paraventricular nucleus, but selectively reduces preferred diet intake following administration into the central nucleus of the amygdala (47). Whereas general and mu, but not delta opioid antagonism in the nucleus accumbens shell produce modest decreases in sucrose intake (48, 49), delta-2 receptor antagonism in the ventral tegmental area marginally decrease sucrose intake (50). Accumbal, but not systemic administration of naltrexone decreases consumption of preferred flavors associated with nutritionally-identical pellets (51).

20.2.2 Molecular Role of General and Specific Opioid Antagonists

Palatable sugar solutions increase hypothalamic dynorphin protein and mRNA levels (52), and enhance naloxone's ability to increase c-fos activity in the central nucleus of the amygdala (53). However, mice lacking the preproenkephalin gene display deficits in emotional responses, but no changes in sensitivity to sucrose (54). Consumption of a palatable food (Fonzies) stimulates dopamine release in the accumbens in a mu-1 antagonist-sensitive manner, and in the medial prefrontal cortex in a mu-1 antagonist-insensitive manner (55). High fat diets increase hypothalamic mu opioid receptors (56), but reduce ventral striatal enkephalin gene expression (57).

20.3 Opioid Antagonist Effects upon Homeostatic Regulatory Challenges

20.3.1 Behavioral Role of General and Specific Opioid Antagonists

20.3.1.1 General Opioid Antagonist Effects

Following the initial observation that naloxone significantly decreased food intake in food-deprived rats (1), this inhibitory effect was observed in deprived and nondeprived rats and mice (58–62), in genetically-obese rats (63), in animals in operant paradigms (64), and across species (e.g., 65–67). Its inhibition is enhanced in both diabetic animals (68) and ovariectomized females (69). General opioid antagonists also block the ingestive following other homeostatic challenges as well, reducing sodium chloride water intake in water-deprived and in hypophysectomized rats (70–74) as well as water intake following angiotenisin II and hypertonic saline (61, 75). Naloxone potently reduces intake following glucoprivation induced by 2-deoxy-D-glucose (2DG) (76), but was less effective in reducing insulin-induced feeding (77–79).

20.3.1.2 Opioid Receptor Subtype Antagonist Effects

Ventricular administration of selective mu, mu-1, and kappa, but not delta-1 opioid antagonists reduces feeding elicited by food deprivation (40, 80–85). Further, ventricular administration of mu and kappa, but not mu-1, delta, or delta-1 antagonist reduces glucoprivic feeding elicited by either 2DG (40, 80–82, 85, 86) or insulin (87). Ventricular pretreatment with either general, mu, delta, or kappa opioid receptor antagonists also reduce lipoprivic feeding induced by the free fatty acid oxidation inhibitor, mercaptoacetate (88).

20.3.1.3 Central Sites of Action of General and Specific Opioid Antagonists

General opioid antagonism decreases food intake in deprived and nondeprived rats following direct injections into the ventromedial and lateral hypothalamic nuclei and the ventral tegmental area (89, 90), but fails to alter deprivation-induced intake in animals with ventromedial hypothalamic cuts (91). The inhibitory effects of naloxone on deprivation-induced intake persists following globus pallidus, striatal, hippocampal, or pineal lesions, and is reduced in adrenalectomized animals (92–95). Paraventricular hypothalamic naloxone injections decrease water deprivation-induced intake (96).

Deprivation-induced feeding is reduced by mu and kappa, but not delta or mu-1 opioid antagonists administered into the paraventricular hypothalamus or nucleus accumbens shell, but not the ventral tegmental area (48–50, 97). The same site-specific inhibitory pattern of effective mu and kappa antagonist effects upon 2DG-induced feeding was observed as well (48–50).

20.3.2 Molecular Role of General and Specific Opioid Antagonists

20.3.2.1 Neurochemical Changes

Acute short-term (e.g., 24–48 h) food deprivation increases paraventricular hypothalamic enkephalin levels and midbrain (3H) naloxone binding (98–101), but decreases OFQ/N and NOP receptor mRNA (102). Chronic (over 2 weeks) food restriction decreases mu opioid binding in the amygdala, parabrachial and habenula nuclei, but respectively decreases (habenula) and increases (stria terminalis, ventral pallidal, medial preoptic, and parabrachial nuclei) kappa opioid binding (103, 104). Chronic food restriction and an induced diabetic state increase dynorphin (1–17) in the dorsomedial, ventromedial, and paraventricular hypothalamus, and dynorphin (1–8) in the accumbens, stria terminalis, cortex, striatum, midbrain, and lateral hypothalamus (105–107). General, mu, and kappa antagonists in food-restricted rats increase c-fos immunoreactivity in the stria terminalis, amygdala, and accumbens (108, 109). Whereas chronic food restriction and an induced diabetic state decrease hypothalamic endorphin (110–112), the combination of food restriction with exercise increases supraoptic hypothalamic dynorphin and arcuate hypothalamic endorphin (113). General, mu, and kappa antagonism block food restriction-induced lowering of thresholds for rewarding lateral hypothalamic stimulation (114, 115). Both an induced diabetic state and food restriction increase kappa binding in the medial preoptic area and decrease mu binding in the lateral habenula (116).

20.3.2.2 Knockout and Antisense Effects

Glucoprivic feeding induced by 2DG is markedly reduced by AS probes directed against coding exons 1 and 2 of the *MOR-1* gene and coding exon 2 of the *KOR-1* gene, but is minimally affected by probes directed against coding exon 3 of either the *KOR-3/ORL-1* or the *DOR-1* genes (117). Lipoprivic feeding induced by Mercaptoacetate is markedly reduced by AS probes directed against coding exons 1, 2, or 3 of the *MOR-1* gene, coding exon 3 of the *KOR-1* gene, coding exons 1 or 2 of the *KOR-3/ORL-1* gene, and coding exon 1 of the DOR-1 gene (88). Thus, opioid AS modulation of glucoprivic and lipoprivic effects paralleled opioid antagonist actions. Like kappa and delta antagonism, an AS probe directed against exon 2 of the *KOR-1* gene decreases deprivation-induced intake, whereas AS probes directed against exon 1 of the *DOR-1* gene, and exon 1 of the *KOR-3/ORL-1* gene produce more modest effects. In contrast, AS probes directed against exons 2, 3, 4, and other extended exons of the *MOR-1* gene and its isoforms produce only modest reductions in deprivation-induced feeding, in contrast to marked mu antagonist effects (118, 119).

20.4 Opioid Antagonist Effects upon Body Weight Regulation

20.4.1 Behavioral Role of General and Specific Opioid Antagonists in Chronic and Obesity Studies

20.4.1.1 General Opioid Antagonist Effects

Whereas acute administration of long-acting general opioid antagonists like beta-chlornaltrexamine and LY255582 decrease intake and weight (120, 121), chronic administration of naloxone and naltrexone transiently decrease food intake and weight in normal rats (78, 122–124), and in rats made obese by a cafeteria diet (16, 125). Naloxone also dose-dependently and time-dependently decreases water intake over a 15-day regimen (126). General opioid antagonists such as naloxone, nalfemene, and LY255582 also decrease feeding, drinking, and weight in obese Zucker rats (127–129) as well as obese ob/ob mice (130). Yet, animals made obese by dorsolateral tegmental lesions, 5-HT neurotoxin treatment, ventromedial hypothalamic lesions, or parasagittal hypothalamic knife cuts display normal patterns of naloxone-induced anorexia (131, 132). Naloxone also potently reduces intake following glucoprivation induced by electrical stimulation of the lateral hypothalamus (133, 134) as well as increasing feeding thresholds elicited by rewarding lateral hypothalamic electrical stimulation (135). Streptozotocin-induced diabetes decreases the threshold necessary to elicit feeding following lateral hypothalamic stimulation in a naltrexone-sensitive manner (136). Naloxone also reduces stress-induced feeding induced by tail-pinch (76, 137, 138).

20.4.1.2 Opioid Receptor Subtype Antagonist Effects

Whereas acute administration of the selective mu opioid antagonist, beta-funaltrexamine, significantly reduces spontaneous food and water intake, body weight, and core body temperature over 48 h (139, 140), acute treatment with a putative functional antagonist of the ORL-1 receptor, nocistatin, inhibits food intake (141). Whereas mu opioid antagonism reduces drinking induced by water deprivation, angiotensin II and isoproterenol (41, 142, 143), mu, mu-1, delta-1, and delta-2 antagonism decrease drinking in water-deprived and sham-drinking rats (46). General and mu receptor antagonism decrease intake of dilute sodium chloride solutions (144), but none of the antagonists alter intake of either hypotonic or hypertonic saline solutions in water-deprived rats (145).

Chronic mu-1 opioid antagonism significantly decreases both food intake and body weight in adult animals and in adolescent animals undergoing dynamic weight gain (125). Chronic mu, mu-1, delta-1, and delta-2 opioid antagonists also significantly decrease weight and intake of a fat source in rats during development of dietary obesity without systematically altering chow or milk intake (146). Normal rats placed on high-energy diets that are either high in carbohydrates or fat gain more weight with the fat diet, and display greater magnitudes of weight loss following chronic mu, delta-2, or kappa-1 antagonists (147). Weight loss and intake reductions following mu, mu-1, delta-1, delta-2, or kappa-1 opioid antagonism are also observed in lean heterozygote and obese homozygote Zucker rats (148).

Mu and kappa antagonists decrease feeding elicited by lateral hypothalamic electrical stimulation (149, 150) with kappa antagonism of the parabrachial nucleus reducing its feeding, but not reinforcement effects (151, 152). Moreover, antibodies raised against dynorphin, but not endorphin increase lateral hypothalamic thresholds necessary to elicit feeding (153–156). In contrast, only mu and mu-1 antagonists reduce feeding elicited by tail-pinch stress (157, 158).

20.4.2 Molecular Role of General and Specific Opioid Antagonists in Chronic and Obesity Studies

20.4.2.1 Neurochemical Changes

Whereas beta-endorphin levels are associated with overeating in genetically obese ob/ob mice and fa/fa rats (159), they are unchanged in genetically-obese Zucker rats (160). Increased hypothalamic dynorphin is observed during nocturnal intake (161, 162) and in obese Zucker rats, whereas decreased amygdala dynorphin occurs following chronic naltrexone infusions in the nucleus tractus solitarius (163).

20.4.2.2 Knockout and Antisense Effects

Mice deficient in beta-endorphin are hyperphagic, obese, and display reduced progressive ratio operant responses for food reinforcement, yet show intact normal orexigenic responses to exogenous opioids as well as normal anorectic responses to naloxone (164, 165). The sensitivity of spontaneous control of body weight and food intake to AS ODN probes targeting coding exons 1, 2, 3, and 4 of the *MOR-1* gene suggests that the receptor responsible for these ingestive effects is completely encoded by this gene (166).

20.5 Opioid Antagonist Effects upon Pharmacologically Elicited Feeding Responses

20.5.1 Behavioral Role of General and Specific Opioid Antagonists

20.5.1.1 General Opioid Antagonist Effects

Both naloxone and naltrexone decrease intake stimulated by mu, delta, or kappa opioid agonist treatment (see reviews: 10, 12) as well as feeding induced by the ORL-1 receptor (167, 168). Naltrexone pretreatment blocks the long-term increases in intake induced by agouti gene-related peptide (169, 170) and the short-term increases in intake elicited by neuropeptide Y (171, 172), peptide YY (173), the serotonin1A receptor agent, 8-OH-DPAT (174), the alpha-2-adrenoceptor antagonist, idazoxan (175), and orexin-A, but not melanin-concentrating hormone (176).

20.5.1.2 Opioid Receptor Subtype Antagonist Effects

Selective opioid antagonists block feeding responses induced by agonists at their respective receptors. Thus, morphine-induced feeding is blocked by general and selective mu-1 opioid antagonism (177). Whereas the general delta opioid antagonist, ICI174864 decreases feeding elicited by a general delta agonist (178), delta-1 agonist-induced feeding is blocked by general and delta-2 antagonists, and delta-2 agonist-induced feeding is blocked by delta-1 and delta-2 antagonists (179). Kappa-1 antagonism eliminates feeding induced by kappa-1, but not kappa-3 opioid agonists (180, 181).

Selective opioid antagonists block feeding responses induced by agonists at other opioid receptors as well. Thus, mu opioid antagonism reduces feeding elicited by mu, delta, and kappa agonists (83), and kappa opioid antagonism reduces feeding elicited by kappa, delta, and mu agonists as well (84, 182). Beta-endorphin-induced feeding was markedly reduced by pretreatment with general, mu, and kappa opioid antagonists and minimally by delta opioid antagonism in rats (183) and goldfish (184). In contrast, dynorphin-induced feeding was most potently reduced by pretreatment by kappa opioid antagonism, and by only high doses of general and mu, but not delta opioid antagonism (185). Whereas neuropeptide Y-induced feeding is reduced by mu and kappa antagonists pretreatment (186, 187), galanin-induced feeding is reduced by mu, but not kappa opioid antagonism (188). Combined mu and kappa antagonism reduced AGRP-induced feeding (189). Mu antagonism reduced feeding elicited by the melanocortin MC3/4 receptor antagonist, SHU-9119, and the melanocortin MC3/4 receptor agonist, MTII reduced beta-endorphin-induced feeding (190).

20.5.1.3 Central Sites of Action of General and Specific Opioid Antagonists

Within-site opioid agonist–antagonist effects have been observed such that OFQ/N-induced feeding elicited from the paraventricular hypothalamus or accumbens was blocked by naloxone (167, 168, 191). General opioid antagonists in the paraventricular hypothalamus and nucleus tractus solitarius reduce NPY-induced feeding as well (192, 193). Whereas mu, but not delta-1 agonist-induced conditioned feeding elicited from the nucleus accumbens is blocked by naltrexone (194), mu and delta-1 agonists in the accumbens elicited feeding that is blocked by mu, delta-1, delta-2, and kappa-1 opioid antagonists. In contrast, delta-2 agonist-induced feeding elicited from the accumbens is largely unaffected by delta-2 antagonism, and actually enhanced by mu and kappa antagonists (195). Mu agonist-induced feeding in the ventral tegmental area is reduced by general, mu, and kappa-1, but not delta antagonists (196). Whereas naltrexone blocked feeding elicited by GABA-A but not GABA-B agonists in the accumbens (197), it blocked feeding elicited by GABA-B but not GABA-A agonists in the ventral tegmental area (198). Such differential general opioid antagonist effects appear to be due to differential involvement of opioid receptor subtypes. Thus, muscimol-induced feeding elicited from the ventral tegmental area is differentially enhanced (mu or delta) and reduced (kappa) by opioid antagonists, whereas baclofen-induced feeding elicited from the ventral tegmental area is significantly reduced by mu or kappa, but not delta antagonists. Further, muscimol-induced feeding elicited from the accumbens is reduced by all three antagonist subtypes, whereas baclofen-induced feeding elicited from the accumbens was significantly reduced by either kappa or delta, but not mu antagonists (199).

Between-site regional opioid–opioid and other agonist–antagonist interactions have been observed as well. Thus, general, mu, and kappa antagonists in the ventral tegmental area block mu agonist-induced feeding elicited from the accumbens, whereas general, mu, delta, and, to a lesser degree, kappa antagonists in the accumbens block mu agonist-induced feeding elicited from the ventral tegmental area (200, 201). Other bidirectional opioid–opioid signaling pathways between the ventral tegmental area and paraventricular hypothalamus, and between the nucleus tractus solitarius and the central nucleus of the amygdala have been demonstrated using the same mu agonist–general antagonist approach (202, 203). One unidirectional opioid–opioid interaction was identified such that mu agonist-induced feeding elicited from the central nucleus of the amygdala is blocked by naltrexone pretreatment in the paraventricular hypothalamus (204).

20.5.2 Molecular Role of General and Specific Opioid Antagonists

Whereas AS probes targeted against coding exons 1 and 4, but not coding exons 2 and 3 of the *MOR-1* gene reduce feeding induced by morphine and the selective mu agonist, DAMGO, feeding elicited by the morphine metabolite, M6G was blocked by AS probes targeted against either coding exons 2 and 3, but not coding exons 1 or 4 of the *MOR-1* gene (205, 206). Importantly, missense probes were ineffective. These data indicate that different isoforms of the *MOR-1* gene mediate different aspects of feeding elicited by activation of the mu opioid receptor. Receptor-selective effects have been observed as well with AS probes directed against the *DOR-1* gene reducing delta-2 agonist-induced feeding, AS probes directed against the *KOR-1* gene reducing kappa agonist-induced feeding, and AS probes directed against the *KOR-3/ORL-1* gene reducing feeding elicited by OFQ/N, but not M6G (205, 207). Beta-endorphin-induced feeding is blocked by AS probes directed against coding exons 1, 3, or 4 of the *MOR-1*, but not *KOR-1, KOR-3/ORL-1* or *DOR-1* genes (183). In contrast, AS probes directed against coding exons 1 and 2 of either the *KOR-1* or *KOR-3/ORL-1* opioid receptor genes reduce dynorphin-induced feeding (185). Therefore, the pharmacological profile using general and selective opioid antagonists, and the molecular profile using AS probes directed against particular exons of the opioid receptor genes provide converging and complementary evidence in establishing which opioid receptor subtypes participate in feeding responses elicited by endogenous opioid peptides, and the molecular approach extends the pharmacological approach in establishing the underlying mechanisms of action of opiate drugs and opioid peptide agonists.

20.6 Conclusions

As indicated in this chapter, the use of general and selective opioid receptor subtype antagonists has clearly demonstrated the role of the endogenous opioid system in virtually every facet of ingestive behavior from modulating the hedonic responses to palatable macronutrient sources (e.g., sugars and fats), through regulating major homeostatic challenges to the organism (e.g., deprivation, glucoprivation, and lipoprivation), through controlling intake in spontaneous food intake and body weight regulation in normal-weight as well as genetic and dietary obesity, and finally through modulating the ingestive responses elicited by major orexigenic systems in the brain. The use of molecular knock-out and knock-down approaches to regulating opioid receptors provide complementary and converging evidence for the aforementioned antagonist effects. Such pervasive effects of opioid antagonists on the different aspects of feeding behavior make the development of more selective antagonists attractive target systems for the treatment of obesity and diabetes and intake of macronutrients associated with these important dysfunctions.

References

1. Pert, C.B., Snyder, S.H. Opiate receptor: demonstration in nervous tissue. Science 1973;179: 1011–1014.
2. Simon, E.J., Hiller, J.M., Edelman, I. Stereospecific binding of the potent narcotic analgesic (3H)etorphine to rat brain homogenate. Proc. Natl. Acad. Sci. (USA) 1973;70:1947–1949.
3. Terenius, L. Stereospecific interaction between narcotic analgesia and a synaptic plasma membrane fraction of rat cerebral cortex. Acta Pharmacol. Toxicol. 1973;32:317–320.
4. Holtzman, S.G. Behavioral effects of separate and combined administration of naloxone and d-amphetamine. J. Pharmacol. Exp. Ther. 1974;189:51–60.
5. Grandison, L., Guidotti, A. Stimulation of food intake by muscimol and beta-endorphin. Neuropharmacology 1977;16:533–536.
6. Tepperman, F.S., Hirst, M. Effects of intrahypothalamic injection of D-Ala-2, D-Leu-5-enkephalin on feeding and temperature in the rat. Eur. J. Pharmacol. 1983;96:243–249.
7. McLean, S., Hoebel, B.G. Feeding induced by opiates injected into the paraventricular hypothalamus. Peptides 1983;4:287–292.
8. Morley, J.E., Levine, A.S. Dynorphin (1–13) induces spontaneous feeding in rats. Life Sci. 1981;29:1901–1903.
9. Walker, J.M., Katz, R.J., Akil, H. Behavioral effects of dynorphin (1–13) in the mouse and rat: initial observations. Peptides 1980;1:341–345.
10. Morley, J.E., Levine, A.S., Yim, G.K.W., Lowy, M.T. Opioid modulation of appetite. Neurosci. Biobehav. Rev. 1983;7:281–305.
11. Glass, M.J., Billington, C.J., Levine, A.S. Opioids and food intake: distributed functional neural pathways? Neuropeptides 1999;33:360–368.
12. Levine, A.S., Morley, J.E., Gosnell, B.A., Billington, C.J., Bartness, T.J. Opioids and consummatory behavior. Brain Res. Bull. 1985;14:663–672.
13. Cooper, S.J., Jackson, A., Kirkham, T.C., Turkish, S. Endorphins, opiates and food intake. Rodgers, R.J., Cooper, S.J., eds. Endorphins, opiates and behavioral processes. New York: John Wiley and Sons 1988:143–186.
14. Kelley, A.E. Neural integrative activities of nucleus accumbens subregions in relation to learning and motivation. Psychobiology 1999;27:198–213.
15. Kelley, A.E., Bakshi, V.P., Haber, S.N., Steininger, T.L., Will, M.J., Zhang, M. Opioid modulation of taste hedonics within the ventral striatum. Physiol. Behav. 2002;76:365–377.
16. Apfelbaum, M., Mandenoff, A. Naltrexone suppresses hyperphagia induced in the rat by a highly palatable diet. Pharmacol. Biochem. Behav. 1981;15:89–91.
17. Lynch, W.C., Libby, L. Naloxone suppresses intake of highly preferred saccharin solutions in food deprived and sated rats. Life Sci. 1983;33:1909–1914.

18. Cooper, S.J. Effects of opiate agonists and antagonists on fluid intake and saccharin choice in the rat. Neuropharmacology 1983;22:323–328.
19. Levine, A.S., Murray, S.S., Kneip, J., Grace, M., Morley, J.E. Flavor enhances the antidipsogenic effect of naloxone. Physiol. Behav. 1982;28:23–25.
20. Shide, D.J., Blass, E.M. Opioid mediation of odor preferences induced by sugar and fat in 6-day-old rats. Physiol. Behav. 1991;50:961–966.
21. Shabir, S., Kirkham, T.C. Diet-induced enhancement of naloxone sensitivity is independent of changes in body weight. Pharmacol. Biochem. Behav. 1999;62:601–605.
22. Glass, M.J., Grace, M.K., Cleary, J.P., Billington, C.J., Levine, A.S. Naloxone's effect on meal microstructure of sucrose and cornstarch diets. Am. J. Physiol. 2001;281:R1605–R16012.
23. Kirkham, T.C., Blundell, J.E. Dual action of naloxone on feeding revealed by behavioral analysis: separate effects on initiation and termination of eating. Appetite 1984;5:45–52.
24. Clarkson, D.B., King, B.M., Hemmer, R.C., Olson, G.A., Kastin, A.J., Olson, R.D. Naloxone decreases consumption of liquid and solid sucrose in vagotomized rats. Physiol. Behav. 1982; 29:927–930.
25. Kirkham, T.C., Cooper, S.J. Naloxone attenuation of sham feeding is modified by manipulation of sucrose concentration. Physiol. Behav. 1988;44:491–494.
26. Rockwood, G.A., Reid, L.D. Naloxone modifies sugar-water intake in rats drinking with open gastric fistulas. Physiol. Behav. 1982;29:1175–1178.
27. Levine, A.S., Weldon, D.T., Grace, M., Cleary, J.P., Billington, C.J. Naloxone blocks that portion of feeding driven by sweet taste in food-restricted rats. Am. J. Physiol. 1995;268: R248–R252.
28. Parker, L.A., Maier, S., Rennie, M., Crebolder, J. Morphine- and naltrexone-induced modification of palatability: analysis by the taste reactivity test. Behav. Neurosci. 1992;106: 999–1010.
29. Glass, M.J., Grace, M., Cleary, J.P., Billington, C.J., Levine, A.S. Potency of naloxone's anorectic effect in rats is dependent on diet preference. Am. J. Physiol. 1996;271:R217–R221.
30. Weldon, D.T., O'Hare, E., Cleary, J., Billington, C.J., Levine, A.S. Effect of naloxone on intake of cornstarch, sucrose and polycose diets in restricted and nonrestricted rats. Am. J. Physiol. 1996;270:R1183–R1188.
31. Dym, C.T., Pinhas, A., Ginzberg, M., Kest, B., Bodnar, R.J. Genetic variance contributes to naltrexone-induced inhibition of sucrose intake in inbred and outbred mouse strains. Brain Res. 2007;1135:136–145.
32. Yu, W.-Z., Sclafani, A., Delamater, A.R., Bodnar, R.J. Pharmacology of flavor preference conditioning in sham-feeding rats: effects of naltrexone. Pharmacol. Biochem. Behav. 1999;64: 573–584.
33. Baker R.M., Li Y., Lee M., Sclafani A., Bodnar R.J. Naltrexone does not prevent acquisition or expression of flavor preferences conditioned by fructose in rats. Pharmacol. Biochem. Behav. 2004;78:239–246.
34. Azzara, A.V., Bodnar, R.J., Delamater, A.R., Sclafani, A. Naltrexone fails to block the acquisition or expression of a flavor preference conditioned by intragastric carbohydrate infusions. Pharmacol. Biochem. Behav. 2000;67:545–557.
35. Delamater, A.R., Sclafani, A., Bodnar, R.J. Pharmacology of sucrose-reinforced place preference conditioning: effects of naltrexone. Pharmacol. Biochem. Behav. 2000;65:697–704.
36. Levine, A.S., Grace, M.K., Cleary, J.P., Billington, C.J. Naltrexone infusion inhibits the development of preference for a high-sucrose diet. Am. J. Physiol. 2002;283(5):R1149–R1154.
37. Marks-Kaufman, R., Kanarek, R. Modifications of nutrient selection by naloxone in rats. Psychopharmacology 1981;74:321–324.
38. Marks-Kaufman, R., Plager, A., Kanarek, R. Central and peripheral contributions of endogenous opioid systems to nutrient selection in rats. Psychopharmacology 1985;85:414–418.
39. Higgs, S., Cooper, S.J. Evidence for early opioid modulation of licking responses to sucrose and intralipid: a microstructural analysis in the rat. Psychopharmacology 1998;139:342–355.
40. Arjune, D., Bodnar, R.J. Suppression of nocturnal, palatable and glucoprivic intake in rats by the kappa opioid antagonist, nor-binaltorphamine. Brain Res. 1990;534:313–316.

41. Beczkowska, I.W., Bowen, W.D., Bodnar, R.J. Central opioid receptor subtype antagonists differentially alter sucrose and deprivation-induced water intake in rats. Brain Res. 1992;589: 291–301.
42. Calcagnetti, D.J., Calcagnetti, R.L., Fanselow, M.S. Centrally administered opioid antagonists, nor-binaltorphamine, 16-methyl cyrenorphine and MR2266 suppress intake of a sweet solution. Pharmacol. Biochem. Behav. 1990;35:69–73.
43. Islam, A.K., Bodnar, R.J. Selective opioid receptor antagonist effects upon intake of a high-fat diet in rats. Brain Res. 1990;508:293–296.
44. Leventhal, L., Kirkham, T.C., Cole, J.L., Bodnar, R.J. Selective actions of central mu and kappa opioid antagonists upon sucrose intake in sham-feeding rats. Brain Res. 1995;685: 205–210.
45. Beczkowska, I.W., Koch, J.E., Bostock, M.E., Leibowitz, S.F., Bodnar, R.J. Central opioid receptor subtype antagonists differentially reduce intake of saccharin and maltose dextrin solutions in rats. Brain Res. 1993;618:261–270.
46. Leventhal, L., Bodnar, R.J. Different central opioid receptor subtype antagonists modify maltose dextrin and deprivation-induced water intake in sham feeding and sham drinking rats. Brain Res. 1996;741:300–308.
47. Glass, M.J., Billington, C.J., Levine, A.S. Naltrexone administered to central nucleus of amygdala or PVN: neural dissociation of diet and energy. Am. J. Physiol. 2000;279:86–92.
48. Bodnar, R.J., Glass, M.J., Ragnauth, A., Cooper, M.L. General, mu and kappa opioid antagonists in the nucleus accumbens alter food intake under deprivation, glucoprivic and palatable conditions. Brain Res. 1995;700:205–212.
49. Kelley, A.E., Bless, E.P., Swanson, C.J. Investigation of the effects of opiate antagonists infused into the nucleus accumbens on feeding and sucrose drinking in rats. J. Pharmacol. Exp. Ther. 1996;278:1499–1507.
50. Ragnauth, A., Ruegg, H., Bodnar, R.J. Evaluation of opioid receptor subtype antagonist effects in the ventral tegmental area upon food intake under deprivation, glucoprivic and palatable conditions. Brain Res. 1997;767:8–16.
51. Woolley, J.D., Lee, B.S., Fields, H.L. Nucleus accumbens opioids regulate flavor-based preferences in food consumption. Neuroscience 2006;143:309–317.
52. Welch, C.C., Kim, E.-M., Grace, M.K., Billington, C.J., Levine, A.S. Palatability-induced hyperphagia increases hypothalamic dynorphin peptide and mRNA levels. Brain Res. 1996; 721:126–131.
53. Pomonis, J.D., Jewett, D.C., Kotz, C.M., Briggs, J.E., Billington, C.J., Levine, A.S. Sucrose consumption increases naloxone-induced c-fos immunoreactivity in limbic forebrain. Am. J. Physiol. 2000;278:R712–R719.
54. Ragnauth, A., Schuller, A., Morgan, M., Chan, J., Ogawa, S., Pintar, J., Bodnar, R.J., Pfaff, D.W. Female preproenkephalin-knockout mice display altered emotional responses. Proc. Natl. Acad. Sci. (USA) 2001;98:1958–1963.
55. Tanda, G., DiChiara, G. A dopamine-mu1 opioid link in the rat ventral tegmentum shared by palatable food (Fonzies) and the non-psychostimulant drugs of abuse. Eur. J. Neurosci. 1998; 10:1179–1187.
56. Barnes, M.J., Lapanowski, K., Conley, A., Rafols, J.A., Jen, K.L., Dunbar, J.C. High fat feeding is associated with increased blood pressure, sympathetic nerve activity and hypothalamic mu opioid receptors. Brain Res. Bull. 2003;61:511–519.
57. Kelley, A.E., Will, M.J., Steininger, T.L., Zhang, M., Haber, S.N. Restricted daily consumption of a highly palatable food (chocolate Ensure(R)) alters striatal enkepahlin gene expression. Eur. J. Neurosci. 2003;18:2592–2598.
58. Brown, D.R., Holtzman, S.J. Suppression of deprivation induced food and water intake in rats and mice by naloxone. Pharmacol. Biochem. Behav. 1979;11:567–583.
59. Cooper, S.J. Naloxone: effects on food and water consumption in the non-deprived and deprived rat. Psychopharmacology 1980;71:1–6.
60. Frenk, H., Rogers, G.H. The suppressant effects of naloxone on food and water intake in the rat. Behav. Neural. Biol. 1979;26:23–40.

61. Holtzman, S.G. Effects of narcotic antagonists on fluid intake in the rat. Life Sci. 1975;16: 1465–1470.
62. Maickel, R.P., Braude, M.C., Zabik, J.E. The effects of various narcotic agonists and antagonists on deprivation-induced fluid consumption. Neuropharmacology 1977;16:863–866.
63. Glass, M.J., O'Hare, E., Cleary, J.P., Billington, C.J., Levine, A.S. The effect of naloxone on food-motivated behavior in the obese Zucker rat. Psychopharmacology 1999;141:378–384.
64. Rudski, J.M., Billington, C.J., Levine, A.S. Naloxone's effects on operant responding depend upon level of deprivation. Pharmacol. Biochem. Behav. 1994;49:377–383.
65. Billington, C.J., Morley, J.E., Levine, A.S., Wright, F., Seal, U.S. Naloxone induced suppression of feeding in tigers. Physiol. Behav. 1985;34:641–643.
66. Morley, J.E., Levine, A.S., Plotka, E.D., Seal, U.S. The effect of naloxone on feeding and spontaneous locomotion in the wolf. Physiol. Behav. 1983;30:331–334.
67. Nizielski, S.E., Morley, J.E., Gosnell, B.A., Seal, U.S., Levine, A.S. Opioid modulation of ingestive behaviors in woodchucks and raccoons. Physiol. Behav. 1985;34:171–176.
68. Levine, A.S., Morley, J.E., Brown, D.M., Handwerger, B.S. Extreme sensitivity of diabetic mice to naloxone-induced suppression of food intake. Physiol. Behav. 1982;28:987–989.
69. Morley, J.E., Levine, A.S., Grace, M., Kneip, J., Gosnell, B.A. The effect of ovariectomy, estradiol and progesterone on opioid modulation of feeding. Physiol. Behav. 1984;33:237–241.
70. Brown, D.R., Blank, M.S., Holtzman, S.G. Suppression by naloxone of water intake induced by deprivation and hypertonic saline in intact and hypophysectomized rats. Life Sci. 1980;26:1535–1542.
71. Brown, D.R., Holtzman, S.G. Evidence that opiate receptors mediate suppression of hypertonic saline-induced drinking in the mouse by narcotic antagonists. Life Sci. 1980;26: 1543–1550.
72. Cooper, S.J., Gilbert, D.B. Naloxone suppresses fluid consumption in tests of choice between sodium chloride solutions and water in male and female water-deprived rats. Psychopharmacology 1984;84:362–367.
73. Czech, D.A., Stein, E.A. Naloxone suppresses osmoregulatory drinking in rats. Pharmacol. Biochem. Behav. 1980;12:987–989.
74. Siviy, S.M., Bermudez-Rattoni, F., Rockwood, G.A., Dargie, C.M., Reid, L.D. Intracerebral administration of naloxone and drinking in water-deprived rats. Pharmacol. Biochem. Behav. 1981;15:257–262.
75. Rowland, N. Comparison of the suppression by naloxone of water intake induced in rats by hyperosmolarity, hypovolemia and angiotensin. Pharmacol. Biochem. Behav. 1982;16:87–91.
76. Lowy, M.T., Maickel, R.P., Yim, G.K.W. Naloxone reduction of stress-related feeding. Life Sci. 1980;26:2113–2118.
77. Levine, A.S., Morley, J.E. Peptidergic control of insulin-induced feeding. Peptides 1981;2: 261–264.
78. Ostrowski, N.L., Rowland, N., Foley, T.L., Nelson, J.L., Reid, L.D. Morphine antagonists and consummatory behaviors. Pharmacol. Biochem. Behav. 1981;14:549–559.
79. Rowland, N., Bartness, T.J. Naloxone suppresses insulin-induced food intake in novel and familiar environments, but does not affect hypoglycemia. Pharmacol. Biochem. Behav. 1982; 16:1001–1003.
80. Arjune, D., Bowen, W.D., Bodnar, R.J. Ingestive behavior following central (D-Ala2,Leu5, Cys6)-enkephalin (DALCE), a short-acting agonist and long-acting antagonist at the delta opioid receptor. Pharmacol. Biochem. Behav. 1991;39:429–436.
81. Arjune, D., Standifer, K.M., Pasternak, G.W., Bodnar, R.J. Reduction by central beta-funaltrexamine of food intake in rats under freely-feeding, deprivation and glucoprivic conditions. Brain Res. 1990;535:101–109.
82. Koch, J.E., Bodnar, R.J. Selective alterations in macronutrient intake of food-deprived or glucoprivic rats by centrally-administered opioid receptor subtype antagonists in rats. Brain Res. 1994;657:191–201.
83. Levine, A.S., Grace, M., Billington, C.J. B-funaltrexamine (B-FNA) decreases deprivation and opioid-induced feeding. Brain Res. 1991;562:281–284.

84. Levine, A.S., Grace, M., Billington, C.J., Portoghese, P.S. Nor-binaltorphamine decreases deprivation and opioid-induced feeding. Brain Res. 1990;534:60–64.
85. Simone, D.A., Bodnar, R.J., Goldman, E.J., Pasternak, G.W. Involvement of opioid receptor subtypes in rat feeding behavior. Life Sci. 1985;36:829–833.
86. Jackson, H.C., Sewell, R.D.E. Hyperphagia induced by 2-deoxy-D-glucose in the presence of the delta-opioid antagonist, ICI174864. Neuropharmacology 1985;24:815–817.
87. Beczkowska, I.W., Bodnar, R.J. Mediation of insulin hyperphagia by specific central opiate receptor antagonists. Brain Res. 1991;547:315–318.
88. Stein, J.A., Znamensky, V., Baumer, F., Rossi, G.C., Pasternak, G.W., Bodnar, R.J. Mercaptoacetate induces feeding through central opioid-mediated mechanisms in rats. Brain Res. 2000;864: 240–251.
89. Segall, M.A., Margules, D.L. Central mediation of naloxone-induced anorexia in the ventral tegmental area. Behav. Neurosci. 1989;103:857–864.
90. Thornhill, J.A., Saunders, W. Ventromedial and lateral hypothalamic injections of naloxone or naltrexone suppress the acute food intake of food-deprived rats. Appetite 1984;5:25–30.
91. Gosnell, B.A., Romsos, D.R., Morley, J.E., Levine, A.S. Opiates and medial hypothalamic knife cuts cause hyperphagia through different mechanisms. Behav. Neurosci. 1985;99:1181–1191.
92. Gosnell, B.A., Morley, J.E., Levine, A.S. Lesions of the globus pallidus and striatum attenuate ketocyclazocine-induced feeding. Physiol. Behav. 1984;33:349–355.
93. Gosnell, B.A., Morley, J.E., Levine, A.S., Kneip, J., Frick, M., Elde, R.P. Opiate induced feeding is not dependent on the hippocampus. Physiol. Behav. 1984;33:27–30.
94. Gosnell, B.A., Waggoner, D.W., Morley, J.E., Levine, A.S. The pineal gland and opiate-induced feeding. Physiol. Behav. 1985;34:1–6.
95. Levine, A.S., Morley, J.E. Adrenal modulation of opiate induced feeding. Pharmacol. Biochem. Behav. 1983;19:403–406.
96. Ukai, M., Holtzman, S.G. Suppression of deprivation-induced water intake by opioid antagonists: central sites of action. Psychopharmacology 1987;91:279–284.
97. Koch, J.E., Glass, M.J., Cooper, M.L., Bodnar, R.J. Alterations in deprivation, glucoprivic and sucrose intake following general, mu and kappa opioid antagonists in the hypothalamic paraventricular nucleus of rats. Neuroscience 1995;66:951–957.
98. Majeed, N.H., Lason, W., Przewlocka, B., Przewlocki, R. Brain and peripheral opioid peptides after changes in ingestive behavior. Neuroendocrinology 1986;42:267–272.
99. Takahashi, H., Motomatsu, T., Nawata, H., Kato, K., Ibayashi, H., Nobunaga, M. Influences of feeding and drinking on circadian rhythms of opioid peptides in plasma, hypothalamus and pituitary gland in rats. Physiol. Behav. 1986;37:609–614.
100. Tsujii, S., Nakai, Y., Fukata, J., Koh, T., Takahashi, H., Usui, T., Imura, H. Effects of food deprivation and high fat diet on opioid receptor binding in rat brain. Neurosci. Lett. 1986;72:169–173.
101. Vaswani, K.K., Tejwani, G.A. Food-deprivation-induced changes in the level of opioid peptides in the pituitary and brain. Life Sci. 1986;38:197–201.
102. Rodi, D., Polidori, C., Bregola, G., Zucchini, S., Simonato, M., Massi, M. Pro-nociceptin/orphanin FQ and NOP receptor mRNA levels in the forebrain of food deprived rats. Brain Res. 2002;957(2):354–361.
103. Wolinsky, T.D., Carr, K.D., Hiller, J.M., Simon, E.J. Effects of chronic food restriction on mu and kappa opioid binding in rat forebrain: a quantitative autoradiographic study. Brain Res. 1994;656:274–280.
104. Wolinsky, T.D., Carr, K.D., Hiller, J.M., Simon, E.J. Chronic food restriction alters mu and kappa opioid receptor binding in the parabrachial nucleus of the rat: a quantitative autoradiographic study. Brain Res. 1996;706:333–336.
105. Berman, Y., Devi, L., Carr, K.D. Effects of chronic food restriction on prodynorphin-derived peptides in rat brain regions. Brain Res. 1994;664:49–53.
106. Berman, Y., Devi, L., Carr, K.D. Effects of streptozotocin-induced diabetes on prodynorphin-derived peptides in rat brain regions. Brain Res. 1995;685:129–134.

107. Berman, Y., Devi, L., Spangler, R., Kreek, M.J., Carr, K.D. Chronic food restriction and streptozotocin-induced diabetes differentially alter prodynorphin mRNA levels in rat brain regions. Mol. Brain Res. 1997;46:25–30.
108. Carr, K.D., Kutchukhidze, N., Park, T.H. Differential effects of mu and kappa opioid antagonists on Fos-like immunoreactivity in extended amygdala. Brain Res. 1999;822:34–42.
109. Carr, K.D., Park, T.H., Stone, E.A. Neuroanatomical patterns of Fos-like immunoreactivity induced by naltrexone in food-restricted and ad libitum fed rats. Brain Res. 1998;779: 26–32.
110. Kim, E.-M., Grace, M.K., Welch, C.C., Billington, C.J., Levine, A.S. STZ-induced diabetes decreases and insulin normalizes POMC mRNA in arcuate nucleus and pituitary in rats. Am. J. Physiol. 1999;276:R1320–R1326.
111. Kim, E.-M., Welch, C.C., Grace, M.K., Billington, C.J., Levine, A.S. Chronic food restriction and acute food deprivation decrease mRNA levels of opioid peptides in the arcuate nucleus. Am. J. Physiol. 1996;270:R1019–R1024.
112. Locatelli, V., Petraglia, F., Tirloni, N., Muller, E.E. Beta-endorphin concentrations in the hypothalamus, pituitary and plasma of streptozotocin-diabetic rats with and without insulin substitution therapy. Life Sci. 1986;38:379–386.
113. Aravich, P.F., Rieg, T.S., Lauterio, T.J., Doerries, L.E. Beta-endorphin and dynorphin abnormalities in rats subjected to exercise and restricted feeding: relationship to anorexia nervosa? Brain Res. 1993;622:1–8.
114. Carr, K.D., Papadouka, V. The role of multiple opioid receptors in the potentiation of reward by food restriction. Brain Res. 1994;639:253–260.
115. Carr, K.D., Simon, E.J. Potentiation of reward by hunger is opioid mediated. Brain Res. 1984;297:369–373.
116. Wolinsky, T.D., Abrahamsen, G.C., Carr, K.D. Diabetes alters mu and kappa opioid binding in rat brain: comparison with effects of food restriction. Brain Res. 1996;738:167–171.
117. Burdick, K., Yu, W.-Z., Ragnauth, A., Moroz, M., Pan, Y.X., Rossi, G.C., Pasternak, G.W., Bodnar, R.J. Antisense mapping of opioid receptor clones: effects upon 2-deoxy-D-glucose-induced hyperphagia. Brain Res. 1998;794:359–363.
118. Hadjimarkou, M.M., Khaimova, E., Pan, Y.-X., Rossi, G.C., Pasternak, G.W., Bodnar, R.J. Feeding induced by food deprivation is differentially reduced by opioid receptor antisense oligodeoxynucleotide probes in rats. Brain Res. 2003;987:223–232.
119. Hadjimarkou, M.M., Singh, A., Kandov, Y., Israel, Y., Pan, Y.-X., Rossi, G.C., Pasternak, G.W., Bodnar, R.J. Opioid receptor involvement in food deprivation-induced feeding: evaluation of selective antagonist and antisense oligodeoxynucleotides probe effects in mice and rats. J. Pharmacol. Exp. Ther. 2004;311:1188–1202.
120. Gosnell, B.A., Grace, M., Levine, A.S. Effects of beta-chlornaltrexamine on food intake, body weight and opioid-induced feeding. Life Sci. 1987;40:1459–1467.
121. Levine, A.S., Grace, M., Billington, C.J., Zimmerman, D.M. Central administration of the opioid antagonist LY255582 decreases short- and long-term food intake in rats. Brain Res. 1991;566:193–197.
122. Brands, B.J., Thornhill, J.A., Hirst, M., Gowdey, C.W. Suppression of food intake and body weight by naloxone in rats. Life Sci. 1979;24:1773–1778.
123. Marks-Kaufman, R., Balmagiya, T., Gross, E. Modifications in food intake and energy metabolism in rats as a function of chronic naltrexone infusions. Pharmacol. Biochem. Behav. 1984;20:911–916.
124. Shimomura, Y., Oku, J., Glick, Z., Bray, G.A. Opiate receptors, food intake and obesity. Physiol. Behav. 1982;28:441–445.
125. Mann, P.E., Pasternak, G.W., Hahn, E.F., Curreri, G., Lubin, E., Bodnar, R.J. Comparison of chronic naloxone and naloxonazine effects upon food intake and body weight maintainance in rats. Neuropharmacology 1988;27:349–355.
126. Olson, G.A., DeLatte, S.W., Kastin, A.J., McLean, J.H., Phillpott, D.F., Olson, R.D. Naloxone and fluid consumption in rats: dose-response relationship for 15 days. Pharmacol. Biochem. Behav. 1985;23:1065–1068.

127. McLaughlin, C.L., Baile, C.A. Nalmefene decreases meal size, food and water intake and weight gain in Zucker rats. Pharmacol. Biochem. Behav. 1983;19:235–240.
128. McLaughlin, C.L., Baile, C.A. Feeding behavior responses of Zucker rats to naloxone. Physiol. Behav. 1984;32:755–761.
129. Shaw, W.N., Mitch, C.H., Leander, J.D., Zimmerman, D.M. Effect of phenylpiperidine opioid antagonists on food consumption and weight gain of the obese Zucker rat. J. Pharmacol. Exp. Ther. 1990;253:85–89.
130. Recant, L., Voyles, N.R., Luciano, M., Pert, C.B. Naltrexone reduced weight gain, alters beta-endorphin and reduces insulin output from pancreatic islets of genetically obese mice. Peptides 1980;1:309–313.
131. Gunion, M.W., Peters, R.H. Pituitary beta-endorphin, naloxone and feeding in several experimental obesities. Am. J. Physiol. 1981;241:R173–R184.
132. King, B.M., Castellanos, F.X., Kastin, A.J., Berzas, M., Mauk, D., Olson, G.A., Olson, R.D. Naloxone-induced suppression of food intake in normal and hypothalamic obese rats. Pharmacol. Biochem. Behav. 1979;11:729–732.
133. Carr, K.D., Simon, E.J. Effects of naloxone and its quatenary analogue on stimulation-induced feeding. Neuropharmacology 1983;22:127–130.
134. Jenck, F., Gratton, A., Wise, R.A. Opioid receptor subtypes associated with ventral tegmental facilitation and periaqueductal gray inhibition of feeding. Brain Res. 1986;423:39–44.
135. Carr, K.D., Wolinsky, T.D. Regulation of feeding by multiple opioid receptors in cingulate cortex; follow-up to an in vivo autoradiographic study. Neuropeptides 1994;26:207–213.
136. Carr, K.D. Streptozotocin-induced diabetes produces a naltrexone-reversible lowering of threshold for lateral hypothalamic self-stimulation. Brain Res. 1994;664:211–214.
137. Bertiere, M.C., Mame Sy, T., Baigts, F., Mandenoff, A., Apfelbaum, M. Stress and sucrose hyperphagia: role of endogenous opiates. Pharmacol. Biochem. Behav. 1984;20:675–679.
138. Morley, J.E., Levine, A.S. Stress-induced eating is mediated through endogenous opiates. Science 1980;209:1259–1261.
139. Millan, M.J., Morris, B.J. Long-term blockade of mu-opioid receptors suggests a role in control of ingestive behavior, body weight and core temperature in the rat. Brain Res. 1988; 450:247–258.
140. Ukai, M., Holtzman, S.G. Effects of beta-funaltrexamine on ingestive behaviors in the rat. Eur. J. Pharmacol. 1988;153:161–165.
141. Olszewski, P.K., Shaw, T.J., Grace, M.K., Billington, C.J., Levine, A.S. Nocistatin inhibits food intake in rats. Brain Res. 2000;872:181–187.
142. Glass, M.J., Hahn, B., Joseph, A., Bodnar, R.J. Central opioid receptor subtype mediation of isoproterenol-induced drinking in rats. Brain Res. 1994;657:310–314.
143. Ruegg, H., Hahn, B., Koch, J.E., Bodnar, R.J. Differential modulation of angiotensin II and hypertonic saline-induced drinking by opioid receptor subtype antagonists in rats. Brain Res. 1994;635:203–210.
144. Gosnell, B.A., Majchrzak, M.J. Effects of a selective mu opioid receptor agonist and naloxone on the intake of sodium chloride solutions. Psychopharmacology 1990;100:66–71.
145. Bodnar, R.J., Glass, M.J., Koch, J.E. Analysis of central opioid receptor subtype antagonism of hypotonic and hypertonic saline intake in water-deprived rats. Brain Res. Bull. 1995; 36:293–300.
146. Cole, J.L., Leventhal, L., Pasternak, G.W., Bowen, W.D., Bodnar, R.J. Reductions in body weight following chronic central opioid receptor subtype antagonists during development of dietary obesity in rats. Brain Res. 1995;678:168–176.
147. Cole, J.L., Ross, A., Bodnar, R.J. Dietary history affects the potency of chronic opioid receptor subtype antagonist effects upon body weight in rats. Nutr. Neurosci. 1999;1:405–418.
148. Cole, J.L., Berman, N., Bodnar, R.J. Evaluation of chronic opioid receptor antagonist effects upon weight and intake measures in lean and obese Zucker rats. Peptides 1997;18:1201–1207.
149. Carr, K.D., Bak, T.H., Simon, E.J., Portoghese, P.S. Effects of the selective K opioid antagonist, nor-binaltorphamine, on electrically-elicited feeding in the rat. Life Sci. 1989;45: 1787–1792.

150. Papadouka, V., Carr, K.D. The role of multiple opioid receptors in the maintenance of stimulation-induced feeding. Brain Res. 1994;639:42–48.
151. Carr, K.D., Aleman, D.O., Bak, T.H., Simon, E.J. Effects of parabrachial opioid antagonism on stimulation-induced feeding. Brain Res. 1991;545:283–286.
152. Carr, K.D., Papadouka, V., Wolinsky, T.D. Norbinaltorphamine blocks the feeding but not the reinforcing effect of lateral hypothalamic electrical stimulation. Psychopharmacology 1993;111:345–350.
153. Carr, K.D. Effects of antibodies to dynorphin A and beta-endorphin on lateral hypothalamic self-stimulation in ad libitum fed and food-deprived rats. Brain Res. 1990;534:8–14.
154. Carr, K.D., Bak, T.H. Rostral and caudal ventricular infusion of antibodies to dynorphin A (1–17) and dynorphin A (1–8): effects on electrically-elicited feeding in the rat. Brain Res. 1990;507:289–294.
155. Carr, K.D., Bak, T.H., Gioannini, T.L., Simon, E.J. Antibodies to dynorphin A(1–13) but not beta-endorphin inhibit electrically-elicited feeding in the rat. Brain Res. 1987;422: 384–388.
156. Schulz, R., Wilhelm, A., Dirlich, G. Intracerebral microinjection of different antibodies against the endogenous opioids suggests alpha-neoendorphin participation in control of feeding behavior. Naunyn Schmiedebergs Arch. Pharmacol. 1984;326:222–226.
157. Hawkins, M.F., Cubic, B., Baumeister, A.A., Bartin, C. Microinjection of opioid antagonists into the substantia nigra reduces stress-induced eating in rats. Brain Res. 1992;584: 261–265.
158. Koch, J.E., Bodnar, R.J. Involvement of mu-1 and mu-2 opioid receptor subtypes in tail-pinch feeding in rats. Physiol. Behav. 1993;53:603–605.
159. Margules, D.L., Moisset, B., Lewis, M.J., Shibuya, H., Pert, C.B. Beta-endorphin is associated with overeating in genetically-obese mice (ob/ob) and rats (fa/fa). Science 1978;202: 988–991.
160. Kim, E.M., O'Hare, E., Grace, M.K., Welch, C.C., Billington, C.J., Levine, A.S. ARC POMC mRNA and PVN alpha-MSH are lower in obese relative to lean Zucker rats. Brain Res. 2000;1000:11–16.
161. Przewlocki, R., Lason, W. The opioid peptide dynorphin, circadian rhythms and starvation. Science 1982;219:71–73.
162. Takahashi, H., Motomatsu, T., Nobunaga, M. Influences of water deprivation and fasting on hypothalamic, pituitary and plasma opioid peptides and prolactin in rats. Physiol. Behav. 1986;37:603–608.
163. Glass, M.J., Briggs, J.E., Billington, C.J., Kotz, C.M., Levine, A.S. Opioid receptor blockade in rat nucleus tractus solitarius alters amygdala dynorphin gene expression. Am. J. Physiol. 2002;283:R161–R167.
164. Appleyard, S.M., Haywood, M., Young, J.I., Butler, A.A., Cone, R.D., Rubinstein, M., Low, M.J. A role for the endogenous opioid beta-endorphin in energy homeostasis. Endocrinology 2003;144:1753–1760.
165. Haywood, M.D., Pintar, J.E., Low, M.J. Selective reward deficit in mice lacking beta-endorphin and enkephalin. J. Neurosci. 2002;22:8251–8258.
166. Leventhal, L., Cole, J.L., Rossi, G.C., Pan, Y.X., Pasternak, G.W., Bodnar, R.J. Antisense oligodeoxynucleotides against the MOR-1 clone alter weight and ingestive responses in rats. Brain Res. 1996;719:78–84.
167. Pomonis, J.D., Billington, C.J., Levine, A.S. Orphanin FQ, agonist of orphan opioid receptor ORL1, stimulates feeding in rats. Neuroreport 1996;8:369–371.
168. Stratford, T.R., Holahan, M.R., Kelley, A.E. Injections of nociceptin into nucleus accumbens shell or ventromedial hypothalamic nucleus increase food intake. Neuroreport 1997;8: 423–426.
169. Hagan, M.M., Rushing, P.A., Benoit, S.C., Woods, S.C., Seeley, R.J. Opioid receptor involvement in the effect of AgRP-(83–132) on food intake and food selection. Am. J. Physiol. 2001;280:R814–R821.

170. Olszewski, P.K., Wirth, M.M., Grace, M.K., Levine, A.S., Giraudo, S.Q. Evidence of interactions between melanocortin and opioid systems in regulation of feeding. Neuroreport 2001;12:1727–1730.
171. O'Hare, E., Levine, A.S., Semotuk, M.T., Tierney, K.J., Shephard, R.A., Grace, M.K., Cleary, J. Utilization of a novel model of food reinforced behavior involving neuropeptide Y, insulin, 2-deoxy-D-glucose and naloxone. Behav. Pharmacol. 1996;7:742–753.
172. Rudski, J.M., Grace, M., Kuskowski, M.A., Billington, C.J., Levine, A.S. Behavioral effects of naloxone on neuropeptide Y-induced feeding. Pharmacol. Biochem. Behav. 1996;54:771–777.
173. Hagan, M.M., Moss, D.E. Effect of naloxone and antidepressants on hyperphagia produced by peptide YY. Pharmacol. Biochem. Behav. 1993;45:941–944.
174. Fletcher, P.J. Opiate antagonists inhibit feeding induced by 8-OH-DPAT: possible mediation in the nucleus accumbens. Brain Res. 1991;560:260–267.
175. Jackson, H.C., Griffin, I.J., Nutt, D.J. Endogenous opioids may be involved in idazoxan-induced food intake. Neuropharmacology 1992;31:771–776.
176. Clegg, D.J., Air, E.L., Woods, S.C., Seeley, R.J. Eating elicited by orexin-a, but not melanin-concentrating hormone, is opioid-mediated. Endocrinology 2002;143:2995–3000.
177. Mann, P.E., Arjune, D., Romero, M.T., Pasternak, G.W., Hahn, E.F., Bodnar, R.J. Differential sensitivity of opioid-induced feeding to naloxone and naloxonazine. Psychopharmacology 1988;94:330–341.
178. Jackson, H.C., Sewell, R.D.E. Are delta opioid receptors involved in the regulation of food and water intake? Neuropharmacology 1985;24:885–888.
179. Yu, W.-Z., Ruegg, H., Bodnar, R.J. Delta and kappa opioid receptor subtypes and ingestion: antagonist and glucoprivic effects. Pharmacol. Biochem. Behav. 1997;56:353–361.
180. Koch, J.E., Pasternak, G.W., Arjune, D., Bodnar, R.J. Naloxone benzoylhydrazone, a kappa-3 opioid agonist, stimulates food intake in rats. Brain Res. 1992;581:311–314.
181. Sipols, A.J., Bayer, J., Bennett, R., Figlewicz, D.P. Intraventricular insulin decreases kappa opioid-mediated sucrose intake in rats. Peptides 2002;23:2181–2187.
182. Jewett, D.C., Grace, M.K., Jones, R.M., Billington, C.J., Portoghese, P.S., Levine, A.S. The kappa-opioid antagonist GNTI reduces U50,488-, DAMGO-, and deprivation-induced feeding, but not butorphanol- and neuropeptide Y-induced feeding in rats. Brain Res. 2001; 909:75–80.
183. Silva, R.M., Hadjimarkou, M.M., Rossi, G.C., Pasternak, G.W., Bodnar, R.J. Beta-endorphin-induced feeding: pharmacological characterization using selective opioid antagonists and antisense probes in rats. J. Pharmacol. Exp. Ther. 2001;297:590–596.
184. DePedro, N., Cespedes, M.V., Delgado, M.J., Alonso-Bedate, M. Mu-opioid receptor is involved in beta-endorphin-induced feeding in goldfish. Peptides 1996;17:421–424.
185. Silva, R.M., Grossman, H.C., Hadjimarkou, M.M., Rossi, G.C., Pasternak, G.W., Bodnar, R.J. Dynorphin A1-17-induced feeding: pharmacological characterization using selective opioid antagonists and antisense probes in rats. J. Pharmacol. Exp. Ther. 2002;301:513–518.
186. Kotz, C.M., Grace, M.K., Billington, C.J., Levine, A.S. The effect of nor-binaltorphamine, beta-funaltrexamine and naltrindole on NPY-induced feeding. Brain Res. 1993;631: 325–328.
187. Israel, Y., Kandov, Y., Kest, A., Lewis, S.R., Bodnar, R.J. Neuropeptide Y-induced feeding: pharmacological characterization using selective opioid antagonists and antisense probes in rats. Peptides 2005;26:1167–1175.
188. Barton, C., York, D.A., Bray, G.A. Opioid receptor subtype control of galanin-induced feeding. Peptides 1996;17:237–240.
189. Brugman, S., Clegg, D.J., Woods, S.C., Seeley, R.J. Combined blockade of both micro- and kappa-opioid receptors prevents the acute orexigenic action of Agouti-related protein. Endocrinology 2002;143:4265–4270.
190. Grossman, H.C., Hadjimarkou, M.M., Silva, R.M., Giraudo, S.Q., Bodnar, R.J. Interrelationships between mu opioid and melanocortin receptors in mediating food intake in rats. Brain Res. 2003;991:240–244.

191. Polidori, C., deCaro, G., Massi, M. The hyperphagic effect of nociceptin/orphanin FQ in rats. Peptides 2000;21:1051–1062.
192. Kotz, C.M., Glass, M.J., Levine, A.S., Billington, C.J. Regional effect of naltrexone in the nucleus of the solitary tract in blockade of NPY-induced feeding. Am. J. Physiol. 2000;278:R499–R503.
193. Kotz, C.M., Grace, M.K., Briggs, J., Levine, A.S., Billington, C.J. Effects of opioid antagonists naloxone and naltrexone on neuropeptide Y-induced feeding and brown fat thermogenesis in the rat. J. Clin. Invest. 1995;96:163–170.
194. Kelley, A.E., Bakshi, V.P., Fleming, S., Holahan, M.R. A pharmacological analysis of the substrates underlying conditioned feeding induced by repeated opioid stimulation of the nucleus accumbens. Neuropsychopharmacology 2000;23:455–467.
195. Ragnauth, A., Moroz, M., Bodnar, R.J. Multiple opioid receptors mediate feeding elicited by mu and delta opioid receptor subtype agonists in the nucleus accumbens shell in rats. Brain Res. 2000;876:76–87.
196. Lamonte, N., Echo, J.A., Ackerman, T.F., Christian, G., Bodnar, R.J. Analysis of opioid receptor subtype antagonist effects upon mu opioid agonist-induced feeding elicited from the ventral tegmental area of rats. Brain Res. 2002;929:96–100.
197. Znamensky, V., Echo, J.A., Lamonte, N., Christian, G., Ragnauth, A., Bodnar, R.J. GABA receptor subtype antagonists differentially alter opioid-induced feeding in the shell region of the nucleus accumbens. Brain Res. 2001;906:84–91.
198. Echo, J.A., Lamonte, N., Ackerman, T.F., Bodnar, R.J. Alterations in food intake elicited by GABA and opioid agonists and antagonists administered into the ventral tegmental area region of rats. Physiol. Behav. 2002;76:107–116.
199. Khaimova, E., Kandov, Y., Israel, Y., Cataldo, G., Hadjimarkou, M.M., Bodnar, R.J. Opioid receptor subtype antagonistas differentially alter GABA agonist-induced feeding elicited from either the nucleus accumbens shell or ventral tegmental area region in rats. Brain Res. 2004;1026:284–294.
200. MacDonald, A.F., Billington, C.J., Levine, A.S. Effects of the opioid antagonist naltrexone on feeding induced by DAMGO in the ventral tegmental area and in the nucleus accumbens shell region in the rat. Am. J. Physiol. 2003;285:R999–R1004.
201. Bodnar, R.J., Lamonte, N., Israel, Y., Kandov, Y., Ackerman, T.F., Khaimova E. Reciprocal opioid–opioid interactions between the ventral tegmental area and nucleus accumbens regions in mediating mu agonist-induced feeding in rats. Peptides 2005;26:621–629.
202. Quinn, J.G., O'Hare, E., Levine, A.S., Kim, E.M. Evidence for a mu-opioid-opioid connection between the paraventricular nucleus and ventral tegmental area in the rat. Brain Res. 2003;991:206–211.
203. Giraudo, S.Q., Kotz, C.M., Billington, C.J., Levine, A.S. Association between the amygdala and the nucleus of the solitary tract in mu opioid induced feeding in the rat. Brain Res. 1998;802:184–188.
204. Giraudo, S.Q., Billington, C.J., Levine, A.S. Effects of the opioid antagonist naltrexone on feeding induced by DAMGO in the central nucleus of the amygdala and in the paraventricular nucleus in the rat. Brain Res. 1998;782:18–23.
205. Leventhal, L., Silva, R.M., Rossi, G.C., Pasternak, G.W., Bodnar, R.J. Morphine-6beta-glucuronide-induced hyperphagia: characterization of opioid action by selective antagonists and antisense mapping in rats. J. Pharmacol. Exp. Ther. 1998;287:538–544.
206. Leventhal, L., Stevens, L.B., Rossi, G.C., Pasternak, G.W., Bodnar, R.J. Antisense mapping of the MOR-1 opioid receptor clone: modulation of hyperphagia induced by DAMGO. J. Pharmacol. Exp. Ther. 1997;282:1402–1407.
207. Leventhal, L., Mathis, J.P., Rossi, G.C., Pasternak, G.W., Bodnar, R.J. Orphan opioid receptor antisense probes block orphanin FQ-induced hyperphagia. Eur. J. Pharmacol. 1998; 349:R1–R3.

Chapter 21
CNS Opiate Systems and Eating Disorders

Elliot D. Luby and David Koval

Abstract Anorexia nervosa resembles drug dependence because of the apparent pattern of starvation abuse. The self-starvation behavior of anorexic subjects is compulsive, self-gratifying, and persistent, despite life-threatening consequences. Opioid systems are activated by food deprivation and may induce the euphoria of self-starvation. Opioids act upon μ-receptors, resulting in a hedonic response, which can be powerfully reinforcing. Opiate blockade using naltrexone was shown to be effective in some anorexic and bulimic subjects. Research utilizing more powerful opioid blockers might show promise in the treatment of this resistant and potentially lethal disorder.

Keywords: Addiction; Anorexia; Bulimia; CNS; Eating disorder; Endogenous; Endorphin; Naltrexone; Opiate; Starvation

21.1 Definitions

Anorexia nervosa is a disorder in which patients refuse to eat as a result of a morbid fear of obesity. They lose weight through caloric restriction, ritualistic exercising, and abuse of laxatives and diuretics. Some patients become involved in bulimic bingeing and purging cycles in which they transiently lose control of disciplined dieting but avoid weight gain through vomiting. In a related disorder, bulimia nervosa, the binge–purge cycle occurs without caloric restriction and a normal body weight is maintained.

E.D. Luby (✉) and D. Koval
Comprehensive Psychiatric Services, 28800 Orchard Lake Road,
Suite 250, Farmington Hills, MI 48334
e-mail: elliot10@aol.com

R. Dean et al. (eds.), *Opiate Receptors and Antagonists*,

21.2 Incidence and Prevalence

The incidence of eating disorders is highest between ages 15 and 30, and is 10 to 20 times greater in females than males (1). The prevalence is highest in middle-class Caucasian families but African-American patients are increasingly diagnosed with these disorders. The disorder occurs in as many in 1 in 200 adolescent girls in British schools, and the rate is rising (2). Eating disorders can be lethal, with a mortality rate approaching 20% found in two populations of anorexic patients over an ~20-year period (3, 4).

21.3 Diagnostic Criteria

21.3.1 Anorexia Nervosa

The diagnostic criteria for anorexia nervosa include the following:

- Weight loss of at least 25% of original body weight or at least 15% below ideal body weight over a 6-month period;
- Distorted body image, such as a morbid fear of obesity and distorted attitudes toward food and body image;
- Amenorrhea of at least 3 months' duration;
- Physical signs, such as lanugo, bradycardia, and hypothermia;
- Excessive exercising, vomiting, laxative abuse, and/or bingeing episodes; and
- Absence of known physical or other psychiatric illness to account for weight loss.

21.3.2 Bulimia Nervosa

The diagnostic criteria for bulimia nervosa include the following:

- Recurrent episodes of binge eating;
- At least three of the following:
  - consumption of high-calorie, easily ingested food during a binge;
  - termination of a binge by abdominal pain, sleep, or self-induced vomiting;
  - surreptitious eating during a binge;
  - repeated attempts to lose weight; and
  - frequent weight fluctuations greater than 10 lb.
- Awareness of abnormal eating patterns and fear of not being able to stop eating voluntarily (in contrast to the marked denial seen in anorexia nervosa);
- Depressed mood after binges; and
- Absence of physical disorders or anorexia nervosa.

In bulimia, body weight stays in a normal range.

21.4 Anorexia Versus Starvation

There are differences between anorexia nervosa and starvation. In anorexia, initiative is high, mood can be elated but is often labile, and patients are strong-willed and take pride in their personal appearance. They do not fatigue easily. In starvation, there is a lack of initiative, a labile, quarrelsome mood, indecisiveness, and deterioration of personal appearance. Anorexic patients continue to exercise, while those in starvation avoid physical exercise as they attempt to conserve resources. However, a number of endocrinologic and metabolic abnormalities of anorexia nervosa are indistinguishable from those of starvation and return to normal when body weight is restored.

- Thyroid function is low.
- Serum triiodothyronine is low.
- Thyroxine is preferentially converted to inactive reverse T3, rather than to active T3.
- The level of thyroid-stimulating hormone (TSH), the response to thyroid-releasing hormone (TRH), and the absolute levels of T4, however, remain normal.
- Glucose tolerance tends to decrease as in diabetes. Anorexia nervosa patients are slightly resistant to insulin but recover from the resultant hypoglycemia more slowly than normal (5, 6).
- The basal level of growth hormone (GH) may be elevated, but its response to some secretagogues such as dopaminergic agonists and insulin, hypoglycemia is reduced (7).
- There are also changes in the hypothalamic pituitary adrenal axis. Cortisol levels in plasma are markedly elevated and escape dexamethasone suppression (8).
- The diurnal rhythm of plasma corticoids is reduced or absent.
- Cushingoid signs of hypercortisolism are not present, perhaps because anorexia patients lack the necessary substrate for lipogenesis and fat deposition, even if stimulated by cortisol.
- Primary or secondary amenorrhea is a cardinal and often the initial presenting sign of anorexia nervosa in a significant number of patients. The secretion of reproductive hormones returns to a prepubertal pattern.
- Luteinizing hormone (LH) and follicle-stimulating hormone (FSH) are low, resulting in low, noncyclic secretion of the ovarian hormones. The changes are at the hypothalamic level (9).
- Norepinephrine levels fall, as heart rate and blood pressure decrease.

21.5 Clinical Research on Anorexia and Opioids

Our particular interest is in the endogenous opioids. Increased endogenous opioid activity in the cerebral spinal fluid of anorexia nervosa patients has been recorded by Kaye et al. (10). It was found only in patients who were severely underweight at the time, and not in those in whom body weight was being maintained or restored.

Total endogenous opioid activity was measured by a radio-receptor assay in which the endogenous opioids compete with labeled enkephalamide for binding to opioid receptors and crude brain membranes. Gerner and Sharpe found normal β-endorphin levels in the cerebrospinal fluid (CSF) of anorexia nervosa patients (11). They used a radioimmunoassay specific for β-endorphin, but the weight of the patients was not recorded, and the results were too difficult to interpret.

However, Marrazzi and Luby, et al., found that the endogenous plasma alkaloids, codeine and morphine, were elevated in patients with anorexia nervosa and bulimia nervosa compared to control subjects. The means for codeine levels were significantly elevated in all patient groups compared to control subjects. Many more anorexic and bulimic subjects had elevated levels compared to the control subjects. For morphine, this was true for the bulimics compared to the control subjects but not for the anorexic or combined patient groups compared to controls (12).

21.6 Anorexia Nervosa: An Addictive Disorder?

Marrazzi and Luby hypothesized that anorexia nervosa was an addiction to dieting, mediated by endogenous opioids (13). According to this hypothesis, endogenous opioids released during an initial period of dieting produce a positively reinforcing sense of elation eventually leading to an addiction to dieting. Evidence in support of the hypothesis consists of the following:

- the addictive characteristics of the clinical behavior;
- changes in endogenous opioid levels in anorexia nervosa;
- changes in endogenous opioid levels and systems induced by food deprivation;
- relevant opioid actions;
- theoretical considerations regarding the relationship of anorexia nervosa and abnormal opioid function; and
- therapeutic benefits derived from the interruption of the addictive cycle with narcotic antagonists.

The World Health Organization (WHO) defines drug dependence as "a state, psychic and sometimes physical, resulting from the interaction between a living organism and a drug, characterized by behavioral and other responses, that always includes a compulsion to take the drug on a continuous or periodic basis in order to experience its psychic effects, sometimes to avoid discomfort." One needs only to substitute "dieting" and "weight loss" for "drug" to realize how closely the anorexic behavior fits the WHO definition of drug dependence.

Behavior in anorexia nervosa is similar in many respects to that observed in the addictive disorders. The similarities include strong denial, compulsiveness, that is, the organization of one's life around dieting and excessive exercise, and persistence despite severe social and life-threatening medical consequences of dieting. Many patients describe feelings of "demonic possession," powerlessness over the weight loss, and a family history of addiction. Patients become experts in nutrition and know the caloric content of every food on their trays. The devotion to dieting and weight loss continues to the exclusion of virtually all other interests, much like an alcoholic or heroin-dependent person becomes preoccupied with the acquisition and use of the addictive substance. Like the addicted, the anorexic patients use denial as a major defense, and frequently refuse hospitalization and treatment until overpowered by physical disease or pressure from the family or an employer. They perceive their eating disorder in an idiosyncratic framework as a necessary discipline or even healthful achievement. Thus two conflicting ego states may coexist: the patient may candidly state that she knows that she cannot wear clothing which reveals her arms and legs because people appear shocked by her wasted appearance, while a moment later she will insist that she is not anorexic and that she still has not achieved her ideal body weight. In therapy, anorexic patients will frequently identify others as having the disorder but will deny its existence in themselves. A 60-lb girl described a 100-lb patient as anorexic, while firmly denying the disorder in herself. When confronted with this apparent paradox, she became angry and refused to discuss the matter further.

There are changes in endogenous opioids in opioid systems induced by food deprivation. In animal studies, food deprivation alters the opioid content of various tissues, as measured by specific radioimmunoassay, although the changes vary greatly, depending on the tissue, the opioid, and the conditions of starvation. It is generally held that the level of opioids in the CSF reflects their production by the brain, whereas the plasma level reflects the production by the pituitary. The study of Knuth and Friesen is of particular interest, because caloric intake was restricted only to 50% of normal, which may resemble the initial dieting that according to our hypothesis triggers anorexia nervosa (14). Female animals were used in this study, and most of the changes in β-endorphin were observed during the starvation-induced anestrus, a possible model of anorexia nervosa-induced amenorrhea. Two studies found that starvation-induced changes in opioid levels could be reversed by refeeding. Increases in opioid action, that is, increases in naloxone-sensitive analgesia and hypotension provide additional if indirect evidence of opioid release during food deprivation lasting as long as 4 days (15, 16).

21.7 Metabolic Response to Caloric Restriction

In addition to food restriction, the metabolic glucopenia-induced blocking either by glycolysis with 2-deoxyglucose (2-DG) or by insulin hypoglycemia (to a degree which would induce feeding) results in an increase in plasma β-endorphin and in opioid analgesia (17, 18). Moreover, there is evidence that opioids are involved in insulin-induced feeding in animals (19, 20), and that naloxone blocks the increase in food intake by 2-DG in human, albeit without reducing the subjective feeling of hunger (21). The assumption is that food restriction induces fluctuations in endogenous opioid activity, as previously discussed. Indeed food restriction capable of maintaining rats at 80–90% of their normal body weight alters their behavioral response to addictive drugs and to the opiate antagonists naloxone and naltrexone (22–31). Two categories of opioid actions appear useful to the starving animal: first, stimulation of food intake to correct starvation; and second, when food is not available, adaptation to starvation, and improved survival. Narcotics and the endogenous opioid peptides increase food intake when injected systemically or directly into the CSF or the hypothalamus. This action appears to be mediated – at least in rats – by multiple subtypes of opiate receptors, including the μ-, κ-, and σ-receptors as demonstrated using a variety of preferential agonists. The endogenous opioid peptides dynorphin and β-endorphin have the same effect (32–43). The suggestion that endogenous endorphins mediate homeostatic adaptations to starvation is based on the similarities between the actions of the opiates and the physiologic changes which take place in starvation and in anorexia nervosa. They result in the conservation of energy and increased survival of the individual. These changes are as follows:

1. Constipation – This slows the transit through the gastrointestinal tract, hence increasing the extraction of nutrients and water;
2. Water retention and famine edema – This is promoted via release of vasopressin and reduction of the digestive secretions (interestingly, vasopressin in the CSF is increased in anorexia nervosa);
3. Decreased body temperature;
4. Decreased release of thyroid hormone and decreased calorigenesis;
5. Decreased blood pressure and vascular sympathetic tone;
6. Depressed respiration and decreased sensitivity of the respiratory center to carbon dioxide and hypoxia;
7. Decreased intensity of emotional reactions, that is, fear and rage;
8. Lethargy, drowsiness, and passivity;
9. Inhibition of reproductive activities, as secretion of FSH and LH are reduced by opioids.

Responses 1 and 2 conserve bodily resources. Responses 3 through 8 decrease the metabolic rate and hence the metabolic need. Response 9 reduces species survival function to those necessary for self-preservation. Margules argues that after the initial response of the sympathetic nervous system and glucagon, the endorphinergic system assumes responsibility for the prolonged adjustment to fuel shortage. Indeed, it is known that starvation-related enduring metabolic changes are not dependent upon the sympathetic nervous system (44).

Opioids downregulate metabolism and enhance food intake. Therefore, it is logical that opiate agonists can cause anorexia as well as hyperphagia. Both responses can be blocked by the development of tolerance or by opiate blockade. Opiate peptides may also have a glucoregulatory mechanism of action. Morphine induces hyperglycemia. Opiate peptides modulate the release of glucoregulatory hormones from the pancreas, including insulin, glucagon, somatostatin, and pancreatic polypeptide, along with other glucoregulatory hormones, such as adrenocorticotropin hormone (ACTH)-enhanced cortisol, GH, and thyroid hormone. The direction of the effects may vary, but all indicate endorphin effects upon glucose regulation. Opioid peptides modulate insulin action and may redistribute glucose during stress. They also enhance glycogenolysis and gluconeogenesis by stimulating glucagon and ACTH release.

There is evidence that the efficiency of food utilization is increased after food deprivation. Thus body weight can be restored with a lower caloric intake. Sometimes body weight is not fully restored after food deprivation, particularly under circumstances of "activity-induced self-starvation." Rats deprived of food for a limited time of day initially lose weight but then recover after adjusting to a new feeding schedule. When allowed to run on a wheel, they ignore the food and run themselves to death (45). This phenomenon has striking similarities with anorexia nervosa, in that a possible role of the opioids should be considered.

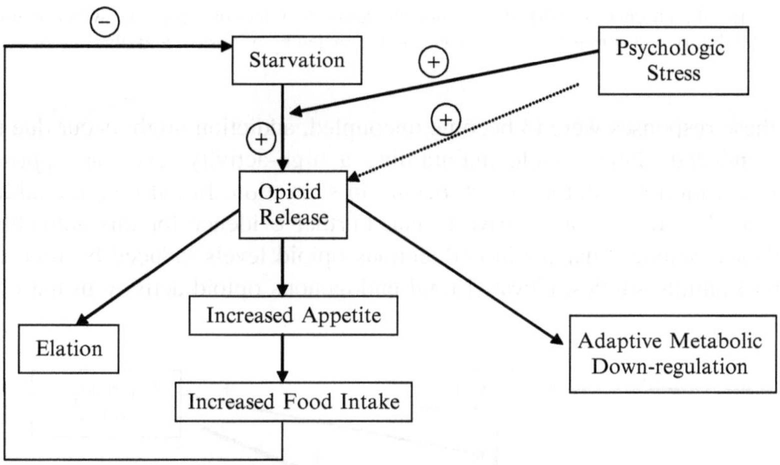

Fig. 21.1 Normal pattern. The thickness of the line suggests the intensity of the response. A broken line indicates the absence or marked reduction in eating disorders of a pathway which is normally present. Inhibitory and stimulatory influences are designated by minus (–) and plus (+), respectively

Marrazzi and Luby developed an opioid model for eating disorders (46). They hypothesized that the opioids play a dual role in responding to starvation in the following manner: they either increase food intake to correct it or adapt for survival in the face of starvation until it is corrected by downregulating metabolic function to an essential minimum.

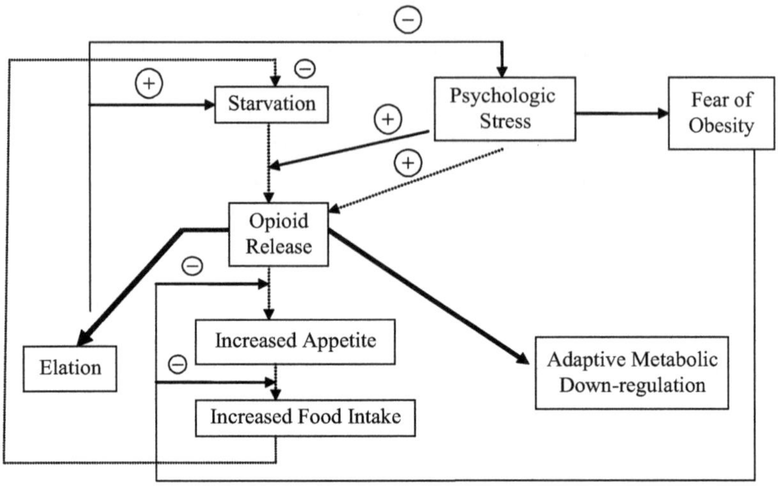

Fig. 21.2 Anorexia nervosa. The thickness of the line suggests the intensity of the response. A broken line indicates the absence or marked reduction in eating disorders of a pathway which is normally present. Inhibitory and stimulatory influences are designated by minus (–) and plus (+), respectively

If these responses were to become uncoupled, addiction might occur due to the opioid-induced elation while maintaining a high-activity level, as opposed to the preservation of calories which occurs in starvation. In bulimia, the addiction would be due to the opioid drive to eat. Further evidence for this autoaddiction hypothesis includes changes in endogenous opioid levels induced by food deprivation in animal studies, elevated total endogenous opioid activity in the CSF of

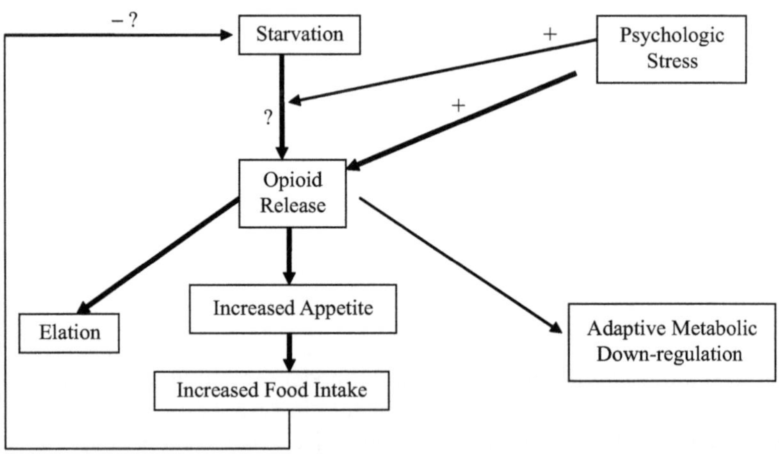

Fig. 21.3 Bulimia. The thickness of the line suggests the intensity of the response. A broken line indicates the absence or marked reduction in eating disorders of a pathway which is normally present. Inhibitory and stimulatory influences are designated by minus (–) and plus (+), respectively

anorexia nervosa patients, the addiction characteristics of the clinical behavior, and the effectiveness of narcotic antagonists in some patients. According to the autoaddiction hypothesis, opiate blockade should be beneficial in the treatment of anorexia nervosa and bulimia by interrupting the addictive cycle.

21.8 Case Studies and Clinical Trials

Narcotic antagonists may be useful in treating bulimia. We treated five bulimic women ranging in age from late adolescence to postmenopause. Four had a classic binge–purge cycle. They were given naltrexone 50 mg twice daily for as little as 2 days. Three of these patients became less obsessively preoccupied by food and were able to control almost completely their bingeing and purging. Two patients discontinued the drug soon after discharge from the hospital and experienced a rapid recurrence of their symptoms.

Marrazzi et al. studied two groups of patients (47). One group was diagnosed with bulimia nervosa and the other with anorexia nervosa. Each group was treated with naltrexone 100 mg b.i.d. for 6 weeks and then in a crossover design with placebo for the same period. A smaller group was treated with open-label naltrexone 200 mg b.i.d. Subjects were drug-free other than for the occasional use of antibiotics or antihistamines. There was an antidepressant washout period 1 month prior to subject participation. At the start and end, electrolytes, liver function studies, weight on a hospital scale, the Eating Disorder Inventory, and a Body Image Test, in which the ratio between the subject's estimate of body size and the actual measurement, was calculated. All but one subject met DSM-IIIR criteria for either anorexia nervosa or bulimia nervosa. That subject had a binge-eating disorder similar to the binge eating of obesity. For 18 of 19 subjects, symptom reduction was evident in the naltrexone period. The data were analyzed blindly. Subjects often thought they knew when they were on the active drug. Binges, purges, urges to binge, urges to purge, daily food intake, and binge–purge ratio all showed statistically significant differences. The therapeutic improvement appeared more in the execution of the urge to binge or purge. The effectiveness of naltrexone was in accord with the autoaddiction hypothesis where the drug appeared to interrupt the addictive cycle. Some underweight anorexics did not gain weight but showed impressive improvement in bulimic behavior. Side effects of naltrexone were minimal; some subjects experienced nausea and headache. Liver function studies never became elevated throughout the study.

Marrazzi et al. also studied the effects of naltrexone in binge-eating disorder. In these patients, binge eating is not compensated for through purging or the use of laxatives. A single subject was studied using naltrexone at a dose of 100 mg b.i.d. in a crossover design with placebo during three 6 to week periods. The subject was a recovering alcoholic, a 36-year-old Caucasian female who had 7-year history of binge eating without purging. Symptoms were reduced during the naltrexone period compared to placebo. When the double-blind coding of drug versus placebo was broken, the assessments of the experimenter based upon the data analyzed blindly and of the subject and her therapist were confirmed.

Luby et al. studied eight subjects diagnosed with anorexia nervosa. Seven of these subjects had been treatment resistant in the past, and six had a history of the disorder ranging from 4 to 10 years. In six patients who were chronically ill, naltrexone in doses from 25 to 75 mg daily associated with the use of total parenteral nutrition (TPN) reduced the obsessive preoccupation with dieting, anxiety about weight gain, resistance to treatment, and positively reinforcing starvation-induced elation. Naltrexone also relieved the opioid-induced abdominal distension and constipation. These results were comparable to a study by Moore et al. when naloxone was given by intravenous infusion to a group of 12 hospitalized anorexic patients, producing a tenfold increase in weight gain per week. The investigators proposed that naloxone was an antilipolytic agent; later they suggested the drug also had antiobsessional properties.

All eight patients were treated with naltrexone in addition to TPN, individual psychotherapy, and family therapy. In seven of these patients, previous treatment had been ineffective. In six patients who had been chronically ill, the drug appeared to have some beneficial effect. There was a diminution in the obsessive preoccupation with dieting, anxiety about weight gain, resistance to treatment and the positively reinforcing elation of starvation decreased. Naltrexone also relieved the constipation and abdominal distension probably through blockage of opioid-mediated mechanisms. Two subjects continued taking naltrexone as outpatients and gained more weight. One maintained her ideal body weight for over 2 years. Naltrexone may have increased the efficiency of food utilization.

Of interest was a 44-year-old anorexic woman who weighed 77 lb on admission (48). She had a 20-year history of the disorder, with multiple prior treatment failures. She entered the hospital in a state of some emaciation and consented to participate in a research project using the new opiate blocker, nalmefene, which is long acting and orally active, like naltrexone, and is 2.5 times more potent. Twenty-four hours after the nalmefene was started at a dose of 20 mg twice daily, the patient awoke from a sound sleep in a classic panic attack. She reported a sense of impending doom, heart palpitations, diaphoresis, depersonalization, and derealization. She had no prior history of panic disorder. We hypothesized that she may have experienced endogenous opiate withdrawal. Presynaptic opiate receptors in the noradrenergic system inhibit norepinephrine release. Their blockade in this patient might have resulted in the massive norepinephrine release precipitating a panic attack. The opioid noradrenergic interactions may be disturbed in panic disorder and this patient may have experienced an endogenous opiate withdrawal very similar to that which occurs in exogenous opiate-dependent patients.

Psychological factors may initiate the acute stages of eating disorders; however, they are insufficient to account for their chronicity and stubborn resistance to treatment. The autoaddiction hypothesis proposes that endogenous opioid systems somehow mediate this autoaddiction, and clinical experience and animal data have been marshaled to support this hypothesis. Total endogenous opioid activities increased in the cerebral spinal fluid of anorexia nervosa patients. Food deprivation alters the level of endogenous opioid peptides and endogenous opioid systems.

Biederman and Vessel proposed that perceptual pleasure is based on release of endorphins in the brain. Their hypothesis is based on the visual system, but they suspect that "other sensory systems may have a similar arrangement." They proposed that μ-opioid receptors are the mediators of pleasure and that they do so by inhibiting GABAergic neurons which are inhibitory in their action. That inhibition of inhibition allows for greater neural excitation, which may ultimately cause the release of dopamine within the corpus striatum, creating the experience of pleasure (49).

The elevated total endogenous opioid activity in the cerebral spinal fluid of anorexia nervosa patients who are markedly cachectic may result from starvation-induced opioid release. It is proposed that these endogenous opiates are the substrates for an autoaddictive state that reinforces anorexic behavior and perpetuates it over time. Opioids downregulate metabolism and adaptation to starvation while the anorexic suppresses their concomitant appetite stimulating properties. The hyperactivity of anorexic patients does not appear to fit the opioid addiction hypothesis; however, physical exercise is known to stimulate endorphin secretion which may be additive to the opioid release from dieting. Chronic anorexic nervosa seems unresponsive to the spectrum of psychotherapeutic modalities. An autoaddiction model may not only provide a basis for further biological research but also contribute to alternative therapeutic approaches utilizing opiate blockers. More selective receptor blockers than those currently available may prove more efficacious.

DeMarines et al. demonstrated opioid dysregulation in anorexia nervosa by feeding subjects an 800-Cal meal at lunchtime. In normal subjects there is an inhibition of GH release in response to growth hormone-releasing hormone (GH-RH). This inhibition does not occur in anorexic subjects, and it was not influenced by an infusion of naloxone as it was in obese subjects (50).

Carr and Papadouka, using rats with electrodes planted in the lateral hypothalamus, found that self-stimulation increased significantly after food deprivation. They assumed that food restriction and weight loss trigger μ- and possibly κ-receptors that facilitate brain stimulation reward "from triggered reward." They cited other observations which indicated that opioid activity is a compensatory response to starvation. Such a response in their opinion might trigger the autoaddiction state in anorexia nervosa, as proposed by Marrazzi and Luby (51). However, Melchior et al. found a reduced anhedonic response to weight loss in anorexic patients (52). The authors used the term "negative allesthesia" to describe the decreased pleasure "related to alimentary stimulation" after a subject is given a caloric glucose load. In normal subjects, glucose-induced negative allesthesia or reduced hedonic response disappears upon weight loss; yet it persisted in six anorexic patients despite major weight loss. In normal and obese subjects 25 mg of naloxone did not increase glucose-induced negative allesthesia, suggesting to the investigators that the maximum effect had occurred to the glucose alone. They concluded that naloxone had acted upon a weaker endogenous opiate system in anorexic subjects. In seeming contradiction, they found that basal plasma levels of β-endorphin were higher in the anorexic group versus the control group. They assumed that there was a dissociation between plasma and central nervous system (CNS) endorphin levels. The persistence of negative allesthesia in anorexia subjects may reset body weight at a lower level and, in their opinion, the mechanism might involve diminished central endorphin activity.

Jonas and Gold observed the association between eating disorders and substance abuse, stating that 25–50% of individuals with anorexia nervosa and bulimia have a history of substance abuse. They proposed that endogenous opioids played a role in the compulsion to binge eat. They successfully used naltrexone in the treatment of these disorders (53).

In a similar vein, Sternbach et al. reported two detoxified heroin addicts who had lost their appetite following treatment with naltrexone. The investigators hypothesized reduced central β-endorphin activity in starvation, rather than an increase. They proposed that a subtype of anorexia nervosa may occur which has an endorphin abnormality as its pathophysiology (54).

DeZwaan and Mitchell reviewed several studies on the effects of opioid blockade in eating disorders. They acknowledged that "endogenous opioid peptides are involved in the regulation of food intake." They reported a 30% reduction in food consumption after a single dose of an opiate blocker versus placebo in normal weight as well as obese and bulimic subjects. Open studies of naltrexone in bulimia nervosa were positive for diminishing binge eating frequency while control studies showed no effect other than for a reduction in the "duration of binge eating episodes and preoccupation with food." There was no beneficial effect of naltrexone on weight reduction in obese subjects. They posited a suppressant effect on the ingestion of "highly palatable food," possibly related to an association between opioids and reward systems. They were troubled by the adverse effects of opiate blockade, including headache, nausea, and the elevation of liver-function studies (55). Marrazzi and Luby did not find liver function studies to be increased in their naltrexone subjects (56).

21.9 Summary

Anorexia nervosa is a disorder of self-starvation in which patients have such a distorted body image and fear of obesity that they fast, even to the point of death. The endocrinologic, metabolic, and physical consequences of the disorder are comparable to those found in obligatory starvation; however, the behavioral changes which occur in anorexia nervosa and in starvation are widely dissimilar. Bulimia nervosa is a disorder of binge eating and purging, in which patients maintain a normal weight.

In this chapter, we reviewed clinical and experimental evidence suggesting hypothalamic or neurotransmitter dysfunction in the pathogenesis of anorexia nervosa and proposed a novel autoaddiction hypothesis. We believe that the evidence supports this hypothesis because in self-starvation endogenous opioids are released in an initial phase of dieting, which powerfully reinforce the process. The endorphinergic reinforcement of dieting and weight loss then lowers the threshold to other reward or hedonic stimuli beyond dieting itself. Prolonged food restriction has been shown to cause a naltrexone-reversible increase in self-stimulation in rats with electrodes placed on the perifornical area of hypothalamus. All pleasure systems in brain may be based on endorphin-related mechanisms. The work of Biederman and Vessel would propose that the experience of reward or pleasure is activated by the release of endorphins acting on μ-receptors. μ-receptors mediate pleasure by inhibiting GABAergic neurons that are inhibitory in their action. Inhibition of inhibition ultimately activates the release of dopamine within the corpus striatum, creating the reinforcing experience of pleasure as it might relate to dieting and weight loss. It is possible that some anorexics who become chronic have weakened endorphin systems prior to the onset of the disorder and that the prolonged weight loss may strengthen them over time, thus enhancing hedonic responses. Bulimics have a powerful drive to eat and purge to control weight. In the anorexic, the opioid drive to eat would be suppressed by the greater reinforcement of opioid-induced elation. On the contrary, in the bulimic, the opioid drive to eat would not be suppressed, resulting in the classic binge–purge cycle. Our model would formulate a treatment plan for both of these disorders based upon interrupting the addictive cycle through opioid blockade.

We recognize that other neurotransmitters and neuropeptides, some not yet discovered, also play roles in the regulation of appetite. Only preliminary results were presented to support the hypothesis. There are contradictory findings in the literature which we reviewed. Much more work is needed, particularly double-blind studies, and the consideration that other, more powerful opiate blockers might become available. Marrazzi believed that there might be underlying differences in endogenous opioid systems which would predispose an individual to anorexia nervosa. Eating disorders, when they become chronic, are stubbornly resistant to treatment. Any possibility of developing a better understanding of their neurobiology might lead to more efficient approaches, relieving the anguish of the patients and their families.

References

1. Halmi KA. Anorexia nervosa: recent investigations. Ann Rev Med 1978;29:137–148.
2. Crisp AH, Palmer RL, Kalucy RS. How common is anorexia nervosa? A prevalence study. Br J Psychiatry 1976;128:549–554.
3. Hsu KLG. Outcome of anorexia nervosa. A review of the literature (1954–1978). Arch Gen Psychiatry 1980;37:1041–1046.
4. Theander S. Long-term prognosis of anorexia nervosa: a preliminary report. In: Darby PL, Garfinkel PE, Garner DM, Coscina DV (eds.) Anorexia Nervosa: Recent Developments in Research. New York: Alan R. Liss, 1983:441–442.
5. Brown, GM. Endocrine alterations in anorexia nervosa In: Darby PL, Garfinkel PE, Garner DM, Coscina DV (eds.) Anorexia Nervosa: Recent Developments in Research. New York: Alan R. Liss, 1983:231–248.
6. Warren, MP, Vande Wiele R. Clinical and metabolic features of anorexia nervosa. Am J Obstet Gynecol 1973;117:435–449.

7. Mecklenberg RS, Loriaux DL, Thompson RH et al. Hypothalamic dysfunction in patients with anorexia nervosa. Medicine 1974;53:147–159.
8. Weiner H, Katz JL. The hypothalamic-pituitary-adrenal axis in anorexia nervosa: a reassessment. In: Darby PL, Garfinkel PE, Garner DM, Coscina DV (eds.) Anorexia Nervosa: Recent Developments in Research. New York: Alan R. Liss, 1983:249–270.
9. Nillius SJ, Wide L. The pituitary responsiveness to acute and chronic administration of gonadotropin-releasing hormone in acute and recovering stages of anorexia nervosa. In: Viegersky RA (ed.) Anorexia Nervosa. New York: Raven Press, 1977:177–188.
10. Kaye WH, Pickar DM, Naber D et al. Cerebrospinal fluid opioid activity in anorexia nervosa. Am J Psychiatry 1982;139:643–645.
11. Gerner RH, Sharp B. CSF β-endorphin immunoreactivity in normal, schizophrenic, depressed, manic, and anorexic subjects. Brain Res 1982;237:244–247.
12. Marrazzi MA, Luby ED et al. Endogenous codeine and morphine in anorexia nervosa and bulimia nervosa. Life Sci 1987;60:1741–1747.
13. Marrazzi MA, Luby ED. An auto-addiction opioid model of chronic anorexia nervosa. Int J Eat Disord 1986;5:191–208.
14. Knuth UA, Friesen HG. Changes in beta-endorphin and somatostatin concentrations in different hypothalamic areas of female rats after chronic starvation. Life Sci 1983;33:827–833.
15. Bodnar RJ, Kelly DD, Spiaggia A et al. Biphasic alterations of nociceptic thresholds induced by food deprivation. Physiol Psychol 1978;6:391–395.
16. McGivern R, Berka C, Bernston GC et al. Effect of naloxone on analgesia induced food deprivation. Life Sci 1979;25:885–888.
17. Davis JM, Lowy MT, Yim GKW et al. Relationship between plasma concentrations of immunoreactive beta-endorphin and food intake in rats. Peptides 1982;4:79–83.
18. Yim, GKW, Lowy MT, Davis JM et al. Opiate involvement in glucoprivic feeding. In: Hoebel B, Novin D (eds.) The Neural Basis of Feeding and Reward. Brunswick, ME: Haer Institute, 1982:485–498.
19. Bodnar RJ, Kelly DD, Brutus M et al. Chronic 2-deoxy-D-glucose treatment adaptation of its analgesic, but not hyperphagic properties. Pharmacol Biochem Behav 1978;9:763–768.
20. Kramer E, Sperber ES, Bodnar RJ. Age-related decrements in the analgesic and hyperphagic responses to 2-deoxy-D-glucose. Physiol Behav 1986;35:929–934.
21. Thompson DA, Welle SL, Lilavivat U et al. Opiate receptor blockade in man reduces 2-deoxy-D-glucose induced food intake but not hunger, thirst and hypothermia. Life Sci 1982;31:847–852.
22. Atrens DM, Marfaing-Jallat P, LeMagnen J. Ethanol preference following hypothalamic stimulation: relation to stimulation parameters and energy balance. Pharmacol Biochem Behav 1983;19:571–575.
23. Carroll ME, Boe IN. Effect of dose on increased etonitazene self-administration by rats due to food deprivation. Psychopharmacology 1984;82:151–152.
24. Carroll ME, France CP, Meisch RA. Intravenous self-administration of etonitazene, cocaine and phencyclidine in rats during food deprivation and satiation. J Pharmacol Exper Therap 1981;217:241–247.
25. Meisch RA, Kliner DJ. Etonitazene as a reinforcer for rats: increased etonitazene-reinforced behavior due to food deprivation. Psychopharmacology 1979;63:97–98.
26. Oei TPS. Effect of body weight reduction and food deprivation on cocaine self-administration. Pharmacol Biochem Behav 1983;19:453–455.
27. Carroll ME, Lac ST, Walker MJ, Kragh R, Newman T. Effects of naltrexone on intravenous cocaine self-administration in rats during food satiation and deprivation. J Pharmacol Exper Therap 1986;238:1–7.
28. Carroll ME. The role of food deprivation in the maintenance and reinstatement of cocaine-seeking behavior in rats. Drug Alcoh Depend 1985;16:85–109.
29. Snell D, Feller D, Bylund D et al. Sensitization produced by repeated administration of naloxone is blocked by food deprivation. J Pharmacol Exper Therap 1982;221:444–452.
30. Takahashi RN, Singer G. Self-administration of tetrahydrocannabinol by rats. Pharmacol Biochem Behav 1979;11:737–740.

31. Carroll ME, Pederson MC, Harrison RG. Food deprivation reveals strain differences in opiate intake of Sprague-Dawley and Wistar rats. Pharmacol Biochem Behav 1985;11:1095–1099.
32. Morley JE, Levine AS. Pharmacology of eating behavior. Ann Rev Pharmacol Toxicol 1985;25: 127–146.
33. Gosnell BA, Levine AS, Morley JE. *N*-Allylnormetozocine (SKF-10,047): the induction of feeling by a putative sigma agonist. Pharmacol Biochem Behav 1983;19:737–742.
34. Morley JE, Levine AS. Dynorphin (1–13) induces spontaneous feeding in rats. Life Sci 1981;29: 1901–1903.
35. Morley JE, Levine AS. Involvement of dynorphin and the kappa opioid receptor in feeding. Peptides 1983;4:797–800.
36. Morley JE, Levine AS, Kneip J et al. The effect of peripherally administered satiety substance on feeding induced by butorphanol tartrate. Pharmacol Biochem Behav 1983;19:577–582.
37. Morley JE, Levine AS, Yim GK et al. Opioid modulation of appetite. Neurosci Biobehav Rev 1983;8:281–305.
38. Sanger DJ. Endorphinergic mechanisms in the control of food and water intake. Appetite: J Intake Res 1981;2:193–208.
39. Sanger DJ, MaCarthy PS. Increased food and water intake produced by rats in opiate receptor agonists. Psychopharmacol 1981;74:217–220.
40. Tannenbaum MG, Pivorun EB. Effect of naltrexone on food intake and hoarding in white-footed mice. Pharmacol Biochem Behav 1984;20:35–37.
41. Morley JE, Levine AS, Gosnell BA et al. Peptides and feeding. Peptides 1985;6(2):181–192.
42. Baile CA, McLaughlin CL, Della-Fera MA. Role of cholecystokinin and opioid peptides in control of food intake. Physiol Rev 1986;66:172–234.
43. Yim GK, Lowy MT. Opioids, feeding and anorexias. Fed Proc 1984;43:2893–2897.
44. Margules DL. Beta-endorphin and endoloxone: hormones of the autonomic nervous system for the conservation or expenditure of bodily resources and energy in anticipation of famine or feast. Neurosci Biobehav Rev 1979;3:155–162.
45. Kanarek R, Collier GH. Self-starvation: a problem of overriding the satiety signal? Physiol Behav 1983;30:307–311.
46. Marrazzi MA, Luby ED. The neurobiology of anorexia nervosa: an auto-addiction? In: Cohen M, Foa P (eds.) The Brain as an Endocrine Organ. New York: Springer-Verlag, 1990:46–95.
47. Luby ED, Marazzi MA. A panic attack precipitated by opiate blockade – a case study. J Clin Psychopharm 1987;October:361–362.
48. Luby ED, Marrazzi MA, Kinzie J. Case reports – treatment of chronic anorexia nervosa with opiate blockade. J Clin Psychopharmacol 1987;7:52–53.
49. Beiderman I, Vessel E. Perceptual pleasure and the brain. Amer Scientist 2006;94:247–253.
50. DeMarinis L, Mancini A, Zuppi P, Fiumara C, Fabrizi ML, Sammartano L, Conte G, Valle D, Daini S, Ferro FM. Opioid dysregulation in anorexia nervosa, naloxone effects on preprandial and postgrandial growth hormone response to growth hormone releasing hormone. Metabolism 1994;43(2):140–143.
51. Carr KD, Papadouka V. The role of multiple opiate receptors in the potentiation of reward by food restriction. Brain Res 1994;639(21):253–260.
52. Melchior JC, Rigaud D, Colas-Linhart N, Rozen R, Fantino M, Apfelbaum M. Negative allesthesia and decreased endogenous opiate system activity in anorexia nervosa. Pharmacol Biochem Behav 1990;35:885–888.
53. Jonas JM, Gold MS. Naltrexone treatment of bulimia. Adv Alcohol Substance Abuse 1987; 7(1):29–37.
54. Sternbach HA, Annitto W, Pottash AL, Gold MS. Anorexic effects of naltrexone in man. Lancet 1982 February 13;1(8268):388–389.
55. DeZwaan H, Mitchell JE. Opiate antagonists and eating behavior in humans: a review. Clin Pharmacol 1992;32(12):1060–1072.
56. Marrazzi MA, Wrobleski JM, Kinzie J, Luby, ED. High dose naltrexone and liver function safety. Am J Addict 1997;6(1):21–29.

Part V
Behavioral Disorders

Chapter 22
Potential Utility of Kappa Ligands in the Treatment of Mood Disorders

William A. Carlezon, Jr. and Bruce M. Cohen

Abstract The biological basis of mood is not understood. The vast majority of present day research on mood and affective states focuses on the roles of brain systems containing monamines (e.g., dopamine, norepinephrine, and serotonin). This focus is logical, since drugs with mood-elevating effects have various and numerous interactions with these systems. However, endogenous opioid systems in the brain may also be involved in regulation of mood. We have become particularly interested in how kappa opioid receptors affect mood states. We will focus here on the potential utility of kappa ligands in the study and treatment of psychiatric conditions. Specifically, research from our groups and others suggests that kappa antagonists might be useful for depression, kappa agonists might be useful for mania, and kappa partial agonists might be useful for bipolar disorder. We will trace the history of our interests, describe our working hypotheses, and review evidence that is consistent and inconsistent with these hypotheses. In addition, we will identify issues that currently represent potential problems for the use of these agents as therapeutics, and plot a course for future work.

Keywords: Depression; Antidepressant; Dynorphin; Kappa opioid; Dopamine; Model; Rat; Mouse

22.1 Background

The biological basis of mood is not understood. The vast majority of present day research on mood and affective states focuses on the roles of brain systems containing monamines, such as dopamine (DA), norepinephrine (NE), and serotonin (5-hydroxytryptamine [5HT]). This focus is logical, since drugs with mood-elevating effects have various and numerous interactions with these systems, and in general they increase extracellular concentrations of monoamines and prolong

W.A. Carlezon (✉) and B.M. Cohen
Department of Psychiatry, McLean Hospital, Belmont, MA 02478
e-mail: bcarlezon@mclean.harvard.edu

R. Dean et al. (eds.), *Opiate Receptors and Antagonists*,

their actions (1). In the brain, increased DA is most often associated with rewarding (pleasurable) mood states: major drugs of abuse (including opiates, stimulants, nicotine, and ethanol) have the common effect of increasing neurotransmission in midbrain DA systems (2), and antipsychotic drugs (which have prominent DA antagonist properties) block reward, lower abnormally-elevated mood, and can produce anhedonia (3). Reduced NE is most often associated with depression, since one of the earliest classes of antidepressant drugs (tricyclic antidepressants [TCAs]) has prominent effects in blocking the synaptic reuptake of this transmitter (4, 5). Recently, the role of brain NE systems in mood states has received reduced attention due to the advent of antidepressant drugs that are selective serotonin reuptake inhibitors (SSRIs), such as fluoxetine (Prozac™). The commercial success of SSRIs as antidepressants – which appear to be safer than tricyclics, although differences in clinical efficacy are negligible (6) – has led to discoveries of fundamental alterations in brain 5HT systems (e.g., the association of stress-induced depression with polymorphisms of the gene coding for the serotonin transporter; 7, 8) that may explain vulnerability to depressive disorders in some individuals. Research on the role of NE systems in depression may be on the verge of a renaissance, however, with the introduction of new antidepressant drugs, such as duloxetine (Cymbalta™), that have dual actions on brain NE and 5HT systems. As such, studies of how brain monoamine systems regulate mood – and how they can be manipulated to control mood – have dominated the field for decades.

Endogenous opioid systems in the brain may also be involved in regulation of mood, although they have received far less attention than monoamine systems. Anecdotally, there is widespread appreciation for the fact that endogenous opioids can cause mood-elevated states such as "runner's high." Based upon studies in laboratory animals, it is clear that such effects involve, at least in part, monoamines: indeed, some of the reward-related effects of opiates such as morphine appear to depend upon their ability to activate DA systems (9) via inhibition of neurons that normally inhibit the activity of midbrain DA neurons (10). Considering that opioid systems are interwoven with monoamine systems in the brain (see 11), it should not be surprising that some effects of opioid receptor stimulation involve monoamine neurotransmitters. However, there is also evidence that rewarding effects of opiates are DA-independent (12). Such findings suggest that the major consequence of activation of endogenous opioid receptors – stimulation of inhibitory G-proteins (see 11) – could be sufficient to alter mood states. Regardless of whether the effects of endogenous opioids or exogenous opiates are a consequence of direct and widespread actions upon cell signal transduction pathways or indirectly involve alterations in monoamine function – or some combination of the two – the fact that these agents can affect mood raises the possibility that drugs that target endogenous opioid systems could be utilized in the treatment of debilitating psychiatric conditions.

We have become particularly interested in how kappa opioid receptors – so-named for the prototype kappa agonist ketocyclazocine (13) – contribute to regulation of mood. Our interest in kappa agents has evolved from what began as two disparate lines of research. The idea that kappa antagonists might be useful for

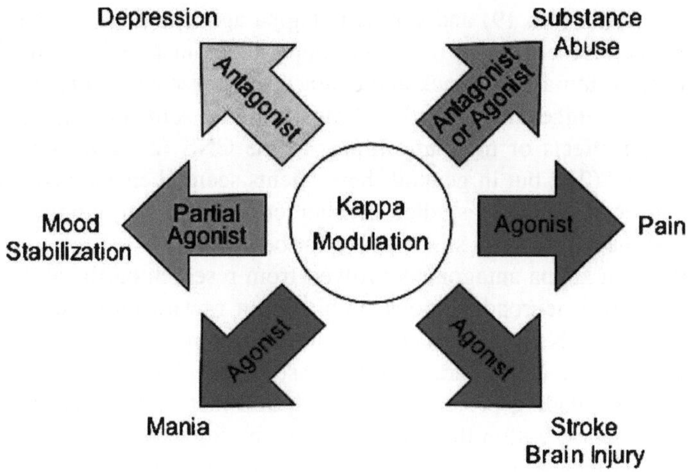

Fig. 22.1 Although this chapter focuses on potential uses for kappa ligands in psychiatry, these agents could prove to have many applications (*see Color Plates*)

the treatment of depression can be traced back to studies of the neurobiological consequences of long-term exposure to addictive drugs such as cocaine (14). The idea that kappa agonists might be useful for the treatment of bipolar disorder or mania can be traced back to studies of the molecular mechanisms of action of antipsychotic drugs (15), which are often used to manage the symptoms of these conditions. In addition, studies of the antidepressant-like effects of kappa antagonists led directly to studies of the prodepressant-like effects of kappa agonists (16). This chapter is designed to serve several purposes: to describe the history of our interests, to articulate our working hypotheses, to review evidence that is consistent and inconsistent with these hypotheses, to identify issues that currently represent potential problems for the use of these agents as therapeutics, and to plot a course for future work. We will focus here on the potential utility of kappa ligands in the study and treatment of psychiatric conditions, although theoretically these agents have broad applications, ranging from the treatment of pruritis to AIDS-related illness (Fig. 22.1).

22.2 Kappa Antagonists

22.2.1 History

Until recently, the prospects for clinical applications of kappa antagonists seemed limited. One consequence of the discovery of endogenous opioid receptors (see 11) and their agonists – including dynorphin, an endogenous agonist at brain kappa receptors (17) – was an interest in developing analgesic agents with reduced abuse liability. Dynorphin (18, 19) and synthetic kappa agonists (e.g., bremazocine; 20) have antinociceptive effects in rats, and kappa antagonists were primarily developed and utilized initially to block and characterize these actions (21). There were scattered reports suggesting potential clinical uses for kappa antagonists, such as minimizing the effects of traumatic injury to the CNS (22, 23) or manipulating feeding behavior (24), but in general these agents seemed envisioned primarily as "molecular probes" (21) for studies of interactions between agonists and kappa receptors and their functional significance for behavior.

Our interest in kappa antagonists evolved from research on the ability of drugs of abuse to induce neuroadaptations within brain reward circuits, including the nucleus accumbens (NAc). Repeated intermittent administration of stimulant drugs such as amphetamine causes dramatic increases in the function of CREB (cAMP response element binding protein), a transcription factor that controls expression of a variety of genes, within the NAc (25). The biological significance (if any) of this change was unclear; conceivably, it could contribute to drug tolerance or drug sensitization (reverse tolerance), two processes thought to play significant roles in the development and maintenance of addictive behaviors. In an attempt to establish causal relationships between drug-induced alterations in CREB function in the NAc and complex (drug-motivated) behaviors, we engineered viral vectors that would enable us to elevate CREB expression (thereby modeling one consequence of drug exposure) or block CREB function specifically within this region. In tests of sensitivity to the rewarding effects of cocaine, elevated expression of CREB in the NAc caused complex alterations in behavior: it made low doses of the drug aversive, and higher doses less rewarding than normal (14). Only through the use of additional models, such as the forced swim test (FST) (26), did it become apparent that elevation of CREB function in the NAc was eliciting the rodent equivalent of signs of major depression: dysphoria, anhedonia, and despair. In addition, it became clear that stress, a common trigger for both depressive and addictive disorders (27), can also activate CREB in the NAc (26). Remarkably, disruption of CREB function in the NAc caused opposite effects to those induced by elevated CREB, and had antidepressant-like effects that were indistinguishable from those of standard antidepressants. Together, these findings led to the working hypothesis that activation of CREB in the NAc is a molecular trigger for aversive (14) or depressive-like (26) symptoms.

Because CREB is a transcription factor that regulates expression of a variety of genes, it seemed likely that the aversive effects of elevated CREB function in the NAc were actually mediated by CREB-regulated target genes. Significant evidence already in the literature implicated dynorphin: the gene for dynorphin contains CREB-sensitive response elements (28), and both in vitro and in vivo studies indicated that CREB regulates expression of the gene (prodynorphin) encoding the peptide precursor of dynorphin (29, 30). In addition, it was already known that kappa agonists can cause aversive and depressive-like signs (including dysphoria) in humans (31) and rodents (32). We found that viral vector-mediated elevations in CREB function within the NAc caused increased prodynorphin expression, whereas disruption of CREB function reduced it (14). This work suggested that the ability of CREB activation in the NAc to trigger aversive states could be related to increased transcription of dynorphin and subsequent elevations in kappa receptor activity in this brain region. This hypothesis was supported by a series of experiments demonstrating that intracerebroventricular (ICV) administration of the kappa antagonist nor-binaltorphimine (nor-BNI) blocked the aversive-like effects of elevated CREB on cocaine reward (14) as well as depressive-like behavior in the FST (26). Importantly, the effects of kappa antagonists are not limited to conditions in which CREB function has been artificially boosted using viral vectors: nor-BNI and related derivatives (GNTI, ANTI) have antidepressant-like effects of their own in the FST (16), a test well documented in its ability to identify in rats treatments with clinical antidepressant efficacy in humans (33). The antidepressant-like effects of kappa antagonists has since been confirmed by other researchers, who have extended these finding to other protocols (34–36) and structurally dissimilar drugs (e.g., JDTic; 37).

22.2.2 Mechanisms

The mechanisms by which kappa antagonists produce antidepressant-like effects are not well understood. There is compelling evidence that alterations in DA function mediated in the NAc are involved, which is the basis for our working model (Fig. 22.2). A key difference between kappa receptors and mu and delta receptors is their anatomical localization in the NAc: kappa receptors are located primarily on the terminals of inputs to the mesolimbic system (38, 39), whereas mu and delta receptors are on the cell bodies of GABAergic medium spiny neurons or interneurons (40). Thus despite common (inhibitory) effects on signal transduction, stimulation of kappa receptors often causes effects opposite to those caused by stimulation of mu or delta receptors. For example, whereas mu and delta agonists increase extracellular concentrations of DA in the NAc (9, 41), kappa agonists decrease them (41, 42). These effects appear to be mediated, at least in part, within the NAc: microinfusions of kappa agonists into this region decrease local DA concentrations (43, 44), most likely by stimulating presynaptic kappa receptors that inhibit DA release from ventral tegmental area (VTA) neurons (38). Thus CREB-mediated increases in dynorphin expression within the NAc could result in local decreases in DA release, which triggers signs of depression (particularly those reflecting altered motivation). Although these effects might occur predominately within the NAc, kappa ligands could also have effects within other parts of the reward circuitry where kappa receptors are expressed, such as the VTA and prefrontal cortex (PFC) (39, 45). According to this model, kappa antagonists have antidepressant effects because they block the consequences of CREB-mediated upregulation of dynorphin function in the NAc by blocking kappa receptors in the NAc (or other regions), leading to restored function of the mesolimbic DA system. Another possibility – which is not mutually exclusive – is that kappa antagonists reduce activation of CREB in the NAc, which normally contributes to elevated dynorphin function. There is

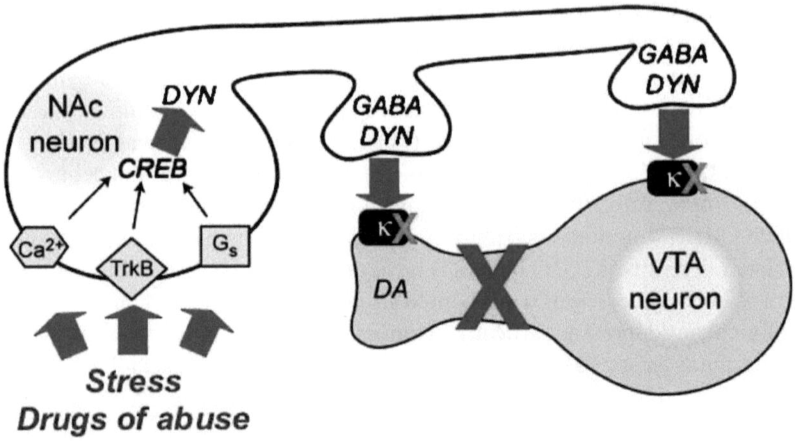

Fig. 22.2 Highly simplified hypothetical scheme by which CREB induction of dynorphin (*DYN*) in the nucleus accumbens (*NAc*) contributes to key symptoms of depression. CREB is activated by D_1 dopamine (*DA*) receptors (through activation of the cAMP pathway) or by Ca^{2+}- or TrkB-regulated signal transduction pathways (see 101), which leads to increased expression of DYN. In turn, DYN feeds back on kappa receptors located on the terminals and cell bodies of ventral tegmental area (*VTA*) DA neurons. Stimulation of these kappa receptors inhibits the VTA neurons (large red X), which may contribute to anhedonia and related symptoms of depression. This outcome may be beneficial in the treatment of some abnormal states, such as types of mania. Antagonists of kappa receptors (small green X's) may thus block the consequences of CREB-induced increases in DYN activity, and exert antidepressant activity in some individuals. Artwork by Christine Konradi (*see Color Plates*)

evidence that antidepressants may, in fact, interfere with CREB function under some circumstances. A variety of antidepressants decrease CREB phosphorylation and CREB-mediated gene transcription in certain in vitro preparations (46). In addition, chronic antidepressant treatment can increase expression of cAMP phosphodiesterases (PDEs) – which metabolize cAMP – in the NAc (47). These findings raise the possibility that molecular processes involving CREB and kappa receptors in the NAc play an underappreciated role in the therapeutic actions of many types of antidepressants. Still another possibility is that kappa antagonists work through yet-to-be described interactions with brain 5HT or NE systems, which appear to be critically involved in the therapeutic effects of SSRIs and TCAs, the most widely prescribed current and older classes of antidepressant drugs.

22.2.3 Complexities

The possibility that the antidepressant-like effects of kappa antagonists are related to an ability to boost the function of brain DA systems adds an additional level of complexity to the development of these drugs for mood disorders. Virtually all addictive drugs facilitate brain DA function (2, 48), an effect often associated with their abuse liability. Standard antidepressant drugs have no abuse liability, so kappa antagonists would not represent an improved therapeutic approach if they posed a risk for misuse. To address the possibility that kappa antagonists have properties that might lead to misuse – or would cause mania-like effects – we examined their effects in the intracranial self-stimulation (ICSS) test, which identifies drugs with reward-altering actions (49). We observed that the selective kappa antagonist ANTI does not alter ICSS behavior at doses eight times higher than those with antidepressant effects in the FST (50), but we have since extended this finding to doses 32 times higher (W.A. Carlezon Jr., unpublished observations). These data suggest that although kappa antagonists may be able to reverse reductions in DA caused by increased kappa tone, they have a limited ability to enhance DA function to the degree that would make the drugs rewarding, or produce mania-like states. Indeed, the effects of kappa antagonists on DA appear to be modest: direct administration of kappa antagonists into the NAc increases local concentrations of DA to ~175% of baseline (51), whereas psychostimulants such as cocaine and amphetamine can cause increases ranging from 500 to 1,000% of baseline (48, 51). Modest increases in DA concentrations within the NAc may be sufficient to cause antidepressant-like effects in the FST without producing rewarding effects. As such, it appears unlikely that kappa antagonists would have abuse liability, at least on their own. Another factor that complicates studies of kappa antagonists in these species is the long-time course of these agents: a single injection of these drugs can block the effects of kappa agonists for as long as 56 days (52). The reasons for this extraordinarily long (but reversible) time course are not understood; this issue is addressed in more detail in another chapter of this edition (53). Regardless, such a long time course can make preclinical studies difficult to design, and it is less than optimal for studies in humans, at least at the early stages of drug development.

22.2.4 Clinical Studies

As yet, the antidepressant-like effects of kappa antagonists have not been examined thoroughly in nonhuman primates or humans. Studies in nonhuman primates are complicated by the fact that there are no widely-accepted models of depression or antidepressant efficacy in this species. Instead, kappa antagonists have been examined in drug self-administration studies in monkeys, and mainly in the context of their ability to block the effects of kappa agonists (54, 55). Selective kappa antagonists have not been examined in humans, although mixed agents with some ability to disrupt kappa function have been tested. One example is buprenorphine, which reportedly has antidepressant effects in certain individuals (56). Buprenorphine is often described as a mixed mu agonist/kappa antagonist (56), although there is compelling evidence that it is actually a kappa partial agonist: it causes low efficacy stimulation of $[^{35}S]GTP\text{-}\gamma S$ in cells engineered to express human kappa receptors, whereas true antagonists (e.g., nor-BNI) are without effect in this assay (57). Thus although reports that buprenorphine can have antidepressant effects in humans are encouraging, it is difficult at this time to attribute them to antagonism of kappa receptors, considering the complex pharmacologic profile of this drug. Similarly, the mixed mu/kappa antagonists naltrexone and nalmephene have been used in clinical trials of substance use and impulse disorders, which have a high degree of comorbid depression. At human opioid receptors, naltrexone and nalmephene have roughly equal binding affinity for mu and kappa receptors (58, 59); nalmephene may be a weak partial agonist at the kappa receptor (60). While naltrexone is FDA approved for use in alcohol dependence and nalmephene appears to have some efficacy for pathological gambling (61), neither has been explicitly tested for depression, and the interpretation of their effects on depression would be made difficult by their dual actions at two opioid receptors. At the present time, we are unaware of any active or planned clinical trials in which more selective kappa antagonists are being studied.

22.2.5 Summary

The idea that kappa antagonists might be useful for the treatment of depression has emerged from basic research demonstrating that stress or repeated exposure to drugs of abuse – two stimuli that can trigger depressive conditions in humans – can activate endogenous dynorphin function. Considering that many treatments for mood disorders were discovered serendipitously over a half century ago (62), the development of kappa antagonists for depressive conditions would represent a rare example of rational drug design in psychiatry. In rodent models, kappa antagonists block signs of anhedonia, dysphoria, and despair. The mechanisms that mediate these effects are not clear, but they may depend upon secondary alterations in the function of brain DA systems. Fortunately, despite actions on brain DA systems, currently available evidence suggests that kappa antagonists do not cause behavioral effects that normally accompany drugs with abuse potential. A great deal of additional work is required to further characterize these agents, with particular emphasis on how chronic kappa receptor blockade would ultimately affect behavior. Studies in rodents, nonhuman primates, and humans are complicated by the fact that all currently available selective kappa antagonists appear to have exceptionally long durations of action for reasons that are not understood (see 53). The development of new classes of kappa antagonists with shorter durations of action is needed, because these ligands would enable the design of studies to address all of these issues.

22.3 Kappa Agonists

22.3.1 History

Initially it was believed that kappa agonists could be utilized as nonaddictive analgesics, since these drugs had antinociceptive properties but lower abuse potential than mu agonists (63). Pentazocine, which is a relatively specific kappa partial agonist (being nearly a full agonist at kappa receptors and having low affinity for mu receptors, at which it is mostly an antagonist; 58) is still clinically available. It is used predominantly for obstetrical pain, where its minimal effects to depress respiration compared to mu agonists is valued. Administration of more selective kappa agonists (such as MR2033) elicited unwanted side effects in humans characterized by derealization and depersonalization and, sometimes, the emergence of depressive-like signs, including dysphoria (31). These observations precluded further development of these agents for clinical use. Trials of kappa agonists for psychiatric conditions have been very limited, and they have shown only mixed success: the kappa agonist spiradoline produced sedation and decreased the frequency of tics in individuals with Tourette's Syndrome at low doses but produced altered perception and increased dysphoria at high doses (64). In clinical studies of substance abusers, the kappa agonist enadoline was observed to reduce some of the effects of cocaine, but it, too, caused sedation, depersonalization, visual distortions, confusion and, at high doses, paranoia (65, 66). Perhaps the most interesting evidence on the effects of kappa agonists in humans comes from experience with salvinorin A, the active component of the plant *Salvia divinorum*, used by the Mazatec peoples of Oaxaca, Mexico, in spiritual and healing rituals. Salvinorin A appears to be the most selective and potent kappa agonist known (67). Its effects are highly situation dependent (68), but it can induce perceptual distortions, depersonalization, and feelings of spatiotemporal dislocation (69, 70). Occasional reports suggest it can cause not only derealization, but euphoria, rather than dysphoria (71), and it is used recreationally by some, although it does not appear to be addictive (i.e., used compulsively; Mendelson et al., manuscript submitted). Of course, humans will take other substances which are aversive in other species, such as lysergic acid diethylamide (LSD). Nonetheless, despite evidence that kappa agonists should lower mood, there are case reports of salvinorin A leading to improved mood and even having antidepressant effects (72). Until recently, however, there has been little consideration of the potential kappa agonists might have for the treatment of mood disorders.

The idea that kappa agonists could play an important role in the study and treatment of mood disorders is derived from two sets of preclinical studies. Antipsychotic drugs are all potent antimanic agents and all induce activation of similar populations of cells in the NAc (as well as in medial thalamic nuclei and central nucleus of the amygdala) (73), regions that may be responsible for mediating many of the symptoms of bipolar disorder. While these studies were performed in rats, similar regional effects of antipsychotic drugs may occur in human subjects (74). Double label immunohistochemistry identified the cells responding to antimanic/antipsychotic drugs as dynorphinergic/GABAergic neurons (15), implying that antipsychotic drugs may increase dynorphin release, leading to an antimanic or mood-lowering effect. The mechanism of this activation of dynorphinergic cells is likely inhibition of multiple monoamine receptors at which antipsychotic drugs are potent antagonists (75).

In parallel, the effects of kappa agonists were studied as comparison drugs in experiments in rats designed to evaluate the antidepressant-like effects of kappa antagonists. These studies demonstrated that U69,593 (a selective kappa agonist) increases immobility behavior in the FST (16). This effect is identical to that caused by elevation of CREB in the NAc (26), drug withdrawal (76), or administration of antimanic agents (77), and opposite of that caused by standard antidepressant drugs. As such, elevated immobility behavior in the FST is a putative indicator of prodepressive or mood-lowering effects. U69,593 also elevated ICSS thresholds (50), an effect similar to that caused by drug withdrawal (78) and antimanic agents (77), and thus is a putative indicator of motivational deficits that often accompany affective disorders. An identical pattern of effects was caused by salvinorin A (42). When considered together, these molecular and behavior studies are consistent with the conclusion that stimulation of brain kappa receptors causes behavioral signs that closely resemble those that characterize depressive disorders.

22.3.2 Mechanisms

Kappa receptors are located throughout the brain (40), in areas often associated with motivation and emotion, including the mesocorticolimbic system, PFC, amygdala, and septum. All of these areas have been associated with motivation and emotion, and it is easy to imagine that each plays a role in the regulation of normal (and abnormal) mood and affective states (see 62). As described above, our work has tended to focus on the mesolimbic DA system, because of our historical interest in its role in motivated behavior. Kappa receptors are located in both ends of the mesolimbic DA system – in its cell body region within the VTA, and its terminal region within the NAc (38, 45) – and stimulation of kappa receptors in either region decreases DA function. For example, administration of kappa agonists into the NAc decrease local DA concentrations (43, 44), most likely by stimulating presynaptic kappa receptors that inhibit DA release from VTA neurons (38). Kappa agonists also have VTA-dependent inhibitory effects on the mesolimbic DA neurons, and both direct and indirect circuits may contribute to drug-induced decreases in the function of this system (45, 79, 80). Future studies involving brain region-specific microinfusions will determine if stimulation of kappa receptors in these other brain areas synergize with – or detract from – the general prodepressive consequences of systemic administration of kappa agonists (16, 42, 50).

22.3.3 Complexities

Of course, the effects of kappa agonists are not limited to the mesolimbic DA system. They affect other pathways, including other neurotransmitter systems that may be important in regulating mood. Indeed, NE release is reduced by kappa agonists, as studied in rat synaptosomes (81) and rabbit hippocampal slices (82). In addition, effects on monoamine turnover may differ by brain region (83).

Although a decrease in DA neurotransmission, at least in limbic regions, is well documented as the immediate response to kappa agonists, less is known about the consequences of repeated or long term drug administration. In monkeys, single doses of kappa agonists reduce cocaine intake, but this effect wanes over time (84). Similarly, in the rat, acute administration of kappa agonists reduces the locomotor-stimulating effects of cocaine, although these same effects are increased after kappa agonists are given repeatedly and then withdrawn, suggesting the development of tolerance (E.H. Chartoff, B.M. Cohen, and W.A. Carlezon Jr., unpublished observations).

Few kappa agonists are entirely selective and full agonists at kappa receptors. Thus the often used U50,488 and U69,593 are not as selective nor do they cause as full an activation of kappa receptors as salvinorin A (85). Also, both U50,488 and U69,593 cause more kappa receptor internalization than salvinorin A (86) or its derivatives (e.g., herkinorin; 87). Therefore, each of these drugs may have different effects with long term administration.

There are sex, strain, and age differences in response to kappa agonists noted even within rats (88, 89), and caution needs to be applied in generalizing between results in rodents, monkeys, and humans. Receptor densities differ by species (90), as does turnover of DA in response to kappa agonists (91, 92) and phosphorylation and desensitization of kappa receptors (93).

Lastly, kappa receptors may not exist as monomers in tissue. Rather, they may often reside in receptor complexes as heterodimers or oligomers. This association may contribute to differences in effects of kappa agonists by region, species, and over time of treatment as receptor associations change (see 94).

22.3.4 Clinical Studies

Under some circumstances, the ability of kappa απηα agonists to decrease DA function in the basal forebrain might have clinical utility. The most obvious indication to us was treatment of mania. This speculation arose in part from our own observation that antipsychotic drugs – which are frequently used to treat mania – activate dynorphinergic neurons (15). Also, although salvinorin A and other kappa agonists can produce psychotomimetic effects under some conditions (especially at high doses) (67, 85, 95), it is conceivable that administration of a derivative or related compound under more carefully controlled conditions might be useful for the treatment of disorders characterized by hyperfunction of DA systems (e.g., mania). In this regard, it is notable that the effects of kappa agonists on DA turnover in the mesolimbic system are state-dependent, with reduction of release greatest when DA cells are most active (96), as they may be in mania or mood elevation.

We tested the possibility that kappa agonists might have mood normalizing effects for patients in manic episodes of bipolar disorder. The relative kappa specific agents spiradoline (used in clinical trials in Tourette's syndrome; 64) and enadoline (used in trials of subjects with substance abuse; 65, 66) were not available. Salvinorin A was not initially chosen for study because it is very short acting and difficult to administer: it is often used by means that achieve absorption from the buccal or nasal mucosa, and is apparently not reliably absorbed following ingestion. Rather, we performed our first studies with commercially available pentazocine, which has been safely given to patients and is approved for pain relief. Pentazocine is nearly a full agonist at kappa receptors, with lower affinity for mu receptors, at which it is predominantly an antagonist. In an initial open-label study in ten patients with mania, two sequential doses of pentazocine (50 mg, as often used for pain) given 2 h apart, reduced manic symptoms transiently but substantially and significantly in each subject without causing notable sedation or affecting concomitant psychotic symptoms (Cohen and Murphy, manuscript submitted). While preliminary, these results are consistent with the implications of studies in rats, which suggest that kappa agonists may decrease mood, especially when mood is abnormally elevated.

22.3.5 Summary

The development of kappa agonists as possible antimanic agents was suggested by the results of parallel studies in rats, one of which observed that clinically used antimanic agents increase the activity of dynorphinergic neurons, while the other directly documented mood lowering effects of kappa agonists. Further support for this research direction comes from evidence in human subjects that both naturally occurring and synthetic kappa agonists can lower mood with acute dosing. Against this background, the finding that pentazocine may reduce manic symptoms is promising. However, these results should not be taken to imply that pentazocine or other kappa agonists will be useful therapeutic agents for the treatment of mania. Much more work is needed, including controlled blinded trials with repeated dosing to gauge the tolerability and longer-term efficacy of this or similar agents. As with kappa antagonists, the development of highly selective, orally active kappa agonists, with half-life durations suitable for clinical use, would be valuable. Work is underway at this and other sites to produce such agents (see 53).

While most synthetic chemistry has been devoted to developing kappa receptor-specific agonists and antagonists, many agents are or will turn out to be partial agonists or mixed agonist/antagonists. These agents may also be clinically useful, especially in the treatment of bipolar disorder, as they may produce a relatively constant signal through kappa receptors, thereby helping to restrict to a limited range the activity of DA and other monoamine neurons thought to be responsible for regulation of mood. Thus, it is possible that partial agonists will have mood stabilizing, rather than simply antidepressant or antimanic, effects in patients with bipolar disorder.

22.4 The Future of Kappa Ligands in the Study and Treatment of Mood Disorders

Psychiatry needs drugs that are safer, act faster, and have fewer side effects. Virtually all existing medications for psychiatric disorders are based on serendipitous discoveries made decades ago (see 97–100). Despite great efforts, the field has not succeeded in developing fundamentally new treatments – with distinct mechanisms of action – for mood disorders. One reason for this state of affairs is that much research focuses on the mechanisms by which currently available psychotropic drugs act, rather than on the abnormal states that are treated by these drugs. Indeed, much of what is believed about the molecular basis of mood disorders is based upon our understanding of the most prominent and immediate neurochemical actions of standard psychotropic medications (62). As such, an improved understanding of normal brain function and the pathophysiology of abnormal mood should hasten the development of new generations of innovative treatments.

In preclinical studies of how the brain adapts to experience, we have discovered that environmental stimuli such as stress and drugs of abuse activate CREB in the NAc. Molecular manipulations that mimic this effect produce a variety of depressive-like behaviors. Although CREB regulates many genes (101), we have found that CREB-mediated increases in dynorphin function within the NAc contribute importantly to the development and expression of depressive-like signs. Elevated dynorphin tone, in turn, may cause depressive-like signs by decreasing the activity of the mesolimbic DA system. Decreased DA function in the NAc has long been presumed to contribute to core depressive symptoms, including anhedonia (3) (Fig. 22.3; 102). Clearly, kappa mediated alterations in the function of other neurotransmitter systems (including NE and 5HT) may also contribute to these effects through yet-to-be identified mechanisms. In addition, CREB may have other molecular actions that are independent of dynorphin and kappa receptors. As only one example, elevated CREB expression in NAc shell increases firing rates of local medium spiny neurons, whereas expression of mCREB decreases them (103). These effects may be due to regulation, by CREB, of the expression or function of channels that control ion flux. When considered together, all of these effects are broadly consistent with the very simple working hypothesis that treatments that reduce the excitability of the NAc are rewarding (or antidepressant), whereas treatments that increase its excitability are aversive (or prodepressant) (104–106). Rigorous tests of this hypothesis will have important implications for our understanding of the biological basis of motivation, which is dysregulated in mood disorders.

Our ability to test these working hypotheses more rigorously in animal models and humans will be facilitated by the discovery and development of improved kappa ligands. Considering the specificity of salvinorin A for kappa receptors, one approach is to use medicinal chemistry techniques to modify this molecule

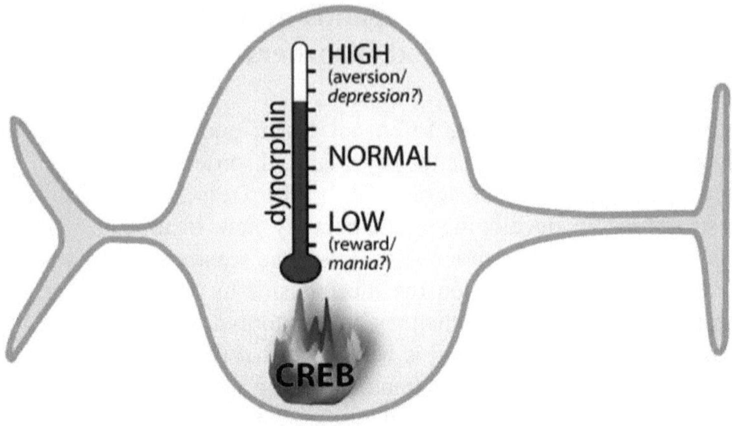

Fig. 22.3 Schematic depiction of how CREB activity in the nucleus accumbens (*NAc*) shell may act as a "hedonic thermostat." Elevated expression of CREB increases transcription of dynorphin, which in turn causes aversive and/or depressive-like states (including dysphoria and anhedonia). Conversely, disruption of CREB activity decreases dynorphin transcription, enabling hedonic processes. Artwork by Christine Konradi; reprinted from Carlezon and Konradi (102), with permission (*see Color Plates*)

with the goal of discovering ligands with characteristics that make them more suitable for clinical trials. For example, it would be useful to have kappa agonists that possess the selectivity of salvinorin A for kappa receptors together with a longer duration of action. Salvinorin A derivatives with reduced propensity to cause receptor internalization (e.g., 87) might have longer time courses and less drug tolerance. Similarly, clinical studies of kappa antagonists appear to depend on the discovery of new ligands that do not have effects that change over time or endure for weeks (or months) after a single injection. The advent of high-throughput small molecule screening techniques provides a hypothesis-free complement to our work with salvinorin A derivatives. Regardless of whether kappa ligands are ever utilized in the treatment of mood disorders, the study of endogenous kappa opioid systems has led to work that has increased our understanding of some of molecular events in the brain that cause dysregulation of mood states. As has been the case with other disease states, understanding how the organs of the body function normally can be the first step toward designing innovative treatments that prevent or reverse the pathophysiology underlying these debilitating disorders.

Acknowledgments Supported by the National Institute of Mental Health (MH63266, to WC), the Stanley Medical Research Institute (to BMC), and donations from John A. Kaneb.

References

1. Ritz MC, Lamb RJ, Goldberg SR, Kuhar MJ (1987) Cocaine receptors on dopamine transporters are related to self-administration of cocaine. Science 237: 1219–1223.
2. Wise RA, Bozarth MA (1987) A psychomotor stimulant theory of addiction. Psych Rev 94: 469–492.
3. Wise RA (1982) Neuroleptics and operant behavior: the anhedonia hypothesis. Behav Brain Sci 5: 39–87.
4. Frazer A (1997) Pharmacology of antidepressants. J. Clin. Psychopharmacol 17 [Suppl 1]: 2S–18S.
5. Koch S, Perry KW, Nelson DL, Conway RG, Threlkeld PG, Bymaster FP (2002) R-fluoxetine increases extracellular DA, NE, as well as 5-HT in rat prefrontal cortex and hypothalamus: an in vivo microdialysis and receptor binding study. Neuropsychopharmacol 27: 949–959.
6. Fawcett J, Barkin RL (1997) Efficacy issues with antidepressants. J. Clin. Psychiatry 58: 32–39.
7. Caspi A, Sugden K, Moffitt TE, Taylor A, Craig IW, Harrington H, McClay J, Mill J, Martin J, Braithwaite A, Poulton R (2003) Influence of life stress on depression: moderation by a polymorphism in the 5-HTT gene. Science 301: 386–389.
8. Vergne DE, Nemeroff CB (2006) The interaction of serotonin transporter gene polymorphisms and early adverse life events on vulnerability for major depression. Curr Psychiatr Rep 8: 452–457.
9. Leone P, Pocock D, Wise RA (1991) Morphine-dopamine interaction: ventral tegmental morphine increases nucleus accumbens dopamine release. Pharmacol Biochem Behav 39: 469–472.
10. Johnson SW, North RA (1992) Opioids excite dopamine neurons by hyperpolarization of local interneurons. J Neurosci 12: 483–488.
11. Snyder SH, Pasternak GW (2003) Historical review: opioid receptors. Trends Pharmacol Sci 24: 198–205.
12. Olds ME (1982) Reinforcing effects of morphine in the nucleus accumbens. Brain Res 237: 429–440.
13. Martin WR, Eades CG, Thompson JA, Huppler RE, Gilbert PE (1976) The effects of morphine- and nalorphine-like drugs in the nondependent and morphine-dependent chronic spinal dog. J Pharmacol Exp Ther 197: 517–532.
14. Carlezon WA Jr, Thome J, Olson VG, Lane-Ladd SB, Brodkin ES, Hiroi N, Duman RS, Neve RL, Nestler EJ (1998) Regulation of cocaine reward by CREB. Science 282: 2272–2275.
15. Ma J, Ye N, Lange N, Cohen BM (2003) Dynorphinergic GABA neurons are a target of both typical and atypical antipsychotic drugs in the nucleus accumbens shell, central amygdaloid nucleus and thalamic central medial nucleus. Neuroscience 121: 991–998.
16. Mague SD, Pliakas AM, Todtenkopf MS, Tomasiewicz HC, Zhang Y, Stevens WC Jr, Jones RM, Portoghese PS, Carlezon WA Jr (2003) Antidepressant-like effects of κ-opioid receptor antagonists in the forced swim test in rats. J Pharmacol Exp Ther 305: 323–330.
17. Chavkin C, James IF, Goldstein A (1982) Dynorphin is a specific endogenous ligand of the kappa opioid receptor. Science 215: 413–415.
18. Han JS, Xie CW (1982) Dynorphin: potent analgesic effect in spinal cord of the rat. Life Sci 31: 1781–1784.
19. Han JS, Xie GX, Goldstein A (1984) Analgesia induced by intrathecal injection of dynorphin B in the rat. Life Sci 34: 1573–1579.
20. Pazos A, Tristan C, Florez J (1983) A comparative study of the respiratory depressant and analgesic effects of bremazocine, a kappa-agonist. Life Sci 33 [Suppl 1]: 579–581.
21. Portoghese PS, Lipkowski AW, Takemori AE (1987) Binaltorphimine and nor-binaltorphimine, potent and selective kappa-opioid receptor antagonists. Life Sci 40: 1287–1292.
22. Faden AI, Takemori AE, Portoghese PS (1987) Kappa-selective opiate antagonist norbinaltorphimine improves outcome after traumatic spinal cord injury in rats. Cent Nerv Syst Trauma 4: 227–237.

23. Vink R, Portoghese PS, Faden AI (1991) kappa-Opioid antagonist improves cellular bioenergetics and recovery after traumatic brain injury. Am J Physiol 261: R1527–R1532.
24. Carr KD, Bak TH, Simon EJ, Portoghese PS (1989) Effects of the selective kappa opioid antagonist, nor-binaltorphimine, on electrically-elicited feeding in the rat. Life Sci 45: 1787–1792.
25. Turgeon SM, Pollack AE, Fink JS (1997) Enhanced CREB phosphorylation and changes in c-Fos and FRA expression in striatum accompany amphetamine sensitization. Brain Res 749: 120–126.
26. Pliakas AM, Carlson R, Neve RL, Konradi C, Nestler EJ, Carlezon WA Jr (2001) Altered responsiveness to cocaine and increased immobility in the forced swim test associated with elevated cAMP response element binding protein expression in nucleus accumbens. J Neurosci 21: 7397–7403.
27. Kendler KS, Karkowski LM, Prescott CA (1999) Causal relationship between stressful life events and the onset of major depression. Am J Psychiatry 156: 837–841.
28. Douglass J, McKinzie AA, Pollock KM (1994) Identification of multiple DNA elements regulating basal and protein kinase A-induced transcriptional expression of the rat prodynorphin gene. Mol Endocrinol 8: 333–344.
29. Cole RL, Konradi C, Douglass J, Hyman SE (1995) Neuronal adaptation to amphetamine and dopamine: molecular mechanisms of prodynorphin gene regulation in rat striatum. Neuron 14: 813–823.
30. Daunais JB, Roberts DC, McGinty JF (1995) Short-term cocaine self administration alters striatal gene expression. Brain Res Bull 37: 523–527.
31. Pfeiffer A, Brantl V, Herz A, Emrich HM (1986) Psychotomimesis mediated by kappa opiate receptors. Science 233: 774–776.
32. Bals-Kubik R, Herz A, Shippenberg TS (1989) Evidence that the aversive effects of μ-opioid antagonists and κ-agonists are centrally mediated. Psychopharmacology 98: 203–20.
33. Willner P (1984) The validity of animal models of depression. Psychopharmacology 83: 1–16.
34. Newton SS, Thome J, Wallace T, Shirayama Y, Dow A, Schlesinger L, Duman CH, Sakai N, Chen JS, Neve R, Nestler EJ, Duman RS (2002) Inhibition of CREB or dynorphin in the nucleus accumbens produces an antidepressant-like effect. J Neurosci 22: 10883–10890.
35. McLaughlin JP, Marton-Popovici M, Chavkin C (2003) κ. opioid receptor antagonism and prodynorphin gene disruption block stress-induced behavioral responses. J Neurosci 23: 5674–5683.
36. Shirayama Y, Ishida H, Iwata M, Hazama GI, Kawahara R, Duman RS (2004) Stress increases dynorphin immunoreactivity in limbic brain regions and dynorphin antagonism produces antidepressant-like effects. J Neurochem 90: 1258–1268.
37. Beardsley PM, Howard JL, Shelton KL, Carroll FI (2005) Differential effects of the novel kappa opioid receptor antagonist, JDTic, on reinstatement of cocaine-seeking induced by footshock stressors vs cocaine primes and its antidepressant-like effects in rats. Psychopharmacology 183: 118–126.
38. Svingos AL, Colago EE, Pickel VM (1999) Cellular sites for dynorphin activation of kappa-opioid receptors in the rat nucleus accumbens shell. J Neurosci 19: 1804–1813.
39. Svingos AL, Colago EE (2002) Kappa-Opioid and NMDA glutamate receptors are differentially targeted within rat medial prefrontal cortex. Brain Res 946: 262–271.
40. Mansour A, Watson SJ, Akil H (1995) Opioid receptors: past, present and future. Trends Neurosci 18: 69–70.
41. Devine DP, Leone P, Pocock D, Wise RA (1993) Differential involvement of ventral tegmental mu, delta and kappa opioid receptors in modulation of basal mesolimbic dopamine release: in vivo microdialysis studies. J Pharmacol Exp Ther 266: 1236–1246.
42. Carlezon WA Jr, Beguin C, DiNieri J, Baumann MH, Richards M, Todtenkopf MS, Rothman RB, Ma Z, Lee DY, Cohen BM (2006) Depressive-like effects of the κ-opioid receptor agonist salvinorin A on behavior and neurochemistry in rats. J Pharmacol Exp Ther 314: 440–447.
43. Donzanti BA, Althaus JS, Payson MM, Von Voigtlander PF (1992) Kappa agonist-induced reduction in dopamine release: site of action and tolerance. Res Commun Chem Pathol Pharmacol 78: 193–210.

44. Spanagel R, Herz A, Shippenberg TS (1992) Opposing tonically active endogenous opioid systems modulate the mesolimbic dopaminergic pathway. Proc Natl Acad Sci USA 89: 2046–2050.
45. Margolis EB, Hjelmstad GO, Bonci A, Fields HL (2003) κ-.opioid agonists directly inhibit midbrain dopaminergic neurons. J Neurosci 23: 9981–9986.
46. Schwaninger M, Schofl C, Blume R, Rosswig L, Knepel W (1995) Inhibition by antidepressant drugs of cyclic AMP response element binding protein/cyclic AMP response element-directed gene transcription. Mol Pharmacol 47: 1112–1118.
47. Takahashi M, Terwilliger R, Lane C, Menzes PS, Conti M, Duman RS (1998) Chronic antidepressant administration increases the expression of cAMP phosphodiesterase 4A and 4B isoforms. J Neurosci 19: 610–618.
48. Di Chiara G, Imperato A (1988) Drugs abused by humans preferentially increase synaptic dopamine concentrations in the mesolimbic system of freely moving rats. Proc Natl Acad Sci USA 85: 5274–5278.
49. Wise RA (1996) Addictive drugs and brain stimulation reward. Ann Rev Neurosci 19: 319–340.
50. Todtenkopf MS, Marcus JF, Portoghese PS, Carlezon WA Jr (2004) Effects of κ-opioid receptor ligands on intracranial self-stimulation in rats. Psychopharmacol 172: 463–470.
51. Maisonneuve IM, Archer S, Glick SD (1994) U50,488, a κ-opioid receptor agonist, attenuates cocaine-induced increases in extracellular dopamine in the nucleus accumbens of rats. Neurosci Lett 181: 57–60.
52. Spanagel R, Shippenberg TS (1993) Modulation of morphine-induced sensitization by endogenous kappa opioid systems in the rat. Neurosci Lett 153: 232–236.
53. Beguin C, Cohen BM (2007) Medicinal chemistry of kappa opioid receptor antagonists. In: Opioid Receptors and Antagonists: From Bench to Clinic. R.L. Dean III, E.J. Bilsky, and S.S. Negus III (eds), Humana Press, Totowa, NJ.
54. Negus SS, Mello NK, Linsenmayer DC, Jones RM, Portoghese PS (2002) Kappa opioid antagonist effects of the novel kappa antagonist 5′-guanidinonaltrindole (GNTI) in an assay of schedule-controlled behavior in rhesus monkeys. Psychopharmacology 163: 412–419.
55. Negus SS (2004) Effects of the kappa opioid agonist U50,488 and the kappa opioid antagonist nor-binaltorphimine on choice between cocaine and food in rhesus monkeys. Psychopharmacology 176: 204–213.
56. Bodkin JA, Zornberg GL, Lukas SE, Cole JO (1995) Buprenorphine treatment of refractory depression. J Clin Psychopharmacol 15: 49–57.
57. Zhu J, Luo LY, Li JG, Chen C, Liu-Chen LY (1997) Activation of the cloned human kappa opioid receptor by agonists enhances [35S]GTPgammaS binding to membranes: determination of potencies and efficacies of ligands. J Pharmacol Exp Ther 282: 676–684.
58. Toll L, Berzetal-Gurske IP, Polgar WE, Brandt SR, Adapa D, Rodrigues L, Schwarts RW, Haggart D, O'Brien A, White A, Kennedy JM, Craymer K, Farrington L, Auh JS (1997) Standard binding and functional assays related to medications development division testing for potential cocaine and opiate narcotic treatment medications. NIDA Res Mono 178: 440–466.
59. Bart G, Schluger JH, Borg L, Ho A, Bidlack JM, Kreek MJ (2005) Nalmefene induced elevation in serum prolactin in normal human volunteers: partial kappa opioid agonist activity? Neuropsychopharmacology 30: 2254–2262.
60. Remmers AE, Clark MJ, Mansour A, Akil H, Woods JH, Medzihradsky F (1999) Opioid efficacy in a C6 glioma cell line stably expressing the human kappa opioid receptor. J Pharmacol Exp Ther 288: 827–833.
61. Grant JE, Potenza MC, Hollander E, Cunningham-Williams R, Nurminen T, Smits G, Kallio A (2006) Multicenter investagation of the opioid antagonist nalmefene in the treatment of pathological gambling. Am J Psychiatry 163: 303–312.
62. Nestler EJ, Carlezon WA Jr (2006) The mesolimbic dopamine reward circuit in depression. Biol Psychiatry 59: 1151–1159.

63. Fraser HF, Rosenberg DE (1964) Studies on the human addiction liability of 2′-hydroxy-5, 9-dimethyl-2-(3,3-dimethylally)-6, 7-benzomorphan (WIN 20, 228): a weak narcotic antagonist. J Pharmacol Exp Ther 143: 149–156.
64. Chappell PB, Leckman JF, Scahill LD, Hardin MT, Anderson G, Cohen DJ (1993) Neuroendocrine and behavioral effects of the selective kappa agonist spiradoline in Tourette's syndrome: a pilot study. Psychiatry Res 47: 267–280.
65. Walsh SL, Geter-Douglas B, Strain EC, Bigelow GE (2001a) Enadoline and butorphanol: evaluation of kappa-agonists on cocaine pharmacodynamics and cocaine self-administration in humans. J Pharmacol Exp Ther 299: 147–158.
66. Walsh SL, Strain EC, Abreu ME, Bigelow GE (2001b) Enadoline, a selective kappa opioid agonist: comparison with butorphanol and hydromorphone in humans. Psychopharmacology 157: 151–162.
67. Roth BL, Baner K, Westkaemper R, Siebert D, Rice KC, Steinberg S, Ernsberger P, Rothman RB (2002) Salvinorin A: a potent naturally occurring nonnitrogenous kappa opioid selective agonist. Proc Natl Acad Sci USA 99: 11934–11939.
68. Valdes LJ 3rd (1994) Salvia divinorum and the unique diterpene hallucinogen, alvinorin (divinorin) A. J Psychoactive Drugs 26: 277–283.
69. Siebert DJ (1994) Salvia divinorum and salvinorin A: new pharmacologic findings. J Ethnopharmacology 43: 53–56.
70. Yan F, Roth BL (2004) Salvinorin A: a novel and highly selective kappa-opioid receptor agonist. Life Sci 75: 2615–2619.
71. Gonzalez D, Riba J, Bouso JC, Gomes-Jarabo G, Barbanoj MJ (2006) Pattern of use and subjective effects of salvia divinorum among recreational users. Drug Alcohol Depend 85: 157–162.
72. Hanes K (2003) Salvia divinorum: clinical and research potential. Maps xiii(1): 18–20.
73. Cohen BM, Wan W, Froimowitz MP, Ennulat DJ, Cherkerzian S, Konieczna H (1998) Activation of midline thalamic nuclei by antipsychotic drugs. Psychopharmacology 135: 37–43.
74. Cohen BM, Yurgelun-Todd D (2001) Alterations of thalamic activity in schizophrenia and in response to antipsychotic drugs: studies in the legacy of Seymour S. Kety. Neuropsychopharmacol 25: 305–312.
75. Ma J, Ye N, Cohen BM (2006) Expression of noradrenergic α1, serotoninergic 5HT2a and dopaminergic D2 receptors on neurons activated by typical and atypical antipsychotic drugs. Prog Neuropsychopharmacol Biol Psychiatry 30: 647–657.
76. Cryan JF, Markou A, Lucki I (2002) Assessing antidepressant activity in rodents: recent developments and future needs. Trends Pharmacol Sci 23: 238–245.
77. Tomasiewicz HC, Mague SD, Cohen BM, Carlezon WA Jr (2006) Behavioral effects of acute and sub-acute administration of lithium and valproic acid in rats. Brain Res 1093: 83–94.
78. Markou A, Hauger RL, Koob GF (1992) Desmethylimipramine attenuates cocaine withdrawal in rats. Psychopharmacology 109: 305–314.
79. Margolis EB, Hjelmstad GO, Bonci A, Fields HL (2005) Both kappa and mu opioid agonists inhibit glutamatergic input to ventral tegmental area neurons. J Neurophysiol 93: 3086–3093.
80. Margolis EB, Lock H, Chefer VI, Shippenberg TS, Hjelmstad GO, Fields HL (2006) Kappa opioids selectively control dopaminergic neurons projecting to the prefrontal cortex. Proc Natl Acad Sci USA 103: 2938–2942.
81. Adamson P, Mantzouridis T, Xiang J-Z, Hajimohammadreza I, Brammer MJ, Campbell IC (1989) α2-adrenergic, κ-opiate, and P1-purinergic autoreceptors have mutually antagonistic effects: a new regulatory mechanism? J Neurochem 53: 1077–1082.
82. Allgaier C, Daschmann B, Sieverling J, Hertting G (1989) Presynaptic kappa-opioid receptors on noradrenergic nerve terminals couple to G proteins and interact with the alpha 2-adrenoceptors. J Neurochem 53: 1629–1635.
83. Ford CP, Mark GP, Williams JT (2006) Properties and opioid inhibition of mesolimbic dopamine neurons vary according to target location. J Neurosci 26: 2788–2797.

84. Mello NK, Negus SS (1998) Effects of kappa opioid agonists on cocaine- and food-maintained responding by rhesus monkeys. J Pharmacol Exp Ther 286: 812–824.
85. Chavkin C, Sud S, Jin W, Stewart J, Zjawiony JK, Siebert DJ, Toth BA, Hufeisen SJ, Roth BL (2004) Salvinorin A, an active component of the hallucinogenic sage salvia divinorum is a highly efficacious kappa-opioid receptor agonist: structural and functional considerations. J Pharmacol Exp Ther 308: 1197–1203.
86. Wang Y, Tang K, Inan S, Siebert D, Holzgrabe U, Lee DY, Huang P, Li JG, Cowan A, Liu-Chen LY (2005) Comparison of pharmacological activities of three distinct kappa ligands (salvinorin A, TRK-820 and 3FLB) on kappa opioid receptors in vitro and their antipruritic and antinociceptive activities in vivo. J Pharmacol Exp Ther 312: 220–223.
87. Groer CE, Tidgewell K, Moyer RA, Harding WW, Rothman RB, Prisinzano TE, Bohn LM (2006) An opioid agonist that does not induce mu opioid receptor-arrestin interactions or receptor internalization. Mol Pharmacol, in press.
88. Barrett AC, Smith ES, Picker MJ (2002) Sex-related differences in mechanical nociception and antinociception produced by mu- and kappa-opioid receptor agonists in rats. Eur J Pharmacol 452: 163–173.
89. Smith MA, French AM (2002) Age-related differences in sensitivity to the antinociceptive effects of kappa opioids in adult male rats. Psychopharmacology 162: 255–264.
90. Mansour A, Khachaturian H, Lewis ME, Akil H, Watson SJ (1988) Anatomy of CNS opioid receptors. Trends Neurosci 11: 308–314.
91. Barber A, Gottschlich R (1997) Novel developments with selective, non-peptidic kappa-opioid receptor agonists. Expert Opin Investig Drugs 6: 1351–1368.
92. Fantegrossi WE, Kugle KM, Valdes LJ 3rd, Koreeda M, Woods JH (2005) Kappa-opioid receptor-mediated effects of the plant-derived hallucinogen, salvinorin A, on inverted screen performance in the mouse. Behav Pharmacol 16: 627–633.
93. Li J, Li J-G, Chen C, Zhang F, Liu-Chen L-Y (2002) Molecular basis of differences in (-)(trans)-3,4-Dichloro-N-methyl-N-[2-(1-pyrrolidiny)-cyclohexyl]benzeneacetamide-induced desensitzation and phosphorylation between human and rat κ-opioid receptors expressed in Chinese hamster ovary cells. Mol Pharmacol 61: 73–84.
94. Devi LA (2001) Heterodimerization of G-protein-coupled receptors: pharmacology, signaling and trafficking. Trends Pharmacol Sci 22(10): 532–537.
95. Bucheler R, Gleiter CH, Schwoerer P, Gaertner I (2005) Use of nonprohibited hallucinogenic plants: increasing relevance for public health? A case report and literature review on the consumption of Salvia divinorum (Diviner's Sage). Pharmacopsychiatry 38: 1–5.
96. Manzanares J, Lookingland KJ, Moore KE (1991) Kappa opioid receptor-mediated regulation of dopaminergic neurons in the rat brain. J Pharmacol Exp Ther 256: 500–505.
97. Ressler KJ, Nemeroff CB (2000) Role of serotonergic and noradrenergic systems in the pathophysiology of depression and anxiety disorders. Depress Anxiety 12 [Suppl 1]: 2–19.
98. Manji HK, Drevets WC, Charney DS (2001) The cellular neurobiology of depression. Nat Med 7: 541–547.
99. Nestler EJ, Gould E, Manji H, Buncan M, Duman RS, Greshenfeld HK, Hen R, Koester S, Lederhendler I, Meaney M, Robbins T, Winsky L, Zalcman S (2002) Preclinical models: status of basic research in depression. Biol Psychiatry 52: 503–528.
100. Morilak DA, Frazer A (2004) Antidepressants and brain monoaminergic systems: a dimensional approach to understanding their behavioural effects in depression and anxiety disorders. Int J Neuropsychopharmacol 7: 193–218.
101. Carlezon WA Jr, Duman RS, Nestler EJ (2005) The many faces of CREB. Trends Neurosci 28: 436–445.
102. Carlezon WA Jr, Konradi C (2004) Understanding the neurobiological consequences of early exposure to psychotropic drugs: linking behavior with molecules. Neuropharmacology 47 [Suppl 1]: 47–60.
103. Dong Y, Green T, Saal D, Marie H, Neve R, Nestler EJ, Malenka RC (2006) CREB modulates excitability of nucleus accumbens neurons. Nat Neurosci 9: 475–477.

104. Carlezon WA Jr, Wise RA (1996) Rewarding actions of phencyclidine and related drugs in nucleus accumbens shell and frontal cortex. J Neurosci 16: 3112–3122.
105. Carlezon WA Jr, Wise RA (2003) Unmet expectations: the brain minds. Nature Med 9: 15–16.
106. Todtenkopf MS, Parsegian A, Neve RL, Carlezon WA Jr (2006) Brain reward regulated by glutamate receptor subunits in the nucleus accumbens shell. J Neurosci 26: 11665–11669.

Chapter 23
Opioid Antagonists in the Treatment of Pathological Gambling and Kleptomania

Jon E. Grant

Abstract This chapter reviews the current knowledge of the clinical characteristics, associated psychopathology, family history, and neurobiology of pathological gambling and kleptomania. This chapter also presents study results of the pharmacological use of opioid antagonists in treating these disorders.

Keywords: Impulse control disorders; Pathological gambling; Behavioral addiction; Kleptomania

23.1 Introduction

In DSM-IV-TR, pathological gambling and kleptomania are currently included within the category of Impulse Control Disorders Not Elsewhere Classified, which also includes intermittent explosive disorder, pyromania, and trichotillomania. Other disorders have been proposed for inclusion based on perceived phenomenological, clinical, and possibly biological similarities: neurotic excoriation (skin-picking), compulsive buying, compulsive internet use, and nonparaphilic compulsive sexual behavior. The extent to which these impulse control disorders share clinical, genetic, phenomenological, and biological features is incompletely understood. Because rigorous research is limited on several of these disorders, this chapter will focus on pathological gambling and kleptomania, two impulse control disorders that have received increasing attention from clinicians and researchers. In particular, this chapter will focus on what is known regarding the neurobiology of these disorders and the role of opioid antagonists in the treatment of these behaviors.

Despite relatively high prevalence rates and significant morbidity associated with pathological gambling and kleptomania (1–2), the neurobiological basis and treatment of these behaviors are still poorly understood. Although originally

J.E. Grant
University of Minnesota, 2450 Riverside Avenue, Minneapolis, MN 55454
e-mail: grant045@umn.edu

R. Dean et al. (eds.), *Opiate Receptors and Antagonists*,

conceptualized as disorders within an obsessive–compulsive spectrum (3), recent research on the clinical characteristics of these disorders, patterns of familial transmission, and responses to pharmacological and psychosocial treatments suggest that pathological gambling and kleptomania may actually share more features with substance dependence (4). Thus, both pathological gambling and kleptomania may more aptly be described as "behavioral addictions" (4). It is this conceptualization of pathological gambling and kleptomania as addictions that has led to the examination of anticraving medication in their treatment.

23.2 Clinical Presentation

23.2.1 Pathological Gambling

Pathological gambling, a chronic, recurring condition characterized by persistent and recurrent maladaptive patterns of gambling behavior, is associated with impaired functioning, reduced quality of life, and high rates of bankruptcy, divorce, and legal difficulties (e.g., stealing, embezzlement, and writing bad checks) (5). Pathological gambling usually begins in early adulthood, with males tending to start at an earlier age (6). Epidemiological studies suggest that women represent ~32% of the pathological gamblers in the United States (7).

Male pathological gamblers appear more likely than females to report problems with strategic forms of gambling, for example, blackjack or poker. Female pathological gamblers tend to report problems with nonstrategic, less interpersonally interactive forms of gambling (e.g., slot machines or bingo) (8–9). Both female and male gamblers report that advertisements are a common trigger of their urges to gamble, although females are more likely to report that feeling bored or lonely may also trigger their urges to gamble (10). Financial and marital problems are common (5).

23.2.2 Kleptomania

Kleptomania is characterized by repetitive, uncontrollable stealing of items not needed for their personal use. Kleptomania, a chronic disorder, begins most often in late adolescence or early adulthood (11, 12). Women appear twice as likely to suffer from kleptomania as men (13, 14). The vast majority of individuals with kleptomania steal from stores (11). As in substance addiction, tolerance has been seen in kleptomania. One study found that 68.2% of individuals reported the value of stolen items had increased over the duration of the disorder (14). Individuals with kleptomania frequently keep, hoard, discard, or return stolen items (12).

Because most individuals with kleptomania try unsuccessfully to stop stealing, feelings of shame and guilt are always present (14). In fact, only 41.7% of married kleptomania subjects had told their spouses about their behavior due to the embarrassment (14). The majority of individuals with kleptomania (64–87%) have been apprehended at some time due to their stealing behavior (12, 13), but only a small percentage (15–23%) have been jailed (14).

23.3 Addiction Model and Etiological Issues

23.3.1 Addiction Model

The model of pathological gambling and kleptomania as behavioral addictions has strong support from recent research. Pathological gambling and kleptomania share certain distinct features with substance use disorders: (1) an urge to engage in a behavior with negative consequences, (2) mounting tension unless the behavior is completed, (3) rapid but temporary reduction of the urge after completion of the behavior, and (4) hedonic feeling early in the addiction (4). In addition, the symptoms of tolerance and withdrawal have analogies in pathological gambling and kleptomania (14, 15). Individuals with pathological gambling or kleptomania spend increasing amounts of time thinking about, planning, and engaging in the behaviors as the disorders progress. They may require more or larger forms of the behavior to produce the same result. Gamblers may spend increasing time and money on their gambling. Kleptomaniacs may steal larger or more valuable items with time.

23.3.2 Genetics of Addiction

Consistent with the notion that pathological gambling may be a behavioral addiction, studies have demonstrated the high comorbidity of pathological gambling with nicotine dependence (41–50%) (16, 17), alcohol abuse or dependence (50–75%) (4, 18), and drug use disorders (40%) (4, 18). In addition, individuals with substance use disorders have a tenfold risk of developing pathological gambling (19). High rates of other psychiatric disorders have also been described, especially mood, attention deficit, and antisocial personality disorders (4). These findings may suggest an underlying neurobiological overlap between pathological gambling and substance use disorders as well as other psychiatric disorders. Similarly, studies have found that 23–50% of kleptomania subjects have a co-occurring substance use disorder (12, 13) and that 15–20% of the first-degree relatives of individuals with kleptomania appear to suffer from substance use disorders (13, 20).

Investigations into the possible shared genetic basis for pathological gambling and substance use disorders have used genetic model-fitting methods to quantify the extent to which genetic and environmental risk might explain the risk for alcohol dependence in adult male twin pairs from the Vietnam Era Twin Registry. The risk for alcohol dependence accounts for a significant but modest proportion of the genetic and environmental risk for pathological gambling (21).

Molecular genetic studies also have provided evidence for the addictive aspects of pathological gambling. The Taq-A1 allele of the dopamine D2 receptor has been implicated in substance use disorders, and a statistically significant association between the Taq-A1 allele and pathological gambling compared to controls has been found (22). Considerable additional research is needed to determine further genetic associations between pathological gambling, kleptomania, and substance use disorders.

And finally, pathological gambling and kleptomania have both demonstrated response to naltrexone, an opioid antagonist that is FDA approved for opiate and alcohol use disorders (see Sect. 23.5 below). These findings that pathological gambling and kleptomania may be responsive to anti-addiction medications may support the inclusion of these disorders within an addictive spectrum.

23.4 Neurobiology

23.4.1 Dopamine

A large body of animal work has established the importance of dopaminergic inputs into the nucleus accumbens and ventral striatum in the prediction and reinforcement of rewarding behavior. Dopamine appears to play a crucial role in the reinforcement and learning of motivationally relevant reward, and in particular, unexpected reward (23). In particular, midbrain dopamine neurons display a phasic mode of activation in response to the probability of a reward (24). Midbrain dopamine neurons also appear to encode a second discriminatory response based upon both the magnitude and the prediction of reward (25). In fact, sustained activation in midbrain dopaminergic neurons has been found to display the highest activation after visual cues that correspond to the most uncertain probability of reward (24). Furthermore, this sustained activation was found to modulate with the expected magnitude of reward, such that dopamine neurons responded differentially to trials in which the reward magnitude was varied from small to moderate, moderate to large, and small to large. The highest sustained activation was discovered in trials in which the magnitude of reward had the highest variability (24).

Human studies with individuals with cocaine dependence have shown mesocorticolimbic dopamine activation after viewing cocaine-related videotapes (26, 27), and occupancy of the dopamine transporter has been correlated with cocaine's euphorigenic effects (28). Dopamine may also mediate some of the rewarding or reinforcing aspects of gambling. One study measured the levels of 3,4-dihydroxyphenylacetic acid (DOPAC) and homovanillic acid (HVA), two dopamine metabolites in the cerebral spinal fluid, and found decreased levels of dopamine and increased levels of DOPAC and HVA in pathological gambling subjects compared to controls, concluding that these findings were consistent with an increased rate of DA neurotransmission (29).

A common process implicated in drug priming is release of dopamine in the nucleus accumbens (30). Similarly, gambling has been shown to produce priming-like effects in problem gamblers (31). Additionally, drugs with similar mechanisms of action can "cross-prime" for reinstatement of other drugs within that class (i.e., amphetamine for cocaine) (32). One study examined whether amphetamine might prime motivation to gamble, and found that amphetamine increased motivation for gambling in gamblers, which could be predicted by the severity of reported gambling problems, though few effects were seen in motivational priming for alcohol in drinkers (33). Additionally, slowing in reading speed to motivationally irrelevant words found to be slowed in the gambling group given amphetamine, but undifferentiated improvement in reading speed for nongamblers. These results suggest that amphetamine can cross-prime for gambling behavior, lending further evidence for the involvement of dopaminergic and/or other aminergic pathways in the pathophysiology of pathological gambling.

23.4.2 Opioid System

The endogenous opioid system influences the experiencing of pleasure and is intimately linked to the dopaminergic system. Opioids modulate mesolimbic dopamine pathways via disinhibition of gamma-aminobutyric acid (GABA) input in the ventral tegmental area (34). Gambling or related behaviors have been associated with elevated blood levels of the endogenous opioid β-endorphin (35). Given their mechanism of action and their efficacy in the treatment of alcohol and opiate dependence (36), opioid receptor antagonists have also demonstrated efficacy in the treatment of pathological gambling. In addition to their possible utility in the treatment of pathological gambling and kleptomania, these studies suggest that the opioid system plays an important role in the pathophysiology of these disorders.

23.4.3 Neuroimaging Studies

While it is not possible to directly correlate these studies with the neuropathology of pathological gambling, discriminatory dopaminergic responses are present in reward probability and magnitude prediction, two key components of any gambling task. In an functional magnetic resonance imaging (fMRI) study of ventral striatal and prefrontal activation in normal volunteers, with no gambling history, who engaged in a gambling task, Dreher et al. found a temporal activation in midbrain regions in the interval between prediction and reward that correlated with reward error prediction (37). This midbrain activation also transiently activated a frontal network that included the left dorsal–lateral prefrontal cortex (DLPFC), superior frontal gyrus, and right anterior cingulated cortex (ACC) (37). Sustained activation in the ventral striatum was found to correlate with maximal uncertainty in the magnitude of a monetary reward (37).

In an fMRI study of ten pathological gambling subjects and age-matched controls imaged while watching gambling-related video, DLPFC activation was found to be significantly elevated in pathological gambling (38). These finding were significantly correlated with cue-induced craving in gambling subjects, and the findings suggest that DLPFC activation represents preferential attention and reward predictability to gambling cues. In contrast to the hyperactivation of the DLPFC, pathological gambling subjects were shown by fMRI to have hypoactive striatal and ventral medial prefrontal cortex (VMPFC) activation compared to controls in response to a gambling task (39). Hypoactivation negatively correlated with pathological gambling severity, and this correlation remained robust after corrections for comorbid depression and tobacco use (39). Another study described decreased VMPFC in gambling subjects compared to controls when engaged in a stroop task, a paradigm known to evoke VMPFC activation in normal volunteers (40).

These studies suggest that dysfunction in the cortico-striatal networks from the prefrontal cortex to midbrain may underlie pathological gambling. This pattern of activation closely resembles a proposed "final common pathway" for drug-seeking and -craving behavior in human models of drug addiction (30). In this proposed circuit, glutamatergic projections from the prefrontal cortex and anterior cingulate cortex initiate drug-seeking behavior through cue-induced craving. Interestingly, substance-addicted individuals display a resting state hypoactivation of the prefrontal cortex, in which craving-associated prefrontal hyperactivation is superimposed (30, 41, 42). Furthermore, the magnitude of change in prefrontal activity has been shown to positively correlate with the severity of cue-induced craving in addicted individuals (30). This cue-induced craving activates dopaminergic neurons in the core of the nucleus accumbens, which output to the ventral pallidum and, ultimately, basal ganglia motoric areas (30).

Future studies are required to determine the extent of shared neuropathology between pathological gambling and substance use disorders. Mechanisms of sustained dopamine release seen in response to a reward of varying magnitude, as in pathological gambling, may mimic the exogenous manipulation of dopamine through substances of abuse.

23.5 Treatment

The treatment of pathological gambling and kleptomania has traditionally been complicated by high rates comorbidity with affective and substance use disorders and high rates of treatment discontinuation (43). Emerging evidence suggests, however, that these disorders can be successfully treated with pharmacotherapy. Although multiple classes of medications have been studied in the treatment of impulse control disorders (e.g., antidepressants, antiepileptics, lithium), some of the most promising results have stemmed from the use of opioid antagonists in the treatment of these disorders.

23.5.1 *Opioid Antagonists*

Because of the possible relationship of pathological gambling and kleptomania to addictive disorders, studies have examined the efficacy of opioid antagonists in the treatment of these behaviors. Opioid antagonists inhibit dopamine neurons within the ventral tegmental area and diminish dopamine function within the nucleus accumbens and the basal brain region (44). Dopamine function within these regions has been implicated in the subjective experience of pleasure and urges (45). The core symptom of uncontrolled urges triggered by a potential reward may be the modifiable component of both pathological gambling and kleptomania (46).

Opioid receptor antagonists inhibit dopamine release in the nucleus accumbens and ventral pallidum through the disinhibition of GABA input to the dopamine neurons in the ventral tegmental area (47–49). The hypothesis underlying the use of opioid antagonists was that decreased dopamine in the nucleus accumbens and motivation circuit would dampen excitement and cravings related to gambling behavior (46). Although modulation of drive and subsequent behavioral output by dopamine, endorphin, and GABA has been investigated, the specific mechanisms remain incompletely understood, particularly as related to pathological gambling (50).

Pathologic gamblers frequently report urges and cravings to gamble similar to symptoms experienced by patients with substance use disorders. Crockford and colleagues reported a case of a patient suffering from both pathological gambling and alcohol dependence whose gambling improved during naltrexone treatment (51). Additional case reports of naltrexone have suggested its beneficial use for kleptomania and other behavioral addictions such as compulsive shopping (46).

An initial 6-week open label, flexible dose trial of naltrexone in 17 subjects with pathological gambling showed statistically significant improvement in gambling urges, thoughts, and behaviors. Doses from 50 to 250 mg/day were used with a mean effective dose of 157 mg/day (52). A follow-up 12-week double-blind placebo-controlled naltrexone trial demonstrated superiority to placebo. Eighty-three subjects were enrolled with 38 subjects terminating early due to inability to tolerate the study drug, large placebo response during the 1-week placebo run-in or noncompliance. Of the 45 remaining subjects, 20 received naltrexone 100–250 mg/day and 25 received placebo. An intent-to-treat analysis demonstrated naltrexone's superiority to placebo, particularly for those gamblers reporting more severe urges to gamble (53). Clinical use of high-dose naltrexone, however, has been limited by the possible occurrence of liver enzyme elevations, especially in patients taking nonsteroidal anti-inflammatory drugs (54).

A recently completed multicenter study further demonstrated the efficacy of another opioid antagonist, nalmefene, in the treatment of pathological gambling. In a sample of 207 subjects, nalmefene demonstrated statistically significant improvement in gambling urges, thoughts, and behavior compared to placebo (55). This 16-week, randomized, dose-ranging, double-blind, placebo-controlled trial was conducted at 15 outpatient treatment centers across the United States between March 2002 and April 2003. Two hundred and seven persons with DSM-IV pathological gambling were randomized to nalmefene (25 mg/day, 50 mg/day, or 100 mg/day) or placebo. Using estimated regression coefficients, the 25 mg/day and 50 mg/day groups showed significant difference from placebo (p = .007 and p = .016, respectively). 59.2% of subjects assigned to 25 mg/day were "much improved" or "very much improved" at the last evaluation, compared to 34.0% of those taking placebo (odds ratio = 2.79; 95% CI: 1.21–6.41; p = 0.033). Adverse experiences included nausea, dizziness, and insomnia.

The only formal medication trial in kleptomania also used the opioid antagonist, naltrexone (56). A 12-week open-label study of naltrexone in ten subjects with kleptomania demonstrated significant improvement in urges to shoplift and shoplifting behavior. The mean effective naltrexone dose was 145 mg/day and resulted in a significant decline in the intensity of urges to steal, stealing thoughts and stealing behavior in nine of the ten subjects compared to baseline symptoms.

A chart review of 17 patients with kleptomania treated in an outpatient clinic with naltrexone for up to 3 years examined effectiveness of medication intervention (57). Comparison of baseline symptoms with most recent follow-up visit showed 76.5% of patients reported decreased urges to steal, and 41.1% reported no stealing behavior at all. In addition, 52.9% of patients were rated as either "not ill at all" or having "very mild" symptoms. Mean effective dose was 135.3 mg/day (57).

23.5.2 Safety of Opioid Anatgonists

One issue raised in the use of opioid antagonists has been potential hepatotoxicity. Naltrexone has earned a black box warning for doses greater than 50 mg/day due to potential liver damage. This warning was based on trials of naltrexone in obesity and dementia (58, 59) when the dose was titrated up to 300 mg/day. In the double-blind trial of naltrexone in pathological gambling, ~25% of subjects receiving active drug experienced liver function abnormalities following naltrexone dosing (up to 200 mg/day), and these enzyme level elevations returned to normal following discontinuation of the drug (53). The findings are consistent with a black box warning regarding a dose-dependent relationship between naltrexone and liver function abnormalities. These trials, however, did not monitor over the counter concomitant medications.

Recent research suggests that naltrexone increases the risk of hepatic transaminase elevations when used concurrently with acetaminophen, aspirin, or nonaspirin (nonsteroidal anti-inflammatory drugs, NSAID) (54). A recent study examining hepatic transaminase profiles in outpatients treated with a mean dose of naltrexone of 142 mg/day for ~1-year duration found no elevations in transaminase levels when concomitant medications (acetaminophen, aspirin, and nonaspirin NSAIDs) were restricted (60). Unlike the data regarding naltrexone, the trial of nalmefene in pathological gambling demonstrated no elevations in hepatic transaminase levels (55).

23.6 Conclusions

Behavioral addictions, such as pathological gambling and kleptomania, have historically received relatively little attention from clinicians and researchers. As such, our understanding of the basic features of these disorders is relatively primitive. Future research investigating these disorders and their relationship to substance use disorders may hold significant promise in advancing prevention and treatment strategies for addiction in general. Emerging data from controlled clinical trials, however, suggest that pathological gambling and kleptomania may respond to opioid antagonists.

Approaches reviewed in this chapter represent significant advances only from several years ago. It is hoped that progress in the treatment of pathological gambling and kleptomania will continue to be made at the rate recently witnessed. More definitive treatment recommendations await completion of additional, large-scale controlled treatment studies for these disorders and comparative investigations of pharmacological agents. Advances in these areas hold the potential for significantly improving the lives of individuals with these disorders and those directly or indirectly affected by their conditions.

References

1. Cunningham-Williams RM, Cottler LB, Compton III WM, Spitznagel EL. Taking chances: problem gamblers and mental health disorders – results from the St. Louis Epidemiologic Catchment Area study. Am J Pub Health 1998; 88:1093–1096.
2. Grant JE, Potenza MN, Levine L, Kim D. Prevalence of impulse control disorders in adult psychiatric inpatients. Am J Psychiatry (in press).
3. Hollander E. Obsessive-compulsive spectrum disorders: an overview. Psychiatr Ann 1993; 23:355–358.
4. Grant JE, Potenza MN. Pathological gambling and other "behavioral addictions." In: Frances RJ, Miller SI, Mack AH, eds. Clinical Handbook of Addictive Disorders (3rd edn.); New York: Guilford Press, 2005, pp. 303–320.
5. Argo TR, Black DW. Clinical characteristics. In: Grant JE, Potenza MN, eds. Pathological Gambling: A Clinical Guide to Treatment; Washington, DC: American Psychiatric Publishing, 2004, pp. 39–53.
6. Ibanez A, Blanco C, Moreyra P, Saiz-Ruiz J. Gender differences in pathological gambling. J Clin Psychiatry 2003; 64:295–301.
7. Volberg RA. The prevalence and demographics of pathological gamblers: implications for public health. Am J Public Health 1994; 84:237–240.
8. Potenza MN, Steinberg MA, McLaughlin SD, Wu R, Rounsaville B, O'Malley SS. Gender-related differences in the characteristics of problem gamblers using a gambling helpline. Am J Psychiatry 2001; 158:1500–1505.

9. Ladd GT, Petry NM. Gender differences among pathological gamblers seeking treatment. Exp Clin Psychopharmacol 2002; 10:302–309.
10. Grant JE, Kim SW. Demographic and clinical features of 131 adult pathological gamblers. J Clin Psychiatry 2001; 62:957–962.
11. Goldman MJ. Kleptomania: making sense of the nonsensical. Am J Psychiatry 1991; 148:986–996.
12. McElroy SL, Pope HG, Hudson JI, Keck PE, White KL. Kleptomania: a report of 20 cases. Am J Psychiatry 1991; 148:652–657.
13. Presta S, Marazziti D, Dell'Osso L, Pfanner C, Pallanti S, Cassano GB. Kleptomania: clinical features and comorbidity in an Italian sample. Compr Psychiatry 2002; 43:7–12.
14. Grant JE, Kim SW. Clinical characteristics and associated psychopathology of 22 patients with kleptomania. Compr Psychiatry 2002; 43:378–384.
15. Blanco C, Moreyra P, Nunes EV, Saiz-Ruiz J, Ibanez A. Pathological gambling: addiction or compulsion? Semin Clin Neuropsychiatry 2001; 6:167–176.
16. Crockford DN, el-Guebaly N. Psychiatric comorbidity in pathological gambling: a critical review. Can J Psychiatry 1998; 43:43–50.
17. Petry NM, Oncken C. Cigarette smoking is associated with increased severity of gambling problems in treatment-seeking gamblers. Addiction 2002; 97:745–753.
18. Petry NM. Pathological Gambling: Etiology, Comorbidity, and Treatment. Washington, DC: American Psychological Association, 2005.
19. Spunt B, Lesieur H, Hunt D, Cahill L. Gambling among methadone patients. Int J Addict 1995; 30:929–962.
20. Grant JE. Family history and psychiatric comorbidity in persons with kleptomania. Compr Psychiatry 2003; 44:437–441.
21. Slutske WS, Eisen S, True WR, Lyons MJ, Goldberg J, Tsuang M. Common genetic vulnerability for pathological gambling and alcohol dependence in men. Arch Gen Psychiatry 2000; 57:666–673.
22. Comings DE, Rosenthal RJ, Lesieur HR, Rugle LJ, Muhleman D, Chiu C, Dietz G, Gade R. A study of the dopamine D2 receptor gene in pathological gambling. Pharmacogenetics 1996; 6:223–234.
23. Kelley AE. Memory and addiction: shared neural circuitry and molecular mechanisms. Neuron 2004; 44:161–179.
24. Tobler, PN, Fiorillo CD, Schultz W. Adaptive coding of reward by dopamine neurons. Science 2005; 307:1642–1645.
25. Fiorillo CD, Tobler PN, Schultz W. Discrete coding of reward probability and uncertainty by dopamine neurons. Science 2003; 299:1898–1902.
26. Kosten TR, Scanley, BE, Tucker KA, Oliveto A, Prince C, Sinha R, Potenza MN, Skudlarski P, Wexler BE. Cue-induced brain activity changes and relapse in cocaine-dependent patients. Neuropsychopharmacology 2006; 31:644–650.
27. Wexler BE, Gottschalk CH, Fulbright RK, Prohovnik I, Lacadie CM, Rounsaville BJ, Gore JC. Functional magnetic resonance imaging of cocaine craving. Am J Psychiatry 2001; 158:86–95.
28. Volkow ND, Wang GJ, Fowler JS, Logan J, Gatley SJ, Hitzemann R, Chen AD, Dewey SL, Pappas N. Decreased striatal dopaminergic responsiveness in detoxified cocaine-dependent subjects. Nature 1997; 386:830–833.
29. Bergh C, Eklund T, Sodersten P, Nordin C. Altered dopamine function in pathological gambling. Psychol Med 1997; 27:473–475.
30. Kalivas PW, Volkow ND. The neural basis of addiction: a pathology of motivation and choice. Am J Psychiatry 2005; 162:1403–1413.
31. Loba P, Stewart SH, Klein RM, Blackburn JR. Manipulations of the features of standard video lottery terminal (VLT) games: effects in pathological and non-pathological gamblers. J Gambl Stud 2001; 17:297–320.
32. Shalev U, Grimm JW, Shaham Y. Neurobiology of relapse to heroin and cocaine seeking: a review. Pharmacol Rev 2002; 54:1–42.

33. Zack M, Poulos CX. Amphetamine primes motivation to gamble and gambling-related semantic networks in problem gamblers. Neuropsychopharmacology 2004; 29:195–207.
34. Johnson SW, North RA. Opioids excite dopamine neurons by hyperpolarization of local interneurons. J Neurosci 1992; 12:483–488.
35. Shinohara K, Yanagisawa A, Kagota Y, Gomi A, Nemoto K, Moriya E, Furusawa E, Furuya K, Terasawa K. Physiological changes in Pachinko players; beta-endorphin, catecholamines, immune system substances and heart rate. Appl Human Sci 1999;18:37–42.
36. Tamminga CA, Nestler EJ. Pathological gambling: focusing on the addiction, not the activity. Am J Psychiatry 2006; 163:180–181.
37. Dreher JC, Kohn P, Berman KF. Neural coding of distinct statistical properties of reward information in humans. Cereb Cortex 2006; 16:561–573.
38. Crockford DN, Goodyear B, Edwards J, Edwards J, Quickfall J, el-Guebaly N. Cue-induced brain activity in pathological gamblers. Biol Psychiatry 2005; 58:787–795.
39. Reuter J, Raedler T, Rose M, Hand I, Glascher J, Buchel C. Pathological gambling is linked to reduced activation of the mesolimbic reward system. Nature Neurosci 2005; 8:147–148.
40. Potenza MN, Leung HC, Blumberg HP, Peterson BS, Fulbright RK, Lacadie CM, Skudlarski P, Gore JC. An FMRI Stroop task study of ventromedial prefrontal cortical function in pathological gamblers. Am J Psychiatry 2003; 160:1990–1994.
41. Jentsch JD, Taylor JR. Impulsivity resulting from frontostriatal dysfunction in drug abuse: implications for the control of behavior by reward-related stimuli. Psychopharmacology (Berl) 1999; 146:373–390.
42. Goldstein RZ, Volkow ND. Drug addiction and its underlying neurobiological basis: neuroimaging evidence for involvement of the frontal cortex. Am J Psychiatry 2002; 159:523–528.
43. Sood ED, Pallanti S, Hollander E. Diagnosis and treatment of pathologic gambling. Curr Psychiatry Rep 2003; 5:9–15.
44. Brahen LS, Capone T, Wiechert V, Desiderio D. Naltrexone and cyclazocine. A controlled treatment study. Arch Gen Psychiatry 1977; 34:1181–1184.
45. Berridge KC, Robinson TE What is the role of dopamine in reward: hedonic impact, reward learning, or incentive salience? Brain Res Brain Res Rev 1998; 28:309–369.
46. Kim SW. Opioid antagonists in the treatment of impulse control disorders. J Clin Psychiatry 1998; 59:159–162.
47. Broekkamp CL, Phillips AG. Facilitation of self-stimulation behavior following intracerebral microinjections of opioids into the ventral tegmental area. Pharmacol Biochem Behav 1979; 11:289–295.
48. Stewart J. Reinstatement of heroin and cocaine self-administration behavior in the rat by intracerebral application of morphine in the ventral tegmental area. Pharmacol Biochem Behav 1984; 20:917–923.
49. van Wolfswinkel L, van Ree JM. Effects of morphine and naloxone on thresholds of ventral tegmental electrical self-stimulation. Naunyn-Schmiedebergs Arch Pharmacol 1985; 330:84–92.
50. Koob GF. Drugs of abuse: anatomy, pharmacology and function of reward pathways. Trends Pharmacol Sci 1992; 13:177–184.
51. Crockford DN, el-Guebaly N. Naltrexone in the treatment of pathological gambling and alcohol dependence. Can J Psychiatry 1998; 43:86 [letter].
52. Kim SW, Grant JE. An open naltrexone treatment study in pathological gambling disorder. Int Clin Psychopharmacol 2001; 16:285–289.
53. Kim SW, Grant JE, Adson DE, Shin YC. Double-blind naltrexone and placebo comparison study in the treatment of pathological gambling. Biol Psychiatry 2001; 49:914–921.
54. Kim SW, Grant JE, Adson DE, Remmel RP. A preliminary report on possible naltrexone and nonsteroidal analgesic interactions. J Clin Psychopharmacol 2001; 21:632–634 [letter].
55. Grant JE, Potenza MN, Hollander E, Cunningham-Williams R, Nurminen T, Smits G, Kallio A. A multicenter investigation of the opioid antagonist nalmefene in the treatment of pathological gambling. Am J Psychiatry 2006; 163:303–312.

56. Grant JE, Kim SW. An open-label study of naltrexone in the treatment of kleptomania. J Clin Psychiatry 2002; 63:349–356.
57. Grant JE. Outcome study of kleptomania patients treated with naltrexone: a chart review. Clin Neuropharmacol 2005; 28:11–14.
58. Pfohl DN, Allen JI, Atkinson RL, Knopman DS, Malcolm RJ, Mitchell JE, Morley JE. Naltrexone hydrochloride (Trexan): a review of serum transaminase elevations at high dosage. NIDA Res Monogr 1986; 67:66–72.
59. Verebey KG, Mule SJ. Naltrexone (Trexan): a review of hepatotoxicity issues. NIDA Res Monogr 1986; 67:73–81.
60. Kim SW, Grant JE, Yoon G, Williams KA, Remmel RP. Safety of high-dose naltrexone treatment: hepatic transaminase profiles among outpatients. Clin Neuropharmacol 2006; 29:77–79.

Chapter 24
Efficacy of Opioid Antagonists in Attentuating Self-Injurious Behavior

Curt A. Sandman

Abstract Self-injurious behavior (SIB) is a primary reason that individuals either are retained in restrictive environments or are administered psychotropic medication. There are no known causes and no universally accepted treatments for this complex behavior. There is developing evidence, however, that individuals exhibiting SIB have a disturbance of the opiate-mediated pain and pleasure system. For instance, many self-injurious individuals do not exhibit the usual signs of pain after their "injurious" behavior. Moreover, for some individuals the addictive properties of elevated endogenous opiates (euphoria) may be responsible for maintaining their SIB. A review [Symons, Thompson & Rodriguez, (2004)] of the recent scientific literature concluded that 80% of the subjects were reported to significantly reduce their SIB after acute treatment with opiate blockers (naltrexone). Although the long term effects of opiate blockers on SIB are unknown, reduction in SIB following acute treatment provides support that a specific biological system may be dysregulated in a subgroup of patients. Reports that levels of endogenous opiates at rest and after SIB episodes predict positive responses to opiate blockers provide further support for opiate-mediated SIB and form the basis for a rational treatment strategy. It is concluded that naltrexone produces a clinically significant reduction in the serious and life-threatening behavior of self injury for individuals who have not been responsive to any other type of treatment. Several suggestions and cautions are provided for regimens of naltrexone treatment of SIB.

Keywords: Opiates; Endorphin; Opiate blockers; POMC; Naltrexone; Self-injurious behavior; SIB

C.A. Sandman
Department of Psychiatry, University of California, Irvine College of Medicine, 333 City Drive Blvd West, Suite 1200, Orange, CA 92868-3205
Preparation of this chapter was supported in part by award HD-48947 from the National Institute of Child Health and Human Development
e-mail: casandma@uci.edu

24.1 Introduction

Despite considerable research effort, self-injurious behavior (SIB) continues to be a primary reason, together with aggression toward others, that individuals either are retained in institutional (restrictive) environments or are administered psychotropic medication. Today, SIB remains unmanageable, expensive [$150,000–$500,000/year/patient in institutional settings, with national costs well over $3,000,000,000 (1)], and often is life threatening. It is surprisingly prevalent, occurring in ~30% of individuals with developmental neurological complications, including those with autistic disorder (2, 3).

Twenty-five experts invited by the National Institute of Child Health and Human Development (NICHD) to discuss the relations among the genetic, neurobiological, and behavioral causes and treatments for SIB reached two general conclusions. Intentional acts of harm to self, evident in many species, (a) have no known cause and (b) no agreed upon treatment (4). The apparent absence of visible progress in understanding or treating SIB is not because of a lack of interest or effort. Studies of self-injury have increased eightfold in the past 10 years with over 1,000 studies reported between 1999 and 2006 (Fig. 24.1).

One major obstacle in understanding the mechanisms of SIB and developing coherent treatment plans is the absence of distinctive behavioral phenotypes. Despite the consensus that SIB has variable expression with no known cause, the group of NICHD experts agreed that SIB could be defined, perhaps with greater precision than most complex human behaviors. SIB is a directly observable behavior that can be reliably counted. The NICHD group argued that data collection and analysis had advanced so that complex patterns of SIB should replace or supplement measures of rate and frequency (5, 6). Two distinct patterns of SIB were proposed

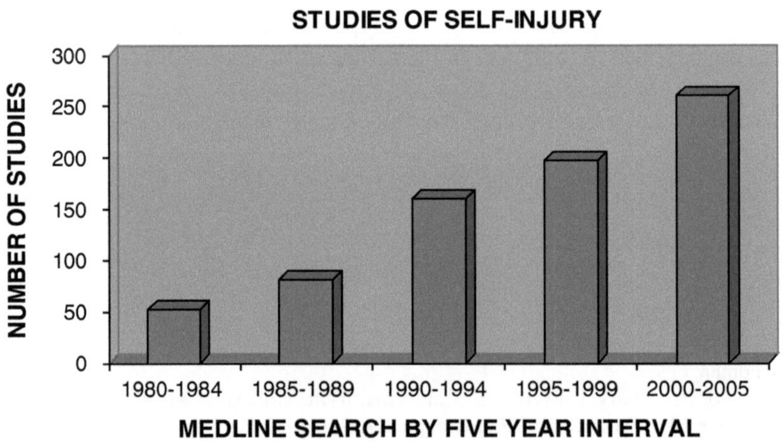

Fig. 24.1 Number of studies of self-injurious behavior (*SIB*) conducted in 5-year intervals from 1980 to the present (*see Color Plates*)

as possible guides. One pattern consists of bouts that are most likely maintained by environmental contingencies. The second pattern involves protracted periods of SIB that are most likely under the primary influence of biological factors. The vast majority of existing studies, however, have reported frequencies or rates of occurrence of SIB often linked to a single environmental manipulation. It is a significant advantage that many forms of SIB can be counted and time-stamped enabling contemporary studies to use sequential and time series procedures to define their structure and their relations with other behaviors and the environment. We subjected extensive and lengthy observations of maladaptive behavior in its natural environmental context to time series analysis and discovered unique temporal and sequential patterns of these severe maladaptive behaviors (2, 3, 7–10).

Specifically, we found for a large majority of the individuals studied, SIB was predicted only by its own recent history. In our cohort of severely self-injurious patients, SIB was expressed consistently in successive occurrences revealing a unique pattern of sequential dependence compatible with a "contagious" distribution. Application of time-series methods of analysis that controlled for chance pairings of events indicated that the contagious patterns of SIB were independent from frequency and rate of occurrence. That is, the temporally dependent patterns we observed were not a function of high rates of occurrence. Moreover, and surprisingly, SIB was not associated consistently with other behaviors or with the several staff activities or environmental conditions recorded in these studies. Thus, in a significant majority of these individuals, SIB episodes were self-perpetuating and not related to antecedent or subsequent environmental circumstances, events, or other recorded behaviors.

This novel and surprising finding was consistent with conclusions of the NICHD group that some expressions of SIB may have an underlying biological basis because a solely self-perpetuating behavior is most parsimoniously explained by internal (i.e., biological) motives (2, 11–13). The vast majority of individuals in our cohort exhibited the most primitive level of internally regulated behavioral patterns despite years of behavioral interventions and treatment with various medications (8, 9). Anecdotal and clinical observations of these individuals also strongly suggested a biological basis for their behavior and specifically involvement of the pain and pleasure systems. Typically, SIB is repetitious consisting of hourly, daily, weekly, monthly, or even yearly cycles (14). Some individuals who repeatedly injure themselves appear immune to the normal experience of pain (12). They abuse and injure their bodies, hitting or biting themselves, hurling themselves to the ground, and banging their head against solid objects resulting in broken bones, disfigurement, blindness, and even loss of life (2, 15, 16). They often work to overcome interventions designed to decrease self-injury in a manner that is consistent with seeking positive reward. For instance, protective devices (such as helmets) may result in individuals exerting greater effort and exhibiting greater rates of behavior to hit and harm themselves (17).

Because many medications that treat pain or induce pleasure are addicting, it is interesting that SIB, in addition to the obvious involvement of pain systems, shares features of addiction such as compulsive and ritualistic (or stereotypic) patterns that either comprise or surround the self-injuring acts. One biological system that has been implicated in SIB and the modulation of pain and pleasure is the hypothalamic–pituitary–adrenal (HPA) stress axis and specifically the proopiomelanocortin (POMC) molecule (3, 18, 19).

24.2 Overview

24.2.1 The Biological Stress System Pain, Pleasure, and SIB

Thompson and Caruso (6) recognized that some forms of SIB were "neurochemically driven and independent of environmental events." Early studies either of basal or of resting levels of a variety of peptides, proteins, transmitters, and amines in plasma or cerebrospinal fluid from patients exhibiting SIB, however, generated inconclusive results. This was not surprising because there was little consistency among studies regarding the rigor of diagnosis, the molecule measured, the tissue assayed, or the conditions assessed (20–26).

24.2.2 Pain and the Endogenous Opioid System

Although it is not a universal observation, most self-injurious individuals do not exhibit the usual signs of pain after their "injurious" behavior. Despite inflicting serious physical damage to their bodies, many of these individuals do not grimace, cry, or show other symptoms that they are experiencing pain. It has been suggested that this absence of response to self-inflicted injury reflects insensitivity to pain and general sensory depression induced either by elevated endogenous opiates or by supersensitive opiate receptors (11, 27–29). This possibility is supported by classical findings that opiate receptor blockers (a) reverse congenital insensitivity to pain (30), (b) normalize hypothalamic-peptide dysfunction coexisting with elevated pain threshold (31), and (c) increase brain responses to sensory information (32). These observations are consistent with a venerable animal literature proving that opiate blockers lower pain threshold (e.g., 33). In summary, these findings support an analgesia (or pain) hypothesis that implies that self-injurious individuals do not feel pain because of *chronically* elevated endogenous opiates and/or opiate receptor downregulation.

24.2.3 Pleasure (Addiction) and the Endogenous Opioid System

It is also possible that the addictive properties of elevated endogenous opiates are responsible for maintaining SIB. If it is presumed SIB does result in pain and that the experience of pain results in the release of opiates, then it can be argued that individuals commit self-inflicted harm to receive the euphoric (pleasurable) effects of increased circulating opiates. From this perspective, SIB is an "addiction" to the endogenous opiate system because its consequences supply a "fix." It has been known for over 25 years that endogenous opiates have addictive properties as indicated by the development of tolerance (34), physical dependence (35), and euphoric-like effects (36) after repeated administration. The repetitive, often compulsive, and ritualistic patterns of SIB (i.e., injury to one area of head or body, stereotyped patterns of behavior, and catastrophic responses if the environment is slightly changed) are similar to rituals and compulsive patterns often associated with addictive behaviors. The addiction hypothesis maintains that individuals with SIB may endure the pain to enjoy the pleasure it produces as well as to avoid a withdrawal effect. The addiction hypothesis predicts that SIB may be reinforced both positively and negatively because it gains the individual access to the narcotic effect of endorphins while simultaneously allowing the individual to escape the unpleasant sensory consequences commonly associated with the absence of opiates following chronic and sustained access.

24.2.4 Stress and the Endogenous Opioid System

The endogenous opioid system is tightly coupled with the general stress response. Evidence from several laboratories indicates that functioning and processing of a stress-related molecule (POMC) in the HPA axis may be perturbed among subgroups of individuals exhibiting SIB (15, 19, 21, 37–43). In humans, most POMC is produced in the pars distalis of the anterior pituitary but also by hypothalamic neurons and neurons in the amygdala and pituitary stalk. POMC, is a well-characterized 31-K dalton, bioinactive protein-like molecule that is post-translationally converted by enzymes (e.g., PC1 and PC2) into biologically active fragments, including B-endorphin (BE) and adrenocorticotropic hormone (ACTH) (15, 44–48). Normally, BE is coreleased from the anterior pituitary with ACTH in response to a variety of stressors. However, elevated BE but not ACTH is associated with SIB either at rest or after an episode of SIB (3, 12, 18). This suggests that one consequence of SIB is the disregulation of the arousal system.

The validity of these hypotheses is not known but they have encouraged treatments, including opiate receptor blockers, designed to regulate the opiate/stress system as means to control SIB.

24.3 Efficacy of Opiate Blockers in the Treatment of SIB

24.3.1 Acute Effects of Naltrexone

In a review of pre-1991 studies (49), six of eight published studies reported that injectable naloxone significantly reduced SIB. In these eight studies, naloxone was tested in a total of ten individuals with SIB. A decrease in SIB was reported

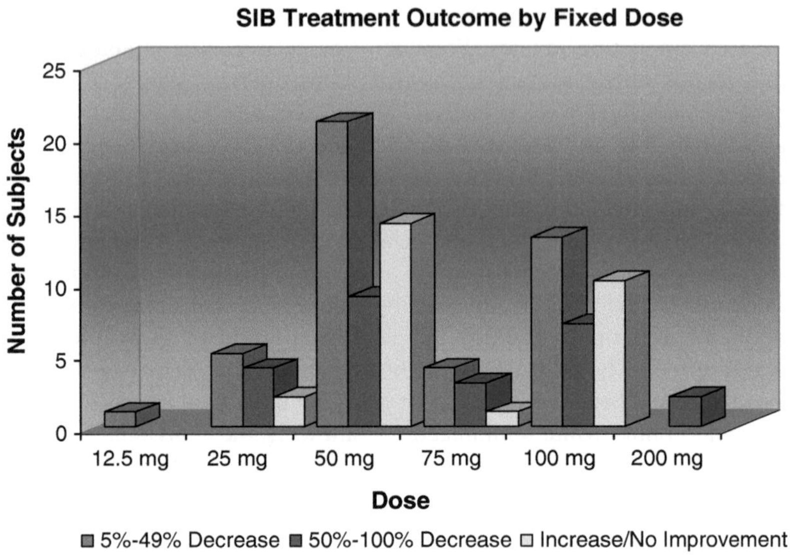

Fig. 24.2 Number of subjects in fixed dose studies with positive responses to naltrexone [adapted from Symons et al. (53)] (*see Color Plates*)

for seven individuals. In that same review, 12 published studies of naltrexone (Naltrexone) in MR/DD individuals were summarized. Most of the studies either were case studies or were studies with very small samples. At that time, 45 MR/DD individuals (at least 28 with SIB) had been treated with naltrexone and 38 individuals had positive responses of various degrees including a reduction in SIB in 24 of the 28 patients. A separate review of 13 studies [including several in the Sandman review (49)] concluded that about one-third of the patients tested with Naltrexone had a decrease in their SIB (50). Several studies in this later review included juvenile patients under the age of 8 years (51) and patients with primary behavioral problems related to aggression and agitation (52). Aggression toward others and agitation are not equivalent to SIB on any obvious dimension except, perhaps, exertion, and the fact that opiate blockers were ineffective in the control of these behaviors adds inferential support to the argument that the opioid system is uniquely implicated in SIB and not in other maladaptive behaviors. The effects of opiate blockers in children who self-injure may be similar to the effects observed in adults but there are too few reports to make that conclusion.

Most recently, a thorough review of the recent scientific literature employing stringent and appropriate criteria for inclusion concluded that the effects of opiate blockers on SIB could be evaluated in a total of 86 patients (53). Eighty percent of the subjects were reported to improve relative to baseline (i.e., SIB reduced) during naltrexone administration (Fig. 24.2). Of the subjects who improved, 47% exhibited a reduction in SIB by 50% or greater. In studies reporting dose levels in milligrams (Fig. 24.3), males were more likely than females to respond. No significant relations were found between treatment outcomes and autism status or form of self-injury.

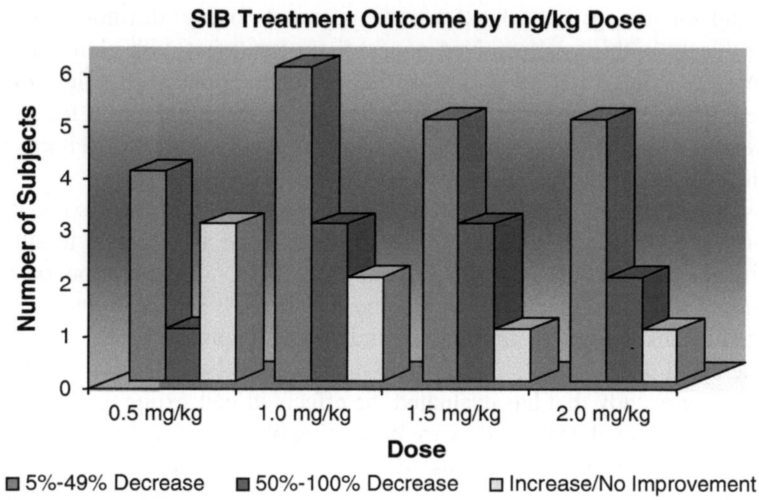

Fig. 24.3 Number of subjects with positive responses to doses of naltexone controlling for weight (mg/kg) [adapted from Symons et al. (53)] (*see Color Plates*)

Two relatively large, placebo-controlled studies (16, 54) included in this review of naltrexone came to very similar conclusions. In a double-blind, placebo-controlled, dose-finding study, Sandman et al. (54) reported that 18 of 21 individuals exhibiting SIB responded favorably to at least one dose (range of 0.5–2.0 mg/kg) of naltrexone (time-sampled video records provided direct observations of the subjects). Acute treatment (1 week at each of three doses) with naltrexone reduced the frequency of SIB without major side-effects. Activity, stereotypy, involuntary movement, and neurological status were not influenced by naltrexone. There were two central findings. First, the highest dose (2 mg/kg) was the most effective, confirming earlier results in this population (55, 56). Seven of the eight patients responding best at the highest dose, also responded favorably to the 1 mg/kg dose. Six of these eight patients also responded at the 0.5 mg/kg dose. Eleven subjects responded positively to both the 1 and 2 mg/kg doses. Second, subjects with the most frequent SIB were the most positive responders to higher doses of naltrexone, consistent with earlier reports (55, 56). A small minority of subjects responded most favorably to lower doses. These results confirmed that at least 50% of the individuals with SIB responded favorably to treatment with opiate blockers.

Another double-blind, placebo-controlled, fixed dose study of eight, severe to profoundly retarded adults included in the review (16), reported that treatment with naltrexone reduced head hitting, head banging, and self-biting. The eight individuals evaluated displayed 18 forms of SIB. Improvement was observed in 77% of the head hitting and head banging episodes and 100% of the self-biting forms. Episodes of high frequency SIB also were more sensitive to treatment with naltrexone. The 100-mg (high) dose was more effective than the 50-mg (low) dose in reducing SIB. For several individuals, some forms of SIB decreased after naltrexone (e.g., head hitting and self-biting) but other forms (e.g., throat poking) did not change. Four of the subjects in this trial received concomitant treatment with clonidine (alpha-2-adrenergic agonist) but no effects on SIB or interactions with naltrexone were observed. These findings compliment previous studies and caution that although naltrexone is effective in reducing SIB, not all forms of self-inflicted harm may be controlled by blocking the opioid system.

These two relatively large studies of *acute treatment* with naltrexone came to very similar conclusions. Opiate blockers appear to be an effective treatment for a significant number of individuals exhibiting SIB. Administration of naltrexone reduces high frequency SIB and some, but not all, self-destructive behavior. Both studies acknowledged that not all individuals expressing SIB were positive responders and that a small minority may increase SIB [see also Barrett (57)].

In the single study that has evaluated the effects of naltrexone using time-series analysis, Symons et al. (58) made very interesting observations. First, they reported that three of the four patients evaluated had at least a 33% reduction in their SIB. (The fourth patient had a 17% reduction in SIB.) Second, and most interesting, they discovered that in addition to the improvement with naltrexone, there was an increase in the sequential dependence between staff behavior and the manifestation of SIB. During treatment with naltrexone, but not during placebo conditions, there was a significant increase in the probability that staff would "prompt" individuals proximal in time and sequence to an SIB event. That is, during treatment with naltrexone, there were more social interactions between staff and patient. One possible conclusion from these findings is that naltrexone exerts its effects on SIB, in part by the opioid-mediated reinforcing influences of social interactions.

24.3.2 Long-Term Effects of Naltrexone Treatments

The long-term effects and consequences of continued treatment with naltrexone is not completely known because most studies reporting treatment of individuals with SIB have been short-term demonstrations or acute trials. Most published long-term studies have been either case studies or open-label designs and they have generated mixed results. Two types of studies comprise the long-term evaluations of naltrexone, either prolonged treatment with naltrexone or extended observations following brief periods of treatment. With these procedures, investigators have reported that about six of eight patients examined in several studies exhibited long-term benefits in varying degrees from treatment with naltrexone (57–59). In the first report, a total of 24 days of naltrexone treatment resulted in elimination of SIB in a 12-year-old girl that persisted for at least 22 months (57). A similar finding was reported after 1 year of continuous treatment with naltrexone in a 28-year-old woman with severe SIB. Not only did treatment eliminate SIB but also the near-zero rate persisted through placebo and no-drug phases of the study (59). In their retrospective study of 56 patients, Casner et al. (60) discovered that 57% of their patients treated with naltrexone between 3 and 878 months were considered to be positive responders and 25% of these met objective criteria as responders.

We (61) examined the long-term (12 month) effects following acute treatment with naltrexone and then we assessed the effects of subsequent long-term treatment with naltrexone. To accomplish this, we enrolled 15 subjects in a double-blind, placebo-controlled acute dose-finding study. Each acute dose was evaluated for a 1-week period with placebo weeks interspersed. Subjects were followed for a 12-month period and then they were enrolled in a multiple baseline design with a single most effective dose (determined in the acute phase) administered to each subject for 2-, 3-month periods over an 18-month interval with placebo periods appropriately separating the treatment phases. Again, time-sampled video records were scored using a computer-assisted program (62).

The primary finding from our study was that a subgroup of patients exhibited persisting effects (decreased SIB) in the 12 months after acute treatment with naltrexone. Seven patients exhibited decreased SIB over the 12-month period and five of these had a 75% reduction in SIB compared to the placebo control period. These five patients, each with at least a 75% reduction in SIB, increased their SIB when administered naltrexone in the long-term treatment protocol. The largest decrease in SIB which was observed in patients with acute exposure, increased their SIB during the 12-month hiatus and then readministered naltrexone several times in the 18-month double-blind, placebo-controlled study.

24.4 Endogenous Opioid Levels Predict Response to Opiate Blockers

In our initial study to examine the relation between circulating endogenous opioids and response to naltrexone, we collected blood samples from ten patients within 2–5 min of a self-injuring act and during a control period (18). At least 1 month later patients were administered three different doses of naltrexone in a double-blind, placebo-controlled crossover study over a 10-week period. All patients were videotaped during the study and behavior was coded with a computer-assisted program. Patients with the highest change in plasma levels of BE after SIB had the most and statistically significant positive response to naltrexone. These results were consistent with several other reports. First, Ernst et al. (21) reported that baseline levels of BE were positively related to changes in behavior (clinical global impressions, CGI) after treatment with naltrexone in five young autistic children. Second, Bouvard et al. (38) found that C-terminal BE decreased after naltrexone only in good responders. Third, Scifo et al. (63) found that increases in SIB and response to naltrexone in some patients, were related to high levels of endogenous opiates (i.e., good responses to naltrexone were observed in patients with high levels of BE). Fourth, Cazzullo et al. (64) reported that patients responding with decreased BE levels after treatment with naltrexone had better and more pervasive behavioral improvement than patients who did not have physiological changes after naltrexone.

In a follow-up study of nine additional patients (total of nineteen), we (3) found that plasma BE was uncoupled from the usually coreleased ACTH (65–71) after an episode of SIB. This unusual pattern was not a function of time of day that blood was sampled, and it confirmed our earlier observations (7, 18) and provided additional support for this specific biological marker among a diverse group of subjects who share a behavioral aberration. In addition, stronger support was generated for the effectiveness of naltrexone in reducing SIB.

Positive responses to low doses of naltrexone were observed in subjects *who did not* exhibit increased BE after SIB. That is, low doses of naltrexone were effective in reducing only SIB in subjects either who did not exhibit a surge in BE after SIB or whose baseline level exceeded the level after SIB. The relation between BE and response to the lowest dose of naltrexone was consistent with our earlier results, and statistically significant with the addition of nine subjects. Previously we (3) suggested that SIB had functional significance because it increased endogenous opiates and thereby delivered positive consequences (i.e., pleasure/euphoria/pain modulation). We argued that the highest dose of naltrexone most effectively blocked this mechanism in subjects with the highest levels of BE after SIB. The results from the follow-up study suggested an alternative possibility related to baseline levels of, or baseline relations between, POMC peptides. Because the lowest dose of naltrexone was most effective in subjects with the highest (morning) baseline (relative to post-SIB) levels, we speculated that the association between baseline ACTH and BE could influence the response to naltrexone (based on evidence that supported reciprocal functions of BE and ACTH (72)). If our speculations were accurate, subjects with the greatest difference between morning BE and ACTH levels would be the most responsive to low doses of naltrexone (because there would be less attenuation of the opioid influence). The test of this possibility confirmed our speculations because we found that subjects with high levels of morning (chronic) BE *and* low levels of ACTH were associated with positive responses to the low dose of naltrexone. This possibility may be compatible with findings that chronic exposure to opioids resulted in supersensitivity to the effects of low doses of opiate antagonists (73, 74).

We have made similar observations in our long-term studies of naltrexone and SIB (19). POMC fragments were measured in twelve self-injurious patients before and after long-term (3-month) treatment with naltrexone, as described in Fig. 24.4. POMC fragments were sampled from blood collected at the end of the baseline and placebo-controlled treatment phases of the study. Two patterns emerged. One group (responders) displayed persisting improvement in SIB and lower relative levels of BE after initial exposure to naltrexone. Chronic administration of naltrexone to this

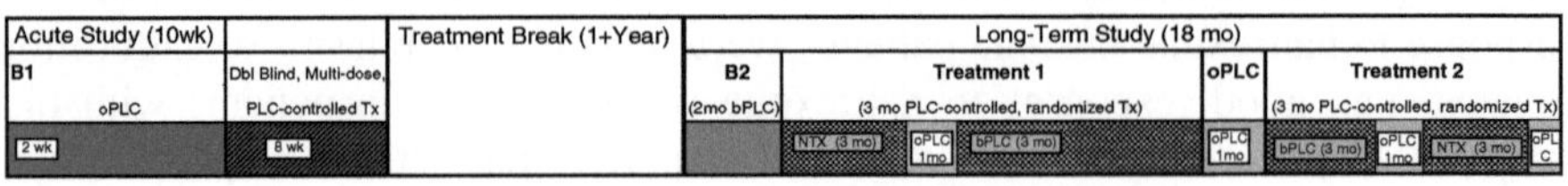

Fig. 24.4 Time-line of treatment protocol for naltrexone. The current study assessed the effects of acute (10-week) exposure to naltrexone, followed by a year without medication, and then a period of long-term treatment with naltrexone (18 months). *NTX* naltrexone, *oPLC* open placebo, *bPLC* baseline placebo, B_1 open placebo (2 weeks), B_2 open placebo (2 months)

group was associated with increased SIB and elevated relative levels of BE. Return to placebo improved their behavior (reduced SIB) and their levels of BE returned to basal levels. The second group (nonresponders) was characterized by absence of persisting improvement after acute treatment with naltrexone and by elevated basal BE levels. Chronic treatment with naltrexone improved their behavior but did not alter their BE levels. Long-term positive responders to acute doses of naltrexone were associated with less disregulation of ACTH and BE.

24.5 Conclusions

When it was established that the body had its own opiate system (75), the endogenous opiates became prime suspects responsible for maintaining SIB. Perhaps individuals who self-injure have elevated thresholds for pain or derive pleasure from painful stimulation. Exposure to, or levels of, endogenous opiates could explain these possibilities. Reduction in SIB following treatment with opiate blockers would provide evidence for the opiate hypothesis of self-injury. Results from studies to test these possibilities, however, are complex. The complexity is related primarily to the fact that patients exhibiting SIB and evaluated after treatment comprise a mixture of etiologies, pathologies, and motivations. Despite the tremendous amount of error introduced with a heterogeneous population, there is substantial evidence that opiate blockers are efficacious in reducing SIB.

The observations that opiate blockers reduce SIB are important for at least two reasons. First, naltrexone produces a clinically significant reduction in a serious and life-threatening behavior for some individuals typically who have not been responsive to any other type of treatment. We have observed startling improvements in individuals who have failed all rational treatments. Some adults in our studies have had protective headgear discontinued for the first time since early childhood. Others have developed adaptive skills and have acquired the ability (or the privilege) to leave institutions for the first time in their lives after treatment with naltrexone. Second, the results with naltrexone are important because they suggest that a *specific biological system* may be disregulated in a subgroup of patients. Because the opiate blockers have few effects in the absence of opiates (76), effective treatment with these drugs must engage the endogenous opioid system. Reports that resting levels of endogenous opiates or levels of endorphin after an SIB episode predict positive responses to opiate blockers provides support for this assumption and the foundation for rational treatment strategies based on biological criteria.

From this chapter we can draw several conclusions. There is consensus in the literature that doses between 1.0 and 2.0 mg/kg or a fixed dose of 100 mg are the most effective for reducing SIB (16, 53, 54). At these doses, at least half of the chronically self-injuring patients exhibit at least a 25% reduction in their behavior. It is important to acknowledge that the studies that have reported reductions of 25% or greater, typically conducted direct observations of the patients and did not rely on global clinical ratings. There is consensus that naltrexone is a safe drug without major or contraindicating side effects. Most individuals entered into naltrexone trials exhibited the most severe SIB for which all other forms of treatment had been ineffective. Often their behavior presented life-threatening consequences and *always* their SIB prevented them from enjoying a less restrictive environment. Against this background, the possible benefits of reduced SIB by treatment with naltrexone exceed the risk of side-effects. We are aware of clinical decisions to treat SIB with naltrexone even when patients presented with risk factors such as chronic hepatitis (77). To our knowledge, there have not been serious side effects *solely* due to administration of naltrexone among MR/DD clients. There is consensus among the studies that naltrexone is an effective treatment because the endogenous opioid system is engaged by SIB (3, 16, 18, 19, 57). SIB has characteristics that resemble addictive behavior (compulsive, ritualistic, destructive) and altered pain threshold. Both of these characteristics implicate the opioid system and support the logic of opiate blockers as reasonable treatments. There is consensus that long-term treatment of SIB with naltrexone apparently is not harmful and may be effective. There is consensus that generally, treatment with naltrexone appears to be effective in about half of the adult patients examined. There is consensus that naltrexone should be avoided during periods when patients are known to be in pain requiring narcotic analgesics, such as surgeries or with bone fractures. Alternately, nonnarcotic analgesics should be administered to patients receiving naltrexone (78).

References

1. Symons, F.J. & Danov, S.E. (2005). A prospective clinical analysis of pain behavior and self-injurious behavior. Pain, 117(3), 473–477.
2. Sandman, C.A. & Touchette, P. (2002). Opioids and the maintenance of self-injurious behavior. In: Schroeder, S.R., Oster-Granite M.L., Thompson T., eds. Self-Injurious Behavior: Gene-Brain-Behavior Relationships. Washington, DC: American Psychological Association, 191–204.
3. Sandman, C.A., Touchette, P., Lenjavi, M., Marion, S. & Chicz-DeMet, A. (2003). B-endorphin and ACTH are dissociated after self-injury in adults with developmental disabilities. American Journal on Mental Retardation, 108, 414–424.
4. Schroeder, S.R., Oster-Granite, M.L. & Thompson, T. (2002). Self-injurious Behavior: Gene-Brain-Behavior Relationships. Washington, DC: American Psychological Association.
5. Bodfish, J.W. & Lewis, M.H. (2002). Self-Injury and Comorbid Behaviors in Developmental, Neurological, Psychiatric, and Genetic Disorders. Washington, DC: American Psychological Association, 23–39.
6. Thompson, T. & Caruso, M. (2002). Self-injury: Knowing what we are looking for. In: Schroeder S.R., Oster-granite M.L., Thompson T., eds. Self-Injurious Behavior: Gene-Brain-Behavior Relationships. Washington, DC: American Psychological Association, 3–21.
7. Sandman, C.A., Touchette, P., Marion, S., Lenjavi, M. & Chicz-DeMet, A. (2002). Disregulation of proopiomelanocortin and contagious maladaptive behavior. Regulatory Peptides, 108, 179–185.
8. Kroeker, R. Touchette, P.E., Engleman, L. & Sandman, C.A. (2004). Quantifying temporal distributions of self-injurious behavior: Defining bouts vs discrete events. American Journal on Mental Retardation, 109, 1–8.
9. Marion, S., Touchette, P. & Sandman, C.A. (2003). Lag sequential analysis reveals a unique structure for self-injurious behavior. American Journal on Mental Retardation, 108, 301–313.

10. Marion, S.D., Touchette, P.E., Kroeker, R. & Sandman, C.A. (2005). Response to "Self-injury and sequential analysis: Context matters". American Journal on Mental Retardation, 110, 326–329.
11. Sandman, C.A. (1988). B-endorphin disregulation in autistic and self-injurious behavior: A neurodevelopmental hypothesis. Synapse, 2, 193–199.
12. Sandman, C.A. & Hetrick, W.P. (1995). Opiate mechanisms in self-injury. Mental Retardation and Developmental Disabilities Research Reviews, 1, 1–7.
13. Iwata, B.A., Roscoe, E.M., Zarcone, J.R. & Richman, D.M. (2002). Environmental determinants of self-injurious behavior. In: Schroeder S.R., Oster-Granite M.L., Thompson T., eds. Self Injurious Behavior: Gene-Brain-Behavior Relationship. Washington, DC: American Psychological Association, 93–103.
14. Fisher, W.W., Piazza, C.C. & Roane, H.S. (2002). Sleep and cyclical variables related to self injurious and other destructive behaviors. In: Schroeder S.R., Oster-Granite M.L., Thompson T., eds. Self Injurious Behavior: Gene-Brain-Behavior Relationship. Washington, DC: American Psychological Association, 205–221.
15. Sandman, C.A., Spence, M.A. & Smith, M. (1999). Proopiomelanocortin (POMC) disregulation and response to opiate blockers. Mental Retardation and Developmental Disabilities Research Reviews, 5, 314–321.
16. Thompson, T., Hackenberg, T., Cerutti, D., Baker, D. & Axtell, S. (1994). Opioid antagonist effects on self-injury in adults with mental retardation: Response form and location as determinants of mediation effects. American Journal on Mental Retardation, 99, 85–102.
17. Newell, K.M., Challis, J.H. & Boros, R. (2002). Further evidence on the dynamics of self-injurious behaviors: Impact forces and limb motions. American Journal on Mental Retardation, 107(1), 60–68.
18. Sandman, C.A., Hetrick, W.P., Taylor, D.V. & Chicz-DeMet, A. (1997). Dissociation of POMC peptides after self-injury predicts responses to centrally acting opiate blockers. American Journal on Mental Retardation, 102, 182–199.
19. Sandman, C.A., Hetrick, W., Taylor, D., Marion, S. & Chicz-DeMet, A. (2000). Uncoupling of proopiomelanocortin (POMC) fragments is related to self-injury. Peptides, 21, 785–791.
20. Coid, J., Allolio, B. & Rees, L.H. (1983). Raised plasma metenkephalin in patients who habitually mutilate themselves. Lancet, 2, 545–546.
21. Ernst, M., Devi, L., Silva, R.R., Gonzalez, M.N., Small, A.M., Malone, R.P. & Campbell, M. (1993). Plasma beta-endorphin levels, naltrexone, and haloperidol in autistic children. Psychopharmacology Bulletin, 29, 221–227.
22. Gillberg, C., Terenius, L.G. & Lonnerhom, G. (1985). Endorphin activity in childhood psychosis. Archives of General Psychiatry, 42, 780–783.
23. Gillberg, C., Terenius, L.G., Hagberg, B., Witt-Engerstom, I. & Eriksson, I. (1990). CSF beta-endorphins in childhood neuropsychiatric disorders. Brain and Development, 12, 88–92.
24. Ross, D.L., Klykylo, W.M. & Hitzemann, R. (1987). Reduction of elevated CSF b-endorphin by fenfluramine in infantile autism. Pediatric Neurology, 3, 83–86.
25. Sandman, C.A., Barron, J.L., Chicz-DeMet, A. & DeMet, E. (1991). Brief Report: Plasma b-endorphin and cortisol levels in autistic patients. Journal of Autism and Developmental Disorders, 21, 83–87.
26. Weizman, R., Weitman, A., Tyano, S., Szekely, B.A. & Sarne, Y.H. (1984). Humoral-endorphin blood levels in autistic, schizophrenic and healthy subjects. Psychopharmacology, 82, 368–370.
27. Sandman, C. A., Datta, P., Barron, J. L., Hoehler, F., Williams, C. & Swanson, J. (1983). Naloxone attenuates self-abusive behavior in developmentally disabled clients. Applied Research in Mental Retardation, 4, 5–11.
28. Cataldo, M. & Harris, J. (1982). The biological basis for self-injury in the mentally retarded. Analysis and Intervention in Developmental Disabilities, 2, 21–39.
29. Deutsch, S.I. (1986). Rationale for the administration of opiate antagonists in treating infantile autism. American Journal on Mental Retardation, 90, 631–635.
30. Dehen, H., Willer, J.C., Boureau, F. & Cambier, J. (1977). Congenital insensitivity to pain, and endogenous morphine-like substances. Lancet, 2(8,032), 293–294.

31. Dunger, D.B., Leonard, J.V., Wolff, O.H. & Preece, M.A. (1980). Effect of naloxone in a previously undescribed hypothalamic syndrome. A disorder of the endogenous opioid peptide system? Lancet, 1(8,181), 1277–1281.
32. Arnsten, A.F., Segal, D.S., Neville, H.J., Hillyard, S.A., Janowsky, D.S., Judd, L.L., et al. (1983). Naloxone augments electrophysiological signs of selective attention in man. Nature, 304(5,928), 725–727.
33. Sandman, C.A., McGivern, R.F., Berka, C., Walker, J.M., Coy, D.H. & Kastin, A.J. (1979). Neonatal administration of beta-endorphin produces "chronic" insensitivity to thermal stimuli. Life Science, 25(20), 1755–1760.
34. Madden, J. IV, Akil, H., Patrick, R.L. & Barchas, J.D. (1977). Stress-induced parallel changes in central opioid levels and pain responsiveness in the rat. Nature, 265(5,592), 358–360.
35. Wei, E. & Loh, H. (1976). Physical dependence of opiate-like peptides. Science, 193(4,259), 1262–1263.
36. Belluzzi, J.D. & Stein, L. (1977). Enkephaline may mediate euphoria and drive-reduction reward. Nature, 266(5,602), 556–558.
37. Gillberg, C. (1995). Endogenous opioids and opiate antagonists in autism: Brief review of empirical findings and implications for clinicians. Developmental Medicine and Child Neurology, 37, 88–92.
38. Bouvard, M.P., Leboyer, M., Launay, J.M., Recasens, C., Plumet, M.H., Waller-Perotte, D., et al. (1995). Low-dose naltrexone effects on plasma chemistries and clinical symptoms in autism: A double-blind, placebo-controlled study. Psychiatry Research, 58, 191–201.
39. Leboyer, M., Bouvard, M.P., Recasens, C., Philippe, A., Guilloud-Bataille, M., Bondoux, D., et al. (1994). Difference between plasma N- and C-terminally directed beta-endorphin immunoreactivity in infantile autism. The American Journal of Psychiatry, 151, 1797–1801.
40. Leboyer, M., Philippe, A., Bouvard, M., Guilloud-Bataille, M., Bondoux, D., Tabuteau, F., et al. (1999). Whole blood serotinin and plasma beta-endorphin in autistic probands and their first degree relatives. Society of Biological Psychiatry, 45, 158–163.
41. Verhoeven, W.M, Tuinier, S., van den Berg, Y.W., Coppus, A.M., Fekkes, D., Pepplinkhuizen, L. & Thijssen, J.H. (1999). Stress and self-injurious behavior; hormonal and serotonergic parameters in mentally retarded subjects. Pharmacopsychiatry, 32(1), 13–20.
42. Sandman, C.A., Barron, J.L., DeMet, E., Chicz-DeMet, A. & Rothenburg, S. (1990b). Opioid peptides and development: Clinical implications. In: Koob G.F., Sandman C.A., Strand F.L., eds. A Decade of Neuropeptides, Past, Present and Future. Annals of the New York Academy of Sciences, 91–107.
43. Sandman, C.A., Barron, J.L., Chicz-DeMet, A. & DeMet, E. (1990a). Plasma b-endorphin levels in patients with self-injurious behavior and stereotypy. American Journal of Mental Retardation, 95, 3–10.
44. Bertagna, X. (1994). Proopiomelanocortin-derived peptides. Endocrinology and Metabolism Clinics of North America, 23(3), 467–485.
45. Bicknell, A.B., Savva, D. & Lowry, P.J. (1996). Pro-opiomelanocortin and adrenal function. Endocrine Research, 22(4), 385–393.
46. Boutillier, A.L., Monnier, D., Koch, B. & Loeffler, J.P. (1994). Pituitary adenyl cyclase-activating peptide: A hypophysiotropic factor that stimulates proopiomelanocortin gene transcription, and proopiomelanocortin-derived peptide secretion in corticotropic cells. Neuroendocrinology, 60(5), 493–502.
47. Seidah, N.G. & Chretien, M. (1992). Propreotein and prohormone convertases of the subtilisin family. Trends in Endocrinology and Metabolism, 3, 133–140.
48. Seidah, N.G., Marcinkiewicz, M., Benjannet, S., Gaspar, L., Beaubien, G., Mattei, M.G., et al. (1991). Cloning and primary sequence of a mouse candidate prohormone convertase PC1 homologous to PC2, Furin, and KEX 2: Distinct chromosomal localization and messenger RNA distribution in brain and pituitary compared to PC2. Molecular Endocrinology, 5, 111–122.
49. Sandman, C.A. (1990–1991). The opiate hypothesis in autism and self-injury. Journal of Child and Adolescent Psychopharmacology, 1, 235–246.

50. Verhoeven, W.M. & Tuinier, S. (1996). The effect of buspirone on challenging behaviour in mentally retarded patients: An open prospective multiple-case study. Journal of Intellectual Disability Research, 40(Pt. 6), 502–508.
51. Campbell, M., Anderson, L.T., Small, A.M., Adams, P., Gonzalez, N.M. & Ernst, M. (1993). Naltrexone in autistic children: Behavioral symptoms and attentional learning. Journal of the American Academy of Child and Adolescent Psychiatry, 32(6), 1283–1291.
52. Zingarelli, G., Ellman, G., Hom, A., Wymore, M., Heidorn, S. & Chicz-DeMet, A. (1992). Clinical effects of naltrexone on autistic behavior. American Journal of Mental Retardation, 97(1), 57–63.
53. Symons, F.J., Thompson, A. & Rodriguez, M.C. (2004). Self-injurious behavior and the efficacy of naltrexone treatment: A quantitative synthesis. Mental Retardation and Developmental Disabilities Research Reviews, 10(3), 193–200.
54. Sandman, C.A., Hetrick, W.P., Taylor, D.V., Barron, J.L., Touchette, P., Lott, I., Crinella, F. & Martinazzi, V. (1993). Naltrexone reduces self-injury and improves learning. Experimental and Clinical Psychopharmacology, 13, 46.
55. Sandman, C.A., Datta, P.C., Barron-Quinn, J., Hoehler, F.K., Williams, C. & Swanson, J.M. (1983). Naloxone attenuates self-abusive behavior in developmentally disabled clients. Applied Research in Mental Retardation, 4, 5–11.
56. Sandman, C.A., Barron, J.L. & Colman, H. (1990). An orally administered opiate blocker, naltrexone attenuates self-injurious behavior. American Journal of Mental Retardation, 95, 93–102.
57. Barrett, R.P., Feinstein, C. & Hole, W.T. (1989). Effects of naloxone and naltrexone on self-injury: A double-blind, placebo-controlled analysis. American Journal of Mental Retardation, 93(6), 644–651.
58. Symons, F.J., Tapp, J., Wulfsberg, A., Sutton, K.A., Heeth, W.L. & Bodfish, J.W. (2001). Sequential analysis of the effects of naltrexone on the environmental mediation of self-injurious behavior. Experimental and Clinical Psychopharmacology, 9(3), 269–276.
59. Crews, W.D. Jr., Bonaventura, S., Rowe, F.B. & Bonsie, D. (1993). Cessation of long-term naltrexone therapy and self-injury: A case study. Research in Developmental Disabilities, 14(4), 331–340.
60. Casner, J.A., Weinheimer, B. & Gualtieri, C.T. (1996). Naltrexone and self-injurious behavior: A retrospective population study. Journal of Clinical Psychopharmacology, 16(5), 389–394.
61. Sandman, C.A., Hetrick, W.P., Taylor, D.V., Marion, S., Touchette, P., Barron, J.L., Martinazai, V., Steinberg, R. & Crinella, F.M. (2000). Long-term effects of Naltrexone on self-injurious behavior. American Journal of Mental Retardation, 105, 103–117.
62. Hetrick, W.P., Isenhart, R.C., Taylor, D.V. & Sandman, C.A. (1991). ODAP: A stand-alone program for observational data acquisition. Behavior Research Methods, Instruments and Computer, 23, 66–71.
63. Scifo, R., Cioni, M., Nicolosi, A., Batticane, N, Tirolo, C., Testa, N, et al. (1996). Opioid – Immune interactions in autism: Behavioral and immunological assessment during a double-blind treatment with naltrexone. Annali dell'Istituto Superiore di Sanita, 32, 351–359.
64. Cazzullo, A.G., Musetti, M.C., Musetti, L., Bajo, S., Sacerdote, P. & Panerai, A. (1999). Beta-endorphin levels in peripheral blood mononuclear cells and long-term naltrexone treatment in autistic children. European Neuropsychopharmacology, 9(4), 361–366.
65. Forman, L.J., Harwell, M.F. & Cater, J. (1990). Beta-endorphin in the male rat pituitary: Testosterone influences the effect of cocaine. Brain Research Bulletin, 25(1), 65–68.
66. Giuffre, K.A., Udelsman, R., Listwak, S. & Chrousos, G.P. (1988). Effects of immune neutralization of corticotropin-releasing hormone, adrenocorticotropin, and beta endorphin in the surgically stressed rat. Endocrinology, 122(1), 306–310.
67. Holson, R.R., Scallet, A.C., Ali, S.F., Sullivan, P. & Gough, B. (1988). Adrenocortical, beta-endorphin and behavioral responses to graded stressors in differentially reared rats. Physiology and Behavior, 42(2), 125–130.
68. Knigge, U., Matzen, S., Bach, F.W., Bang, P. & Warberg, J. (1989). Involvement of histaminergic neurons in the stress-induced release of pro-opiomelanocortin-derived peptides in rats. Acta Endocrinologica (Copenh), 120(4), 533–539.

69. Oltras, C.M., Mora, F. & Vives, F. (1987). Beta-endorphin and ACTH in plasma: Effects of physical and psychological stress. Life Science, 40(17), 1683–1686.
70. Recher, H., Willis, G.L., Smith, G.C. & Copolov, D.L. (1988). i.r. Beta-endorphin, corticosterone, cholesterol and triglyceride concentrations in rat plasma after stress, cingulotomy or both. Pharmacology, Biochemistry, and Behavior, 31(1), 75–79.
71. Shutt, D.A., Smith, A.I., Wallace, C.A., Connell, R. & Fell, L.R. (1988). Effect of myiasis and acute restraint stress on plasma levels of immunoreactive beta-endorphin, adrenocorticotrophin (ACTH) and cortisol in the sheep. Australian Journal of Biological Sciences, 41(3), 297–301.
72. Sandman, C.A. & Kastin, A.J. (1990). Neuropeptide modulation of development and behavior: Implications for psychopathology In: Deutsch S, ed. Application of Basic Neuroscience to Child Psychiatry. Washington, DC: Plenum Publishing, 101–124.
73. Shen, K.F. & Crain, S.M. (1992). Chronic selective activation of excitatory opioid receptor functions in sensory neurons results in opioid "dependence" without tolerance. Brain Research, 597(1), 74–83.
74. Crain, S.M. & Shen, K.F. (1995). Ultra-low concentrations of naloxone selectively antagonize excitatory effects of morphine on sensory neurons, thereby increasing its antinociceptive potency and attenuating tolerance/dependence during chronic cotreatment. Proceedings of the National Academy of Sciences of the United States of America, 92(23), 10540–10544.
75. Pert, C.B. & Snyder, S.H. (1973). Opiate receptor: Demonstration in nervous tissue. Science, 179(77), 1011–1014.
76. Reisine, T. & Pasternak, G. (1996). Opioid analgesics and antagonists. In Hardman J.G., Limbird L.E., Molinoff P.B., Ruddon R.W., & Gilman A.G., eds. The Pharmacological Basis of Therapeutics. New York, NY: McGraw-Hill, 521–556.
77. Hetrick, W.P., Krutzik, M.N., Taylor, D.V., Sandman, C.A., Rusu, L. & Martinazzi, V.P. (1993). Naltrexone has no hepatotoxic effects in a self-injurious patient with chronic hepatitis. Journal of Clinical Psychopharmacology, 13(6), 453–454.
78. Sandman, C.A., Thompson, T., Barrett, R.P., Verhoeven, W.M.A., McCubbin, J.A., Schroeder, S.R. & Hetrick, W.P. (1998). Opiate blockers. In Reiss S., & Aman M.G., eds. The Consensus Handbook of Psychopharmacology. Columbus, OH: The OSU Nisonger Center.

Chapter 25
Pharmacotherapeutic Effects of Opioid Antagonists in Alcohol-Abusing Patients with Schizophrenia

Ismene Petrakis

Abstract Schizophrenia is a devastating clinical disorder that affects ~1% of the general population. The prevalence of alcohol use disorders among schizophrenic patients is greater than the rate observed in the general population. While behavioral treatments have been developed to treat patients with comorbid schizophrenia and substance use, pharmacologic management may provide another therapeutic option for these patients. The opioid antagonist naltrexone was developed and approved by the Food and Drug Administration (FDA) to treat alcohol use disorders in noncomorbid patients. More recently, there has been interest in the use of opioid antagonist treatment for patients with schizophrenia and comorbid alcohol dependence. The evidence supporting the use of naltrexone in this group is from data from heterogeneous samples of dually diagnosed patients including those with schizophrenia and schizoaffective disorder and from one randomized trial in patients with schizophrenia and schizoaffective disorder. The controlled clinical trial in patients with schizophrenia and alcohol use/dependence compared naltrexone to placebo augmentation of neuroleptic in 31 outpatients. Outcomes focused on alcohol use and craving, but also rigorously evaluated symptoms of psychosis, cognitive symptoms and side effects. The results consistently suggest that naltrexone is both safe and effective in this group of patients. Taken together, the data suggest that the opioid antagonist naltrexone may be a good therapeutic option to treat alcohol use disorders in patients with schizophrenia.

Keywords: Opioid antagonist; Schizophrenia; Alcohol abuse; Comorbidity

25.1 Introduction

Schizophrenia is a devastating clinical disorder that affects ~1% of the general population (44). The prevalence of substance use disorders (SUDs) among schizophrenic patients is greater than the rate observed in the general population (44) and

I. Petrakis
West Haven Veterans Administration Medical Center,
#116-A, 950 Campbell Avenue, West Haven, CT 06516
e-mail: ismene.petrakis@yale.edu

has been associated with a number of clinical issues including increased psychotic symptoms (11), an increased rate of medication noncompliance (16), more frequent and longer hospitalizations (16), a higher rate of crisis-oriented service utilization, and consequently a higher cost of care (16). Social problems associated with substance abuse in patients with schizophrenia are similar to the problems in patients without comorbid schizophrenia and include legal entanglements, housing instability, lower rates of employment, and poor money management (11).

While there is evidence that certain psychosocial approaches can be effective in the treatment of comorbid substance abuse disorders [e.g., (6)], these require highly trained staff and may not be feasible in traditional mental health treatment settings, where most patients are treated. In addition, substance-dependent patients with comorbid schizophrenia may have reluctance to participate in traditional substance abuse treatments and self-help groups (such as Alcoholics Anonymous) where members do not have comorbid psychotic disorders (32). The cognitive deficits associated with schizophrenia may interfere with the ability to fully participate in psychosocial treatments and negative symptoms may undermine patients' motivation. In contrast, pharmacological treatments are generally familiar to dually diagnosed patients, require less new learning than psychosocial treatments, and dose scheduling can be readily integrated into treatment. Therefore, effective medications to treat SUDs should have a positive clinical impact in the treatment of patients with schizophrenia and comorbid substance abuse.

After nicotine, the most common drug of abuse in patients with schizophrenia is alcohol. There are four compounds approved by the Food and Drug Administration (FDA) to treat alcohol dependence, but there are no medications approved by the FDA for the specific treatment of patients with alcohol dependence and schizophrenia. However, a growing literature has evaluated the potential of medications to treat alcohol dependence in patients with comorbid schizophrenia [e.g., (29, 3, 37, 40)].

25.2 Opioid Antagonist Use in Schizophrenia

Interest in the morphine-like peptides, or endorphins, and their involvement in behavior and psychological events led to the suggestion that they be important in some mental illnesses (34). Animal models of psychosis have suggested an interaction between opioid peptides and schizophrenic behavior. However, data from humans is inconsistent. For example, although some reports have suggested levels of opioids in cerebrospinal fluid samples (CSF) varied with the severity of the disease, other studies were equivocal. Clinical evidence has suggested that opiates may have a prophylactic or therapeutic effect on mental illness; specifically, the psychoactive properties of opiates may include reduction in rage, aggression, and paranoia (34).

The preclinical and clinical data suggesting a role for the endogenous opiates in the pathophysiology of schizophrenia led to studies evaluating the use of opiate antagonists for treatment in nondually diagnosed patients with schizophrenia.

While opiate *agonists*, such as methadone had no effect, when compared to placebo (21), a promising report suggested the opioid antagonist naloxone temporarily reduced hallucinations in four case of schizophrenic patients (18). Naloxone was subsequently given to many patients and was found to decrease the perceptive and delusional symptoms (41). However, naloxone is limited by a short half-life and must be given intravenously. The oral antagonist naltrexone was also evaluated, using doses ranging from 50 to 800 mg, both as adjunctive medication and as monotherapy with mixed results in treating positive symptoms of schizophrenia [reviewed in (28, 47)]. While it was hypothesized that naltrexone may be effective as an augmentation predominately for negative symptoms (28), results from a crossover augmentation trial of naltrexone failed to find an effect on positive *or* negative symptoms (47). Using a cross-over design, nalmefene was found to decrease positive but not negative symptoms (43).

There has been some interest in the use of opioid antagonists for the treatment of other related symptoms of schizophrenia such as stereotypic behaviors like polydypsia (5). After a pilot study suggested naloxone may be effective in improving polydipsia (31), naltrexone was evaluated in an open trial in patients with severe hyponatremia due to polydipsia (5). While other symptoms decreased from baseline, there was no significant effect on polydipsia. The opioid antagonists may also have a role in treating some of the consequences of schizophrenia. Laboratory studies with preclinical animals have suggested that opioid antagonist therapy may be effective in dyskinesia (53). A few clinical studies have evaluated antagonist treatment for tardive dyskinesia. They include several studies with naloxone (50, 7, 46, 8) but again the limitations of naloxone did not encourage further evaluation. In a randomized study with oral naltrexone, naltrexone in combination with clonazepam significantly improved symptoms of tardive dyskinesia, suggesting that the opioid antagonist naltrexone may have a role in combination therapy for tardive dyskinesia (53).

25.3 Opioid Antagonist Treatment in Alcohol Dependence

The μ-opioid antagonist naltrexone has been FDA-approved for treatment of alcohol dependence since 1994. There is a rich preclinical literature suggesting that opioid antagonists reliably reduce alcohol consumption under a variety of circumstances (12). Naltrexone was clinically tested first by Volpicelli and colleagues (51), who used naltrexone as an adjunctive treatment to standard psychotherapy in a placebo-controlled, double-blind, study of recently detoxified alcoholic volunteers. Naltrexone-treated individuals reported lower levels of alcohol craving, fewer drinks and drinking days, and lower rates of relapse than did placebo-treated patients. Volpicelli's initial findings were then replicated and extended by others (33, 1). Three meta-analyses of the placebo-controlled trials each concluded that naltrexone has a modest effect on drinking measures (24, 49, 48). In all these clinical studies, naltrexone was effective in the context of a standard effective psychosocial intervention.

The largest study to date of naltrexone is the multisite COMBINE trial, which evaluated natlrexone, acamrosate, the combination and behavioral interventions for alcohol dependence (2). Subjects who received medical management with naltrexone had better alcohol use outcomes than those in most other groups, and there was no advantage to combination with acamprosate. The results suggested that naltrexone may be effectively utilized in nonspecialty healthcare settings. Recently, a few studies have suggested that "targeted" naltrexone, that is naltrexone not taken in the traditional daily dosage as a relapse prevention, but taken when experiencing craving, may be effective in reducing heavy drinking in nonabstinent individuals (20, 26). Further, a depot preparation of naltrexone has also been shown to be effective in the treatment of alcohol dependence (14) and has recently been approved for use by the FDA.

There are negative studies of naltrexone for alcohol dependence as well (25, 15). The largest of these studies is a multisite Veterans Administration (VA) cooperative trial of 627 alcohol-dependent veterans, in which there was no effect of naltrexone on the percentage of relapse days, drinking days, and drinks per drinking days (27). It has been hypothesized that the VA cooperative study results may not be generalizable to all patients manifesting alcohol dependence, as the veterans were overwhelmingly male, older and with longer duration of alcoholism than the subjects enrolled in previous trials with naltrexone (13). Another factor may be comorbidity with mental disorders since subjects manifesting comorbid major psychiatric disorders, such as posttraumatic stress disorder, major depression, and generalized anxiety disorders, were not excluded (patients with psychotic disorders *were* excluded) but did not receive psychotropics. In contrast, naltrexone was effective in reducing alcohol use in patients manifesting comorbid psychiatric disorders in another study where subjects with comorbid diagnoses were included, but only if treated with psychotropic medications at stable doses for at least 3 months prior to randomization (30). Therefore, patients with better-controlled psychiatric conditions may find naltrexone effective, or naltrexone may work synergistically with psychotropic medications in improving drinking outcomes.

25.4 Opiate Antagonist Treatment in Patients with Alcohol Dependence and Psychiatric Comorbidity

There is some evidence that clinicians who treat patients with alcohol dependence do in fact preferentially prescribe naltrexone to dually diagnosed individuals. In evaluating the utilization of naltrexone in the VA system nationally, despite a very low rate of prescribing (2% of patients with alcohol dependence were prescribed naltrexone), the presence of a comorbid mental disorder was one of the clinical factors associated with an increase likelihood of being prescribed naltrexone (36). It may be that those patients with comorbid psychiatric disorders have more experience with medications and are more willing to embrace pharmacotheraputic treatments or that pharmacotherapeutic treatments are particularly effective in this group. Nevertheless, rigorous studies to evaluate this question have only recently been undertaken (see Table 25.1).

Table 25.1 Studies evaluating naltrexone in alcohol-dependent patients with comorbid psychotic spectrum disorders

Authors	Population, *n*	Intervention	Type of study	Results
Brown et al. (10)	Subjects ($n = 34$) with bipolar disorder and alcohol dependence	Naltrexone 50 mg/day	Sixteen-week open-label add-on study	Reduction in heavy drinking and alcohol craving
Maxwell and Shinderman (29)	Mentally ill outpatients ($n = 72$) with alcohol use disorders	Clinical treatment with naltrexone	Retrospective chart review	Reduction in drinking by ≥75% in 81.9% of subjects
Petrakis et al. (36)	Subjects ($n = 31$) with schizophrenia or schizoaffective disorder and alcohol abuse/dependence	Naltrexone/placebo 50 mg/day	Twelve-week, double-blind randomized controlled trial	Fewer heavy drinking days and lower craving on naltrexone compared to placebo. No effect of naltrexone on psychotic symptoms
Ralevski et al. (42)*	Subjects ($n = 30$) with schizophrenia or schizoaffective disorder and alcohol dependence	Naltrexone/placebo 50 mg/day	Twelve-week, double-blind randomized controlled trial and open label follow-up	No effect of naltrexone on cognitive functioning
Petrakis et al. (38)	Subjects ($n = 254$) with major Axis I disorder and alcohol dependence	Four cells: disulfiram 250 mg/day and placebo, disulfiram 250 mg/day and naltrexone 50 mg/day, naltrexone 50 mg/day alone, and placebo alone	Twelve-week double-blind randomized controlled trial of disulfiram, naltrexone alone and in combination	More consecutive days of abstinence on active medication compared to placebo. No advantage of the combination
Petrakis et al. (39)**	Subjects ($n = 67$) with psychotic level disorder and alcohol dependence	Four cells: disulfiram and placebo, disulfiram and naltrexone, naltrexone alone, and placebo alone	Twelve-week double-blind randomized controlled trial of disulfiram, naltrexone alone, and in combination	Fewer heavy drinking days on active medication compared to placebo. No advantage of the combination

[a]The data from this study was collected as part of the main trial reported in Petrakis et al. (36)

There are a few pilot studies evaluating naltrexone in dually diagnosed patients. In a retrospective study on 72 psychiatric patients treated with naltrexone for alcohol use disorders, 82% of them significantly reduced their drinking (29). This sample included subjects with psychotic spectrum disorders, including schizophrenia, schizoaffective disorder, and bipolar disorder (n = 35). A small add on open-label study of naltrexone in patients with bipolar disorder suggested that naltrexone was well tolerated and decreased alcohol use and craving (10). Two related studies evaluated naltrexone in depression. Naltrexone decreased alcohol use and improved depressive symptoms in an open-label study with patients manifesting alcohol dependence (45). In a study in elderly outpatients with depression and alcohol dependence, naltrexone augmentation of sertraline did not add benefit in terms of depressive symptoms or alcohol use outcomes (35).

The first large-scale study (n = 254) in dually diagnosed individuals was conducted in order to compare disulfiram and naltrexone, alone and in combination, as treatment for alcohol dependence in a veteran population with a heterogeneous set of comorbid mental disorders, many of whom were concurrently receiving pharmacotherapy for their symptoms (38). The results showed that only the most stringent drinking outcomes were significantly better in individuals assigned to active medication versus placebo. In particular, individuals on active medication had more consecutive weeks of abstinence compared to those on placebo. There was no overall advantage of one medication over the other, and no advantage of the combination of both medications. There was a high rate of abstinence overall, with 177 subjects (69.7%) of all subjects achieving *complete* abstinence during the 12-week trial. These medications, including the combination, had tolerable side effects consistent with those seen in nondually diagnosed patients.

25.5 Opiate Antagonist Treatment in Patients with Alcohol Dependence and Schizophrenia

Secondary analysis of the above-mentioned 12-week randomized clinical trial of disulfiram and naltrexone alone and in combination for individuals with Axis I disorders and alcohol dependence was conducted to evaluate the effect of a psychotic spectrum disorder on alcohol use outcomes (39). In this 12-week outpatient study, individuals were randomized to one of four groups: (1) naltrexone alone, (2) placebo alone, (3) disulfiram and naltrexone, or (4) disulfiram and placebo. The study also evaluated the effect these medications had on the symptoms of psychosis. Because of the relatively small number of subjects who had schizophrenia alone, all subjects with disorders within the psychotic spectrum (n = 66), including schizophrenia, schizoaffective disorder, and bipolar disorder, were included in this psychotic spectrum group.

Individuals with a psychotic spectrum disorder had worse alcohol outcomes, including fewer days of consecutive abstinence, fewer total days of abstinence and more heavy drinking days than those without a psychotic spectrum disorder.

However, there were significant interactions between the diagnosis of a psychotic spectrum disorder and medication condition on several alcohol use outcomes. In each case, subjects with psychotic spectrum disorders that were treated with active medication (disulfiram or naltrexone) had significantly better outcomes when compared to subjects on placebo. Specifically, those with psychotic spectrum disorders who were treated with active medication had significantly more days of abstinence and fewer total heavy drinking days when compared to placebo. There were no significant differences in outcome in those treated with naltrexone compared to those with disulfiram, and no advantage of the combination compared to either alone. Within the group with psychotic spectrum disorders, there were no significant changes in psychotic symptoms over time or due to treatment condition. This study supported the use of these medications for the treatment of alcohol dependence in individuals with comorbid psychotic-spectrum disorders.

Only a few studies have evaluated opiate antagonist medications in alcohol-abusing schizophrenic patients. The first randomized controlled, clinical trial with naltrexone patients with schizophrenia, and alcohol dependence was conducted in 31 outpatients who were also stabilized on neuroleptic treatment (37). Individuals were treated for 12 weeks with naltrexone 50 mg or placebo in conjunction with weekly behavioral therapy with relapse prevention strategies combined with skills training. Outcome measures included alcohol use outcomes, craving, psychotic symptoms, side effects, and cognitive measures.

The results were quite promising. Of the 31 subjects randomized, 25 subjects reached follow-up and there was not a significant difference between the placebo-treated group and the naltrexone-treated group on retention. Those individuals on naltrexone had significantly fewer drinking days and therefore more days of abstinence, fewer heavy drinking days, and significantly lower self-reported craving compared to those on placebo. Overall, naltrexone was well tolerated and did not cause a worsening of psychosis. The results of the study suggested naltrexone is safe and effective in conjunction with standard psychosocial and pharmacological treatments in patients manifesting schizophrenia. These results are consistent with most published studies that have found that naltrexone has a modest effect on alcohol consumption (24). A modest effect on alcohol consumption is likely to be a clinically significant finding in individuals with serious mental illness, since individuals with mental illness may suffer the consequences of alcohol use at a lower rate of alcohol consumption than individuals without mental illness (22), so even small changes in alcohol consumption may have a big clinical impact.

An important finding from this study is that naltrexone did not worsen symptoms of schizophrenia. Subjects' positive and negative symptoms were largely unchanged during the study, and there was no effect of naltrexone on these symptoms. This is consistent with existing literature that has shown opiate antagonists do not worsen psychosis in nonalcohol abusing schizophrenic patients (41, 47) and in alcohol-abusing schizophrenic patients (3).

In a second phase of this study, the effect of naltrexone treatment on cognition in patients with schizophrenia and comorbid alcohol dependence was also evaluated (42). Thirty of the 31 subjects were included in the analysis; after the initial

12 weeks of treatment subjects were offered the option of open-label naltrexone for an additional 12 weeks. Fourteen opted to continue, eight patients continued on naltrexone, and six switched from placebo to naltrexone. Outcome measures included alcohol use; symptoms of schizophrenia, memory and attention were assessed at baseline, week 12 and week 24.

Results showed that naltrexone treatment had no effect on cognitive functioning for patients with alcohol dependence and schizophrenia at 12 weeks and at 24 weeks. In evaluating naltrexone as a potentially effective treatment for alcohol misuse in dually diagnosed individuals, the absence of any adverse effects on cognitive function is clinically important. Cognitive deficits associated with schizophrenia are associated with clinical sequelae such as worsening prognosis, increased rates of hospitalization, reduced socioeconomic status, increased mortality, and poorer adaptive functioning (19, 17, 54). The standard treatment for schizophrenia, the neuroleptic medications, can have adverse cognitive effects (9). In recommending an adjunctive medication for these patients, a careful evaluation of potential adverse effects, including effect on cognition, is important.

These results are in the context of a standard clinical dose (50 mg) and good medication compliance (37). In this trial, compliance may have been high because of the low rate of side effects reported. Of note, only two subjects reported nausea; this low rate may be due to the antiemetic effects of the neuroleptic medications. Nevertheless, compliance with naltrexone has been reported to be an issue in other clinical trials (52). Currently, a larger study is underway evaluating directly-observed naltrexone in patients with schizophrenia. While alcohol use outcomes are not yet known, some information is available on the kinds of patients referred to this study. The majority have been referred by a mental health profession, rather than self-referred and the subject group has been characterized as having low levels of alcohol drinking, low levels of recognition of alcohol problems but moderately high levels of alcohol use severity and high levels of ambivalence (4). This is consistent with the hypothesis that in patients with schizophrenia, relatively lower levels of alcohol drinking leads to clinical impairment and highlights the need for effective treatments for this group of patients.

25.6 Conclusions

Taken together, results from these studies suggest that opiate antagonist treatment may be an effective treatment for alcohol misuse in patients with comorbid schizophrenia. In fact, individuals with schizophrenia may be particularly suited for treatment with medications for alcohol dependence in general and with opiate antagonist treatment in particular. This may be in part because patients with schizophrenia may not be able to benefit as fully from the forms of treatments that have been developed for noncomorbid alcohol-dependent individuals, so medication effects may be more readily apparent. Nevertheless, even with effective psychosocial treatments that are available (6), finding effective pharmacotherapies increases therapeutic options for patients. Results from the recent COMBINE trial suggest patients may be able to be treated effectively with naltrexone with a primary-care-based intervention, or may be referred to a specialty clinic for psychotherapy (2). Although not yet tested, giving patients choices will likely lead to a greater number of individuals getting the treatment they need. In extrapolating to patients with schizophrenia, pharmacotherpeutic options may be more readily integrated into existing mental health treatment and appropriate for patients who do not have access to specialty clinics.

Opioid-antagonist treatments, such as natlrexone, may also be particularly suited for this group of patients. While there are only a few studies, the findings have been consistent and in the case of the one randomized clinical trial, robust. There was a significant difference in alcohol use outcomes despite a relatively small sample size and concurrent treatment with an active psychosocial treatment. Further, the high rate of compliance and the low rate of side effects suggest that it may be particularly well tolerated in this group of patients. Nevertheless, these conclusions should be interpreted with caution since they are based on small studies. Larger definitive studies are still indicated. Of particular interest may also be what effect the depot preparation of naltrexone has and whether this can be best integrated into existing mental health treatment for this group of patients.

References

1. Anton, R. F., D. H. Moak, et al. (1999). "Naltrexone and cognitive behavioral therapy for treatment of outpatient alcoholics: result a placebo-controlled trial." *American Journal of Psychiatry* 156(11): 1758–64.
2. Anton, R. F., S. S. O'Malley, et al. (2006). "Combined pharmacotherapies and behavioral interventions for alcohol dependence: the COMBINE study: a randomized controlled trial [see comment]." *Journal of the American Medical Association* 295(17): 2003–17.
3. Batki, S., J. Dimmock, et al. (2002). "Directly observed naltrexone treatment of alcohol dependence in schizophrenia: preliminary analysis." *Alcoholism: Clinical and Experimental Research* 26: 83A.
4. Batki, S., J. Dimmock, et al. (2005). "Recruitment and characteristics of alcohol dependent patients with schizophrenia." *Alcoholism: Clinical and Experimental Research* 29: 78A.
5. Becker, J. A., M. B. Goldman, et al. (1995). "Effects of naltrexone on mannerisms and water imbalance in polydipsic schizophrenics: a pilot study." *Schizophrenia Research* 17(3): 279–82.
6. Bellack, A., M. Bennett, et al. (2006). "A randomized clinical trial of a new behavioral treatment for drug abuse in people with severe and persistent mental illness." *Archives of General Psychiatry* 63: 426–32.
7. Blum, I., H. Munitz, et al. (1984). "Naloxone may be beneficial in the treatment of tardive dyskinesia." *Clinical Neuropharmacology* 7(3): 265–7.
8. Blum, I., P. F. Nisipeanu, et al. (1987). "Naloxone in tardive dyskinesia." *Psychopharmacology* 93(4): 538.
9. Blyler, C. R. and J. M. Gold (2000). Cognitive effects of typical antipsychotic medication treatment: another look. In T. Sharma and P. D. Harvey (eds.) *Cognition in Schizophrenia.* Oxford, Oxford University Press: 241–265.
10. Brown, E. S., L. Beard, et al. (2006). "Naltrexone in patients with biopolar disorder and alcohol dependence." *Depression and Anxiety* 23(8): 492–5.

11. Dixon, L. (1999). "Dual diagnosis of substance abuse in schizophrenia: prevalence and impact on outcomes." *Schizophrenia Research* 35(Suppl.): S93–100.
12. Froehlich, J., S. O'Malley, et al. (2003). "Preclinical and clinical studies on naltrexone: what have they taught each other?" *Alcoholism: Clinical and Experimental Research* 27(3): 533–9.
13. Fuller, R. and E. Gordis (2001). "Naltrexone treatment for alcohol dependence." *The New England Journal of Medicine* 345(24): 1770–1.
14. Garbutt, J. C., H. R. Kranzler, et al. (2005). "Efficacy and tolerability of long-acting injectable naltrexone for alcohol dependence: a randomized controlled trial. [see comment] [erratum appears in JAMA. 2005 April 27; 293(16):1978]." *Journal of the American Medical Association* 293(13): 1617–25.
15. Gastpar, M. T., U. Bonnet, et al. (2002). "Lack of efficacy of naltrexone in the prevention of alcohol relapse: resultes from a German multicenter study." *Journal of Clinical Psychopharmacology* 22(6): 592–8.
16. Gerding, L. B., L. A. Labbate, et al. (1999). "Alcohol dependence and hospitalization in schizophrenia." *Schizophrenia Research* 38(1): 71–5.
17. Green, M. F., R. S. Kern, et al. (2000). "Neurocognitive deficits and functional outcome in schizophrenia: are we measuring the "right stuff"?" *Schizophrenia Bulletin* 26(1): 119–36.
18. Gunne, L. M., L. Lindstrom, et al. (1977). "Naloxone-induced reversal of schizophrenic hallucinations." *Journal of Neural Transmission General Section* 40(1): 13–9.
19. Harvey, P. D., E. Howanitz, et al. (1998). "Symptoms, cognitive functioning, and adaptive skills in geriatric patients with lifelong schizophrenia: a comparison across treatment sites." *American Journal of Psychiatry* 155(8): 1080–6.
20. Heinala, P., H. Alho, et al. (2001). "Targeted use of naltrexone without prior detoxification in the treatment of alcohol dependence: a factorial double-blind, placebo-controlled trial." *Journal of Clinical Psychopharmacology* 21(3): 287–92.
21. Judd, L. L., D. S. Janowsky, et al. (1981). "Behavioral effects of methadone in schizophrenic patients." *American Journal of Psychiatry* 138(2): 243–5.
22. Kavanagh, D., J. McGrath, et al. (2002). "Substance misuse in patients with schizophrenia: epidemiology and management." *Drugs* 62(5): 743–55.
23. Ko, G. (1984). "A double blind trial of chronic methadone in schizophrenia."
24. Kranzler, H. and J. Van Kirk (2001). "Efficacy of naltrexone and acamprosate for alcoholism treatment: a meta-analysis." *Alcoholism: Clinical and Experimental Research* 25: 1335–41.
25. Kranzler, H., V. Modesto-Lowe, et al. (2000). "Naltrexone vs nefazodone for treatment of alcohol dependence. A placebo-controlled trial." *Neuropsychopharmacology* 22(5): 493–503.
26. Kranzler, H. R., S. Armeli, et al. (2003). "Targeted naltrexone for early problem drinkers." *Journal of Clinical Psychopharmacology* 23(3): 294–304.
27. Krystal, J. H., J. Cramer, et al. (2001). "Naltrexone in the treatment of alcohol dependence." *The New England Journal of Medicine* 345(24): 1734–9.
28. Marchesi, G. F., G. Santone, et al. (1995). "The therapeutic role of naltrexone in negative symptom schizophrenia." *Progress in Neuro Psychopharmacology and Biological Psychiatry* 19(8): 1239–49.
29. Maxwell, S. and M. S. Shinderman (2000). "Use of naltrexone in the treatment of alcohol use disorders in patients with concomitant major mental illness." *Journal of Addictive Diseases* 19(3): 61–9.
30. Morris, P. L., M. Hopwood, et al. (2001). "Naltrexone for alcohol dependence: a randomized controlled trial [comment]." *Addiction* 96(11): 1565–73.
31. Nishikawa, T., A. Tsuda, et al. (1994). "Naloxone attenuates drinking behavior in psychiatric patients displaying self-induced water intoxication." *Progress in Neuro Psychopharmacology and Biological Psychiatry* 18(1): 149–53.
32. Noordsy, D. L., B. Schwab, et al. (1996). "The role of self-help programs in the rehabilitation of persons with severe mental illness and substance use disorders." *Community Mental Health Journal* 32(1): 71–81; discussion 83–6.
33. O'Malley, S., A. Jaffe, et al. (1992). "Naltrexone and coping skills therapy for alcohol dependence. A controlled study." *Archives of General Psychiatry* 49(11): 881–7.

34. Olson, G. A., R. D. Olson, et al. (1984). "Endogenous opiates: 1983." *Peptides* 5(5): 975–92.
35. Oslin, D. W. (2005). "Treatment of late-life depression complicated by alcohol dependence." *American Journal of Geriatric Psychiatry* 13(6): 491–500.
36. Petrakis, I. L., D. Leslie, et al. (2003). "Use of naltrexone in the treatment of alcoholism nationally in the Department of Veterans Affairs." *Alcoholism: Clinical and Experimental Research* 27 (11): 1780–4.
37. Petrakis, I. L., S. O'Malley, et al. (2004). "Naltrexone augmentation of neuroleptic treatment in alcohol abusing patients with schizophrenia." *Psychopharmacology* 172: 291–7.
38. Petrakis, I. L., J. Poling, et al. (2005). "Naltrexone and disulfiram in patients with alcohol dependence and comorbid psychiatric disorders." *Biological Psychiatry* 57: 1128–37.
39. Petrakis, I., C. Nich, et al. (2006b). "Psychotic spectrum disorders and alcohol abuse: a review of pharmacotherapeutic strategies and a report on the effectiveness of naltrexone and disulfiram." *Schizophrenia Bulletin* 32(4): 644–54.
40. Petrakis, I. L., D. Leslie, et al. (2006a). "Atypical antipsychotic medication and substance use-related outcomes in treatment of schizophrenia." *The American Journal on Addictions* 15: 44–9.
41. Pickar, D., W. Bunney, et al. (1989). "Repeated naloxone administration in schizophrenia: a phase II world Health Organization study." *Biology of Psychiatry* 25: 440–8.
42. Ralevski, E., K. Balachandra, et al. (2006). "Effects of naltrexone on cognition in a treatment study of patients with schizophrenia and comorbid alcohol dependence." *Journal of Dual Diagnosis* 2(4): 53–69.
43. Rapaport, M. H., O. Wolkowitz, et al. (1993). "Beneficial effects of nalmefene augmentation in neuroleptic-stabilized schizophrenic patients." *Neuropsychopharmacology* 9(2): 111–5.
44. Rieger, D. A., M. E. Farmer, et al. (1990). "Comorbidity of mental disorders with alcohol and other drug abuse. Results from the Epidemiological Catchment Area (ECA) study." *Journal of the American Medical Association* 264(19): 2511–8.
45. Salloum, I., J. Cornelius, et al. (1998). "Naltrexone utility in depressed alcoholics." *Psychopharmacology* 34(1): 111–5.
46. Sandyk, R. and S. R. Snider (1985). "Naloxone and tardive dyskinesia." *Biological Psychiatry* 20(12): 1335–6.
47. Sernyak, M. J., W. M. Glazer, et al. (1998). "Naltrexone augmentation of neuroleptics in schizophrenia." *Journal of Clinical Psychopharmacology*. Volume 18, Issue 3, pages 248–51.
48. Srisurapanont, M. and N. Jarusuraisin (2005). "Naltrexone for the treatment of alcoholism: a meta-analysis of randomized controlled trials." *International Journal of Neuropsychopharmacology* 8(2): 267–80.
49. Streeton, C. and G. Whelan (2001). "Naltrexone, a relapse prevention maintenance treatment of alcohol dependence: a meta-analysis of randomized controlled trials." *Alcohol and Alcoholism* 36(6): 544–52.
50. Volavka, J., B. Anderson, et al. (1982). "Naloxone and naltrexone in mental illness and tardive dyskinesia." Annals of the New York Academy of Sciences 398: 97–102.
51. Volpicelli, J., A. Alterman, et al. (1992a). "Naltrexone in the treatment of alcohol dependence." *Archives of General Psychiatry* 49(11): 876–80.
52. Volpicelli, J.R., K.C. Rhines, et al. (1997). "Naltrexone and alcohol dependence: role of subject compliance." Archives of General Psychiatry 54(8): 737–42.
53. Wonodi, I., H. Adami, et al. (2004). "Naltrexone treatment of tardive dyskinesia in patients with schizophrenia." *Journal of Clinical Psychopharmacology* 24(4): 441–5.
54. Ziedonis, D., M. L. Steinberg, et al. (2003). Co-occurring addictive and psychotic disorders. In A. W. Graham, T. K. Schultz and M. F. Mayo-Smith (eds.) *Principles of Addiction Medicine, Third Edition*. Chevy Chase, MD, American Society of Addiction Medicine: 1297–1298.

Part VI
Medical Indications

Chapter 26
Current Issues in the Use of Opioid Antagonists (Naltrexone for Opiate Abuse: A Re-Educational Tool as Well as an Effective Drug)

Colin Brewer and Emmanuel Streel

Abstract The increasing availability in the past decade of largely unlicensed but clinically effective implant and depot preparations of naltrexone has greatly reduced the compliance problems that limited oral naltrexone's usefulness in opioid dependence. This chapter describes the evolution of these preparations, reviews the growing literature and discusses the new clinical issues and problems that their effectiveness can create. We describe a new phenomenon, 'pseudo-breakthrough', as well as clinical examples of true opioid breakthrough and show that blood naltrexone levels well above the conventional effective minimum (around 2 ng/ml) may occasionally fail to block opioids. The history of naltrexone's alleged hepatotoxicity is explained and demolished. Durable and effective opiate blockade makes psycho-social components of treatment easier to deliver and facilitates lasting cognitive and behavioural changes. Other topics covered include tissue reactions, other side effects, opioid receptor up-regulation and the conceptual and practical similarities between using naltrexone for opioid abuse and disulfiram for alcohol abuse. Finally, we stress the urgent need to use and improve the various rapid, humane and effective techniques of naltrexone induction. Otherwise, the generally low true completion rates of conventional opioid withdrawal techniques will prevent many suitable patients from initiating naltrexone treatment and thus benefiting from its new formulations.

Keywords: Naltrexone; Implants; Depot; Heroin; Addiction; Hepatotoxicity; Treatment; Blockade

---

C. Brewer (✉) and E. Streel
The Stapleford Centre, 25a Eccleston Street, London SW1W 9NP, UK
e-mail: cbrewer@doctors.net.uk

26.1 Introduction

In the notably uncrowded field of effective medications for addiction treatment, naltrexone (NTX) has several useful and desirable features. Unlike opiate agonists, it has no problems of abuse, legislative restriction or diversion. Over 30 years of clinical experience have shown that it is remarkably safe in overdose and apparently lacking in serious, clinically important organ toxicity. When adequate blood levels are maintained, it is also much more effective than opiate maintenance at preventing illicit opiate use. Indeed, there are few other drugs in any field that will so unfailingly 'do what it says on the packet'. Unlike its only current competitors in alcoholism treatment though it is significantly less effective than disulfiram (DSF) and of similar effectiveness to acamprosate (ACP) in most studies the pharmacokinetics and relatively low daily dose-requirement of NTX make it suitable for clinically useful depot preparations. Poor compliance undermined its potential until these depot preparations started to appear some 10 years ago, though it must be said that most clinicians showed a depressing lack of imagination and awareness of the several validated and common-sense techniques for improving oral compliance. This chapter will review the main areas of agreement and disagreement in the current and potential use of NTX (and by implication at least, of other opioid antagonists) in the management of opioid and alcohol abuse. We shall also discuss some conceptual and political issues in treatment and describe some little-known clinical techniques that, between us, we have found helpful since first using oral NTX in treatment in 1985 and implantable NTX since 1997.

26.2 Overview and History

Like abortion and contraception (neither of which are exclusively medical or even professional issues) addiction treatment usually carries a large amount of moral and even religious baggage, which is no less important for being often denied or passed off as something else. Particularly in the United States, the prescribing of medicines for addiction treatment has many opponents, especially in the case of maintenance with methadone or other opioid agonists. There is no gain, it is widely asserted, without pain and therefore prescribing medications that claim to increase the former while implicitly reducing the latter may be inconsistent with this philosophy. A recent survey (1) puts the prescribing of drugs such as NTX and DSF for alcohol abuse at no more than about 15% of cases *even when a physician is in charge of treatment*. It is sometimes argued that to prescribe medication for addiction is to 'medicalise' the problem and that this is inappropriate for such a complex psychobiosocial condition. Few people raise such objections over medical interventions in fertility control, even though pregnancy is also a complex psychobiosocial condition and not a 'disease'. (We shall not attempt to tackle the paradox that chief among the objectors to medication are 'Twelve-Step' advocates who are so insistent that addiction *is* a 'disease'.)

Ambivalence about pharmacological interventions for addiction affects patients as well as physicians. Because NTX is a relapse-prevention drug, its use may not be consonant with the belief of some patients that despite several previous relapses, this time round, *things will be different.* They have learned their lesson, or have a new job or partner, or have too much to lose, or have found God, etc., and so are not going to relapse. To such people, one can only point out that while of course many people fully recover from pneumonia without antibiotics, their chances of doing so are greatly increased with appropriate antibacterial therapy. The unfortunate fact is that relapse – and often *early* relapse – is distressingly common following opiate detoxification, even for the small minority (in most 'intention to treat' studies) who actually manage to withdraw completely from opiates – only 27% in a recent study (2) from a British 'centre of excellence' - and get through the often difficult first month or two thereafter. This problem is possibly even more marked after long-term methadone maintenance treatment (MMT) even when patients have volunteered for detoxification, have largely or completely abstained from illicit opiate use for many years, have been living essentially unremarkable lives apart from their methadone, are well motivated to become opiate-free and do not need 'rehabilitation' (3). However, in our experience, there is no shortage of patients who are genuinely keen to liberate themselves from opiates, are only too aware of the risks of relapse after opiate detoxification, know how difficult it can be to resist the temptation to use heroin again and value the protection against relapse that NTX can provide.

Many of these patients also recognise how easy it is to be tempted to discontinue oral NTX. Direct supervision of oral NTX consumption greatly improves compliance. Indeed, it remains an important technique if, for example, tissue reactions or the temporary unavailability of physician or implant make seamless implant or depot treatment difficult, and we shall return to it later. However, evading supervision is a challenge to which many patients seem to feel obliged to rise. Indeed, as was pointed out in the context of DSF (a drug which can be very effective in the treatment of another and much commoner addiction and to which we will also return later). 'For any drug which has to be taken daily on a chronic basis and for which compliance is a problem, administration in depot form as an implant is an obvious solution (4).' This became obvious to most researchers as soon as NTX began to be used clinically in the early 1970s and that was when the first studies of possible depot preparations were published (5, 6). Human studies, under the aegis of National Institute on Drug Abuse (NIDA), with a range of implant formulations, such as esterification and NTX microspheres covered with biodegradable plastics, were published in the 1980s (7). The implants were small enough to be inserted with a trocar and cannula (i.e. a modified wide-bore needle) and showed that NTX levels could be maintained for several weeks with minimal or acceptable levels of tissue reaction. Attempts to make a commercially viable depot preparation appear to have started in the early 1990s but despite the obvious need for it, nothing had become available by the mid-1990s even for 'named patient' use. Phase II studies did not appear until 1998, and then for alcohol rather than heroin abuse (8).

In 1996, responding to requests from a few physicians wanting to improve compliance with NTX treatment of opiate addicts, George Malmberg of Wedgwood Pharmacy, Sewell, NJ, produced some experimental implants based on standard implant technology as applied to a number of other drugs, consisting of NTX powder compacted with a small amount of magnesium stearate. The first, small implants contained only 100 mg of NTX and were inserted subcutaneously using a trocar and cannula. Early studies with volunteers, including one of the physicians, indicated that tissue tolerance was acceptable and that clinically effective blood levels were achievable, as judged by the ability of the implants to block the effects of challenge doses of opiates.

To achieve longer duration of action, larger implants containing 1 g of NTX were manufactured. They were cylindrical in shape but at ~9-mm diameter (and about 20 mm long) they needed to be inserted through a small (10 mm) incision under local analgesia. They appeared to provide blockade for 5–7 weeks on average and completely prevented relapse during the first 4 weeks after detoxification in a consecutive series of the first 54 patients treated in Britain (9). All patients were made aware that these implants had not passed through any of the usual testing and licensing procedures (or indeed, any animal studies), but both patients and physicians could draw some reassurance from previous NTX implant studies and from the very low organ toxicity of NTX (see below) as demonstrated in over a decade of oral use.

Despite their immediately obvious value in preventing early relapse (which quite often meant the prevention of later relapse as well), it was also soon obvious, as it had been with oral NTX, that most patients needed the protection of NTX implants for much longer than the 7–8 weeks which was the best that the Malmberg implants could usually manage. If they did not have further implants, relapse often – but by no means invariably – tended to follow, sometimes quite soon after the blockade had worn off. This problem would also have occurred with the injectable, microsphere depot preparations that Kranzler et al. had been using, had they been available for treating opiate abusers, since they only provided adequate blockade (as do later formulations now available) for 4–5 weeks (10). It is true that one has more time before opiate antagonism disappears to persuade a reluctant patient of the need to have a further NTX implant than of the need to take another NTX tablet. However, given that ambivalence about treatment is the norm with all addictions, it is inevitable that, for reasons we will discuss shortly, the uptake of repeated implants will decline over time, unless treatment is tied to, for example, a probation order (another issue we shall discuss.)

Accordingly, thoughts turned to alternative manufacturing techniques and formulations to extend the blockade of the implants not just by a few weeks but by several months. By 2001, a ‘second generation’ NTX implant became available, produced by Dr. George O’Neill in Australia. It used some of the technology studied by Chiang et al. in the early 1980s, in that the NTX was contained in biodegradable (poly-lactate or poly-glycolate) plastic-covered microspheres. However, instead of being suspended in an inert vehicle, as with depot-injections, the microspheres were compressed with additional biodegradable plastic into pellets for subcutaneous (s.c.) insertion about 8 mm in diameter, so that diffusion – and hence duration of action – could be prolonged almost at will, depending on microsphere size, the rate of biodegradation, the proportion of NTX to matrix and – most importantly – the number of pellets that were inserted. From the earliest publications about the O'Neill implant, it appeared that effective blockade could be maintained for over 6 months (11, 12).

26.3 Testing-Out and Other Aspects of Naltrexone's Ability to Block Opiates

Apart from the already-mentioned ambivalence about giving up a particular pattern of drug-using behaviour, users of illicit drugs are often very curious about the effects of both psychoactive drugs and of medication prescribed to treat their drug problem. Also, and particularly in private practice, patients may wonder whether doctors are deceiving them for therapeutic or financial reasons. When starting oral or depot NTX for the first time, a significant proportion of patients will thus smoke, sniff or inject heroin at the earliest opportunity after their first dose. This is often taken as a bad sign but more often than not, it is actually a good sign. Typically, these patients are merely checking that NTX really will block opiates as effectively as they have been told it does (13). Often, this message is somewhat equivocal, because patients are usually also told routinely that they could kill themselves if they were to take very large amounts of heroin; packet inserts generally reinforce this point. Naturally, this makes some of them wonder how much heroin they would have to take to get at least a partial effect. Fortunately, apart from a small number of patients who need larger than average NTX doses or who metabolise NTX unusually quickly, these experiments nearly always have the effect of convincing the patient of the reality and the power of the opiate blockade, provided that NTX is taken regularly. As we discuss later, it does not necessarily matter much if the patient is not entirely pleased to find that NTX really does what it is supposed to do.

Just how much heroin NTX can block is an important question and one which at the moment, we can only partially answer. The early published studies describing opiate challenges usually involved no more than 25 mg of diamorphine, which is the equivalent of barely 60 mg of typical 40% pure British street heroin, representing a heroin habit in the range of 0.25–0.3 g daily. While there are many patients who do not normally use more than this in a whole day, such modest daily totals are much less than quite a few patients take in a single dose. Average heroin habits of between 0.5 g and 0.75 g daily are common and habits of 2–3 g daily are by no means rare. Clearly, clinicians need to know whether, and at what blood levels, NTX and 6-beta-naltrexole (6BNT) will block these higher heroin intakes. In the absence of objective data, our information about the opiate-blocking ability of implants initially consisted largely of reports by patients of their unsuccessful attempts to overcome the blockade with varying amounts of heroin and other opiates. It was naturally impossible to be certain that these accounts and dose estimates were accurate and the purity of street heroin can vary considerably. However, collectively, they represented an impressive amount of information, which it was difficult to ignore or discount. Some patients with access to large amounts of heroin – usually dealers, pop-stars or other well-funded users – interpreted the term 'opiate challenge' quite literally and smoked or injected several grams of heroin to test the blockade to the limit, rather as they might put a new car through its paces. It was reassuring to the prescribing doctor when patients said things like: 'I gave up after smoking six grams, doc, because nothing was happening'. Such experience reassured the patients too.

The first objective report of the ability of implanted (or indeed, oral) NTX to block the larger opiate doses more typical of heroin addicts, showed that the Malmberg implants could produce blood levels 2 weeks after insertion that were sufficient to block the effects of 1,000 mcg of fentanil administered in 50 mcg doses over the course of 20 min (14). This total dose is equivalent to about 1,000 mg of pethidine (ten times the usual maximum analgesic dose in opiate-naïve patients) or between 0.3 g and 0.5 g of British street heroin. However, because no laboratory in Britain was able to measure routinely blood levels of NTX and its pharmacologically active metabolite 6BNT, we did not know whether at the time of the fentanil challenge, the patient had relatively high or low NTX and 6BNT levels.

Once it became possible for us to have NTX and 6-beta-naltrexol (6BNTX) measured through the University of Oslo (see below) we could start to answer these questions more precisely. If we saw patients who reported the results of self-administration within a few days of their experiment, we could take blood samples on the assumption that blood levels would not have changed much in the preceding few hours or days and that if they had changed, they would almost certainly have fallen rather than risen in the interim. Here are two previously unpublished case histories of patients who claimed to have taken known amounts of pharmaceutical opiates and from whom blood samples were taken shortly afterwards.

Case 1. Forty-nine days after the insertion of a Malmberg implant, this patient claimed to have injected intravenously (i.v.) a 50 mg ampoule of methadone. This equates approximately to the injection of 75 mg of morphine or 30–35 mg of diamorphine. He experienced no opiate effects. A very recent injection track was clearly visible when blood was taken 4 h later. Serum NTX and 6BNT levels were 3 ng/ml and 9 ng/ml, respectively.

Case 2. Twenty-one days after a similar implantation, a female patient claimed to have injected 300 mg of dissolved and filtered instant-release morphine tablets i.v. (≅125 mg diamorphine) with no opiate effects; 24 h later, blood was taken and her serum NTX and 6BNT were found to be 5 ng/ml and 51 ng/ml, respectively. We still had no case with objective data about both opiate dose and NTX blood level but an opportunity soon presented itself.

Case 3. A patient who normally smoked 1 g/day of heroin had rapid opiate detoxification (ROD) under oral sedation in hospital and a 1 g Malmberg implant was inserted during the procedure under local analgesia. Three weeks later, the patient used heroin and claimed that he was 'feeling it'. It seemed important to discover whether or not this was a true opiate effect. Three weeks after implantation, blood was taken and the patient was challenged with 100 mg of diamorphine i.v. injected over ~3 min. This amount was consistent with his pre-detox habit and equates approximately to 250 mg of morphine or – assuming 4 × daily dosing and a typical 24 h morphine/methadone equivalent of 5:1 - to over 100 mg of methadone. No objective opiate effects were observed but he reported a slight feeling of relaxation. He was then given 50 mg of crushed NTX by mouth under direct observation. Four hours later, another blood sample was taken and the challenge was repeated with a further 100 mg of i.v. diamorphine. He reported similar mild subjective sensations but again, no objective changes were noted. Serum NTX levels before and 4 h after the oral NTX were 5 ng/ml and 15 ng/ml, respectively. The 6BNT levels were 12 ng/ml and 56 ng/ml, respectively. For comparison, blood levels of NTX and 6BNT in another patient 10 h after swallowing 50 mg of NTX were 5 ng/ml and 28 ng/ml, respectively (15).

It was still not known whether it was possible to override conventional oral doses of NTX if a sufficiently large dose of opiates were administered. Unpublished data suggested that Malmberg implants typically gave NTX levels reaching or exceeding 6–7 ng/ml, which was similar to typical NTX levels between peak and trough after oral NTX (16). However, half-lives of NTX and 6BNT are as short as 4 h and 12 h, respectively, in some studies (17). 6BNT levels may therefore be more relevant than NTX. Mean trough levels of NTX and 6BNT as low as 2.1 ± 0.47 ng/ml and 17.6 ± 5 ng/ml have been reported 24 h after a single 100 mg dose of NTX (18) and a 6BNT level of 9.8 ng/ml was recorded 16 h after 50 mg of NTX (15) One patient needed a single dose of 200 mg of oral NTX to achieve complete opiate blockade with 25 mg of diamorphine at 24 h (19). It seemed probable that at peak NTX blood levels an hour or two after an oral dose (and for several hours or tens of hours afterwards, depending on the size of that dose); the blockade could not be overcome even by considerably more than 6 g of street heroin, but it was important to know what happens when blood NTX levels typically fall, 24 h after a standard oral dose, to nearer the 1–2 ng/ml levels that most current depot preparations aim to reach or exceed and that are 'the concentration [of NTX] *thought to produce* opioid antagonist effects (8)' (Our italics) The following three cases, the last two of which are also previously unreported, began to give us some answers.

Case 4. This patient, who travelled extensively, claimed to be snorting up to 10 g of heroin daily. Even this very large dose was evidently blocked by a series of Malmberg implants but he relapsed after about 7 months. Because of the relapse and his peripatetic lifestyle, he seemed a particularly suitable early candidate for a longer-acting implant. However, with such high levels of daily use, it was important to reassure ourselves (and him) that the new implant could give comparable levels of blockade. Prior to a further detoxification and following a supervised test dose to confirm his tolerance, he was maintained for a week on 200 mg of prescribed oral morphine four times daily. During ROD under general anaesthesia, an O'Neill implant containing 3.4 g NTX was inserted subcutaneously. Six days later, blood was taken. The next day, he snorted 500 mg of pharmaceutical diamorphine under medical supervision over a period of 40 min. There were no changes in pupil size or respiratory rate during this period or subsequently. The serum NTX was 2.8 ng/ml and 6BNT was 9.0 ng/ml. Serum levels of morphine and 6-monoacetyl morphine were 525 ng/ml and 164 ng/ml, respectively. (The levels were so high that the laboratory enquired whether the sample was taken post mortem). This case, like the previous one, has been published (14).

Case 5. The first patient in Britain to receive an O'Neill implant had previously been opiate-free for 3 years, protected by 20 consecutive Malmberg implants. Eighty-two days after the insertion of the O'Neill implant, blood was taken and 500 mcg of fentanyl was given i.v. during a period of 10 min. No opiate effects were seen or experienced. The NTX level was 1.5 ng/ml. For technical reasons, the 6BNT level could not be measured but on a previous occasion his 6BNT:NTX ratio had been 1.36:1.

Case 6. About 8 weeks after an O'Neill implant, the patient had an argument with his partner and not only took an overdose of temazepam but also injected some heroin. His reported behaviour subsequently seemed more typical of benzodiazepine than of opiate intoxication and his pupils were apparently not pin-point. However, he had once nearly died from an opiate overdose and his family wanted reassurance that the implant was still working. A few days later, 61 days post-implantation, he attended for blood sampling and an opiate challenge. After 300 mcg of fentanyl i.v. over 5 min, no opiate effects were seen or felt. NTX and 6BNT levels were 2.2 ng/ml and 3.6 ng/ml, respectively.

It hardly needs to be said that such challenges need to be done in an appropriate setting with at least basic resuscitation equipment available and adequate supplies of naloxone ready to inject if necessary. However, in practice, we have never needed to resort to either facility. Further reassurance came from preliminary Australian reports (initially personal communications) that no deaths from opiate overdose had been recorded within the 9 months after the insertion of an O'Neill implant. This experience has been extended, confirmed, and recently published (20, 21).

However, we have also learned that for some patients, the 'conventional' lowest effective blood NTX levels of 1–2 ng/ml or even 3 ng/ml are not sufficient in practice to block the effects of opiates, even at relatively modest intakes. Such instances are uncommon. A paper reporting our experience to date is in preparation but it is clear that in one patient, a blood NTX level of 4.3 ng/ml was insufficient to prevent obvious opiate effects after he smoked no more than about 200 mg of street heroin. It has also become clear recently that buprenorphine may, as is not unexpected, have a greater ability than other opiates to displace NTX from opiate receptors. O'Neill (22) has reported that patients may be only partially protected by NTX implants, even with serum levels of NTX above 4 ng/ml, when large doses of buprenorphine (e.g. 32 mg) are injected intravenously. However, it also appears that when breakthrough does occur, as in the case just mentioned, it is the euphoric effects that are the soonest and most likely to be experienced and not the much more serious respiratory depressant effects. Very low levels of

NTX seem to confer disproportionate protection against death from this cause, a finding that may be linked to recent suggestions that incorporating microdoses of NTX with opiates used for analgesia may both enhance analgesic effects and prevent the development of tolerance.

26.4 Breakthrough and Pseudo-Breakthrough

The previous section should give a reasonable indication of how much heroin, or other opiates, current implants can be expected to block in most patients. However, the matter is more complex than it appears, because although breakthrough is obviously possible at inadequate NTX levels, not everything that sounds like breakthrough, from the patient's description, is the genuine article.

First of all, there is much more to opiate dependence than the pharmacological effects of the drug in question. There is a large psycho-social component of most forms of drug dependence and of course, some addictions – for example, to food or sex – involve no external pharmacology at all. That the ritual of drug-taking can be even more important than the pharmacology is shown by case reports of addiction to placebos, including an apparent withdrawal syndrome. This is especially the case when heroin is injected, partly because a separate 'needle addiction' has been convincingly documented and partly because the 'rush' or 'pharmacological orgasm' that follows i.v. injection is probably more rapid and more intense that that obtainable by slower means of putting relatively large doses of intoxicants into the cerebral blood supply.

Another possible factor is that when heroin is injected i.v., it causes – as do other opiates to a greater or lesser extent – histamine release. This presumably accounts for the local or generalised flushing that is often seen after i.v. heroin or morphine and since histamine release is not mediated through opiate receptors, it is not blocked by opiate antagonists. We speculate that it may contribute to the problem posed by a small but particularly interesting group of patients who continue to inject heroin despite the absence of any apparent true opiate effects following appropriate test doses of morphine or diamorphine. (We have not yet seen such consistent patterns of use with smokers or snorters.) A detailed report of two such cases is also in preparation but we can provide brief details of one of them.

Case 7. A young woman with a history of anxiety preceding the onset of i.v. heroin abuse and of much failed treatment received a Malmberg implant. She resumed injecting heroin occasionally during the first month after implantation but following a third consecutive implant started to inject almost daily. She insisted that she was getting typical heroin effects but there was no objective opiate response to an appropriate test dose of i.v. diamorphine and no reaction to high doses of i.v. naloxone either. On two occasions, NTX and 6BNT levels were well above conventional minimally effective antagonist levels. Fortunately, with appropriate counselling and support, she was able to abandon this behaviour. Six years later (at the time of writing) she remains opiate-free and leads a full and fairly conventional life.

26.5 Toxicity and Side Effects: The Myth of Serious Hepatotoxicity

In nearly 40 years of clinical use – more than 20 of them following its general release in the United States and almost as many in Britain and other countries – NTX has yet to be associated with any serious organ toxicity that might limit its use. The only one which is regularly cited as having any importance is hepatotoxicity and a special warning to this effect appears in the prescribing handbooks and product information in most countries where NTX is used. However, these warnings are very misleading; the reason for their existence (and persistence) is not widely known and needs to be told. According to a personal communication from H. Kleber, who was involved in some of the early 1970s clinical studies, there was much pressure to change the status of NTX from a highly experimental 'Phase 1' compound to one that could at least be used without too much bureaucratic hassle in clinical trials. This pressure was the direct result of the large number of US servicemen who had started abusing heroin while in Vietnam and who were expected to need treatment when they returned home. As has been widely documented, and to general surprise, most of these heroin abusers actually abandoned their habit when they returned to the United States and relatively few needed treatment. However, not being able to foretell the future, the relevant authorities and clinicians naturally wanted the addicted servicemen to have access to the new and promising drug that was an alternative to MMT. Full safety and toxicity trials had not been concluded but the available evidence was reassuring. Accordingly, the responsible government department agreed in 1972 to easing the restrictions on its use, provided that a 'black box' warning about possible hepatotoxicity was included, because some studies had raised concerns on that point. Having got into the official literature, the warning has stayed there, even though the justification for it is now very questionable.

The most convincing evidence for this statement is probably not the numerous toxicity studies carried out since 1972 but the fact that for over a decade, oral NTX has been used – often in daily doses much higher than the 50 mg usual in addiction treatment – to relieve the intense and demoralising pruritus that is a common manifestation of severe jaundice. The high bilirubin levels are due, in most cases, to serious liver disease, sometimes life-threatening. Even if the jaundice is secondary to obstruction, severe biliary stasis itself often causes significant disturbance of liver function tests (LFTs). We first became interested in this issue when a patient became jaundiced due to acute Hepatitis B infection, apparently acquired during a single episode of sharing injecting equipment about 6 weeks before he detoxified. The jaundice appeared about a week after he received a Malmberg NTX implant. Previous exposure to NTX had not caused him any ill-effects and the attending physician decided to resist the temptation to remove the implant immediately and merely observed his progress as an in-patient instead. The jaundice increased a little as expected and then waned, the LFTs returning to normal in the usual way and the usual time. Our subsequent review of the literature (23) revealed the otherwise little-known use of NTX in the jaundice of pruritus (24). Studies since then have been equally reassuring. While, NTX use may occasionally be associated with moderately abnormal LFTs (especially, according to some studies, if non-steroidal anti-inflammatory drugs (NSAIDs) are used concomitantly) and while the association may sometimes be causative, it seems that in none of the reported cases did abnormal LFTs reflect any obvious deterioration in the health of the patient or lead to any clinical alarm. All abnormalities disappeared rapidly when NTX was discontinued and sometimes even when it was not. It therefore seems safe to say that where there is a strong indication for NTX treatment in either opiate or alcohol abuse, the existence of even serious liver disease should not be an automatic contra-indication and the appearance of LFT abnormalities after starting NTX treatment should lead to observation and frequent review rather than to reflex termination or change of treatment.

The one toxic effect of NTX that may be relevant is that like very many other drugs, it may occasionally cause skin eruptions. In over 20 years, including many implanted patients where compliance with NTX was not in doubt, we have seen only two cases verified by skin-testing with NTX. Both involved implanted patients with generalised, rather than local, rashes and it may be that implantation slightly increases the risk of sensitisation. However, even with implants, such rashes are rare and with appropriate management, may not even require the removal of the implant.

26.6 Side Effects or Withdrawal Effects?

If it is not used to precipitate withdrawal as part of a ROD programme, NTX is usually – indeed, ideally – initiated as soon as possible after opiate withdrawal. This means that NTX will very often be started in patients who are still experiencing varying degrees of withdrawal distress and discomfort. These may be at least transiently aggravated by NTX and it is hardly surprising if some patients attribute the discomfort to the NTX. Unfortunately, the prolonged abstinence syndrome that Eklund described as being quite common following planned MMT withdrawal is also seen in an unfortunate minority of patients after withdrawal from any other opiate as well. However, in most cases, these symptoms will have largely or completely disappeared within 2–3 months. That is to say, by that time, most patients can expect to be sleeping reasonably well without hypnotics and not to be experiencing lethargy, sweating, arthralgia, colic and/or diarrhoea, pilo-erection and generalised unhappiness. The corollary is that until enough time has passed for this recovery to occur, it may be both difficult and unwise to make a confident diagnosis of NTX side effects or of an underlying psychiatric or physical condition. Vigorous treatment of persistent withdrawal symptoms with, for example, alpha-adrenergic agonists for sweating, non-opioid analgesics and hypnotics may clarify the supposed 'dual diagnosis' as well as producing some very grateful patients. Our unfashionable belief that the small risks of significant dependence from prescribing benzodiazepine (BDZ) or other hypnotics are more than balanced by improvements in well-being and rehabilitation has recently been supported in a randomised controlled trial (RCT) (25).

Both depression and anxiety are possibly even more common after opiate withdrawal than they are before it. Whether they are best conceptualised as illnesses or as understandable reactions to life events and frustrated aspirations, and thus the best ways of managing them, are beyond the scope of this chapter. Since NTX – especially depot/implanted NTX – can greatly increase the proportion of patients who succeed in becoming opiate-free and staying that way for more than just a few days, there will naturally be many anxious and depressed patients among those in NTX treatment. However, it seems clear that NTX does not by itself cause significant depression (26) and indeed usually improves it if patients thereby remain opiate-free.

One patient experienced very troublesome diarrhoea for 10 weeks following ROD and NTX implantation. Only s.c. injections of octreotide 2–3 × daily (27) controlled it but it gradually diminished and was most likely a prolonged withdrawal effect. Had the patient been taking oral NTX, she would probably have quickly discontinued it, relieved the diarrhoea and other withdrawal symptoms by resuming opiates and been reluctant to detoxify again.

In many studies of NTX in alcoholism (from which patients with any history of opiate abuse are usually excluded), about 10–15% of patient experience diarrhoea, nausea and/or vomiting following the first NTX dose. Following the second dose, the incidence is much less and usually soon falls to zero. However, this experience may put some patients off continuing with treatment. Since these symptoms are so similar to those of opiate withdrawal, we suggest that they may represent the acute displacement by NTX of endogenous opioids from their presumed receptors, provoking a kind of short-lived 'internal' withdrawal in a genetically susceptible minority.

26.7 Receptor Up-Regulation and Supersensitivity After Naltrexone Discontinuation

In the neurobiology of addiction, the neuroadaptive changes, and especially the cyclic adenosine 3′,5′-monophosphate (cAMP) up-regulation induced by chronic exposure, have been extensively studied (28, 29); cross-tolerance of drugs like morphine and clonidine even lead some researchers to consider the up-/down-regulation of receptors as a new therapeutic approach. Indeed, Streel et al. (30) showed in opiate-dependent rats that pre-treatment with the noradrenergic antagonist yohimbine could potentiate the efficiency of noradrenergic agonist clonidine in reducing opiate withdrawal. These results are explained through an up-/down-regulation of noradrenergic receptors using a combination of antagonists/agonists. This apparent up-regulation of opiate receptors has been questioned by researchers as the use of opiate antagonists became more established in opiate dependence management. Golovko et al. (31) showed that chronic administration of naloxone or NTX increased the density of opioid receptors and their sensitivity to agonists like morphine or heroin. These neuroadaptative changes could increase the risk of overdose after the discontinuation of NTX treatment following chronic antagonist exposure. However, even the simple interruption of chronic opiate intake is also associated with neuroadaptative changes that could lead to a higher risk of overdose. It has been clearly demonstrated that individuals leaving *all* the major pharmacotherapies for opioid dependence (whether methadone, morphine, buprenorphine, levo-alpha-acetyl-methadol or NTX) experience higher overdose and death rates compared with those in treatment (32). Therefore, all patients, not only those treated with NTX, show a hypersensitivity to opiate agonists after discontinuation of chronic treatment, or of illicit use.

Furthermore, as is clearly shown in several studies, naloxone and NTX act as inverse agonists in morphine-dependent rats (33, 34), while in opiate-naive animals, naloxone and NTX act as antagonists. This explains why naloxone is more potent in precipitating withdrawal the more dependent the animal becomes during morphine exposure (35) regardless of how much morphine is present. The same authors also conclude that even a single dose of morphine can turn naloxone into an inverse agonist (36). The interactions between opiates agonists and antagonists are thus more complex than previously supposed and there is a need for a better understanding of opiate receptor activity in the presence of antagonists, inverse agonists, partial antagonists and agonists. Moreover studies also suggest that changes in the social environment can increase the effects of opiates. Smith et al. (37) showed that the kappa-opioid receptor system is sensitive to social and environmental manipulations. Zachariou et al. (38) also highlighted some interesting findings about the behavioural and neural plasticity associated with chronic opiate exposure and the essential role of regulators of G-protein signalling (RGS). They also demonstrated that the deletion of the RGS9 gene caused a dramatic increase of sensitivity to morphine and that, more specifically, RGS9-2 was a regulator of behavioural response to opiates.

However, other factors may be involved, since neurobiology cannot totally explain the potential adverse consequence of discontinuing opiate-dependence pharmacotherapies. As McGregor et al. showed (39), some patients are unrealistically optimistic about the risks of overdosing if they resume heroin use even sporadically after a significant period of abstinence. Fortunately, although the education of patients and their families is clearly important, the large and well-documented protective effect of O'Neill long-acting implants against admission and – presumably – death due to opiate overdose in abstinent patients for many months after their full opiate blocking effect has faded appears to be much more powerful, consistent and truly life-saving than any amount of exhortation or information (20, 21). It constitutes a very powerful reason for accelerating their availability and for further studies.

26.8 Local Tissue Reactions

Local reactions to depot NTX injections have been reported, even though the total NTX dose is relatively small, and since no incision is involved, the risk of introducing infections is presumably much smaller. None of the reports seems to involve more than minor and transient discomfort, usually requiring no active treatment. The inclusion of magnesium stearate in Malmberg-type implants, though apparently hallowed by implant-making tradition, seems to cause typical giant cell tissue reactions in some cases, perhaps as many as 10%. Often these present as painless sterile cysts, which settle spontaneously in 2-3 months though sometimes, incision, drainage and the removal of the implant are unavoidable (40).

The biodegradable plastic used in O'Neill implants and in Vivitrol has a long and excellent record of safety and tissue tolerance. Nevertheless, reactions (other than those due primarily to local infection) can occasionally occur. Typically, they start several weeks after insertion and well after the wound has healed. Short, high-dose courses of oral steroids may abort the reactions, as may antihistamines.

Golz and Partecke (41) used a unique type of implant, made in a Berlin hospital pharmacy from pure NTX base, compacted without any additives. This model seems to have a very low incidence of tissue reactions despite giving adequate blood levels, and we used them successfully in one patient who had unacceptable skin reactions to both Malmberg and O'Neill implants. NTX base alone may thus have little potential for irritating tissues.

26.9 Scheduled and Unscheduled Removal of Implants and Dealing with Severe Pain in Patients with Active Depot Naltrexone

One of the myths of implant treatment is that patients can easily remove implants as often do so. In reality, such removal is very rare. If it happens at all, it is most likely during the first few days after rapid detoxification when patients may still be affected by sedative drugs, or when adequate symptom control has not yet been achieved. Such patients often soon recognise that their behaviour was unwise and request another implant as soon as possible. We have sometimes suggested that the next implant be sited where it cannot easily be reached. Removal may also suggest – sometimes with the benefit of hindsight – that the patient was not suitable for abstinence-based treatment and that resuming or instituting agonist maintenance is urgently needed.

Clearly, an intramuscular depot cannot be removed. However, there are times when removal of an implant may be urgently considered in order to deal with severe pain. Alternatively, the presence of an implant, or of an active depot injection, or indeed the recent administration of 150 mg or 200 mg of oral NTX providing antagonism for 3–4 days, may require special techniques to overcome pain. These include regional nerve blocks and the intensive use of non-opioid analgesics, including sub-anaesthetic doses of oral or parenteral ketamine, which is not blocked by NTX.

26.10 Compliance

It may be thought obvious that compliance with a particular treatment is crucial to the outcome of that treatment but that is too simplistic an approach. First of all, it is now clear from several studies – though common sense would surely have suggested it if the studies had not – that patients who comply with treatment not only have better outcomes but also differ in several other important respects from patients who do not. Compliance, in essence, means following medical instructions. People who do not follow medical instructions may have several reasons for their lack of cooperation, ranging from failure or inability to understand the instructions, to various beliefs and attitudes which make them actively hostile to the proffered advice. They may also be generally disorganised in their lives, or affected by short-term stress or distress that distracts them from their usual efficiency.

However, at a strictly therapeutic level, compliance with a particular pharmacological or psychological treatment only matters if the treatment in question actually has a specific positive effect over and above any placebo or non-specific effects that it may have. To comply perfectly with an ineffective treatment confers, by definition, no benefit over equally perfect compliance with an appropriate placebo treatment. Conversely, even partial compliance with a significantly effective treatment may give better outcomes than good compliance with an ineffective one. Since NTX is a highly effective opiate antagonist, it follows that maximising compliance is more than usually important, and the most recent review (42) confirms that without supervised administration, the effectiveness of oral NTX in opiate abuse is modest at best.

That is why it is so depressing that the effectiveness of supervised oral NTX was neglected or ignored for so long by so many clinicians. Many patients could probably have been helped and many clinicians might have been less unenthusiastic about NTX had they realised this. Naturally, one must always be cautious about studies whose design falls short of the 'gold standard' of the RCT. However, when childhood acute leukaemia almost invariably meant death within a few weeks or months, even a few reports of long remissions were likely to be important and significant. So it was with some early studies of the effects of supervised NTX on people imprisoned for heroin-related offences. Such prisoners were normally regarded as 'poor clinical material' and nearly always relapsed to opiate use very quickly when released. Their position in the prisoner hierarchy was right at the bottom of the 'trust ladder'. Despite these poor prognostic factors, Brahen et al. (43) showed as early as 1984 that when the ingestion of oral NTX was closely supervised as part of a day-release parole programme to prepare them for the end of their sentences, the majority of parolees complied with treatment and thus remained heroin-free during their time out of prison on parole. Furthermore, they rose rapidly on the 'trust ladder' to become some of the most responsible inmates.

Similar results were obtained in a parole-release programme in Singapore but in this study (44) (which unfortunately does not show up readily in Medline searches and is thus rarely cited) it was possible to make a persuasive comparison of outcomes in an otherwise identical comprehensive treatment and testing programme without NTX. The programme that included NTX was considerably more effective at preventing relapse and re-incarceration. Confirmation was finally obtained in an RCT (45).

26.11 Comparisons with Disulfiram

Despite very different modes of pharmacological action, NTX and DSF are rather similar in that provided they are taken consistently at an adequate dose, both drugs can effectively prevent the target behaviour – opiate use in the case of NTX, alcohol use in the case of DSF. (The less effective behavioural antagonism of NTX in alcoholism is discussed elsewhere.) Even more than with NTX, the strong evidence-base for the effectiveness of DSF when compliance is addressed has been ignored but in the last few years, recognition – albeit often rather grudging – has arrived (46, 47). This is important because for various reasons, DSF does not currently lend itself to a pharmacologically active depot or implant preparation and supervision is thus currently the only way to improve compliance. However, compared with NTX, there have been many studies of supervised administration with DSF going back to the 1960s, nearly all of them positive and quite often very positive. We may thus be able to get some useful ideas for NTX treatment by reading the DSF literature.

What it shows – consistently – is that time and effort devoted to optimising supervision and compliance are not wasted and that in general, the better the supervision, the better the compliance and the better the outcome. Furthermore, these results are obtained with less additional counselling/psychotherapy because achieving sustained sobriety means that the patients have fewer problems that need counselling. Azrin (48), one of the first to write about DSF supervision in detail, has spelled out some of the basic principles. Supervision sounds, and is, a simple enough concept but 'as with many simple procedures, such as giving an intramuscular injection, measuring the blood pressure or taking the temperature with an oral thermometer, there are right and wrong ways of doing it and attention to detail is important' (49). Azrin's suggestions are designed mainly for family-supervision of purely voluntary patients but it is not difficult to work out the small modifications needed for treatment linked to parole or probation. Many recurrent offenders could have been given greatly improved chances of abstaining for useful periods from both alcohol and opiates had these studies been more widely heeded. We believe that one of the most important and beneficial uses of depot NTX preparations is likely to be as a probation- or parole-linked treatment for recurrent heroin-related offenders. It remains to be seen whether such preparations will be as effective in recurrent alcohol-related offenders. We suspect that they will not, because studies comparing supervised oral DSF with supervised or compliant patients taking oral NTX or acamprosate (ACP) consistently show DSF to be much more effective, with an average effect size of 0.52 against about 0.25 for both NTX and ACP (50–54).

26.12 Special Techniques for Maximising Success and Minimising Distress and Drop-Out in the Transition from Opiates to Naltrexone

We briefly mentioned the conventional aim of starting NTX – whether oral or depot – as soon as possible after opiate ingestion has ceased and withdrawal symptoms have largely subsided. In practice, this means a gap of at least 5 days after the last dose of heroin or other short-acting opiates and a week or more after methadone. Giving NTX too soon after the last dose can precipitate very unpleasant acute withdrawal that can, and often does, put patients off further treatment with NTX. However, despite its long half-life, buprenorphine, with its partial antagonist activity may prove to be the least troublesome 'transitional' opioid.

Detoxification phobia, usually based on previous unpleasant experience, is real and quite common and prevents or deters many patients from contemplating or actively seeking 'detox' even though many of them are in other respects well-motivated and well-suited for abstinence-based management. However, even when patients get as far as entering a clinic for in-patient withdrawal, the Biblical adage that 'many are called but few are chosen' applies. We have mentioned the 27% success rate of Strang and McCambridge (2) in a conventional programme where patients received a 10-day methadone reduction to zero and were expected to stay for 28 days in all. A more detailed reading of this study indicates that the mean length of stay was only 12 days and the median about 10. In other words, most patients discharged themselves around or before the time that they received their last dose of methadone, when withdrawal symptoms are usually at a peak. Only 27% of patients stayed for the full 28 days. The others left not because they had managed to detoxify but declined the additional psycho-social components of the programme; they left before anything that could truthfully be called 'detoxification' had been achieved, a fact obliquely recognised by the authors. It also appears that when NTX was accepted by patients in this unit, it was usually administered on the day before planned discharge. Since this would be expected to produce precipitated withdrawal in some patients, it is hardly surprising that very few patients accepted a second dose.

Because such poor true completion rates (and hence rates of transition to NTX) are the norm for conventional programmes, clinicians started as early as the mid 1970s to devise ways of accelerating the transition and of making it more tolerable. Blachley et al. (55) were the first to suggest that naloxone could be used to precipitate withdrawal, with anaesthesia or i.v. sedation to get the patient through the shortened but intensely unpleasant acute abstinence syndrome, though they did not put the idea into practice. Resnick et al. (56) in 1977 used repeated small s.c. naloxone injections to precipitate a milder syndrome, which could be ameliorated with oral sedatives. The discovery in 1980 that clonidine (and other α-adrenergic agonists) had a useful and specific effect on some withdrawal symptoms, aided these developments. By the late 1980s, small and repeated doses of oral NTX had largely replaced naloxone as the precipitation agent, several protocols using clonidine and oral sedation had been published (57–59), and Loimer et al. in Vienna had shown that general anaesthesia with i.v. thiopentone could indeed be used to prevent awareness of the acute process (60, 61).

The blatant commercialisation of this process by some corporate bodies – notably the Spanish-Israeli CITA Centro de Investigacien y Tratamiento de Adicciones group (62) – as well as many excessive claims for long-term abstinence rates caused an understandably angry and sceptical reaction in many quarters. However, a decade or so later, it is clear that rapid methods can give NTX induction rates close to 100%, even using 'intention to treat' analysis, while conventional methods continue to limp behind at around 30–40% or less (63). The main argument now is about whether the reduction in fear and distress obtained by using general anaesthesia or i.v. sedation justifies the possible increase in risk. It has certainly been safely used in infants with severe heart disease who became therapeutically addicted after surgery (64).

26.13 Psychological Aspects of Treatment with Naltrexone Implants

A question commonly asked about treatment with NTX implants is: What happens when the patient stops having implants? The implication is that as soon as the patient is not protected by NTX, relapse becomes very likely. Fortunately, both clinical experience and psychological theory suggest that this is not usually the case. We have already referred to the large behavioural component in all addictions. Right from the start, NTX was seen as an aid to reconditioning patients (65) and that is how it works in practice. After returning to his normal environment, if a patient is able - thanks to a NTX implant - to walk past the dealers that he sees every day and to resist the cues and temptations that his normal social milieu will inevitably present, then there is a better chance that eventually he or she will stop automatically associating these cues and situations with heroin use. By practising abstinence in a real-life situation, addicts can eventually change their self-image from that of a person who is likely to use in such situations to that of a person who is likely not to use (66).

As we have pointed out before, learning to abstain successfully is very similar in principle to learning to speak a foreign language fluently (67). It is not enough simply to know the foreign words, or – in managing addictions - the social and psychological techniques for resisting temptation (68, 69). What matters is the amount of real-life practice and the ability to use those words or techniques not just correctly and appropriately but *automatically,* without having to think about them. It appears that consistent opiate blockade with NTX can aid this acquisition of automaticity and we have suggested as a testable hypothesis that the outcome at 12 months after detoxification would be better after a single implant lasting 6 months than after a single implant lasting only 1 month. If this were found to be the case, then clearly it could not be due to a persisting pharmacological effect of the NTX, which would have largely worn off before 12 months, but most probably to the ability of NTX over a period of several months to facilitate and consolidate cognitive and behavioural changes. Recently, a study of long-term supervised DSF in very chronic alcoholics has indicated that after 18 months continuous DSF, it became significantly more likely that patients would be able to abstain successfully without DSF (70). It seems reasonable to suggest that pending further studies, a similar minimum period of NTX implant treatment should be encouraged.

Unfortunately, not all heroin addicts make life easy for their treatment team by confining their taste for intoxication to opiates alone. Poly-drug abuse – including, most certainly, alcohol abuse - is common. It is often present before opiate detoxification and may indeed be a powerful reason for preferring MMT, or other agonist maintenance, to NTX treatment. Conversely, it may become prominent only after the initiation of depot NTX treatment makes recourse to opiates impossible. Fortunately, this is often a transient phenomenon and may be seen as a mixture of self-medication for residual opiate withdrawal symptoms and the persistence of the habit of getting intoxicated with *something*, if only occasionally. However, there are many patients for whom opiates are the only problem, or by far the largest and when opiate use ceases after NTX initiation, the use of substitute intoxicants does not occur once withdrawal is complete, or at all, or else it happens only occasionally in a non-problematic way. Such patients may need little therapeutic input and are a pleasure to treat – and they are not rare, especially if they have had several years of MMT and need no 'rehabilitation' because they are working, integrated into the mainstream community and reasonably content.

Conversely, there are patients for whom even the effective removal of opiate abuse from their repertoire of intoxication or dependence will have a relatively small impact on their overall recovery because they have multiple problems and either continue using other drugs - or start (or resume) using them - heavily when opiates are blocked. Even if their subsequent drug use is modest or absent, years of unemployment (and unemployability), poor or absent education, crime and incarceration, dysphoria and dys-socialisation may have left serious and refractory deficits. Such patients may well need the long-term help of a good residential unit with an intensive post-discharge programme. Unfortunately, the antagonism of many such units to medical treatments, already mentioned, means that patients with depot or implanted NTX may be excluded, or subject to hostility if they are accepted. Attitudes like this are irrational. There is nothing about treatment with NTX or other medications that conflicts with the basic aim of all addiction treatment programmes, which is to aid the extinction of undesirable habits of thought and behaviour and to replace them with more appropriate ones.

26.14 Naltrexone Politics

This is an appropriate place to mention, briefly, some unseemly arguments that the availability and use of NTX – oral or depot/implanted – have engendered. Apart from those who are unhappy about *any* pharmacological treatments for addiction, NTX has been used by the quite large number of people, professional and otherwise, who are opposed to MMT and other substitution programmes, which they typically categorise as 'simply giving drugs to addicts'. Conversely, those who support MMT – including, not surprisingly, some physicians who obtain a large part of their income from agonist prescribing – have sometimes perceived NTX as a threat to their prominence and/or income. In our view, neither response is helpful to our patients, who should be our main concern and who deserve – as in most other fields of medicine – to be offered a range of treatments to suit their particular needs, circumstances and attitudes.

26.15 The Future

This concept of treatment relying heavily but not exclusively on pharmacological antagonists and which we have suggested should be called 'Antagonist-Assisted Abstinence' (59, 71) is likely to become more important as antagonists for other drugs of abuse are developed. There already exist antagonists for cannabis (72) and, still in development, vaccines for nicotine and cocaine, which will not need to be produced in depot format because they will have very prolonged effects (73). In principle, monoclonal antibodies can be produced that will block the effect of almost any drug. They have already been used successfully in the treatment of poisoning with digitalis alkaloids (74) and tricyclic antidepressants (75). Cocaine presents certain problems because it does not act through a single receptor and because the amount used is in grams rather than milligrams, requiring correspondingly large amounts of active or passive antibodies. However, once effective and acceptably safe medications of sufficient potency have been developed, their incorporation into an implant or depot preparation will be as essential for good compliance as it has been for NTX. Let us hope their development and availability will be on a much shorter timescale.

References

1. Mark TL, Kranzler HR, Song X, Bransberger P, Poole V, Crosse S. Physicians' opinions about medications to treat alcoholism. Addiction 2003 May;98(5):617–26.
2. Strang J, McCambridge J, Best D, Beswick T, Bearn J, Rees S, Gossop M. Loss of tolerance and overdose mortality after inpatient opiate detoxification: follow up study. BMJ 2003;326:959–60.
3. Eklund C. Withdrawal from methadone maintenance treatment in Sweden. Introduction, pp. 9–10. Uppsala University Press, 1996.
4. Gessner P, Gessner N. Disulfiram and its metabolites. Buffalo, 1992.
5. Martin WR, Sandquist V. A sustained release depot for narcotic antagonists. Arch Gen Psychiatry 1974;30(1):31–3.
6. Sullivan M, Kalkwarf DR. Sustained release of naltrexone from glyceride implants. NIDA Res Monogr 1976 January;4:27–32.

7. Chiang CN, Hollister LE, Kishimoto A, Barnett G. Kinetics of naltrexone sustained-release preparation. Clin Pharmacol Ther 1984;36(5):704–8.
8. Kranzler HB, Modesto-Lowe V, Nuwayser E. Sustained-release naltrexone for alcoholism treatment: a preliminary study. Alcohol Clin Exp Res 1998;22:1074–9.
9. Foster J, Brewer C. Naltrexone implants completely prevent early (one month) relapse after opiate detoxification (abstract). Addict Biol 1999;4:232.
10. Comer S, Collins E, Kleber HD, Nuwayser E, Kerrigan J, Fischman M. Depot naltrexone: long-lasting antagonism of the effects of heroin in humans. Psychopharmacology 2002;159: 351–60.
11. Hulse GK, O'Neil G. Using naltrexone implants in the management of the pregnant heroin user. Aust N Z J Obstet Gynaecol 2002;42(5):102–6.
12. Hulse GK, Arnold-Reed DE, O'Neil G, Chan CT, Hansson RC. Achieving long-term continuous blood naltrexone and 6-beta-naltrexol coverage following sequential naltrexone implants. Addict Biol 2004;9:67–72.
13. Foster J, Brewer C, Steele T. Naltrexone implants can completely prevent early (1-month) relapse after opiate detoxification: a pilot study of two cohorts totalling 101 patients with a note on naltrexone blood levels. Addict Biol 2003;8:211–7.
14. Brewer C, Gastfriend DR. Rapid opioid detoxification. JAMA 1998;279(23):1872.
15. Brewer C. Serum naltrexone and 6-beta-naltrexol levels from naltrexone implants can block very large amounts of heroin: a report of two cases. Addict Biol 2002;7:321-3.
16. Meyer M, Straughn A, Lo M, Schary W, Whitney C. Bioequivalence, dose-proportionality and pharmacokinetics or naltrexone after oral administration. J Clin Psychiat 1984;45(9): 15–9.
17. McCaul M, Wand S, Rohde C, Lee S. Serum 6-beta-naltrexol levels are related to alcohol responses in heavy drinkers. Alcohol Clin Exp Res 2000;24(9):1385–91.
18. Verebey K, Volavka J, Mule S, Resnick R. Naltrexone: disposition, metabolism and effects after acute and chronic dosing. Clin Pharmacol Ther 1976;20:315–28.
19. Resnick RB, Volavka J, Freedman A, Thomas M. Studies of EN-1639A (Naltrexone): a new narcotic antagonist. Am J Psychiat 1974;131(6):646–50.
20. Hulse G. Tait R. A pilot study to assess the impact of naltrexone implant on accidental opiate overdose in 'high risk' adolescent heroin users. Addict Biol 2003;8(3):337–42.
21. Hulse G, Tait R, Comer S. et al. Reducing hospital presentations in opioid overdose in patients treated with sustained release naltrexone implants. Drug Alcohol Depend 2005;79(3):351–7.
22. O'Neill G, Parsons Z, Hulse G. The problem of intravenous buprenorphine injection with naltrexone implants. Paper presented at the 3rd Stapleford Berlin Conference, March 18–20, 2006. Abstract and Powerpoint slides viewable at http://www.staplefordcentre.co.uk
23. Brewer C, Wong V-S. Naltrexone: a case report of lack of hepatotoxicity in acute viral hepatitis, with a review of the literature. Addict Biol 2004;9:81–7.
24. Terg R, Coronel E, Sorda J, Munoz AE, Findor J. Efficacy and safety of oral naltrexone treatment for pruritus of cholestasis, a crossover, double blind, placebo controlled study. J Hepatol 2002;37(6):717–22.
25. Stella L, D'Ambra C, Mazzeo F. et al. Naltrexone plus benzodiazepine aids abstinence in opioid-dependent patients. Life Sci 2005;77:2717–22.
26. Dean AJ, Saunders JB, Jones RT, Young RM, Connor JP, Lawford BR. Does naltrexone treatment lead to depression? Findings from a randomized controlled trial in subjects with opioid dependence. J Psychiatry Neurosci 2006 January;31(1):38–45.
27. Brewer C, La octreotida en la desintoxicacion rapida de opiaceos. Revista Espanola de Drogodependencias 1999;24:426–7.
28. Aghajanian GK. Tolerance of locus coeruleus neurons to morphine and suppression of withdrawal response by clonidine. Nature 1978;276:186–8.
29. Nestler E. Molecular mechanisms of drug addiction. J Neurosci 1992;12:2439–50.
30. Streel E, Dan B, Campanella S, Meyvaert A, Hanak C, Pelc I, Verbanck P. A pharmacological modulation of opiate withdrawal using an up-/down-modulation of the noradrenergic system in opiate-dependent rats. Int J Neuropsychopharmacol 2005;7:1–6.

31. Golovko AI, Golovko SI, Leont'eva LV, Romanenko OI, Konoplin DA. Molecular aspects of pharmacological activity of naltrexone and naloxone. Eksp Klin Farmakol 2003;66(1): 71–8.
32. Digiusto E, Shakeshaft A, Ritter A, O'Brien S, Mattick RP. NEPOD research group. Serious adverse events in the Australian national evaluation of pharmacotherapies for opioid dependence (NEPOD). Addiction 2004;99:450–60.
33. Cruz SL, Villarreal JE, Volkow ND. Further evidence that naloxone acts as an inverse opiate agonist: implications for drug dependence and withdrawal. Life Sci 1996;58(26):PL381–9.
34. Wang D, Raehal KM, Bilsky EJ, Sadee W. Inverse agonists and neutral antagonists at mu opioid receptor (MOR): possible role of basal receptor signaling in narcotic dependence. J Neurochem 2001;77(6):1590–600.
35. Sadée W, Wang D, Bilsky EJ. Basal opioid receptor activity, neutral antagonists, and therapeutic opportunities. Life Sci 2005;76:1427–37.
36. Wang Z, Bilsky EJ, Porreca F, Sadee W. Constitutive mu opioid receptor activation as a regulatory mechanism underlying narcotic tolerance and dependence. Life Sci 1994;54(20): PL339–50.
37. Smith MA, Bryant PA, McLean JM. Social and environmental enrichment enhances sensitivity to the effects of Kappa opioids: studies on antinociception, diuresis and conditioned place preference. Pharmacol Biochem Behav 2003;76:93–101.
38. Zachariou V, Georgescu D, Sanchez N, Rahman Z, DiLeone R, Berton O, Neve RL, Sim-Selley LJ, Selley DE, Gold S, Nestler E. Essential role for RGS9 in opiate addiction. PNAS 2003;100(23):13656–61.
39. McGregor C, Darke S, Ali R, Christie P. Experience of non-fatal overdose among heroin users in Adelaide, Australia: circumstances and risk perceptions. Addiction 1998;93(5):701–11.
40. Waal H, Christophersen A, Frogopsahl G, Olsen L, Morland J. Implantasjon av naltrexonkapsler. Tidsskr Nor Laegeforen. 2003;123(12):1660–1.
41. Gölz J, Partecke G. Katamnesticher entwicklung opiatabhängiger nach naltrexon-induzierten entzug unter narcose, naltrexongestutzter rückfallprophylaxe und ambulanter psychosozialer nachsorge. Süchttherapie 2000;1:166–72.
42. Johansson BA, Berglund M, Lindgren A. Efficacy of maintenance treatment with naltrexone for opioid dependence: a meta-analytical review. Addiction 2006;101:491–503.
43. Brahen L, Henderson R, Capone T. Naltrexone treatment in a jail work-release program. J Clin Psychol 1984;45:49–52.
44. Chan KY. The Singapore naltrexone community-based project for heroin addicts compared with a drug-free community-based programme: the first cohort. J Clin Forensic Med 1996;3:87–92.
45. Cornish J, Metzger D, Woody G, Wilson D, Mclellan T, Vandergrift B, O'brien C. Naltrexone pharmacotherapy for opioid dependent federal probationers. J Subst Abuse Treat 1997; 14(6):529–34.
46. Fuller R, Gordis E. Does disulfiram have a role in alcoholism treatment today? Addiction 2004;99:21–4.
47. Ehrenreich H, Krampe H. Does disulfiram have a role in alcoholism treatment today? Not to forget about disulfiram's psychological effects. Addiction 2004;99:25–8.
48. Azrin NH. Disulfiram and behaviour therapy: a social-biochemical model of alcohol abuse and treatment. In: Treatment Options in Addiction - Medical Management of Alcohol and Opiate Abuse, Brewer C. (Ed.), London Gasreu 1993:19–28.
49. Brewer C, Meyers RJ, Johnsen J. Does disulfiram help to prevent relapse in alcohol abuse? (invited review). CNS Drugs 2000;14:329–41.
50. Brewer C. Supervised disulfiram is more effective in alcoholism than naltrexone or acamprosate - or even psychotherapy: how it works and why it matters (editorial) Adicciones 2005;17(4):285–96.
51. De Sousa A, De Sousa A. Naltrexone vs disulfiram. A one year follow up of alcohol dependence treatment. Alcohol Alcohol. 2004 November–December;39(6):528–31.

52. De Sousa A, De Sousa A. An open randomized study comparing disulfiram and acamprosate in the treatment of alcohol dependence. Alcohol Alcohol 2005 November–December; 40(6):545–8.
53. Berglund M, Johansson BA. The SBU report on treatment of alcohol and drug problems. In: Maintenance Treatment of Heroin Addiction, Waal H and Haga E (Eds.), Oslo, Norway, Cappelen Akademisk Forlag, 2003:76–90.
54. Alho H, Laaksonen E. A randomized, comparative study of evidence-based alcohol dependence treatments: disulfiram, naltrexone, and acamprosate in the treatment of alcohol dependence. A randomized, multicentre, open-label, comparative trial of disulfiram, naltrexone and acamprosate in the treatment of alcohol dependence, Alcohol Alcohol. 2008 Jan-Feb; 43(1):53–61.
55. Blachly P, Casey D, Marcel L et al. Rapid detoxification from heroin and methadone using naloxone. A model for study of the treatment of the opiate abstinence syndrome. In: Development in the Field of Drug Abuse, Senay E, Shorty V, and Alkesne H (Eds.), Cambridge, MA, Schenkman Publishing, 1975:327–36.
56. Resnick RB, Kestenbaum RS, Washton A, Poole D. Naloxone-precipitated withdrawal: a method for rapid induction onto naltrexone. Clin Pharmacol Ther 1977;21:409–13.
57. Charney DS, Riordan CE, Kleber HD et al. Clonidine and naltrexone: a safe, effective and rapid treatment of abrupt withdrawal from methadone therapy. Arch Gen Psychiatry 1982;39:1327–32.
58. Brewer C. Blood pressure monitoring at home for rapid opioid withdrawal with clonidine and naltrexone. Lancet 1987;1:621.
59. Brewer C, Rezae H, Bailey C. Opiate withdrawal and naltrexone induction in 48–72 hours with minimal dropout using a modification of the clonidine-naltrexone technique. Br J Psychiatry 1988;153:340–43.
60. Loimer N, Schmid R, Presslich O, Lenz K. Continuous naloxone administration suppresses opiate withdrawal symptoms in human opiate addicts during detoxification treatment. J Psychiatry Res 1988;23:81–6.
61. Brewer C. Ultra-rapid, antagonist-precipitated opiate detoxification under general anaesthesia or sedation. Addict Biol 1997;2:291–302.
62. Brewer C, Williams J, Carreño JE, Bobes J. Unethical promotion of rapid opiate detoxification under anaesthesia (RODA). Lancet 1998;351:218.
63. Laheij RJF, Krabbe PFM, De Jong CAJ. Rapid heroin detoxification under general anaesthesia. JAMA 2000;283:1143.
64. Greenberg M. Ultra rapid opioid detoxification of two children with congenital heart disease. J Addict Dis 2000;19:53–8.
65. Wickler A. Opioid Dependence: Mechanisms and Treatment. New York, Plenum Press, 1980.
66. Murphy S, Hoffman A. An empirical description of phases of maintenance following treatment for alcohol dependence. J Subst Abuse 1993;5:131–43.
67. Brewer C, Streel E. Learning the language of abstinence in addiction treatment: some similarities between relapse-prevention with disulfiram, naltrexone and other pharmacological antagonists and intensive 'immersion' methods of foreign language teaching. Subst Abuse 2003;24(3):157–73.
68. Brewer C. Resisting temptation: a psychological analysis. Br J Addict 1989;84:1371–2.
69. Brewer C. Combining pharmacological antagonists and behavioural psychotherapy in treating addictions: why it is effective but unpopular. Br J Psychiatry 1990;157:34–40.
70. Krampe H, Stawicki S, Wagner T, Bartels C, Aust C, Rüther E, Poser W. Follow-up of 180 alcoholic patients for up to seven years after outpatient treatment: impact of alcohol deterrents on outcome. Alcohol Clin Exp Res 2006; 30(1):86-95.
71. Streel E, Verbanck P. Ultra-rapid opiate detoxification: from clinical applications to basic science (invited review). Addict Biol 2003;8:123–8.
72. Croci T, Landi M, Galzin AM, Marini P. Role of cannabinoid CB1 receptors and tumor necrosis factor-alpha in the gut and systemic anti-inflammatory activity of SR 141716 (Rimonabant) in rodent. Br J Pharmacol 2003;140(1):115–22.

73. Kosten TR, Biegel D. Therapeutic vaccines for substance dependence. Expert Rev Vaccines 2002;1(3):363–71.
74. Eddleston M, Rajapakse S, Rajakanthan et al. Anti-digoxin Fab fragments in cardiotoxicity induced by ingestion of yellow oleander: a randomised controlled trial. Lancet 2000;355: 967–72.
75. Heard K, O'Malley G, Dart R. Treatment of amitriptyline poisoning with ovine antibody to tricyclic antidepressants. Lancet 1999;354:1614–5.

Chapter 27
Emergency Room Use of Opioid Antagonists in Drug Intoxication and Overdose

Simon F.J. Clarke, Rob Török, Paul I. Dargan, and Alison L. Jones

Abstract Opioid receptor antagonists are effective at reversing the clinical features of opioid toxicity; however, if administered overenthusiastically, they can precipitate acute withdrawal symptoms (AWS) in regular opioid users. These symptoms may cause the patients to discharge themselves against medical advice and they are in danger of renarcotization either due to the effect of the antagonists wearing off or because of the patients seek further opioids, often in larger doses, to overcome AWS. Clinicians treating opioid overdose are therefore walking a clinical tightrope between undertreating the patient and precipitating AWS.

The three opioid antagonists that have been licensed for clinical use are naloxone, naltrexone, and nalmefene. Unfortunately, the latter two have long durations of action which may cause prolonged AWS, and they are not recommended for Emergency Department treatment of acute opioid toxicity. The evidence base for the appropriate dose, route of administration, and observation of opioid-intoxicated patients is presented, and a clinical algorithm has been developed. Optimal therapy includes careful titration of intravenous boluses of naloxone so that patients are able to maintain their own airway and breathe adequately, without precipitating AWS, followed by at least 2-h observation. The subcutaneous and intramuscular routes should only be used if intravenous access cannot be established.

Keywords: Naloxone; Naltrexone; Nalmefene; Acute withdrawal symptoms (AWS); Intravenous; Intramuscular; Subcutaneous

27.1 Introduction

Opioids are chemicals (both endogenous and exogenous) that act at specific membrane-bound receptors. There are four subclasses of opioid receptor which have undergone a series of nomenclature changes in recent years by the International

S.F.J. Clarke, R. Török, P.I. Dargan, and A.L. Jones
Department of Emergency Medicine, Frimley Park Hospital, Portsmouth Road, Camberley, Surrey GU16 7UJ, UK
e-mail: sfjclarke@doctors.org.uk

Union of Pharmacology (IUPHAR) and International Narcotics Research Conference (INRC) (1–5), although clinical studies still tend to use the classical receptor terms, mu, delta, kappa, and ORL1 (orphan-opioid receptor).

Opioid receptors are coupled to G-proteins and stimulation causes a number of cellular effects:

- inhibition of adenyl cyclase, which reduces intracellular cyclic adenosine-3′,5′-monophosphate (cAMP) levels;
- activation of potassium channels or closure of calcium channels which hyperpolarizes the cell membrane.

These reduce neurotransmitter release [acetylcholine, noradrenaline, glutamate, and gamma-aminobutyric acid (GABA)] from nerve terminals (4, 6) and the variety of clinical effects produced by stimulation of different receptor subtypes is a product

Table 27.1 Classifications of opioid receptors (3–5, 7)

Classical	IUPHAR 1996	IUPHAR 2000	INRC	Receptor distribution	Clinical manifestations
Mu	OP3	MOP	MOR	Cortex (lamina IV), basal ganglia, thalamus, limbic system, midbrain, pons, medulla	Central and spinal analgesia Respiratory depression Bradycardia
				Dorsal horn of spinal cord	Sedation Euphoria
				Other (gut, vas deferens, immune cells)	GI dysmotility Prolactin and growth hormone release
Kappa	OP2	KOP	KOR	Basal ganglia, thalamus, hypothalamus, limbic system, pons, medulla	Central and spinal analgesia Miosis Dysphoria Psychomimetic effects
Delta	OP1	DOP	DOR	Cortex (olfactory), basal ganglia Dorsal horn of spinal cord Other (vas deferens, lymphocyte)	Spinal analgesia Modulation of mu receptor function
ORL1	OP4	NOP	NOR	Cortex, thalamus, hypothalamus, limbic system, midbrain, pons Presynaptic (sympathetic, parasympathetic, sensory nerves) Postsynaptic (spinal nerves)	Antagonism of central analgesia

IUPHAR International Union of Pharmacology, *INRC* International Narcotics Research Conference, *ORL1* orphan-opioid receptor, *MOR* mu-opioid receptor, *KOR* kappa-opioid receptor, DOR delta-opioid receptor, NOR neuron-derived orphan receptor, *GI* gastrointestinal, *MOP* mu-opioid peptide, *KOP* kappa-opioid peptide, Dop delta-opioid peptide, *NOP* nociceptin-opioid peptide.

of their differential anatomical distribution (Table 27.1) rather than differences in receptor signal transduction (3, 4, 7).

Stimulation of each receptor type produces specific physiological changes, some of which may be used therapeutically (analgesia and sedation), while others produce unwanted effects (respiratory depression). In addition, opioids have psychotropic activity and may cause dysphoria, euphoria, and hallucinations which have led to them being used recreationally as drugs of abuse; people taking them regularly for such purposes may become psychologically and physically dependent on them. Chronic misuse may also result in desensitization and tolerance due to a combination of:

- reduced receptor-ligand affinity;
- downregulation of the receptors (receptors undergo structural change before internalization);
- loss of receptors both on and in the cells;
- alterations in G-protein secondary messengers; and
- changes in phosphorylation sites (6, 8).

This means that over time, chronic recreational users need increasing doses to achieve the same effect. If they abruptly stop taking opioids they undergo an acute withdrawal syndrome (AWS) due to development of supranormal levels of cAMP, which occurs as soon as 12 h after stopping opioids or almost immediately when opioid antagonists are given (3, 6). This induces increased neurotransmitter release which leads to the features of hyperexcitability that characterize AWS; this starts with yawning, lacrimation, salivation, rhinorrhoea, shivering, and piloerection ("cold turkey") and progress to diarrhoea, vomiting, agitation, and transient fluctuations in blood pressure. Although it is not generally life-threatening (9), there is a risk of aspiration pneumonitis if emesis occurs before conscious levels rise. Controlled detoxification programs involve sedation with benzodiazepines, or even general anesthesia for ultrarapid techniques.

The constellation of clinical effects produced by individual opioids is the result of differential affinity for receptor subtypes; some agents are predominantly agonists (such as morphine and fentanyl), others (such as buprenorphine and pentazocine) have a mixture of agonist action at some receptors while antagonizing others, and a small number antagonize all opioid receptors. The amount of these effects depends on the degree of receptor occupancy which, in turn, depends upon the dose of drug administered and the individual patient's tolerance of the drug. At high doses, opioids will produce stronger effects at receptors at which they would have a weak action at lower doses, adverse effects such as respiratory depression become more pronounced, and therapeutic effects may also become so exaggerated as to become potentially harmful, such as excess sedation. Thus, the clinical profile of individual opioids varies with the dose used and the clinical features of many opioids in overdose are so similar.

Opioid antagonists have been known about since the second decade of the last century (10); however, unlike their predecessors, such as nalorphine and levallorphan which had some agonist activity and caused respiratory depression (11), the current antagonists naloxone, naltrexone, and nalmefene act as competitive inhibitors at all opioid receptors. They prevent binding of agonists and agonist–

antagonists, and they seem to be devoid of any innate clinical effect except for reversal of the effects of the opioid agonists. Animal studies have suggested that naloxone may also inhibit GABA release and stimulate cholinergic activity, but no human studies have confirmed this (12, 13).

The Emergency Department (ED) use of opioid antagonists is almost exclusively for the treatment of opioid toxicity, most of which is related to inadvertent overdose during recreational use, or to an opioid ingestion in deliberate-self harm. In the past, animal studies and the finding of opioid endogenous peptides in the adrenal medulla (14) suggested that opioid antagonists might have a role in the treatment of shock states and spinal cord injury; however, clinical trials did not consistently confirm the theories so opioid antagonists have not become accepted therapies in the circumstances (15–17). Similarly, studies have found that naloxone does not reverse the clinical effects of ethanol (18–20).

Acute opioid intoxication and overdose are common causes of presentation to EDs around the developed world; opioids account for 5% of toxic exposures to pharmaceuticals reported to Poison Control Centers in the United States (21). In the North-West region of the United Kingdom, opioids are involved in nearly 10% of instances of overdose (personal communication with Jane Cooper, Project Coordinator, Manchester and Salford Self-Harm group).

27.2 Naloxone

27.2.1 Pharmacology

Naloxone (*n*-allylnoroxymorphone) is a synthetic derivative of oxymorphone and acts as an antagonist at all opioid receptors (22); it seems to be devoid of any agonist activity. Naloxone is highly lipid soluble and can reach a brain to serum ratio up to 15 times greater than that of morphine (23), with a distribution half-life of 4–5 min (24). The first clinical effects can be seen within 1–2 min of intravenous (IV) injection and 15 min of intramuscular (IM) administration, although the latter can be much slower in the presence of hypotension (23). Naloxone is rapidly metabolized in the liver by a number of pathways: conjugation with glucuronic acid and excretion in the urine accounts for 65% of the elimination of naloxone (25, 26). First pass metabolism of naloxone results in an oral bioavailability of 3% and therefore oral administration is clinically ineffective and naloxone needs to be administered parenterally. Other metabolic processes include *N*-dealkylation, and reduction of the 6-keto portion produces 6-beta-naloxol which has opioid antagonist activity (22) and there is some evidence that the action of naloxone is prolonged in renal failure (27).

The elimination half-life is ~65 min (range 30–100 min) and metabolites can be found in the urine for up to 72 h of an IV dose. However, the clinical effects may be shorter than would be suggested by this basic pharmacokinetic data; the high lipid solubility results in a rapid increase in levels in the brain after administration.

This sets up a steep concentration gradient between the brain and the serum, down which naloxone moves and this means that naloxone is removed from its site of action, and hence its clinical effect diminishes (28–32), before significant metabolism occurs. Naloxone undergoes significant first pass metabolism which strictly mitigates against oral administration (26).

27.2.2 Therapeutic Uncertainties

Naloxone was introduced into clinical practice in the early 1960s (28, 33). In spite of long experience in its use, there is still considerable confusion about the appropriate dose and route of administration; for example, Poisindex suggests 0.4–2 mg boluses and in the United Kingdom the British National Formulary recommends 0.8–2 mg boluses, repeated as necessary up to 10 mg for adults (10 mcg/kg followed by 100 mcg/kg boluses for children). The route of administration is also subject to significant variation: IV, IM, and SC routes have all been advocated and it is still common practice to give naloxone by both IV and IM routes (34, 35). More recently, intranasal (IN) instillation (36, 37) and nebulized administration (38) have been advocated to reduce the risk of needle-stick injuries and transmission of infections to healthcare workers.

There are a number of possible reasons for this variation in practice:

- Uncertainties over the dose of opioid ingested or injected; this influences the amount of naloxone needed to displace the opioid agonist from the receptors.
- Concerns over acute complications and precipitation of AWS if too much naloxone is given.
- Concerns about the risk of recurrence of opioid toxicity if insufficient naloxone is given.
- The potential difficulty in gaining IV access in IV-drug users.

27.2.2.1 Receptor Binding

Opioids exert their effect by binding to a series of receptors. Naloxone has antagonist activity at all of the receptor types and the amount needed to provide such an effect depends upon the number of receptors occupied. It has been estimated that 13 mcg/kg naloxone (1 mg in an 80-kg man) produces 50% receptor occupancy (39); however, this will be reduced in the presence of opioid agonists. This, in turn, is directly related to the dose of opioid ingested or injected and the individual patient's tolerance to opioids which are unfortunately seldom known in clinical practice (40). Instances have been reported where up to 20 times the recommended doses of naloxone have been needed to counteract massive opioid overdoses (41–43), even more with body-packers with up to 50 mg used in a single patient over 24 h (authors' personal experiences). Numerous case histories have revealed a 96-fold variation in rate of naloxone infusions (0.125–12 mg/h) given for prolonged overdoses (44–53).

27.2.2.2 Acute Complications

Over the years, a number of reports have been published that highlighted potential concerns over the safety of naloxone. Since its introduction, numerous cases have described other possible adverse effects of naloxone. Pulmonary edema has been reported, although most of these cases occurred either following reversal of opioid anesthesia (often for cardiac surgery) (54–60) or in the presence of preexisting cardiorespiratory disease (61). Opioid agonists have been known to cause noncardiogenic pulmonary edema by, as yet, unidentified mechanisms, since it was first noted by William Osler in the 1880s (62–73) and it seems likely that naloxone unmasks this edema by reversing the opioid-induced respiratory depression (74). In addition, the effect of coadministered myocardial depressants such as propoxyphene or cardiorespiratory pathology could not be ruled out in these cases.

Seizures (75) and arrhythmias (76–80) have also been noted, but again could have other causes, such as hypoxia (77), the opioids themselves (66, 78, 81), their coingestants (most notably cocaine or scopolamine), (80, 82) or preexisting disease (76, 79).

A number of episodes of severe hypertensive reactions have been reported following administration of naloxone to patients with preexisting simple hypertension, (83–87) and one report showed a significant rise in serum catecholamine concentrations in a patient with a phaeochromocytoma following administration of naloxone without prior exposure to exogenous opioids (88). Currently, a great deal of research is being focused on the interaction between opioids and the autonomic nervous system and it would seem reasonable to postulate that naloxone antagonizes opioid-mediated inhibition of noradrenaline release from nerve endings (4). Other interactions have yet to be defined. Canine experiments have indicated that reducing hypoxia and hypercapnia lowers serum catecholamine concentrations, and it has been proposed that hyperventilating patients prior to administration of naloxone would reduce the risk of sympathetic-mediated adverse effects (81, 89), but this has not been verified in humans. In contrast, Estilo and Cottrel (90) found no changes in blood pressure, heart rate, and plasma catecholamine levels when naloxone was given to normotensive patients.

A number of observational studies looked at complications within a short period of time of administration of naloxone (Table 27.2). Yealy (101) found that a 0.7% complication rate within 5 min of naloxone administration (0.4–2.4 mg), which included mild, transient fluctuations in blood pressure. Smith (96) noted 8% complications all within 20 min of 2–4 mg boluses. Similarly, Osterwalder (34) observed a 5% complication rate within 15 min of naloxone but the doses were not mentioned; one patient (0.6%) further died of pulmonary edema 8 h after naloxone but further exposure to opioid could not be ruled out. In a second study (89), the same author reported a 6.6% complication rate within 10 min of small doses of

Table 27.2 Studies of complications

Author and study type	Methods	Key results	Study limitations
Barton (36) Prospective observational study 2 mg IN	95 patients with altered mental status given 2 mg IN naloxone; a 2 mg IV rescue dose was administered if the patient failed to regain consciousness by the time cannulation was achieved Data was collected prospectively on EMS sheets	Response rate 45% responded after IN administration. 9% more responded after the IV rescue dose (i.e., 20% of the responders did not improve with IN naloxone); 56% of these were reported to have a nasal abnormality (epistaxis, rhinitis, deviated septum) Time to Response Response was relatively rapid (mean 9.9 ± 4.4 min) Complications AWS No patients were noted to suffer AWS Renarcotization 16% of those who responded to the IN dose required a subsequent dose on naloxone	No comment was made about any nasal abnormalities in the IN responder group (i.e., are these abnormalities absolute or partial contraindications to the IN route?) Short-study period; patients were not followed up beyond transport to the ED
Buajordet (35) Prospective observational study	1,192 cases of suspected opioid overdose given naloxone (0.4–0.8 mg IM + 0.4 mg IV boluses up to 1.6 mg) by EMS personnel	Adverse events occurred in 45% AWS 32% Nausea, vomiting 9% Aggressiveness 8% Tachycardia 6% Shivering 5% Sweating 3% Tremor 1% Miscellaneous complications Confusion 32% Headache 22% Seizures 4% Miscellaneous 9%	Short follow up (until the patient left the scene or was taken to the ED). Renarcotization may have been missed The IV doses were given rapidly

(continued)

Table 27.2 (continued)

Author and study type	Methods	Key results	Study limitations
Christenson (91) Prospective, observational study	573 patients who had been were given naloxone (0.8 mg SC or 0.4 mg IV boluses) in the prehospital setting or ED over a 1-year period Patients were contacted after discharge to ascertain if they had suffered any complications within the following 24 h. A list of those who could not be contacted was matched with the databases of attendances in all of the hospitals in the city and with the coroner's records Relevant ED and in-patient records from the index visit were scrutinized to identify any factors that may be predictive of these complications	1. 16% suffered an adverse event within 24 h: • Supplemental oxygen for hypoxia (12.4%) • Repeat naloxone (8.8%) • IV antibiotics (2.4%) • IPPV (2.2%) • IV fluids for hypotension (2%) 2. The following factors were found to be predictive of complications if they were present 1 h after administration of naloxone: • Inability to mobilise • SpO2 ≤ 92% on air • RR ≤ 10/min or ≥20/min • Temperature ≤35°C or ≥37.5°C • HR ≤50/min or ≥100/min • GCS <15 3. One patient was misclassified; he fulfilled the criteria for discharge but was inadvertently kept in and subsequently needed a second dose of naloxone	Most of the study population had taken heroin overdoses and the rule needs to be validated with other opioids, particularly long-acting agonists.
Goldfrank (92) Two-phase study: 1. Prospective, observational; 2. Cohort study. Variable dose by IV infusion	Phase 1. Seven patients presenting to an ED with symptoms consistent with opioid OD Patients were given naloxone (6 × 2 mg/1 × 0.8 mg IV) then levels were taken at intervals for up to 1¼ h	Naloxone was found to be eliminated from the plasma in two phases: rapid over the first 15 min and second, slower phase over 2 h The measured levels were higher than predicted. The revised dosing regime suggested an initial bolus dose should be titrated, followed by an infusion at 2/3 of the bolus/h. A second bolus of half the initial bolus should be considered after 15 min	Small study The revised dosing regime has not been tested on volunteers and has not been validated clinically in the ED setting The pharmacokinetic equations were not explained

	This data was used to calculate the rate at which naloxone leaves the central compartment using specified but undefined pharmacokinetic equations. A nomogram was constructed to predict plasma levels from a bolus followed by an infusion of naloxone, at different doses Phase 2. Ten healthy volunteers Volunteers were given either a 2 mg or a 4 mg bolus IV followed by an infusion at 75% of the bolus dose/h. Blood samples were drawn at intervals up to 3 h and the levels were compared with those predicted by the nomogram The levels were entered into defined pharmacokinetic equations to adjust the nomogram		
Kelly (37) Unblinded RCT 2 mg IM 2 mg IN	155 unrousable patients with suspected opioid toxicity and RR < 10/min; they were given 2 mg naloxone either IM (n = 71) or IN (n = 84). If they failed to respond after 8 min they were given a rescue dose of 0.8 mg naloxone IM	Response rate There was no significant difference in efficacy between groups (87% IM vs 74% IN) Time to response IM was statistically significantly faster than IN at increasing RR > 10/min (6 min vs 8 min [$p = 0.006$]). The clinical significance of this difference is doubtful No significant difference in time to increased GCS > 11 between routes Complications AWS IN group had half the rate of AWS as the IM group (12% IN vs 24% IM) but this did not reach statistical significance	No record was made of the renarcotization rate No mention of other factors in those who failed to respond to the relatively high doses of naloxone (e.g., coingestants in both groups or nasal abnormalities in the IN route)

(continued)

Table 27.2 (continued)

Author and study type	Methods	Key results	Study limitations
Loimer (93) Nonrandomized controlled trial	30 consecutive patients admitted to a prison hospital. 22 were opioid addicts while 8 nonaddicts acted as controls. All were given 1 mg naloxone	AWS 100% in addicts (within 1 min and lasted for at least 30 min) 0% in nonaddicts	Small study Limited external validity; patients were not being treated for acute opioid toxicity
Loimer (94) Nonrandomized controlled trial 1 mg IV 1 mg IM 1 mg IN	17 consecutive opioid-dependent patients admitted to a psychiatry unit for detoxification. All patients were given 1 mg naloxone, either IM, IV, or IN	Response rate All patients developed AWS Time to response IN route precipitated AWS as rapidly as IV IM was slower than the other routes	Small study Limited external validity; patients were not being treated for acute opioid toxicity
Osterwalder (34) Prospective, observational study	169 patients attending an ED with suspected heroin/heroin mixture intoxication. 84% given naloxone although dosing regime not recorded Data collected prospectively in ED In-patient notes were reviewed on discharge and coroner's list of drug deaths was scrutinized retrospectively	Overall complications 95% were discharged from the ED • 70% < 1 h • 83% < 2 h • 5% > 8 h One patient died 7 h post discharge of pulmonary oedema (0.2 mg IV + 0.2 mg IM naloxone given and observed for 1.5 h). Further heroin use cannot be ruled out in this case This gives a delayed complication rate of 0.6% Complications after naloxone administration 47% self-discharged within 30 min of being given naloxone; none was found to have died or returned to the ED in the following 24 h Nine patients were admitted (5%). All complications were apparent at of within 15 min of arrival in the ED: • 4 cardiac arrests • 3 pulmonary edema • 2 seizures	Doses of naloxone were not mentioned Long-acting/orally ingested opioids were not studied

Osterwalder (89) Prospective, observational study	453 patient episodes of OD of IV heroin/heroin mixtures with increase in GCS and RR after naloxone treatment in an ED 0.1–2.8 mg IV or 0.1–0.9 mg IM (median 0.2 mg both routes) Prospective data collection in the ED	AWS 1. Case described (0.2%) Miscellaneous complications 51 (11.3%) complications were encountered within 10 min of naloxone: • 10 cardiac arrest • 9 pulmonary edema • 8 delayed response • 5 aspiration • 4 hyperthermia • 6 seizures (after prolonged hypoxia or in known epileptics) • 3 rhabdomyolysis • 2 pneumonia • 2 hypoglycemia • 2 hypothermia	There was no attempt made to ascertain the effect of route and dose on complication rate Long-acting/orally ingested opioids were not studied No record of self-discharge rate Did not look for delayed complications A temporal relationship between naloxone administration and onset of complications does not necessarily imply a causal relationship
Robertson (95) Nonrandomized, consecutive cohort study Dose not specified IV IN	154 patients with suspected opioid overdose who were given naloxone by prehospital paramedics both before and after introduction of a protocol for IN administration. Prior to the IN protocol, naloxone were given IV • IV $n = 104$ • IN $n = 50$ Retrospective review of EMS records	Response rate No significant difference (58% IV vs 66% IN [$p = 0.3$]). Time to response No significant difference in time of arrival at patient's side to clinical effect (20.3 min IV vs 20.7 min IN [$p = 0.9$]). Time from administration to clinical effect was longer with IN but it was quicker to administer Complications Renarcotization Significantly more patients needed a second dose of naloxone in the IN group (34% IN vs 18% IV [$p = 0.05$])	Naloxone doses were not specified Acute withdrawal symptoms were not reported Renarcotization rates were not reported Confounding factors such as coingestants could not be ruled out

(continued)

Table 27.2 (continued)

Author and study type	Methods	Key results	Study limitations
Smith (96) Retrospective observational study	124 patients presenting to an ED with heroin intoxication. Patients were given 2–4 mg boluses of naloxone IV/IM in the ED Review of ambulance service and ED records; death certificates issued by the coroner during the study period; and the in-patient notes of those who were admitted	AWS 49% self-discharged from the ED Renarcotization None of the self-discharged patients was retransported by the ambulance service and none died within 6 days of treatment Miscellaneous complications Five patients died (4%); all in cardio-respiratory arrest before naloxone was administered Ten (8%) admitted for complications, all apparent at or within 20 min of arrival in the ED: • 2 hypoxic encephalopathy • 3 pulmonary edema • 1 aspiration pneumonia • 3 effects of coingestants • 1 AWS	Long-acting/orally ingested opioids were not studied Retrospective data review: patients traveling by other means of transport, or to other destinations may have been missed No note was made of dose/route of naloxone given in each of the cases described
Sporer (97) Retrospective, observational. 2 mg IV 2 mg IM	625 patients with presumed opioid OD, given naloxone by paramedics and transported to an ED • 2 mg IV • 2 mg IM Review of ambulance and hospital notes and coroner's records	Response rate There was no significant difference in response rates (defined by an improvement in RR and GCS within 5 min of naloxone) of different routes: • 94% IM • 90% IV • 98% IM + IV Complications Renarcotization 35% required a second dose of naloxone but it was not possible to differentiate between routes AWS	There was no data given to correlate AWS and renarcotisation with route of administration of naloxone No follow-up of patients discharged from the ED was attempted

		7% required restraint for AWS + 0.8% escaped from the ambulance post naloxone Miscellaneous 74% were followed up to hospital: • 97% were discharged after 2h observation • 3% admitted (pulmonary edema, infections or complications of coingestants)	
Vilke (98) Retrospective, observational study	998 patients with presumed opioid OD who responded to naloxone (2mg IM or IV or 4mg ET boluses) that had been given by paramedics and who refused transport to hospital over a 1-year period Patients were identified from the EMS database. The coroner's records were reviewed to identify patients who tested positive for morphine after death	AWS 998/8,366 (12%) of patients given naloxone were released against medical advice Renarcotization None of the 998 patients was found to have died within 12h of initial treatment Miscellaneous complications Not recorded	Patients who were transported to an ED at a later stage either due to recurrence of toxicity or due to other delayed complications would have been missed Patients who died but were given an alternative cause of death (e.g., trauma) or those who died of nonmorphine opioid poisoning, would also have been missed The retrospective collection of data assumes that the demographic details given to the ambulance crews were always correct; incorrect details would have meant that patients who had died would have been missed
Wanger (99) Cohort study 0.4mg IV 0.8mg SC	196 consecutive patients with suspected opioid OD who were given naloxone by paramedics • First 4 weeks, 74 patients given 0.4mg IV • Subsequent 8 weeks, 122 were given 0.8mg SC In both phases, 0.4mg IV was used as a second, rescue dose after 5min as needed	Response rate There was no significant difference between routes to time of effect (defined as an increase in RR to ≥10/min) Time to response SC took longer to work from time of administration but was quicker to give as IV cannulation was not required Complications	Not randomized All of the patients had normal BP; theoretically, SC would be less effective in the presence of hypotension Confounding factor is difference in dose used between groups; double dose was associated with half the need for a rescue dose in the SC route No follow up was performed

(continued)

Table 27.2 (continued)

Author and study type	Methods	Key results	Study limitations
		Renarcotization A second dose was needed in: • 35% IV • 15% SC AWS Anecdotal impression that opioid antagonism was smoother in SC route, but AWS rate was not formally recorded	
Watson (100) Urban ED, USA Retrospective, observational study	84 patients who attended an ED with presumed opioid toxicity over an 8-year period, and who were treated with naloxone 2 mg boluses All IV except 1 IM and 1 via ET tube ED notes reviewed by an expert panel	50% responded to naloxone AWS 12% of responders suffered AWS Renarcotization 31% of responders developed signs of renarcotisation; 14% required a second dose of naloxone • Renarcotization was more likely to occur with long-acting opioids (58% vs 20% with short-acting agents [$p = 0.04$]), and was found to occur up to 2 h after naloxone administration • Opioid route and use of coingestants had no influence on recurrence of toxicity Miscellaneous complications Not recorded	Small study There are concerns regarding the relevance of the study population; first, the large number of nonresponders, in spite of relatively large bolus doses, suggests that many of these patients were not poisoned with opioids or had ingested large doses of other CNS-depressant drugs. Second, the numbers do not add up (42 responders + 17 nonresponders + 22 indeterminate response + 9 lost documentation = 90, more than the 84 enrolled in the study)

Yealy (101) Retrospective, observational study	813 patients with AMS given 0.4–2.4 mg of naloxone by paramedics: • 800 IV • 7 intratracheal • 4 sublingual • 1 IM • 1 SC Review of ambulance charts to assess response rate to naloxone and adverse events occurring within 5 min of naloxone administration	60 patients (7.4%) responded within 5 min of naloxone, suggesting opioid excess as a cause of AMS Miscellaneous complications 1. Complication occurred in the responder group (1.7%): • Vomiting after 0.8 mg IV In the nonresponders, five had various complications (0.7%): • Vomiting after 0.8 mg IV; had previously been given an emetic • Grand-mal fit in a known epileptic after 0.8 mg IV • Hypertension after 1.2 mg • 2 cases of hypotension after 0.8 mg	Late complications (e.g., recurrent toxicity) would have been missed Retrospective data collection

IN intranasal, *IM* intramuscular, *IV* intravenous, *AMS* altered mental status, *BP* blood pressure, *EMS* emergency medical service, *OD* oral dose, *ET* endotracheal tube, *HR* hazard ratio, *CNS* central nervous system, *GCS* gamma-glutamylcysteine synthetase, *RR* relative risk, *ED* emergency department, *RCT* randomized controlled trial

naloxone (0.1–2.8 mg, median 0.2 mg). Although all of the reported complications occurred soon after naloxone was administered, it does not mean that naloxone was the cause of the complications. As with the case reports, all of the complications mentioned in these studies could have been the result of other factors such as preexisting illness (seizures in known epileptics), the overdose itself (opioid-induced pulmonary edema or seizures due to hypoxia), or coingestant use (reversal of opioid inhibition of cocaine arrhythmias). In addition, a number of studies were undertaken where extremely high doses (up to 5.4 mg/kg boluses and 4 mg/kg/h infusions) of naloxone were given to nonopioid-dependent subjects without any reported adverse effects and with little obvious alterations to sympathetic function (15–17, 102–104). This would seem to suggest that naloxone is intrinsically safe. However, it would be prudent to titrate the dose of naloxone carefully in the presence of stimulant coingestants such as cocaine or preexisting hypertension (105, 106).

27.2.2.3 Acute Withdrawal Symptoms

Opioid antagonists can precipitate AWS in chronic opioid users (30, 40, 107), provoking an often-violent reaction that can include effects such as hyperexcitability, yawning, lacrimation, salivation, shivering, pilo-erection, diarrhea, and vomiting (108–110); for this reason the dose of naloxone used in chronic opioid users should be closely titrated to reverse clinical features such as respiratory depression and coma. Interestingly, in one early study on the use of naloxone to reverse morphine anesthesia in nonopioid-dependent, general surgical patients, mild acute withdrawal-like symptoms were observed to occur after the administration of 15 mcg/kg naloxone (31). Also, in a group of opioid-naïve volunteers, symptoms resembling AWS (behavioral changes, sweating, and yawning) were reported when they were given extremely high doses (2–4 mg/kg) of naloxone (111).

27.2.2.4 Renarcotization

The effects of naloxone last for a briefer period than all but the most short-acting opioids (28–32) because it is rapidly redistributed away from its site of action, due to its high lipid solubility (23). Repeated doses of naloxone may be needed for long-acting agents (112–118) and large doses of shorter-acting opioids (40, 119), and so infusions have been used.

Patients may suffer harm if they become renarcotized having self-discharged from medical care early, particularly, if they seek further opioid to overcome the effects of AWS.

27.2.2.5 Summary

Clearly clinicians are on a therapeutic knife edge between giving a sufficient dose of naloxone to overcome the initial opioid toxicity and reduce the risk of renarcotization while using a small enough dose to avoid AWS and other theoretical adverse effects. The next sections assess the evidence regarding the optimal dose and route of administration of naloxone and the appropriate period of observation after treatment. Table 27.2 contains summaries of the papers identified for this purpose.

27.2.3 Effect of Dose and Route of Naloxone on Response Rate

Five papers compared routes of administration (36, 37, 95, 97, 99). The studies used different criteria to define opioid intoxication (in terms of history and clinical findings), different definitions of what constituted a response to naloxone (in terms of improvements in respiratory rate and Glasgow Coma Scale), and times of observation before failure to respond was deemed to have occurred [ranging from 5 min (97, 99), 8 min (37), and time to achieve cannulation (36); Robertson (95) did not report a time].

Sporer (97) showed that 2 mg naloxone works intramuscularly (IM) as well as 2 mg intravenously (IV) (94% and 90% response rates, respectively); this is perhaps not surprising considering the relatively large dose given and it was not possible to distinguish differences in complication rate between the study groups.

Wanger's study (99) revealed that 0.8 mg naloxone subcutaneously (SC) worked as rapidly as 0.4 mg IV from time of arrival at the patient's side to time of clinical effect; the IV route was faster from administration to effect but this was offset by the time needed to achieve cannulation. Neither of these studies settles concerns about unpredictable and erratic absorption from the IM/SC injection sites in those patients who are hypotensive, but they may be useful alternative routes when IV access is difficult to obtain. No studies have evaluated the absorption kinetics of IM administration of naloxone in detail. It is likely that variables – including depth of injection, dose given, muscle blood flow, site, and so forth – would all alter the rate of absorption, particularly in the opioid-poisoned patient with hypotension.

Three studies have assessed the reliability of IN administration. Barton (36) noted that 20% of the patients with altered mental state, who responded to naloxone, did not improve after the initial IN bolus but did so after IV dosing. More than half of this group was discovered to have a problem with their nose, such as epistaxis, rhinitis, or a deviated septum. Kelly (37) found no clinically significant difference in response rate or time to response when patients with presumed opioid overdose were given 2 mg naloxone either IM or IV (response rate 87% IM vs 74% IN and time to response 6 min IM vs 8 min IN). Robertson (95) found a lower overall rate of response in his patient population who were given unspecified doses of naloxone IV or IN; however, there was no significant difference in response rate between routes (58% IV vs 66% IN). The authors found that the IV route was significantly quicker from time of administration to response, but this was offset by the time taken to gain IV cannulation, as Sporer (97) found for the SC route. This would suggest that SC or IN routes could be considered if the patient has no IV access, but not once cannulation has been achieved.

Goldfrank's landmark study (92) provides a good practical dosing guide for patients who require prolonged opioid antagonism. It was a small study where the end point measured plasma naloxone levels and not clinical effect; however, it claimed only to be an initial guide to treatment, and stressed the importance of close observation of the patient and titration of dose as necessary. This makes sense because of individual tolerance and susceptibility to opioids – for example, clinical observation has shown that corpulent patients will absorb opioids into fatty tissues from which it is expected to redistribute out more slowly and such patients tend to need more prolonged naloxone infusions.

27.2.4 Effect of Dose and Route of Naloxone on AWS

Reported rates of AWS-related complications vary widely from 7.8% to 49% with 2–4 mg boluses (34, 96–98, 100) to 0.2% with a median of 0.2 mg (range 0.1–2.4 mg) (89), although it is not clear from this last study if all AWS was recorded. Precise definitions for AWS were not given in the papers so it is uncertain if the actual outcome measures were directly comparable. Two studies recorded AWS [0.2% (89) and 12% (100)], with another paper (97) quoting the number of patients (7%) who required restraint; these were presumably the most severely affected patients. The other studies described the proportion of patients who discharged against medical advice (18–47%) (34, 96, 98). Patients self-discharge for many reasons – for example, fear of police involvement or anger at losing the opioid-induced psychotropic high – so that the number of absconders does not necessarily equate to those who experience AWS. Buajordet (35) reported rates of individual symptoms suggestive of AWS (ranging from 1% for tremor to 9% for nausea and vomiting), but unfortunately it is not possible to ascertain from the data how many patients were affected. Wanger et al. (99) reported that the paramedics who administered naloxone had the impression that patients given 0.8 mg SC has a smoother emergence than those who had received 0.4 mg IV, but they did not formally report AWS rates.

The IN route has been advocated in an attempt to reduce the risk of needle-stick injuries to healthcare workers as a result of AWS. Loimer (93) gave 1 mg to nonoverdosed opioid addicts and noted that all displayed signs of withdrawal. This is perhaps not surprising because these patients will have had lower opioid receptor occupancy than patients who had overdosed which provides less competition for naloxone. In a subsequent study (94), the authors noted that 1 mg IN naloxone produced AWS as rapidly as IV, with IM significantly slower. Kelly (37) noted a trend toward reduced AWS when opioid toxicity was treated with 2 mg IN when compared with 2 mg IV (12% vs 24%), but this did not reach statistical significance and Barton (36) did not report any AWS after 2 mg IN.

It is difficult to interpret the data for a number of reasons:

- The lack of information comparing absolute doses and rates of administration of naloxone with AWS, the precise drugs and coingestants taken in overdose, and the state of drug dependency/tolerance prior to AWS.
- The study design may influence the results, with retrospective studies being more likely to miss data. Lack of blinding is a potential source of bias; for example, Wanger's (99) anecdotal comments about smoother emergence with the SC route may be a genuine finding indicative of slower increase in naloxone concentrations at the receptors, but it may also simply reflect paramedics' preference for an easier route of administration.

The published data does not allow a dose–response relationship to be defined between naloxone and AWS; however, pharmacologically it would make sense that AWS should occur with higher receptor occupancy, therefore, using a dose just sufficient to overcome the acute toxic effects of opioids should, in theory, minimize the risk of precipitation of AWS. Further research is needed to try to define the precise relationship between AWS and route, dose and rate of administration of naloxone.

27.2.5 Effect of Dose and Route of Naloxone on Recurrence of Toxicity

The observational studies that described the number of patients who required second doses of naloxone showed a wide degree of variation. Christenson (91) reported 8.8% after 0.4 mg (IV) or 0.8 mg (SC) whereas Watson (100) noted 14% after 2 mg (IM), Barton (36) 16% after 2 mg (IN), and Sporer (97) 35% after 2 mg IV or IM. This variation is likely to be partly due to differences between the study populations. Also the criteria for giving further doses may have differed between individual clinicians with some possibly being more inclined to treat signs of recurrence of opioid toxicity conservatively. Only Watson's paper quoted both rates of renarcotization (31%) and numbers of patients who were actually given second doses of naloxone (14%); it would be informative if future studies similarly quoted both of these figures. Watson also found that recurrence of toxicity was significantly more likely when long-acting opioids were ingested, although route of opioid administration and use of coingestants surprisingly did not have any noticeable effect.

Two cohort studies attempted to compare renarcotization rates for different routes or doses. Wanger (99) reported that 0.4 mg IM naloxone was associated with double the recurrence rate (35%) of 0.8 mg SC (15%) which is perhaps not surprising considering the smaller dose. Robertson (95) noted that IN administration was associated with a higher rate of renarcotization than the IV route (34% vs 18%) although the doses given were not mentioned, so it is not clear if they were comparable. In neither study was the number of patients who were given subsequent doses of naloxone reported.

Smith (96), Osterwalder (34), and Vilke (98) all studied patients who absconded having received naloxone. None of them found any patient to have required further medical treatment or to have died in the following few hours (12 h Vilke, 24 h Osterwalder, and 6 days Smith). All of the studies retrospectively collected data from the local coroners, Emergency Medical Services and EDs; it is possible that some patients who suffered harm at a later stage might have been missed. Patient details are not always given correctly, for a multitude of reasons, and therefore subsequent attendances may be missed. Patients may also seek medical attention in different locations.

A dose–response relationship between naloxone dose and recurrence of opioid toxicity cannot be defined from the available data; however, renarcotization should be anticipated when patients have taken long-acting opioids, especially, if they are regular users because they develop an adipose reservoir which can leach out slowly. Avoidance of AWS by careful titration of the original bolus of naloxone should, in theory, reduce the chances of renarcotization occurring away from medical care, and close monitoring of the patients should allow prompt treatment of recurrent opioid toxicity.

27.2.6 Timing of Complications

Christenson et al. (91) suggested that if patients fulfilled certain criteria 1 h after administration of naloxone then they could be discharged safely; however, one of their patients who had taken heroin needed further naloxone after 2 h. Watson (100) similarly noted that patients who had taken long-acting opioids developed renarcosis up to 2 h after their initial treatment. Since the half-life of naloxone is 60–90 min, it would seem logical to observe patients for signs of recurrent toxicity for at least 2 h after the last dose of naloxone, because at this point, it is likely that the clinical effects of naloxone will have worn off. However, further studies are needed to validate this. Interestingly, Osterwalder (34) quoted one patient who was discharged after 1.5 h then found dead 7 h later; the patient had been seen after he returned home and seemed to be well before going to bed. He was found to have died from pulmonary edema which may have represented a late complication, but also could have been the result of further heroin exposure. Unfortunately, postmortem concentrations of morphine and its metabolites were not reported so it is not possible to ascertain whether further opioid was taken in this case. It would not be practicable to recommend observation for longer periods because most patients discharge themselves when they feel better and in our clinical experience it can be difficult to persuade them to remain even for 2 h.

27.2.7 Research Difficulties

Whyte and colleagues (120) have recently highlighted the particular difficulties in conducting research in clinical toxicology. Legal, political, and ethical difficulties, particularly in the context of obtaining consent, often hinder the recruitment of adequate numbers of patients. There are also a number of significant methodological difficulties to be overcome.

- It is difficult to eliminate confounding factors, such as the wide range of different opioids, coingestants, and adulterants that can be taken, the variety of routes by which they can be taken (orally, intravenously, subcutaneously, nasally, or by smoking), and the complex treatment regimes that are given. It is often difficult to determine what individual patients have taken because usually they do not know. It is also difficult to predict patient tolerance related to previous chronic opioid use.
- The outcomes being measured in many trials are relatively rare so that trials would have to be prohibitively large to achieve sufficient power.
- Blinding of treatments is extremely difficult because patients are often in the ED for such a short period before they are discharged that the clinician who administers the treatment is usually the one who has to review the response to that treatment.
- The external validity of the studies can be questioned because many are undertaken in regional poisons centers whereas most patients are treated in general hospitals where there is limited access to specialized toxicology laboratory facilities. Similarly, it could be argued that patients who agree to participate in research are not representative of the whole population of opioid overdose patients.
- Follow up of patients is difficult; Smith et al. (96) managed to contact only 32% of the patients who had been discharged. Other studies compared the lists of patients discharged with ambulance service records and death certificates issued by the local coroners. As was noted above, there are a number of reasons why some patients may have been lost to follow up.

Comparing different studies can be difficult because different criteria are often used for when to use naloxone or, as previously described, when to determine that naloxone therapy has failed. In addition, the variability in confounding factors makes direct comparison between studies unreliable. As a result of these difficulties, the backbone of research undertaken into the treatment of opioid intoxication consists of observational studies; therefore, it is not possible to undertake formal systematic reviews or meta-analyses. An algorithm (Fig. 27.1) has been devised by the authors (121) to attempt to summarize the research in a way that is clinically useful. Where there are gaps in the evidence base, consensus derived from the clinical experience of Medical Toxicology Units in the USA, Europe, and Australia have been used.

27.2.8 Summary

Paracelsus (1493–1541) stated that "all substances are poisons … the right dose differentiates a poison and a remedy" and naloxone is no exception. There are a number of circumstances where it may cause harm, most notably by precipitating

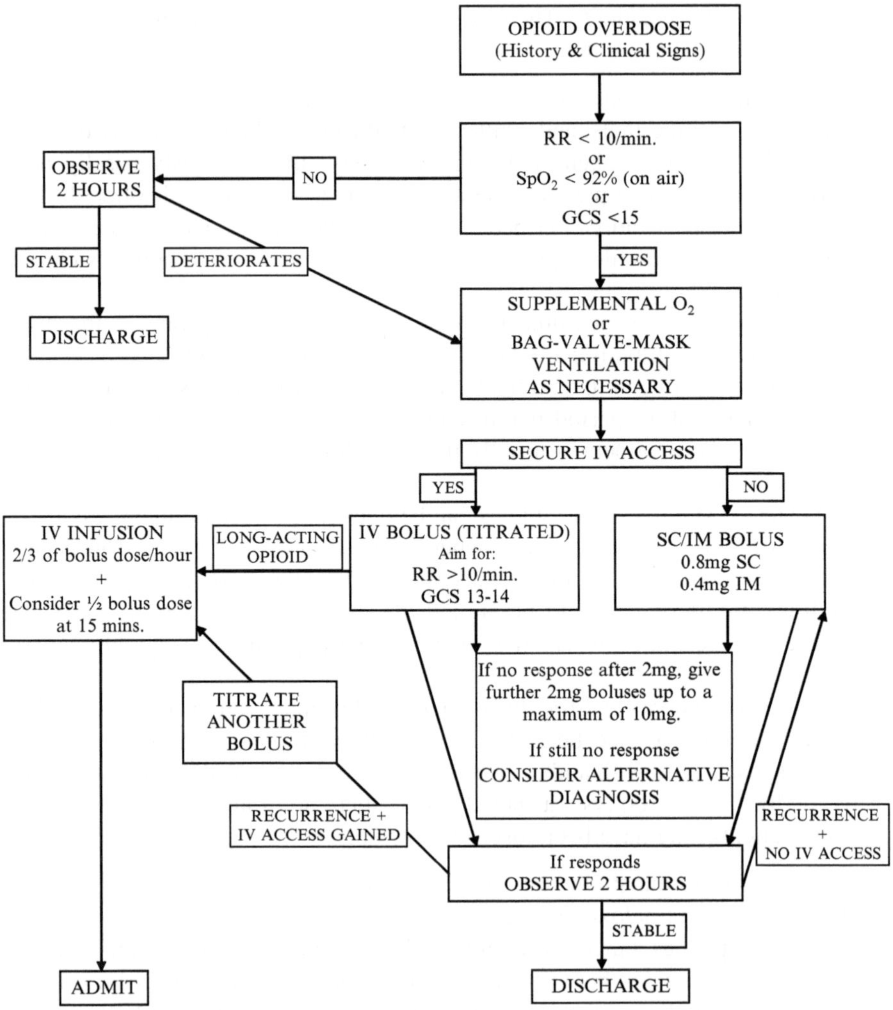

Fig. 27.1 Algorithm of treatment of opioid poisoning (121)

AWS if excessive doses are used in chronic opioid users, but also when autonomic-stimulating drugs have been coingested, and in the presence of untreated hypertension. The aim of treatment is to use the lowest dose of naloxone to increase respiratory rate and conscious level in an opioid-poisoned patient without precipitating AWS or dramatic changes in pulse rate and blood pressure. Clinical experience would suggest that careful titration can be best achieved by giving small boluses of IV naloxone whilst reserving the IM and SC routes for those patients in whom IV cannulation is difficult (not uncommon in long-term, regular IV drug users). The IN route seems to show potential because the onset of effect seems to be similar to IV administration. However, all of the studies have used single boluses of relatively large doses of naloxone (1–2 mg) and the authors do not think that it can be recommended as a route of administration until further research is undertaken to determine its efficacy when small doses are titrated.

27.3 The Long-Acting Opioid Antagonists: Nalmefene and Naltrexone

Nalmefene and naltrexone were introduced in the 1980s. They have a significantly longer duration of action than naloxone; this is due to a combination of longer half-lives [elimination $t_{1/2}$ is 60–90 min for naloxone compared to 10 h for naltrexone (29) and 8–9 h for nalmefene (122)] and lower lipid solubility which means that they are redistributed away from their sites of action more slowly (123) and in the case of naltrexone the active metabolite β-naltrexone (124).

This prolonged action means that nalmefene and naltrexone can be used for controlled, rapid detoxification of chronic opioid use, and to help former addicts to abstain from further opioid use (125); it has also been suggested that they can be used to reverse procedural sedation using opioids (123, 126, 127), as long as no need for ongoing opioid analgesia is anticipated. They have been advocated for the reversal of noniatrogenic opioid toxicity because it has been suggested that there is a lower risk of renarcotization; however, a number of significant problems have become apparent.

1. The evidence for lack of renarcotization is slim; first, in both Phase II and III studies on naltrexone, Kaplan and Marx (128, 129) noted no cases of renarcotization, in patients given nalmefene for presumed opioid intoxication but the subjects were only followed up for 4 h (recurrence of sedation and respiratory depression would not be expected to occur until 2–4 h later). Second, Konieczko and colleagues (130) found that 0.4 mg nalmefene was no better than either 0.4 mg or 1.6 mg naloxone at reversing respiratory depression up to 6 h postadministration of 10 mg morphine. Lastly, some opioid agonists have a longer duration of action than nalmefene and naltrexone, notably methadone, levorphanol and propoxyphene (131).
2. AWS occur in chronic opioid users and with the long-acting antagonists these can be severe and prolonged (126); a number of case reports have been published which describe some marked reactions where the patients have required heavy sedation (131–135) and, in some cases, general anesthesia (136–138), to control their symptoms. Most reported cases of AWS have lasted for 24–48 h, but in one episode, the patient remained confused for 7 days, although other contributory factors such as hypoxia could not be ruled out (135).
3. If opioids are subsequent needed, the doses may need to be much higher; it may be extremely difficult to achieve adequate analgesia for up to 72 h afterwards (139, 140). In opioid addicts who abscond after being given long-acting

antagonists for the treatment of acute overdose, they may attempt to overcome the AWS using high doses of opioid, with the theoretical risk of overdosing again (131).

Although the evidence suggests that both nalmefene and naltrexone are at least as effective as naloxone at treating both acute and chronic opioid toxicity (129), the potential risks of their long-term action make them less useful in Emergency Room practice. If long-term opioid antagonism is required then naloxone infusions, using the Goldfrank dosing regime (92) has the advantage of better control.

References

1. Dhawan BN, Cesselin F and Raghubir R. International union of pharmacology. XII. Classification of opioid receptors. *Pharmacol Rev*. 1996; 48; 567–592.
2. Calo G, Guerrini R, Rizzi A, Salvadori S and Regoli D. Pharmacology of nociceptin and its receptors. *Br J Pharmacol*. 2000; 129; 1261–1283.
3. Corbett AD, Henderson G, McKnight AT and Paterson SJ. 75 years of opioid research: the exciting but vain quest for the Holy Grail. *Br J Pharmacol*. 2006; 147; S153–S162.
4. Johnson EE and Lambert DG. Molecular pharmacology of the opioid/nociceptin system. *Curr Anaesth Crit Care*. 2002; 13; 305–312.
5. Nelson LS. Opioids. In Goldfrank LR, Flomenbaum NE, Lewin NA, Howland MA, Hoffman RS and Nelson LS. Goldfrank's Toxicological Emergencies (7th Ed). 2002. McGraw-Hill., New York
6. Jordan B and Devi LA. Molecular mechanisms of opioid receptor signal transduction. *Br J Anaesth*. 1998; 81; 12–19.
7. Pasternak GW. Multiple morphine and enkephalin receptors and the relief of pain. *JAMA*. 1988; 259; 1362–1367.
8. Williams JT, Christie MJ and Manzoni O. Cellular and synaptic adaptations mediating opioid dependence. *Physiol Rev*. 2001; 81; 299–343.
9. Chiang WK and Goldfrank LR. Substance withdrawal. *Emerg Clin North Am*. 1990; 8; 613–632.
10. Martin WR. Naloxone. *Ann Intern Med*. 1976; 85; 765–768.
11. Evans JM, Hogg MIJ, Lunn JN and Rosen M. A comparat ive study of the narcotic agonist activity of naloxone and levallorphan. *Anaesthesia*. 1974; 29; 721–727.
12. Dingledine R, Iversen LL and Breuker E. Naloxone as a GABA antagonist; evidence from iontophoretic, receptor binding and convulsant studies. *Eur J Pharmacol*. 1978; 47; 19–27.
13. Gruol DL, Barker JL and Smith TG. Naloxone antagonism of GABA-evoked membrane polarizations in cultured mouse spinal cord neurons. *Brain Res*. 1980; 198; 323–332.
14. Smith G and Pinnock C. Naloxone – paradox or panacea? *Br J Anaesth*. 1985; 57; 547–549.
15. Gurll NJ, Reynolds DG, Vargish T and Lechner R. Naloxone without transfusion prolongs survival and enhances cardiovascular function in hypovolaemic shock. *J Pharmacol Exp Ther*. 1982; 220; 621–624.
16. Groeger JS and Inturrisi CE. High-dose naloxone: pharmacokinetics in patients in septic shock. *Crit Care Med*. 1987; 15; 751–756.
17. Bracken MB, Shepard MJ, Collins WF, Holford TR, Young W, Baskin DS, Eisenberg HM, Flamm E, Leo-Summers L, Maroon J, Marshall LF, Perot PL, Peipmeier J, Sonntag VKR, Wagner FC, Wilberger JE, and Winn HR. A randomized, controlled trial of methylprednisolone or naloxone in the treatment of acute spinal-cord injury. *N Engl J Med*. 1990; 322; 1405–1411.
18. Mattila MJ, Nuotto E and Seppala. Naloxone is not an effective antagonist of ethanol. *Lancet*. 1981; 1; 775–776.

19. Nuotto E, Palva ES and Lahdenranta U. Naloxone fails to counteract heavy alcohol intoxication. *Lancet*. 1983; 2; 167.
20. Nuotto E, Palva ES and Seppla T. Naloxone-ethanol interaction in experimental and clinical situations. *Acta Pharm Toxicol*. 1984; 54; 278–284.
21. Watson WA, Litovitz TL, Rodgers GC Jr, Klein-Schwartz W, Reid N, Youniss J, Flanagan A and Wruk KM. 2004 Annual report of the american association of poison control centers, toxic exposure surveillance system. *Am J Emerg Med*. 2005; 23; 589–666.
22. Handal KA, Schauben JL and Salamone FR. Naloxone. *Ann Emerg Med*. 1983; 12; 438–445.
23. Berkowitz BA. The relationship of pharmacokinetics to pharmacological activity: morphine, methadone and naloxone. *Clin Pharmacokinet*. 1976; 1; 219–230.
24. Ngai SH, Berkowitz BA, Yang JC, Hempstead J and Spector S. Pharmacokinetics of naloxone in rats and in man; basis for potency and short duration of action. *Anesthesiology*. 1976; 44; 398–401.
25. Weinstein SH, Pfeffer M, Schor JM, Indindoli L and Mintz M. Metabolites of naloxone in human urine. *J Pharm Sci*. 1971; 60; 1567–1568.
26. Fishman J, Roffwarg H and Hellman L. Disposition of naloxone in normal and narcotic dependant men. *J Pharmacol Exp Ther*. 1973; 187; 575–580.
27. Hanes SD, Franklin M, Kuhl DA and Headley AS. Prolonged opioid antagonism with naloxone in chronic renal failure. *Pharmacotherapy*. 1999; 19; 897–901.
28. Sadove MS, Balagot RC, Hatano S and Jobgen EA. Study of a narcotic antagonist – n-allyl-noroxymorphone. *JAMA*. 1963; 183; 666–668.
29. Howland MA. Opioid antidotes. In Goldfrank LR, Flomenbaum NE, Lewin NA, Howland MA, Hoffman RS and Nelson LS. Goldfrank's Toxicological Emergencies (7th Ed). 2002. McGraw-Hill, New York
30. Evans LEJ, Roscoe P, Swainson CP and Prescott LF. Treatment of drug overdosage with naloxone, a specific narcotic antagonist. *Lancet*. 1973; 1; 452–455.
31. Longnecker DE, Grazis PA and Eggers GWN. Naloxone for antagonism of morphine-induced respiratory depression. *Anesth Analg*. 1973; 52; 447–452.
32. Evans JM, Hogg MIJ, Lunn JN and Rosen M. Degree and duration of reversal by naloxone of effects of morphine in conscious subjects. *Br Med J*. 1974; 2; 589–591.
33. Foldes FF, Lunn JN, Moore J and Brown IM. N-allylnoroxymorphone: a new potent narcotic antagonist. *Am J Med Sci*. 1963; 245; 23–30.
34. Osterwalder JJ. Patients intoxicated with heroin or heroin mixtures: how long should they be monitored? *Eur J Emerg Med*. 1995; 2; 97–101.
35. Buajordet I, Næss A-C, Jacobsen D and Brørs O. Adverse events after naloxone treatment of episodes of suspected acute opioid overdose. *Eur J Emerg Med*. 2004; 11; 19–23.
36. Barton ED, Colwell CB, Wolfe T, Fosnocht D, Gravitz C, Bryan T, Dunn W, Benson J and Bailey J. Efficacy of intranasal naloxone as a needleless alternative for treatment of opioid overdose in the prehospital setting. *J Emerg Med*. 2005; 29; 265–271.
37. Kelly A-M, Kerr D, Dietze P, Patrick I, Walker T and Koutsogiannis Z. Randomised trial of intranasal versus intramuscular naloxone in prehospital treatment for suspected opioid overdose. *Med J Australia*. 2005; 182; 24–27.
38. Mycyk MB, Szyszko AL and Aks SE. Nebulized naloxone gently and effectively reverses methadone intoxication. *J Emerg Med*. 2003; 24; 185–187.
39. Melichar JK, Nutt DJ and Malizia AL. Naloxone displacement at opioid receptor sites measured in vivo in the human brain. *Eur J Pharmacol*. 2003; 459; 217–219.
40. Allen SC. Problems with naloxone (letter). *Br Med J*. 1975; 3(5980); 434.
41. Moore RA, Rumack BH, Conner CS and Peterson RG. Naloxone after narcotic poisoning. *Am J Dis Child*. 1980; 134; 156–158.
42. Schneir AB, Vadeboncoeur TF, Offerman SR, Barry JD, Ly BT, Williams SR and Clark RF. Massive OxyContin ingestion refractory to naloxone therapy. *Ann Emerg Med*. 2002; 40; 425–428.
43. Gober AE, Kearns GL, Yokel RA and Danziger L. Repeated naloxone administration for morphine overdose in a 1-month-old infant. *Pediatrics*. 1979; 63; 606–608.

44. Waldron VD, Klimt CR and Seibel JE. Methadone overdose treated with naloxone infusion. *JAMA*. 1973; 225; 53.
45. Bradberry JC and Raebel MA. Continuous infusion of naloxone in the treatment of narcotic overdose. *Drug Intell Clin Pharm*. 1981; 15; 945–950.
46. Redfern N. Dihydrocodeine overdose treated with naloxone infusion. *Br Med J*. 1983; 287; 751–752.
47. Gourlay GK and Coulthard K. The role of naloxone infusions in the treatment of overdoses of long half-life narcotic agonists: application to nor-methadone. *Br J Clin Pharm*. 1983; 15; 269–272.
48. Lewis JM, Klein-Schwartz W, Benson BE, Oderda GM and Takai S. Continuous naloxone infusion in pediatric narcotic overdose. *AJDC*. 1984; 138; 944–946.
49. Tenenbein M. Continuous naloxone infusion for opiate poisoning in infancy. *J Pediatr*. 1984; 105; 645–648.
50. Romac DR. Safety of prolonged, high-dose infusion of naloxone hydrochloride for severe methadone overdose. *Clin Pharm*. 1986; 5; 251–254.
51. Hendra TJ, Gerrish SP and Forrest ARW. Fatal methadone overdose. *Br Med J*. 1996; 313; 481–482.
52. Sachdeva DK and Jolly BT. Tramadol overdose requiring prolonged opioid antagonism. *Am J Emerg Med*. 1997; 15; 217–218.
53. Johnstone RE, Jobes DR, Kennell EM, Behar MG and Smith TC. Reversal of morphine anesthesia with naloxone. *Anesthesiology*. 1974; 41; 361–367.
54. Flacke JW, Flacke WE and Williams GD. Acute pulmonary edema following naloxone reversal of high-dose morphine anesthesia. *Anesthesiology*. 1977; 47; 376–8.
55. Taff RH. Pulmonary edema following naloxone administration in a patient without heart disease. *Anesthesiology*. 1983; 59; 576–577.
56. Prough DS, Roy R, Bumgarner J and Shannon G. Acute pulmonary edema in healthy teenagers following conservative doses of intravenous naloxone. *Anesthesiology*. 1984; 60; 485–486.
57. Partridge BL and Ward CF. Pulmonary edema following low-dose naloxone administration. *Anesthesiology*. 1986; 65; 709–710.
58. Harrington LW. Acute pulmonary edema following use of naloxone: a case study. *Crit Care Nurs*. 1988; 8; 69–73.
59. Wride SRN, Smith RER and Courtney PG. A fatal case of pulmonary oedema in a healthy young male following naloxone administration. *Anaaesth Intens Care*. 1989; 17; 374–377.
60. Brimacombe J, Archdeacon J, Newell S and Martin J. Two cases of naloxone-induced pulmonary oedema – possible use of phentolamine in management. *Anaesth Intens Care* 1991; 19; 578–580.
61. Schwartz JA and Koenigsberg MD. Naloxone-induced pulmonary edema. *Ann Emerg Med* 1987; 16; 1294–1296.
62. Larpin R, Vincent A and Perret C. Hospital morbidity and mortality of acute opiate intoxication. *Presse Méd*. 1990; 19; 1403–1406.
63. Louria DB, Hensle T and Rose J. The major medical complications of heroin addiction. *Ann Intern Med* 1967; 67; 1–22.
64. Steinberg AD and Karliner JS. The clinical spectrum of heroin pulmonary edema. *Arch Intern Med*. 1968; 122; 122–127.
65. Gopinathan K, Saroja D, Spears JR, Gelb A and Emmanuel GE. Hemodynamic studies in heroin induced acute pulmonary edema. *Circulation*. 1970; 42(Suppl); 44.
66. Duberstein JL and Kaufman DM. A clinical study of an epidemic of heroin intoxication and heroin-induced pulmonary edema. *Am J Med*. 1971; 51; 704–714.
67. Fraser DW. Methadone overdose: illicit use of pharmaceutically prepared parenteral narcotics. *JAMA*. 1971; 217; 1387–1389.
68. Bogartz LJ and Miller WC. Pulmonary edema associated with propoxyphene intoxication. *JAMA*. 1971; 215; 259–262.
69. Frand UI, Shim CS and Williams MH. Methadone-induced pulmonary edema. *Ann Intern Med*. 1972; 76; 975–979.

70. Katz S, Aberman A, Frand U, Stein I and Fulop M. Heroin pulmonary edema. Evidence for increased pulmonary capillary permeability. *Am Rev Res Dis*. 1972; 106; 472–474.
71. Robin ED, Cross CE and Zelis R. Pulmonary edema. *N Eng J Med*. 1973; 288; 292–302.
72. Lusk JA and Maloley PA. Morphine-induced pulmonary edema (letter). *Am J Med*. 1988; 84; 367–368.
73. Dettmeyer R, Schmidt P, Musshoff F, Dreisvogt C and Madea B. Pulmonary edema in fatal heroin overdose: immunohistological investigations with IgE, collagen IV and laminin – no increase of defects of alveolar-capillary membranes. *Forensic Sci Int*. 2000; 110; 87–96.
74. Allen T. No adverse reaction (letter). *Ann Emerg Med*. 1989; 18; 116.
75. Mariani PJ. Seizure associated with low-dose naloxone (letter). *Am J Emerg Med*. 1989; 7; 127–128.
76. Michaelis LL, Hickey PR, Clark TA and Dixon WM. Ventricular irritability associated with the use of naloxone hydrochloride. *Ann Thorac Surg*. 1974; 18; 608–614.
77. Lawrence JR and Lee FR. Ventricular fibrillation after narcotic withdrawal (letter). *Lancet*. 1975; 2; 717.
78. Andree RA. Sudden death following naloxone administration. *Anesth Analg*. 1980; 59; 782–784.
79. Cuss FM, Colaço CB and Baron JH. Cardiac arrest after reversal of effects of opioids with naloxone. *Br Med J*. 1984; 288; 363–364.
80. Merigian KS. Cocaine-induced ventricular arrhythmias and rapid atrial fibrillation temporally related to naloxone administration. *Am J Emerg Med*. 1993; 11; 96–97.
81. Labi M. Paroxysmal atrial fibrillation in heroin intoxication. *Ann Intern Med*. 1969; 71; 951–959.
82. Horowitz Z. Subcutaneous naloxone: a less rude awakening? *Acad Emerg Med*. 1998; 5; 283–285.
83. Tanaka GY. Hypertensive reaction to naloxone (letter). *JAMA*. 1974; 228; 25–26.
84. Azar I and Turndorf H. Severe hypertension and multiple atrial premature contractions following naloxone administration. *Anesth Analg*. 1979; 58; 524–525.
85. Estilo AE and Cottrell JE. Naloxone, hypertension, and ruptured cerebral aneurysm (letter). *Anesthesiology*. 1981; 54; 352.
86. Ward S and Corall IM. Hypertension after naloxone (letter). *Anaesthesia*. 1983; 83; 1000–1001.
87. Levin ER, Sharp B, Drayer JIM and Weber MA. Case report: severe hypertension induced by naloxone. *Am J Med Sci*. 1985; 290; 70–72.
88. Mannelli M, Maggi M, De Feo ML, Cuomo S, Forti G, Moroni F and Giusti G. Naloxone administration releases catecholamines (letter). *N Engl J Med* 1983; 308; 645–646.
89. Osterwalder JJ. Naloxone – for intoxications with intravenous heroin and heroin mixtures – harmless or hazardous? A prospective clinical study. *J Toxicol Clin Toxicol*. 1996; 34; 409–416.
90. Estilo AE and Cottrell JE. Hemodynamic and catecholamine changes after administration of naloxone. *Anesth Analg*. 1982; 61; 349–353.
91. Christenson J, Etherington J, Grafstein E, Innes G, Pennington S, Wanger K, Fernandes C, Spinelli JJ and Gao M. Early discharge of patients with presumed opioid overdose: development of a clinical prediction rule. *Acad Emerg Med*. 2000; 7; 1110–1118.
92. Goldfrank L, Weisman RS, Errick JK and Lo M-W. A dosing nomogram for continuous infusion intravenous naloxone. *Ann Emerg Med*. 1986; 15; 566–570.
93. Loimer N, Hofmann P and Chaudhry HR. Nasal administration of naloxone for detection of opiate dependence. *J Psychiatry*. 1992; 26; 39–43.
94. Loimer N, Hofmann P and Chaudhry HR. Nasal administration of naloxone is as effective as the intravenous route in opiate addicts. *Int J Addict*. 1994; 29; 819–827.
95. Robertson TM, Hendey GW, Stroh G and Shalit M. Intranasal versus intravenous naloxone for prehospital narcotic overdose. *Acad Emerg Med*. 2005; 12(Suppl 1); 166–167.
96. Smith DA, Leake L, Loflin JR and Yealy DM. Is admission after intravenous heroin overdose necessary? *Ann Emerg Med* 1992; 21; 1326–1330.
97. Sporer KA, Firestone J and Isaacs M. Out-of-hospital treatment of opioid overdoses in an urban setting. *Acad Emerg Med*. 1996; 3; 660–667.

98. Vilke GM, Sloane C, Smith AM and Chan TC. Assessment for deaths in out-of-hospital heroin overdose patients treated with naloxone who refuse transport. *Acad Emerg Med.* 2003; 10; 893–896.
99. Wanger K, Brough L, Macmillan I, Goulding J, MacPhail I and Christenson JM. Intravenous vs subcutaneous naloxone for out-of-hospital management of presumed opioid overdose. *Acad Emerg Med.* 1998; 5; 293–299.
100. Watson WA, Steele MT, Muelleman RL and Rush MD. Opioid toxicity recurrence after an initial response to naloxone. *J Toxicol Clin Toxicol.* 1998; 36; 11–17.
101. Yealy DM, Paris PM, Kaplan RM, Heller MB and Marini SE. The safety of prehospital naloxone administration by paramedics. *Ann Emerg Med.* 1990; 19; 902–905.
102. Jasinski DR, Martin WR and Haertzen CA. The human pharmacology and abuse potential of N-allylnoroxymorphone (naloxone). *J Pharmacol Exp Ther.* 1967; 157; 420–426.
103. Flamm ES, Young W, Collins WF Piepmeier J, Clifton GL and Fischer B. A phase I trial of naloxone treatment in acute spinal cord injury. *J Neurosurg.* 1985; 63; 390–397.
104. Hara K, Senn BN and Floras JS. Evaluation of acute haemodynamic response to high-dose naloxone in young hypertensive and normotensive humans. *Clin Invest Med.* 1995; 18; 108–113.
105. Buchwald A. Naloxone use: side-effects may occur (letter). *Ann Emerg Med.* 1988; 17; 765.
106. Neal JM. Complications of naloxone (letter). *Ann Emerg Med.* 1988; 17; 765–766.
107. Wikler A, Fraser HF and Isbell H. N-allylnormorphone: effects of single doses and precipitation of acute "abstinence syndromes" during addiction to morphine, methadone or heroin in man (post-addicts). *J Pharmacol Exp Ther.* 1953; 109; 8–20.
108. Freitas PM. Narcotic withdrawal in the emergency department. *Am J Emerg Med.* 1985; 3; 456–460.
109. Popper C, Kelen GD and Cunningham G. Naloxone hazard in a drug abuser (letter). *Lancet.* 1989; 2; 446.
110. Gaddis GM and Watson WA. Naloxone-associated patient violence: an overlooked toxicity? *Ann Pharmacother.* 1992; 26; 196–198.
111. Cohen MR, Cohen RM, Pickar D, Weingartner H, Murphy DL and Bunney WE. Behavioural effects after high dose naloxone administered to normal volunteers (letter). *Lancet.* 1981; 2; 1110.
112. Sesso AM and Rodzvilla JP. Naloxone therapy in a seven-month-old with methadone poisoning. *Clin Pediatr.* 1975; 14; 388–389.
113. Simons PS. The treatment of methadone poisoning with naloxone (Narcan). *J Pediatr.* 1973; 83; 846–847.
114. Buchner LH, Cimino JA, Rabin HW and Stewart B. Naloxone reversal of methadone poisoning. *N Y State J Med.* 1972; 72; 2305–2309.
115. Kersch ES. Treatment of propoxyphene overdosage with naloxone. *Chest.* 1973; 63; 112–114.
116. Lovejoy FH, Mitchell AA and Goldman P. The management of propoxyphene poisoning. *J Pediatr.* 1974; 85; 98–100.
117. Vlasses PH and Fraker T. Naloxone for propoxyphene overdosage (letter). *JAMA.* 1974; 229; 1167.
118. Hantson P, Evenepoel M, Ziade D, Hassoun A and Mahieu P. Adverse cardiac manifestations following dextropropoxyphene overdose: can naloxone be helpful? *Ann Emerg Med.* 1995; 25; 263–266.
119. Kaufman DM, Hegyl T and Duberstein JL. Heroin intoxication in adolescents. *Pediatrica.* 1972; 50; 746–753.
120. Whyte IM, Buckley NA and Dawson AH. Data collection in clinical toxicology: are there too many variables. *J Toxicol Clin Toxicol.* 2002; 40; 223–230.
121. Clarke SFJ, Dargan PI and Jones AL. Naloxone in opioid poisoning: walking the tightrope. *Emerg Med J.* 2005; 22; 612–616.
122. Dixon R, Howes J, Gentile J, Hsu HB, Hsiao J, Garg D, Weidler D, Meyer M and Tuttle R. Nalmefene: intravenous safety and kinetics of a new opioid antagonist. *Clin Pharmacol Ther.* 1986; 39; 49–53.

123. Kim S, Wagner HN, Villemagne VL, Kao PF, Dannals RF, Ravert HT, Joh T, Dixon RB and Civelek AC. Longer occupancy of opioid receptors by nalmefene compared to naloxone as measured in vivo by a dual-detector system. *J Nucl Med.* 1997; 38; 1726–1731.
124. Verebey K, Volavka J, Mule SJ and Resnick RB. Naltrexone: disposition, metabolism and effects after acute and chronic dosing. *Clin Pharmacol Ther.* 1976; 20; 315–328.
125. Robinson CP. Naltrexone hydrochloride. *Drugs Today.* 1985; 21; 257–276.
126. Wang DS, Sternbach G and Varon J. Nalmefene: a long-acting opioid antagonist. Clinical applications in emergency medicine. *J Emerg Med.* 1998; 16; 471–475.
127. Chumpa A, Kaplan RL, Burns MM and Shannon MW. Nalmefene for elective reversal of procedural sedation in children. *Am J Emerg Med.* 2001; 19; 545–548.
128. Kaplan JL and Marx JA. Effectiveness and safety of intravenous nalmefene for Emergency Department patients with suspected narcotic overdose: a pilot study. *Ann Emerg Med.* 1993; 22; 187–190.
129. Kaplan JL, Marx JA, Calabro JJ, Gin-Shaw SL, Spiller JD, Spivey WL, Gaddis GM, Zhao N and Harchelroad FP. Double-blind, randomized study of nalmefene and naloxone in Emergency Department patients with suspected narcotic overdose. *Ann Emerg Med.* 1999; 34; 42–50.
130. Konieczko KM, Jones JG, Barrowcliffe MP, Jordan C and Altman DG. Antagonism of morphine-induced respiratory depression with nalmefene. *Br J Anaesth.* 1988; 61; 318–323.
131. Gaeta TJ, Capodano RJ and Spevack TA. Potential danger of nalmefene use in the emergency department (letter). *Ann Emerg Med.* 1997; 29; 193–194.
132. Bristow K, Meek M and Clark N. Acute opioid withdrawal in the emergency department: inadvertent naltrexone abuse? *Emerg Med.* 2001; 13; 359–363.
133. Quigley MA and Boyce SH. Unintentional rapid opioid detoxification. *Emerg Med J.* 2001; 18; 494–495.
134. Yeo M, Campbell V, Bonomo Y and Sawyer SM. Acute opioid withdrawal on accidental injection of naltrexone. *J Paediatr Child Health.* 2003; 39; 315–317.
135. Das PP, Grover S and Kumar S. Naltrexone-precipitated delirium. *German J Psychiat.* 2005; 8; 101–103.
136. Mannelli P, De Risio S, Pozzi G, Janiri L and De Giacomo M. Serendipitous rapid detoxification from opiates: the importance of time-dependent processes. *Addiction.* 1999; 94; 589–591.
137. De Giacomo M, Gaspari R, Stefanelli A, Barelli A and Mannelli P. Emergency therapeutic approach simulating ultrarapid opioid detoxification in methadone withdrawal precipitated by erroneous administration of naltrexone. *Eur J Emerg Med.* 1999; 6; 153–155.
138. Boyce SH, Armstrong PAR and Stevenson J. Effect of inappropriate naltrexone in a heroin misuser. *Emerg Med J.* 2003; 20; 381–382.
139. Gal TJ, Di Fazio CA and Dixon R. Prolonged blockade of opioid effect with oral nalmefene. *Clin Pharmacol Ther.* 1986; 40; 537–542.
140. Vickers AP and Jolly A. Naltrexone and problems in pain management. *Br Med J.* 2006; 332; 132–133.

Chapter 28
Kappa-Opioid Antagonists as Pruritogenic Agents

Alan Cowan and Saadet Inan

Abstract Norbinaltorphimine (norBNI), the prototype kappa-opioid receptor antagonist, *N*-benzylnorBNI, and 5′-guanidinonaltrindole (GNTI) precipitate stereotyped scratching after subcutaneous injection behind the neck of Swiss-Webster mice. The intensity of the behavioral activation and its repetitive nature represent one of the most arresting sights in preclinical psychopharmacology. The rank order for both potency and efficacy was GNTI > norBNI > *N*-benzylnorBNI. Although nalfurafine, the clinically tested kappa-opioid receptor agonist, decreased the incidence of GNTI-induced compulsive scratching in a dose-related manner, it is likely that this antagonism is mediated by mechanisms additional to a possible direct interaction with kappa receptors.

The robust syndrome will be of interest to basic scientists as a compelling behavior in its own right, as well as providing an experimental model for potential drug discovery in psycho- and dermatopharmacology.

Keywords: Pruritus; Itch; Stereotyped scratching; norBNI; GNTI; Nalfurafine

28.1 Introduction

Medical students are taught that opioids can induce pruritus in patients. Well, perhaps not every opioid and certainly not all to the same extent, but the association is instilled at an early stage in their careers (1). Those students specializing in anesthesiology learn subsequently that pruritus is a well-recognized side effect when morphine is given either epidurally or intrathecally for postoperative and obstetric analgesia. Experienced clinicians can infuse naloxone intravenously to specifically counter the itching (2) but reversal of analgesia is often an unwanted consequence (3).

Naloxone, naltrexone, and nalmefene are the three nonselective opioid antagonists that reduce scratching activity in a variety of pruritic states (4–7). Most notably,

A. Cowan (✉) and S. Inan
Department of Pharmacology, Temple University School of Medicine,
3420 North Broad Street, Philadelphia, PA 19140
e-mail: acowan@temple.edu

R. Dean et al. (eds.), *Opiate Receptors and Antagonists*,

these agents are providing a potential treatment for the pruritus of cholestasis which was to be expected given that increased opioidergic tone has been implicated in this condition (8, 9). So, with this background, it is reasonable to suppose that the typical pain investigator, with any interest at all in the nascent, yet overlapping research area of pruritus (10), would accept the following general statement: opioids cause itching while opioid antagonists are antipruritic.

With the advent of receptor-selective opioid antagonists, this assertion needs to be reviewed and updated. One aim of this chapter is to call attention to the remarkable scratch-inducing properties of antagonists that show selectivity for kappa-opioid receptors. On the one hand, we contend that such standard kappa-receptor antagonists as norbinaltorphimine (norBNI) (11) and 5′-GNTI (12, 13) precipitate immediate behavioral activation (especially stereotyped scratching) in mice as impressive as any drug-induced overt syndrome in psychopharmacology. Yet, almost all researchers studying these antagonists in mice have seemingly neither observed nor commented formally on this most visually impressive compulsive behavior. Mice responding to norBNI or GNTI with around 400 bouts of frenzied scratching in 30 min captures a picture of animals "on fire" with synapses aglow and a measurable behavior (1) of interest in its own right, as well as (2) providing an experimental model for potential drug discovery in psycho- and dermatopharmacology.

28.2 Effects of Kappa Antagonists on Overt Behavior

28.2.1 Initial Observations with norBNI

Kamei and Nagase (14) were the first to report that "when norBNI is injected subcutaneously into the rostral back, (ICR) mice scratched the skin around the injection site with their paws." This factual sentence, by itself, gives no hint of the stereotyped nature, and focused intensity and fervor, of the behavior. The incidence of scratching bouts increased with increasing dose of norBNI (3–30 mg/kg) and far exceeded that in corresponding vehicle-control mice, even at +90 min. Numerous pharmacologists, pretreating animals with norBNI [perhaps at different subcutaneous (s.c.) injection sites, or intraperitoneally] at various times before challenge with a kappa agonist, have made no mention of excessive scratching by mice (15–17), rats (18), or monkeys (19).

28.2.2 Findings with GNTI

GNTI was first synthesized by Portoghese and colleagues and characterized, using smooth muscle preparations, as a potent and selective antagonist at kappa-opioid receptors (20) despite being an analogue of naltrindole, the well-known delta-receptor antagonist. Initial publications from in vivo work with GNTI appeared in 2001–2002 and described interactional studies with opioids using food intake in rats (21) and operant behavior in monkeys (22) as bioassays. By itself, GNTI did not appear to affect gross behavior in these two species. Subsequent studies with rodents described the use of the more selective and potent GNTI relative to norBNI in terms of enhancing allodynia after sciatic nerve ligation (23), and countering immobility in the forced swim test, often claimed to predict antidepressant potential (24).

Our own experiments with GNTI (25) have extended the original observations of Kamei and Nagase (14) to a second, selective kappa antagonist and have confirmed the ability of such compounds to precipitate immediate and vigorous body scratching in a second strain of mouse (26). A summary of these studies is presented below.

28.3 Experimental Protocol

The behavioral effects of GNTI were compared with those of norBNI and *N*-benzyl-norBNI (BnorBNI), originally considered as "the first peripherally selective kappa antagonist" (27). The three structures are shown in Fig. 28.1.

Groups of 8–10 male Swiss-Webster mice (24–27 g) were used. Each animal was weighed and allowed to acclimate for at least 1 h in individual, rectangular observation boxes. GNTI dihydrochloride (Tocris), norBNI dihydrochloride (Research

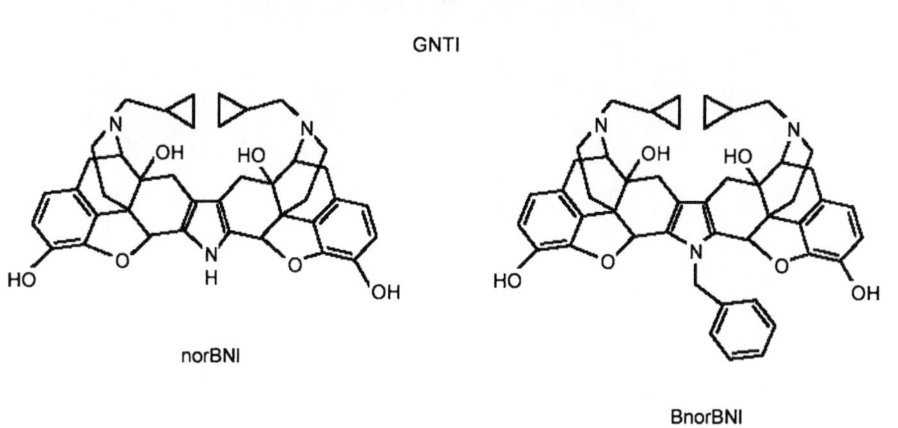

Fig. 28.1 Chemical structures of test compounds

Biochemicals International), and BnorBNI (courtesy of Drs. Husbands and Lewis, University of Bath, UK) were injected subcutaneously (0.25 ml/25 g) to the back of the neck of each mouse (Fig. 28.2) and the number of bouts of hind leg scratching movements directed at the head and neck (Fig. 28.3) was counted for 30 min. Doses

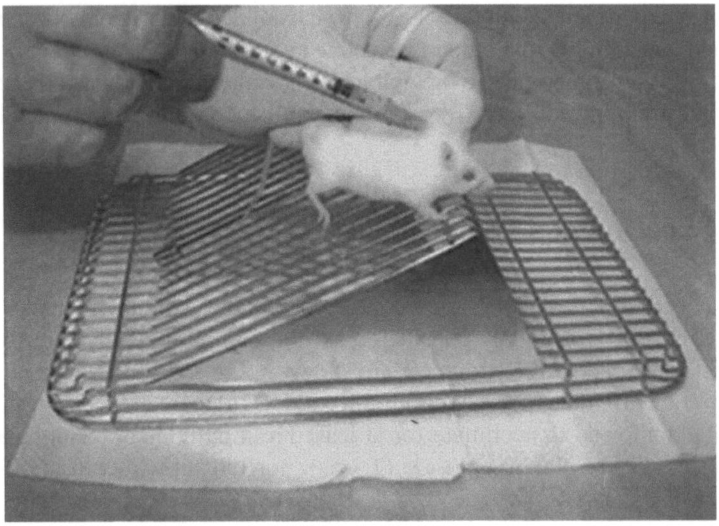

Fig. 28.2 Injecting 5′-guanidinonaltrindole (GNTI) subcutaneously to the back of the neck of a Swiss-Webster mouse

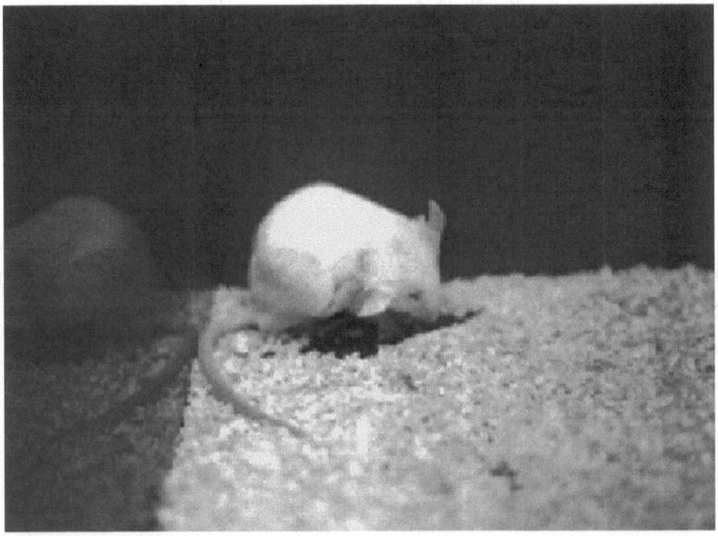

Fig. 28.3 Repetitive scratching of the neck area after injection of 5′-guanidinonaltrindole (GNTI)

of the test compounds were calculated in terms of the respective salt. Potencies (D_{50} values) were determined by linear regression analysis.

28.4 Results

Compulsive, vigorous scratching began within 5 min of injecting each test compound and the rank order of both potency and efficacy was GNTI > norBNI > BnorBNI (Fig. 28.4). Potencies (and 95% confidence levels) were 0.16 (0.08–0.30) mg/kg for GNTI and 7.0 (5.5–9.8) mg/kg for norBNI. A D_{50} value for BnorBNI could not be calculated. With a dose of 0.30 mg/kg of GNTI, peak scratching occurred between 10 and 30 min and tapered off gradually between 30 and 80 min. Tolerance did not develop to the excessive scratching when GNTI (0.30 mg/kg, s.c.) was given to mice once daily for eight consecutive days.

When groups of eight mice were pretreated with nalfurafine (0.01, 0.02, and 0.03 mg/kg, s.c. at −20 min), the structurally novel kappa-opioid receptor agonist (28–30), the incidence of scratching was decreased in a dose-related manner. For example, the 579 ± 74 bouts caused by (saline + 1 mg/kg of GNTI) in 30 min fell markedly to only 66 ± 29 bouts in corresponding animals receiving (30 µg/kg of nalfurafine + 1 mg/kg of GNTI). In this experiment, antagonism by nalfurafine was

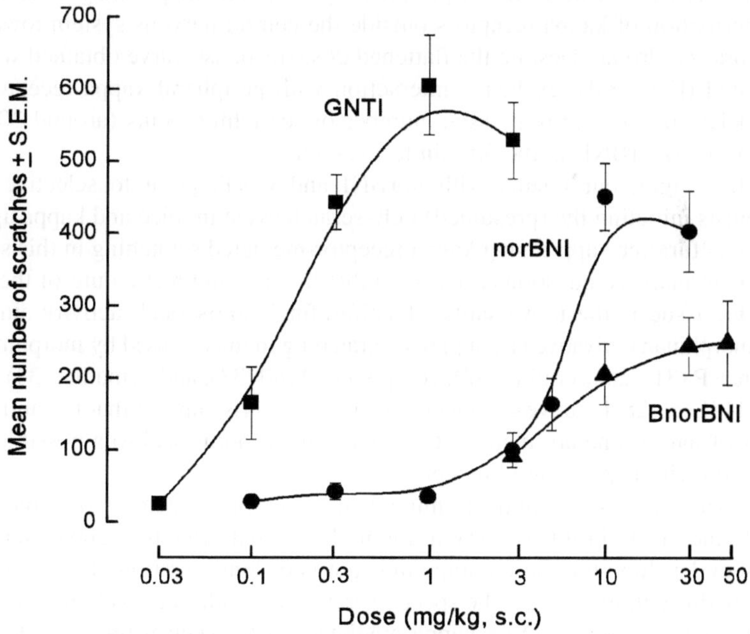

Fig. 28.4 Dose–response relationships for test compounds in eliciting scratching in mice ($n = 8–10$) for 30 min

substantial (90%) but not complete. The residual level of stimulant scratching activity argues against the antagonism being merely a consequence of mild sedation in the mice.

28.5 Perspective

Our preliminary structure–activity study has established that norBNI, the prototype kappa-receptor antagonist, and GNTI, a recently introduced, structurally novel kappa antagonist, both induce frenzied scratching when injected subcutaneously in the back of the neck of Swiss-Webster mice. GNTI is ~44 times more potent than norBNI in this respect and reliably precipitates the following repetitive syndrome: momentary licking of a hind paw followed immediately by a bout of compulsive scratching (with that hind paw) of neck and head areas. This behavioral activation is not observed when GNTI is delivered to mice either by intrathecal or by intracerebroventricular routes of administration and, additionally, Sprague–Dawley rats are essentially unaffected by standard s.c. doses (0.30 and 3 mg/kg) of the kappa antagonist (unpublished results).

It would appear that the *selective* antagonism of kappa receptors associated with norBNI and GNTI is a prerequisite for the scratching that we observed since naloxone, the nonspecific opioid antagonist, does not elicit the stimulant behavior in mice. Our use of BnorBNI, the peripherally restricted kappa antagonist, targeted the contribution of kappa receptors outside the central nervous system toward the behavioral syndrome. Despite the flattened dose–response curve obtained with this compound (Fig. 28.4), exclusive interaction with peripheral kappa receptors can nevertheless provide an impressive number of scratching bouts (around 200 with 10 mg/kg of BnorBNI) in the 30-min test session.

At first sight, our results with norBNI and GNTI point to selective kappa antagonists initiating the (presumed) itch–scratch cycle in mice and kappa agonists such as nalfurafine suppressing kappa receptor-mediated scratching in this species. On further analysis, questions arise as to the direct or indirect nature of the kappa link. One issue is the universality of nalfurafine's antiscratch activity since this epoxymorphinan derivative can suppress scratching in mice caused by morphine (31), substance P (31), chloroquine (32), compound 48/80 (33), and agmatine (34) as well as GNTI (Sect. 28.4, above). Collectively, these reports suggest that the antiscratch actions of nalfurafine are mediated by mechanisms additional to a possible direct interaction with kappa-opioid receptors.

Another issue is the almost immediate onset of scratching precipitated by norBNI and GNTI in mice. Current dogma has it that selective kappa antagonism is slow to develop with these compounds but is of long duration (16, 22, 35). It is therefore difficult to attribute the speedy scratching syndrome solely to antagonism at kappa-opioid receptors. Non-kappa-mediated events, such as the possible release of various scratch-inducing substances (e.g., histamine, 14) by norBNI and GNTI, need to be examined experimentally.

Our results with BnorBNI also require careful interpretation. This is particularly so since a recent publication (36) describes an *additive* action for this agent with U69593 (a kappa agonist) after s.c. administration in the mouse tail withdrawal assay. In contrast, selective antagonism of U69593 could be demonstrated in this assay when BnorBNI was given intracerebroventricularly (36). Our most recent work further complicates the picture: pretreatment of mice with BnorBNI (10 mg/kg, s.c.), 30 min before a diuretic dose (0.10 mg/kg, s.c.) of U50488H (the standard kappa agonist), significantly suppressed the expected diuresis over the following 5 h. In other words, BnorBNI seems to be acting as a kappa-receptor antagonist in this assay after s.c. injection in mice.

The aforementioned caveats notwithstanding, the key fact remains that norBNI and GNTI, widely classified as selective kappa-receptor antagonists, can markedly stimulate the overt behavior of Swiss-Webster mice. It seems that induction of excessive scratching (mood elevation?) has gone essentially unreported by the many biologists who have used norBNI and GNTI as pharmacological tools for eventual (next day?) analysis of blunted kappa receptor function. Be that as it may, a number of outstanding questions remain to be addressed by behavioral pharmacologists. Here are a few: (1) Do chemically diverse kappa antagonists, such as JDTic (37), arodyn analogs (38), and regioisomers of GNTI also precipitate frenzied scratching in mice?; (2) Since nalfurafine suppresses GNTI-induced scratching in mice, and is being developed clinically to treat uremic pruritus in dialysis patients (39), can this animal model be used to evaluate "new generation" antipruritics even though the pathophysiology of itch states is ill-defined?; and (3) If the repetitive scratching movements elicited by GNTI in mice happen to reflect responses to stimuli other than itching, does the syndrome offer an animal model of human compulsive/perseverative behavior?

Acknowledgments It is a pleasure to thank Drs. S.M. Husbands and J.W. Lewis for the sample of BnorBNI and Drs. G.B. Kehner and A.V. Rilling for their technical help.

References

1. Gutstein HB, Akil H. Opioid analgesics. In: Goodman and Gilman's The Pharmacological Basis of Therapeutics, 11th Edn., Brunton LL, Lazo JS and Parker KL (eds.), 2006, McGraw-Hill, New York, pp. 547–590.
2. Bovill JG. Opioids and NSAIDs. In: Pharmacology for Anesthesiologists, Howard FJP and Bovill JG (eds.), 2005, Taylor and Francis, London, pp. 105–123.
3. Wang J-J, Ho S-T, Tzeng J-I. Comparison of intravenous nalbuphine infusion versus naloxone in the prevention of epidural morphine-related side effects. Reg. Anesth. Pain Med. 1998;23:479–484.
4. Metze D, Reimann S, Beissert S, Luger T. Efficacy and safety of naltrexone, an oral opiate receptor antagonist, in the treatment of pruritus in internal and dermatological diseases. J. Am. Acad. Dermatol. 1999;41:533–539.
5. Jones EA, Zylicz Z. Treatment of pruritus caused by cholestasis with opioid antagonists. J. Palliat. Med. 2005;8:1290–1294.

6. Ikoma A, Steinhoff M, Ständer S, Yosipovitch G, Schmelz M. The neurobiology of itch. Nat. Rev. Neurosci. 2006;7:535–547.
7. Paus R, Schmelz M, Bíró T, Steinhoff M. Frontiers in pruritus research: scratching the brain for more effective itch therapy. J. Clin. Invest. 2006;116:1174–1185.
8. Bergasa NV, Jones EA. Pruritus complicating liver disease. In: Itch: Basic Mechanisms and Therapy, Yosipovitch G, Greaves MW, Fleischer AB and McGlone F (eds.), 2004, Marcel Dekker, New York, pp. 205–218.
9. Bergasa NV. The pruritus of cholestasis. J. Hepatol. 2005;43:1078–1088.
10. Ständer S, Schmelz M. Chronic itch and pain – similarities and differences. Eur. J. Pain. 2006;10:473–478.
11. Takemori AE, Ho BY, Naeseth JS, Portoghese PS. Nor-binaltorphimine, a highly selective kappa-opioid antagonist in analgesic and receptor binding assays. J. Pharmacol. Exp. Ther. 1988;246:255–258.
12. Jones RM, Portoghese PS. 5′-Guanidinonaltrindole, a highly selective and potent κ-opioid receptor antagonist. Eur. J. Pharmacol. 2000;396:49–52.
13. Portoghese PS. From models to molecules: opioid receptor dimers, bivalent ligands, and selective opioid receptor probes. J. Med. Chem. 2001;44:2259–2269.
14. Kamei J, Nagase H. Norbinaltorphimine, a selective κ-opioid receptor antagonist, induces an itch-associated response in mice. Eur. J. Pharmacol. 2001;418:141–145.
15. Cowan A, Murray CW. Effect of nor-binaltorphimine on the behavior of mice and rats receiving multiple injections of U-50,488. Prog. Clin. Biol. Res. 1990;328:303–306.
16. Broadbear JH, Negus SS, Butelman ER, de Costa BR, Woods JH. Differential effects of systemically administered nor-binaltorphimine (nor-BNI) on κ-opioid agonists in the mouse writhing assay. Psychopharmacology 1994;115:311–319.
17. McCurdy CR, Sufka KJ, Smith GH, Warnick JE, Nieto MJ. Antinociceptive profile of salvinorin A, a structurally unique kappa opioid receptor agonist. Pharmacol. Biochem. Behav. 2006;83:109–113.
18. Takemori AE, Schwartz MM, Portoghese PS. Suppression by nor-binaltorphimine of kappa opioid-mediated diuresis in rats. J. Pharmacol. Exp. Ther. 1988;247:971–974.
19. Ko MCH, Lee H, Song MS, Sobczyk-Kojiro K, Mosberg HI, Kishioka S, Woods JH, Naughton NN. Activation of κ-opioid receptors inhibits pruritus evoked by subcutaneous or intrathecal administration of morphine in monkeys. J. Pharmacol. Exp. Ther. 2003;305: 173–179.
20. Stevens WC, Jones RM, Subramanian G, Metzger TG, Ferguson DM, Portoghese PS. Potent and selective indolomorphinan antagonists of the kappa-opioid receptor. J. Med. Chem. 2000;43:2759–2769.
21. Jewett DC, Grace MK, Jones RM, Billington CJ, Portoghese PS, Levine AS. The kappa-opioid antagonist GNTI reduces U50,488-, DAMGO-, and deprivation-induced feeding, but not butorphanol- and neuropeptide Y-induced feeding in rats. Brain Res. 2001;909:75–80.
22. Negus SS, Mello NK, Linsenmayer DC, Jones RM, Portoghese PS. Kappa opioid antagonist effects of the novel kappa antagonist 5′-guanidinonaltrindole (GNTI) in an assay of schedule-controlled behavior in rhesus monkeys. Psychopharmacology 2002;163:412–419.
23. Obara I, Mika J, Schäfer MK-H, Przewlocka B. Antagonists of the κ-opioid receptor enhance allodynia in rats and mice after sciatic nerve ligation. Br. J. Pharmacol. 2003;140:538–546.
24. Mague SD, Pliakas AM, Todtenkopf MS, Tomasiewicz HC, Zhang Y, Stevens WC, Jones RM, Portoghese PS, Carlezon WA. Antidepressant-like effects of κ-opioid receptor antagonists in the forced swim test in rats. J. Pharmacol. Exp. Ther. 2003;305:323–330.
25. Cowan A, Inan S, Kehner GB. GNTI, a kappa receptor antagonist, causes compulsive scratching in mice. The Pharmacologist 2002;44 (Suppl. 1):A51.
26. Green AD, Young KK, Lehto SG, Smith SB, Mogil JS. Influence of genotype, dose and sex on pruritogen-induced scratching behavior in the mouse. Pain 2006;124:50–58.
27. Srivastava SK, Chauvignac C, Miller CN, Traynor JR, Husbands SM, Lewis JW. Benzylnorbinaltorphimine, a peripherally active selective κ-antagonist? Fourth Eur. Opioid Conf. (Uppsala, Sweden) 2002;P1.

28. Endoh T, Matsuura H, Tajima A, Izumimoto N, Tajima C, Suzuki T, Saitoh A, Suzuki T, Narita M, Tseng L, Nagase H. Potent antinociceptive effects of TRK-820, a novel κ-opioid receptor agonist. Life Sci. 1999;65:1685–1694.
29. Togashi Y, Umeuchi H, Okano K, Ando N, Yoshizawa Y, Honda T, Kawamura K, Endoh T, Utsumi J, Kamei J, Tanaka T, Nagase H. Antipruritic activity of the κ-opioid receptor agonist, TRK-820. Eur. J. Pharmacol. 2002;435:259–264.
30. Wakasa Y, Fujiwara A, Umeuchi H, Endoh T, Okano K, Tanaka T, Nagase H. Inhibitory effects of TRK-820 on systemic skin scratching induced by morphine in rhesus monkeys. Life Sci. 2004;75:2947–2957.
31. Umeuchi H, Togashi Y, Honda T, Nakao K, Okano K, Tanaka T, Nagase H. Involvement of central μ-opioid system in the scratching behavior in mice, and the suppression of it by the activation of κ-opioid system. Eur. J. Pharmacol. 2003;477:29–35.
32. Inan S, Cowan A. Kappa opioid agonists suppress chloroquine-induced scratching in mice. Eur. J. Pharmacol. 2004;502:233–237.
33. Wang Y, Tang K, Inan S, Siebert D, Holzgrabe U, Lee DYW, Huang P, Li J-G, Cowan A, Liu-Chen L-Y. Comparison of pharmacological activities of three distinct κ ligands (salvinorin A, TRK-820 and 3FLB) on κ opioid receptors in vitro and their antipruritic and antinociceptive activities in vivo. J. Pharmacol. Exp. Ther. 2005;312:220–230.
34. Inan S, Cowan A. Agmatine-induced stereotyped scratching in mice is antagonized by nalfurafine, a kappa opioid agonist. The Pharmacologist 2006;48:38.
35. Endoh T, Matsuura H, Tanaka C, Nagase H. Nor-binaltorphimine: a potent and selective κ-opioid receptor antagonist with long-lasting activity in vivo. Arch. Int. Pharmacodyn. 1992; 316:30–42.
36. Chauvignac C, Miller CN, Srivastava SK, Lewis JW, Husbands SM, Traynor JR. Major effect of pyrrolic *N*-benzylation in norbinaltorphimine, the selective κ-opioid receptor antagonist. J. Med. Chem. 2005;48:1676–1679.
37. Carroll I, Thomas JB, Dykstra LA, Granger AL, Allen RM, Howard JL, Pollard GT, Aceto MD, Harris LS. Pharmacological properties of JDTic: a novel κ-opioid receptor antagonist. Eur. J. Pharmacol. 2004;501:111–119.
38. Bennett MA, Murray TF, Aldrich JV. Structure-activity relationships of arodyn, a novel acetylated kappa opioid receptor antagonist. J. Peptide Res. 2005;65:322–332.
39. Wikström B, Gellert R, Ladefoged SD, Danda Y, Akai M, Ide K, Ogasawara M, Kawashima Y, Ueno K, Mori A, Ueno Y. κ-Opioid system in uremic pruritus: multicenter, randomized, double-blind, placebo-controlled clinical studies. J. Am. Soc. Nephrol. 2005;16:3742–3747.

Chapter 29
Clinical Effect of Opioid Antagonists on Clinical Pruritus

Nora V. Bergasa

Abstract Increased opioidergic tone is associated with pruritus. Evidence suggests that in cholestasis there is increased opioidergic tone. The amelioration of the pruritus of cholestasis and its behavioral manifestation, scratching activity, by opiate antagonists supports the idea that this type of neurotransmission contributes at least in part, to the pruritus experienced by patients with liver disease. Opiate antagonists have been reported to decrease pruritus associated with other conditions including malignancy and kidney disease, suggesting that increase in opioidergic tone contributes to the pathophysiology of chronic pruritus.

Keywords: Pruritus; Cholestasis; Naloxone; Naltrexone; Uremia; Scratching behavior

29.1 Introduction

Pruritus or itch is a complication of several diseases including those pertaining to the skin and some systemic, sometimes organ-specific disorders including malignancy, renal failure and liver disease. The etiology of pruritus is most conditions is unknown. In this chapter, current ideas on the pathophysiology of pruritus and the use of opiate antagonist to treat this maddening symptom as a complication of disease are discussed. Pruritus is a side effect of some medications including those with affinity for the mu opioid receptor (i.e., morphine). The use of opiate antagonists to treat this complication is not discussed in this chapter.

29.1.1 *The Sensation of Pruritus*

Pruritus or itch is defined as an unpleasant sensation that triggers the need to scratch (1). In a study of 100 patients with atopic dermatitis, a condition of unknown etiology

N.V. Bergasa
Metropolitan Hospital Center, Department of Medicine, New York, NY 10029
e-mail: bergasan2@nychhc.org

R. Dean et al. (eds.), *Opiate Receptors and Antagonists*,

characterized by chronic pruritus, the majority of the patients reported that their need to scratch ceased in association with a sensation of satisfaction and the appearance of pain (2).

29.1.2 Neurophysiology of Pruritus

The neurophysiology of pruritus and the scratch reflex is not well studied because, in part, of limited methodology. The behavior that results from pruritus, scratching, has been interpreted as a reflex aimed to protect from a potentially harmful stimulus. Stimulation of polymodal polymodal (i.e., that respond to more than one type of stimuli) nociceptors (i.e., sensory fibers that respond to nociceptive stimuli) can result in pruritus. The identification of neurons that respond to histamine alone have been defined as itch transmitting (3).

Studies that incorporated positron emission tomography (PET) (4–7) and functional magnetic resonance imagings (fMRIs) (8–11) to identify the activation of brain areas in response to pruritogenic stimuli, including histamine and allergens, have been conducted. The results from these studies may not be comparable because the experimental paradigms were not consistent among them, and the imaging techniques are not the same; however, they are a start in the exploration of brain activity in the symptom of pruritus. The administration of histamine to the skin of volunteers was associated with activation of certain brain areas that included the anterior cingular cortex, areas of the insula, and the posterior cingular cortex, which concern emotional processing, and of the basal ganglia, and supplemental and pre-motor areas, which concern the planning of movement. These data have been interpreted as a reflection of the sensory aspect of pruritus, and the expected movement that results from that sensation, scratching activity, consistent with the definition of pruritus; however, the areas of the brain that are involved in the spontaneous sensation of pruritus, such as that experienced by patients with malignancy, uremia, and cholestasis are unknown. The study of pruritus in these clinical conditions is challenged by the sophistication of the design, which should mimic the sensation of pruritus in the absence of external cutaneous stimulation.

29.1.3 Pathophysiology of Pruritus

The origin of pruritus can be peripheral, as that secondary to primary pruritic skin conditions, or central as that associated with cerebral strokes (12, 13) and multiple sclerosis (14). The neurotransmission system that has been identified to be relevant in the perception of pruritus is the endogenous opioid system. In this context, increased central opioidergic neurotransmission can be associated with pruritus, as exemplified by the effect of the central administration of morphine. Morphine is an alkaloid that binds to opioid receptors, preferentially the mu type, to exert its effect and it is widely used for the treatment of pain. The increased in opioidergic tone by the central administration of morphine is associated with pruritus in human beings (15–18). This type of pruritus can be prevented or relieved by the administration of opiate antagonists (e.g., naloxone), suggesting that it is an opioid-receptor mediated complication (19, 20).

An idea in evolution in the mechanism of chronic pruritus is central sensitization for this symptom. Allodynia is defined as a state in which a non-painful stimulus around an injured area is perceived as painful. This condition is believed to result from central sensitization to pain (21). Studies done in patients with chronic pruritus secondary to atopic dermatitis, have suggested that there is central sensitization for itch in these patients. Noxious stimuli such as heat and mechanical, electrical and chemical stimulation were perceived as itch in patients with atopic dermatitis, in contrast to the painful perception reported by the control subjects (22). In addition, the perfusion of histamine into a defined area of the skin to mimic chronic itch allowed a chemical stimulus to be perceived not only as pain, as expected, but also as itch; these results suggest that chronic pruritogenic stimuli may allow non-pruritogenic stimuli to be perceived as pruritus (22). The central sensitization for itch would result from constant pruritogenic (i.e., pruriceptive) input, which would not allow nociceptive stimuli to inhibit itch but to facilitate it. The timing of the appearance of itch in these studies is consistent with neurotransmission via C-nociceptors (22).

It is plausible that conditions characterized by chronic pruritus such as chronic renal failure and cholestasis, which are considered to result in the accumulation of some pruritogenic substances, also result in central sensitization for itch, leading to the perception of itch by non-pruritogenic stimuli that would result from the constant stimuli of C-pruriceptors by retained pruritogens. Microneurographic recordings in a patients with chronic pruritus and prurigo nodularis secondary to chronic scratching have identified spontaneously active itch fibers (23).

29.1.4 Is Central Sensitization for Itch a Common Pathway in Diseases Characterized by this Symptom

Morphine inhibits pain and induces pruritus by a central mechanism. In contrast to pain transmitting neurons, spinal neurons that transmit pruritus information to the thalamus are not spontaneously activated (24). Spontaneous activation of the pain pathway inhibits the activity of the pruritus pathway (25). It has been suggested that morphine-mediated pruritus results from the desinhibition of the pruritus pathway, associated with the inhibition of the pain pathway by that drug. In cholestasis, increased central opioidergic tone, which would be analogous to the effect of morphine, may suppress the stimulation of pain-transmitting neurons and activate the central pruritus pathway (i.e. desinhibition). In this model (26), the administration of opiate antagonists would decrease pruritus. In this context, the administration of opiate antagonists to patients with the pruritus of cholestasis is associated with amelioration of the pruritus, supporting the idea that increased opioidergic tone mediates this type of pruritus, at least in part (27–30). In addition, the accumulation of pruritogens, as it is believed to occur in cholestasis, may result in constant stimulation of C-pruriceptors and lead to central sensitization for itch. This phenomenon would allow for non-pruritogenic stimuli to be perceived as pruritogenic. This model of pruritus has two components, central and peripheral, and could represent a therapeutic possibility by changing opioidergic tone to the non-pruritic mode (i.e. central mechanism) and to increase the threshold to the perception of pruritus (i.e. peripheral mechanism).

29.2 Opioidergic Neurotransmission and Pruritus

The rationale to use opiate antagonists in the treatment of pruritus appears to have developed from the experience that morphine causes pruritus; however, reports on the use of opiate antagonists to treat pruritus have yielded equivocal results. Some of the reasons for this inconsistency may relate to the methodology used to obtain data on the effects of opiate antagonists on this symptom, and from different mechanisms of pruritus in different conditions. In this context, the use of opiate antagonists for the treatment of pruritus secondary to liver disease has been supported by a clear rationale, which concerns increased opioidergic tone in cholestasis.

29.2.1 Etiology of the Pruritus of Cholestasis

Cholestasis is defined as impaired secretion of bile (31). It is a complication of liver disease, in particular, those characterized by injury or obstruction of the intra and extrabiliary system. One of the most common symptoms of cholestasis, and perhaps the most devastating is pruritus (32). The etiology of the pruritus of cholestasis is unknown (26). It has been inferred that it results from the accumulation of substances that normally are excreted in bile and, as a result of cholestasis, accumulate in plasma and other tissues and cause pruritus. The nature of this substance(s) is unknown. In support of the idea that the pruritogen(s) is made in the liver is that in patient with chronic cholestasis, as the liver disease progresses and the liver funtion decreases, the pruritus tends to cease (33). Furthermore, patients in whom pruritus is a prominent problem or the indication for liver transplantation report disappearance of the pruritus immediately after their operation.

29.2.2 Opioidergic Neurotransmission in Cholestasis

Three lines of evidence suggest that central opioidergic tone is increased in cholestasis: (i) patients with cholestasis can experience a constellation of symptoms and signs similar to those of an opiate withdrawal reaction after the administration of opiate antagonists (28, 34). In the original report (34), this reaction included increased blood pressure, abdominal pain, tachycardia, and insomnia. This reaction stood in sharp contrast to the absence of any symptoms when the drug was given to normal volunteers at dose 60 times higher than what the patients had received, (ii) a stereospecific naloxone reversible state of antinociception (analgesic) can be displayed by rats with cholestasis secondary to bile duct resection (35); mice with cholestasis secondary to bile duct resection are also reported to exhibit a state of opioid-mediated antinociception (36, 37), and (iii) there is downregulation of mu opioid receptors in rats with cholestasis secondary to bile duct resection (38).

It is hypothesized that increased opioidergic tone in cholestasis mediates the pruritus; a central mechanism was proposed (39). In this hypothesis, the pruritus of cholestasis would be analogous to the pruritus that results from the pharmacological increase in opioidergic tone by central morphine (15–18). That the pruritus of cholestasis is mediated, at least in part, by endogenous opioids, is supported by the amelioration of the pruritus by opiate antagonists (40) (27–30, 34, 40, 41–46).

29.2.3 The Liver as a Source of Endogenous Opioids in Hepatic Disease

The reasons there is increased opioidergic tone in cholestasis is unknown; however, the serum concentration of Met-enkephalin and Leu-enkephalin, two of the endogenous opioids are reported to be higher in patients with cholestasis (34, 47). In this context, Met-enkephalin immunoreactivity is expressed by the liver of rats with cholestasis secondary to bile duct resection, and by the liver of patients with liver disease including primary biliary cirrhosis (48), and chronic hepatitis C (49). One question that arises is whether the enhanced expression of Met-enkephalin immunoreactivity (MEIR) in liver disease, is related in any way to the increased central opioidergic tone. In this context, however, some transport proteins that can transport opiates in vitro are common to the basolateral domain of the hepatocyte, to the choroid plexus, and to the blood brain barrier (50); accordingly, it is plausible that they can also transport periphery-derived opioids into the central nervous system (CNS). Furthermore, it has been reported that increased availability of opioid peptides in the periphery may facilitate their entrance into the CNS (51).

29.3 Fundamental Studies Towards Clinical Trials of Opiate Antagonists for the Treatment of the Pruritus of Cholestasis

In the landmark paper of Thornton and Losowsky it was reported that patients with pruritus (and fatigue) secondary to cholestasis developed an opiate-withdrawal like reaction after the administration of nalmefene, an opiate antagonist (34). In addition, nalmefene was associated with a relief of their pruritus, as assessed by a visual analogue scale (34). Two reports on the use of opiate antagonist for the treatment of pruritus and liver disease had been published several years prior to that publication (40, 52); however, studies on the potential role of endogenous opioids in the pruritus of cholestasis did not follow until much later (39).

The ameliorating effect of the pruritus by nalmefene was interpreted as a result of the blockade of the release of pruritogenic substances by this drug (34); however, an alternative interpretation was proposed as a hypothesis, which stated that the increase in opioidergic tone, suggested by the opiate withdrawal-like syndrome, mediated at least in part the pruritus of cholestasis, thus explaining the reported relief of the pruritus after the patients of the opiate antagonists (39). The successful testing of this hypothesis required the availability of reliable methodology for application in clinical studies of pruritus.

29.3.1 Behavioral Methodology to Study Scratching

Pruritus is defined as the need to scratch (4, 53, 54). Pruritus is a sensation, and as a sensation, it cannot be directly measured; however, the behavior that results from pruritus, scratching, can be directly measured provided there is methodology to record such behavior (39). One of the limitations in studies of pruritus had been the lack of objective data provided by clinical trials of therapeutic interventions to treat pruritus. Indeed, the need for the development of objective methodology has been recognized for many years by investigators in the field (55, 56). A specification of methodology necessary to study pruritus is that it differentiates scratching behavior from gross body movements. This challenge was met and behavioral methodology has been available for use in clinical trials for more than a decade (57).

29.3.2 Instruments to Study Scratching Behavior

In response to the need to provide behavioral methodology to include in clinical trials of pruritus, a scratching activity monitoring system was developed. The scratching activity monitoring system consists of a scratch transducer, a frequency modulate (FM) transmitter and receiver, a digital counter and a personal computer (57). The scratch transducer is a piece of piezoelectric (polyvinyldiende fluoride) film, 1 cm^2 in area, 28 μm thick and metalized on both sides with aluminum–nickel alloy, to create an electrical contact to the film. The sensor is permanently glued to a Polyform cast custom made for each patient and the cast is placed on the patient's finger (the middle finger of the dominant hand, because it was observed in pilot studies that people tend to scratch more with their dominant hand). Deflection of the film by scratching generates an electrical signal. The signal from the film is telemetered by a small battery-powered FM transmitter ($2 \times 7 \times 6$ cm) strapped to the patient's arm, to a receiver located several meters away from the patient.

A signal processor produces a signal proportional to the duration and intensity of scratching. The signal processor is a frequency counter that incorporates a threshold detector and a bandpass filter to inhibit extraneous counts not directly related to scratching from being counted. Fourier analysis of the demodulated signals revealed that frequencies associated with vibrations of the fingernail derived from the act of scratching were between 30 and 1,000 Hz. The number of times the filtered signal exceeds a fixed threshold within a 30-second interval is counted, and the count values are logged by a computer. The threshold level is adjusted such that approximately 90% of the scratching signal is captured, while the signal associated with the gentle rubbing or incidental contact of the sensor is excluded. This device allows continuous recording of scratching activity over prolonged periods of time. The counts recorded by the system correlate with independent assessments of scratching activity. The data can be plotted as average scratching activity for each successive 1-hr period as the scratching activity index or as hourly scratching activity.

Portable systems based on the principle used to develop. The scratching activity monitoring system (57) have also been developed (58, 59). Thus, the incorporation of behavioral methodology in clinical trials has been possible for several years (27–30, 60).

29.3.3 *Insight from Behavioral Studies in Pruritus*

The use of objective methodology is not intended to ignore oral reports by the subjects on the perception of their pruritus, which may provide insight into this symptom (27–30, 60), but efforts to understand the neuropsychological physiology and pathophysiology that mediates the perception of pruritus and how it translates into scratching behavior, a universal reaction to pruritus, seems necessary. In this context, important observations have been made thanks to the use of the scratching activity monitoring system . In a double-blind randomized placebo controlled study of naloxone infusion in patients with the pruritus of cholestasis, it was discovered that scratching behavior in some patients displays a 24-hour rhythm (Fig. 29.1) (29). Although the appropriate experiments to study whether this rhythm is circadian, the duration suggests that it may be, and if so, it suggests that scratching behavior may be centrally regulated, as many circadian rhythms are (29). Another observation made from a placebo-controlled trial of the drug gabapentin in patients with liver disease and pruritus has identified a new area of study that might have been completely missed if only subjective methodology had been applied (61). In this study, the administration of gabapentin was associated with an increase in hourly scratching activity; in contrast, the administration of placebo was associated with a significant decrease in scratching behavior. These results have emphasized the role of the placebo effect in studies of pruritus and have led to insights into the neurotransmission of the placebo effect (61). In addition, and relevant to this chapter, is the fact that the administration of opiate antagonists is associated with a decrease in scratching; these studies, which will be discussed in another section of this chapter, have provided, for the first time, behavioral and not anecdotal data on

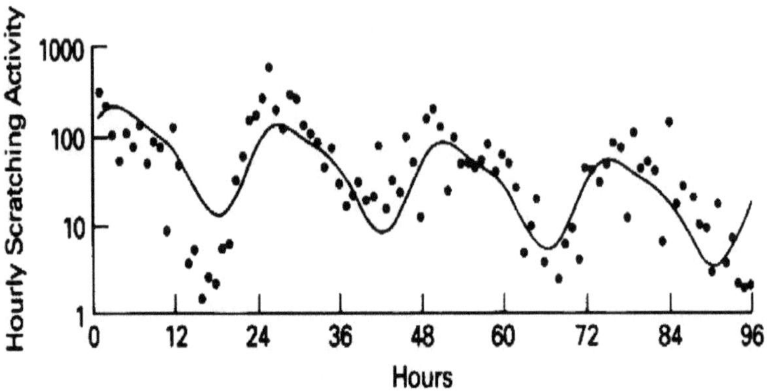

Fig. 29.1 Mean hourly scratching activity during the 96-h study period of a patient with cholestasis and pruritus. The continuous line indicates the 24-h rhythm that best fits the observations; this line has a significant downward linear trend (slope = –0.0081 ± 0.0021) ($P < 0.001$), which is consistent with the sequence of treatments (placebo, placebo, naloxone, naloxone, the latter being associated with a decrease in hourly scratching activity). Reproduced with permission from Bergasa et al. (28)

the ameliorating effect of a specific type of drugs on pruritus, and therefore have helped to identify for the first time a specific type of neurotransmission with clinical relevance to human health and disease. In the absence of the behavioral data that are now available, the ameliorating effect of opiate antagonists on the pruritus of cholestasis, may have remained ignored as it did for many years (39).

29.3.4 Behavioral Studies from Animal Models of Scratching

Studies of scratching behavior in laboratory animals have provided insight on the neurotransmission underlying scratching, which may be relevant to pruritus and scratching in human beings.

Behavioral animal studies support the existence of an opioid-mediated pathway that results in scratching behavior. The central administration of morphine and the opiate agonist ligand D-ala2-MePhe4,gly-ol5-enkephalin is associated with scratching behavior in laboratory animals (62, 63, 64). Recordings from neurons located in the superficial dorsal horn in rats identified neurons that, when exposed to low doses of morphine, facilitated neuronal response to peripheral stimuli from histamine, a substance recognized as pruritogenic in human beings, and from noxious heat (24).

Very interesting data emerging from a model of opiate-induced scratching in monkeys may provide some insight into central opioid-mediated pruritus and scratching behavior (64, 65). The scratching behavior associated with the administration of morphine into the medullary dorsal horn of monkeys was decreased by the co-administration of U50488H, a selective kappa agonist (64, 65). In addition, the administration of a kappa agonist prevented mu opioid receptor-mediated scratching in mice (66). Furthermore, in animal model of estrogen-induced cholestasis, the administration of nalfurafine, a kappa opioid receptor agonist, inhibited scratching behavior (67). Taken together, these data suggest that stimulation of the mu opioid receptor, to which morphine binds preferentially, is associated with scratching, which can be prevented or decreased by the administration of opiate antagonists (e.g. naloxone) and furthermore, they suggest that the stimulation of kappa receptor may decrease opioid-mediated scratching and pruritus in human beings.

29.4 Clinical Trials of Opiate Antagonists for the Treatment of Pruritus

29.4.1 Opiate Antagonists for the Treatment of the Pruritus of Cholestasis

The ameliorating effect of the pruritus of cholestasis by the administration of opiate antagonists including nalmefene (28, 30, 34), naloxone (27, 29, 40, 68), and naltrexone (41, 42, 44, 45) supports the hypothesis that endogenous opioids contribute to the pruritus. The administration of continuous infusions of the opiate antagonists naloxone (0.2 μg/kg/hr) preceded by 0.4 mg administered as an intravenous bolus was associated with a significant decrease in mean hourly scratching activity in two controlled clinical trials (27, 29), one of which was double-blind randomized placebo-controlled (Fig. 29.2) (27, 29). In a controlled randomized study, oral nalmefene was also associated with a significant decrease in hourly scratching activity (28, 30); this drug is not available for use at the present time. Naltrexone, another opiate antagonist with oral bioavailability has been studied in several populations of patients with liver disease and pruritus in clinical trials that used subjective methodology (41, 42, 44, 45). In these studies, naltrexone at doses of 50 mg by mouth daily was associated with a decrease in the perception of pruritus as assessed by the visual analogue scale.

An opiate withdrawal-like reaction (28, 30, 34) is a potential complication of the treatment of patients with cholestasis with opiate antagonists; accordingly, concern regarding the use of opiate antagonists in patients with cholestasis and pruritus exists. This reaction can be avoided by introducing opioid antagonism as intravenous naloxone at very low doses (e.g. 0.002 μg/kg/min) by continuous infusion, gradually increasing the dose to 0.8 μg/kg/min depending on the patients' response (69, 70) and to start oral naltrexone at the lowest possible dose (12.5 mg/day to be increased to 50–100 mg over several days, if needed). Except for the potential development of an opiate withdrawal-like syndrome, naltrexone has been well tolerated by patients with liver disease (46) and it has a good safety profile (71).

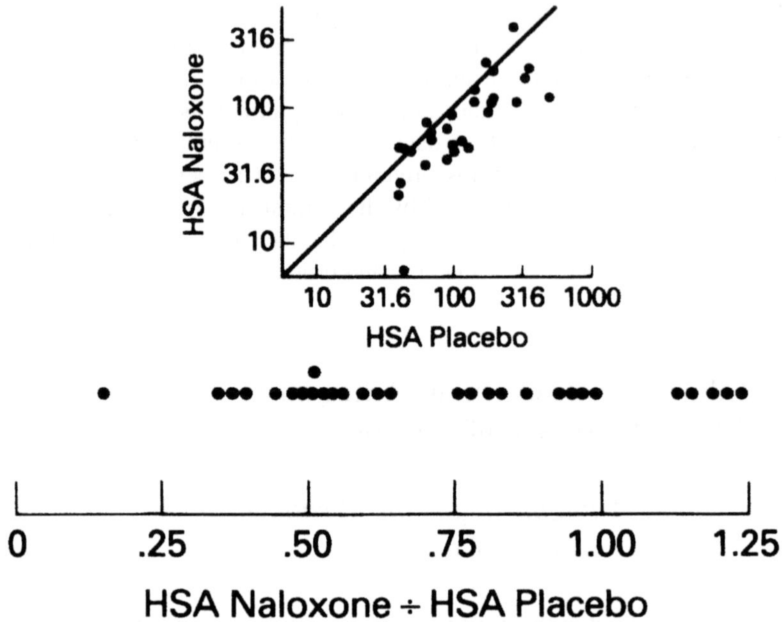

Fig. 29.2 Distribution of naloxone–placebo ratios of hourly scratching activities (*HSA*). The geometric mean HSA recorded by each patient during naloxone infusions was divided by the corresponding mean HSA during placebo infusions. Inset: mean HSA recorded during naloxone infusions plotted as a function of the mean HSA during placebo infusions. The ratio of the geometric mean HSA during naloxone infusions to that during placebo infusions was 0.727 (CI, 0.612–0.842; $P<0.001$) and was greater than 1.0 only in five patients. The therapeutic advantage of naloxone over placebo is indicated by values of the ratio below 1.0 in the horizontal plot and data points below the 45-degree line in the inset graph. Reproduced with permission from Bergasa et al. (28)

29.4.2 Opiate Antagonists for the Treatment of the Pruritus of Uremia

The rationale for the use of opiate antagonists for the treatment of pruritus secondary to uremia appears to have evolved from experiences on the use of this type of medications in other types of pruritus (72). A subsequent publication reported from group of patients on hemodialysis serum levels of Met-enkephalin equivalents were higher in patients with pruritus than in patients without pruritus (73); furthermore, the serum concentrations of Met-enkephalin equivalents were higher in the group of patients who had a partial response to the treatment with the opiate antagonists naltrexone, than in those who responded to the drug with amelioration of the pruritus. In addition, it was reported that the severity of the pruritus prior to treatment correlated with plasma concentration of Met-enkephalin equivalents. The authors proposed that endogenous opioids (e.g. Met-enkephalins) may induce basophil degranulation leading to histamine release, and that the opiate antagonist prevented the effect of enkephalins on this type of cell. This proposition has to be reconciled with the lack of effect of antihistamines in the treatment of the pruritus associated uremia (73). In the context of clinical trials of pruritus in uremia, opiate antagonists have not been consistently associated with an amelioration of the pruritus of uremia (Table 29.1), which may be related to the methodology used (i.e., subjective) and the heterogeneity of the patients studied; however, the use of a kappa opioid receptor agonist was reported to be associated with a decrease in this type of pruritus (74). These data suggest that the endogenous opioid system may be involved in the pruritus of uremia, and perhaps in other forms of systemic pruritus, in ways that go beyond traditional opiate antagonist drugs.

29.4.3 Opiate Antagonists for the Treatment of the Pruritus of Skin Diseases

Pruritus is the most common symptom in patients with skin diseases. A role of the endogenous opioid system in the mediation of the pruritus secondary to skin diseases has also been considered; however, there are few published clinical trials on the use of opiate antagonists for these conditions (Table 29.2) (75, 76). Recently, the use of topical 1% naltrexone cream was studied to treat pruritus. In the open label study reported in the publication and which included twelve patients with pruritus secondary to skin disease, the cream was associated with a decrease in this symptom (76). In addition, the administration of naltrexone cream was associated with an increase in the expression of mu opioid receptor in the epidermis (76), which correlated with the ameliorating effect of the cream In the placebo-controlled trial 40 patients with pruritus were studied but the causes of the pruritus were not provided. It is important to note, nevertheless, that it is reported that the relief of the pruritus associated with topical naloxone required a median of 46 min to be experienced; however, the placebo cream was not without an effect, although the placebo-associated relief took a median of 74 min to be experienced. It is this strong placebo effect that concerns investigators in clinical trials of pruritus. Accordingly, it is emphasized that the use of behavioral methodology, which is already available, in studies of pruritus should be considered at the time of study design. Furthermore, the placebo effect itself may reveal important pathophysiological mechanism on the neurotransmission of pruritus.

29.5 Summary

Clinical observations in human beings, behavioral studies in animals, and data from basic neurophysiology experiments support an association between opioid receptors and pruritus.

Table 29.1 Clinical trials of opiate antagonists for the treatment of the pruritus of uremia in patients on hemodialysis or peritoneal dialysis

Study design	Duration	No. of patients	Medication/dose/route	Methods	Results	Reference
Multicenter randomized double-blind placebo-controlled cross-over with 7 day wash-out period between treatments	7 days	15	NTX/50 mg per day/orally	VAS	Decrease in VAS by 79% in the NTX–P sequence and by 90% in the P–NTX sequence	(78)
Randomized double-blind placebo-controlled cross over with 7 day wash-out period between treatment	4 weeks	23	NTX/50 mg per day/orally	VAS and pruritus score	No significant change in VAS or pruritus score	(79)
Multicenter, randomized comparison between two drugs	2 weeks	52 $n = 26$ NTX $n = 26$ loratadine	NTX/50 mg per day/orally	VAS	No significant change in the mean VAS on either treatment	(80)

VAS visual analogue scale, *NTX* naltrexone, *P* placebo

Table 29.2 Clinical trials of opiate antagonists for pruritus in which patients with skin diseases were included

Study design	Duration	No. of patients with skin conditions[a]	Medication/dose/ route	Methods	Results	Reference
Open label	2 to 48 weeks	18 mixed causes	NTX/50 mg/orally (2 patients with PN required 100 mg per day orally)	VAS	Mixed causes group: in four patients the VAS decreased by 100%, in seven by a range from 20% to 80%, and in 7 there was no change	(75)**
		17 PN			PN group: in 8 patients the VAS decreased by 100%; in 7 by a range from 10% to 80%, and in 4, there was no change	
Study1: multicenter open label	15 days	14	1% naloxone cream to areas of pruritus twice a day		Relief of pruritus within 15 min of application lasting about 4 hours and decrease in the VAS at days 8 and 15	(76)**

Number of patients*:
Reference 75: 18 of 50 patients had pruritus secondary to various skin conditions and seventeen had prurigo nodularis.
Reference 76: 12 patients had pruritus secondary to skin disease. Forty patients were included in a controlled study reported in the same publication but the causes of pruritus were not listed. In this study (Study I), naloxone cream had a therapeutic advantage over the placebo.
VAS visual analogue scale, *NTX* naltrexone, *PN* prurigo nodularis

One of the behavioral manifestations associated with nalmefene in patients with cholestasis was an opiate withdrawal-like reaction. This reaction was interpreted as evidence for increased opioidergic tone in cholestasis, and it is an example on how a change in behavior contributed to the scientific exploration of the opioid system in the pruritus of cholestasis; however, there were concerns regarding the methodology in the study of pruritus existed (56, 57). The need to develop methodology that delivered objective has been met. Accordingly, the stage is set for further studies on the pathophysiology of pruritus, a maddening complication of disease, which continues to escape understanding and for which effective treatment is desperately needed.

References

1. Greaves MW, Wall PD: Pathophysiology of itching. Lancet 1996; 348(9032): 938–40.
2. Aoki T: Pleasure of "scratch" is a complex sensation of itch and pain. Second International Workshop for hte Study of Itch, Toyama, 2003.
3. Schmelz M, Schmidt R, Bickel A, Handwerker HO, Torebjörk HE: Specific c-receptrs for Itch in Human Skin. J Neurosci 1997; 17: 8003–8008.
4. Hsieh JC, Hagermark O, Stahle-Backdahl M, et al.: Urge to scratch represented in the human cerebral cortex during itch. J Neurophysiol 1994; 72(6): 3004–8.
5. Mochizuki H, Tashiro M, Kano M, Sakurada Y, Itoh M, Yanai K: Imaging of central itch modulation in the human brain using positron emission tomography. Pain 2003; 105(1–2): 339–46.
6. Drzezga A, Darsow U, Treede RD, et al.: Central activation by histamine-induced itch: analogies to pain processing: a correlational analysis of O-15 H2O positron emission tomography studies. Pain 2001; 92(1–2): 295–305.
7. Darsow U, Drzezga A, Frisch M, et al.: Processing of histamine-induced itch in the human cerebral cortex: a correlation analysis with dermal reactions. J Invest Dermatol 2000; 115: 1029–1033.
8. Walter B, Sadlo MN, Kupfer J, et al.: Brain activation by histamine prick test-induced itch. J Invest Dermatol 2005; 125(2): 380–2.
9. Leknes SG, Bantick S, Willis CM, Wilkinson JD, Wise RG, Tracey I: Itch and motivation to scratch: an investigation of the central and peripheral correlates of allergen- and histamine-induced itch in humans. J Neurophysiol 2007; 97(1): 415–22.
10. Mochizuki H, Sadato N, Saito DN, et al.: Neural correlates of perceptual difference between itching and pain: a human fMRI study. Neuroimage 2007; 36(3): 706–17.
11. Valet M, Pfab F, Sprenger T, et al.: Cerebral processing of histamine-induced itch using short-term alternating temperature modulation--an FMRI study. J Invest Dermatol 2008; 128(2): 426–433.
12. Massey E: Unilateral neurogenic pruritus following stroke. Stroke 1984; 15: 901–3.
13. Shapiro P, Braun C: Unilateral pruritus after a stroke. Arch Dermatol 1987; 123: 1521–530.
14. Osterman P: Paroxysmal itching in multiple sclerosis. Br J Dermatol 1976; 95: 555–8.
15. Ballantyne JC, Loach AB, Carr DB: Itching after epidural and spinal opiates. Pain 1988; 33(2): 149–60.
16. Ballantyne JC, Loach AB, Carr DB: The incidence of pruritus after epidural morphine. Anaesthesia 1989; 44(10): 863.
17. Finley RS: Pain management with spinally administered opioids. American Journal of Hospital Pharmacy 1990.
18. Ruan X: Drug-related side effects of long-term intrathecal morphine therapy. Pain Physician 2007; 10(2): 357–66.

19. Dailey PA, Brookshire GL, Shnider SM, et al.: The effects of naloxone associated with the intrathecal use of morphine in labor. Anesth Analg 1985; 64(7): 658–66.
20. Abbound TK, Lee K, Zhu J, et al.: Prophylactic oral naltrexone with intrathecal morphine for cesarean section: effects on adverse reactions and analgesia. Anesth Analg 1990; 71(4): 367–70.
21. LaMotte RH: Subpopulations of "Nocifensor Neurons" Contributing to Pain and Allodynia, Itch and Alloknesis. Am Pain Soc J 1992; 1: 115–26.
22. Ikoma A, Fartasch M, Heyer G, Miyachi Y, Handwerker H, Schmelz M: Painful stimuli evoke itch in patients with chronic pruritus: central sensitization for itch. Neurology 2004; 62(2): 212–7.
23. Schmelz M, Hilliges M, Schmidt R, et al.: Active "itch fibers" in chronic pruritus. Neurology 2003; 61(4): 564–6.
24. Andrew D, Craig AD: Spinothalamic lamina I neurons selectively sensitive to histamine: a central neural pathway for itch. Nat Neurosci 2001; 4(1): 72–7.
25. Ikoma A, Rukwied R, Stander S, Steinhoff M, Miyachi Y, Schmelz M: Neurophysiology of pruritus: interaction of itch and pain. Arch Dermatol 2003; 139(11): 1475–8.
26. Bergasa NV: The pruritus of cholestasis. J Hepatol 2005; 43(6): 1078–88.
27. Bergasa NV, Talbot TL, Alling DW, et al.: A controlled trial of naloxone infusions for the pruritus of chronic cholestasis. Gastroenterology 1992; 102(2): 544–9.
28. Bergasa NV, Talbot TL, Schmitt JP, et al.: Open label trial of oral nalmefene therapy for the pruritus of cholestasis. Hepatology 1998; 27: 679–84.
29. Bergasa NV, Alling DW, Talbot TL, et al.: Naloxone ameliorates the pruritus of cholestasis: results of a double-blind randomized placebo-controlled trial. Annals of Internal Medicine 1995; 123(3): 161–167.
30. Bergasa NV, Alling DW, Talbot TL, Wells M, Jones EA: Oral nalmefene therapy reduces scratching activity due to the pruritus of cholestasis: a controlled study. Journal of the American Academy of Dermatology 1999; 41(3): 431–34.
31. Reichen J, Simon F: Cholestasis. In: Arias IM JW, Popper H, Schachter D, Schafritz DA, ed. The liver: Biology and pathobilogy, Second ed. New York: Raven Press, 1988; 1105–1124.
32. Sherlock S, Dooley J: Primary Biliary Cirrhosis. Diseases of the Liver and Biliary System. London: Blackwell, 1991; 236–248.
33. Lloyd-Thomas HG, Sherlock S: Testosterone therapy for the pruritus of obstructive jaundice. Br Med J 1952; 2(4797): 1289–91.
34. Thornton JR, Losowsky MS: Opioid peptides and primary biliary cirrhosis. British Medical Journal 1988; 297(6662): 1501–4.
35. Bergasa NV, Alling DW, Vergalla J, Jones EA: Cholestasis in the male rat is associated with naloxone-reversible antinociception. Journal of Hepatology 1994; 20: 85–90.
36. Dehpour AR, Akbarloo N, Ghafourifar P: Endogenous nitric oxide modulates naloxone-precipitated withdrawal signs in a mouse model with acute cholestasis. Behav Pharmacol 1998; 9(1): 77–80.
37. Ghafourifar P, Dehpour AR, Akbarloo N: Inhibition by L-NA, a nitric oxide synthase inhibitor, of naloxone- precipitated withdrawal signs in a mouse model of cholestasis. Life Sci 1997; 60(19): 265–70.
38. Bergasa NV, Rothman RB, Vergalla J, Xu H, Swain MG, Jones EA: Central mu-opioid receptors are down-regulated in a rat model of cholestasis. Journal of Hepatology 1992; 15(1–2): 220–4.
39. Jones EA, Bergasa NV: The pruritus of cholestasis: from bile acids to opiate agonists. Hepatology 1990; 11(5): 884–7.
40. Bernstein JE, Swift R: Relief of intractable pruritus with naloxone. Archives of Dermatology 1979; 115: 1366–67.
41. Carson KL, Tran TT, Cotton P, Sharara AI, Hunt CM: Pilot study of the use of naltrexone to treat the severe pruritus of cholestatic liver disease. American Journal of Gastroenterology 1996; 91: 1022–3.

42. Wolfhagen FHJ, Sternieri E, Hop WCJ, Vitale G, Bertolotti M, van Buuren HR: Oral naltrexone treatment for cholestatic pruritus: a double-blind, placebo-controlled study. Gastroenterology 1997; 113(4): 1264–69.
43. Neuberger J, Jones EA: Liver transplantation for intractable pruritus is contraindicated before an adequate trial of opiate antagonist therapy. Eur J Gastroenterol Hepatol 2001; 13(11): 1393–4.
44. Terg R, Coronel E, Sorda J, Munoz AE, Findor J: Efficacy and safety of oral naltrexone treatment for pruritus of cholestasis, a crossover, double blind, placebo-controlled study. J Hepatol 2002; 37(6): 717–22.
45. Mansour-Ghanaei F, Taheri A, Froutan H, et al.: Effect of oral naltrexone on pruritus in cholestatic patients. World J Gastroenterol 2006; 12(7): 1125–8.
46. Tandon P, Rowe BH, Vandermeer B, Bain VG: The efficacy and safety of bile Acid binding agents, opioid antagonists, or rifampin in the treatment of cholestasis-associated pruritus. Am J Gastroenterol 2007; 102(7): 1528–36.
47. Spivey J, Jorgensen R, Gores G, Lindor K: Methionine-enkephalin concentrations correlate with stage of disease but not pruritus in patients with primary biliary cirrhosis. American Journal of Gastroenterology 1994; 89(11): 2018–2032.
48. Bergasa NV, Liau S, Homel P, Ghali V: Hepatic Met-enkephalin immunoreactivity is enhanced in primary biliary cirrhosis. Liver 2002; 22(2): 107–13.
49. Boyella VD, Nicastri AD, Bergasa NV: Human hepatic met-enkephalin and delta opioid receptor-1 immunoreactivities in viral and autoimmune hepatitis. Ann Hepatol 2008; 7(3): 221–6.
50. Dagenais C, Ducharme J, Pollack GM: Uptake and efflux of the peptidic delta-opioid receptor agonist. Neurosci Lett 2001; 301(3): 155–8.
51. Banks WA, Kastin AJ: Peptide transport systems for opiates across the blood-brain barrier. Am J Physiol 1990; 259(1 Pt 1): E1–10.
52. Summerfield J: Naloxone modulates the perception of itch in man. Br J Clin Pharmacol 1980; 10: 180–182.
53. Wall PD, Melzack R: Textbook of pain. 3rd ed. Edinburgh: Curchill Lingstone, 1995.
54. Greaves MW, Wall PD: Pathophysiology of itching. The Lancet 1996; 348(9041): 938–940.
55. Savin J, Paterson W, Oswald I: Scratching during sleep. Lancet 1973; ii: 296–297.
56. Savin J, Paterson W, Oswald I, Adam K: Further studies of scratching during sleep. Br J Dermatol 1975; 93: 297–302.
57. Talbot TL, Schmitt JM, Bergasa NV, Jones EA, Walker EC: Application of piezo film technology for the quantitative assessment of pruritus. Biomedical Instrumentation and Technology 1991; 25(5): 400–3.
58. Stein H, Bijak M, Heerd E, et al.: [Pruritometer 1: Portable measuring system for quantifying scratching as an objective measure of cholestatic pruritus]. Biomed Tech (Berl) 1996; 41(9): 248–52.
59. Bijak M, Mayr W, Rafolt D, Tanew A, Unger E: Pruritometer 2: portable recording system for the quantification of scratching as objective criterion for the pruritus. Biomed Tech (Berl) 2001; 46(5): 137–41.
60. O'Donohue JW, Haigh C, Williams R: Ondansetron in the treatment of the pruritus of cholestasis: a randomised controlled trial. Gastroenterology 1997; 112: A 1349.
61. Bergasa NV, McGee M, Ginsburg IH, Engler D: Gabapentin in patients with the pruritus of cholestasis: a double-blind, randomized, placebo-controlled trial. Hepatology 2006; 44: 1317–1323.
62. Thomas DA, Williams GM, Iwata K, Kenshalo DJ, Dubner R: Effects of central administration of opioids on facial scratching in monkeys. Brain Research 1992; 585(1–2): 315–7.
63. Thomas DA, Hammond DL: Microinjection of morphine into the rat medullary dorsal horn produces a dose-dependent increase in facial scratching. Brain Research 1995; 695(2): 267–70.
64. Ko MC, Song MS, Edwards T, Lee H, Naughton NN: The role of central mu opioid receptors in opioid-induced itch in primates. J Pharmacol Exp Ther 2004; 310(1): 169–76.

65. Ko MC, Lee H, Song MS, et al.: Activation of kappa-opioid receptors inhibits pruritus evoked by subcutaneous or intrathecal administration of morphine in monkeys. J Pharmacol Exp Ther 2003; 305(1): 173–9.
66. Togashi Y, Umeuchi H, Okano K, et al.: Antipruritic activity of the kappa-opioid receptor agonist, TRK-820. Eur J Pharmacol 2002; 435(2–3): 259–64.
67. Inan S, Cowan A: Nalfurafine, a kappa opioid receptor agonist, inhibits scratching behavior secondary to cholestasis induced by chronic ethynylestradiol injections in rats. Pharmacol Biochem Behav 2006; 85(1): 39–43.
68. Ilagan MB, Garcia L, Rothstein K, Manzarbeitia C, MuÒoz S: Naloxone infusions for management of intractable pruritus in cholestatic liver transplant candidates. Hepatology 1996; 24: 696.
69. Jones EA, Dekker LR: Florid opioid withdrawal-like reaction precipitated by naltrexone in a patient with chronic cholestasis. Gastroenterology 2000; 118(2): 431–2.
70. Jones EA: Trials of opiate antagonists for the pruritus of cholestasis: primary efficacy endpoints and opioid withdrawal-like reactions. J Hepatol 2002; 37(6): 863–5.
71. Krystal JH, Cramer JA, Krol WF, Kirk GF, Rosenheck Ra: Naltrexone in the treatment of alcohol dependence. New England Journal of Medicine 2001; 345: 1734–1739.
72. Andersen LW, Friedberg M, Lokkegaard N: Naloxone in the treatment of uremic pruritus: a case history. Clin Nephrol 1984; 21(6): 355–6.
73. Odou P, Azar R, Luyckx M, Brunet C, Dine T: A hypothesis for endogenous opioid peptides in uraemic pruritus: role of enkephalin. Nephrol Dial Transplant 2001; 16(9): 1953–4.
74. Wikstrom B, Gellert R, Ladefoged SD, et al.: Kappa-opioid system in uremic pruritus: multicenter, randomized, double-blind, placebo-controlled clinical studies. J Am Soc Nephrol 16, 3742-7. 2005; 16: 3742–47.
75. Metze D, Reimann S, Luger TA: Effective treatment of pruritus with naltrexone, an orally active opiate antagonist. Ann N Y Acad Sci 1999; 885: 430–2.
76. Bigliardi PL, Stammer H, Jost G, Rufli T, Buchner S, Bigliardi-Qi M: Treatment of pruritus with topically applied opiate receptor antagonist. J Am Acad Dermatol 2007; 56(6): 979–88.

[illegible]

Chapter 30
Effects of Opioid Antagonists on L-DOPA-Induced Dyskinesia in Parkinson's Disease

Susan H. Fox, Tom H. Johnston, and Jonathan M. Brotchie

Abstract Long-term treatment of Parkinson's disease with the dopamine precursor 3,4-dihydroxyphenylalanine (L-DOPA) is compromised by the development of motor complications, including involuntary movements termed dyskinesia. The neural mechanisms underlying L-DOPA-induced dyskinesia (LID) involve altered activity of GABAergic striatal output pathways resulting, directly and indirectly, in underactivity of the output regions of the basal ganglia. These GABAergic striatal efferents employ, as co-neurotransmitters, a variety of opioids produced from the large molecular weight opioid precursors pre-proenkephalin-A and -B (PPE-A and PPE-B).

Preclinical studies in the 6-hydroxydopamine (6-OHDA)-lesioned rat and 1-methyl-4-phenyl-1,2,3,6-tetrahydropyridine-lesioned primate models of parkinsonism have consistently demonstrated increased striatal expression of PPE-A and PPE-B in models of dyskinesia compared with the non-dyskinetic state. These, and data from studies in humans, suggest that enhanced opioid peptide transmission is associated with the expression of LID. Behavioural studies using non-selective and subtype-selective opioid receptor antagonists in animal models have shown conflicting results but suggest that, under certain circumstances, opioid antagonists are able to alleviate LID. On balance, studies in PD patients suggest that non-subtype-selective opioid receptor antagonists will not significantly reduce LID. Recent data suggest that the μ-subtype opioid receptor may be the most promising target for novel therapeutics to suppress the expression of LID in patients, though, to date, subtype-selective opioid receptor antagonists have not been assessed in the clinic.

Keywords: Parkinson's disease; Opioid antagonists; Dyskinesia; Clinical trial; MPTP-primate; 6-Hydroxydopamine-lesioned rat

---

S.H. Fox (✉), T.H. Johnston, and J.M. Brotchie
Division of Neurology, Movement Disorders Clinic MCL7-421,
Toronto Western Hospital, 399, Toronto, Ontario, Canada, M5V 2S8
e-mail: sfox@uhnresearch.ca

R. Dean et al. (eds.), *Opiate Receptors and Antagonists*,

30.1 Introduction

30.1.1 L-DOPA-Induced Dyskinesia

Parkinson's disease (PD) is a common neurodegenerative disorder characterized by slowness of movement, bradykinesia, as well as rigidity, rest tremor, and postural instability (1). The cause of PD is unknown but the diagnostic pathological changes include a progressive loss of midbrain dopaminergic neurons. The mainstay of symptomatic therapy for PD is dopamine replacement in the form of the dopamine precursor 3,4-dihydroxyphenylalanine (L-DOPA). L-DOPA can provide adequate control of parkinsonian symptoms for several years. However, with time, complications in response to L-DOPA emerge which can significantly compromise the therapeutic benefits of such therapy. In particular, prolonged L-DOPA therapy is associated with reduced, and increasingly unpredictable, efficacy, termed 'wearing off' and 'on–off' motor fluctuations and, with the appearance of involuntary movements, L-DOPA-induced dyskinesia (LID) (2, 3). LID can occur at variable times in response to L-DOPA. Thus, LID most commonly occurs at the peak dose of L-DOPA action ('peak-dose dyskinesia'), and consists of choreiform and dystonic movements in the limbs and neck (4). Less common is LID occurring at the beginning and end of dose, when the levels of L-DOPA are rising and falling, respectively, known as 'diphasic dyskinesia' (5).

In recent years, significant progress has been made in defining the neural mechanisms by which L-DOPA elicits dyskinesia once it has been established (in general, studies relate to peak-dose dyskinesia). The principal abnormalities responsible for this expression of peak-dose dyskinesia are changes in the patterning and a net underactivity of basal ganglia outputs, that is, the internal globus pallidus (GPi) and substantia nigra pars reticulata (SNr) with subsequent overactivity of thalamocortical pathways (6–9). Underactivity of GPi/SNr may be secondary to increased inhibition from the 'direct' GABAergic striatal output pathway that projects from the striatum to the GPi/SNr (7, 10–12). Other basal ganglia pathways are probably also involved; thus, underactivity of projections from the striatum involved in the 'indirect' pathway with subsequent overactivity of the external globus pallidus (GPe) and underactivity of subthalamic nucleus have been suggested to play a role in the pathophysiology of LID and other forms of dyskinesia (7, 10, 13).

30.2 Enhanced Opioid Neurotransmission is Associated with L-DOPA-Induced Dyskinesia

The neural mechanisms responsible for altering the activity of basal ganglia pathways in LID involve changes in both dopaminergic and non-dopaminergic neurotransmitters systems (14). In particular, opioid peptides are found within the basal ganglia and there is a body of evidence to suggest that enhanced transmission by opioid peptides in striatal output pathways may underlie the pathophysiology of LID.

The GABAergic striatal projection neurons are classically considered to be broadly segregated with respect to the opioid peptides they use as co-transmitters. Thus, the GABAergic striatopallidal projection neurons of the direct pathway express opioids derived from the precursor pre-proenkephalin-B (PPE-B; including several dynorphins, leu- and met-enkephalin, and α-neoendorphin), while the striatopallidal neurons of the indirect pathway express leu- and met-enkephalins derived from pre-proenkephalin-A (PPE-A) (15–22).

30.2.1 PPE-B Expression

In animal models of untreated parkinsonism, PPE-B mRNA and dynorphin peptide levels are reduced within the striatum (23–28). In the 6-hydroxydopamine (6-OHDA)-lesioned rat model of parkinsonism, following long-term L-DOPA treatment and the development of L-DOPA-induced motor complications, there is a marked up regulation of both PPE-B expression and dynorphin peptide levels in the striatum (24, 25, 29–33). Conversely, in animals treated with the dopaminergic drugs, lisuride, bromocriptine, and ropinirole, agents that induce less LID than L-DOPA in the clinic when given as monotherapy, there is no significant increase in PPE-B expression (32, 34, 35). In addition, in the 1-methyl-4-phenyl-1,2,3,6-tetrahydropyridine (MPTP) non-human primate model of parkinsonism, striatal PPE-B mRNA expression is significantly increased by 185% in the MPTP-lesioned macaque exhibiting LID, compared with parkinsonian, non-dyskinetic MPTP-lesioned macaques (36). In human PD, studied in brains postmortem, no change has been demonstrated in striatal dynorphin levels (37, 38); however, striatal PPE-B mRNA expression is significantly increased by 172% in dyskinetic PD patients compared to age-matched controls (36). Thus, in established, stable LID, there is enhanced PPE-B expression in the striatum.

In addition, striatal PPE-B expression has been shown to progressively increase over time and follow the time course of development of LID in 6-OHDA-lesioned rat, suggesting that elevated PPE-B is associated not only with the expression of LID, once established, but also with the development of LID over time, 'priming' (30).

30.2.2 PPE-A Expression

In rat and non-human primate animal models of untreated parkinsonism, there is a consistent finding of a significant increase in PPE-A in striatal neurons projecting the GPe (25, 29, 39–42). Following long-term L-DOPA therapy and the development of

LID, the most consistent findings have been a lack of normalization and even further elevation in levels of PPE-A. For instance, in 6-OHDA-lesioned rat after long-term L-DOPA and associated LID, there is a further significant increase in PPE-A levels in the striatum compared to parkinsonism (32, 43). Similar findings have been reported in the MPTP-lesioned primate (44–47) and marmosets with a unilateral 6-OHDA lesion (48). However, other studies have shown no significant change in PPE-A mRNA levels following long-term L-DOPA-treatment in MPTP monkeys with LID compared with non-dyskinetic (40, 49). In normal primates given very high doses of L-DOPA which lead to subsequent development of LID, a significant increase in PPE-A expression has been demonstrated (50). Postmortem studies from patients with PD who had received long-term L-DOPA use have also demonstrated increased striatal PPE-A compared to age-matched controls, but there was no specific correlation to the presence of LID (51, 52). The association of elevated, compared to normal, PPE-A with the behavioural expression of LID is further demonstrated by the finding that agents that do not induce dyskinesia significantly reduce PPE-A caused by dopamine depletion. Thus, in 6-OHDA-lesioned rats, where repeated treatment with bromocriptine results in less dyskinesia than L-DOPA, there was a significant reduction in levels of PPE-A compared with L-DOPA-treated animals (34). Similarly, in the MPTP-lesioned marmoset, chronic treatment with cabergoline, bromocriptine, and ropinirole caused no or minimal dyskinesia and reversed the increase in PPE-A induced by dopamine depletion (44, 49). Furthermore, in animal models, co-treatment with L-DOPA and glutamate receptor antagonists that are known to reduce LID, including the AMPA-receptor antagonist LY293558 and the NMDA antagonist CI-1041, also normalize PPE-A expression (46, 47).

Thus, the evidence from animal models of LID as well as human postmortem studies suggest that enhanced expression of PPE-A and PPE-B is associated with the expression and possibly the development of LID in PD. In humans, further evidence of this association comes from positron emission tomography studies that have shown significantly reduced striatal and thalamic [^{11}C]diprenorphine binding in dyskinetic, but not in non-dyskinetic, PD patients, suggesting enhanced opioid transmission in PD patients with LID (53). These findings suggest that increased opioid neuropeptides accompany and thus may be involved in the pathophysiology of LID. However, these data can be interpreted in many ways. Enhanced opioid transmission may be:

1. responsible for, or at least contribute to, the expression of LID once it has been established,
2. necessary for the processes by which LID develops, that is how the brain becomes primed by repeated dopaminergic stimulation to express dyskinesia when challenged by subsequent dopaminergic drugs, and
3. a response to the expression of LID.

The relative importance of each of these mechanisms as they relate to the products of PPE-A and PPE-B is still being defined. However, most progress has been made in defining the situation in which opioid transmission might, or might not, contribute to the expression of LID once it has been established.

30.3 A Role for Opioid Transmission in the Expression of Established LID

The potential mechanisms whereby enhanced opioid peptides might contribute to the expression of LID relate predominantly to the role that opioid peptides play as modulators of dopamine, GABA, and glutamate neurotransmission in the basal ganglia. Both PPE-A and PPE-B can be processed to produce a range of peptides having different activities at μ-, δ-, and κ-opioid receptors. These peptides can be transported and released not only at the site of the synthesis, the striatum, but also at the regions receiving inputs from the striatum (54, 55). Possible mechanisms that have been proposed to underlie LID include:

1. enhanced enkephalin release in the GPe that may reduce GABA release via activation of δ-opioid receptors and
2. opioids released from the terminals of the direct pathway that may activate κ- or μ-opioid receptor to decrease glutamate or increase GABA release, respectively.

All these actions would be expected to reduce firing in the output regions of the basal ganglia and so result in dyskinesia. On the other hand, some actions of opioids within the basal ganglia, for example, κ-opioid stimulation reducing striatal glutamate release (56), might be expected to reduce LID.

To date, it has not been clear how PPE-A and PPE-B are processed in parkinsonism or LID and whether the relative synthesis of one particular product, over another, changes in these disease conditions. Furthermore, it is not clear whether active peptides generated by a precursor synthesized in the striatum are differentially trafficked to the target regions of the direct and indirect pathway. Additionally, opioid peptides other than those synthesized from PPE-A and PPE-B, including endomorphin-1 and β-endorphin, are present within the basal ganglia circuitry; the role of these in LID is unknown. Using high-performance liquid chromatography coupled with radioimmunoassay to assess the levels of opioid peptides throughout the basal ganglia in macaques, we have shown that α-neoendorphin levels are selectively elevated by 43% and 60% in GPi and SN, respectively, of MPTP-lesioned macaques with LID compared with non-dyskinetic (57). Activation of μ- and δ-opioid receptors by enhanced α-neoendorphin release in these regions may contribute to the pathophysiology of LID.

Further evidence for a role of μ-opioid receptors in LID comes from a recent finding that μ-opioid receptor-mediated G-protein activation is significantly enhanced in the basal ganglia and cortex of L-DOPA-treated dyskinetic monkeys, whereas δ- and κ-receptor-induced increases are limited to only a few regions (58). In addition, an association has been reported between PD patients who develop early-onset LID and the presence of the A118G single-nucleotide polymorphism (SNP) in the μ-opioid receptor (59). This SNP is carried by 20% of the Caucasian population and increases binding affinity and potency of β-endorphin (60).

30.4 Preclinical Studies Using Opioid Receptor Antagonists to Suppress the Expression of L-DOPA-Induced Dyskinesia in Animal Models of PD

Several studies have been performed to test the hypothesis that the enhanced opioid transmission underlies the expression of peak-dose LID. Studies in the long-term, L-DOPA-treated 6-OHDA-lesioned rat have shown that non-subtype-selective opioid receptor antagonists, naloxone and naltrindole, significantly reduce L-DOPA-induced rotations (an action which can be equated with an anti-dyskinetic effect) (34, 61). In addition, δ- and κ-subtype-selective opioid receptor antagonists, naltrindole and norbinaltorphimine (*nor*-BNI), respectively, but not the μ-opioid receptor antagonist, cyprodime, significantly reduced behaviours equivalent to LID in rats (34). The effect of *nor*-BNI in rats is probably mediated via antagonism of κ-receptors in the output regions of the basal ganglia as infusion of *nor*-BNI into the SNr-reduced LID-related behaviours in 6-OHDA-lesioned rat (62).

Studies in MPTP-lesioned primates with LID have produced data that contradict each other as well as the studies in rats. The non-subtype-selective opioid receptor antagonists, naloxone and naltrexone, have been shown either to have no effect in macaques (63) or significantly reduce, in marmosets, LID, without affecting parkinsonian disability (64, 65). More recently, using similar doses of naloxone and naltrexone, an exacerbation of LID was noted in macaques (66). The difference in findings may relate to different species of primate used, differences in dose of L-DOPA used to induce dyskinesia or other aspects of the details of experimental design such as time since induction of dyskinesia, or each animal's treatment history. To date, there has only been one study using subtype-selective opioid receptor antagonists in non-human primates. This study showed that μ- and δ-subtype-selective opioid receptor antagonists, but not κ-antagonists, significantly reduced the expression of LID in the MPTP-lesioned marmoset, without affecting parkinsonism (64).

Preclinical studies on the involvement of opioid transmission in the expression of LID once established can be summarized in the following ways:

1. It is clear that in rodent and primate models of LID, enhanced opioid transmission can under some, though not all, circumstances contribute to the expression of LID.
2. It is likely that the relative contribution of different opioids to LID is complex and that while some opioids may contribute to the expression of LID, others might have no role or even act to suppress the expression of LID.
3. It may be necessary to selectively target individual opioid receptor systems to deliver effects to suppress the expression of LID.
4. The relative involvement of subtypes of opioid receptors is likely to be different in rodents versus primate species.
5. Studies in primates suggest that the μ-opioid receptor is likely the subtype most critically involved in the expression of LID.

30.5 Clinical Studies of Potential of Opioid Receptor Antagonists to Reduce Expression of LID in PD Patients

Early, small-scale reports suggested an anti-dyskinetic action of naloxone in PD. Thus, in two PD patients with bothersome LID, acute treatment with iv naloxone (2.4 mg) reduced symptoms without affecting parkinsonian symptoms (67). In six PD patients with on–off fluctuations, naloxone (8 mg) resulted in an increase in the percentage on time by 44% and reduction in LID compared to saline (68). Neither of the above-mentioned studies were double-blind. Double-blind, randomized placebo-controlled clinical trials using the longer acting, orally active non-subtype-selective opioid antagonist, naltrexone, have also been performed. Low-dose oral naltrexone (~1 mg/kg) failed to show any effect on LID (69), whereas a higher dose of naltrexone (5 mg/kg) had a minimal effect in reducing LID as recorded in patient diaries, with no effect on parkinsonian disability (70).

In an attempt to clarify the situation with regard to the potential for opioid antagonists to reduce LID, we performed an additional double-blind, randomized placebo-controlled, crossover trial in 14 PD patients (71) employing methodology with demonstrated ability to block central opioid receptors (72). Patients were assessed for parkinsonism and dyskinesia during a standard L-DOPA challenge test and a concurrent infusion of iv infusion of 0.3 mcg/kg/min naloxone, or placebo. This study failed to demonstrate any reduction in LID, but did show an extension in the duration of action of L-DOPA by 18% without any effect on parkinsonism (71). In this latter respect confirming the initial finding of Trabucchi et al. (68). The current data suggest that in patients, non-subtype-selective opioid receptor antagonists do not provide robust and consistent reductions in LID; however, this may relate to an action on multiple subtypes of opioid receptor which may have result in both pro-dyskinetic as well as anti-dyskinetic effects (see also earlier discussion related to conflicting data in MPTP-lesioned primates) and thus may mask any potential benefit. To date, no subtype-selective opioid receptor antagonists have been investigated in LID in PD patients.

30.6 Role of Opioid Peptides in Development ('Priming') of LID

In recent years, the possibility that enhanced opioid peptide transmission might contribute to mechanisms by which the brain becomes sensitized to L-DOPA and thus primed to express LID when challenged with subsequent dopaminergic therapies has gained credence. Indeed, it is consistent with several of the findings of elevation in opioid peptide expression described above. It appears that an elevation in striatal PPE-A expression may dramatically enhance, if not be necessary for, the ability of L-DOPA to elicit LID. Thus, in MPTP-lesioned primates, the lesion-induced elevation of PPE-A is transient if animals are left untreated, that is parkinsonian for more than 4–6 months (73). If L-DOPA therapy is initiated during a period when PPE-A is elevated, LID evolves rapidly; if L-DOPA therapy is initiated later, it is extremely difficult to generate LID (73). This finding supports a potential for opioid antagonists to suppress the priming process and thus the development of LID if they were given in combination with L-DOPA de novo. However, studies in 6-OHDA-lesioned rat have shown no effect of naloxone, daily *nor*-BNI, nor the κ-receptor agonist U-50, 488H, treatment in preventing the development of LID (61, 74, 75). This suggests that in rats at least, modulation of κ-receptors does not alter the mechanisms underlying the development of LID. However, to date, no studies have been performed with selective μ- or δ-opioid receptor antagonists nor have been conducted in primates. Given the species differences in the relative involvement of opioid subtypes in the expression of LID, evaluation of their role in priming might also require primate studies (76).

30.7 The Future for Opioid Receptor Antagonists in LID?

While it is clear that levels of several opioids are elevated in the basal ganglia in LID, there is currently conflicting preclinical and clinical data with respect to the contribution they play to LID. Changes in opioid peptide expression may not necessarily reflect a causative role in the expression of LID and could also be consistent with roles in the priming process or a secondary response to motor behaviour of LID, possibly an unsuccessful compensatory response, attempting to suppress LID. However, several opportunities exist for opioid receptor antagonists to have a therapeutic role in LID. On balance, it appears that blockade of opioid transmission, in a way that is not selective for subtypes of opioid receptor, has little anti-dyskinetic potential when administered as an adjunct to L-DOPA. However, the μ-opioid receptor subtype appears to be a promising target- and subtype-selective agents need to be assessed in the clinical setting as to their ability to reduce LID in PD.

References

1. Lang AE, Lozano AM. Parkinson's disease. First of two parts. N Engl J Med 1998;339: 1044–1053.
2. Nutt JG. Clinical pharmacology of levodopa-induced dyskinesia. Ann Neurol 2000;47: S160–S164; discussion S164–S166.
3. Rajput AH, Fenton ME, Birdi S, Macaulay R, George D, Rozdilsky B, Ang LC, Senthilselvan A, Hornykiewicz O. Clinical-pathological study of levodopa complications. Mov Disord 2002;17: 289–296.
4. Luquin MR, Scipioni O, Vaamonde J, Gershanik O, Obeso JA. Levodopa-induced dyskinesias in Parkinson's disease: clinical and pharmacological classification. Mov Disord 1992;7: 117–124.

5. Muenter MD, Sharpless NS, Tyce GM, Darley FL. Patterns of dystonia ("I-D-I" and "D-I-D-") in response to L-DOPA therapy for Parkinson's disease. Mayo Clin Proc 1977;52: 163–174.
6. Brotchie JM, Lee J, Venderova K. L-DOPA-induced dyskinesia. J Neural Transm 2005; 112:359–91.
7. Bezard E, Brotchie JM, Gross CE. Pathophysiology of levodopa-induced dyskinesia: potential for new therapies. Nat Rev Neurosci 2001;2: 577–588.
8. Calon F, Grondin R, Morissette M, Goulet M, Blanchet PJ, Di_Paolo T, Bedard PJ. Molecular basis of levodopa-induced dyskinesias. Ann Neurol 2000;47: S70–S78.
9. Calon F, Morissette M, Rajput AH, Hornykiewicz O, Bedard PJ, Di_Paolo T. Changes of GABA receptors and dopamine turnover in the postmortem brains of parkinsonians with levodopa-induced motor complications. Mov Disord 2003;18: 241–253.
10. Crossman AR. A hypothesis on the pathophysiological mechanisms that underlie levodopa- or dopamine agonist-induced dyskinesia in Parkinson's disease: implications for future strategies in treatment. Mov Disord 1990;5: 100–108.
11. Gnanalingham KK, Smith LA, Hunter AJ, Jenner P, Marsden CD. Alterations in striatal and extrastriatal D-1 and D-2 dopamine receptors in the MPTP-treated common marmoset: an autoradiographic study. Synapse 1993;14: 184–194.
12. Mitchell IJ, Boyce S, Sambrook MA, Crossman AR. A 2-deoxyglucose study of the effects of dopamine agonists on the parkinsonian primate brain. Implications for the neural mechanisms that mediate dopamine agonist-induced dyskinesia. Brain 1992;115: 809–824.
13. Matsumura M, Tremblay L, Richard H, Filion M. Activity of pallidal neurons in the monkey during dyskinesia induced by injection of bicuculline in the external pallidum. Neuroscience 1995;65: 59–70.
14. Brotchie JM, Lee J, Venderova K. Levodopa-induced dyskinesia in Parkinson's disease. J Neural Transm 2005;112: 359–391.
15. Cuello AC, Paxinos G. Evidence for a long Leu-enkephalin striopallidal pathway in rat brain. Nature 1978;271: 178–180.
16. Haber S, Elde R. Correlation between Met-enkephalin and substance P immunoreactivity in the primate globus pallidus. Neuroscience 1981;6: 1291–1297.
17. Gerfen CR. The neostriatal mosaic: multiple levels of compartmental organization. Trends Neurosci 1992;15: 133–139.
18. Cuello AC, Emson PC, Paxinos G, Jessell T. Substance P containing and cholinergic projections from the habenula. Brain Res 1978;149: 413–429.
19. Gerfen CR. The neostriatal mosaic: compartmentalization of corticostriatal input and striatonigral output systems. Nature 1984;311: 461–464.
20. Beckstead RM, Kersey KS. Immunohistochemical demonstration of differential substance P-, met-enkephalin-, and glutamic-acid-decarboxylase-containing cell body and axon distributions in the corpus striatum of the cat. J Comp Neurol 1985;232: 481–498.
21. Del Fiacco M, Paxinos G, Cuello AC. Neostriatal enkephalin-immunoreactive neurones project to the globus pallidus. Brain Res 1982;231: 1–17.
22. Vincent S, Hokfelt T, Christensson I, Terenius L. Immunohistochemical evidence for a dynorphin immunoreactive striato-nigral pathway. Eur J Pharmacol 1982;85: 251–252.
23. Carta A, Fenu S, Morelli M. Alterations in GAD67, dynorphin and enkephalin mRNA in striatal output neurons following priming in the 6-OHDA model of Parkinson's disease. 2001;22: 59–60.
24. Gerfen CR, Engber TM, Mahan LC, Susel Z, Chase TN, Monsma FJ, Sibley DR. D1 and D2 dopamine receptor-regulated gene expression of striatonigral and striatopallidal neurons. Science 1990;250: 1429–1432.
25. Gerfen CR, McGinty JF, Young WS. Dopamine differentially regulates dynorphin, substance P, and enkephalin expression in striatal neurons: in situ hybridization histochemical analysis. J Neurosci 1991;11: 1016–1031.
26. Zamir N, Skofitsch G, Bannon MJ, Helke CJ, Kopin IJ, Jacobowitz DM. Primate model of Parkinson's disease: alterations in multiple opioid systems in the basal ganglia. Brain Res 1984;322: 356–360.

27. Jiang HK, McGinty JF, Hong JS. Differential modulation of striatonigral dynorphin and enkephalin by dopamine receptor subtypes. Brain Res 1990;507: 57–64.
28. Parent A, Asselin MC, Cote PY. Dopaminergic regulation of peptide gene expression in the striatum of normal and parkinsonian monkeys. Adv Neurol 1996;69: 73–77.
29. Engber TM, Susel Z, Kuo S, Gerfen CR, Chase TN. Levodopa replacement therapy alters enzyme activities in striatum and neuropeptide content in striatal output regions of 6-hydroxydopamine lesioned rats. Brain Res 1991;552: 113–118.
30. Duty S, Brotchie JM. Enhancement of the behavioral response to apomorphine administration following repeated treatment in the 6-hydroxydopamine-lesioned rat is temporally correlated with a rise in striatal preproenkephalin-B, but not preproenkephalin-A, gene expression. Exp Neurol 1997;144: 423–432.
31. Cenci MA, Lee CS, Bjorklund A. L-DOPA-induced dyskinesia in the rat is associated with striatal overexpression of prodynorphin- and glutamic acid decarboxylase mRNA. Eur J Neurosci 1998;10: 2694–2706.
32. Henry B, Crossman AR, Brotchie JM. Effect of repeated L-DOPA, bromocriptine, or lisuride administration on preproenkephalin-A and preproenkephalin-B mRNA levels in the striatum of the 6-hydroxydopamine-lesioned rat. Exp Neurol 1999;155: 204–220.
33. Andersson M, Hilbertson A, Cenci MA. Striatal fosB expression is causally linked with L-DOPA-induced abnormal involuntary movements and the associated upregulation of striatal prodynorphin mRNA in a rat model of Parkinson's disease. Neurobiol Dis 1999;6: 461–474.
34. Henry B, Brotchie JM. Potential of opioid antagonists in the treatment of levodopa-induced dyskinesias in Parkinson's disease. Drugs Aging 1996;9: 149–158.
35. Ravenscroft P, Chalon S, Brotchie JM, Crossman AR. Ropinirole versus L-DOPA effects on striatal opioid peptide precursors in a rodent model of Parkinson's disease: implications for dyskinesia. Exp Neurol 2004;185: 36–46.
36. Henry B, Duty S, Fox SH, Crossman AR, Brotchie JM. Increased striatal pre-proenkephalin B expression is associated with dyskinesia in Parkinson's disease. Exp Neurol 2003;183: 458–468.
37. Sivam SP. Dopamine dependent decrease in enkephalin and substance P levels in basal ganglia regions of postmortem parkinsonian brains. Neuropeptides 1991;18: 201–207.
38. Taquet H, Javoy_Agid F, Giraud P, Legrand JC, Agid Y, Cesselin F. Dynorphin levels in parkinsonian patients: Leu5-enkephalin production from either proenkephalin A or prodynorphin in human brain. Brain Res 1985;341: 390–392.
39. Augood SJ, Emson PC, Mitchell IJ, Boyce S, Clarke CE, Crossman AR. Cellular localisation of enkephalin gene expression in MPTP-treated cynomolgus monkeys. Brain Res Mol Brain Res 1989;6: 85–92.
40. Herrero MT, Augood SJ, Hirsch EC, Javoy_Agid F, Luquin MR, Agid Y, Obeso JA, Emson PC. Effects of L-DOPA on preproenkephalin and preprotachykinin gene expression in the MPTP-treated monkey striatum. Neuroscience 1995;68: 1189–1198.
41. Young WS, 3rd, Bonner TI, Brann MR. Mesencephalic dopamine neurons regulate the expression of neuropeptide mRNAs in the rat forebrain. Proc Natl Acad Sci U S A 1986;83: 9827–9831.
42. Asselin MC, Soghomonian JJ, Cote PY, Parent A. Striatal changes in preproenkephalin mRNA levels in parkinsonian monkeys. Neuroreport 1994;5: 2137–2140.
43. Duty S, Henry B, Crossman AR, Brotchie JM. Topographical organization of opioid peptide precursor gene expression following repeated apomorphine treatment in the 6-hydroxydopamine-lesioned rat. Exp Neurol 1998;150: 223–234.
44. Morissette M, Grondin R, Goulet M, Bedard PJ, Di_Paolo T. Differential regulation of striatal preproenkephalin and preprotachykinin mRNA levels in MPTP-lesioned monkeys chronically treated with dopamine D1 or D2 receptor agonists. J Neurochem 1999;72: 682–692.
45. Morissette M, Goulet M, Soghomonian JJ, Blanchet PJ, Calon F, Bedard PJ, Di_Paolo T. Preproenkephalin mRNA expression in the caudate-putamen of MPTP monkeys after chronic treatment with the D2 agonist U91356A in continuous or intermittent mode of administration: comparison with L-DOPA therapy. Brain Res Mol Brain Res 1997;49: 55–62.

46. Perier C, Marin C, Bonastre M, Tolosa E, Hirsch EC. AMPA receptor antagonist LY293558 reverses preproenkephalin mRNA overexpression in the striatum of 6-OHDA-lesioned-rats treated with L-dopa. Eur J Neurosci 2002;16: 2236–2240.
47. Morissette M, Dridi M, Calon F, Tahar AH, Meltzer LT, Bedard PJ, Di Paolo T. Prevention of levodopa-induced dyskinesias by a selective NR1A/2B N-methyl-D-aspartate receptor antagonist in parkinsonian monkeys: implication of preproenkephalin. Mov Disord 2006;21: 9–17.
48. Pirker W, Tedroff J, Ponten H, Gunne L, Andren PE, Hurd YL. Coadministration of (–)-OSU6162 with L-DOPA normalizes preproenkephalin mRNA expression in the sensorimotor striatum of primates with unilateral 6-OHDA lesions. Exp Neurol 2001;169: 122–134.
49. Tel BC, Zeng BY, Cannizzaro C, Pearce RK, Rose S, Jenner P. Alterations in striatal neuropeptide mRNA produced by repeated administration of L-DOPA, ropinirole or bromocriptine correlate with dyskinesia induction in MPTP-treated common marmosets. Neuroscience 2002;115: 1047–1058.
50. Zeng BY, Pearce RK, MacKenzie GM, Jenner P. Alterations in preproenkephalin and adenosine-2a receptor mRNA, but not preprotachykinin mRNA correlate with occurrence of dyskinesia in normal monkeys chronically treated with L-DOPA. Eur J Neurosci 2000;12: 1096–1104.
51. Nisbet AP, Foster OJ, Kingsbury A, Eve DJ, Daniel SE, Marsden CD, Lees AJ. Preproenkephalin and preprotachykinin messenger RNA expression in normal human basal ganglia and in Parkinson's disease. Neuroscience 1995;66: 361–376.
52. Calon F, Birdi S, Rajput AH, Hornykiewicz O, Bedard PJ, Di PT. Increase of preproenkephalin mRNA levels in the putamen of Parkinson disease patients with levodopa-induced dyskinesias. J Neuropathol Exp Neurol 2002;61: 186–196.
53. Piccini P, Weeks RA, Brooks DJ. Alterations in opioid receptor binding in Parkinson's disease patients with levodopa-induced dyskinesias. Ann Neurol 1997;42: 720–726.
54. Seizinger BR, Grimm C, Hollt V, Herz A. Evidence for a selective processing of proenkephalin B into different opioid peptide forms in particular regions of rat brain and pituitary. J Neurochem 1984;42: 447–457.
55. Breslin MB, Lindberg I, Benjannet S, Mathis JP, Lazure C, Seidah NG. Differential processing of proenkephalin by prohormone convertases 1(3) and 2 and furin. J Biol Chem 1993;268: 27084–27093.
56. Hill MP, Brotchie JM. Control of glutamate release by calcium channels and kappa-opioid receptors in rodent and primate striatum. Br J Pharmacol 1999;127: 275–283.
57. Zhou S, Wang G, Crossman AR, Brotchie JM. Concurrent analysis of seven opioid neuropeptides in brain tissue by reversed phase high-performance liquid cromatography combined with radioimmunoassay (in preparation).
58. Chen L, Togasaki DM, Langston JW, Di Monte DA, Quik M. Enhanced striatal opioid receptor-mediated G-protein activation in L-DOPA-treated dyskinetic monkeys. Neuroscience 2005;132: 409–420.
59. Strong JA, Dalvi A, Revilla FJ, Sahay A, Samaha FJ, Welge JA, Gong J, Gartner M, Yue X, Yu L. Genotype and smoking history affect risk of levodopa-induced dyskinesias in Parkinson's disease. Mov Disord 2006;21: 654–659.
60. Bond C, LaForge KS, Tian M, Melia D, Zhang S, Borg L, Gong J, Schluger J, Strong JA, Leal SM, Tischfield JA, Kreek MJ, Yu L. Single-nucleotide polymorphism in the human mu opioid receptor gene alters beta-endorphin binding and activity: possible implications for opiate addiction. Proc Natl Acad Sci U S A 1998;95: 9608–9613.
61. Carey RJ. Naloxone reverses L-dopa induced overstimulation effects in a Parkinson's disease animal model analogue. Life Sci 1991;48: 1303–1308.
62. Newman DD, Rajakumar N, Flumerfelt BA, Stoessl AJ. A kappa opioid antagonist blocks sensitization in a rodent model of Parkinson's disease. Neuroreport 1997;8: 669–672.
63. Gomez-Mancilla B, Bedard PJ. Effect of nondopaminergic drugs on L-dopa-induced dyskinesias in MPTP-treated monkeys. Clin Neuropharmacol 1993;16: 418–427.
64. Henry B, Fox SH, Crossman AR, Brotchie JM. Mu- and delta-opioid receptor antagonists reduce levodopa-induced dyskinesia in the MPTP-lesioned primate model of Parkinson's disease. Exp Neurol 2001;171: 139–146.

65. Klintenberg R, Svenningsson P, Gunne L, Andren PE. Naloxone reduces levodopa-induced dyskinesias and apomorphine-induced rotations in primate models of parkinsonism. J Neural Transm 2002;109: 1295–1307.
66. Samadi P, Gregoire L, Bedard PJ. Opioid antagonists increase the dyskinetic response to dopaminergic agents in parkinsonian monkeys: interaction between dopamine and opioid systems. Neuropharmacology 2003;45: 954–963.
67. Sandyk R, Snider SR. Naloxone treatment of L-dopa-induced dyskinesias in Parkinson's disease. Am J Psychiatry 1986;143: 118.
68. Trabucchi M, Bassi S, Frattola L. Effect of naloxone on the "on-off' syndrome in patients receiving long-term levodopa therapy. Arch Neurol 1982;39: 120–121.
69. Rascol O, Fabre N, Blin O, Poulik J, Sabatini U, Senard JM, Ane M, Montastruc JL, Rascol A. Naltrexone, an opiate antagonist, fails to modify motor symptoms in patients with Parkinson's disease. Mov Disord 1994;9: 437–440.
70. Manson AJ, Katzenschlager R, Hobart J, Lees AJ. High dose naltrexone for dyskinesias induced by levodopa. J Neurol Neurosurg Psychiatry 2001;70: 554–556.
71. Fox S, Silverdale M, Kellett M, Davies R, Steiger M, Fletcher N, Crossman A, Brotchie J. Non-subtype-selective opioid receptor antagonism in treatment of levodopa-induced motor complications in Parkinson's disease. Mov Disord 2004;19: 554–560.
72. Ngai SH, Berkowitz BA, Yang JC, Hempstead J, Spector S. Pharmacokinetics of naloxone in rats and in man: basis for its potency and short duration of action. Anesthesiology 1976;44: 398–401.
73. Schneider JS, Decamp E, Wade T. Striatal preproenkephalin gene expression is upregulated in acute but not chronic parkinsonian monkeys: implications for the contribution of the indirect striatopallidal circuit to parkinsonian symptomatology. J Neurosci 1999;19: 6643–6649.
74. Newman DD, Rajakumar N, Flumerfelt BA, Stoessl AJ. A kappa opioid antagonist blocks sensitization in a rodent model of Parkinson's disease. Neuroreport 1997;8: 669–672.
75. Marin C, Bove J, Bonastre M, Tolosa E. Effect of acute and chronic administration of U50, 488, a kappa opioid receptor agonist, in 6-OHDA-lesioned rats chronically treated with levodopa. Exp Neurol 2003;183: 66–73.
76. Anderson DW, Neavin T, Smith JA, Schneider JS. Neuroprotective effects of pramipexole in young and aged MPTP-treated mice. Brain Res 2001;905: 44–53.

Chapter 31
Endocrine Effects of Opioid Antagonists

Jack H. Mendelson and Nancy K. Mello

Abstract The hypothalamic–pituitary–gonadal (HPG) axis and the hypothalamic–pituitary–adrenal (HPA) axis are regulated in part by endogenous opioid peptides. The endogenous opioid system has primarily inhibitory actions on the HPG and the HPA axis hormones. Exogenous opioid antagonists block endogenous opioid inhibition, usually resulting in stimulation of hormone release. This chapter summarizes the effects of a series of opioid antagonists (naltrexone, naloxone, nalmefene, and nalbuphine) on HPG and HPA axis hormones and on prolactin. Clinical studies and preclinical studies in nonhuman primates are discussed. Interestingly, stimulation of hormone release by opioid antagonists has been useful for the treatment of a number of endocrine disorders including infertility, hypothalamic amenorrhea, and male impotence and as tests of HPA axis function.

Keywords: Opioid antagonists; Opioid agonists; Naltrexone; Naloxone; Nalmefene; Nalbuphine; Prolactin; HPA axis hormones; HPG axis hormones

31.1 Introduction

The opioid antagonists have a wide range of experimental and medical applications. In addition to their value as pharmacological tools, they have proved clinically effective for reversal of opioid overdose (1) and are variably effective for treatment of disorders ranging from substance abuse and alcoholism (2–4) to anxiety, depression, and bulimia (5) (see also reviews in this volume). The focus of this chapter is on the effects of opioid antagonists on the neuroendocrine system. This topic is of interest, in part, because endogenous opioid peptides are involved in the regulation of many aspects of the neuroendocrine system. We will first describe studies of the effects of opioid antagonists on the hypothalamic–pituitary–gonadal (HPG) axis. In the second part of this chapter, we will discuss the effects of naltrexone, naloxone, nalmefene, and nalbuphine

J.H. Mendelson and N.K. Mello (✉)
Alcohol and Drug Abuse Research Center, McLean Hospital-Harvard Medical School, Belmont, MA 02478

on the hypothalamic–pituitary–adrenal (HPA) axis. Finally, we will describe the interactions of opioid antagonists with the anterior pituitary hormone prolactin. We will emphasize studies in humans and nonhuman primates throughout this chapter.

Our early research in this area was conducted in the context of evaluating the safety and effectiveness of naltrexone for the treatment of opioid abuse and dependence (6, 7). In the early 1970s, the Nixon administration established the Special Action Office for Drug Abuse Prevention (SAODAP) program under the leadership of Jerome Jaffe. One goal of the SAODAP program was to identify safe and effective alternatives to methadone for the treatment of opioid addiction. There was considerable evidence of illicit diversion of methadone and overdose deaths, and this prompted the search for safer treatment medications with relatively low abuse liability. The pharmacology of naltrexone suggested that it might be an ideal candidate treatment medication (8, 9). Inpatient clinical trials confirmed that this long-acting opioid antagonist significantly reduced operant response-contingent self-administration of heroin in opioid-dependent men, and had minimal adverse side effects (6, 7). However, translation of these findings into outpatient naltrexone maintenance treatment has proved problematic. Patient compliance was poor, in part, because naltrexone had no agonist effects. Moreover, when patients chose to use opioids, they could discontinue naltrexone without any adverse consequences, a pattern often observed with antabuse treatment for alcoholism. Although naltrexone remains useful for the treatment of a highly motivated group of opioid-dependent patients, such as nurses, physicians, and other professionals (10), its early promise as a treatment medication for heroin addiction was not fulfilled (11).

At periodic intervals during our inpatient evaluations of naltrexone, we collected blood samples for analysis of anterior pituitary, adrenal, and gonadal hormones. One unexpected finding from these early studies was that naltrexone increased the amplitude and frequency of the pulsatile release of luteinizing hormone (LH). The possible biological significance of this finding was not apparent at that time. Although it was known that a mid-cycle surge in LH was necessary to trigger ovulation, the critical role of the *frequency* of pulsatile LH release patterns for normal ovulatory menstrual cycles was not appreciated until the seminal studies of Ernst Knobil in the early 1970s (12, 13). The importance of the frequency of pulsatile infusion of synthetic LH-releasing hormone (LHRH) for restoring normal patterns of LH and follicle-stimulating hormone (FSH) secretory activity was first demonstrated in ovariectomized female rhesus monkeys (12, 13). Lesions of the arcuate nucleus and the median eminence disrupted hypothalamic release of endogenous LHRH, and abolished LH and FSH secretory activity. Pulsatile administration of synthetic LHRH restored LH and FSH secretory patterns, whereas continuous administration of synthetic LHRH did not (12, 13). This fundamental discovery was rapidly translated into clinical practice where it was found that disorders of the menstrual cycle are often characterized by abnormal LH secretory patterns (14–16). Administration of LHRH at a normal physiological frequency restored normal menstrual cycle function and fertility in some women (14–17). Interestingly as described below, naltrexone also proved useful for the treatment of infertility disorders because of its stimulatory effects on LH pulsatile release (18–20).

31.2 Opioid Antagonist Effects on the HPG Axis

The HPG axis controls reproductive function and regulates the changes in the pituitary gonadotropins (LH and FSH) and the gonadal steroid hormones (estradiol and progesterone) that define the phases of the menstrual cycle and determine ovulation in women. The hormonal regulation of the HPG axis is very complex and a complete description is beyond the scope of this chapter (21–23). However, it is generally accepted that the HPG axis is under inhibitory endogenous opioid control. The endogenous opioid peptides inhibit the release of hypothalamic LHRH (21, 22, 24). LHRH stimulates the release of LH and FSH from the gonadotropes in the anterior pituitary. Exogenous opioid agonists act like endogenous opioid peptides to inhibit LHRH release and subsequent release of LH and FSH. Antagonism of endogenous opioid tone stimulates LHRH pulsatile release and subsequent release of LH and FSH. Details of the studies demonstrating the effects of opioid antagonists on the HPG axis are described below in Section 31.2.1.

In women, LH and FSH are also regulated by the gonadal steroid hormones, estradiol and progesterone (22). The gonadotropin and ovarian steroid hormone levels are controlled by a complex pattern of reciprocal stimulation and inhibition that changes across the menstrual cycle. The successive phases of the menstrual cycle are defined by changes in the relative ovarian steroid hormone levels and the frequency of LH and FSH pulsatile release (23). After menopause or surgical ovariectomy, the inhibitory influence of the ovarian steroid hormones is removed, and LH and FSH remain at high levels similar to levels measured at ovulation in a normal menstrual cycle. In men, testosterone and estradiol come from the testes, and disruption of the hypothalamic–pituitary–testicular axis results in elevated LH levels (25, 26). LH stimulates increased secretion of testosterone, and testosterone in turn inhibits LH pulsatile release (25, 26). It is thought that estrogens and/or progesterone may inhibit pituitary gonadotropins through their interactions with endogenous opioid peptides. Consistent with this view, preclinical studies reported that administration of estrogen and progesterone increased the concentration of β-endorphin in hypophyseal blood in monkeys (27–29).

31.2.1 Naltrexone Stimulates Release of LH

31.2.1.1 Clinical Studies of the HPG Axis

Chronic opioid dependence is often associated with disorders of sexual function that are usually attributed to the inhibitory effects of opioids on testosterone and LH (30, 31). In a clinical laboratory study, two detoxified opioid-dependent men were given saline, heroin (10 mg, IV) and heroin + naltrexone (50 mg, PO) on different days, and blood samples were collected for analysis of LH and testosterone (32). Heroin immediately decreased LH levels and subsequently decreased testosterone whereas saline control administration had no effect. Pretreatment with

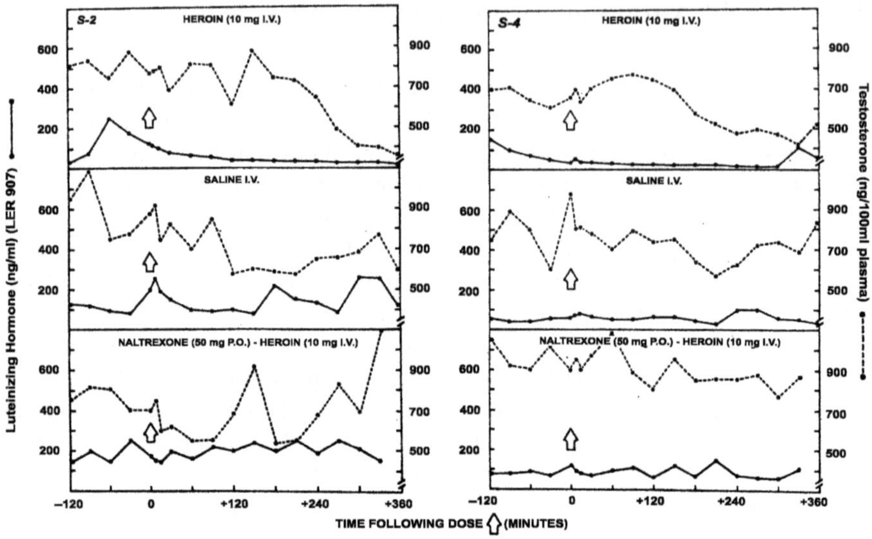

Fig. 31.1 The effect of intravenous heroin on plasma luteinizing hormone (*LH*) and testosterone, before and after antagonist blockade (subjects S2 and S4). *Abscissa*: time after IV administration of heroin, saline, or heroin plus oral naltrexone. *Left ordinate*: LH (ng/ml). *Right ordinate*: testosterone (ng/100 ml). Reprinted with permission from Mirin et al. (32)

the opioid antagonist naltrexone blocked the suppressive effect of heroin on LH and increased the number of LH secretory pulses. Illustrative data are shown in Fig. 31.1. These findings were replicated in another group of heroin-dependent men studied on a clinical research ward (33). Heroin (10 mg, IV) significantly reduced LH and testosterone after acute administration. After 10 days of heroin self-administration (10 mg, IV, every 6 h), the degree of LH and T suppression was equivalent to that after the first acute dose. These data were interpreted to suggest that the tolerance developed to the chronic effects of heroin on the HPG axis. Acute naltrexone administration (50 mg, PO) significantly increased LH levels but not testosterone levels. After 22 days of naltrexone maintenance, LH and testosterone levels were in the low and high normal range, respectively. These data suggested that the stimulatory effects of naltrexone are modulated by the negative steroid feedback effects of testosterone on LH release (33).

We also studied the effects of naltrexone or placebo on LH in eight healthy men who had no history of opioid or other drug abuse (34). Naltrexone (50 mg, PO) or placebo was given in a counterbalanced order and integrated plasma samples were collected during consecutive 20-min periods over 8 h. Figure 31.2 shows the effects of naltrexone and placebo on LH in individual subjects. LH levels were significantly higher after naltrexone than after placebo administration. During interviews conducted at the end of the study, subjects described the effects of naltrexone as unpleasant and complained of fatigue, dysphoria, nausea, feelings of lightheadedness and faintness, sweating, and occasional feelings of unreality. One subject left

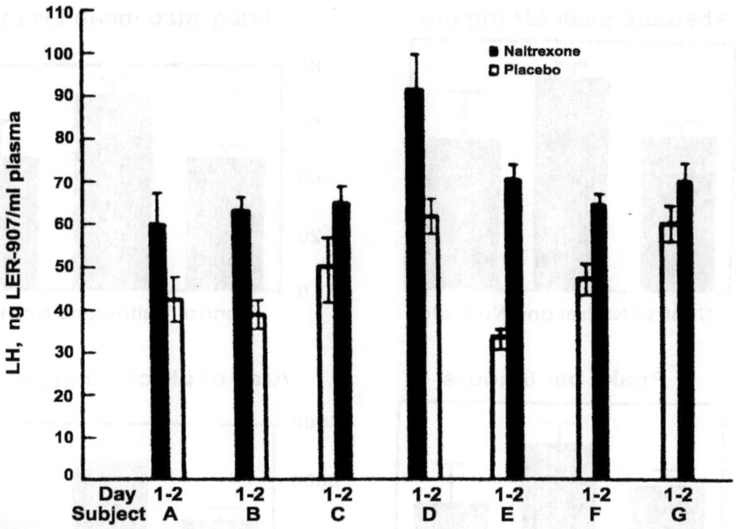

Fig. 31.2 Integrated plasma luteinizing hormone (*LH*) levels for seven adult males following naltrexone or placebo administration. LH levels are shown on the left ordinate, and the study day (1–2) and the subject number are shown on the abscissa. Mean values were calculated from the true mean integrated values of 20 sampling times; therefore, variability in plasma levels of the hormone during the 8-h period is already accounted for in the calculated means since these means represent integrated plasma values. The brackets on each bar represent the meaningful experimental variability, that is the mean standard error for analysis of duplicate samples at each 20-min interval. Reprinted with permission from Mendelson et al. (34)

the study because the dysphoric effects of naltrexone were so unpleasant. Three subjects reported uncontrollable penile erections, and naltrexone dose-related penile erections were also observed in nonhuman primates (35). A quantitative analysis of the effects of naltrexone and placebo on pulsatile LH secretion confirmed and extended the earlier clinical findings (36). Normal men given placebo did not differ from a cohort of 38 normal men in any of the LH pulsatile parameters examined. In contrast, men given naltrexone had significantly more LH peaks in 8 h, higher absolute LH peaks, a higher area of the LH curve (ng/ml/min), and a higher integrated mean LH. These data are summarized in Fig. 31.3.

In clinical endocrinology, a number of compounds have been used to assess the status of pituitary function (38). Synthetic LHRH and thyroid-releasing hormone are often used as provocative tests of anterior pituitary hormone function. On the basis of our discovery that naltrexone stimulated LH release in men, we postulated that it might be useful as a provocative test of anterior pituitary function in women. Naltrexone (50 mg, PO) was given to women during the early-follicular phase or during the mid- or late-follicular phase of the menstrual cycle (39, 40). Figure 31.4 shows that naltrexone significantly increased LH levels in women studied during the early-follicular phase. Baseline LH levels were higher in women studied during the mid- and late-follicular phase and the greatest naltrexone-induced

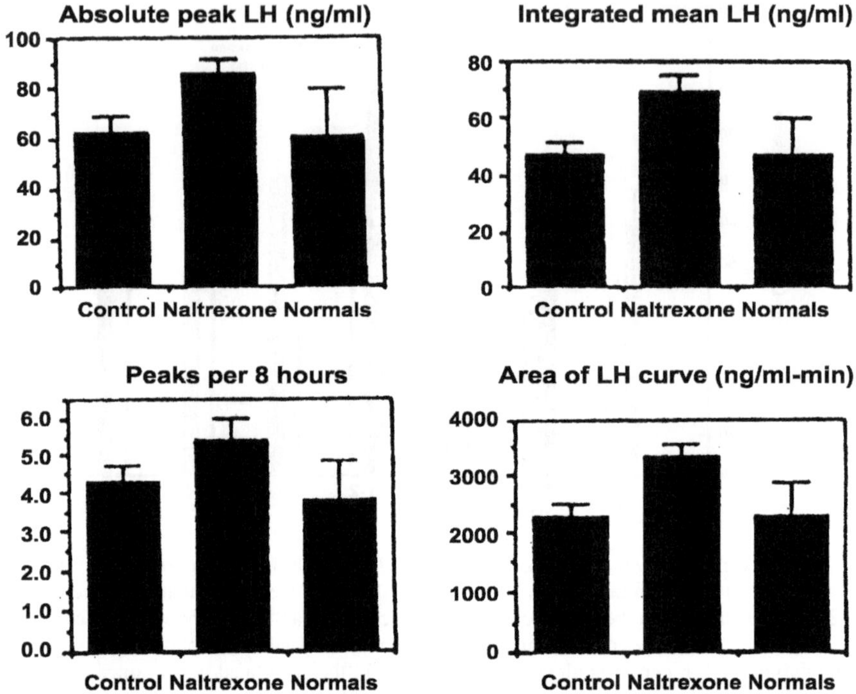

Fig. 31.3 Quantitative analysis of luteinizing hormone (*LH*) pulsatile release after saline control and naltrexone administration. The absolute peak LH and the integrated mean LH (*top row*), the number of LH peaks per hour, and the area of the LH curve after naltrexone (50 mg, PO) administration (*second row*) in subjects who served as their own control when they received placebo naltrexone. In addition, data are shown for 38 normal males who did not receive naltrexone or naltrexone placebo. Reprinted with permission from Mendelson et al. (39)

increase in LH release occurred in the preovulatory phase of the menstrual cycle. This preliminary study was replicated in 14 women studied during the early-follicular phase of the menstrual cycle (days 2–4) (41). Naltrexone (50 mg, PO) significantly increased LH levels and this increase was enhanced by consumption of alcohol 60 min after naltrexone administration. Alcohol enhancement of naltrexone stimulation of LH occurred during the ascending limb of the blood alcohol curve. Peak blood alcohol levels over 120 mg/dl were detected 90 min after drinking began (41).

Naltrexone stimulation of LH release during the early-follicular phase of the menstrual cycle was inconsistent with earlier studies showing that the opioid antagonist naloxone only stimulated LH release during the mid-follicular and luteal phases of the menstrual cycle (42, 43). This discrepancy probably reflects the difference in duration of action of naloxone ($T_{1/2}$ of 1 h) and naltrexone ($T_{1/2}$ of 10 h) (8, 44). Currently, treatment with naltrexone (20–50 mg, PO/day) remains an effective alternative to pulsatile administration of LHRH for women with hypothalamic ovarian failure (19, 20). Women with hypothalamic amenorrhea

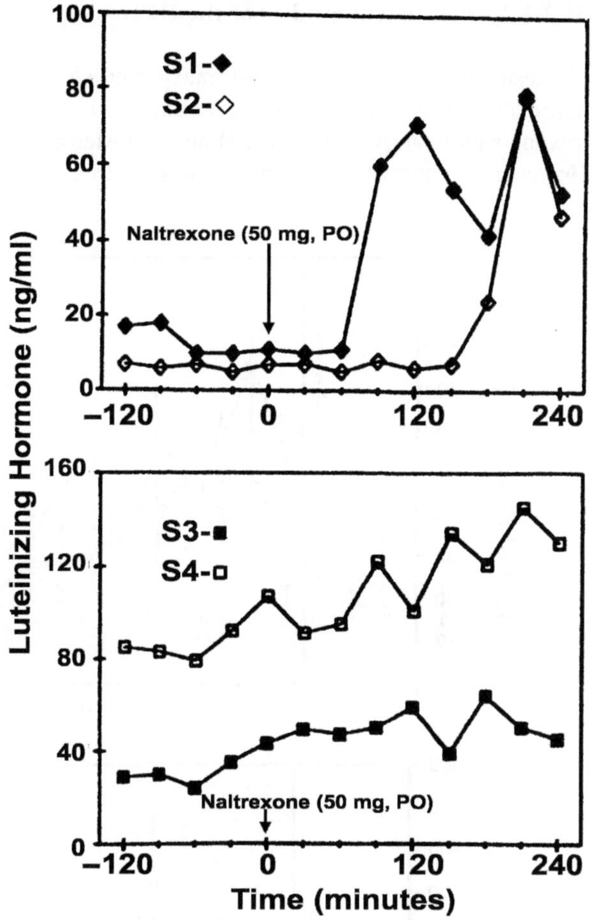

Fig. 31.4 LH levels before and after naltrexone administration. Abscissa: time (min) before and after oral naltrexone administration (50 mg, PO) at time 0. *Ordinate*: Luteinizing hormone (ng/ml). The top panel shows luteinizing hormone (LH) values for two women (S-1, S-2) studied during the early-follicular phase of the menstrual cycle. The bottom panel shows LH values for two subjects (S-3, S-4) studied during the mid- and late-follicular phase of the menstrual cycle. Reprinted with permission from Mendelson et al. (39)

had a significant increase in both the amplitude and the frequency of LH pulsatile release. The pregnancy rate in women treated with naltrexone for infertility was similar to that in a normal population. These findings confirm and extend the earlier reports that naltrexone was an effective treatment for infertility (18). Importantly, daily administration of naltrexone (100 mg, PO) to women during the luteal phase of the menstrual cycle did not disrupt the endocrine characteristics of the luteal phase in comparison to control cycles (45). Women athletes may develop persistent amenorrhea, and the long-acting opioid antagonist nalmefene significantly increased the mean amplitude of LH pulses in comparison to baseline or to placebo administration (46). Subsequent studies with nalmefene also reported significant increases in LH levels and LH pulse frequency in normal men (47) and increases LH and testosterone levels in older men with impotence (48). Taken together, these data illustrate the potential therapeutic value of opioid antagonists for the treatment of infertility, amenorrhea and male impotence.

31.2.1.2 Preclinical Studies of the HPG Axis

In rhesus monkeys, there was an unexpected sex difference in the acute effects of naltrexone on LH and the gonadal steroid hormones (49). Figure 31.5 shows that naltrexone significantly increased LH and testosterone levels in male rhesus monkeys. However, in contrast to human females, naltrexone had no effect on LH in rhesus

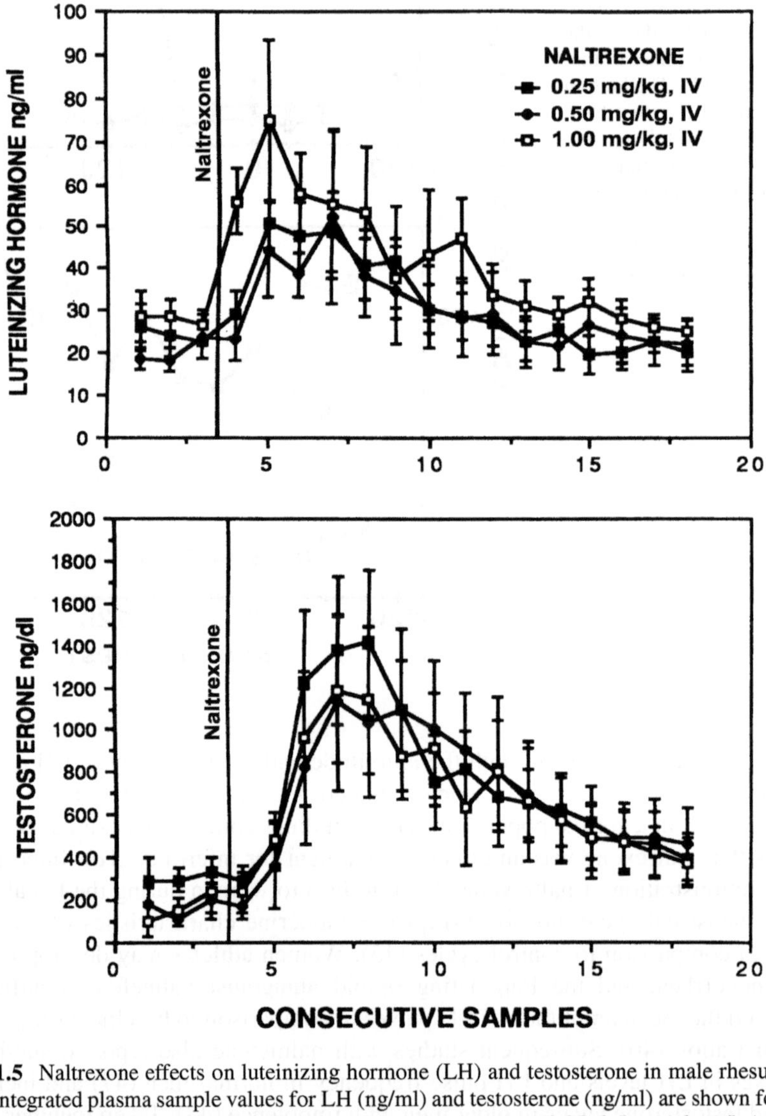

Fig. 31.5 Naltrexone effects on luteinizing hormone (LH) and testosterone in male rhesus monkeys. Integrated plasma sample values for LH (ng/ml) and testosterone (ng/ml) are shown for three consecutive 20-min samples before IV naltrexone administration (0.25, 0.5, or 1.0 mg/kg) and for 15 consecutive 20-min samples after naltrexone administration. Each data point is the mean ± SE of four subjects. Reprinted with permission from Mello et al. (49)

females during the early-follicular phase (cycle days 1–3) or the late-follicular phase (cycle days 10–12) of the menstrual cycle. Moreover, naltrexone significantly suppressed estradiol levels in rhesus females, unlike its effects on testosterone in males. All procedures were identical in males and females. Although baseline gonadal steroid levels were higher in males than in early-follicular-phase females, estradiol levels in late-follicular-phase females were relatively high, consistent with the ascending limb of the periovulatory estradiol surge. The basis for the differences in naltrexone's effects on LH in female rhesus monkeys and in women (39, 41) is unclear. These data suggested that there are sex differences in the endogenous opioid regulation of the LH release in adult rhesus monkeys. The sex differences observed in adult males and females are consistent with sex differences in LH and FSH secretory activity in infant rhesus monkeys after castration at 1 week of age (50).

To examine the generality of the endocrine effects of naltrexone, we also studied the long-acting opioid antagonist nalmefene, a derivative of naltrexone (51). In emergency medicine, nalmefene reverses opioid agonist-induced respiratory depression for 8 h or more (52). Nalmefene, like naltrexone, also stimulated LH release and increased testosterone levels in male rhesus monkeys (53). Figure 31.6 shows the time course of changes in LH and testosterone after IV placebo or nalmefene administration. Peak levels of LH occurred within 50 min after nalmefene, followed by an initial increase in testosterone, and significant increases in testosterone were detected within 40–50 min after LH increased significantly. These data illustrate the well-established reciprocal control of LH and testosterone through negative feedback mechanisms. These findings are also consistent with evidence that regulation of hypothalamic LHRH release and subsequent LH release from the anterior pituitary is under endogenous opioid inhibitory control (13, 21, 54, 55).

31.3 Opioid Antagonist Effects on the HPA Axis

HPA axis hormones integrate physiological responses to stress (56, 57). Corticotropin-releasing hormone (CRH) from the basal hypothalamus stimulates adrenocorticotropic hormone (ACTH) release from corticotrophs in the anterior pituitary. ACTH stimulates the release of cortisol from the adrenal and this facilitates cardiovascular, respiratory, gastrointestinal, and immune system responses to stress. Both CRH and ACTH secretion are under negative feedback control by the adrenal hormone cortisol in humans and nonhuman primates, and by corticosterone in rodents. CRH cannot be measured in peripheral circulation, but increases in CRH can be inferred from increases in plasma ACTH. CRH neurons are widely distributed throughout the central nervous system, and a number of neuronal systems may be involved in the regulation of CRH secretion. Endogenous opioids are also involved in the regulation of the HPA axis and appear to inhibit CRH secretion. Administration of human CRH (hCRH) to ovariectomized rhesus monkeys significantly increased cortisol levels, and this effect was not altered by concurrent administration of naloxone (58). hCRH alone suppressed LH and FSH, and this

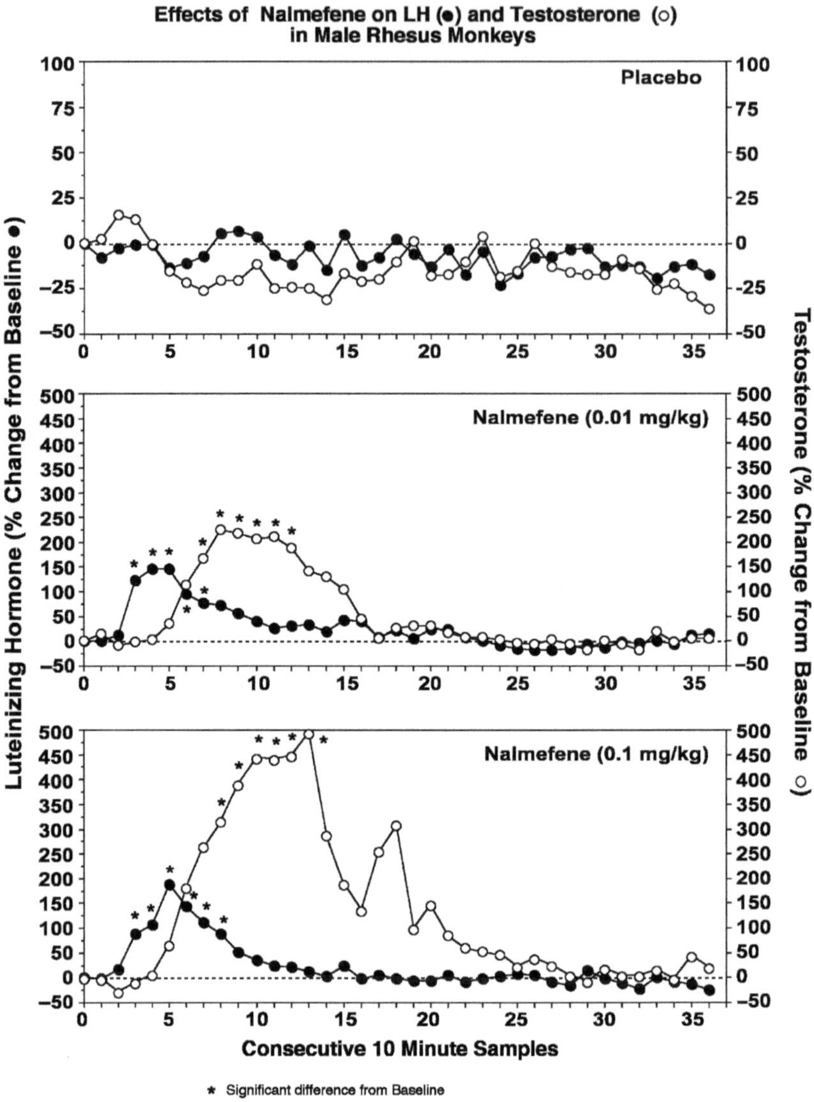

Fig. 31.6 Nalmefene and placebo effects on luteinizing hormone (LH) and testosterone. The abscissas show consecutive samples collected at 10-min intervals after IV placebo and nalmefene (0.01 and 0.10 mg/kg, IV) administration. The left ordinate shows LH levels (ng/ml) expressed as percent change from baseline (closed circles) during each of the three conditions. The right ordinate shows testosterone levels (ng/dl) expressed as percent change from baseline (open circles). Each data point is based on the average (±SEM) LH or testosterone level in four or five monkeys. Statistically significant changes from the pre-placebo or pre-nalmefene baseline are indicated by asterisks ($P < 0.05$). Reprinted with permission from Mello et al. (53)

effect was prevented by concurrent administration of naloxone (22, 58). There is considerable evidence that μ- and κ-selective opioid agonists usually decrease basal and stimulated ACTH and cortisol levels in humans (59–62), whereas stimulant drugs such as cocaine and nicotine stimulate ACTH and cortisol, and by inference, CRH (63, 64).

Dysregulation of the HPA axis has been implicated in a number of psychiatric disorders including depression, anxiety, and posttraumatic stress disorders (65–70) as well as drug abuse (71–74) and alcoholism (75–79). Comorbid substance abuse and psychiatric disorders are often reported (80–82). The appropriate HPA response to "stress" is usually exaggerated in depressive illness (56, 83). Chronic hyperactivity of the HPA axis is associated with elevated CRH secretion (measured in cerebrospinal fluid), a blunted ACTH response to exogenous CRF but a normal cortisol response, and ACTH resistance to suppression by dexamethasone (a synthetic glucocorticoid) (65, 67, 70). Naloxone also stimulated greater ACTH and cortisol release in normal healthy volunteers than in depressed patients (84).

31.3.1 Clinical Studies of Opioid Effects on the HPA Axis

Opioid antagonist stimulation of the HPA axis has been documented in humans, nonhuman primates, and rodents. The short-acting opioid antagonist naloxone consistently stimulates ACTH and cortisol release in clinical studies (85, 86). Recent interest in the use of opioid antagonists for the treatment of alcoholism (2–4, 87, 88) has been paralleled by clinical studies of the effects of opioid antagonists on the HPA axis. It has been suggested that dysregulation of the HPA axis may increase risk for the development of alcoholism. For example, children of alcoholics had a greater ACTH and cortisol response to naloxone than children of nonalcoholics (76–79). The HPA axis response to naloxone was compared in healthy adults with and without a family history of alcoholism. Baseline cortisol and ACTH levels did not differ significantly between the two groups, and there were no significant differences in the ACTH response to naloxone (75). However, the naloxone-stimulated increase in cortisol was significantly greater in subjects with a family history of alcoholism. These data were consistent with earlier findings in the children of alcoholics (76–78), and provide support for the notion that an inherited deficiency in hypothalamic opioid regulation of the HPA axis may be associated with a higher risk for alcoholism.

In clinical studies, the long-acting μ-opioid antagonist naltrexone consistently stimulates ACTH and cortisol under a number of conditions (39–41, 89–91). In women studied during the early-follicular phase of the menstrual cycle, administration of naltrexone (50 mg, PO) significantly increased ACTH levels by 100–200% over baseline values within 120–140 min (39, 40). Cortisol levels increased significantly within 120–180 min after naltrexone administration. A similar time course of increases in cortisol after naltrexone administration was also observed in follicular-phase women (41). Alcohol significantly increased naltrexone-stimulated increases in cortisol during the ascending limb of the blood alcohol curve (41).

The long-acting opioid antagonist nalmefene (10 and 30 mg) also stimulated significant increases in both ACTH and cortisol in normal healthy volunteers (92). The peak levels and duration of the nalmefene-stimulated increases in ACTH were significantly greater than those after administration of naloxone, but the increases in cortisol were similar (92). These data were interpreted to suggest that the increase in ACTH may have produced maximal stimulation of the adrenals. However, the increases in ACTH and cortisol were not nalmefene or naloxone dose-dependent, suggesting that there may have been a ceiling effect. There were no changes in ACTH or cortisol after vehicle control administration (92).

In contrast to naltrexone and nalmefene, the long-acting opioid antagonist nalbuphine did not significantly alter ACTH or cortisol levels in men with a history of cocaine abuse (93). Nalbuphine is usually classified as a mixed-action μ-antagonist/κ-agonist (94, 95), but in vitro studies suggest that nalbuphine may also have μ-agonist activity (96, 97). Naltrexone is primarily a μ-opioid antagonist and nalmefene appears to be a μ-antagonist and a partial agonist at κ-opioid receptors (8, 94, 98, 99). If nalbuphine has both μ- and κ-agonist activity, this could account for the lack of effect on ACTH and cortisol (93).

In clinical endocrinology, the long-acting opioid antagonists are also being used to assess the function of the HPA axis (100). It appears that the opioid antagonist nalmefene has several advantages over the traditional HPA axis function tests (insulin hypoglycemia test and the ACTH stimulation test) insofar as it may be more sensitive to early disorders of adrenal function (100). This application is important insofar as dysregulation of the HPA axis may increase vulnerability to depression and a number of other psychiatric disorders, as well as immune system dysfunction and cardiovascular disease (56, 66, 67, 101, 102).

31.3.2 *Preclinical Studies of Opioid Effects on the HPA Axis*

The pulsatile release patterns of ACTH and cortisol in rhesus monkeys are very similar to those in humans (103–105). ACTH and cortisol releases are circadian in gonadally intact rhesus monkeys (106–108). In males, castration disrupts circadian release patterns of cortisol, suggesting the importance of the steroid milieu in regulating the HPA axis (109). Similarly, ACTH and cortisol did not increase in response to a cocaine challenge in ovariectomized female rhesus monkeys (110) in contrast to gonadally intact rhesus females and males (111–113).

Although a number of studies have shown that cocaine stimulates ACTH and cortisol release in humans, nonhuman primates, and rodents [see for review (63)], there has been less interest in the effects of opioid antagonists on the HPA axis. The effects of a series of antagonists with different opioid receptor selectivity on the HPA axis were studied in nonhuman primates (114). Consistent with the clinical studies described above, the μ-opioid antagonist, naltrexone (0.0032–1.0 mg/kg, IM), produced dose-dependent and significant increases in

ACTH and cortisol. The μ-selective irreversible antagonist, clocinnamox (0.032–0.32 mg/kg, IM), did not produce significant increases in either ACTH or cortisol. The δ-selective opioid antagonist, naltrindole (0.1–0.32 mg/kg, IM), produced a significant increase in ACTH only at the highest dose (3.2 mg/kg, IM) and no significant changes in cortisol. The long-acting κ-antagonist, nor-binaltorphimine (1–3.2 mg/kg, IM), increased both ACTH and cortisol levels in comparison to vehicle controls; however, these increases were significant only for cortisol. In general, the range of changes in cortisol levels was relatively small (10–40 μg/dl), whereas antagonist-induced changes in ACTH levels ranged from 10–160 pg/ml. These data were interpreted to suggest that opioid stimulation of ACTH and cortisol cannot be attributed to only μ-, κ-, or δ-receptors, but rather may involve multiple opioid receptors (114). Further, the adverse effects of naltrexone (tremors, salivation, and vomiting) sometimes observed in nonhuman primates as well as in humans may have contributed to the HPA axis stimulation observed (114).

31.4 Opioid Effects on Prolactin

Prolactin is secreted from the lactotrope cells in the anterior pituitary. Unlike the pituitary gonadotropins and ACTH, prolactin is not regulated by negative feedback from peripheral target sites, that is, the gonadal or adrenal steroid hormones. Rather, prolactin appears to control its own secretion by feedback regulation of hypothalamic dopamine (115, 116). This regulatory system is further complicated by the fact that the dopamine release from tuberoinfundibular dopamine neurons is autoregulated by dopamine itself (117). The dopamine-sensitive lactotropes have primarily D_2 dopamine receptors, and prolactin is under inhibitory dopaminergic control (116, 118). Dopamine agonists with high affinity for dopamine D_2 receptors inhibit prolactin release, and D_2 receptor antagonists stimulate prolactin release (116). Dopamine infusion produced dose-dependent decreases in prolactin in rhesus monkeys (119). After chronic exposure (74–300 days) to cocaine, an indirect dopamine agonist, postdopamine increases in prolactin were significantly enhanced in comparison to precocaine conditions. These data suggested that dopamine infusions could provide a sensitive index of changes in dopaminergic regulation of prolactin as a function of chronic drug exposure (119).

Although prolactin is primarily under inhibitory dopaminergic control, endogenous opioid systems are also important in prolactin regulation as evidenced by the stimulatory effects of μ- and κ-opioid agonists. The mechanisms of underlying opioid agonist stimulation of prolactin release are not fully understood, but it is likely that opioid agonists reduce tonic dopaminergic inhibition of prolactin release. Several studies suggest that endogenous opioid peptides reduce dopamine turnover and release from the hypothalamic tuberoinfundibular dopamine neurons (120–124). Additional evidence for opioid modulation of the dopaminergic systems that control prolactin comes from a study of the interactions between κ-opioid agonists and dopamine agonists in rhesus monkeys (125). Prolactin stimulation by the κ-opioid agonist,

U69,593 was blocked by dopamine D_2-like agonists (quinpirole and 7-OH-DPAT), but not by a dopamine D_1 agonist, SKF 82958 (125). These findings were consistent with the generally accepted view that the dopamine-sensitive lactotropes in the anterior pituitary have primarily D_2 dopamine receptors (116, 118).

31.4.1 Clinical Studies of Opioid Effects on Prolactin

Opioid agonists selective for μ- and κ-receptors consistently stimulate prolactin release in humans. Administration of a single dose of heroin (10mg, IV) increased plasma prolactin levels to over eight times baseline levels, but after 9 days of heroin self-administration, there was some blunting of the prolactin response to an acute dose of heroin (126). $\text{Dynorphin}_{\text{A1–13}}$ has greater affinity for κ- than for μ-opioid receptors (98, 127). In methadone-maintained subjects, the prolactin response to $\text{dynorphin}_{\text{A1–13}}$ was significantly lower than in normal controls (128). Because methadone alone continues to stimulate prolactin release in long-term methadone-maintained subjects (129), these studies began 1h before methadone administration (128). $\text{Dynorphin}_{\text{A1–13}}$ (120 and 500mcg/kg, IV) administration to healthy volunteers stimulated a greater prolactin response in women than in men (130). The basis for this significant sex difference in prolactin stimulation was not clear. Women had significantly higher baseline prolactin levels than men and menstrual cycle phase was not specified (130). Taken together, these data are consistent with the notion that both short-term and chronic exposure to opioid agonists alter dopaminergic tone, resulting in tonic inhibition of prolactin release (126, 128).

The effects of opioid antagonists on prolactin are inconsistent and are influenced by sex, drug use history, and relative activity at μ- and κ-receptors (41, 47, 126, 128, 130). For example, administration of naltrexone did not significantly alter prolactin levels in opioid-dependent men (126), but naltrexone significantly stimulated prolactin in normal women during the early-follicular phase of the menstrual cycle (39, 41). The long-acting opioid antagonist nalmefene did not increase prolactin in men after oral administration (10mg) (47). IV administration of 3 and 10mg nalmefene increased prolactin levels in the normal men and women, but these effects were not nalmefene dose-dependent (98). No sex differences were detected and menstrual cycle phase was not determined (98). These data were attributed to the fact that nalmefene is a partial agonist at κ-opioid receptors as well as a full antagonist at μ-opioid receptors (98).

Nalbuphine is also a long-acting mixed-action μ-antagonist/κ-agonist analgesic (94, 131). Nalbuphine stimulated prolactin release in abstinent male cocaine abusers (93). Figure 31.7 shows prolactin data from a single subject studied at both a low and a high dose of nalbuphine. It is apparent that prolactin levels were nalbuphine dose-dependent. Peak levels of nalbuphine were detected within 10min after IV administration and prolactin levels increased significantly within 20min and reached peak values after 60min (93). Interpretation of these data is complicated by the fact that the highest dose of nalbuphine was also associated with nega-

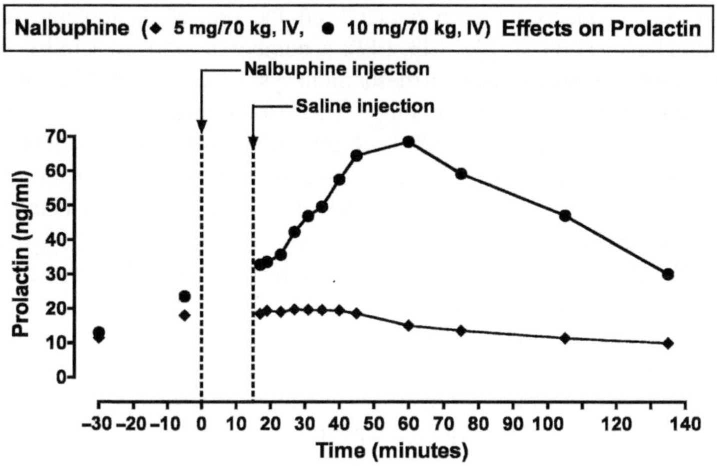

Fig. 31.7 The effects of nalbuphine on prolactin in a male cocaine abuser. *Abscissa*: Time (min) before and after nalbuphine and saline administration. *Ordinate*: Prolactin (ng/ml). The effects of nalbuphine (5 mg/70 kg, IV) are shown as closed diamonds. The effects of nalbuphine (10 mg/70 kg, IV) are shown as closed circles. Reprinted with permission from Goletiani et al. (93)

tive subjective effects and nausea. In healthy normal volunteers, 10 mg/70 kg of morphine and nalbuphine produced similar subjective and physiological effects and were well-tolerated (131–134). However, in men with a history of cocaine abuse, 10 mg/70 kg nalbuphine produced vomiting and sedation (135).

31.4.2 Preclinical Studies of Opioid Effects on Prolactin

A series of studies in nonhuman primates have confirmed and extended clinical reports that both μ- and κ-opioid agonists stimulate prolactin release. μ- and κ-opioid agonists produced similar maximal levels of prolactin release in rhesus monkeys, but a systemically active δ-opioid agonist, SNC-80, did not increase prolactin (136). In contrast, the opioid antagonists naltrexone, nalmefene, and quadazocine did not stimulate prolactin release (49, 53, 137–140). However, there are some exceptions to the general pattern. Nalmefene (0.5–5.09 mg, IV) stimulated prolactin release in gonadally intact but not in ovariectomized rhesus monkeys (141). Naloxone and naltrexone decreased basal prolactin levels after IV administration (49, 142, 143). Under most conditions, naloxone, nalmefene, and quadazocine antagonized the prolactin-stimulating effects of both μ- and κ-opioid agonists as described below. Parallel studies of the effects of κ-antagonists on μ- and κ-stimulation of prolactin have not been possible because short-acting κ-opioid antagonists are not yet available (144, 145).

The μ-opioid agonists morphine and heroin consistently stimulate prolactin release in nonhuman primates (123, 137, 142, 143, 146, 147). The μ-opioid antagonists naloxone, nalmefene, and quadazocine each antagonized the prolactin-stimulating effects of these μ-opioid agonists (137, 142, 143, 147). A number of κ-opioid agonists have been shown to stimulate prolactin release in rhesus monkeys (125, 136, 138–140, 148, 149). For example, the κ-opioid agonists dynorphin$_{A1-17}$, the stable dynorphin$_{A1-8}$ analogue E-2078, salvinorin A, bremazocine, U50, 488, U69, 593, R84, 760, and spiradoline each produced dose-related increases in prolactin levels. Quadazocine antagonized the prolactin-stimulating effects of dynorphin$_{A1-17}$, U69, 593, and E-2078 (138, 139). Naltrexone also antagonized the prolactin-stimulating effects of E-2078 (139), dynorphin$_{A1-17}$, and U69, 593 (136). Similarly, nalmefene antagonized the prolactin-stimulating effects of U50, 488, spiradoline, and salvinorin A (136, 140, 149).

Some studies of μ- and κ-opioid agonist effects on prolactin levels used an innovative cumulative dosing procedure (136–140). In this procedure, several increasing doses of the opioid agonist were administered, and prolactin levels were measured at one or more time points after each dose. Both μ- and κ-opioid agonists produced dose-dependent increases in prolactin under these conditions. One advantage of cumulative-dosing procedures is that a complete drug dose-effect curve can be determined within a single study day. Moreover, when antagonists are used to examine receptor mechanisms that mediate a drug-induced endocrine effect, cumulative dosing procedures are useful to compare the effects of placebo and antagonist treatment. Cumulative dosing procedures are widely used in behavioral pharmacology to study the effects of multiple drug doses in a single session, and these applications suggest the potential usefulness for endocrine studies (85, 134, 137). The alternate procedure, that is, administration of single-drug doses on different days is most appropriate for studies of the time course of drug effects (125, 148).

31.5 Summary of the Effects of Opioid Agonists and Antagonists on the HPG and HPA Axis and Prolactin

The endogenous opioid peptides are involved in regulation of the endocrine systems that control reproduction and responses to stress. These endogenous opioids are one component of a complex regulatory system that includes the neurotransmitters dopamine, CRH, serotonin, acetylcholine, norepinephrine, and epinephrine (150). The endogenous opioid system has primarily inhibitory actions on the HPG and the HPA axis hormones. Accordingly, the opioid antagonists usually stimulate hormone release, in part through antagonism of endogenous opioid inhibition. Opioid agonists usually reduce basal levels of hormones that are under endogenous opioid inhibitory control and attenuate the responses of these hormones to a pharmacological challenge. The specific actions of both opioid agonists and antagonists depend on their relative affinity for μ- and κ-opioid receptors. Considerably less is known about the role of δ-opioid receptors (114, 136).

The HPG and the HPA axes are also under inhibitory feedback control by the gonadal and adrenal target hormones. For example, hypothalamic LHRH stimulation of LH and FSH release may stimulate and be inhibited by the gonadal steroid hormones, estradiol, testosterone, and progesterone. Hypothalamic CRH stimulation of pituitary ACTH release may stimulate and be inhibited by the adrenal steroid hormone cortisol. In contrast, the anterior pituitary hormone prolactin is primarily under inhibitory dopaminergic control by dopamine D_2 receptors. Both μ- and κ- opioid agonists stimulate prolactin release, and μ-opioid antagonists reliably block the prolactin-stimulating effects of μ- and κ- agonists. However, the opioid antagonists alone have inconsistent effects on prolactin depending on their relative activity at μ- and κ-opioid receptors, as well as the sex and drug history of the subject.

The interactions between the endocrine system and the opioid antagonists have led to several health-related applications in clinical endocrinology. Opioid antagonists have been used effectively for the treatment of infertility, hypothalamic amenorrhea, and male impotence. Opioid antagonists have also been used as provocative tests to assess the function of the HPA axis. Dysregulation of this stress-responsive endocrine system is one prominent feature of many affective disorders and may indicate relative risk for substance abuse problems and alcoholism. As more selective opioid antagonists become available, more precise analysis of endocrine regulatory control systems and other clinical applications are likely.

Acknowledgments Preparation of this chapter was supported in part by K05-DA00064, K05-DA00101, and P01-DA14528 from the National Institute on Drug Abuse, NIH. We thank Inge M. Knudson for her excellent assistance in research for this chapter and Rita Head for patient and meticulous preparation of the manuscript.

References

1. Dixon R, Howes J, Gentile J, et al. Nalmefene: Intravenous safety and kinetics of a new opioid antagonist. Clin Pharmacol Ther 1986;39(1):49–53.
2. Anton RF, Pettinati H, Zweben A, et al. A multi-site dose ranging study of nalmefene in the treatment of alcohol dependence. J Clin Psychopharmacol 2004;24(4):421–8.
3. Mason BJ, Ritvo EC, Morgan RO, et al. A double-blind, placebo-controlled pilot study to evaluate the efficacy and safety of oral nalmefene HCl for alcohol dependence. Alcohol Clin Exp Res 1994;18(5):1162–7.
4. Mason BJ, Salvato FR, Williams LD, Ritvo EC, Cutler RB. A double-blind, placebo-controlled study of oral nalmefene for alcohol dependence. Arch Gen Psychiatry 1999;56(8):719–24.
5. Modesto-Lowe V, Van Kirk J. Clinical uses of naltrexone: A review of the evidence. Exp Clin Psychopharm 2002;10:213–27.
6. Mello NK, Mendelson JH, Kuehnle JC, Sellers ML. Operant analysis of human heroin self-administration and the effects of naltrexone. J Pharmacol Exp Ther 1981;216(1):45–54.
7. Meyer RE, Mirin SM. The Heroin Stimulus. New York: Plenum Press; 1979.
8. Jaffe JH, Martin WR. Opioid analgesics and antagonists. In: Gilman AG, Goodman LS, Gilman A, eds. The Pharmacological Basis of Therapeutics, 6th ed. New York: MacMillan Publ. Co., Inc.; 1980:494–534.
9. Martin WR, Jasinski DR, Mansky PA. Naltrexone, an antagonist for the treatment of heroin dependence. Effects in man. Arch Gen Psychiatry 1973;28:784–91.
10. Roth A, Hogan I, Farren C. Naltrexone plus group therapy for the treatment of opiate-abusing health-care professionals. J Subst Abuse Treat 1997;14:19–22.
11. Rothenberg JL, Sullivan MA, Church SH, et al. Behavioral naltrexone therapy: An integrated treatment for opiate dependence. J Subst Abuse Treat 2002;23:351–60.

12. Knobil E. On the control of gonadotropin secretion in the rhesus monkey. Recent Prog Horm Res 1974;30:1–46.
13. Knobil E. The neuroendocrine control of the menstrual cycle. Recent Prog Horm Res 1980; 36:53–88.
14. Crowley WF, Jr., Filicori M, Spratt DI, Santoro NF. The physiology of gonadotropin-releasing hormone (GnRH) secretion in men and women. Recent Prog Horm Res 1985;41:473–526.
15. Santoro N, Filicori M, Crowley J. Hypogonadotropic disorders in men and women: Diagnosis and therapy with pulsatile gonadotropin-releasing hormone. Endocr Rev 1986;7:11–23.
16. Santoro N, Wierman ME, Filicori M. Intravenous administration of pulsatile gonadotropin-releasing hormone in hypothalamic amenorrhea: Effects of dosage. J Clin Endocrinol Metab 1986;62:109–16.
17. Hammond C, Wiebe R, Haney A, Yancy S. Ovulation induction with luteinizing hormone-releasing hormone in amenorrheic infertile women. Am J Obstet Gynecol 1979;135:924–39.
18. Wildt L, Leyendecker G. Induction of ovulation by the chronic administration of naltrexone in hypothalamic amenorrhea. J Clin Endocrinol Metab 1987;64(6):1334–5.
19. Wildt L, Leyendecker G, Sir-Petermann T, Waibel-Treber S. Treatment with naltrexone in hypothalamic ovarian failure: Induction of ovulation and pregnancy. Hum Reprod 1993;8: 350–8.
20. Leyendecker G, Waibel-Treber S, Wildt L. Pulsatile administration of gonadotrophin releasing hormone and oral administration of naltrexone in hypothalamic amenorrhoea. Hum Reprod 1993;8:184–8.
21. Yen SSC, Quigley ME, Reid RL, Ropert JF, Cetel NS. Neuroendocrinology of opioid peptides and their role in the control of gonadotropin and prolactin secretion. Am J Obstet Gynecol 1985;152:485–93.
22. Yen SSC. Neuroendocrinology of reproduction. In: Yen SSC, Jaffe RB, Barbieri RL, eds. Reproductive Endocrinology, 4th ed. Philadelphia, PA: W.B. Saunders Co.; 1999:30–80.
23. Yen SSC. The human menstrual cycle: Neuroendocrine regulation. In: Yen SSC, Jaffe RB, Barbieri RL, eds. Reproductive Endocrinology: Physiology, Pathophysiology, and Clinical Management, 4th ed. Philadelphia: W.B. Saunders Co.; 1999:191–217.
24. Ferin M, Van Vugt D, Wardlaw S. The hypothalamic control of the menstrual cycle and the role of endogenous opioid peptides. Recent Prog Horm Res 1984;40:441–85.
25. Veldhuis JD, Iranmanesh A, Demers LM, Mulligan T. Joint basal and pulsatile hypersecretory mechanisms drive the monotropic follicle-stimulating hormone (FSH) elevation in healthy older men: Concurrent preservation of the orderliness of the FSH release process: A general clinical research center study. J Clin Endocrinol Metab 1999;84(10):3506–14.
26. Veldhuis JD, Iranmanesh A, Mulligan T, Pincus SM. Disruption of the young-adult synchrony between luteinizing hormone release and oscillations in follicle-stimulating hormone, prolactin, and nocturnal penile tumescence (NPT) in healthy older men. J Clin Endocrinol Metab 1999;84(10):3498–505.
27. Wardlaw SL, Thoron L, Frantz AG. Effects of sex steroids on brain beta-endorphin. Brain Res 1982;245:327.
28. Wardlaw SL, Wehrenberg WB, Ferin M, Antunes AL, Franz AG. Effect of sex steroids on beta-endorphin in hypophyseal portal blood. J Clin Endocrinol Metab 1982;55:877.
29. Wehrenberg WB, Wardlaw SL, Franz AG, Ferin M. Beta-endorphin in hypophyseal portal blood: Variations throughout the menstrual cycle. Endocrinology 1982;111:879.
30. Mendelson JE, Meyer RE, Ellingboe J, Mirin SM, McDougle M. Effects of heroin and methadone on plasma cortisol and testosterone. J Pharmacol Exp Ther 1975;195:296–302.
31. Mendelson JH, Mendelson JE, Patch VD. Plasma testosterone levels in heroin addiction and during methadone maintenance. J Pharmacol Exp Ther 1975;192:211–7.
32. Mirin SM, Mendelson JH, Ellingboe J, Meyer RE. Acute effects of heroin and naltrexone on testosterone and gonadotropin secretion: A pilot study. Psychoneuroendocrinology 1976;1:359–69.
33. Mendelson JH, Ellingboe 1, Kuehnle JC, Mello NK. Heroin and naltrexone effects on pituitary-gonadal hormones in man: Interaction of steroid feedback effects, tolerance and supersensitivity. J Pharmacol Exp Ther 1980;214(3):503–6.

34. Mendelson JH, Ellingboe J, Kuehnle JC, Mello NK. Effects of naltrexone on mood and neuroendocrine function in normal adult males. Psychoneuroendocrinology 1979;3:231–6.
35. Braude MC, Morrison JM. Preclinical toxicity studies of naltrexone. NIDA Res Monogr 1976(9):16–26.
36. Ellingboe J, Veldhuis JD, Mendelson JH, Kuehnle JC, Mello NK. Effect of endogenous opioid blockade on the amplitude and frequency of pulsatile luteinizing hormone secretion in normal men. J Clin Endocrinol Metab 1982;54(4):854–7.
37. Mendelson JH, Mello NK, Teoh SK, Ellingboe J. Use of naltrexone for the diagnosis and treatment of reproductive hormone disorders in women. In: LS Harris (ed.) Problems of Drug Dependence 1990. NIDA Research Monograph, No. 105, DHHS Publ. No. (ADM) 91-1753, pp. 161–7. Washington, DC: US Government Printing Office; 1991
38. Rebar RW. Practical evaluation of hormonal status. In: Yen SSC, Jaffe RB, Barbieri RL, eds. Reproductive Endocrinology. Philadelphia: W.B. Saunders Co.; 1999:709–44.
39. Mendelson JH, Mello NK, Cristofaro P, Skupny A, Ellingboe J. Use of naltrexone as a provocative test for hypothalamic-pituitary hormone function. Pharmacol Biochem Behav 1986; 24(2):309–13.
40. Mendelson JH, Mello NK, Teoh SK, Ellingboe J. Use of Naltrexone for the Diagnosis and Treatment of Reproductive Hormone Disorders in Women. Washington, D.C.: U.S. Government Printing Office; 1991.
41. Teoh SK, Mendelson JH, Mello NK, Skupny A. Alcohol effects on naltrexone-induced stimulation of pituitary, adrenal and gonadal hormones during the early follicular phase of the menstrual cycle. J Clin Endocrinol Metab 1988;66:1181–6.
42. Quigley ME, Yen SSC. The role of endogenous opiates on LH secretion during the menstrual cycle. J Clin Endocrinol Metab 1980;51:179–81.
43. Ropert JF, Quigley ME, Yen SS. Endogenous opiates modulate pulsatile luteinizing hormone release in humans. J Clin Endocrinol Metab 1981;52(3):583–5.
44. Verebey K, Volavka J, Mule SJ, Resnick RB. Naltrexone: Disposition, metabolism and effects after acute and chronic dosing. Clin Pharmacol Ther 1976;20:315–28.
45. Rossmanith WG, Monn M, Benz R. Effects of chronic opioid antagonism on gonadotrophin and ovarian sex steroid secretion during the luteal phase. Clin Endocrinol (Oxf) 1998;49(3): 343–51.
46. McArthur JW, Turnbull BA, Pehrson J, et al. Nalmefene enhances LH secretion in a proportion of oligo-amenorrheic athletes. Acta Endocrinol (Copenh) 1993;128(4):325–33.
47. Graves GR, Kennedy TG, Weick RF, Casper RF. The effect of nalmefene on pulsatile secretion of luteinizing hormone and prolactin in men. Hum Reprod 1993;8(10):1598–603.
48. Billington CJ, Shafer RB, Morley JE. Effects of opioid blockade with nalmefene in older impotent men. Life Sci 1990;47(9):799–805.
49. Mello NK, Mendelson JH, Bree MP, Skupny A. Naltrexone effects on pituitary and gonadal hormones in male and female rhesus monkeys. Pharmacol Biochem Behav 1989;31:683–91.
50. Plant TM. A striking sex difference in the gonadotropin response to gonadectomy during infantile development in the rhesus monkey (Macaca mulatta). Endocrinology 1986;119:539–45.
51. Hahn EF, Fishman J, Heilman RD. Narcotic antagonists 4. Carbon-6 derivative of N-substituted noroxymorphones as narcotic antagonists. J Med Chem 1975;18:259–62.
52. Gal TJ, DiFazio CA. Prolonged antagonism of opioid action with intravenous nalmefene in man. Anesthesiology 1986;64(2):175–80.
53. Mello NK, Mendelson JH, Kelly M. Acute effects of nalmefene on LH, prolactin, and testosterone in male rhesus monkeys. Pharmacol Biochem Behav 2000;66:275–84.
54. Crowley WF. Role of endogenous opioid peptides in the physiological regulation of luteinizing hormone and prolactin secretion. In: Negro-Vilar A, Conn PM, eds. Peptide Hormones: Effects and Mechanisms of Action. Boca Raton, FL: CRC Press; 1988:79–118.
55. Veldhuis JD, Rogol AD, Johnson ML. Endogenous opiates modulate the pulsatile secretion of biologically active luteinizing hormone in man. J Clin Invest 1983;72:2031–40.
56. Chrousos GP, Gold PW. The concepts of stress and stress system disorders: Overview of physical and behavioral homeostasis. JAMA 1992;267:1244–52.

57. Tsigos C, Chrousos G. Hypothalamic-pituitary-adrenal axis, neuroendocrine factors and stress. J Psychosom Res 2002;53:865–71.
58. Gindoff PR, Ferin M. Endogenous opioid peptides modulate the effect of corticotropin-releasing factor on gonadotropin release in the primate. Endocrinology 1987;121(3):837–42.
59. Pfeiffer A, Herz A. Endocrine actions of opioids. Horm Metab Res 1984;16(8):386–97.
60. Allolio B, Schulte HM, Deuss U, Kallabis D, Hamel E, Winkelman W. Effect of oral morphine and naloxone on pituitary-adrenal response in man induced by human corticotropin-releasing hormone. Acta Endocrinol (Copenh) 1987;114(4):509–14.
61. Grossman A. Brain opiates and neuroendocrine function. Clin Endocrinol Metab 1983;12(3): 725–46.
62. Rittmaster RS, Cutler GB, Sobel DO, et al. Morphine inhibits the pituitary-adrenal response to ovine corticotropin-releasing hormone in normal subjects. J Clin Endocrinol Metab 1985;60:891–5.
63. Mello NK, Mendelson JH. Cocaine, hormones and behavior: Clinical and preclinical studies. In: Pfaff DW, Arnold AP, Etgen AM, Fahrbach SE, Rubin RT, eds. Hormones, Brain and Behavior. New York: Academic Press; 2002:665–745.
64. Mendelson JH, Sholar MB, Goletiani NV, Siegel AJ, Mello NK. Effects of low and high nicotine cigarette smoking on mood states and the HPA axis in men. Neuropsychopharmacology 2005;30:1751–63.
65. Heit S, Ownes MJ, Plotsky P, Nemeroff CB. Corticotropin-releasing factor, stress, and depression. Neuroscientist 1997;3:186–94.
66. Holsboer D. F. The corticosteroid receptor hypothesis of depression. Neuropsychopharmacology 2000;23(5):477–501.
67. Nemeroff CB. Psychopharmacology of affective disorders in the 21st century. Biol Psychiatry 1998;44(7):517–25.
68. Rupprecht R, Holsboer D. F. Neuroactive steroids: Mechanisms of action and neuropsychopharmacological perspectives. Trends Neurosci 1999;22:410–6.
69. Rupprecht R, Holsboer DF. Neuropsychopharmacological properties of neuroactive steroids. Steroids 1999;64:83–91.
70. Parker KJ, Schatzberg AF, Lyons DM. Neuroendocrine aspects of hypercortisolism in major depression. Horm Behav 2003;43(1):60–6.
71. Koob GF, Le Moal M. Drug addiction, dysregulation of reward, and allostasis. Neuropsychopharmacology 2001;24(2):97–129.
72. Kreek MJ, Koob GF. Drug dependence: Stress and dysregulation of brain reward pathways. Drug Alcohol Depend 1998;51:23–47.
73. Marinelli M, Piazza PV. Interaction between glucocorticoid hormones, stress and psychostimulant drugs. Eur J Neurosci 2002;16(3):387–94.
74. Sinha R. How does stress increase risk of drug abuse and relapse? Psychopharmacology (Berl) 2001;158(4):343–59.
75. Hernandez-Avila CA, Oncken C, Van Kirk J, Wand G, Kranzler HR. Adrenocorticotropin and cortisol responses to a naloxone challenge and risk of alcoholism. Biol Psychiatry 2002;51(8):652–8.
76. Wand GS, Mangold D, El Deiry S, McCaul ME, Hoover D. Family history of alcoholism and hypothalamic opioidergic activity. Arch Gen Psychiatry 1998;55:1114–9.
77. Wand GS, Mangold D, Ali M, Giggey P. Adrenocortical responses and family history of alcoholism. Alcohol Clin Exp Res 1999;23:1185–90.
78. Wand GS, Mangold D, Ali M. Adrenocorticotropin responses to naloxone in sons of alcohol-dependent men. J Clin Endocrinol Metab 1999;84:61–8.
79. Wand G, McCaul ME, Gotjen D, Reynolds J, Lee S. Confirmation that offspring from families with alcohol-dependent individuals have greater hypothalamic-pituitary-adrenal axis activation induced by naloxone compared with offspring without a family history of alcohol dependence. Alcohol Clin Exp Res 2001;25(8):1134–9.
80. Brady KT, Sinha R. Co-occurring mental and substance use disorders: The neurobiological effects of chronic stress. Am J Psychiatry 2005;162(8):1483–93.
81. Contoreggi C, Herning RI, Na P, et al. Stress hormone responses to corticotropin-releasing hormone in substance abusers with severe comorbid psychiatric disease. Biol Psychiatry 2003; 54:873–8.

82. Volkow ND. Drug abuse and mental illness: Progress in understanding comorbidity. Am J Psychiatry 2001;158(8):1181–3.
83. Gold PW, Goodwin FK, Chrousos GP. Clinical and biomedical manifestations of depression: Relationship to the neurobiology of stress (Part II). N Engl J Med 1988;319:413–20.
84. Burnett FE, Scott LV, Weaver MG, Medbak SH, Dinan TG. The effect of naloxone on adrenocorticotropin and cortisol release: Evidence for a reduced response in depression. J Affect Disord 1999;53(3):263–8.
85. Mangold D, McCaul ME, Ali M, Wand GS. Plasma adrenocorticotropin responses to opioid blockade with naloxone: Generating a dose-response curve in a single session. Biol Psychiatry 2000;48(4):310–4.
86. Volavka J, Cho D, Mallya A, Bauman J. Naloxone increases ACTH and cortisol levels in man. N Engl J Med 1979;300:1056–7.
87. O'Malley SS, Jaffe AJ, Chang G, Scottenfeld RS, Meyer RE, Rounsaville B. Naltrexone and coping skills therapy for alcohol dependence. A controlled study. Arch Gen Psychiatry 1992;49:881–7.
88. Volpicelli JR, Alterman AI, Hayashida M, O'Brien CP. Naltrexone in the treatment of alcohol dependence. Arch Gen Psychiatry 1992;49:876–80.
89. Farren CK, O'Malley S, Grebski G, Maniar S, Porter M, Kreek MJ. Variable dose naltrexone-induced hypothalamic-pituitary-adrenal stimulation in abstinent alcoholics: A preliminary study. Alcohol Clin Exp Res 1999;23:502–8.
90. O'Malley SS, Krishnan-Sarin S, Farren C, Sinha R, Kreek MJ. Naltrexone decreases craving and alcohol self-administration in alcohol-dependent subjects and activates the hypothalamo-pituitary-adrenocortical axis. Psychopharmacology 2002; 160:19–29.
91. Morley J. Neuroendocrine effects of endogenous opioid peptides in human subjects: A review. Psychoneuroendocrinology 1983;8:361–79.
92. Schluger JH, Ho A, Borg L, Porter, M., Maniar S, Gunduz M, Perret G, King A and Kreek MV. Nalmefene causes greater hypothalamic-pituitary-adrenal axis activation than naloxone in normal volunteers: Implications for the treatment of alcoholism. Alcohol Clin Exp Res 1998;22:1430–6.
93. Goletiani NV, Mendelson JH, Sholar MB, Siegel AJ, Skupny A, Mello NK (2008). Effects of nalbuphine on anterior pituitary and adrenal hormones and subjective responses in male cocaine abusers. Pharmacol Biochem Behav 2007;86:667–677.
94. Jaffe JH, Martin WR. Opioid analgesics and antagonists. In: Gilman AG, Rall TW, Nies AS, Taylor P, eds. The Pharmacological Basis of Therapeutics. New York: Pergamon Press; 1990: 485–521.
95. Preston KL, Jasinski DR. Abuse liability studies of opioid agonist-antagonists in humans. Drug Alcohol Depend 1991;28(1):49–82.
96. Emmerson PJ, Clark MJ, Mansour A, Akil H, Woods JH, Medzihradsky F. Characterization of opioid agonist efficacy in a C_6 glioma cell line expressing the μ opioid receptor. J Pharmacol Exp Ther 1996;278:1121–7.
97. Gharagozlou P, Demirci H, David Clark J, Lameh J. Activity of opioid ligands in cells expressing cloned mu opioid receptors. BMC Pharmacol 2003;3:1.
98. Bart G, Schluger JH, Borg L, Ho A, Bidlack JM, Kreek MJ. Nalmefene induced elevation in serum prolactin in normal human volunteers: Partial kappa opioid agonist activity? Neuropsychopharmacology 2005;30(12):2254–62.
99. Michel ME, Bolger G, Weissman BA. Binding of a new opiate antagonist, nalmefene, to rat brain membranes. Methods Find Exp Clin Pharmacol 1985;7(4):175–7.
100. Geer EB, Landman RE, Wardlaw SL, Conwell IM, Freda PU. Stimulation of the hypothalamic-pituitary-adrenal axis with the opioid antagonist nalmefene. Pituitary 2005;8(2):115–22.
101. Chrousos GP, Gold PW. A healthy body in a healthy mind - and vice versa - the damaging power of "uncontrollable" stress. J Clin Endocrinol Metab 1998;83(6):1842–5.
102. Heinrichs SC, Menzaghi F, Merlo Pich PE, Britton KT, Koch GF. The role of CRF in behavioral aspects of stress. Ann N Y Acad Sci 1995;771(1):92–104.
103. Iranmanesh A, Lizarralde G, Short E, Veldhuis JD. Intensive venous sampling paradigms disclose high frequency adrenocorticotropin release episodes in normal men. J Clin Endocrinol Metab 1990;71:1276–83.

104. Sarnyai Z, Veldhuis JD, Mello NK, Mendelson, JH, Erös-Sarnyai M, Mercer G, Gelles H, Kelly M (1995). The concordance of pulsatile ultradian release of ACTH and cortisol in male rhesus monkeys. J Clin Endocrinol Metab 80:54–9.
105. Veldhuis JD, Johnson ML. Cluster analysis: A simple, versatile and robust algorithm for endocrine pulse detection. Am J Physiol 1986;250:E486–93.
106. Carnes M, Kalin NH, Lent SJ, Barksdale CM, Brownfield MS. Pulsatile ACTH secretion in rhesus monkeys: Variation with time of day and relationship to cortisol. Peptides 1988;9:325–31.
107. Kalin NH. ACTH in plasma and CSF in the rhesus monkey. Biol Psychiatry 1986;21(2): 124–40.
108. Leshner A, Toivola P, Terasawa E. Circadian variations in cortisol concentrations in the plasma of female rhesus monkeys. J Endocrinol 1978;78:155–66.
109. Smith CJ, Norman RL. Circadian periodicity in circulating cortisol is absent after orchidectomy in rhesus macaques. Endocrinology 1987;121(6):2186–91.
110. Sarnyai Z, Mello NK, Mendelson JH, Nguyen P, Erös-Sarnyai M. Effects of cocaine and corticotropin-releasing factor (CRF) on pulsatile ACTH and cortisol release in ovariectomized rhesus monkeys. J Clin Endocrinol Metab 1995;80(9):2745–51.
111. Broadbear JH, Winger G, Cicero TJ, Woods JH. Effects of self-administered cocaine on plasma adrenocorticotropic hormone and cortisol in male rhesus monkeys. J Pharmacol Exp Ther 1999;289:1641–7.
112. Broadbear JH, Winger G, Cicero TJ, Woods JH. Effects of response contingent and non-contingent cocaine injection on hypothalamic-pituitary-adrenal activity in rhesus monkeys. J Pharmacol Exp Ther 1999;290(1):393–402.
113. Sarnyai Z, Mello NK, Mendelson JH, Eros-Sarnyai M, Mercer G. Effects of cocaine on pulsatile activity of the hypothalamic-pituitary-adrenal axis in male rhesus monkeys: Neuroendocrine and behavioral correlates. J Pharmacol Exp Ther 1996;277(1):225–34.
114. Williams KL, Holden Ko MC, Rice KC, Woods JH. Effect of opioid receptor antagonists on hypothalamic-pituitary-adrenal activity in rhesus monkeys. Psychoneuroendocrinology 2003;28:513–28.
115. Yen SSC. Studies of the role of dopamine in the control of prolactin and gonadotropin secretion in humans. In: Fuxe K, Hokfelt T, Luft R, eds. Central Regulation of the Endocrine System. New York: Plenum Press; 1979:387–416.
116. Yen SSC, Jaffe RB. Prolactin in human reproduction. In: Yen SSC, Jaffe, R. B., Barbieri, R. L., ed. Reproductive Endocrinology: Physiology, Pathophysiology, and Clinical Management. 4th ed. Philadelphia: W.B. Saunders Co.; 1999:257–83.
117. Sarkar DK, Gottschall PE, Meites J, et al. Uptake and release of [3H] dopamine by the median eminence: Evidence for presynaptic dopaminergic receptors and for dopaminergic feedback inhibition. Neuroscience 1983;10(3):821–30.
118. Ben-Jonathan N. Dopamine: A prolactin-inhibiting hormone. Endocr Rev 1985;6(4):564–89.
119. Mello NK, Mendelson JH, Drieze JH, Teoh SK, Kelly ML, Sholar JW. Effects of dopamine on prolactin: Interactions with cocaine self-administration by female rhesus monkeys. J Pharmacol Exp Ther 1994;270(3):1110–20.
120. Annunziato L. Regulation of the tuberoinfundibular and nigrostriatal systems; evidence for different kinds of dopaminergic neurons in the brain. Neuroendocrinology 1979;29: 66–76.
121. Demarest KT, Moore KE. Disruption of 5-hydroxytryptaminergic neuronal functions blocks the action of morphine on tuberoinfundibular dopaminergic neurons. Life Sci 1981; 28:1345–51.
122. Van Loon GR, Ho D, Kim C. b-Endorphin-induced decrease in hypothalamic dopamine turnover. Endocrinology 1980;106:76–80.
123. Wehrenberg WB, McNicol D, Wardlaw SL, Frantz AG, Ferin M. Dopaminergic and serotonergic involvement in opiate-induced prolactin release in monkeys. Endocrinology 1981; 109:544–7.
124. Wilkes MM, Yen SSC. Augmentation by naloxone of efflux of GnRH from superfused medial basal hypothalamus. Life Sci 1980;28:2355–60.

125. Butelman ER, Kreek MJ. Kappa-opioid receptor agonist-induced prolactin release in primates is blocked by dopamine D(2)-like receptor agonists. Eur J Pharmacol 2001; 423(2–3):243–9.
126. Ellingboe J, Mendelson JH, Kuehnle JC. Effects of heroin and naltrexone on plasma prolactin levels in man. Pharmacol Biochem Behav 1980;12:163–5.
127. Mansour A, Fox CA, Akil H, Watson SJ. Opioid-receptor mRNA expression in the rat CNS: Anatomical and functional implications. Trends Neurosci 1995;18:22–9.
128. Bart G, Borg L, Schluger JH, Green M, Ho A, Kreek MJ. Suppressed prolactin response to dynorphin A1–13 in methadone-maintained versus control subjects. J Pharmacol Exp Ther 2003;306(2):581–7.
129. Kreek MJ. Medical complications in methadone patients. In: Kissin B, Lowinson J, Millman R, eds. Recent Developments in Chemotherapy of Narcotic Addiction. New York: Ann. Acad. Sci.; 1978:110–34.
130. Kreek MJ, Schluger J, Borg L, Gunduz M, Ho A. Dynorphin A1–13 causes elevation of serum levels of prolactin through an opioid receptor mechanism in humans: Gender differences and implications for modulation of dopaminergic tone in the treatment of addictions. J Pharmacol Exp Ther 1999;288(1):260–9.
131. PDR. Physicians Desk Reference, 57th ed. Montvale, NJ: Thomson PDR; 2003.
132. Errick JK, Heel RC. Nalbuphine: A preliminary review of its pharmacological properties and therapeutic efficacy. Drugs 1983;26:191–211.
133. Zacny JP, Conley K, Galinkin J. Comparing the subjective, psychomotor and physiological effects of intravenous buprenorphine and morphine in healthy volunteers. J Pharmacol Exp Ther 1997;282(3):1187–97.
134. Walker DJ, Zacny JP, Galva KE, Lichtor JL. Subjective psychomotor, and physiological effects of cumulative doses of mixed-action opioids in healthy volunteers. Psychopharmacology 2001;155:362–71.
135. Mello NK, Mendelson JH, Sholar MB, Jaszyna-Gasior M, Goletiani NV, Siegel AJ. Effects of the mixed mu/kappa opioid nalbuphine on cocaine-induced changes in subjective and cardiovascular responses in men. Neuropsychopharmacology 2005;30:618–32.
136. Butelman ER, Ball JW, Kreek MJ. Comparison of the discriminative and neuroendocrine effects of centrally penetrating kappa-opioid agonists in rhesus monkeys. Psychopharmacology (Berl) 2002;164(1):115–20.
137. Bowen CA, Negus SS, Kelly M, Mello NK. The effects of heroin on prolactin levels in male rhesus monkeys: Use of cumulative-dosing procedures. Psychoneuroendocrinology 2002;27:319–36.
138. Butelman ER, Harris TJ, Perez A, Kreek MJ. Effects of systemically administered dynorphin A(1–17) in rhesus monkeys. J Pharmacol Exp Ther 1999;290(2):678–86.
139. Butelman ER, Harris TJ, Kreek MJ. Effects of E-2078, a stable dynorphin A(1–8) analog, on sedation and serum prolactin levels in rhesus monkeys. Psychopharmacology (Berl) 1999; 147(1):73–80.
140. Butelman ER, Harris TJ, Kreek MJ. Apparent efficacy of k-opioid receptor ligands on serum prolactin levels in rhesus monkeys. Eur J Pharmacol 1999;383:304–9.
141. Van Vugt DA, Webb MY, Reid RL. Naloxone antagonism of corticotropin-releasing hormone stimulation of prolactin secretion in rhesus monkeys. J Clin Endocrinol Metab 1989;68(6):1060–6.
142. Gilbeau PM, Almirrez RG, Holaday JW, Smith CG. Opioid effects on plasma concentrations of luteinizing hormone and prolactin in the adult male rhesus monkey. J Clin Endocrinol Metab 1985;60:299–305.
143. Gold MS, Redmond DE, Jr., Donabedian RK. The effects of opiate agonist and antagonist on serum prolactin in primates: Possible role for endorphins in prolactin regulation. Endocrinology 1979;105:284–9.
144. Butelman ER, Negus SS, Ai Y, de Costa BR, Woods JH. Kappa opioid antagonist effects of systemically administered nor-binaltorphimine (nor-BNI) in a thermal antinociception assay in rhesus monkeys. J Pharmacol Exp Ther 1993;257:1269–76.

145. Negus SS, Mello NK, Linsenmayer DC, Jones RM, Portoghese PS. Kappa opioid antagonist effects of the novel kappa antagonist 5′-guanidinonaltrindole (GNTI) in an assay of schedule-controlled behavior in rhesus monkeys. Psychopharmacology 2002;163:412–9.
146. Belchetz PE, Ridley RM, Baker HF. Studies of the accessibility of prolactin and growth hormone to brain: Effect of opiate agonists on hormone levels in serial, simultaneous plasma and cerebrospinal fluid samples in the rhesus monkey. Brain Res 1982;239:310–4.
147. Van Vugt DA, Webb MY, Reid RL. Comparison of the duration of action of nalmefene and naloxone on the hypothalamic-pituitary axis of the rhesus monkey. Neuroendocrinology 1989;49(3):275–80.
148. Butelman ER, Ball JW, Kreek MJ. Peripheral selectivity and apparent efficacy of dynorphins: Comparison to non-peptidic kappa-opioid agonists in rhesus monkeys. Psychoneuroendocrinology 2004;29(3):307–26.
149. Butelman ER, Mandau M, Tidgewell K, Prisinzano TE, Yuferov V, Kreek MJ. Effects of salvinorin A, a kappa-opioid hallucinogen, on a neuroendocrine biomarker assay in nonhuman primates with high kappa-receptor homology to humans. J Pharmacol Exp Ther 2007; 320(1):300–6.
150. Yen SSC, Jaffe RB, Barbieri RL. Reproductive Endocrinology: Physiology, Pathophysiology and Clinical Management, 4th ed, pp. 839. Philadelphia: W.B. Saunders; 1999.

Chapter 32
Opioid Antagonists in Traumatic Shock: Animal and Human Studies

Liangming Liu

Abstract Since the opioid antagonist, naloxone, was found to be beneficial in reducing the effects of traumatic shock in 1978, a series of work on the roles of endogenous opioid peptides (EOPs) and their antagonists in circulatory shock was conducted. It was demonstrated that EOPs played very important roles in the pathogenesis of circulatory shock. Naloxone, naltrexone, and nalbuphine had positive effect on many types of shock, such as hemorrhagic and endotoxic shock. But these opioid antagonists are not highly selective for specific opioid receptor subtypes. Because they can act on μ-opioid receptors to affect the pain threshold of shock patients, their application has been greatly limited, especially for traumatic shock. To solve this issue, many laboratories studied the type of shock associated with opioid receptors, and attempted to use their specific receptor antagonists to treat them. Research showed thyrotropin-releasing hormone (TRH), a physiological opioid antagonist, and δ- and κ-opioid receptor antagonists ICI 174,864 and nor-binaltorphimine (nor-BNI) have good beneficial effect on shock parameters without affecting the pain threshold of traumatic shock victims.

Keywords: Naloxone; Naltrexone; Nalbuphine; ICI 174,864; Nor-BNI; Antishock; Hemodynamics; Hemorrhagic; Endotoxic

32.1 Introduction

Endogenous opioid peptides (EOPs) consist of enkephalins, endorphins, and dynorphins. They are extensively distributed in the central nervous system and peripheral tissues such as gastrointestinal tract, pancreas, adrenal medulla, sympathetic ganglion, and so on (1, 2). A great deal of research demonstrated that EOPs take part in the regulation of cardiovascular function. The main evidence includes the location

L. Liu
State Key Laboratory of Trauma, Burns and Combined Injury, Research Institute of Surgery, Daping Hospital, The Third Military Medical University, Chongqing 400042, P.R.China
e-mail: liuliangming2002@yahoo.com

of EOPs neuron in central nervous system; their signal pathway is consistent with the antagonistic system that regulates the cardiovascular system; and central and peripheral administration of EOPs produce potential cardiovascular effects (3, 4).

Since Holaday and Faden first reported in 1978 that the opioid antagonist, naloxone, could reverse endotoxic shock, a large amount of research on the role of EOPs in circulatory shock and the antishock effect of opioid antagonists has been conducted (5). It was demonstrated that EOPs played very important roles in the pathogenesis of circulatory shock (6–13). Naloxone, naltrexone, and nalbuphine had beneficial effects in many types of shock such as hemorrhagic and endotoxic shock (6, 9, 10). These opioid antagonists are not highly selective for specific opioid receptor subtypes. They can act on μ-opioid receptor to affect the pain threshold of shock patients while they exert their antishock effects (11, 14, 15). Thus, their application has been greatly limited, especially for traumatic shock.

Traumatic shock, a common clinical syndrome, is often seen in civilian and military situations. It is the major cause of the early death of severely injured patients. The literature shows that it accounts for about 50% of the deaths of battle personnel (16, 17). However, there are no good approaches for its treatment except for fluid resuscitation and organ function support (18, 19). As the research progresses on the pathophysiology of shock, many antishock agents such as calcium channel antagonists (20), the scavenger of oxygen-derived free radicals (21, 22), and opioid receptor antagonists were found (23–25). Among these agents, the opioid receptor antagonists, naloxone, naltrexone, and nalbuphine, expressed a better effect. As mentioned above, however, these opioid receptor antagonists are not highly selective to the different subclasses of opioid receptors. They may antagonize μ-opioid receptors to affect the pain threshold while they antagonize δ- and κ-opioid receptors to exert the antishock effect. Thus, they are not suitable for traumatic shock (11). Therefore, it is very important to elucidate the subtype of opioid receptors involved in the pathogenesis of traumatic shock and to look for their specific antagonists to treat this type of shock. A series of work on this issue has been performed in our laboratory in recent years.

32.2 Role of β-Endorphin in Cardiovascular Function and Immune Depression Following Traumatic Shock

32.2.1 Role of β-Endorphin in Cardiovascular Depression Following Traumatic Shock

The changes of plasma β-endorphin concentration following traumatic shock in rabbits and its role in the cardiovascular depression were investigated in our lab (26). Traumatic shock of rabbits was induced by fracturing the right femur and inducing hemorrhaged to a mean arterial blood pressure (MAP) of 50 mmHg for 45 min. The results indicated that plasma β-endorphin was significantly increased following

Table 32.1 The changes of β-endorphin and hemodynamics following traumatic shock in rabbits (mean ± SD)

	Baseline	Following traumatic shock (min) 0	45	90	180	300
β-EP (ng/L)	69 ± 21	200 ± 52**	94 ± 17	121 ± 25**	215 ± 57**	321 ± 92**
MAP (mmHg)	99.0 ± 11.2	49.5 ± 1.5**	64.5 ± 3.75**	59.2 ± 4.5**	47.2 ± 12.0**	35.2 ± 8.25**
LVSP (mmHg)	157.5 ± 11.2	75.5 ± 7.5**	105.1 ± 12.7**	97.5 ± 8.2**	84.7 ± 12.0**	73.5 ± 24.7**
V_{pm} (1/s)	10.3 ± 2.9	6.3 ± 1.0**	8.0 ± 2.1**	7.6 ± 2.6**	6.2 ± 1.3**	5.0 ± 1.2**
L_0	211.9 ± 57.5	60.8 ± 10.6**	69.4 ± 12.5**	49.7 ± 11.8**	41.2 ± 16.3**	26.8 ± 22.1**
$+dp/dt_{max}$ (mmHg/s)	11,407 ± 2,227.5	5,167 ± 667.5**	6,202 ± 997.5**	4,815 ± 1,125**	4,192 ± 1,222.5**	2,692 ± 1,267.1
$-dp/dt_{max}$ (mmHg/s)	7,402 ± 127.5	3,472 ± 900.2**	4470 ± 1,335.3**	3,667 ± 1,425.5**	3,075 ± 1,117.2**	2,325 ± 682.2**

Traumatic shock was induced by smashed right femur fracture and hemorrhaged to a MAP of 50mmHg for 45min. Zero minute following shock means the end of the hypotensive period

**$P < 0.01$ as compared with baseline

β-EP β-endorphin, *MAP* mean arterial blood pressure, *LVSP* left intraventricular systolic pressure, V_{pm} the maximal physiological velocity, L_0 the area of p – dp/dt vector loop, $\pm dp/d_{tmax}$ the maximal rate of left intraventricular pressure rise or decline

traumatic shock and it was negatively correlated with the decreased hemodynamics (Table 32.1). Intracerebral ventricular (i.c.v.) administration of β-endorphin antiserum could reverse traumatic shock-induced decreased hemodynamics (Table 32.2). It was suggested that β-endorphin was involved in cardiovascular depression following traumatic shock.

32.2.2 *Role of β-Endorphin in Immune Depression Following Traumatic Shock in Rats*

Since EOPs had been discovered over 20 years ago, people have gradually realized that EOPs play important roles not only in analgesia and cardiovascular regulation but also in the regulation of the immune function (27, 28). Animal and human studies demonstrated that the immune function of the host is depressed following severe trauma or shock, but the mechanism for the depression of the immune function after trauma and shock is not clear. Basic research demonstrated that the self stability of the immune system is, except for depending on the mutual regulation of immune cells and humoral factors, also depends on the balance of the neuroendocrine-immune network. EOPs (mainly β-endorphin), as a neuromodulator, exert important regulatory effects on the neuro-endocrine-immune network. Following trauma, shock, or surgical operation, the endogenous opioid system is activated; pituitary and immune cells synthesize and increase release of

Table 32.2 Effects of β-endorphin antiserum on hemodynamics following traumatic shock in rabbits

Index	Group	*N*	Baseline	End of shock	Time after administration of β-EP antiserum (min)				
					5	30	90	180	300
MAP (mmHg)	I	11	94.5 ± 11.3	49.5 ± 1.5	52.5 ± 5.3	54.8 ± 9.8	51.2 ± 17.3	41.3 ± 27.8	23.3 ± 22.5
	II	9	104.3 ± 9.8	49.5 ± 1.5	89.3 ± 8.3**	75.8 ± 9.0**	67.5 ± 15**	55.5 ± 24**	44.3 ± 41.3
LVSP (mmHg)	I	11	154.5 ± 13.5	96.0 ± 7.5	93.8 ± 18.8	93.8 ± 18.8	89.3 ± 20.3	57.8 ± 38.3	393 ± 38.3
	II	9	150.2 ± 30	96.8 ± 18	117.8 ± 26.30*	117.8 ± 21.0*	102.8 ± 21.0*	88.5 ± 39.0*	91.5 ± 21.8*
$+dp/dt_{max}$ (mmHg/s)	I	11	12,262 ± 3,720	5,677 ± 2,010	5,535 ± 1,747	5,160 ± 2,400	4,785 ± 2,497	3,045 ± 2,250	1,710 ± 3,022
	II	9	12,600 ± 2,902	6,397 ± 1,462	8,790 ± 1,860**	7,522 ± 1,905**	6,480 ± 2,437	5,377 ± 3,315	3,780 ± 3,532
$-dp/dt_{max}$ (mmHg/s)	I	11	6,877 ± 885	3,885 ± 907	3,420 ± 510	3,195 ± 1,050	3,240 ± 967	2,437.5 ± 1,635	1,050 ± 1,432
	II	9	7,500 ± 2,250	3,690 ± 780	5,660 ± 1,462**	4,890 ± 1,350**	4,935 ± 2,287**	3,742 ± 1,830*	3,097 ± 2,760*
L_o	I	11	151 ± 41	64 ± 21	63 ± 19	57 ± 27	54 ± 47	27 ± 24	19 ± 34
	II	9	179 ± 45	64 ± 27	156 ± 56**	105 ± 44**	85 ± 48	48 ± 16	57 ± 45

Traumatic shock was induced by smashed right femur fracture and hemorrhaged to a MAP of 50 mmHg for 45 min. End of shock means the end of the hypotensive period. I control group II β-endorphin antiserum group.

*$P < 0.05$; **$P < 0.01$ as compared with baseline

β-EP β-endorphin, *MAP* mean arterial blood pressure, *LVSP* left intraventricular systolic pressure, L_o the area of $p - dp/dt$ vector loop, $\pm dp/dt_{max}$ the maximal rate of left intraventricular pressure rise or decline

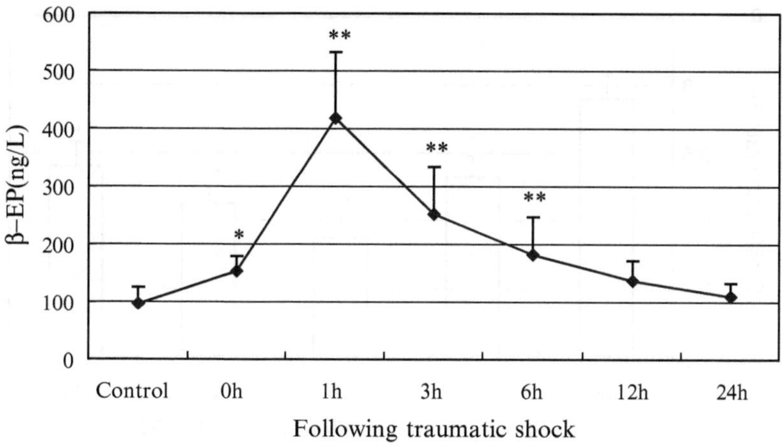

Fig. 32.1 Changes of plasma β-endorphin following traumatic shock in rats. Traumatic shock was induced by crushing right femur fracture and hemorrhaged to a mean arterial blood pressure (*MAP*) of 40 mmHg for 60 min, at the end of hypotensive period, the shed blood was reinfused. $n = 10$, *β-EP* β-endorphine; *$P < 0.05$; **$P < 0.01$ versus control group

β-endorphin, resulting in the increase of β-endorphin in plasma. Regarding the role of β-endorphin in immune depression following traumatic shock, it was previously presumed based mainly from the correlation analyses for changes in β-endorphin and immune function. But, it lacks direct evidence.

With traumatic shock rats, we observed the changes of plasma β-endorphin following shock and its effects on concanavalin A (con A)-induced spleen cell proliferation, IL-2 production, and IL-2 receptor (IL-2R) expression. It was found that plasma β-endorphin was significantly increased following traumatic shock (Fig. 32.1). It peaked up at 1 h and returned to the baseline at 24 h after shock, which was consistent with the report of Levy and Nerlich (29, 30). The plasma from shock rats significantly suppressed con A-induced proliferation of spleen cell from normal rats and suppress IL-2 production and IL-2R expression (Figs. 32.2a and 32.3). Plasma from shock rats pretreated with β-endorphin antiserum or inactivated, however, could not suppress con A-induced proliferation of spleen cell and the production and expression of IL-2 and IL-2R (Figs. 32.2b and 32.4). The results directly demonstrated that β-endorphin was involved in the immune depression following traumatic shock (31, 32).

32.3 Opioid Receptors Associated with Traumatic Shock

Since the opioid receptor was first found in 1973, six subtypes of opioid receptors have since been identified. They are μ, δ, κ, ε, σ, and γ. Studies showed that not all subtypes of opioid receptors are involved in the cardiovascular depression of

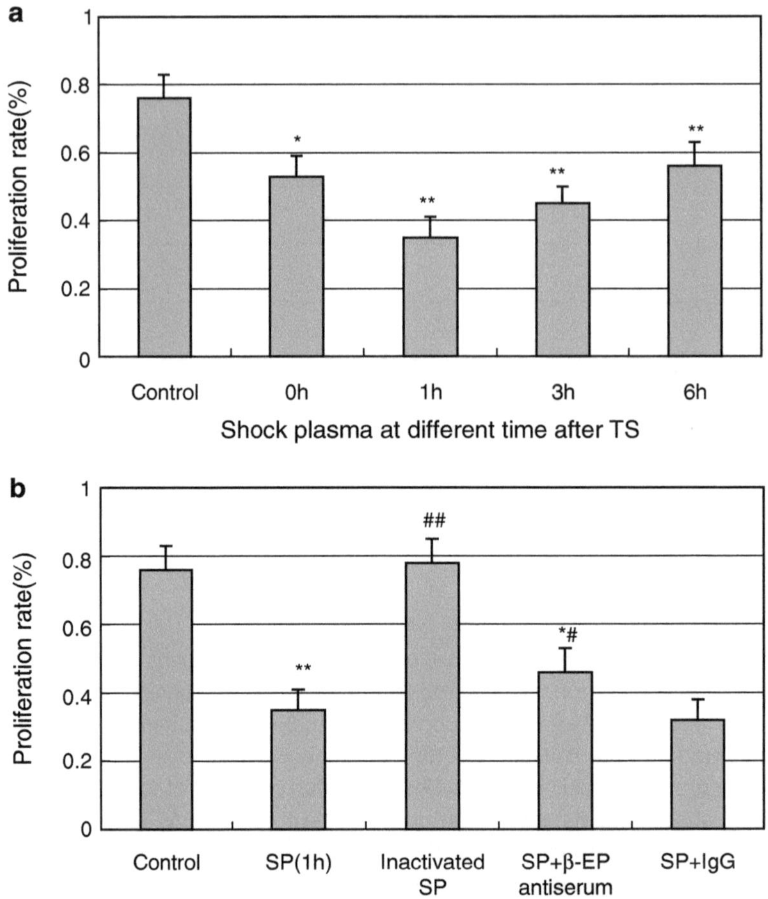

Fig. 32.2 Effect of shock plasma (**a**) and plasma pretreated with β-endorphin antiserum or inactivated (**b**) on concanavalin A (*conA*)-induced spleen cell proliferation of rats. *TS* trauma shock, *SP* shock plasma; $*P < 0.05$; $**P < 0.01$ versus control group; $^{\#}P < 0.05$; $^{\#\#}P < 0.01$ versus SP group

shock. Different types of shock may involve different subtypes of opioid receptors. No consistent conclusion about which opioid receptors participate in the pathogenesis of shock has been reached to date.

For hemorrhagic shock, Feuerstein observed changes in opioid receptors in the brain stem of hemorrhagic shock rats by radioimmunoassay. The results showed that δ- and κ-opioid receptors in brain stem were significantly increased during hemorrhagic shock, but other types of opioid receptors did not change (33). Our lab also found that following hemorrhagic shock, μ-opioid receptors did not change significantly (34). Fan et al. found that i.c.v. administration of δ- and κ-opioid receptor antagonists significantly elevated the MAP of hemorrhagic shock rats, but the μ-opioid receptor antagonist β-funaltrexamine (β-FNA, i.c.v.) was without effect (35). Holaday also found that hemorrhagic shock-induced hypotension could

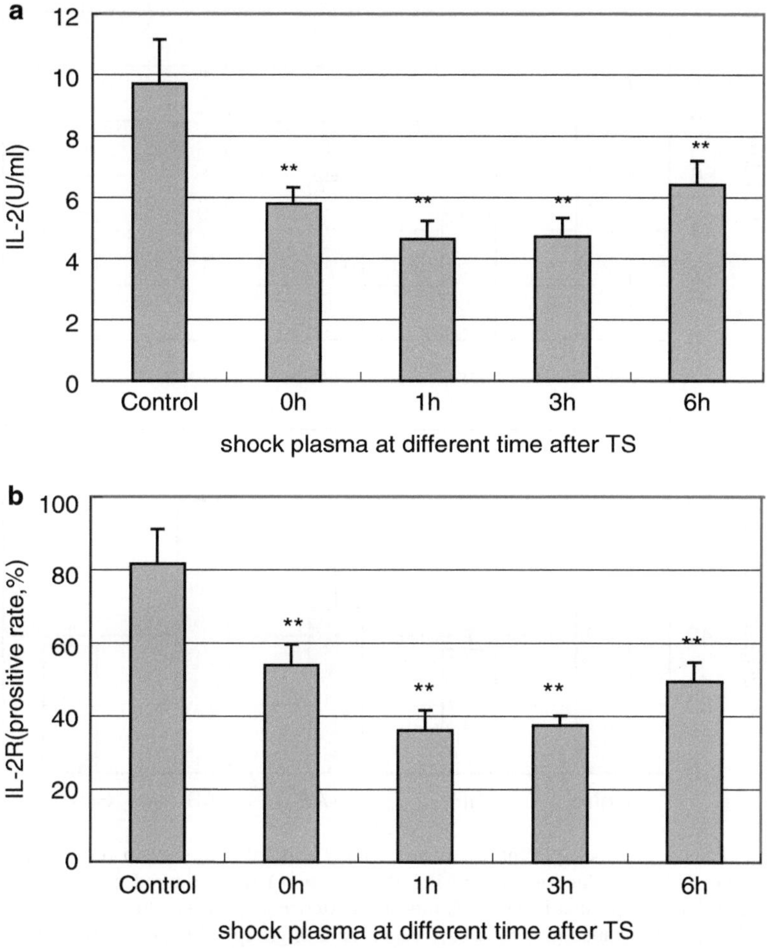

Fig. 32.3 Effects of plasma from shocked rats on concanavalin A (*conA*)-induced IL-2 production (**a**) and IL-2R expression (**b**) (by cytoflowmetry) in normal splenic cells. *TS* traumatic shock; control group means the plasma from normal rats; 0, 1, 3, 6h group means the plasma from shocked rats at 0, 1, 3, 6h after shock; $^{**}P < 0.01$ versus control group

be reversed by the δ-opioid receptor antagonist ICI 154,129, but not by a μ-opioid receptor antagonist. These results suggested that opioid receptors associated with hemorrhagic shock are primarily δ and κ receptors. However, other studies in cats showed that μ- and δ-opioid receptors may be the major opioid receptors involved in the pathogenesis of hemorrhagic shock, and κ receptors playing a minor role (36, 37). Hock observed an intravenous (i.v.) injection of 2mg/kg of nalorphine, the κ- and σ-opioid receptor agonists and μ-opioid receptor antagonist, could increase the MAP in hemorrhagic shock in cats. This result supports the hypothesis that μ-opioid receptors are involved in the pathogenesis of hemorrhagic shock. Curtis found that the δ-opioid receptor antagonist J 7747 elevated MAP in

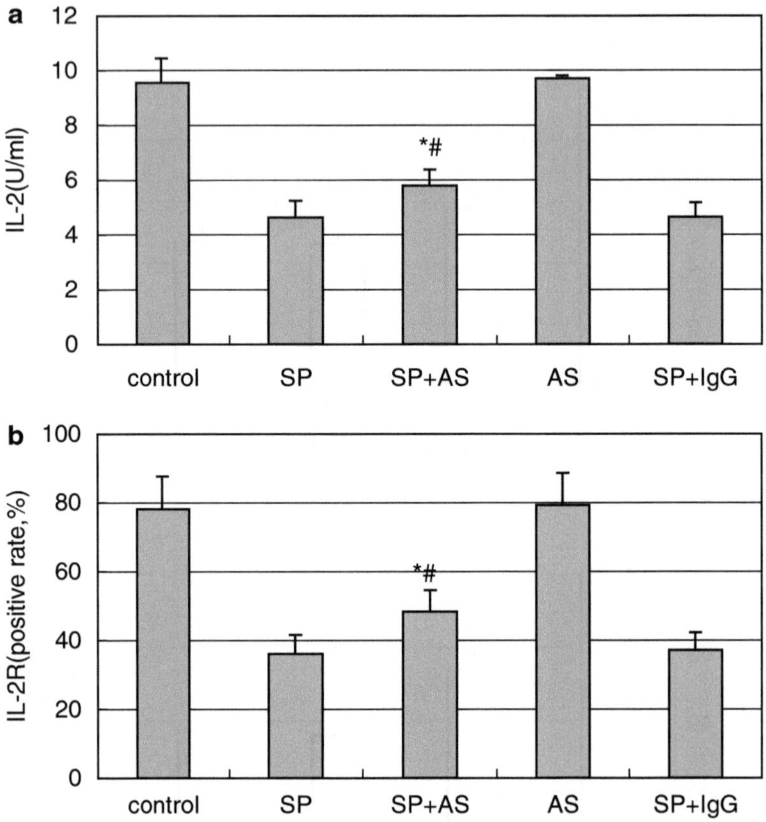

Fig. 32.4 Effects of shock plasma pretreated with β-endorphin antiserum on concanavalin A (*conA*)-induced IL-2 production (**a**) and IL-2R expression (**b**) in cultured normal splenic cells from shocked rats. *SP* plasma from shock rats at 1 h after shock, *AS* β-endorphin antiserum, SP + AS SP + β-endorphin antiserum; $^{*}P < 0.01$ versus control group; $^{\#}P < 0.01$ versus SP group

hemorrhagic-shocked cats, but the κ-opioid receptor antagonist MR 2266 could not. These findings suggested that in cats, the δ-opioid receptor may be closely involved with the pathogenesis of hemorrhagic shock, but κ-opioid receptors may not participate in the pathogenesis of hemorrhagic shock in cats.

For endotoxic shock, Holaday and Long found that the δ-opioid receptor antagonist ICI 154,129 and ICI 174, 864 could improve the hypotension status and cardiovascular depression during shock, but the μ-opioid receptor antagonist naloxazone did not have such an effect (38, 39, 40). These results suggested that the δ-opioid receptor may be associated with the pathogenesis of endotoxic shock, but μ receptor may not. For burn shock, Hong et al. reported that i.c.v. administration of the μ-opioid receptor agonist [D-Ala2, N-MePhe4, Gly-ol]-enkephalin (DAMGO) potentiated the burn shock in rats and accelerated the animal death; its antagonist, naloxone (i.c.v.), conversely improved the cardiovascular function. Similarly, the δ-opioid receptor agonist [D–pen(2), D–Leu(5)]– enkephalin (DPDPE) potentiated the burn shock and its antagonist ICI 174,864 improved the shock symptoms.

But the κ-opioid receptor agonist dynorphin A1-13 did not affect the course of shock and its antagonist nor-binaltorphimine (nor-BNI) did not improve the cardiovascular function (41). These results suggested that burn shock-associated opioid receptors are mainly μ and δ receptors.

Nonetheless, which opioid receptors are involved in traumatic shock remains unclear. By observing the changes of myocardial and brain μ-, δ-, and κ-opioid receptors and the antagonizing effect of i.c.v. administration of specific opioid receptor antagonists, we investigated the subtypes of opioid receptors involved in the pathogenesis of traumatic shock (15, 42). The results showed that myocardial and brain δ- and κ-opioid receptors were significantly increased after traumatic shock. It was negatively associated with decreased cardiovascular function (Tables 32.3 and 32.4). μ-opioid receptors did not change significantly, and were not associated with the changes in the cardiovascular function. The specific δ- and κ-opioid receptor antagonists, ICI 174,864 and nor-BNI, respectively, significantly reversed the decrease of cardiovascular function when administered i.c.v. after traumatic shock, but the μ-opioid receptor antagonist β-FNA did not (Fig. 32.5). These results suggested that δ- and κ-opioid receptors take part in the pathogenesis of traumatic shock, but μ-opioid receptor does not.

32.4 Antishock Effects of Opioid Antagonists

32.4.1 Nonselective Opioid Receptor Antagonists

The antishock property of naloxone, the nonspecific opioid receptor antagonist, has been demonstrated by many studies from our lab and clinical trials. It has beneficial effects on hemorrhagic, endotoxic, burns, and spinal shock (43, 44). Its antishock effects can be summarized as follows: (1) acts at central opioid receptors to abate the inhibitory effect of EOPs on cardiovascular system (45); (2) directly acts at peripheral opioid receptors, especially in heart and blood vessels to antagonize EOPs cardiovascular depression (13, 15, 46, 47); (3) stabilizes lysosome membrane to decrease the release of cathepsin D and myocardium depressing factor (MDF) by nonopioid receptor mechanism (48, 49); and (4) abates the sequestration of neutrophil granulocytes and platelets, reducing the release of free radicals in the lung to lessen the pulmonary injury (50, 51). Some reports showed that early application of naloxone in endotoxic and cardiac shock patients showed a positive effect (52, 53). Li et al. observed the effect of naloxone on 16 refractory septic shock patients. The results demonstrated that after receiving the high dose of naloxone i.v. infusion (6.0 ± 3.5 mg), those patients improved in recovery, the MAP was improved, and dopamine decreased (52). Putterman et al. reported that 0.4–1.2 mg/kg of naloxone administered intravenously significantly increased the MAP and urine output of endotoxic and cardiac shock patients. MAP was increased to 130 ± 24.7 mmHg in 10–60 min after administration from 75 ± 9.8 mmHg before naloxone administration. Urine output was increased to 122 ± 25 ml/h from16 ± 12 ml/h. Nevertheless,

Table 32.3 The alterations of the B_{max} (pmol/mg protein) of myocardial and brain μ-, δ-, and κ-opioid receptors following traumatic shock in rats

	μ			δ			κ		
	T	F	H	T	F	H	T	F	H
Heart									
B		18.9 ± 5.5			19.6 ± 4.7			28.4 ± 7.8	
0	19.4 ± 4.7	18.4 ± 4.3	19.1 ± 3.9	34.5 ± 9.5**	21.3 ± 5.2$^{\#}$	28.2 ± 3.7**	58.3 ± 14.3**	28.9 ± 6.7$^{\#\#}$	41.2 ± 9.2$^{**\#}$
1 h	20.0 ± 7.1	19.1 ± 2.9	19.2 ± 4.1	27.9 ± 8.9*	24.5 ± 4.7*	25.1 ± 4.2*	53.4 ± 16.5**	39.1 ± 7.2$^{*\#}$	40.5 ± 8.7$^{*\#}$
2 h	21.8 ± 6.9	20.5 ± 3.7	21.1 ± 4.2	32.1 ± 10.2*	22.4 ± 5.7$^{\#}$	23.4 ± 3.1$^{*\#}$	50.8 ± 18.4*	32.5 ± 7.4$^{\#\#}$	39.4 ± 7.5$^{*\#}$
3 h	23.9 ± 5.8	21.2 ± 4.5	20.9 ± 3,1	35.2 ± 9.4**	21.1 ± 3.9$^{\#}$	24.0 ± 2.9$^{*\#}$	58.4 ± 17.3**	33.2 ± 6.4$^{\#\#}$	38.1 ± 8.4$^{*\#}$
4 h	23.2 ± 6.4	20.1 ± 3.5	21.1 ± 3.8	28.2 ± 9.9*	20.2 ± 4.7$^{\#}$	23.3 ± 4.5	53.1 ± 14.8**	30.2 ± 7.4$^{\#\#}$	37.5 ± 7.6$^{*\#}$
Brain									
B		28.6 ± 7.8			43 ± 9.9			58.3 ± 12.5	
0	26.5 ± 8.1	27.1 ± 6.3	28.47.2	76.4 ± 17.4**	52.7 ± 8.9$^{*\#}$	60.2 ± 8.9**	100.0 ± 28.1**	69.1 ± 11.2$^{*\#}$	80.5 ± 14.3$^{**\#}$
1 h	31.8 ± 8.7	29.8 ± 5.7	28.5 ± 6.7	64.1 ± 15.3**	51.8 ± 7.4	57.4 ± 9.1*	90.1 ± 21.2**	56.7 ± 10.5$^{\#}$	72.3 ± 13.7**
2 h	30.5 ± 7.6	28.1 ± 6.9	29.2 ± 7.4	68.1 ± 18.1**	52.1 ± 9.2$^{\#}$	59.2 ± 9.4*	89.8 ± 24.3**	57.4 ± 11.9$^{\#}$	75.4 ± 14.9**
3 h	35.0 ± 10.4	29.5 ± 7.7	28.4 ± 8.1	66.5 ± 17.7**	50.6 ± 8.8	54.4 ± 9.9*	87.2 ± 19.5**	55.4 ± 12.1$^{\#}$	74.9 ± 16.1*
4 h	31.8 ± 9.4	29.6 ± 7.5	29.0 ± 6.9	62.3 ± 14.2*	48.6 ± 8.9$^{\#}$	53.1 ± 8.6*	84.2 ± 24.1*	56.7 ± 11.7$^{\#}$	73.2 ± 15.1*

$^{*}P < 0.05$; $^{**}P < 0.01$ as compared to baseline; $^{\#}P < 0.05$ as compared to traumatic shock group mean ± SD, B_{max} the maximal binding site of the plasma receptor to radio ligand, *B* baseline, 0: at the end of hemorrhage, 1 h-4 h: the time point following traumatic shock, *T* traumatic shock (right femur fracture plus hemorrhage at 20 ml/kg), *F* single right femur fracture, *H* single hemorrhage (20 ml/kg)

Table 32.4 The changes of hemodynamic parameters following traumatic shock in rats

		Traumatic shock group				
	Baseline	0	1	2	3	4
Femur fracture plus hemorrhage group						
MAP (mmHg)	105.2 ± 18.2	42.7 ± 12.2**	76.5 ± 10.2**	73.5 ± 19.7**	80.2 ± 11.1**	57.7 ± 17.1**
LVSP (mmHg)	140.2 ± 16.4	78.7 ± 23.0**	119.2 ± 16.5**	112.5 ± 28.5*	108.1 ± 11.3**	99.1 ± 36.4**
$+dp/dt_{max}$ (mmHg/s)	9,750 ± 2,353	4,875 ± 2,586**	7,762 ± 2,304*	7,590 ± 2,446*	6,765 ± 1,326**	6,067 ± 396**
$-dp/dt_{max}$ (mmHg/s)	7,275 ± 2,190	2,665 ± 1,164**	4,807 ± 741**	4,837 ± 1,707**	4,822 ± 1,293**	3,682 ± 2,404**
Femur fracture group						
MAP (mmHg)	104.9 ± 14.8	90.8 ± 10.9*	98.4 ± 14.5	96.7 ± 16.7	94.5 ± 18.9	90.4 ± 17.6
LVSP (mmHg)	143.5 ± 19.5	126.5 ± 20.4*	134.4 ± 19.6	136.1 ± 18.7	135.5 ± 24.1	130.7 ± 21.2
$+dt/dt_{max}$ (mmHg/s)	9,615 ± 2,212	7,125 ± 2,032*	8,234 ± 2,164	8,354 ± 2,232	8,492 ± 2,514	9,105 ± 2,094
$-dt/dt_{max}$ (mmHg/s)	7,073 ± 1,904	6,015 ± 1,824	6,724 ± 1,757	6,635 ± 1,824	6,579 ± 1,736	6,614 ± 1,545
Hemorrhage group						
MAP (mmHg)	106.8 ± 17.4	64.5 ± 12.5**	78.4 ± 13.4**	84.5 ± 16.9**	86.5 ± 17.9**	70.6 ± 14.6**
LVSP (mmHg)	141.5 ± 19.4	82.5 ± 17.6**	124.3 ± 18.4*	125.1 ± 19.2*	129.4 ± 20.1*	119.4 ± 17.6*
$+dp/dt_{max}$ (mmHg/s)	9,557 ± 2,192	5,926 ± 1,124**	6,825 ± 1,635**	7,132 ± 1,524**	6,224 ± 1,735**	6,015 ± 1,349**
$-dp/dt_{max}$ (mmHg/s)	7,315 ± 1,854	4,054 ± 1,514**	5,545 ± 1,459**	5,612 ± 1,671**	5,437 ± 1,438**	5,047 ± 1,424**

*$P < 0.05$; **$P < 0.01$ as compared to baseline

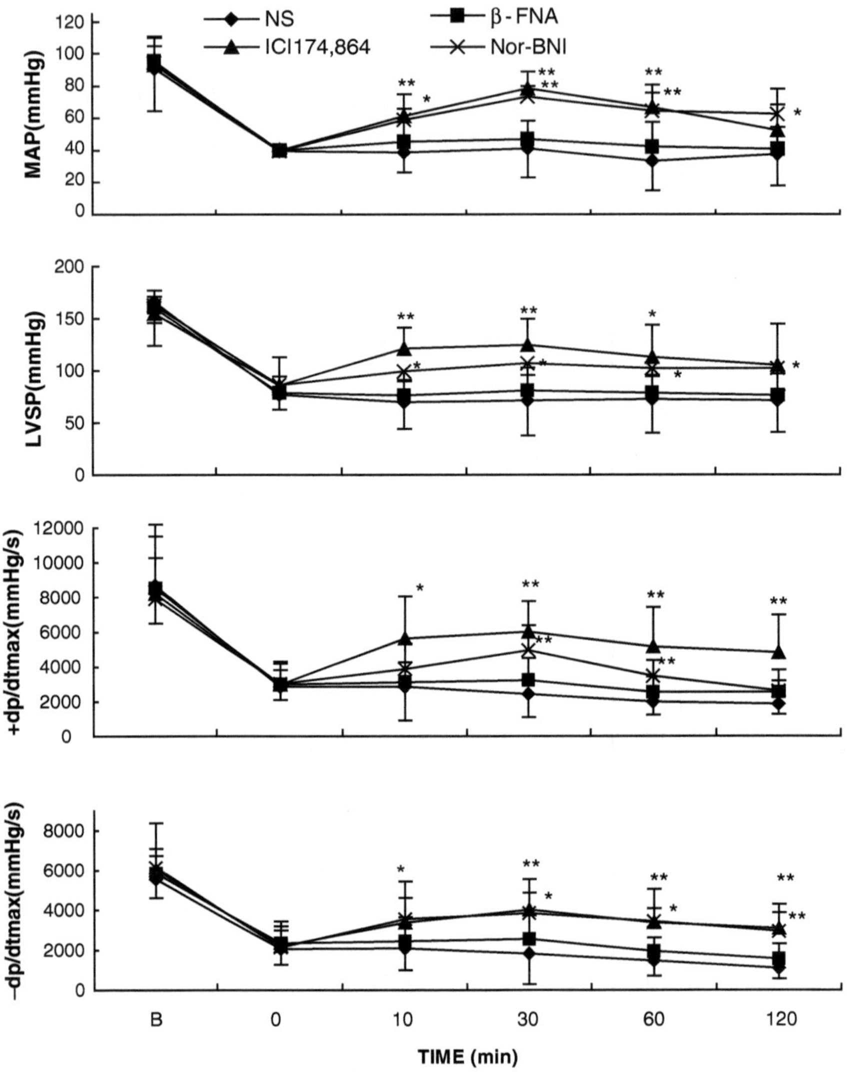

Fig. 32.5 The antagonizing effects of intracerebroventricular (*i.c.v.*) administration of β-funaltrexamine (*β-FNA*), ICI174,864 and norbinaltorphimine (*nor-BNI*) on hemodynamic parameters following traumatic shock in the rat. *B* baseline, Time 0: at the end of shock; Time 10, 30, 60, 120 stand for 10, 30, 60, and 120 min after i.c.v. administration. *$P < 0.05$; **$P < 0.01$, as compared with NS group

the clinical application of naloxone needs further confirmation. Because some reports showed that although naloxone had a positive effect on improving the cardiovascular function for endotoxic shock patients, it did not significantly increase the survival rate (54). In addition, the half-life of naloxone is only 62 min in humans, so the action time is very short. As mentioned above, naloxone can affect the pain threshold of shock patients, so it is not suitable for traumatic shock.

Nabuphine, a partial agonist, not only antagonizes μ-opioid receptor but also stimulates the κ-opioid receptor. Its half-life is 5 h in humans and longer than naloxone. Naltrexone is a long-lasting opioid antagonist. Basic and clinical studies showed that they have a beneficial effect for septic, cardiac, and hemorrhagic shock. But because they can also affect the pain threshold of shock patients, their clinical application is still restricted (55-58).

32.4.2 Specific Opioid Receptor Antagonists

Nonselective opioid receptor antagonists, because they affect the pain threshold of shock patients among other problems, are not suitable for traumatic shock in the clinic. There are two strategies to solve this issue. The first strategy is using thyrotropin-releasing hormone (TRH), a physiological opioid antagonist. Research showed it did not affect the pain threshold of shock victim, but it mainly sensitizes adrenergic receptors and downregulates brain δ-opioid receptors to produce its antishock properties (59, 60). The second strategy is the selection of specific opioid receptor antagonists, such as δ- and κ-opioid receptor antagonists.

32.4.2.1 Effects of TRH on Traumatic Shock

TRH is a three-peptide hormone secreted from hypothalamus. In 1978, Holaday et al. reported it had beneficial effect on shock. A series of work involving its antishock effects and mechanisms has been conducted in our lab (61). The results showed that TRH had a beneficial effect on hemorrhagic, endotoxic, and traumatic shock. Meanwhile, it also had a positive effect on traumatic shock at high altitude (62). For hemorrhagic shock, TRH (5–10 mg/kg, i.v.) significantly improved the MAP and cardiac contractility of hemorrhagic shock rats, rabbits, and dogs and increase their survival time and survival rate. For endotoxic shock, TRH (4 mg/kg, i.v.) significantly increased the MAP and survival rate of endotoxic shock rats. For traumatic shock, TRH (5 mg/kg, i.v.) significantly improved the hemodynamic parameters and cardiac contractility of traumatic shock rats both at sea level and at high altitude, and increased the survival rate.

32.4.2.2 Effects of δ- and κ-Opioid Receptor Antagonists on Traumatic Shock

Effects of δ-Opioid Receptor Antagonist ICI 174,864 and κ-Opioid Receptor Antagonist Nor-BNI on Traumatic Shock

In traumatic shock rats, we observed the effect of δ-opioid receptor antagonist ICI 174,864 and κ-opioid receptor antagonist nor-BNI. The results showed that i.v. administration of δ-and κ-opioid receptor antagonists ICI 174,864 and nor-BNI

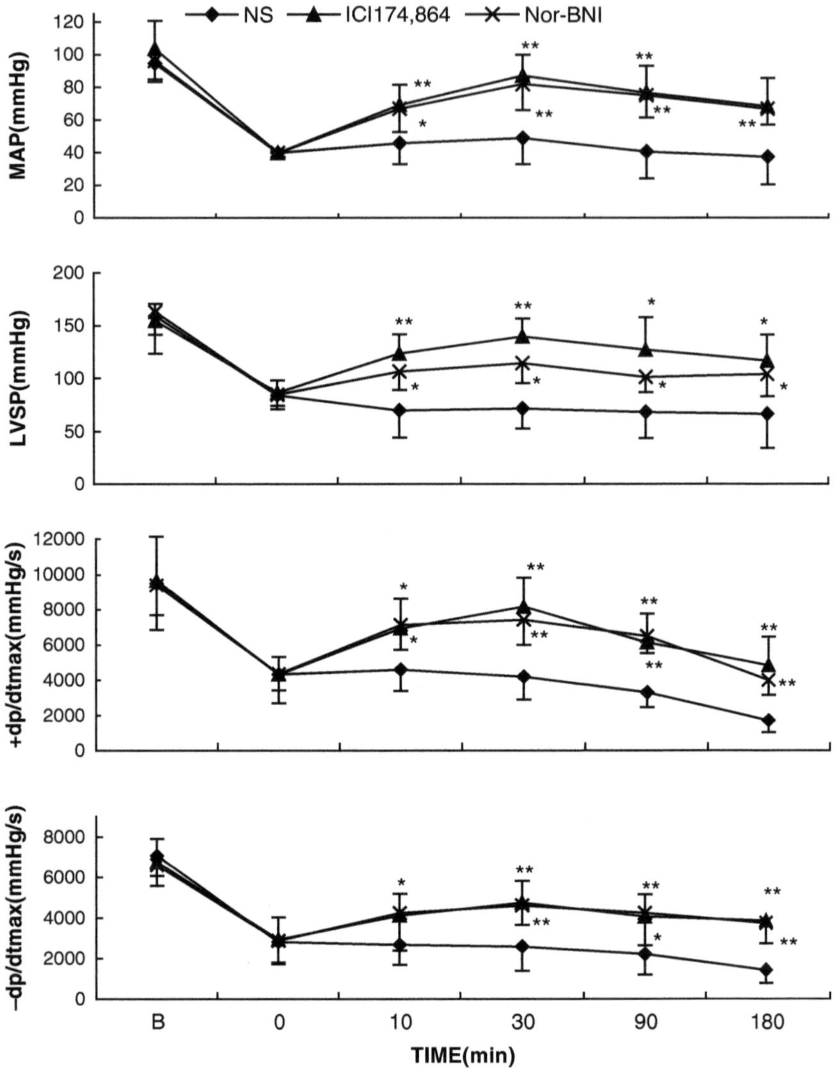

Fig. 32.6 Effects of ICI174,864 and norbinaltorphimine (*nor-BNI*) on hemodynamic parameters after traumatic shock in rats. *B* baseline, Time 0: at the end of shock; Time 10, 30, 90, 180, stand for 10, 30, 90, and 180 min after intravenous (*i.v.*) administration. *$P < 0.05$; **$P < 0.01$, as compared with NS group

(0.5 mg/kg), respectively, significantly increased the MAP and improved the hemodynamic parameters of traumatic shock (Fig. 32.6). The 24-h survival rates were significantly prolonged (80% and 70% in ICI 174,864 and nor-BNI group, respectively, vs 30% in control group) (Fig. 32.7). In addition, we observed the effects of intracerebral administration of ICI 174,864 and nor-BNI on traumatic shock in rabbits and obtained the same results. These results suggest that the

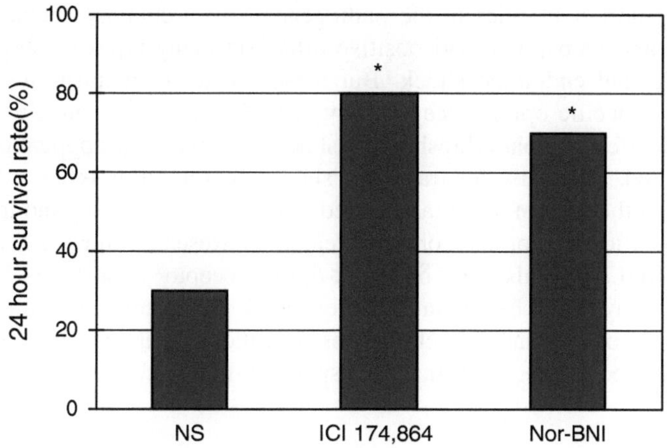

Fig. 32.7 Effect of ICI174,864 and norbinaltorphimine (*nor-BNI*) on 24 h survival rate of rats after traumatic shock. *$P < 0.05$, as compared to NS group

specific δ- and κ-opioid receptor antagonists ICI 174,864 and nor-BNI have a beneficial effect on traumatic shock (13, 63–65).

Effects of δ-Opioid Receptor Antagonist Natrindole and κ-Opioid Receptor Antagonist Nor-BNI on Vascular Hyporeactivity Following Hemorrhagic Shock in Rats

Previous studies have reported that after severe trauma or shock, or associated systemic inflammatory response syndrome (SIRS) and multiple organ dysfunction syndrome (MODS), the vascular reactivity to vasoconstrictors and vasodilators is greatly reduced. This reduced vascular reactivity may play an important role in the incidence, development, and outcome of the shock state and may interfere with the therapy of shock, especially interfere with the application of vasoactive agents (66). Studies in our lab found the δ- and κ-opioid receptor antagonist naltrindole and nor-BNI could significantly improve shock-induced vascular hyporeactivity (67). The mechanism may be related to naltrindole and nor-BNI regulating large conductance calcium-activated potassium channel (BKCa) and calcium channel by opioid receptor (68–70).

32.5 Conclusion and Perspective

Since the opioid antagonist, naloxone, was found to be beneficial in reducing the effects of traumatic shock in 1978, a series of work on the roles of EOPs and their antagonists in circulatory shock was conducted. It was demonstrated that EOPs played very important roles in the pathogenesis of circulatory shock. Naloxone, naltrexone, and nalbuphine had positive effect on many types of shock, such as hemorrhagic and endotoxic shock. But these opioid antagonists are not highly selective for specific opioid receptor subtypes. Because they can act on μ-opioid receptors to affect the pain threshold of shock patients, their application has been greatly limited, especially for traumatic shock. To solve this issue, many laboratories studied the type of shock associated with opioid receptors, and attempted to use their specific receptor antagonist to treat them. Research showed TRH, a physiological opioid antagonist, and δ- and κ-opioid receptor antagonists ICI 174,864 and nor-BNI have good beneficial effect on shock parameters without affecting the pain threshold of traumatic shock victims. But these results are from our lab and their effects need further confirmation, especially in clinic.

References

1. Wilson SP, Klein RL, Chang KJ, Gasparis MS, Viveros OH, Yang WH. Are opioid peptides co-transmitters in neuro-adrenergic vesicles of sympathetic nerve? Nature 1980; 288:707–709.
2. Hughes J, Kosterlitz HW, Smith TW. The distribution of methionine-enkaphalin and leucine-enkaphalin in the brain and periperal tissues. Br J Pharmacol 1977; 61:639–647.
3. Gordon FJ. Central opioid receptors and barreflex control of sympathetic and cardiovascular function. J Pharmacol Exp Ther 1986; 237:428–436.
4. Feuerstein G, Faden AI. Differential cardiovascular effects of μ, δ and κ opiate agonists at discrete hypothalamic sites in the anesthetized rats. Life Sci 1982; 31:2197–2200.
5. Holaday JW, Faden AI. Naloxone reversal of endotoxin hypotension suggests role of endorphins in shock. Nature 1978; 275:450–451.
6. Isoyama T, Tanaka J, Sato T, Shatney CH. Effect of naloxone and morphine in hemorrhagic shock. Circ Shock 1982; 9:375–382.
7. Gurll NJ, Reynolds DG, Holaday JW. Evidence for a role of endorphins in the cardiovascular pathophysiology of primate shock. Crit Care Med 1988; 16:521–530.
8. Murray MJ, Offord KP, Yaksh TL. Physiologic and plasma hormone correlates of survival in endotoxic dogs: effects of opiate antagonists. Crit Care Med 1989; 17:39–47.
9. Reynolds DG, Gurll NJ, Holaday JW, Lechner RB. The therapeutic efficacy of opiate antagonist in hemorrhagic shock. Resuscitation 1989; 18:343–357.
10. Dziki AJ, Lynch WH, Ramsey CB, Law WR. β-adrenergic dependent and independent actions of naloxone on perfusion during endotoxic shock. Circ Shock 1993; 39:29–38.
11. Molina PE. Endogenous opioid analgesia in hemorrhagic shock. J Trauma 2003; 54:S126–S132.
12. Molina PE. Opiate modulation of hemodynamic, hormonal and cytokine response to hemorrhage. Shock 2001; 15:471–478.
13. Liu LM, Hu DY, Pan XK, Lu RQ, Dan FJ. Subclass opioid receptors associated with the cardiovascular depression after traumatic shock and the antishock effects of its specific receptor antagonist. Shock 2005; 24:470–475.
14. Roy S, Charboneau RG, Barke RA. Morphine synergizes with lipopolysaccharide in a chronic endotoxemia model. J Neuroimmunol 1999; 95:107–114.
15. Liu LM, Chen HS, Hu DY, Lu RQ, Chen Y, Dan FJ. Role of opioid receptors in the cardiovascular depression following hemorrhagic shock in rats. Chin J Traumatol 1999; 2:48–52.
16. Bellamy RF. The cause of death in conventional land warfare: implication for combat casualty care research. Mil Med 1984; 149:55–62.

17. Champion HR, Bellamy RF, Roberts CP, Leppaniemi A. A profile of combat injury. J Trauma 2003; 54:S13–S19.
18. Champion HR. Combat fluid resuscitation and overview of conferences. J Trauma 2003; 54: S7–S12.
19. Nolan J. Fluid resuscitation for the trauma patient. Resuscitation 2001; 48:57–69.
20. Horton JW, White J, Maass D, Sanders B, Thompson M, Girroir B. Calcium antagonists improve cardiac mechanical performance after thermal trauma. J Surg Res 1999; 87:39–50.
21. Buttemeyer RA, Schlenzka PW, Mall LJ. Epigallocatechin gallate can significantly decrease free oxygen radicals in the reperfusion injury in vivo. Transpl Proc 2003; 35:3116–3120.
22. Bergman M, Perelman A, Dubinsky Z, Grossman S. Scavenging of reactive oxygen species by a novel glucuronated flavonoid antioxidant isolated and purified from spinach. Phytochemistry 2003; 62:753–762.
23. Chamberlain JM, Klein BL. A comprehensive review of naloxone for the emergency physician. Am Emerg Med 1994; 12:650–660.
24. Akin MZ, Tuncel N, Gurer F, Kural N, Uslu S. Effects of vasoactive intestinal peptide and naloxone combination on urinary *N*-acetyl-*b*-D-glucosaminidase level and kidney histology of rats exposed to severe hemorrhage. Pharmacology 1993; 47:194–199.
25. Greeneltch KM, Haudenschild CC, Keegan AD, Shi YF. The opioid antagonist naltrexone blocks acute endotoxic shock by inhibiting tumor necrosis factor-a production. Brain Behav Immun 2004; 18:476–484.
26. Hu DY, Pan XK, Liu LM, Lu RQ. The effects of δ and κ opioid receptor antagonists on traumatic shock. Chin Crit Care Med. 2000; 12:101–104.
27. Albert EP, Paola S. β-endorphin in the immune system: a role at last. Immunology Today 1997; 18:317–319
28. Refojo D, Kovalovsky D, Young JI, Rubinstein M, Holsboer F, Reul JM, Low MJ, Arzt E. Increased splenocyte proliferative response and cytokine production in beta-endorphin-deficient mice. J Neuroimmunol 2002; 131:126–134.
29. Levy EM, Mcintosh T, Black PH. Elevation of circulating beta-endorphin levels with concomitant depression of immune parameters after traumatic injury. J Trauma 1986; 26:246–249.
30. Nerlich ML, Holch M, Stalp M, Dwenger A, Fauler J. Neuropeptide levels early after trauma: immunomodulatory. J Trauma 1994; 37:759–768.
31. Wen AQ, Liu LM, Hu DY. Role of β-endorphin in con-A induced spleen cell proliferation in rats with traumatic hemorrhagic shock. Acta Acad Med Militaris Tertiae 2001; 23:404–406.
32. Wang J, When AQ, Liu LM. Role of β-endorphin in the regulation of con-A induced IL-2R expression and IL-2 production in rat splenic cells following traumatic hemorrhagic shock. Acta Acad Med Militaris Tertiae 2003; 25:657–659.
33. Feuerstein G, Faden AI, Krumins SA. Alteration in opiate receptors binding after hemorrhagic shock. Eur J Pharmacol 1984; 100:245–246.
34. Liu LM, Chen HS, Hu DY. Effect of TRH on brain μ, δ and κ opioid receptors following hemorrhagic shock in rats. Chin J Pharmacol Toxicol 1995; 47:268–270.
35. Fan L. Role of brain endogenous opioid peptides during hemorrhagic shock in rats. J Beijing Med Univ 1988; 20:5–8.
36. Hock CE, Curtis MT, Jaffe JS, Lefer AM. Beneficial actions of nalorphine during hemorrhagic shock in cats. Pro Soc Exp Bio Med 1983; 173 (1):176–181.
37. Curtis MT, Lefer AM. Actions of opiate antagonist with selective receptor interactions in hemorrhagic shock. Circ Shock 1983; 10:131–145.
38. Holaday JW, D'Amato RJ. Multiple opioid receptors: evidence for mu-delta binding site interactions in endotoxic shock. Life Sci 1983;33:703–706.
39. Long TB, Ruvio BA, Glatt CE, Holaday JW. ICI 174864, a putative delta opioid antagonist, reverses endotoxemic hypotension: pretreatment with dynorphin 1–13, a kappa agonist, blocks this action. Neuropeptides 1984; 5:291–294.
40. Holaday JW, Pasternak GW, D'Amato RJ, Ruvio BA, Faden AI. Naloxazone lacks therapeutic effects in endotoxic shock yet blocks the effects of naloxone. Eur J Pharmacol. 1983; 89: 293–296.

41. Hong XR. Role of β-endorphin in hypothalamic nuclei paraventricularis during burn shock and its receptors mechanisms. Prog Physiol Sci 1993; 24:242–244.
42. Wen AQ, Wang J, Liu LM, Hu DY. Role of opioid receptors δ, K and μ in suppression of cellular immunity following traumatic hemorrhagic shock in rats. Chin J Traumatol 2002; 18:692–695.
43. Holaday JW, Faden AI. Naloxone acts at central opiate receptors to reverse hypotension, hypothermia and hypoventilation in spinal shock. Brain Res 1980;189:295–300.
44. Lin BC. Effects of naloxone on burn shock in rats. Chin J Appl Phsiol 1985; 1:212–216.
45. Faden AI, Jacobs TP, Holaday JW. Endorphin-parasympathetic interaction in spinal shock. J Auton Nerv Syst 1980; 2:295–304.
46. Koyama S, Santiesteban HL, Ammons WS, Manning JW. The effects of naloxone on the peripheral sympathetics in cat endotoxic shock. Circ Shock 1983; 10:7–13.
47. Lechner RB, Gurll NJ, Reynolds DG. Intracoronary naloxone in hemorrhagic shock: dose-dependent sterospecific effects. Am J Physiol 1985; 249 (Pt. 2):H272–H277.
48. Tuggle DW, Horton JW. Naloxone improves myocardial perfusion in hypovolemic shock. Curr Surg. 1985; 42:195–198.
49. Curtis MT, Lefer AM. Protection actions of naloxone in hemorrhagic shock. Am J Physiol 1980; 239:H416–H421.
50. Chen CJ, Cheng FC, Liao SL, Chen WY, Lin NN, Kuo JS. Effects of naloxone on lactate pyruvate, pyruvate metabolism and antioxidant enzyme activity in rat cerebral ischemia/perfusion. Nurosci Lett 2000; 287:113–116.
51. Ekstrom BF, Kuenzig M, Schwartz SI. Pulmonary platelet trapping in escherichia coli endotoxin injected dogs treated with methylprednisolone ibuprofen and naloxone. Acta Chir Scand 1986; 152:181–185.
52. Li SK, Cui ZJ. High dose naloxone in septic shock patients refractory to dopamine. J Postgrad Med 2003; 26:18–19.
53. Putterman C, Halpern P, Leykin Y, Sorkine P, Geller E, Bursztein S. Early use of naloxone in shock: a clinical trial. Resuscitation 1986; 13:185–190.
54. Boeuf B, Gauvin F, Guerguerian AM, Farrell CA, Lacoroix J, Jenicek M. Therapy of shock with naloxone: a meta-analysis. Crit Care Med. 1988; 26:1910–1916.
55. Muldoon SM, McKenzie JE, Collins FJ. Pressor effect of nalbuphine in hemorrhagic shock is dependent on the sympathoadrenal system. Circ Shock 1988; 26:89–98.
56. Reynolds DG, Gurll NJ, Holaday JW, Lechner RB. The therapeutic efficacy of opiate antagonists in hemorrhagic shock. Resuscitation 1989; 18:243–251.
57. Hu YG, Li Z, Guo JX, Cheng MZ, Xu T, Han JS. Clinical study on the antishock effects of naltrexone, a long lasting opioid antagonist. J Beijing Med Univ 1992; 24:81–84.
58. Greeneltch KM, Haudenschild CC, Keegan AD, Shi YF. The opioid antagonist naltrexone blocks acute endotocxic shock by inhibiting tumor necrosis factor-a production. Brain Behav Immun 2004; 18:476–484.
59. Liu LM, Chen HS, Hu DY, Lu RQ, Li TX. Effects of TRH on cardiac adrenoceptors and dopaminergic receptors following hemorrhagic shock in the rat. Shock 1995; 3:430–433.
60. Liu LM, Chen HS, Hu DY, Lu RQ, Wu Y. The importance of δ- and κ-opioid receptor in the property of TRH against hemorrhagic shock. Shock 1997; 7:60–64.
61. Hu DY, Liu LM, Zhou XW, Lu RQ, He FC, Chen HS. The preclinical study of thyrotroping-releasing hormon. Chin J Pharacol Toxicol 2000; 14:241–246.
62. Hu DY, Liu LM, Li P, Liu JC, He XP, Xiao N, Shi QG, Tian KL, Zhou XW. Benefical effect of TRH on hemorrhagic shock with pulmonary edema at high altitude in the rat. Chin J Mod Appl Pharmacol 2004; 21:349-353.
63. Tian KL, Liu LM, Lu RQ. Beneficial effects of ICI174864 on traumatic shock is related to pituitary. Chongqing Med 2003; 32:1340-1342.
64. Tian KL, Liu LM, Lu RQ. Beneficial effects of ICI174864 on traumatic shock is related to adrenal medulla. J Traumatic Surg 2003; 5:52-54.
65. Liu LM, Hu DY, Chen HS, LU RQ, Wu Y, Zhou XW. ICI174,864, nor-binaltorphimine improve the hemodynamics of hypovolemic rabbits. Mod Appl Pharm 1996; 13:1-4.

66. Liu LM, Ward JA, Dubick MA. Hemorrhagic shock induced vascular hyporeactivity to norepinephrine in select vasculatures of rats and the roles of nitric oxide and endothelin. Shock 2003; 19:208–214.
67. Kai L, Hu DY, Liu LM. Effects of opioid antagonists on vascular reactivity following hemorrhagic shock in rats. Acta Acad Med Militaris Tertiae 2002; 24:1185-1188.
68. Kai L, Wang ZF, Hu DY, Shi YL, Liu LM. Opioid receptor antagonists modulate Ca^{2+}-activated K^+ channels in mesenteric arterial smooth muscle cells of rats in hemorrhagic shock. Shock 2003; 19:85–90.
69. Zhou R, Liu LM, Hu DY. Involvement of BKCa α subunit tyrosine phosphorylation in vascular hyporesponsiveness following hemorrhagic shock in rat. Cardiovasc Res 2005; 68: 327-335.
70. Kai L, Hu DY, Liu LM, et al. Modulation of Ca^{2+} by opioid receptor antagonists in mesenteric arterial smooth muscle cells of rats in hemorrhagic shock. J Cardiovasc Pharmacol 2002; 40:618–624.

Chapter 33
The Efficacy of Opioid Antagonists Against Heatstroke-Induced Ischemia and Injury in Rats

Mao-Tsun Lin, Ching-Ping Chang, and Sheng-Hsien Chen

Abstract Prior administration of naltrexone or cyclic D-phe-cys-try-arg-thr-pen-thr-NH_2 (CTAP) (a μ-opioid receptor antagonist), but not nor-binaltorphine (a κ-opioid receptor antagonist) or ICI-174864 (a δ-opioid receptor antagonist), improve heat tolerance in the rat. As compared to those of normothermic controls, all vehicle-pretreated heatstroke rats displayed higher levels of creatinine, blood urea nitrogen, alkaline phosphatase, glutamic oxaloacetic transaminase, glutamic pyruvic transaminase, tumor necrosis factor-alpha, prothrombin time, activated partial thromboplastin time, and D-dimer in the plasma, cellular ischemia and injury markers in brain, and intracranial pressure. In contrast, all vehicle pretreated heatstroke animals had lower levels of mean arterial pressure, cerebral perfusion pressure, cerebral blood flow, brain PO_2, and platelet count and protein C in the plasma. Twenty minutes before the start of heat exposure, prior administration of CTAP or naltrexone improves heat tolerance by reducing the systemic inflammation, hypercoagulable state, and tissue ischemia and injury that occurred during heatstroke. The results show that μ-opioid receptor antagonism is effective for attenuation of heatstroke reactions.

Keywords: Heatstroke; Opioid receptor antagonist; Ischemia; Coagulation; Inflammation; Brain

33.1 Introduction

Heatstroke is characterized by body temperature elevation (over 40°C) and multiple organ dysfunction or failure (in particular, the central nervous system ischemia, hypoxia, and damage) (7, 15). In the rodents, systemic-activated inflammation, hypercoagulable state or disseminated inadequate coagulation (DIC), and tissue

M.-T. Lin (✉), C.-P. Chang, and S.-H. Chen
Department of Medical Research, Chi Mei Medical Center, Tainan, Taiwan 710, Republic of China, 891201
e-mail: @mail.chimei.org.tw

R. Dean et al. (eds.), *Opiate Receptors and Antagonists*,

ischemia and injury all occur during heat stroke (14, 31). DIC or hypercoagulable state is evidenced by increased prothrombin time (PT), activated partial thromboplastin time (aPTT), and D-dimer, and decreased platelet count and protein C in plasma. Tissue ischemia and injury is evidenced by increased blood urea nitrogen (BUN), creatinine, glutamic oxaloacetic transaminase (SGOT), glutamic pyruvic transaminase (SGPT), and alkaline phosphatase (ALP) levels in plasma, as well as increased glycerol, glutamate, and lactate/pyruvate ratio in brain. An increase in intracranial pressure (ICP) is also noted during heatstroke. On the contrary, a decrease in mean arterial pressure (MAP), cerebral perfusion pressure (CPP = MAP − ICP), and cerebral blood flow (CBF) or partial pressure of oxygen (PO_2) is observed after the onset of heatstroke.

Other line of evidence has indicated that opioids in the body are involved in the pathogenesis of heat stroke. Patients with heat stroke display an increase in their serum levels of β-endorphin (2). An increase in the brain levels of β-endorphin (26) or dynorphin A (49) has also been observed in rats with heatstroke. Naltrexone, a broad-spectrum opioid receptor antagonist, is able to ameliorate the severity of heatstroke (26, 45, 46, 50). In fact, naltrexone is a nonselective antagonist of opioid receptors with affinity to μ receptors in low doses. However, at high doses, some effects on κ receptors have been noted previously (47, 29). Indeed, a more recent study has demonstrated that intravenous (IV) administration of cyclic D-phe-cys-try-arg-thr-pen-thr-NH_2 (CTAP; a μ-opioid receptor antagonist) (29), but not norbinaltorphimine (a κ-opioid receptor antagonist) (5), or ICI-174864 (a δ-opioid receptor antagonist) (18), significantly improves survival during heatstroke (16).

In the following sections, we describe the efficacy of opioid antagonists (in particular, the CTAP) against heatstroke-induced activated inflammation, DIC, and tissue ischemia and injury in a rat model.

33.2 Materials and Methods

33.2.1 Experimental Animals

Adult Sprague-Dawley rats (weight 284 ± 9 g) were obtained from the Animal Resource Center of the National Science Council of the Republic of China (Taipei, Taiwan). The animals were housed four in a group at an ambient temperature of 22 ± 1°C, with a 12-h light/dark cycle. All protocols were approved by the Animal Ethics Committee of the Chi Mei Medical Center (Tainan, Tainan) in accordance with the Guide for the Care and use of Laboratory Animals of the National Institutes of Health as well as the guide lines of the Animal welfare Act. Adequate anesthesia was maintained to abolish the corneal reflex and pain reflexes induced by tail pinching throughout all experiments (~8 h) by intraperitoneal doses of sodium pentobarbital (60 mg/kg body weight). At the end of the experiments, control rats and any rats that had survived heatstroke were killed with an overdose of sodium pentobarbital.

33.2.2 Induction of Heatstroke

Before induction of heatstroke, the core temperature of the anesthetized rat was maintained at about 36°C with a folded heating pad, except during heat stress the room temperature was 24°C. Heatstroke was induced by increasing the temperature of the folded heating pad to 43°C with circulating hot water. The moment at which the MAP dropped to 25 mmHg from the peak level was taken as the onset of heatstroke (28, 35, 36). Immediately after the onset of heatstroke, the heating pad was removed, and the animals were allowed to recover at room temperature (24°C). Our pilot study showed that the latency for the onset of heatstroke (interval between the start of heat exposure and the onset of heatstroke) was found to be 59–63 min for the vehicle-treated heatstroke group ($n = 8$). Then, both physiologic parameters and survival times (intervals between the initiation of heat stress and animal death) were observed to about 480 min (or the end of experiments). For comparison with the vehicle-treated heatstroke group, all drug-treated heatstroke group animals were exposed to heat for exactly 61 min and then allowed to recover at room temperature (24°C).

33.2.3 Experimental Group

Five major groups of animals were designated for experiments. (a) In normothermic control rats ($n = 8$), the core temperature (T_{co}) was maintained at about 36°C with a folded heating pad at a room temperature of 24°C throughout the entire experiments. (b) In the vehicle-treated heatstroke group ($n = 8$), the animals were treated with a dose of normal saline intravenously (IV; 1 ml/kg body weight) 20 min before heat stress. (c) In the drug-treated heatstroke groups ($n = 8$ per group), the animals received an IV dose of CTAP (Tocris Cookson, Ltd., UK; 50–200 μg/kg), nor-binaltorphimine (NBO) (Toris Cookson, Ltd., UK; 20–200 μg/kg), ICI-174864 (Tocris Cookson, Ltd., UK; 0.05–1 mg/kg), or naltrexone (phoenix Pharmaceuticals, Inc., Mountain View, CA, USA; 0.1–10 mg/kg) 20 min before the initiation of heat stress, or an IV dose of 200 μg/kg body weight of CTAP or 10 mg/kg body weight of naltrexone at the time of onset of heatstroke.

33.2.4 Physiological and Biochemical Parameter Monitoring

The right femoral artery and vein of rats were cannulated with polyethylene tubing (PE50), under sodium pentobarbital anesthesia, for blood pressure monitoring and drug administration. The animals were positioned in a stereotaxic apparatus (Kopf 1406; Grass Instrument Co., Quincy, MA) to insert probes for measurement of ICP. The ICP was monitored with a Statham P23AC transducer via a 20-gauge stainless-steel needle type (diameter 0.90 mm; 38 mm), which was introduced into the lateral cerebral ventricle according to the stereotaxic coordinates of (42). All recordings were made on a four-channel Gould polygraph. Core temperature was monitored continuously by a thermocouple, and both MAP and heart rate (HR) were continuously monitored with a pressure transducer. Different groups of animals were used for the different sets of experiments: measurement of latency for heatstroke rats; measurement of survival time for vehicle-treated and drug-treated heatstroke rats; measurement of T_{co}, baroreceptor sensitivity (BRS), MAP, ICP, cerebral perfusion pressure (CPP = MAP – ICP), cerebral blood flow (CBF), and brain PO_2; measurement of cerebral levels of glutamate, glycerol, lactate/pyruvate, nitric oxide metabolites (NO_x^-), and 2,3-dihydroxybenzoic acid (DHBA); measurement of plasma levels of aPTT, PT, platelet count, protein C, and D-dimer; measurement of plasma levels of creatinine, BUN, SGOT, SGPT, and ALP; measurement of serum levels of tumor necrosis factor-alpha (TNF-α) and interleukin-10 (IL-10); and measurement of neuronal damage score for normothermic controls, vehicle-treated heatstroke rats, and drug-treated heatstroke rats.

33.2.5 Measurement of Extracellular Glutamate, Glycerol, Lactate/Pyruvate, NO_x^-, and DHBA in the Striatum

Each animal was anesthetized with sodium pentobarbital administered intraperitoneally. The animal's head was mounted in a stereotaxic apparatus (David Kopf Instruments) with the nose bar positioned 3.3 mm below the horizontal line. After a midline incision, the skull was exposed, and a burr hole was made in the skull for the insertion of a dialysis probe (4 mm in length, CMA/12, Carnegie Medicine, Stockholm, Sweden). The microdialysis probe was stereotaxically implanted into the striatum according to the atlas and coordinates of (42). As described previously (17), an equilibrium period of 60 min without sampling was allowed after probe implantation. The microdialysis probes were perfused at a µl/min with a sterile isotonic solution, and the dialysates were sampled in microvials. The dialysates were collected every 10 min in a CMA/140 fraction collector. Aliquots of dialysates (5 µl) were injected into a CMA600 Microdialysis analyzer for measurement of lactate, glycerol, pyruvate, glutamate, NO_x^-, and DHBA.

33.2.6 Measurement of CBF, Brain O_2, and Brain Temperature

A 100-µm-diameter thermocouple and two 230-µm fibers were attached to the oxygen probe. This combined probe measures oxygen, temperature, and microvascular blood flow. The measurement requires OxyLite™ and OxyFlo™ instruments. OxyLite 2000 (Oxford Optronix, Ltd., Oxford, UK) is a two-channel device (measuring PO_2

and temperature at two sites simultaneously), whereas OxyFlo 2000 is a two-channel laser Doppler perfusion monitoring instrument. The combination of these two instruments provides simultaneous tissue blood flow, oxygenation, and temperature data. Laser Doppler signals were recorded in blood perfusion units (BPU), which are a relative unite scale defined using a carefully controlled motility standard.

33.2.7 Measurement of Baroreflex Sensitivity

The method we used for determination of the BRS was detailed by Smyth et al. (51) and Parati et al (41). In our study, because of limitations of research design, one single dose of phenylephrine (20 μg/kg, IV) was used to increase MAP. Both the blood pressure and pulse interval changes were recorded in the PowerLab 4/20 high performance data recording system. The data were analyzed by Microsoft Excel 2000.

33.2.8 Neuronal Damage Score

The extent of cerebral neuronal damage was scored on a scale of 0–3, from the grading system of Pulsinelli et al (43), in which 0 is normal, 1 indicates that ~30% of the neurons are damaged, 2 indicates that ~60% of the neurons are damaged, and 3 indicates that 100% of the neurons are damaged.

33.2.9 Statistical Analysis

Data are presented as means ± SEM. Repeated-measures analysis of variance was conducted to test the treatment-by-time interactions and the effect of treatment over time on each score. The Duncan multiple-range test was used for post hoc multiple comparison among means. Wilcoxon test were used for evaluation of neuronal damage scores. These data were presented as "median" followed by first (Q1) and third (Q3) quartile. $P < 0.05$ was considered evidence of statistical significance.

33.3 Experimental Results

33.3.1 CTAP or Naltrexone Increases both Latency and Survival Time During Heatstroke

As shown in our previous results (26, 16), the vehicle-treated rats had a latency of 61 ± 2 min as well as a survival time of 97 ± 7 min. CTAP (100–200 μg/kg, IV) or naltrexone (0.1–10 mg/kg, IV) administered 20 min before heating, but not immediately at the onset of heatstroke, prolonged both the latency and the survival time dose-dependently. However, pretreatment with nor-binaltoryshine or ICI-174684 20 min before heating affected neither the latency nor the survival time.

33.3.2 CTAP or Naltrexone Attenuates Heatstroke-Induced Cerebrovascular Dysfunction During Heatstroke

As demonstrated in our previous findings, in vehicle-treated heatstroke groups, the T_{co}, ICP, and cellular levels of glutamate, glycerol, and lactate/pyruvate ratio in brain were significantly higher at 71 min after the start of exposure (43°C) than they were for normothermic controls. In contrast, the values for MAP, CPP, BRS, CBF, and brain PO_2 were all significantly lower than those of normothermic controls. Treatment with CTAP (100–200 μg/kg, IV) (16) or naltrexone (0.1–10 mg/kg, IV) 20 min before the start of heat exposure significantly attenuated the heat stress-induced arterial hypotension, intracranial hypertension, cerebral hypoperfusion and hypoxia, decreased BRS, and increased levels of extracellular ischemia (e.g., glutamate, lactate/pyruvate ratio) and damage (e.g., glycerol) markers in brain (17).

33.3.3 CTAP Attenuates Heatstroke-Induced Hypercoagulable State

Table 33.1 summarizes the plasma levels of aPTT, PT, platelet count, protein C, and D-dimer for normothermic controls, vehicle-treated heatstroke rats, and CTAP-treated heatstroke rats. It can be seen from the table that aPTT, PT, and D-dimer values during heatstroke for rats treated with normal saline (1 ml/kg body weight, IV) were all significantly higher at 71 min after the start of heat exposure (43°C) than they were for normothermic controls. In contrast, the values for plasma protein C and platelet count levels were all significantly lower than those of normothermic controls. Pretreatment with CTAP (200 μg/kg, IV) 20 min before initiation of heat exposure significantly attenuated the heat stress-induced increased plasma levels of aPTT, PT, and D-dimers, as well as the decreased plasma levels of protein C and platelet count. It should be noted that the plasma levels of aPTT, PT, platelet count, protein C, and D-dimer measured for normothermic rats treated with CTAP (200 μg/kg, IV) were indistinguishable from those of the normothermic rats without treatment.

33.3.4 CTAP Attenuates Heatstroke-Induced Cellular Injury and Organ Dysfunction

Table 33.2 summarizes the blood urea nitrogen values and plasma levels of creatinine, SGOT, SGPT, and ALP for normothermic controls, vehicle-treated heatstroke

Table 33.1 The plasma levels of aPTT, PT, platelet counts, D-dimer, and protein C for normothermic controls, vehicle-treated heatstroke rats, and CTAP-treated heatstroke rats

Treatment group/ time course	aPTT (s)	PT (s)	Platelet counts (×1,000/μl)	Protein C (μg/L)	D-dimer (μg/ml)
Normothermic controls					
0 min	26 ± 3	9.4 ± 0.2	1,114 ± 81	3.0 ± 0.1	45 ± 2
61 min	25 ± 2	9.6 ± 0.2	1,116 ± 79	3.0 ± 0.1	46 ± 3
71 min	27 ± 2	9.3 ± 0.1	1,110 ± 66	3.1 ± 0.1	45 ± 3
Vehicle-treated heatstroke rats					
0 min	25 ± 2	9.5 ± 2	1,110 ± 79	3.0 ± 0.1	47 ± 2
61 min	83 ± 6*	13.6 ± 0.3*	797 ± 70*	2.0 ± 0.1*	88 ± 3*
71 min	99 ± 8*	14.3 ± 0.3*	710 ± 42*	0.5 ± 0.1*	109 ± 7*
CTAP-treated heatstroke rats					
0 min	25 ± 3	9.3 ± 0.2	1,109 ± 77	3.1 ± 0.1	46 ± 2
61 min	37 ± 7**	9.4 ± 0.3**	991 ± 75**	2.0 ± 0.1	66 ± 3**
71 min	39 ± 6**	9.5 ± 0.3**	995 ± 73**	2.0 ± 0.1**	62 ± 3**

Values are means ± SEM of eight rats per group. Vehicle (normal saline 1 ml/kg, IV) or CTAP (200 μg/kg in 1 ml normal saline, IV) was administered 20 min before heat stress

*$P < 0.05$ compared with normothermic controls; **$P < 0.05$ compared with vehicle-treated heatstroke rats (ANOVA followed by Duncan test)

CTAP cyclic D-phe-cys-try-arg-thr-pen-thr-NH_2, *PT* prothrombin time, *aPTT* activated partial thromboplastin time

Table 33.2 The plasma levels of creatinine, BUN, SGOT, SGPT, and ALP for normothermic controls, vehicle-treated heatstroke rats, and CTAP-treated heatstroke rats

Treatment group/ time course	Creatinine (mg/kg)	BUN (mg/dl)	SGOT (IU/L)	SGPT (IU/L)	ALP (IU/L)
Normothermic controls					
0 min	0.40 ± 0.03	12 ± 2	165 ± 18	78 ± 7	408 ± 39
61 min	0.38 ± 0.02	13 ± 2	168 ± 17	75 ± 6	405 ± 40
71 min	0.37 ± 0.03	14 ± 2	164 ± 16	79 ± 8	409 ± 41
Vehicle-treated heatstroke rats					
0 min	0.38 ± 0.03	13 ± 1	169 ± 17	77 ± 6	401 ± 42
61 min	0.55 ± 0.06*	23 ± 2*	476 ± 21*	202 ± 17*	612 ± 47*
71 min	0.91 ± 0.08*	29 ± 3*	499 ± 25*	225 ± 19*	737 ± 49*
CTAP-treated heatstroke rats					
0 min	0.41 ± 0.03	14 ± 2	167 ± 16	79 ± 7	405 ± 40
61 min	0.43 ± 0.02**	16 ± 2**	293 ± 22**	141 ± 15**	484 ± 38**
71 min	0.39 ± 0.03**	15 ± 1**	261 ± 18**	139 ± 14**	501 ± 39**

Values are means ± SEM of eight rats per group. Vehicle (normal saline 1 ml/kg, IV) or CTAP (200 μg/kg in 1 ml normal saline, IV) was administered 20 min before heat stress

*$P < 0.05$ compared with normothermic controls; **$P < 0.05$ compared with vehicle-treated heatstroke rats (ANOVA followed by Duncan test)

CTAP cyclic D-phe-cys-try-arg-thr-pen-thr-NH_2, *BUN* blood urea nitrogen, *SGOT* glutamic oxaloacetic transaminase, *SGPT* glutamic pyruvic transaminase, *ALP* alkaline phosphatase, *IU* international unit

rats, and CTAP-treated heatstroke rats. It can be seen from the table that the blood urea nitrogen values and plasma levels of creatinine, SGOT, SGPT, and ALP were all significantly higher at 71 min after the start of heat exposure than they were for normothermic controls. Pretreatment with CTAP (200 µg/kg, IV) 20 min before initiation of heat exposure significantly attenuated the heat stress-induced increased plasma levels of BUN, creatinine, SGOT, and ALP. The BUN, creatinine, SGOT, SGPT, and ALP values measured for normothermic controls treated with CTAP were indistinguishable from those of normothermic rats without treatment.

As demonstrated in our previous studies (16), the scores for neuronal damage in heatstroke rats treated with vehicle solutions 20 min before initiation of heat exposure (median [Q1, Q3], 2[2, 2]) were all significantly greater ($P < 0.05$) than those for the normothermic controls (median [Q1, Q3], 0[0, 0]). However, the neuronal damage scores for heatstroke rats treated with CTAP (median [Q1, Q3], 0(0, 0)) were all significantly lower ($P < 0.05$) than those for heatstroke controls. Heatstroke-induced cell body shrinkage, pyknosis of the nucleus, and loss of Nissl substance in the striatum were attenuated with CTAP (16).

33.3.5 CTAP Attenuates Heatstroke-Induced Activated Inflammation

Table 33.3 summarizes the values of serum TNF-α and IL-10 in different groups of rats. The values of serum TNF-α of vehicle-treated heatstroke rats obtained at 71 min after initiation of heat exposure were significantly higher than those at 0 min. CTAP treatment adopted at 20 min before heat stress significantly suppressed the increased levels of serum TNF-α obtained at 71 min during heatstroke. In vehicle-treated heatstroke rats, serum levels of IL-10 were maintained at a negligible level. However, the serum levels of IL-10 were greatly elevated in CTAP-treated heatstroke rats.

33.3.6 CTAP Attenuates Heatstroke-Induced Overproduction of NO_x^- and DHBA

Table 33.4 summarizes the extracellular levels of NO_x^- and DHBA in striatum for normothermic controls, vehicle-treated heatstroke rats, and CTAP-treated heatstroke rats. It can be seen from the table that the extracellular levels of both NO_x^- and DHBA in striatum were all significantly higher at 61–71 min after the start of heat exposure than they were for normothermic controls. Pretreatment with CTAP (200 µg/kg, IV) 20 min before initiation of heat exposure significantly attenuated the heat stress-induced overproduction of both NO_x^- and DHBA in striatum. The NO_x^- and DHBA values obtained for normothermic controls treated with CTAP were indistinguishable from those of normothermic rats without treatment.

Table 33.3 Serum levels of tumor necrosis factor at (TNF)-α and interleukin (IL)-10 for normothermic controls, vehicle-treated heatstroke rats, and CTAP-treated heatstroke rats

Treatment group/time course	Serum TNF-α, pg/mL	Serum IL-10, pg/mL
Normothermic controls		
0 min	1.2 ± 0.5	0.7 ± 0.3
61 min	1.1 ± 0.4	0.5 ± 0.2
71 min	1.4 ± 0.3	0.6 ± 0.2
Vehicle-treated heatstroke rats		
0 min	1.5 ± 0.4	0.8 ± 0.3
61 min	443 ± 32*	1.0 ± 0.2
71 min	587 ± 69*	1.2 ± 0.3
CTAP-treated heatstroke rats		
0 min	1.4 ± 0.4	0.9 ± 0.3
61 min	225 ± 19**	395 ± 32**
71 min	166 ± 17**	506 ± 48**

Values are means ± SEM of eight rats per group. Vehicle (normal saline 1 ml/kg, IV) or CTAP (200 μg/kg in 1 ml normal saline, IV) was administered 20 min before heat stress

*$P < 0.05$ compared with normothermic controls; **$P < 0.05$ compared with vehicle-treated heatstroke rats (ANOVA followed by Duncan test)

CTAP cyclic D-phe-cys-try-arg-thr-pen-thr-NH_2

Table 33.4 Extracellular levels of NO_x^- and DHBA in the striatum for normothermic controls, vehicle-treated heatstroke rats, and CTAP-treated heatstroke rats

Treatment group/time course	NO_x^- (μM)	DHBA (% of baseline)
Normothermic controls		
0 min	2.5 ± 0.4	100 ± 4
61 min	2.7 ± 0.5	99 ± 3
71 min	2.9 ± 0.3	98 ± 3
Vehicle-treated heatstroke rats		
0 min	2.6 ± 0.3	100 ± 3
61 min	11 ± 1*	715 ± 28*
71 min	12 ± 1*	733 ± 33*
CTAP-treated heatstroke rats		
0 min	2.4 ± 0.4	100 ± 4
61 min	3.2 ± 0.5**	211 ± 16**
71 min	3.5 ± 0.6**	194 ± 17**

Values are means ± SEM of eight rats per group. Vehicle (normal saline 1 ml/kg, IV) or CTAP (200 μg/kg in ml normal saline, IV) was administered 20 min before heat stress

*$P < 0.05$ compared with normothermic controls; **$P < 0.05$ compared with vehicle-treated heatstroke rats (ANOVA followed by Duncan test)

DHBA dihydroxybenzoic acid, *NO_x^-* nitric oxide metabolites, *CTAP* cyclic D-phe-cys-try-arg-thr-pen-thr-NH_2

33.4 Discussion, Conclusions, and Perspectives

33.4.1 Discussion

Hall and colleagues (22) have indicated that hyperthermia stimulates production of ROS (radical oxygen species), which activates metals and limits heat tolerance by promoting circulatory and intestinal barrier dysfunction. In addition, overproduction of RNS (radical nitrogen species) may contribute to the splanchnic vasodilation that precedes vascular collapse with heatstroke. In addition, systemic administration of a μ-opioid receptor antagonist (CTAP), but not a δ-opioid receptor antagonist (ICI-174864), or a κ-opioid receptor antagonist (NBO), significantly prolonged both the latency and survival time during heatstroke (16). Furthermore, the hyperthermia exhibited during heatstroke can be reduced by CTAP pretreatment. Evidence has also accumulated to indicate that the hyperthermia or fever induced by central injection of IL-1β, TNF-α, or macrophage inflammatory protein-1 or systemic administration of lipopolysaccharide can be prevented by pretreatment with central administration of CTAP (3, 24, 55, 6). Thus, it appears that prior antagonism of μ-opioid receptors with CTAP or naltrexone attenuates overproduction of ROS and RNS during heatstroke by reducing hyperthermia in the rat.

In our results, the prolongation of survival in heatstroke rats pretreated with CTAP or naltrexone was found to be related to enhancement of MAP and CBF as well as reduction in both ICP and cerebral damage. The maintenance of CBF at an appropriate level in rats pretreated with CTAP or naltrexone was brought about by higher CPP (resulting from lower ICP and higher MAP) during heatstroke. It has been well documented that both circulatory shock and cerebral ischemia are related to increased production of ROS (56, 53, 54) and RNS (11, 30). Pretreatment with free radical scavengers (10, 38, 53) or inducible nitric oxide synthase (iNOS) inhibitors (11) all significantly attenuated heatstroke-induced arterial hypotension, cerebral ischemia, and neuronal damage. Therefore, the neuroprotective effects of CTAP or naltrexone involve attenuation of brain ischemia and damage during heatstroke via attenuating ROS and RNS generation. The contention is supported by several previous findings. For example, naltrexone improves CBF, reduces seizure activity, and enhances survival time in gerbils following temporary occlusion of bilateral common carotid artery (4, 21, 25, 58) as well as in rat cerebral ischemia/reperfusion (13). Pretreatment with naltrexone has also been shown to reduce ischemia-induced suppression of extracellular pyruvate levels and enhancement of lactate/pyruvate ratio as well as cerebral ischemia/reperfusion induced increases of endogenous catalase, glutathione peroxidase, and manganese superoxide dismutase activities (13).

Heatstroke resembles repstic shock in many aspects (7, 15). In rat model, heat stress induces increased levels of cytokines, including TNF-α, IL-6, and IL-1 (33, 38, 27, 34) in the plasma. The arterial hypotension during heatstroke can be mimicked by IV administration of IL-1β (33). Pretreatment with IL-1β (33) or endothelin-1A (35) receptor inhibitors or glucocorticoids (34) are able to improve arterial hypotension during heatstroke. Overproduction of heat shock protein 72 by sublethal heat shock (53, 57) or progressive exercise (27) ameliorates arterial hypotension and cerebral ischemia during heatstroke by reducing TNF-α overproduction. It has also been shown that acute heart failure (37, 48) are related with overproduction of TNF-α in the plasma. Other line of evidence has suggested that IL-10 has important antiinflammatory and immunosuppressive properties through suppression of TNF-α and other proinflammatory cytokines (39). Our results have shown that, after the onset of heatstroke in rats, pretreatment with CTAP produces a significant increase in the serum level of IL-10 accompanied by a reduction of heatstroke reactions as mentioned in the preceding section. Putting these observations together, CTAP or naltrexone may ameliorate arterial hypotension and cerebral ischemia and damage by increasing IL-10 but decreasing TNF-α production.

It has been shown that an endotoxin given systemically is able to elicit an increase of iNOS-dependent NO production in the nucleus tractus solitarii and induce arterial hypotension (32). Under heat stress, in addition to circulatory shock and cerebral ischemia, iNOS-dependent NO overproduction was also noted in both the plasma (47) and the brain (11) of rats. Inhibition of the iNOS-dependent NO formation in the plasma (47) and/or in the brain (26); present results) with naltrexone or CTAP may alleviate arterial hypotension as well as cerebral ischemia exhibited during heatstroke by potentiating BRS as well as reducing hyperthermia and β-endorphin overproduction.

Opioids have been implicated in the pathogenesis of heatstroke (44-46, 49, 50). An increase in the serum concentrations of β-endorphin have also been observed in patients (2) or rats (26) with heatstroke. In addition, it has been shown that (a) hyperthermia has the capacity to upregulate dynorphin immunoreactivity in the brain, (b) inhibition of NOS considerably attenuates the dynorphin immunoreaction following heat stress, and (c) upregulation of dynorphin is somehow contributing to hyperthermia induced brain damage (49). It should be stressed that our results showed that naltrexone attenuated the overproduction of NO following heat stress (26), whereas the results of (49) showed that inhibition of NOS attenuated the dynorphin immunoreactivity following heat stress. The discrepancy between these two groups of results is not apparent now.

In guinea pigs, intensive and prolonged intraperitoneal heating (IPH) caused a pathologic sequela characterized by high mortality (heatstroke) (44). This IPH-induced heat disorder was accompanied by two "paradoxical" thermoregulatory phenomena. First, although cutaneous vasodilation readily occurred at the onset of the IPH-induced hyperthermia, it later changed to vasoconstriction; this phenomenon was termed as "hyperthermia-induced vasoconstriction." Second, when IPH was stopped, the initial hyperthermia was followed by hypothermia; this was termed as "hyperthermia-induced hypothermia." Romanovsky and Blatteis (46) further showed that naltrexone improved survival during heatstroke by attenuating the hyperthermia-induced vasoconstriction and hyperthermia-induced hypothermia in guinea pigs. However, it is not known whether the improved survival of naltrexone-treated or CTAP-treated rats was accompanied by the blockade of the hyperthermia-induced vasoconstriction and attenuation of hyperthermia-induced hypothermia as revealed in guinea pigs (44-46).

The baroreceptor reflex is one of the fundamental mechanisms through which the central nervous system controls peripheral hemodynamic performance. Our findings showed that BRS, MAP, and maximal reflex bradycardia were all diminished with naltrexone (26) or CTAP (16). CTAP or naltrexone confers pivotal protection against circulatory shock during heatstroke by increasing both BRS and maximal reflex bradycardia.

In a rat model of heatstroke, heat stress-induced hypercoagulable state or DIC as evidenced by increased PT, aPTT, and D-dimer and decreased platelet count and protein C. In addition, rats with heatstroke had cellular ischemia and injury as indicated by an increase in blood urea nitrogen, plasma levels of creatinine, SGOT, SGPT, and ALP, and brain levels of ischemia (e.g., glutamate and lactate/pyruvate ratio) and injury (e.g., glycerol) markers (17) (Lee et al., 2005). In fact, hypercoagulable state and overproduction of cytokines may contribute to the multiple organ dysfunction and death (12, 23, 1, 19, 9, 8). Hypercoagulable state was diagnosed in our heatstroke rats by increased PT and aPTT accompanied by raised D-dimer, as well as a low platelet count (40). The occurrence of arterial hypotension and cerebral hypoperfusion, hypoxia, and neuronal damage during heatstroke may be associated with hypercoagulable state. In the present study, CTAP therapy may improve multiple organ dysfunction or failure during heatstroke by attenuating the hypercoagulable state.

Protein C is a key molecule in the coagulation cascade, and reduced levels of protein C are related to poor outcome in rats with sepsis (20) and heatstroke (14). Exogenous administration of activated protein C (14) or CTAP (present result) are shown to be able to reverse the reduced levels of protein C that occurred during heatstroke.

33.4.2 Conclusions

The foregoing statements can be summarized in Fig. 33.1 which shows the proposed scheme of the interacting sequence of events occurring from the beginning of heat exposure to heatstroke development. After onset of heatstroke, cessation, or diminution of blood flow to the brain (resulting from both arterial hypotension and intracranial hypertension) and the visceral organs (resulting from cutaneous vasodilation) induces cerebral and visceral ischemia and hypoxia, respectively. As heat stress continues, reactive nitrogen species (RNS) and reactive oxygen species (ROS) generation can produce multifocal cellular injury and inflammation (22, 53, 54, 11). In the present results, the prolongation of survival in heatstroke rats treated with CTAP or naltrexone was found to be related to reversal of decreased MAP, increased ICP, decreased BRS, tissue ischemia and hypoxia, hypercoagulable state, activated systemic inflammation, and multiple organ dysfunction or failure.

It should be stressed that systemic delivery of CTAP or naltrexone 20 min before the initiation of heat stress, but not at the time point of onset of onset of heatstroke, significantly reduced the cerebral ischemia and injury. Therefore, CTAP or naltrexone can be used as preventive, rather than therapeutic, measure for heatstroke reactions.

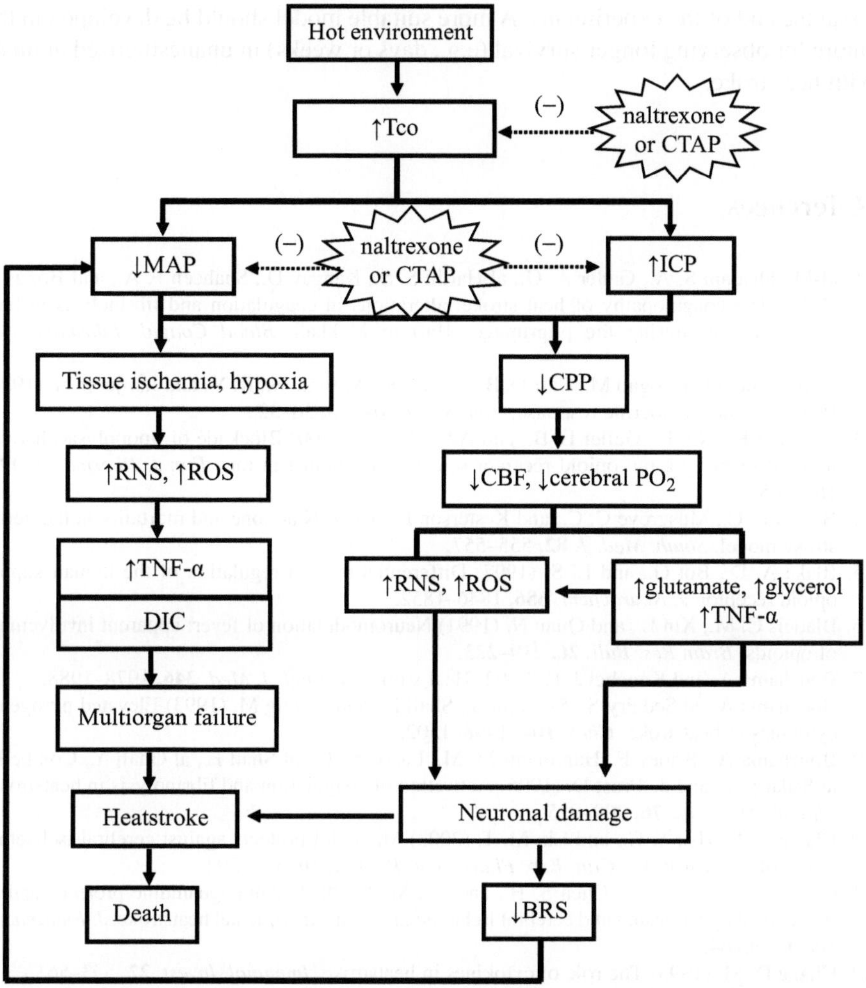

Fig. 33.1 Proposed scheme of the interacting sequence of events occurring from the beginning of heat stress to heatstroke occurrence. Arrows indicate increased (↑) or decreased (↓). T_{co} core temperature, *MAP* mean arterial pressure, *ICP* intracranial pressure, *CPP* cerebral perfusion pressure, *CBF* cerebral blood flow, *ROS* radical oxygen species, *RNS* radical nitrogen species, *TNF-α* tumor necrosis factor-α, *DIC* disseminated inadequate coagulation, *BRS* baroreceptor sensitivity. (–) denotes reversal [modified from (52)]

33.4.3 Perspectives

For humane reasons, all the data presented in the current report were obtained from rats under general anesthesia. Anesthesia or rectal temperature probes all influence the thermoregulatory profiles generated during and after heatstroke. These anesthetized animals have to be terminated ~480 min after the initiation of heat exposure (or at the end of the experiment). A more suitable model should be developed in the future for observing longer survival (e.g., days or weeks) in unanesthetized animals with heatstroke.

References

1. al-Mashhadani S. A., Gader A. G., al Harthi S. S., Kangav D., Shaheen F. A., and Bogus F. (1994) The coagulopathy of heat stroke: alterations in coagulation and fibrinolysis in heat stroke patients during the pilgrimage (Haj) to Makkah. *Blood Coagul. Fibrinolysis* **5,** 731–736.
2. Appenzeller O., Khogali M., Carr D. B., Gumaa K., Mustafa M. K. Y., and Jamjoom A. (1986) Heatstroke and endocrine response. *Ann. Sports Med.* **3,** 30–32.
3. Benamar K., Xin L., Geller E. B., and Adler M. W. (2000) Blockade of lipopolysaccharide-induced fever by a mu-opioid receptor-selective antagonist in rats. *Eur. J. Pharmacol.* **401,** 161–165.
4. Benzel E. C., Musgrove C. C., and Kesterson L. (1989) Naloxone and mortality in the gerbil stroke model. *South. Med. J.* **82,** 555–557.
5. Blake A. D., Bot G., and Li S. (1997) Differential agonist regulation of the human kappa-opioid receptor. *J. Neurochem.* **686,** 1846–1852.
6. Blatteis C. M., Xin L., and Quan N. (1991) Neuromodulation of fever: apparent involvement of opioids. *Brain Res. Bull.* **26,** 219–223.
7. Bouchama A. and Knochel J. P. (2002) Heat stroke. *N. Engl. J. Med.* **346,** 1978–1988.
8. Bouchama A., al Sedairy S., Siddiqui S., Shail E., and Rezeig M. (1993) Elevated pyrogenic cytokines in heatstroke. *Chest* **104,** 1498–1502.
9. Bouchama A., Bridey F., Hammami M. M., Lacombe C., al Shail E., al Ohali Y., Combe F., al Sedairy S., and de Prost D. (1996) Activation of coagulation and fibrinolysis in heatstroke. *Thromb. Haemost.* **76,** 909–915.
10. Chang C. P., Hsu Y. C., and Lin M. T. (2003) Magnolol protects against cerebral ischaemic injury of rat heatstroke. *Clin. Exp. Pharmacol. Physiol.* **30,** 387–392.
11. Chang C. P., Lee C. C., Chen S. H., and Lin M. T. (2004) Aminoguanidine protects against intracranial hypertension and cerebral ischemic injury in experimental heatstroke. *J. Pharmacol. Sci.* **95,** 56–64.
12. Chang D. M. (1993) The role of cytokines in heatstroke. *Immunol. Invest.* **22,** 553–561.
13. Chen C. J., Cheng F. C., Liao S. L., Chen W. Y., Lin N. N., and Kuo J. S. (2000) Effects of naloxone on lactate, pyruvate metabolism and antioxidant enzyme activity in rat cerebral ischemia/reperfusion. *Neurosci. Lett.* **287,** 113–116.
14. Chen C. M., Hou C. C., Chen K. C., Tian R. L., Chang C. P., and Lin M. T. (2006a) Activated protein C therapy in a rat heatstroke model. *Crit. Care Med.* **34,** 1960–1966.
15. Chen S. H., Niu K. C., and Lin M. T. (2006) Cerebrovascular dysfunction is an attractive target for therapy in heatstroke. *Clin. Exp. Pharmacol. Physiol.* **33,** 663–672.
16. Chen Z. C., Kuo J. R., Huang Y. P., and Lin M. T. (2005) Mu-opioid receptor blockade protects against circulatory shock and cerebral ischemia during heatstroke. *J. Cardiovasc. Pharmacol.* **46,** 754–760.
17. Chou Y. T., Lai S. T., Lee C. C., and Lin M. T. (2003) Hypothermia attenuates circulatory shock and cerebral ischemia in experimental heatstroke. *Shock* **19,** 288–393.
18. Cotton R., Giles M. G., Miller L., Shaw J. S., and Timms D. (1984) ICI 174864: a highly selective antagonist for the opioid delta-receptor. *Eur. J. Pharmacol.* **97,** 331–332.
19. el Kassimi F. A., Al Mashhadani S., Abdullah A. K., and Akhtar J. (1986) Adult respiratory distress syndrome and disseminated intravascular coagulation complicating heat stroke. *Chest* **90,** 571–574.

20. Esmon C. T. (2003) The PC pathway. *Chest* **124,** 26s–32s.
21. Faden A. I. (1988) Role of thyrotropin-releasing hormone and opiate receptor antagonists in limiting central nervous system injury. *Adv. Neurol.* **47,** 531–546.
22. Hall D. M., Buettner G. R., Oberley L. W., Xu L., Matthes R. D., and Gisolfi C. V. (2001) Mechanisms of circulatory and intestinal barrier dysfunction during whole body hyperthermia. *Am. J. Physiol Heart Circ. Physiol.* **280,** H509–H521.
23. Hammami M. M., Bouchama A., Al Sedairy S., Shail E., AlOhaly Y., and Mohamed G. E. (1997) Concentrations of soluble tumor necrosis factor and interleukin-6 receptors in heatstroke and heatstress. *Crit Care Med.* **25,** 1314–1319.
24. Handler C. M., Price R. W., Geller E. B., and Adler M. W. (1998) Effect of mu-selective opioid antagonists on MIP-1 beta and IL-1 beta-induced fever. *Ann. N. Y. Acad. Sci.* **856,** 270–273.
25. Hosobuchi Y., Baskin D. S., and Woo S. K. (1982) Reversal of induced ischemic neurologic deficit in gerbils by the opiate antagonist naloxone. *Science* **215,** 69–71.
26. Huang Y. P., Lin M. T., Chen J. S., and Wu P. Y. (2005) Naltrexone protects against hypotension, hyperthermia, and beta-endorphin overproduction during heatstroke in the rat. *J. Pharmacol. Sci.* **97,** 519–524.
27. Hung C. H., Chang N. C., Cheng B. C., and Lin M. T. (2005) Progressive exercise preconditioning protects against circulatory shock during experimental heatstroke. *Shock* **23,** 426–433.
28. Kao T. Y., Chio C. C., and Lin M. T. (1994) Hypothalamic dopamine release and local cerebral blood flow during onset of heatstroke in rats. *Stroke* **25,** 2483–2486.
29. Kramer T. H., Shook J. E., Kazmierski W., Ayres E. A., Wire W. S., Hruby V. J., and Burks T. F. (1989) Novel peptidic mu opioid antagonists: pharmacologic characterization in vitro and in vivo. *J. Pharmacol. Exp. Ther.* **249,** 544–551.
30. Lee I. Y., Lee C. C., Chang C. K., Chien C. H., and Lin M. T. (2005a) Sheng mai san, a Chinese herbal medicine, protects against renal ischaemic injury during heat stroke in the rat. *Clin. Exp. Pharmacol. Physiol.* **32,** 742–748.
31. Lee J. J., Lin M. T., Wang N. L., Lin C. L., and Chang C. K. (2005b) Platonin, a cyanine photosensitizing dye, causes attenuation of circulatory shock, hypercoagulable state, and tissue ischemia during heat stroke. *Shock* **24,** 577–582.
32. Lin H. C., Wan F. J., Kang B. H., Wu C. C., and Tseng C. J. (1999) Systemic administration of lipopolysaccharide induces release of nitric oxide and glutamate and c-fos expression in the nucleus tractus solitarii of rats. *Hypertension* **33,** 1218–1224.
33. Lin M. T., Liu H. H., and Yang Y. L. (1997) Involvement of interleukin-1 receptor mechanisms in development of arterial hypotension in rat heatstroke. *Am. J. Physiol.* **273,** H2072–H2077.
34. Liu C. C., Chien C. H., and Lin M. T. (2000) Glucocorticoids reduce interleukin-1 concentration and result in neuroprotective effects in rat heatstroke. *J. Physiol.* **527,** 333–343.
35. Liu C. C., Chen Z. C., Cheng B. C., and Lin M. T. (2004a) Prior antagonism of endothelin-1A receptors alleviates circulatory shock and cerebral ischemia during rat heatstroke. *J. Pharmacol. Sci.* **96,** 177–187.
36. Liu C. C., Ke D., Chen Z. C., and Lin M. T. (2004b) Hydroxyethyl starch produces attenuation of circulatory shock and cerebral ischemia during heatstroke. *Shock* **22,** 288–294.
37. Nakagawa Y., Homma S., Yamamoto I., Banno M., Nakazato H., Imanaga H., and Yamamoto N. (1993) In vivo and in vitro activation of macrophages with a cyanine photosensitizing dye, platonin. *Cancer Immunol. Immunother.* **37,** 157–162.
38. Niu K. C., Lin K. C., Yang C. Y., and Lin M. T. (2003) Protective effects of alpha-tocopherol and mannitol in both circulatory shock and cerebral ischaemia injury in rat heatstroke. *Clin. Exp. Pharmacol. Physiol.* **30,** 745–751.
39. Oberholzer A., Oberholzer C., and Moldawer L. L. (2000) Cytokine signaling - regulation of the immune response in normal and critically ill states. *Crit. Care Med.* **28,** N3–N12.
40. Okelford P. A. and Carter C. J. (1982) Disseminated intravascular coagulation: the application and utility of diagnostic test. In: Okelford PA, Carter CJ (eds.): Seminars in Thrombosis and Haemostasis. New York: Thieme-Strattom, pp. 198–215.

41. Parati G., Di Rienzo M., and Mancia G. (2000) How to measure baroreflex sensitivity: from the cardiovascular laboratory to daily life. *J. Hypertens.* **18,** 7–19.
42. Paxinos G. and Watson C. (1982) The Rat Brain is Stereotoxic Coordinates. New York: Academic Press.
43. Pulsinelli W. A., Brierley J. B., and Plum F. (1982) Temporal profile of neuronal damage in a model of transient forebrain ischemia. *Ann. Neurol.* **11,** 491–498.
44. Romanovsky A. A. and Blatteis C. M. (1994) Body temperature elevation per se induces the late phase syndrome. In: Milton AS (ed.): Temperature Regulation: Recent Physiological and Pharmacological Advances. Basel: Birkhäuser, pp. 41–46.
45. Romanovsky A. A. and Blatteis C. M. (1996) Heat stroke: opioid-mediated mechanisms. *J. Appl. Physiol.* **81,** 2565–2570.
46. Romanovsky A. A. and Blatteis C. M. (1997) Naltrexone modifies thermoregulatory symptoms and lessens the severity of heat stroke in guinea pigs. *Ann. N. Y. Acad. Sci.* **813,** 548–552.
47. Sachidhanandam S. B., Low K. S., and Moochhala S. M. (2002) Naltrexone attenuates plasma nitric oxide release following acute heat stress. *Eur. J. Pharmacol.* **450,** 163–167.
48. Schirmer W. J., Schirmer J. M., and Fry D. E. (1989) Recombinant human tumor necrosis factor produces hemodynamic changes characteristic of sepsis and endotoxemia. *Arch. Surg.* **124,** 445–448.
49. Sharma H. S. and Alm P. (2002) Nitric oxide synthase inhibitors influence dynorphin A (1–17) immunoreactivity in the rat brain following hyperthermia. *Amino. Acids* **23,** 247–259.
50. Sharma H. S., Westman J., Cervos-Navarro J., Dey P. K., and Nyberg F. (1997) Opioid receptor antagonists attenuate heat stress-induced reduction in cerebral blood flow, increased blood-brain barrier permeability, vasogenic edema and cell changes in the rat. *Ann. N. Y. Acad. Sci.* **813,** 559–571.
51. Smyth H. S., Sleight P., and Pickering G. W. (1969) Reflex regulation of arterial pressure during sleep in man. A quantitative method of assessing baroreflex sensitivity. *Circ. Res.* **24,** 109–121.
52. Tsai C. C., Lin M. T., Yang C. C., Liao J. F., and Lee J. J. (2006) Platonin, a cyaninine photosensitizing dye, is effective for attenuation of heat stroke in rats. *Shock.* **26,** 601–607.
53. Wang J. L., Ke D. S., and Lin M. T. (2005a) Heat shock pretreatment may protect against heatstroke-induced circulatory shock and cerebral ischemia by reducing oxidative stress and energy depletion. *Shock* **23,** 161–167.
54. Wang N. L., Liou Y. L., Lin M. T., Lin C. L., and Chang C. K. (2005b) Chinese herbal medicine, Shengmai San, is effective for improving circulatory shock and oxidative damage in the brain during heatstroke. *J. Pharmacol. Sci.* **97,** 253–265.
55. Xin L., Zhao S. F., Geller E. B., McCafferty M. R., Sterling G. H., and Adler M. W. (1997) Involvement of beta-endorphin in the preoptic anterior hypothalamus during interleukin-1 beta-induced fever in rats. *Ann. N. Y. Acad. Sci.* **813,** 324–326.
56. Yang C. Y. and Lin M. T. (2002) Oxidative stress in rats with heatstroke-induced cerebral ischemia. *Stroke* **33,** 790–794.
57. Yang Y. L. and Lin M. T. (1999) Heat shock protein expression protects against cerebral ischemia and monoamine overload in rat heatstroke. *Am. J. Physiol.* **276,** H1961–H1967.
58. Zabramski J. M., Spetzler R. F., Selman W. R., Roessmann U. R., Hershey L. A., Crumrine R. C., and Macko R. (1984) Naloxone therapy during focal cerebral ischemia evaluation in a primate model. *Stroke* **15,** 621–629.

Chapter 34
A Review of the Opioid System in Cancer Patients and Preliminary Results of Opioid Antagonists in the Treatment of Human Neoplasms

Paolo Lissoni

Abstract Today there is no doubt about the possible influence of the psychological status on cancer growth. In particular, it has been demonstrated that brain opioid system plays a fundamental role in mediating the psychic influence on tumor growth, either by modulating the immune functionless or by regulating cancer cell proliferation. However, the effects of the various opioid agonists on cancer growth are very controversial, since they depend on several variables, including dose, schedule of administration, animal species, and tumor histotype. In any case, the activation of the opioid system tends to stimulate cancer development, particularly through the mu-opioid receptor, directly either by stimulating tumor cell proliferation or by inducing a suppression of the anticancer immunity, due to the inhibition of the antitumor cytokine IL-2 and to the stimulation of IL-10 secretion, which in contrast may suppress the antitumor immunity. Moreover, the stimulatory effect of stress on cancer development is mainly mediated by an activation of the opioid system, since it may be completely abrogated by the opioid antagonists. Naltrexone (NTX) is the most commonly used opioid antagonist, because of its long-acting action and its possibility to be administered orally. At present, only few preliminary clinical studies have been performed to evaluate the possible use of opioid antagonists in the treatment of human neoplasms, as previously demonstrated in experimental conditions. Two fundamental clinical trials have been carried out up till now, by using low- or high-dose NTX, in an attempt to obtain a partial or a complete block of the opioid system. Since tumor regressions have been reported by both schedules of treatment, future-randomized clinical studies with low- or high-dose NTX will be required to establish which may be the optimal schedule of treatment of human neoplasms by opioid antagonists.

Keywords: Beta-endorphin; Dynorphins; Enkephalins; Naloxone; Naltrexone; Opioid antagonists; Opioid system

---

P. Lissoni
Divisione di Radioterapia Oncologica, Ospedale San Gerardo,
20052 Monza, Italy
e-mail: p.lissoni@hsgerardo.org

R. Dean et al. (eds.), *Opiate Receptors and Antagonists*,

34.1 Introduction

The recent advances in the psychoneuroimmunological sciences have demonstrated that the immune functions depend not only on the activities of the immune cells but also on the existence of a physiological neuroendocrine system involved in the regulation of their inhibition (43, 16). The psychological status may influence the immune responses, including the anticancer immunity, by an extremely complex neuroendocrine network. Within the great variety of neuroimmune interactions, the endogenous opioid system has been shown to play a fundamental role in the neuroimmunomodulation (35). The immunomodulatory effects of the different opioid molecules would mainly depend on pharmacological subtype, dose, and schedule of administration (16). However, according to recent experimental observations, the endogenous opioid system and its immunomodulatory activity cannot be studied by in vivo investigations alone, without taking into consideration its fundamental interaction with another essential neuroimmunomodulatory system, the endocannabinoids (15).

The endogenous cannabinoid system has been shown to influence the immune status through the release of at least four endocannabinoid molecules; the most important of them is represented by the anandamide (15). The endocannabinoid system plays an immunostimulatory action, mainly by the activation of dendritic cells, and the inhibition of macrophage-mediated immunosuppressive effects, which is dependent upon the release of proinflammatory immunosuppressant cytokines, such as interleukin (IL)-6 (5). Stress and depression have been proven to be associated with hyperactivation of the endogenous opioid system (45). In contrast, both pleasure and spiritual feeling have appeared to be mediated by a hyperactivity of the endogenous cannabinoid system (27). Despite the existence of a large variety of neuroimmunoactive molecules, the influence of the psychospiritual life on the immune inhibition of the system would depend primarily on a balance between opioid and cannabinoid endogenous systems, and in particular, stress-induced immunosuppression and pleasure-related immunostimulation which are primarily mediated by brain opioid and cannabinoid systems, respectively. In addition, both the opioid and cannabinoid systems are under a physiological neuroendocrine regulation, controlled by the pineal gland (27).

34.2 Opioid Receptors

The opioid receptors may be classified by binding studies in mu, delta, and kappa receptors (14). The mu-opioid receptor has beta-endorphin as an endogenous ligand, while enkephalins and dynorphins are the endogenous ligands for delta and kappa receptors, respectively. Moreover, the existence of another opioid receptor has been demonstrated, the so-called zeta-opioid receptor, also known as the opioid growth factor (OGF) receptor, which has appear to play a potential role in the modulation of cell proliferation (54). Its endogenous ligand is represented by the met-5-enkephalin, also called OGF, which appears to exert an oncostatic action on several cancer cell lines (54). A number of opioid receptor antagonists are currently available. Naloxone (NLX) and the long-acting naltrexone (NTX) are the commonly used mu-opioid receptor antagonists (19). Similarly, naltrindole is a classic delta-opioid receptor antagonist (39). The expression of opioid receptors is influenced by several neurotransmitters and neuromodulators, but in particular it seems to be under a cannabinergic modulation (8), as well as being under a pineal regulatory control (30).

34.3 Opioid-Cannabinergic System Interactions

Endogenous opioid and cannabinoid systems are the two fundamental neuroimmune functional systems involved in mediating the influence of the psychospiritual condition on health status (27). The opioid system mediates anxiety, depression, and stress (43), whereas the cannabinergic system is involved in the perception of pleasure and in the spiritual expansion of mind (15). Endogenous cannabinoid and opioid systems are connected by a bidirectional interaction (11), which plays a fundamental role in the modulation of psychobiology. In addition to their interactions, mediated by several neurotransmitters and neuromodulators, the two mechanisms are connected by the action of cytokines released by the activated immune cells, particularly by IL-10 secreted by TH2-lymphocytes. IL-10 is also the main cytokine utilized by T-regulator lymphocytes to suppress the immune responses, including the anticancer immunity and the autoimmune reactions (42). In addition, IL-10 has been shown to be under a psychoneuroendocrine stimulatory control by the opioid system and noradrenaline (44). IL-10, released in response to an opioid stimulation, would create an unbalanced ratio between opioid and cannabinergic systems. In fact, IL-10 appears to be able to stimulate the action of fatty acid amide hydrolase (FAAH) (31), which is the enzyme responsible for the degradation of the endogenous cannabinoids, with a subsequent decline in blood concentrations as a consequence of their enhanced metabolization. This is confirmed by the evidence of an inverse correlation between FAAH blood concentrations and concentrations of the endogenous cannabinoid, anandamide (21). IL-10 produced in response to an enhanced opioid system activity may induce an endogenous cannabinoid deficiency through a stimulation of FAAH degrading activity.

In contrast, the antitumor cytokine IL-12 may inhibit FAAH activity (31), with an increase in the activity of the endocannabinoid system, as well as documented by the enhanced anandamide blood concentrations. Therefore, the suppression and the stimulation of the anticancer immunity are associated with an opioid system hyperfunction and with an endocannabinoid hyperactivity, respectively. The central role of IL-10 in the suppression of the anticancer immunity is also suggested by the fact that it also constitutes the main cytokine produced by cancer cells themselves to counteract the action of the T-cytotoxic lymphocytes (5). Cytokine modulation of opioid-cannabinergic system interactions is illustrated in Fig. 34.1. On the contrary, from a psychoneuroendocrine point of view, the functional balance between cannabinoid and opioid systems would seem to be mainly mediated by the

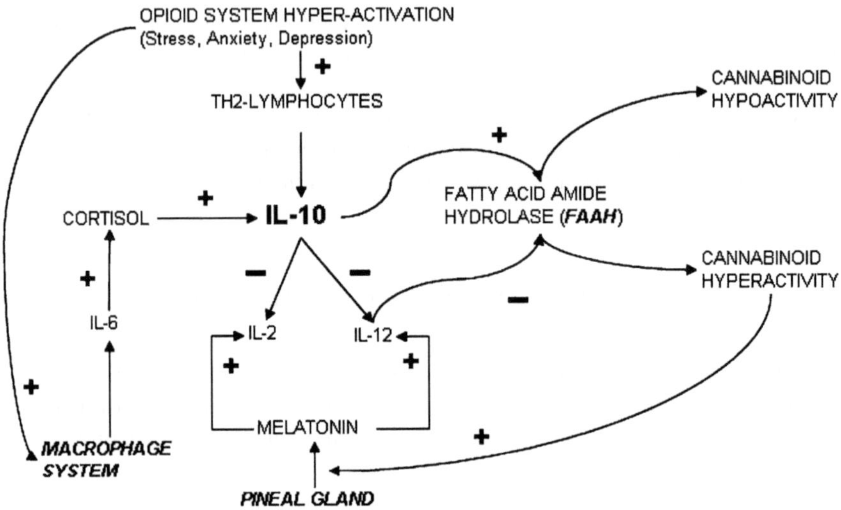

Fig. 34.1 Cytokines modulation of opioid-cannabinergic interactions

pineal gland (32, 27). The functional unit, consisting of opioid-cannabinoid-pineal interactions, would represent the most important neurochemical structure involved in mediating the influence of the psychospiritual status on the anticancer immunity. The opioid system may suppress the anticancer immunity by stimulating the release of IL-10, which has been proven to inhibit the secretion of the two most important anticancer cytokines in humans, IL-2 and IL-12 (44).

The pineal gland has appeared to exert a physiological anticancer role (32), whereas the effect of the endocannabinoid system on the anticancer immunity still needs to be studied. Despite their potential inhibitory action on T-lymphocyte proliferation, cannabinoids may counteract macrophage-mediated immunosuppressive effects (15), which would play an important role in determining cancer-related immunodeficiency (42), with a potential induction of an effective anticancer immune reaction. In fact, the chronic treatment of cannabinoids appears to inhibit cancer growth and dissemination in experimental conditions (15), whereas that of opioids may promote cancer onset and development (40). Thus, opioids and endocannabinoids would constitute the main neurochemical bases to explain the promoting action of stress, anxiety, and depression on cancer growth, as well as the protective action of the psychology of pleasure and spiritual joy on tumor development.

34.4 Opioid System-Pineal Interactions

The pineal cells may express opioid receptors (7), and this evidence represents the biochemical basis for a possible direct opioid influence on the pineal endocrine activity. Both mu-opioid agonists, such as morphine (9), and delta-opioid agonists, such as met-enkephalin analogues (23), appear to stimulate the release of melatonin, which is the most investigated hormone released from the pineal gland. On the contrary, melatonin tends to inhibit the secretion of the mu-opioid receptor agonist, beta-endorphin (24), and to stimulate the production of the delta-opioid agonist, met-enkephalin (20), with a subsequent increase in its brain content. The opioid system exerts a major stimulatory action on the pineal gland, whereas the pineal gland modulates the different opioid functions, by stimulating delta-opioid receptor-mediated activities, and inhibiting those related to the mu-opioid receptor. The promoting effect of the opioid agents on melatonin secretion from the pineal gland is further confirmed by the evidence of an inhibitory action of the mu-opioid antagonist NLX on the nocturnal increase in melatonin blood concentrations (30). Because of the potential modulatory effects of the opioid agonists and antagonists on the pineal function and the well-documented anticancer activity of melatonin (32), the in vivo effects of the opioid agonists and antagonists on cancer development and on the immune responses is mediated, in part, by the pineal gland.

34.5 Immunomodulatory Effects of Opioid Agonists and Antagonists

The immunomodulatory actions of the opioid agents described in the literature are controversial, because the in vitro observations are often contradictory with respect to the in vivo evidences. The immunomodulating effects of the opioid agents mainly depend on their dosage. It has been demonstrated that both endorphins and enkephalins may either stimulate or suppress the immune functions, depending on the dose and schedule of administration, with generally immunosuppressive effects at high doses, and immunostimulatory actions at low doses (17). Further, lymphocytes may express opioid receptors for both endorphins and enkephalins (49). Thus, opioid agonists and antagonists may directly influence lymphocyte functions by acting on specific opioid receptors.

However, opioid agents may also influence the immune system by modulating the secretion and the activity of other immunomodulating neurohormones and neuropeptides, provided by similar or different immune effects with respect to those played by the various opioids. This finding may explain the controversial results observed in vitro and in vivo. In addition to the opioid influence on lymphocyte functions, the action of the opioid agents on immune cells (other than lymphocytes), in particular their stimulatory effect on the macrophages (18), which exerts a dominant suppressive effect on the antitumor immunity despite their potential anticancer cytotoxic activity (42). At present it is known that the anticancer immunity is mainly mediated by T lymphocytes and dendritic cells, whereas it is suppressed by macrophages and T-regulator lymphocytes. Beta-endorphin, a mu-opioid agonist, has been shown to play both immunostimulatory and immunosuppressive effects depending on the different immune parameters experimentally investigated.

The most relevant immunostimulatory action of beta-endorphin would consist of the stimulation of T-lymphocyte proliferation (36), probably by acting in part on NLX-insensitive receptors, and activation of natural killer (NK) cytotoxicity (34). On the contrary, the most evident immunosuppressive effect of beta-endorphin is represented by the stimulation of IL-10 secretion from TH2-lymphocytes, by acting on specific mu-opioid receptors, which is antagonized by NTX (44). Moreover, the mu-opioid agonists appear to inhibit TH1-lymphocyte and dendritic cell functions, with a subsequent decline in the secretion of IL-2 and IL-12, respectively (44), which play a fundamental role in the generation of an effective anticancer immune response. Therefore, despite some potential immunostimulatory effects, such as the activation of NK cytotoxicity (34), the stimulatory action of mu-opioid agonists on IL-10 secretion would reduce and support the clinical relevance of other potential immunostimulatory activities, with the end result of an inhibition of the anticancer immunity. In fact, IL-10 has been proven to be one of the most potent immunosuppressive cytokines because of its inhibitory effect on IL-2 and IL-12 endogenous production. In other words, the in vivo immune effects of the mu-opioid receptor agonists would represent the algebric result of several contradictory actions, and the in vivo end result of the mu-opioid agonists would consist of an immunosuppressive status, at least in terms of anticancer immunity. Stress-induced immunosuppression following stimulation of tumor onset and development appears to be mediated by the action of mu-opioid receptor agonists, because it is blocked by the mu-opioid antagonist NTX and mimicked by the mu-opioid agonist, morphine (22, 45).

Met-enkephalin has also been proven to play an important immunostimulating activity by acting on delta-opioid receptors, consisting of activation of TH1 lymphocytes, with a following enhanced secretion of IL-2 and stimulation of NK cell functions (50, 38). The immunostimulatory property of delta-opioid receptor activation is also confirmed by the fact that the selective delta-opioid receptor antagonist, naltrindole, may play an evident immunosuppressive effect (2). Finally, preliminary results would suggest a potential antitumor immunostimulatory action of kappa-opioid receptor agonists, such as dynorphins, by enhancing the anticancer cytotoxicity played by macrophages (13). Dynorphin has appeared to be able to counteract corticosteroid-induced immunosuppression, whereas the immunostimulatory action of beta-endorphin may be blocked by the concomitant administration of corticosteroids (33).

Despite the controversial results described in the literature, it is possible to affirm that the mu-opioid receptor agonists may play a prevalent immunosuppressive action, at least on the anticancer immunity, whereas delta- and kappa-opioid receptor agonists would play a stimulatory role on the anticancer immune reaction.

34.6 Oncostatic Properties of Opioid Agonists and Antagonists

Several tumor histotypes may express different types of opioid receptors, whose biological and prognostic significance has still to be better characterized (51). The data available in the literature are very controversial, since both opioid agonists and antagonists have been shown to play either inhibitory or stimulatory effects on cancer cell proliferation, depending on cancer cell lines, dose, schedule of administration, and different experimental conditions. The results are particularly controversial for the mu-opioid receptor agonists, such as morphine, which have appeared to exert both stimulatory and inhibitory actions on cancer cell growth (40). In any case, irrespectively of its action on cancer cell proliferation, morphine appears to stimulate tumor angiogenesis (40). Because of the fundamental role of the angiogenesis in determining tumor growth and dissemination, it is probable that morphine may in vivo play a dominant stimulatory action on cancer development.

In the same way, there are controversial results concerning the effects of the opioid antagonists on tumor growth. NTX appears to inhibit the growth of neural tumors (53). However, NTX may inhibit the growth of other solid tumor histotypes. NTX appears to inhibit breast cancer cell growth, even though this inhibitory action was limited only to estrogen receptor-positive tumors (1). A hypothesis to explain the fact that both opioid antagonists and agonists may either stimulate or inhibit cancer cell growth has been proposed (52), which demonstrated that an intermittent blockade of mu-opioid receptors by low-dose NTX may allow an increase in number and sensitivity of opioid receptors for binding by endogenous oncostatic opioids, such as OGF. In contrast, a complete blockade of the mu-opioid receptors with high dose NTX would stimulate cancer growth.

The role of the delta-opioid receptor agonists is also controversial. Despite the potential oncostatic action of met-enkephalin in some experimental conditions, the delta-opioid receptor antagonist naltrindole appears to inhibit cancer cell proliferation (6). Despite the possible expression of different subtypes of opioid receptors by cancer cells (12), including mu-, delta-, kappa-, and zeta-opioid receptors, the clinical and prognostic significance of opioid receptor expression by cancer cells is still unclear. This is because opioid receptors expressed on cancer cell surface may mediate both stimulatory and inhibitory actions on cancer cell proliferation depending on tumor histotypes, as well as on the subtype of opioid receptor. At present, only in few cases has the biological and prognostic significance of opioid receptor expression by cancer cells been clarified. It has been observed that the expression of kappa-opioid receptor is associated with a lower grade of malignancy in brain tumors (37), whereas the biological significance of mu-opioid receptor expression is more controversial (48). The contradictory results concerning the action of the opioid agents on in vivo cancer growth may be explained, in part, by their influence on the clinical history of the neoplastic disease and would depend not only on a direct action on cancer cell proliferation (either stimulatory or inhibitory) but also on their effects on angiogenic processes and anticancer immunity. Therefore, the controversial in vivo results of opioid agents on cancer growth with respect to the in vitro observations may be explained by their effects on several mechanisms involved in the regulation of host-tumor interactions, including cancer cell proliferation, angiogenesis, and anticancer immunity.

In general, the in vivo effects of the mu-opioid agonists tend to play a stimulatory action on cancer growth. Similarly, despite their potential immunostimulatory action, delta-opioid agonists may stimulate tumor cell proliferation because the administration of the delta antagonist naltrindole suppresses cancer growth (6). Finally, the in vivo effects of opioid agents on cancer growth would depend not only on their oncostatic, immunomodulating, and angiogenesis-regulating activities but also on their influence on the secretion of other neurohormones and neuropeptides, namely endogenous cannabinoids and pineal hormones, which produce a great number of bio-oncological effects. It has been demonstrated that the in vivo cancer development and biological malignancy of cancer cells depend not only on the biological characteristics of tumor cells but also on the psychoneuroimmune status of patients through a complex neuroendocrine regulation (41, 47). The possible mediation of opioid influence on tumor growth by other neurochemical systems is also suggested by the evidence that beta-endorphin appears to stimulate metastasis development only in tumor-bearing animals when it is injected in specific brain areas (46), as well as by its controversial results on tumor growth (35).

34.7 Clinical Investigations of Opioid and Cannabinoid Systems

In vivo, brain opioid activity may be investigated by the measurements of beta-endorphin, met-enkephalin, and dinorphin concentrations into the blood and cerebrospinal fluid, as well as by evaluating the endocrine response to the administration of the opioid antagonist NTX, which increases cortisol and luteinizing hormone (LH) blood levels (19). Similarly, the functional status of the brain endocannabinoid may be investigated in vivo by measuring blood or fluid concentrations of different endocannabinoids, such as anandamide, as well as by determining the blood concentrations of the main enzyme responsible for cannabinoid degradation, FAAH (31). High levels of FAAH would reflect a deficiency of the endocannabinoid system, whereas low values of FAAH would be associated with an enhanced cannabinoid functional activity.

34.8 Clinical Investigation of the Opioid System in Cancer Patients

The functional status of brain opioid system activity in cancer patients still needs to be further investigated and established. According to preliminary clinical studies, several alterations of opioid function have been described in patients with advanced cancer, namely, consisting of a progressive disappearance of the physiological opioid circadian secretion with cancer development (3) and an anomalous endocrine response to agonists of different opioid receptors (25). The anomalous endocrine response following the administration of opioid agents may represent an index of hyperactivity of the brain opioid system occurring with the progression of the neoplastic disease. Finally, abnormal opioid system activity has been shown to be associated with a pineal hypofunction, concomitantly to cancer progression (10). Because both the opioid system and the pineal gland may influence cancer cell proliferation and antitumor immunity, cancer-related immunosuppression and the biological malignancy of cancer cells may depend, in part, on an anomalous pineal-opioid system relationship. In any case, it is known that the opioid system is involved in anxiety, stress, and pain conditions. Therefore, the eventual cancer-related opioid hyperfunction in the brain could simply represent the consequence of the clinical and psychological status of the oncologic patients.

34.9 Clinical Studies with Opioid Antagonists in Human Neoplasms

The use of opioid antagonists have been proposed in the treatment of human neoplasms for two main reasons, their immunomodulating activity and their potential antiproliferative action [at least against tumors characterized by possible opioid-dependent growth, such as some brain tumors (48)]. Despite the large number of experiments suggesting a potential anticancer activity of opioid antagonists in relation to the different tumor histotypes, very few clinical studies have been performed up to now to verify the possible anticancer efficacy of their administration in humans.

At present, there is no certain role for opioid system manipulation in the treatment of human neoplasms. The few clinical data available in the literature are generally limited to the use of NTX, which has been utilized as either cytostatic or immunomodulating agent. Moreover, both low- and high-dose NTX have been explored in an attempt to obtain either a partial and transient or a total and prolonged opioid receptor blockade, respectively. The rationale of low-dose NTX (4) is justified by at least three different mechanisms consisting of: (1) an increase in opioid receptor density and number on cancer cell membranes, whose stimulation of the receptors may inhibit tumor cell growth; (2) an enhancement of endorphin and enkephalin concentrations, with their potential cytostatic action; and (3) a stimulation of NK cell cytotoxic activity.

The rationale of high-dose NTX is mainly related to the inhibition of the immunosuppressive status depending on an enhanced brain opioid activity (28, 29), and/or the blockade of mu-opioid receptor in the case of tumors (such as brain glioblastoma) whose growth may be stimulated by the opioid agents (26). Preliminary clinical results with oral administration of low-dose NTX have shown objective tumor regressions in about 20% of advanced cancer patients progressing on standard anticancer therapies, with tumor responses in several cancer histotypes, including breast cancer, ovarian carcinoma, pancreatic cancer, colorectal cancer, prostate cancer, melanoma, and malignant lymphomas (4).

Preliminary results suggest that the therapeutic dosage of NTX ranged from 2 to 5 mg/day every night. Dosages below 1.75 mg/day had no therapeutic effect. Finally, a number of patients, who did not respond to 3 mg, obtained some benefits from a dose of 5 mg/day. These results need to be confirmed by controlled clinical trials.

Randomized studies with high-dose NTX, consisting of an oral dose of 100 mg every 2 days, have shown promising results in the treatment of brain glioblastoma compared with only radiotherapy (RT). Patients treated by RT plus NTX showed a 1-year survival of about 50%, compared to less than 30% in patients treated by with RT only (26).

Interesting results have been also reported by using high-dose NTX as an immunomodulating agent in association with subcutaneous (SC) low-dose IL-2, as an neuroimmunotherapy of cancer. In the first study, pharmacological doses of NTX in association with SC low-dose IL-2 have been shown to induce a greater increase in lymphocyte number to that previously obtained in the same patients with IL-2 alone. In addition, there was a reduction in neoplastic growth in more than 50% of metastatic renal cell cancer patients, whose tumor growth had been progressing under IL-2 alone (28). In a second study, the concomitant administration of IL-2 with high-dose NTX appeared to cause a further amplification of IL-2-induced lymphocytosis compared to that already achieved by the treatment of the pineal indole melatonin, suggesting that a pharmacological blockade of the mu-opioid receptor may amplify the anticancer immunomodulating properties of the pineal hormone (29). According to the results of previous studies (44), NTX may improve IL-2-dependent anticancer immunity by suppressing TH2-lymphocyte activation with a following decline in IL-10 endogenous production that may counteract IL-2 anticancer activity (5).

34.10 Future Perspectives with Opioid Antagonists in Cancer Therapy

The first objective for a rationale application of the opioid antagonists in the treatment of human neoplasms is represented by the exact definition of the prognostic significance of opioid receptor expression in relation to the different tumor histotypes. This objective is particularly relevant for those tumors, whose growth seems to be stimulated by the opioid agents, such as brain neoplasms (48). The evaluation of the therapeutic anticancer efficacy of the opioid antagonists in tumors positive for opioid receptors would constitute the only possible way to propose their use not only on the basis of empiristic criteria but also in relation to a well-defined biological rationale. Moreover, because of the wide variety of biological effects on cancer cell proliferation and anticancer immunity exerted by opioid antagonists and agonists, with both stimulatory and inhibitory effects, it is probable that the optimal clinical application of opioid antagonists in the treatment of human neoplasms requires the concomitant administration of other neuroimmunomodulating molecules. These molecules would be capable of counteracting the eventual undesirable biological effects of opioid antagonists on cancer growth and/or on the anticancer immunity, such as the antiproliferative and immunomodulating actions of the pineal hormones (32) and the cannabinoid agents (15). Opioid antagonists may inhibit cancer cell proliferation, but they may also negatively influence some anticancer immune functions, such as NK cell cytotoxicity, which is stimulated by the mu-opioid agonists (34). In contrast, opioid agonists may induce anticancer immunostimulating effects, but they also tend to stimulate angiogenic mechanisms (40).

Similarly, cannabinoid agents may exert a direct cytostatic action, but they may also counteract T-lymphocyte proliferation (15). Only the pineal hormone melatonin has been shown to constantly induce an inhibition of cancer cell proliferation and a stimulation of the anticancer immunity (32). Therefore, an anticancer neuroimmune therapeutic strategy with opioid antagonists in association with melatonin and other oncostatic pineal hormones, such as methoxytryptamine, and/or cannabinoid agents, may constitute the optimal psychoneuroimmune anticancer strategy to control neoplastic progression. The aim of future clinical trials to treat cancer may require reestablishing the psychoneuroimmune status of health. Preliminary clinical studies with NTX in association with melatonin and the anticancer cytokine IL-2 seem to support this interesting perspective (29).

References

1. Abou-Hissa H., and Tejwani G.A. (1991) Antitumor activity of naltrexone and correlation with steroid hormone receptors. Biochem. Biophys. Res. Commun. 175, 625–630.
2. Arakawa K., Akami T., Okamoto M., Oka T., Nagase H., and Matsumoto S. (1992) The immunosuppressive effect of delta-opioid receptor antagonist on rat renal allograft survival. Transplantation 53, 951–953.
3. Barni S., Lissoni P., Rovelli F., Crispino S., Paolorossi F., Esposti D., et al. (1988) Alteration of opioid peptide circadian rhythm in cancer patients. Tumori 74, 357–360.
4. Bihari B. (1995) Efficacy of low-dose naltrexone as an immune stabilizing agent for the treatment of HIV/AIDS. AIDS. Patient Care 9, 3 (abstract).
5. Blattman J.N., and Greenberg P.D. (2004) Cancer immunotherapy: a treatment for the masses. Science 305, 200–205.
6. Chen Y.L., Law P.Y., and Loh H.H. (2004) Inhibition of Akt/protein kinase B signaling by naltrindole in small cell lung cancer cells. Cancer Res. 64, 8723–8730.
7. Chuchuen U., Ebadi M., and Govitrapong P. (2004) The stimulatory effect of mu- and delta-opioid receptors on bovine pinealocyte melatonin synthesis. J. Pineal Res. 37, 223–229.
8. Devane W.A., Spain J.W., Coscia C.J., and Howlett A.C. (1986) An assessment of the role of opioid receptors in the response to cannabimimetic drugs. J. Neurochem. 46, 1929–1935.
9. Esposti D., Esposti G., Lissoni P., Parravicini L., and Fraschini F. (1988a) Action of morphine on melatonin release in the rat. J. Pineal Res. 5, 35–39.
10. Esposti D., Lissoni P., Tancini G., Barni S., Crispino S., Paolorossi F., et al. (1988b) A study on the relationship between the pineal gland and the opioid system in patients with cancer. Cancer 62, 494–499.
11. Fattore L., Cosso G., Spano M.S., Deiana S., Fadda P., Scherma M., et al. (2004) Cannabinoids and interactions with the opioid system. Crit. Rev. Neurobiol. 16, 147–158.
12. Fichna J., and Janecka A. (2004) Opioid peptides in cancer. Cancer Metastasis Rev. 23, 351–366.
13. Foster J.S., and Moore R.N. (1987) Dynorphin and related opioid peptides enhance tumoricidal activity mediated by murine peritoneal macrophages. J. Leukoc. Biol. 42, 171–174.
14. Grossman A., and Clement-Jones V. (1983) Opiate receptors, enkephalins and endorphins. Clin. Endocrinol. Metab. 12, 31–56.
15. Grotenhermen F. (2004) Pharmacology of cannabinoids. Neuroendocrinol. Lett. 25, 14–23.

16. Jankovic B.D. (1994) Neuroimmunomodulation. Ann. N. Y. Acad. Sci. 741, 379–385.
17. Jankovic B.D., and Maric D. (1987) Enkephalins and immunity. Ann. N. Y. Acad. Sci. 496, 115–125.
18. Koff W.C., and Dunegan M.A. (1985) Modulation of macrophage-mediated tumoricidal activity by neuropeptides and neurohormones. J. Immunol. 135, 350–354.
19. Krabtree B.L. (1984) Review of naltrexone, a long-acting opioid antagonist. Clin. Pharmacol. 3, 237–281.
20. Kumar M.S.A., Chen C.L., Sharp D.L., Liu J.M., Kaira P.S., and Kaira S.P. (1982) Diurnal fluctuation in methionine-enkephalin levels in the hypothalamic and pre-optic area of male rats: effects of pinealectomy. Neuroendocrinology 35, 28–31.
21. Lazzarin N., Valenise H., Bari M., Ubaldi F., Battisti N., Finazzi-Agro A., et al. (2004) Fluctuations of fatty acid amide hydrolase and anandamide levels during the human ovulatory cycle. Gynecol. Endocrinol. 18, 212–218.
22. Lewis J.W., Shavit Y., Terman G.W., Nelson I.R., Gale R.P., and Liebeskind J.C. (1983) Apparent involvement of opioid peptides in stress-induced enhancement of tumor growth. Peptides 4, 635–638.
23. Lissoni P., Esposti D., Esposti G., Mauri R., Resentini M., Morabito F., et al. (1986a) A clinical study on the relationship between the pineal gland and the opioid ststem. J. Neural Transm. 65, 63–73.
24. Lissoni P., Resentini M., Mauri R., Esposti D., Esposti G., Rossi D., et al. (1986b) Effects of tetrahydrocannabinol on melatonin secretion in man. Horm. Metab. Res. 18, 77–78.
25. Lissoni P., Barni S., Garuti F., Astuti R., and Tancini G. (1989) Opioid receptors in human neoplasms. Int. J. Biol. Markers 4, 55–56.
26. Lissoni P., Meregalli S., Fossati V., Barni S., Tancini G., Barigozzi P., et al. (1993) Radioendocrine therapy of brain tumors with the long-acting opioid antagonist naltrexone in association with radiotherapy. Tumori 79, 198–201.
27. Lissoni P., Cangemi P., Pirato D., Roselli M.G., Rovelli F., Brivio F., et al. (2001) A review on cancer-psychospiritual status interactions. Neuroendocrinol. Lett. 22, 175–180.
28. Lissoni P., Malugani F., Bordin V., Conti A., Maestroni G., and Tancini G. (2002a) A new immunotherapeutic strategy of subcutaneous low-dose interleukin-2 plus the long-acting opioid antagonist naltrexone in metastatic cancer patients progressing on interleukin-2 alone. Neuroendocrinol. Lett. 23, 255–258.
29. Lissoni P., Malugani F., Malysheva O., Kozlov V., Laudon M., Conti A., et al. (2002b) Neuroimmunotherapy of untreatable metastatic solid tumors with subcutaneous low-dose interleukin-2: modulation of interleukin-2-induced antitumor immunity by blocking the opioid system. Neuroendocrinol. Lett. 23, 341–344.
30. Lowenstein R.P., Pereyra E.N., Soveyra C.G., and Cardinali D.P. (1984) Effect of naloxone on the nocturnal rise of rat pineal melatonin content. Eur. J. Pharmacol. 98, 261–264.
31. Maccarone M., Valenise H., Bari M., Lazzarin N., Romanini C., and Finazzi-Agro A. (2001) Progesterone up-regulates anandamide hydrolase in human lymphocytes: role of cytokines and implications for fertility. J. Immunol. 166, 7183–7189.
32. Maestroni G.J.M. (1993) The iminunoneuroendocrine role of melatonin. J. Pineal Res. 14, 1–10.
33. Mastroni G.J.M., and Conti A. (1989) Beta-endorphin and dynorphin mimic the circadian immunoenhancing and anti-stress effects of melatonin. Int. J. Immunopharmacol. 11, 393–340.
34. Mathews P.M., Froelich C.W.L. Jr., and Bankhurst A.D. (1983) Enhancement of natural cytotoxicity by beta-endorphin. J. Immunol. 130, 1658–1662.
35. Morley J.E., Kay N., Allin J., Moon T., and Billington C.J. (1985) Endorphins, immune functions and cancer. Psychopharmacol. Bull. 21, 485–488.
36. Novolotskaya E.V., Malkova N.V., Zargarova T.A., Lepikhova T.N., Krasnova S.B., and Lipkin V.M. (2002) Effect of synthetic beta-endorphin-like peptide immunorphin on human T lymphocytes. Biochemistry 3, 357–363.
37. Pan E.C., Bohn L.M., Beleheva M.N., Thomas G.E., Manepalli A.N., Mainone J.Y., et al. (1998) Kappa-opioid receptor binding varies inversely with tumor grade in human gliomas. Cancer 83, 2561–2566.

38. Plotnikoff N.P., Miller G.C., Nimeh N., Faith R.E., Murgo A., and Wybran J. (1987) Met-enkephalin enhances T lymphocytes and T helper/suppressor ratios in cancer patients. Ann. N. Y. Acad. Sci. 496, 608–619.
39. Portoghese P.S., Sultana M., and Takemori A.E. (1988) Naltrindole, a highly selective and potent non-peptide delta-opioid receptor antagonist. Eur. Pharmacol. 146, 185—186.
40. Rassmussen M., Zhy W., Tonnesen J., Cadet P., Tonnesen E., and Stefano G.B. (2002) Effects of morphine on tumor growth. Neuroendocrinol. Lett. 23, 193–198.
41. Riley V. (1981) Psychoneuroendocrine influence on immunocompetence and neoplasia. Science 212, 1100–1109.
42. Rosenberg S.A. (1992) The immunotherapy and gene therapy of cancer. J. Clin. Oncol. 10, 180–199.
43. Rubinow D.R. (1990) Brain, behavior, and immunity: an interactive system. J. Natl. Cancer Inst. Monogr. 10, 79–82.
44. Sacerdote P., and Panerai A.E. (1999) Role of opioids in the modulation of TH1/TH2 responses. Neuroimunomodulation 6, 422–423.
45. Shavit Y., Terman G.W., Martin F.C., Lewis J.W., Liebeskind J.C., and Gaie R.P. (1985) Stress, opioid peptides, the immune system, and cancer. J. Immunol. 135 (Suppl. 2), 834–837.
46. Simon R.H., Arbo T.E., and Lundy J. (1985) Beta-endorphin injected in the nucleus of the raphe magnis facilitates metastatic tumor growth. Brain Res. Bull. 12, 487–491.
47. Vinnitsky V.B. (1988) Neurochemical mechanisms of the formation of antitumor activity. Ann. N. Y. Acad. Sci. 521, 195–214.
48. Westphal M., and Li C.H. (1984) Beta-endorphin: characterization of binding sites specific for the human hormone in human glioblastoma SF 126 cells. Proc. Natl. Acad. Sci. USA 81, 2921–2924.
49. Wybran J., Apelboom T., Famaery J.P., and Covaerts A. (1979) Suggestive evidence for morphine and methionine-enkephalin receptors-like in normal blood lymphocytes. J. Immunol. 123, 1068–1070.
50. Wybran J., Schandené L., von Vooren J.P., Vandermoten G., Latinne D., Sonnet J., et al. (1987) Immunologic properties of methionine-enkephalin and therapeutic implications in AIDS, ARC and cancer. Ann. N. Y. Acad. Sci. 496, 108–114.
51. Zagon I.S., and McLaughiin P.J. (1987) Modulation of murine neuroblastoma in nude mice. J. Natl. Cancer Inst. 78, 141–147.
52. Zagon I.S., and McLaughlin P.J. (1989) Opioid antagonist modulation of murine neuroblastoma: a profile of cell proliferation and opioid peptides and receptors. Brain Res. 20, 16–28.
53. Zagon I.S., McLaughiin P.J., Goodman S.R., and Rhodes R.E. (1987) Opioid receptors and endogenous opioids in diverse human and animal cancers. J. Natl. Cancer Inst. 79, 1059–1065.
54. Zagon I.S., Roesener C.D., Verderame M.F., Ohlsson-Wilhelm B.M., Levin R.J., and McLaughlin P.J. (2000) Opioid growth factor regulates the cell cycle of human neoplasms. Int. J. Oncol. 17, 1057–1061.

Chapter 35
Nonclinical Pharmacology of VIVITROL®: A Monthly Injectable Naltrexone for the Treatment of Alcohol Dependence

Reginald L. Dean, III

Abstract Oral naltrexone is a nonselective opioid antagonist. It is approved for the pharmacological treatment of alcohol and opioid dependence, but the efficacy of oral naltrexone is limited by poor patient compliance. To address this limitation, numerous attempts have been made by many groups to develop an injectable extended-release formulation of naltrexone including. At Alkermes, different formulations of naltrexone, encapsulated into biodegradable polymer microspheres [e.g., Alkermes' Medisorb® extended-release naltrexone (XR-NTX); VIVITROL®], were tested using in vitro assays and in vivo models to select a lead formulation. Pharmacokinetic studies in rats confirmed that the principle formulation produced stable, pharmacologically relevant plasma levels of naltrexone for ~1 month following a single injection. The pharmacodynamic effects (antagonism of morphine antinociception) of XR-NTX corresponded well with the pharmacokinetic profile from the same animals. While brain mu-opioid receptor density was found to increase over time in these rats, it did not appear to affect the ability of naltrexone to suppress morphine antinociception. Additional results in rats suggested that it may be feasible to manage acute pain in XR-NTX-treated patients by titrating typical opioid analgesics upwards to patient comfort under medical observation without causing further sedation or additional respiratory depression. Finally, the pharmacokinetic profile of XR-NTX in monkeys confirmed the long duration of elevated plasma concentrations of naltrexone. Both naltrexone and the poly(d,L-lactide-co-glycolide) (PLG) polymer matrix in which it is encapsulated are well-tolerated. VIVITROL was approved by the Food and Drug Administration (FDA) in 2006 for once-monthly administration for the pharmacological treatment of alcohol dependence.

Keywords: Alcohol dependence; Extended-release; Naltrexone; PLG polymer; Biodegradable microspheres; Pain; Pharmacokinetics

---

R.L. Dean, III
Alkermes, Inc., 88 Sidney Street, Cambridge, MA 02139
e-mail: reggie.dean@alkermes.com

R. Dean et al. (eds.), *Opiate Receptors and Antagonists*,

35.1 Introduction

While most people sensibly drink alcohol, there are a substantial number of drinkers who regularly abuse alcohol or are alcohol dependent, which lead to social, economic, and medical problems. Alcohol dependency is a serious chronic problem seen worldwide. In the United States alone, it is estimated that alcohol-related costs including lost work productivity and health problems are about $185 billion annually (1).

Alcohol dependence is a disease which is characterized by a 1) strong need or compulsion to drink (craving), 2) an inability to limit drinking (loss of control), 3) the need to drink more alcohol in order to feel its euphoric effects (tolerance), and 4) the development of withdrawal symptoms (which may include nausea, shakiness, sweating, anxiety, and, in severe cases, hallucinations and seizures) following the discontinuation of alcohol use after a period of long-time abuse (physical dependence) (2). While the progression of symptoms is similar from person to person, the time course may vary and include periods of remission, controlled or nonproblematic drinking, and relapse (return to heavy drinking). Prognosis for recovery varies depending on a number of factors and the treatment approaches employed (3, 4). However, recovery from alcohol dependence is a life-long process and relapse is always a possibility.

As of 2007 there were four pharmacotherapies approved by the US Food and Drug Administration (FDA) for the treatment of alcohol dependence: disulfiram (Antabuse®), acamprosate (Campral®), oral naltrexone (ReVia®), and extended-release naltrexone injectable suspension (VIVITROL®). Current treatment involves a combination of pharmacotherapy together with some form of psychosocial therapy.

Naltrexone (ReVia®), a nonselective, high affinity opiate antagonist, has been explored to treat both opioid and alcohol dependence. In the mid-1960s, oral naltrexone was first investigated for the treatment of narcotic addiction and was subsequently approved in 1985 for the treatment of opioid dependence. Interest in using opioid antagonists for treating alcohol dependence arose from theories that the endogenous opioid system mediates many of the reinforcing attributes (i.e., rewarding properties) of alcohol through their effect on the dopamine system [animal and human studies in support of this involvement are reviewed in (5–8); also see Chaps. 18 and 19 in this book]. In 1994, oral naltrexone was approved for the treatment of alcohol dependence (9).

Oral administration of 50 mg naltrexone has generally been shown to reduce relapse to heavy drinking in alcohol-dependent patients, decrease the number of drinks consumed when relapse does occur, and promote abstinence [reviewed in (10–12)]. Oral naltrexone is also reported to reduce both the craving for and the reinforcing euphoric qualities of alcohol (13–17). Despite the fact that naltrexone has been available for nearly 15 years and the reported evidence that it is effective in the treatment of alcohol dependence, naltrexone is not widely used in the clinic (18, 19). Oral naltrexone is associated with a number of limitations which may subsequently diminish its efficacy in treating alcohol dependency and could increase the risk of relapse. First, daily dosing of oral naltrexone results in fluctuating plasma concentrations of the drug during the day (Fig. 35.1a), with high concentrations shortly after taking the medication to subeffective concentrations later in the day. This pattern repeats itself daily over the course of multiple months of treatment (Fig. 35.1b).

Second, adherence to the prescribed treatment regimen is a significant problem (20–22). This is compounded by the requirement of daily self-medication of naltrexone. Typically, alcohol-dependent individuals want the euphoria associated with drinking (15) and thus are less willing to take oral medication every day over the course of months of treatment. Often reasons for noncompliance include:

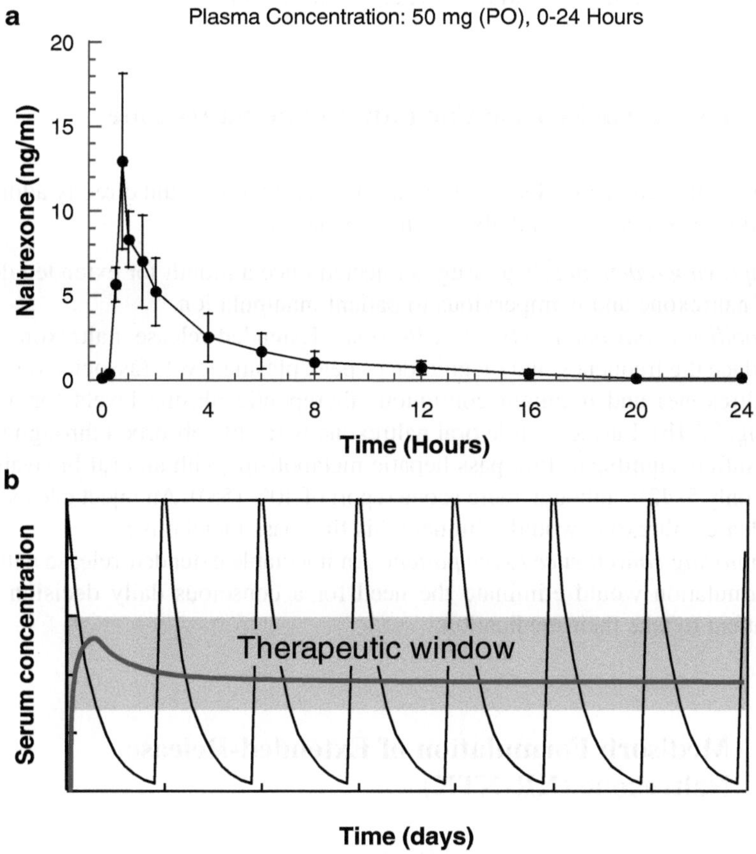

Fig. 35.1 (**a**) Typical profile of plasma naltrexone levels over 24 h following a 50 mg oral dose in humans. Oral naltrexone was given daily to normal healthy volunteers ($N = 6$) for five consecutive days. This graph shows the plasma naltrexone concentrations following the fifth dose. Note the high concentration peak of naltrexone within the first hour of oral dosing followed by a fairly rapid decline in plasma levels to below the minimum therapeutic levels (2 ng/ml) within 8 h of dosing. (**b**) A modeled plasma profile following an injectable, extended-release formulation of naltrexone. An extended-release formulation would reduce repetitive peaks in plasma levels (as illustrated in Fig. 35.1a), extend the duration of the therapeutic plasma levels, eliminate first pass metabolism in the liver, and eliminate the need for daily dosing by the patient

indifference in getting treatment for dependency, harmful social environment, forgetting to take the medication, false impression of being cured and medication no longer necessary, heavy drinking, and the adverse effects associated with oral naltrexone (18, 23, 24). Finally, there is the issue of marginal efficacy as a result of too low a dose of naltrexone. The approved dose of oral naltrexone for treating alcohol dependence is 50 mg daily (25). This dose was chosen because it was found to be effective in the treatment of opiate dependence by blocking abused opioids at the receptor level in the brain (26). However, it is not known whether this is also the optimum dose for treating alcohol dependency. In fact, animal and human studies suggest that the effects of naltrexone on alcohol drinking are dose-dependent, with greater efficacy at higher oral doses (i.e., 100 mg) (27).

35.2 Extended-Release Formulation of Naltrexone

An injectable extended-release formulation of naltrexone could directly address the limitations associated with daily oral naltrexone by

(a) *Improving adherence*. The drug is injected once a month for extended delivery of naltrexone and is impervious to patient manipulation.
(b) *Stabilizing plasma levels of naltrexone*. Extended-release naltrexone would reduce the frequency and magnitude of peak plasma levels (associated with oral naltrexone) and maintain continuous therapeutic plasma levels for a month (Fig. 35.1b). Further, while oral naltrexone is readily absorbed through the gut, it suffers significant first pass hepatic metabolism (with an oral bioavailability of only 5–42% although there is one report of 40% (55)). An injectable extended-release naltrexone would eliminate this first pass metabolism.
(c) *Improving convenience to the patient*. An injectable extended-release naltrexone formulation would eliminate the need for a conscious daily decision by the patient to take their medication.

35.3 Medisorb Formulation of Extended-Release Naltrexone (XR-NTX)

One proven technology for extended release drug delivery is the encapsulation of drug in polymeric microspheres made of poly(D,L-lactide-co-glycolide) (PLG) (28). PLG is a common biodegradable copolymer with a history of safe human usage as sutures, orthopedics, bone plates, and extended-release pharmaceuticals (e.g., Riperdal Consta®, Lupron Depot®, Zoladex®, Decapeptyl® SR, and Sandostatin LAR® Depot). Such polymers can be fabricated into small diameter (<100 microns) injectable microspheres and formulated to provide improved in vivo release of drugs for predefined periods of time ranging from days to months. Drug release from PLG microspheres is governed by water uptake, diffusion of the bioactive molecule through the polymer matrix, and the biodegradation of the polymer (28, 29). Biological degradation of PLG occurs primarily through hydrolysis, with the degradation products being the monomers, lactic acid and glycolic acid (28, 29). These monomers are further metabolized and eliminated from the body as carbon dioxide and water.

35.3.1 Process for Formulating Medisorb Naltrexone Microspheres

A proprietary water-based solvent extraction process is used to make Medisorb naltrexone microspheres (30). In this process, both drug and polymer are dissolved in a common organic cosolvent system. This "oil" phase is then emulsified (oil/water) with an aqueous solution. The emulsion undergoes a partial solvent extraction, via exposure to limited water volume, prior to transfer to a large aqueous "quench" solution. At this point, the oil droplets are precipitated into drug encapsulated microspheres. The microspheres are recovered, dried, and undergo a secondary extraction step to further reduce the residual solvents. They are again recovered and dried a final time. The dried microspheres are aseptically filled into glass vials.

35.3.2 Microsphere Release Mechanism

At the time of administration, the microspheres are suspended in a sterile aqueous microsphere diluent to aid in the suspension and injection of XR-NTX. Following injection, initial release of drug from the microspheres is diffusion controlled. Subsequently, release is controlled by diffusion and polymer degradation (see Fig. 35.2 for a more detailed explanation).

35.3.3 Selection of a Lead Formulation

Drug release is controlled by a number of factors. Among the strongest are drug loading, PLG monomer ratio (lactide: glycolide ratio), and the nature of the polymer chain end-group. These factors not only control the drug release kinetics but also affect the dose volume and polymer degradation rate (28). Different PLG formulations were made in which the lactide:glycolide ratio and the naltrexone loading varied (30).

The formulations were initially characterized with numerous in vitro tests which measured microsphere size, uniformity, release rate, and stability. Several different formulations were tested in rats to provide in vivo pharmacokinetic (PK) data. Of these, selected formulations were tested in nonhuman primates to assess tolerability

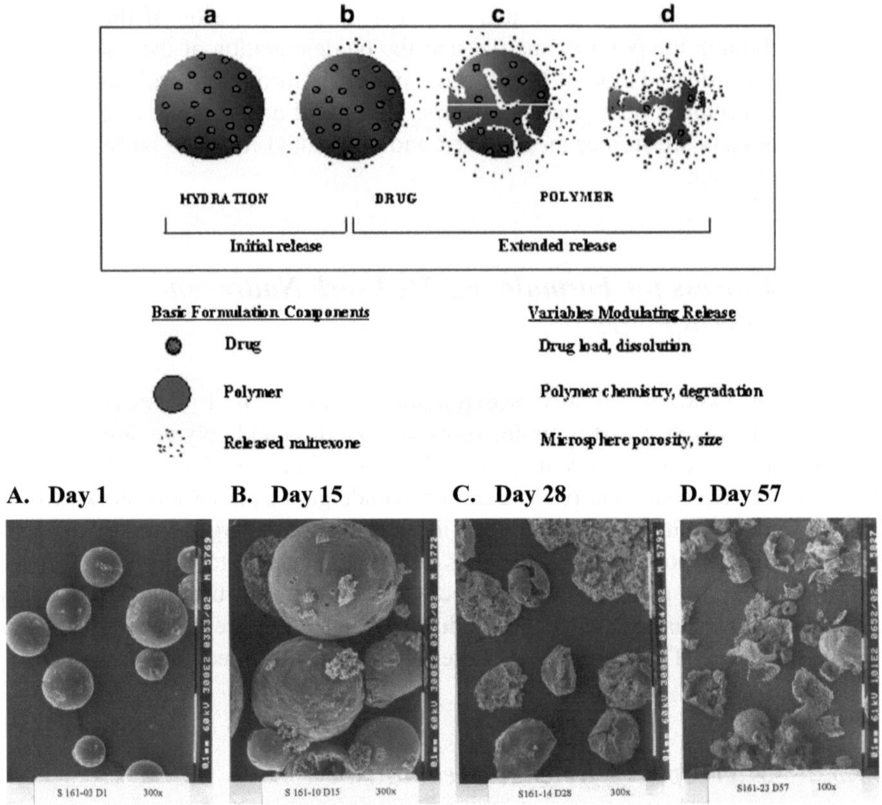

Fig. 35.2 (**a**) Components of extended-release naltrexone and the variables affecting drug release. Upon injection, the microspheres (A) begin to absorb water almost immediately, leading to a swelling of the microspheres (B). This process begins an initial release phase where a small amount of drug at or near the surface of the microspheres is slowly released. As water absorption continues, hydrolysis begins to breakdown the polymer resulting in the gradual collapse and erosion of the microspheres' internal structure (C). This polymer erosion process results in the extended-release of the drug from the microspheres. The polymer matrix eventually breaks down into lactic acid and glycolic acid, which are completely metabolized by the body and eliminated as carbon dioxide and water (D) [from (30)]. (**b**) Scanning electron photomicrographs showing microsphere morphology and degradation of Medisorb naltrexone microspheres during in vitro release at 37 °C in a physiological buffer. (A) Day 2. Note loss of dimpled character commonly associated with hydration and swelling (300×); (B) Day 15. Swelling of microspheres continues (300×); (C) Day 28. Significant erosion of the interior of the microspheres has occurred with the residual polymer shell continuing to degrade (300×); (D) Day 57. Continued degradation of residual polymer matrix after completion of naltrexone release (100x) [from (30)]

and confirm the PK profile observed in rats. One formulation was then selected as the lead. This formulation entered into a formal development program involving safety/toxicokinetics in rats and rabbits to establish a relationship between PK and pharmacodynamics (PD) in rats before progressing to a Phase I safety/PK study in humans.

35.3.3.1 In Vitro Release of Naltrexone from Microspheres

The analytical results indicated high encapsulation efficiency for all the formulations (30). Increasing drug content (% loading) typically resulted in increased drug release within the initial 24 hours and increased the overall rate of release. Increasing the glycolide content also increased the overall rate of release, but to a lesser extent. A representative in vitro release profile of a promising formulation at 37 °C in a physiological buffer is shown in Fig. 35.3 A near linear in vitro release profile was seen which provided an extended release of naltrexone for over 1 month with minimal initial drug release. In addition, there was a simultaneous degradation of the microsphere polymer with the drug release (Fig. 35.2b).

35.3.3.2 In Vivo Pharmacokinetic and Pharmacodynamic Evidence of Efficacy in Rats

Pharmacological blockade of opiate receptors following an acute injection of naltrexone attenuates the antinociceptive effects of morphine in rats (31). With XR-NTX it is necessary to evaluate the extended pharmacological effects of this drug by repeatedly testing the same animal on a behavioral measure of antinociception over the course of several months. The behavioral test employed in this study (32), the morphine-induced antinociception test, is a standard pharmacological means for assessing antinociception by measuring the response of individual rats to a thermal stimulus (33, 34). In this test, rats are placed on a moderately heated

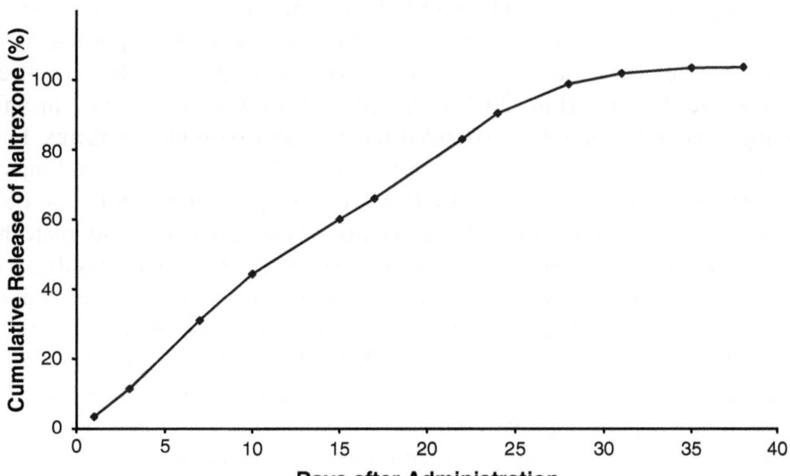

Fig. 35.3 Representative in vitro drug release profile of a promising formulation of Alkermes' Medisorb® extended-release naltrexone (*XR-NTX*) as measured in an aqueous buffer media at physiological pH and temperature [from (30)]

(48 °C) platform (a "hot plate") and after a short period of time, the animals respond to the heat by licking their hind paw. The rats are quickly removed from the hot plate as soon as a response is noted. However, if an opioid analgesic, such as morphine, is first given to the rat, the reaction to the heat is abolished or greatly attenuated (up to a maximum of 60 sec). Pharmacological blockade of opiate receptors in the central nervous system (CNS) by XR-NTX should block the effects of morphine and return the performance of morphine-treated animals to control levels. This test is ideally suited for evaluating the extended release effects of naltrexone because it permits each rat to be tested multiple times over a period of several weeks to months.

Naltrexone-containing or nonloaded (placebo) microspheres were suspended in an aqueous diluent and injected intramuscularly to provide a total of 50 mg/kg or a comparable mass of placebo microspheres. Animals received an intraperitoneal (i.p.) injection of morphine (1 mg/kg) or saline on the hot plate test days. Half the animals receiving XR-NTX were sacrificed 36 days after the injection, a time when the behavioral effects of naltrexone were diminished. The placebo- and the remaining naltrexone-treated rats received a second, identical microsphere injection 34 days after the first injection. These animals were retested on the hot plate and sacrificed on day 37 (following the second injection), a time when the pharmacodynamic effects of naltrexone had completely dissipated. Injections of XR-NTX or placebo were well tolerated by the rats, independent of the number of injections. This was evidenced by the absence of local site reactions, such as redness, swelling, exudation, or scratching, upon in vivo and ex vivo examination.

For quantitation of plasma levels of naltrexone, blood samples were collected via tail vein from all animals immediately after each behavioral test. Concentrations of naltrexone in plasma were determined by liquid chromatography-mass spectrometry/mass spectrometry (LC-MS/MS) and were below the level of quantitation (LOQ ≤ 1 ng/ml) in all rats prior to treatment. Maximum plasma levels were observed by 3 days. Plasma concentrations of naltrexone did not significantly differ from each other between 3 and 14 days, with detectable levels of naltrexone maintained to 35 days (Fig. 35.4a). A similar pattern was observed in animals receiving a second injection of extended-release naltrexone microspheres. Further, naltrexone was no longer quantifiable in plasma 35 days after the second injection.

The pharmacodynamic effects of XR-NTX corresponded well with the PK profile from the same animals (Fig. 35.4b). Animals were tested on the hot plate 30 min following an injection of morphine. Animals receiving placebo microspheres demonstrated a pronounced antinociceptive response to morphine (as determined by their latency to lick one hind paw approaching the maximum allowable duration of 60 sec). In contrast, animals receiving XR-NTX (50 mg/kg total naltrexone) responded at or very near the level of those that received no morphine (i.e., ~35 sec response time), suggesting near complete antagonism of morphine. This response to repeated challenges of morphine continued for ~1 month following a single XR-NTX injection. After 1 month, the XR-NTX treated rats' responses to morphine rapidly returned to that of the rats receiving placebo microspheres. In the groups receiving a second dose of XR-NTX at day 34, morphine continued to be blocked and ineffective through the second month (Fig. 35.6b). Once again, at the

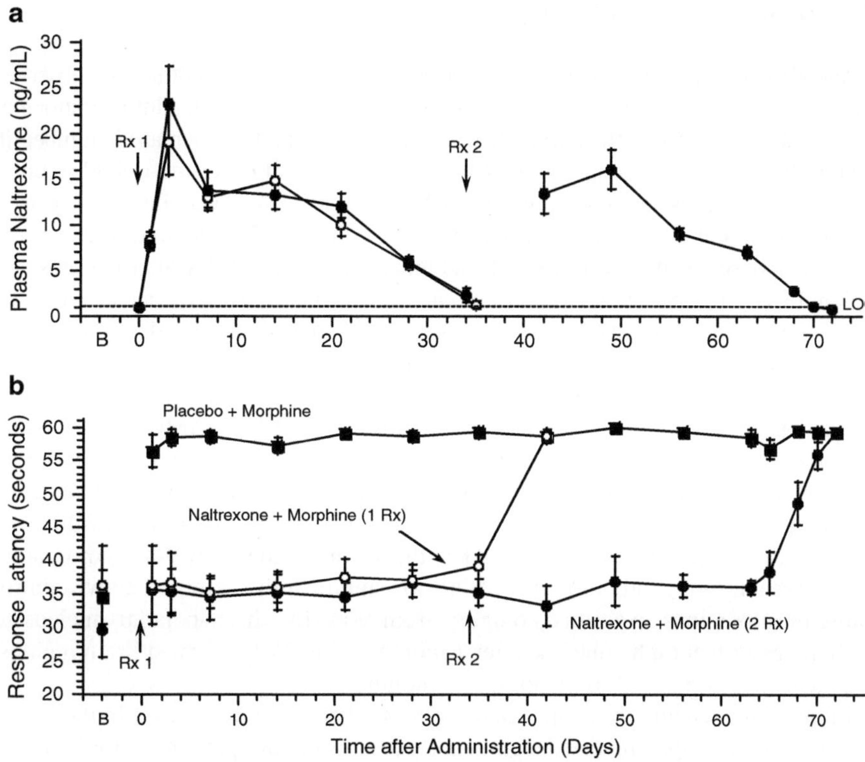

Fig. 35.4 (**a**) Plasma levels of naltrexone in rats following either a single intramuscular (*i.m.*) injection of Alkermes' Medisorb® extended-release naltrexone (*XR-NTX*) (*open circles*) or a second, identical injection 34 days following the first treatment (*closed circles*). Plasma levels of naltrexone were maintained for ~21 days following a single injection. This effect was repeated with a second injection after an additional 34 days. Each point represents the mean ± SEM naltrexone plasma concentration (ng/ml) from nine rats. *LOQ* lower limit of quantitation (<1 ng/ml), *RX 1, 2* time of first and second XR-NTX injection. (**b**) Morphine (1 mg/kg) antinociception following either a single or a second injection of XR-NTX microspheres in the same rats (as above) as measured on the hot plate test. Naltrexone antagonized morphine-induced antinociception, with responses equivalent to those observed under baseline conditions. By 41 days after a single injection of XR-NTX microspheres, the antinociceptive actions increased to levels observed in the placebo + morphine-treated group. In contrast, two naltrexone treatments consistently suppressed morphine-induced antinociception for a total of 68 days. Data represent the mean ± SEM of latency to lick a hind paw by nine rats. **Performance of XR-NTX + morphine group significantly different from placebo + morphine group ($p < 0.01$). [from (32)]

end of that month, the rats' responses rapidly reverted to that of the non-naltrexone microsphere control group. These data demonstrate that following intramuscular (i.m.) injections of XR-NTX, naltrexone is gradually released and successfully blocks the opiate receptors in the brain for a full month, thereby antagonizing the antinociceptive properties of morphine.

Brain Mu-Opioid Receptor Changes

Increases in mu-opioid receptor density (receptor upregulation) are commonly observed in the brains of rodents in response to multiple daily or continuous administrations of opioid antagonists (35–39), although the functionality of this increased number in receptor binding studies is questioned (40). Therefore, the effect of mu-opioid receptor density following the administration of XR-NTX formulation was investigated as a neurochemical measure of the pharmacodynamic efficacy (32). The time course of the changes in these receptors following the administration of XR-NTX microspheres was explored using receptor binding and immunohistochemistry. At the conclusion of the behavioral testing (hot plate) following one or two injections of naltrexone microspheres (spaced 34 days apart), animals were sacrificed and the brains removed.

Frozen brains were cut into 20-μm thick sections and were used for quantitative autoradiography of mu-opioid receptor binding using [^{3}H] DAMGO (39). Brain sections adjacent to those used for receptor binding were processed for mu-opioid receptor immunoreactivity (40) using autoradiography with Ab-1 (Oncogene Research Products) as the primary antibody to mu-opioid receptors (MOR) and [I^{125}] anti-rabbit immunoglobulin G (IgG) as the secondary antibody. Autoradiography revealed that radioligand binding to MOR was significantly increased above control brains in all regions examined, ranging from 90% in the habenular nucleus to 160% in the dorsal raphe nucleus after 1 month (Table 35.1). In most brain regions, these densities continued to increase at 2 months.

Immunohistochemistry using brain sections adjacent to those used in the radioligand autoradiography revealed significant increases in mu-opioid receptor immunoreactivity in only 2 of 15 brain regions examined after 1 month of treatment with extended-release naltrexone (Table 35.2). Following 2 months of treatment, increased immunoreactivity compared to controls was observed in 14 of 15 regions. However, the magnitude of these increases was lower than those observed with receptor binding, ranging from 10% in the perirhinal cortex to 40% in the substania nigra.

To further investigate the increase in mu-opioid receptor density, an independent group of rats was treated with XR-NTX (50 mg naltrexone/kg) and sacrificed at various time points following the injection. The brains were rapidly removed and the cortex, midbrain, and striatum were dissected free and used in a saturation radioligand ([^{3}H]DAMGO)-binding assay (41) to examine the time course of the changes in mu-opioid receptor density. Evidence of increased mu-opioid receptor density (B_{max}) was observed as early as 5 days after administration (Fig. 35.5). By 1 week after the XR-NTX microsphere injection, the B_{max} for DAMGO binding to the midbrain and striatum was significantly increased (110% compared to placebo treatment). These increases in receptor density were sustained throughout the subsequent 33 days, at least 1 week after significant decline in pharmacodynamic efficacy was observed. The density of cortical MOR, however, did not begin to increase until 30 days after the extended-release naltrexone administration and reached significance (120% increase over placebo treated) at 40 days. In contrast to receptor density, no significant changes in mu-opioid receptor affinity (K_d) was observed in any brain region, at any time point.

Table 35.1 Mu-opioid receptor binding in rat brain following Alkermes' Medisorb® extended-release naltrexone (XR-NTX)

	Treatment				
Brain region	Control	Naltrexone (1 month)	Increase (%)	Naltrexone (2 months)	Increase (%)
Central gray	7.48 (0.27)	17.74 (0.74)*	140	19.90 (0.62)*	160
Dentate gyrus	7.10 (0.39)	15.68 (0.82)*	125	17.34 (0.89)*	140
Dorsal raphe nucleus	7.22 (0.86)	18.84 (2.31)*	160	22.92 (1.06)*	220
Habenular nucleus	19.41 (1.41)	36.40 (2.50)*	90	40.92 (2.42)*	120
Hippocampus CA1	4.77 (0.29)	12.03 (0.79)*	150	13.48 (0.75)*	190
Inferior colliculus	10.35 (1.72)	23.15 (1.87)*	130	27.39 (1.54)*	170
Lateral orbital cortex	8.84 (0.72)	20.16 (0.81)*	120	23.68 (1.31)*	170
Nucleus accumbens	12.45 (1.11)	25.05 (2.16)*	90	21.94 (1.31)*	70
Perirhinal cortex	6.41 (0.24)	12.52 (0.51)*	100	14.54 (0.57)*	130
Striatum	8.04 (0.67)	15.23 (0.79)*	80	13.73 (0.38)*	75
Subiculum	20.04 (1.56)	33.77 (2.26)*	70	40.40 (1.75)**	100
Substantia nigra	8.69 (0.77)	17.95 (0.68)*	100	20.54 (1.48)*	140
Superior colliculus	8.90 (1.15)	20.40 (1.57)*	120	20.06 (1.42)*	120
Tenia tecta	9.18 (1.07)	22.67 (1.33)*	150	28.73 (1.71)**	215
Thalamus	11.27 (1.51)	21.46 (1.41)*	100	21.18 (1.07)*	90

Brains from naltrexone-treated animals were processed for quantitative autoradiography of mu-opioid receptor binding using [3H] DAMGO (d-ala2, N-methyl-phe4, glycol5) enkephalin. One group of animals was sacrificed when the behavioral effects of naltrexone were still maximal (i.e., 29 days following treatment). The remaining animals received a second microsphere treatment 34 days following the first injection and were sacrificed after an additional 29 days to gain insight into the relationship between the duration of extended release naltrexone (see Fig. 35.4) and the magnitude of opiate receptor changes. Significant increases in mu-opioid receptor binding were observed in all brain regions examined. Note that these increases were seen within 1 month with only the subiculum and tenia tecta showing further changes with 2 months of naltrexone. Data are presented as mean ± SEM μCi/g. *Naltrexone versus control ($p < 0.05$), **1 versus 2 months naltrexone ($p < 0.05$) (32)

Suppression of Morphine Antinociception by XR-NTX: Extent of Opioid Receptor Blockade

Concurrent with these neurochemical changes in mu-opioid receptor density, XR-NTX was found still to be effective in blocking morphine-induced antinociception for 28 days as measured using the hot plate. However, this study was done with only a single, low challenge dose of morphine (1 mg/kg). To better understand the depth of opioid receptor blockade mediated by XR-NTX microspheres, the antinociceptive response of naltrexone-treated rats to a range of higher doses of morphine (0.5–50 mg/kg) was studied to determine if there is a shift in the antinociceptive potency of morphine (i.e., hypersensitivity). Therefore, rats were injected with XR-NTX (50 mg naltrexone/kg) or placebo microspheres and tested weekly using the hot plate test for assessing antinociception. The latency to lick the hind paw

Table 35.2 Mu-opioid receptor immunoreactivity in rat brain following Alkermes' Medisorb® extended-release naltrexone (XR-NTX)

	Treatment				
Brain region	Control	Naltrexone (1 month)	Increase (%)	Naltrexone (2 months)	Increase (%)
Central gray	2.89 (0.19)	3.22 (0.33)	10	3.98 (0.25)**	40
Dentate gyrus	2.60 (0.18)	2.87 (0.17)	10	3.19 (0.17)*	20
Dorsal raphe nucleus	2.44 (0.13)	2.90 (0.17)	20	3.09 (0.21)*	30
Habenular nucleus	2.90 (0.17)	3.29 (0.18)	10	3.86 (0.24)*	30
Hippocampus CA1	2.57 (0.18)	2.61 (0.13)	0	2.96 (0.18)	15
Inferior colliculus	2.96 (0.16)	3.34 (0.17)	10	3.73 (0.13)*	20
Lateral orbital cortex	2.77 (0.18)	3.05 (0.24)	10	3.37 (0.13)*	20
Nucleus accumbens	2.90 (0.20)	3.54 (0.24)*	20	3.79 (0.11)*	30
Perirhinal cortex	2.49 (0.13)	2.53 (0.18)	0	2.72 (0.07)	10
Striatum	2.82 (0.15)	3.25 (0.20)	30	3.61 (0.20)*	30
Subiculum	3.26 (0.13)	3.82 (0.25)	15	4.26 (0.21)*	30
Substantia nigra	2.50 (0.15)	3.08 (0.16)*	20	3.52 (0.17)*	40
Superior colliculus	2.64 (0.10)	2.72 (0.14)	0	3.17 (0.12)	20
Tenia tecta	2.75 (0.12)	3.03 (0.14)	10	3.31 (0.08)	20
Thalamus	2.79 (0.16)	3.33 (0.16)	20	3.80 (0.16)*	40

Brain sections adjacent to those used in mu-opioid receptor binding (Table 35.1) were processed for immunohistochemical visualization of mu-opioid receptors using a radiolabeled secondary antibody for autoradiographic quantitation. The increases in immunoreactivity following extended-release naltrexone were only seen in selected brain regions and were less robust compared to the changes in receptor binding (Table 35.1). Note that, in contrast to the increases in binding that were relatively constant between 1 and 2 months, the majority of brain regions examined showed increases in immunoreactivity only after 2 months of extended-release naltrexone. Data are presented as mean ± SEM nCi/g. *Naltrexone versus control ($p < 0.05$), **1 versus 2 months naltrexone ($p < 0.05$) (32).

while on the hot plate was measured and dose-response curves for morphine-induced antinociception were generated. These curves allows for the estimation of the morphine dose required to induce antinociception in 50% of the treated rats (ED_{50}). This pharmacological index provides a point of comparison between extended-release naltrexone and placebo-treated rats, quantifying the degree of suppression of morphine-induced antinociception. One week after administration, naltrexone reduced the antinociceptive potency of morphine by 15-fold relative to placebo microspheres (ED_{50} = 2.7, 1.3/6 mg/kg vs 42.0, 21/82 mg/kg, placebo vs XR-NTX treated, mean, 95% CI, $p < 0.05$; Fig. 35.6a). Similar reductions in morphine potency were maintained for the duration of the study (Fig. 35.6b). Only by 4 weeks after the initiation of treatment was the 50 mg/kg dose of morphine capable of inducing full antinociception in the XR-NTX-treated group. Despite the previous observation of naltrexone-induced increase in brain mu-opioid receptor density, no evidence of hypersensitivity to the antinociceptive properties of morphine was observed at any time after XR-NTX administration.

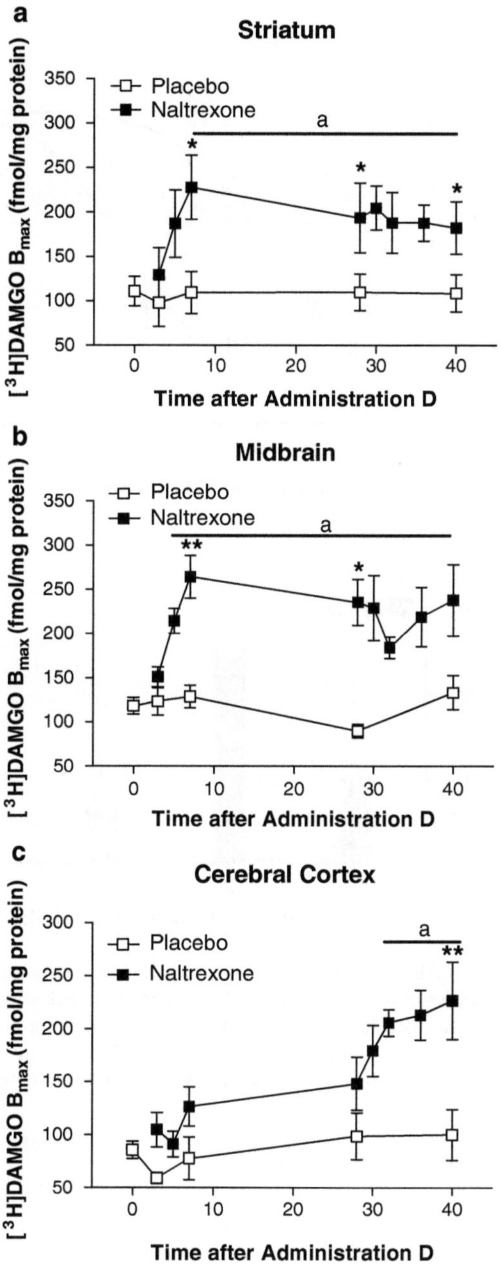

Fig. 35.5 Regional changes in mu-opioid receptor density (B_{max}) in the brain following a single intramuscular (*i.m.*) dose of Alkermes' Medisorb® extended-release naltrexone (*XR-NTX*). Data represents the mean ± SEM of data from eight sets of pooled striata from 16 rats (**a**) or midbrain (**b**) and cerebral cortex (**c**) from eight rats. Significant increases in the density of mu receptors in the cerebral cortex were not observed until 32–40 days after the XR-NTX microspheres injection (**c**). In contrast, receptor density in the striatum (**a**) and midbrain (**b**) and was significantly increased by 7 days (relative to placebo treated), (**a**) significantly different from t_0 control ($p < 0.05$) *, **significantly different from contemporaneous control ($p < 0.05$ and 0.001, respectively) [from (32)]

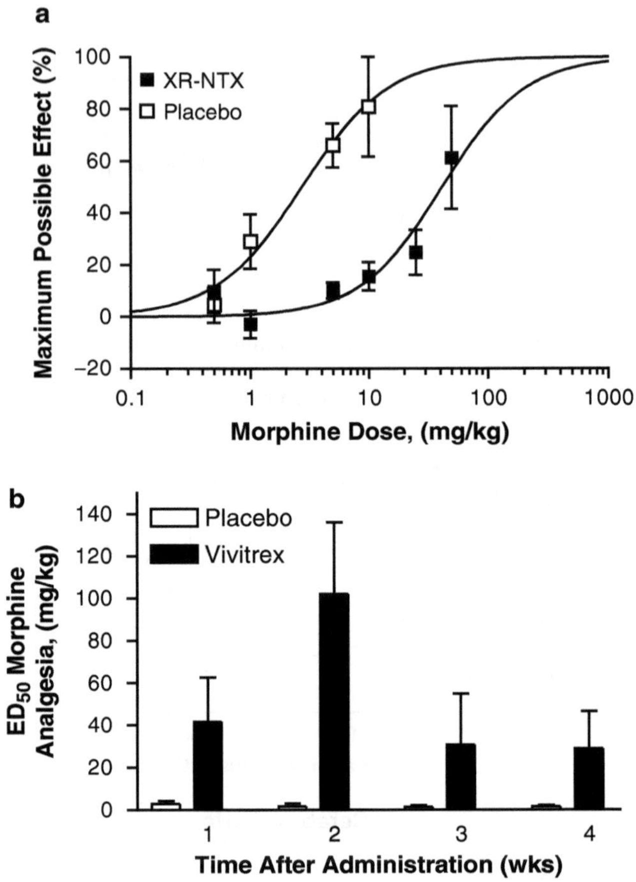

Fig. 35.6 (**a**) The ability of Alkermes' Medisorb® extended-release naltrexone (*XR-NTX*) to suppress the antinociceptive properties of morphine was readily apparent 1 week after administration. While placebo-treated rats demonstrated full antinociception (>120 sec without licking a hind paw) after the administration of 10 mg/kg morphine, the administration of 50 mg/kg morphine to the XR-NTX-treated rats was still not sufficient to produce full antinociception. Data represents the mean ± SEM of data from eight rats.

$$\text{Percent of maximal possible effect} = \frac{\text{morphine latency} - \text{saline latency}}{\text{maximum latency (120 seconds)} - \text{saline latency}}$$

(**b**) The mean ED_{50} values (±SEM) between XR-NTX and placebo groups were significantly different at all time points ($p < 0.05$). Within the placebo-treated or the XR-NTX-treated groups, the ED_{50} values for morphine antinociception over the four weekly time points were not significantly different [adapted from (42)]

Overriding the Blockade of Antinociceptive Actions of Opioids in Rats Treated with XR-NTX

Patients taking naltrexone for alcohol or opioid dependence will be resistant to opioid analgesia, which poses a major therapeutic challenge when treating acute pain (e.g., lower back pain, kidney stones, and bone fracture). The most effective and commonly used drugs to relieve acute pain are opioids, which act at the same receptors that naltrexone blocks. Despite over two decades of clinical experience managing acute pain states in the presence of oral naltrexone, there are only a limited number of published clinical studies regarding the feasibility of overriding naltrexone-induced opioid receptor blockade with high doses of opioid analgesics for pain management (43–45). Adverse effects of opioids are multiple in number, are usually receptor mediated, difficult to separate from the desired analgesic effect and progressively increase as the opioid dose increases (46, 47). One concern with the use of high doses of centrally acting opioid analgesics is their effect on respiration (48). Even at clinically relevant doses, opioid analgesics produce some degree of respiratory depression (43, 49) primarily due to their effect on MOR in the brain stem (43, 47). An additional concern associated with significant dose escalation of opioids is sedation in ambulatory patients (48). Thus, a nonclinical study examining the feasibility to overcome naltrexone-mediated opioid receptor blockade with opioid analgesics, and the relationship between this and the presence/degree of adverse effects, was conducted.

Using the hot plate test after XR-NTX or placebo microsphere administration, rats were treated with an opioid analgesic (morphine, hydrocodone, or fentanyl) to determine the dose required to produce the maximum response latency (MRL) of 60sec. Rats were later treated with higher doses of the same opioid to determine any potential effects on respiration rate or locomotor activity. In naïve rats, 15 mg/kg morphine, 0.1 mg/kg fentanyl, and 8 mg/kg hydrocodone produced MRL. In XR-NTX-treated rats, all the opioid analgesics tested had an effect in reversing the opioid receptor blockade of naltrexone. However, only fentanyl was able to completely overcome naltrexone blockade at the earlier time points associated with the peak and steady release phase of XR-NTX (see Table 35.3). Compared to placebo, these doses did not further depress respiration or alter locomotor activity. The results of this animal study demonstrate that XR-NTX blocks the antinociceptive effects of acute opioids at conventional doses, as expected. The study, however, provides support for the concept of titrating up doses of opioids to produce antinociception by overriding XR-NTX receptor blockade without further depressing respiration or causing sedation. These results suggest that competitive blockade by naltrexone produces a generalized rightward shift in the dose-response curve while maintaining the relative relationship between antinociception, respiratory rate, and locomotor activity – rather than a marked, unpredictable alteration in the pharmacodynamic relationship between these parameters. Furthermore, these results in rats suggest that it may be feasible to manage acute pain in XR-NTX-treated

Table 35.3 Percent reversal of naltrexone-mediated blockade of opioid receptors on hot plate test

Day antinociceptive	4	19	39
Morphine	36% (90 mg/kg)	46% (90 mg/kg)	96% (45 mg/kg)
Fentanyl	100% (2 mg/kg)	100% (2 mg/kg)	100% (0.5 mg/kg)
Hydrocodone	69% (80 mg/kg)	80% (80 mg/kg)	100% (80 mg/kg)

patients by titrating typical opioid analgesics upwards to patient comfort under medical observation without causing sedation or additional respiratory depression. For clinical purposes, it will be important to identify optimal opioid agonists for surmounting the effects of XR-NTX to produce analgesia without clinically relevant adverse effects.

35.3.3.3 Pharmacokinetic Profile of XR-NTX in Nonhuman Primates

The lead formulation of XR-NTX displayed good in vivo release kinetics, as indicated by plasma naltrexone concentrations in rats (see above), but it is known that there is a substantial species variation with regard to the metabolism of naltrexone (50–52). The major urinary metabolite of naltrexone (6β-naltrexol) in the monkey is similar to man, while in the rat no major metabolites have been reported. Thus the PK profile of extended-release naltrexone may be different in rat and nonhuman primates.

Four rhesus monkeys (weighing 6.0-8.9 kg) received a single dose of the XR-NTX formulation (administered subcutaneously in two injections) for a total naltrexone dose of 150 mg per animal (this is equivalent on a weight basis to 20 mg naltrexone/kg in a 7.5 kg monkey). Blood samples for PK analysis were collected at multiple time points out to 48 days following administration of the XR-NTX microspheres. Concentrations of naltrexone and 6β-naltrexol in plasma were determined using a LC-MS/MS method.

No significant clinical observations of the injection sites were seen nor was there any appreciable weight loss in individual monkeys over the course of the study. Table 35.4 summarizes the PK parameters using a normalized dose of 20 mg naltrexone/kg. The plasma profile of 6β-naltrexol paralleled the naltrexone profile, but the plasma concentrations were generally ten times lower then that of naltrexone (Fig. 35.7). These monkey PK data confirm the rat PK profile in that the lead XR-NTX microsphere formulation produced an acceptable naltrexone profile over a 1-month period.

35.3.4 *Preclinical Summary*

The final formulation of XR-NTX maintains stable, pharmacologically relevant plasma levels of naltrexone for at least 28 days. The PK profile in rats and monkeys and the PD performance of the XR-NTX formulation meet the goals set forth early

Table 35.4 Pharmacokinetic parameters following a single dose of extended-release naltrexone in rhesus monkeys (20 mg/kg dose)

	C_{max} (ng/ml)	T_{max} (days)	$AUC_{0-1\ day}$ (ng day/ml)	$AUC_{0\text{-last day}}$ (ng day/ml)
Naltrexone	38.0±6.2	0.08±0.0	22.0±4.1	315±62
6 beta-naltrexol	1.5±0.5	1.2±0.7	1.1±0.2	28.0±3.8

Values are mean ± SD

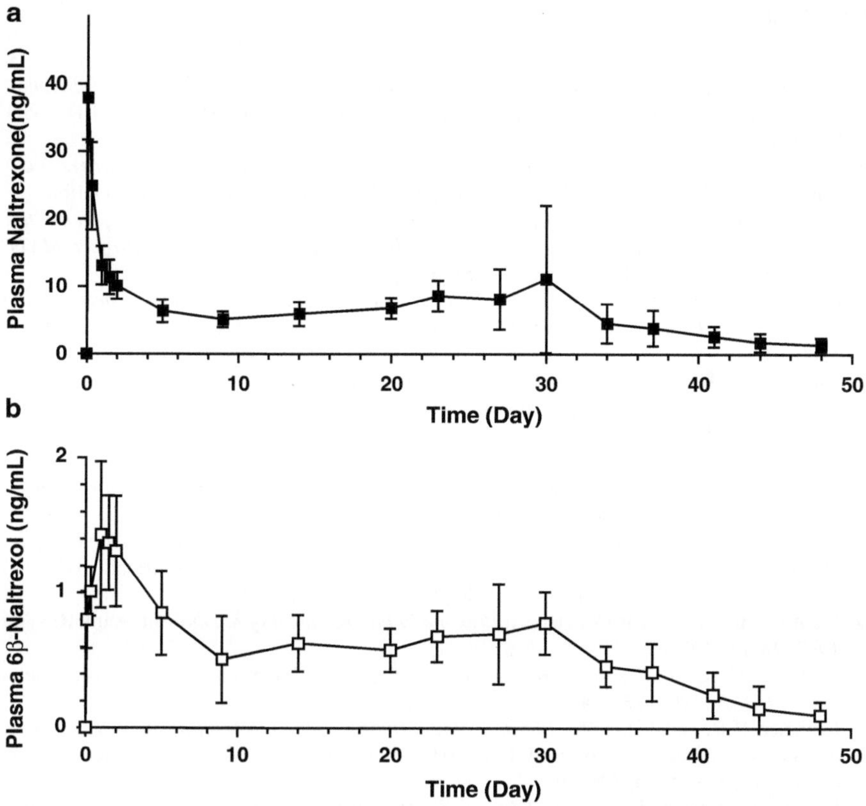

Fig. 35.7 Plasma concentrations of naltrexone (**a**) and its major metabolite, 6 β-naltrexol (**b**) in rhesus monkeys following a single subcutaneous (*s.c.*) dose of Alkermes' Medisorb® extended-release naltrexone (*XR-NTX*) microspheres, normalized to 20 mg/kg. The lower limit of quantitation was 0.2 ng/ml for both. Data represents the mean values ± SD from four monkeys [adapted from (42)]

in the development of this drug. Given that both naltrexone and the PLG polymer matrix in which it is encapsulated are well tolerated locally, XR-NTX was recommended for clinical testing. Based on the nonclinical data, this formulation ought to prove safe and effective in the treatment of alcohol dependence by providing an advanced means for maintaining elevated plasma levels of naltrexone for a 1-month treatment cycle. Therefore, an investigational new drug (IND) application was filed in 2000 for XR-NTX to test in clinical trials with alcohol-dependent patients. Subsequently, based on positive clinical trail results (53, 54), a new drug application (NDA) was filed in 2005 and VIVITROL was approved for the treatment of alcohol dependence in 2006.

Acknowledgments This work was produced as part of the duties of employees of Alkermes, Inc. The author thank all the current and former employees who had made a significant contribution to the XR-NTX research program. Alkermes thank the National Institute on Alcohol Abuse and Alcoholism (NIAAA) for their funding with a Small Business Innovation Research Program grant.

References

1. Harwood, H., *The Economic Costs of Alcohol and Drug Abuse in the United States: Estimates, Update Methods, and Data*. 2000, Washington, DC: U.S. DHHS, PHS, NIH, NIDA, NIAAA.
2. American Psychiatric, A., *Diagnostic and Statistical Manual of Mental Disorders*. Fourth Edition, Text Revision edn. 2000, Washington, DC: American Psychiatric Association.
3. Project MATCH Research, G., *Matching alcoholism treatments to client heterogeneity: treatment main effects and matching effects on drinking during treatment. Project MATCH Research Group*. J Stud Alcohol, 1998. **59**(6): pp. 631–9.
4. Project MATCH Research, G., *Matching alcoholism treatments to client heterogeneity: Project MATCH three-year drinking outcomes*. Alcohol Clin Exp Res, 1998. **22**(6): pp. 1300–11.
5. Ulm, R.R., J.R. Volpicelli, and L.A. Volpicelli, *Opiates and alcohol self-administration in animals*. J Clin Psychiatry, 1995. **56 Suppl. 7**: pp. 5–14.
6. Herz, A., *Endogenous opioid systems and alcohol addiction*. Psychopharmacology (Berl), 1997. **129**(2): pp. 99–111.
7. O'Leary, G., J. Borrow, and R.D. Weiss, *Opioid antagonists in the treatment of alcohol dependence*. Curr Psychiatry Rep, 2001. **3**(6): pp. 484–8.
8. Volpicelli, J.R., S. Krishnan-Sarin, and S.S. O'Malley, *Alcoholism Pharmacotherapy*, in *Neuropsychopharmacology: A Fifth Generation of Progress*, C. Nemeroff, Ed. 2002, Lippincott Williams and Wilkins: Philadelphia, PA. pp. 1445–59.
9. Weinrieb, R.M. and C.P. O'Brien, *Naltrexone in the treatment of alcoholism*. Annu Rev Med, 1997. **48**: pp. 477–87.
10. Garbutt, J.C., et al., *Pharmacological treatment of alcohol dependence: a review of the evidence*. JAMA, 1999. **281**(14): pp. 1318–25.
11. Kranzler, H.R. and J.H. Jaffe, *Pharmacologic Interventions for Alcoholism*, in *Principles of Addiction Medicine*, B.B. Wilford, Ed. 2003, American Society of Addiction Medicine, Inc.: Chevy Chase, MD. pp. 701–19.
12. U.S. Department of Health and Human, S., *Naltrexone and Alcohol Treatment*. Treatment Improvement Protocol Series 28. Vol. DHHS Publication No. (SMA) 98-3206. 1998, Washington, DC: PHS, SAMSHA, CSAT.
13. Jaffe, A.J., et al., *Naltrexone, relapse prevention, and supportive therapy with alcoholics: an analysis of patient treatment matching*. J Consult Clin Psychol, 1996. **64**(5): pp. 1044–53.
14. Swift, R.M., et al., *Naltrexone-induced alterations in human ethanol intoxication*. Am J Psychiatry, 1994. **151**(10): pp. 1463–7.
15. Volpicelli, J.R., et al., *Effect of naltrexone on alcohol "high" in alcoholics*. Am J Psychiatry, 1995. **152**(4): pp. 613–5.
16. Monterosso, J.R., et al., *Predicting treatment response to naltrexone: the influence of craving and family history*. Am J Addict, 2001. **10**(3): pp. 258–68.
17. Davidson, D., et al., *Effects of naltrexone on alcohol self-administration in heavy drinkers*. Alcohol Clin Exp Res, 1999. **23**(2): pp. 195–203.
18. Mark, T.L., et al., *Barriers to the use of medications to treat alcoholism*. Am J Addict, 2003. **12**(4): pp. 281–94.
19. Thomas, C.P., et al., *Research to practice: adoption of naltrexone in alcoholism treatment*. J Subst Abuse Treat, 2003. **24**(1): pp. 1–11.
20. Volpicelli, J.R., et al., *Naltrexone and alcohol dependence. Role of subject compliance*. Arch Gen Psychiatry, 1997. **54**(8): pp. 737–42.
21. Krystal, J.H., et al., *Naltrexone in the treatment of alcohol dependence*. N Engl J Med, 2001. **345**(24): pp. 1734–9.
22. Oncken, C., J. Van Kirk, and H.R. Kranzler, *Adverse effects of oral naltrexone: analysis of data from two clinical trials*. Psychopharmacology (Berl), 2001. **154**(4): pp. 397–402.

23. U.S. Department of Health and Human, S., *10th Special Report to the U.S. Congress on Alcohol and Health*. 2000. PHS, NIH, NIAAA: Washington, DC.
24. Pettinati, H.M., et al., *Improving naltrexone response: an intervention for medical practitioners to enhance medication compliance in alcohol dependent patients*. J Addict Dis, 2000. **19**(1): pp. 71–83.
25. PDR, *Physician's Desk Reference*. 51st ed. 1997. Medical Economics: Montvale, NJ.
26. Verebey, K., et al., *Naltrexone: disposition, metabolism, and effects after acute and chronic dosing*. Clin Pharmacol Ther, 1976. **20**(3): pp. 315–28.
27. Mason, B.J., *Dosing issues in the pharmacotherapy of alcoholism*. Alcohol Clin Exp Res, 1996. **20**(Suppl. 7): pp. 10A-6A.
28. Hutchinson, F.G. and B.J.A. Furr, *Design of biodegradable polymers for controlled release*, in *Drug Delivery Systems: Fundamentals and Techniques*, J.G. Lloyd-Jones, Ed. 1987, VCH: New York. pp. 106–119.
29. Shive, M.S. and J.M. Anderson, *Biodegradation and biocompatibility of PLA and PLGA microspheres*. Adv Drug Deliv Rev, 1997. **28**(1): pp. 5–24.
30. Hotz, J., et al., *Development of Vivitrex: A One Month Extended Release Naltrexone Formulation*, in *26th Annual Meeting of the Research Society on Alcoholism*. June, 2003. Ft. Lauderdale, FL.
31. Heilman, R.D., et al., *An evaluation of the hot plate technique to study narcotic antagonists*. Res Commun Chem Pathol Pharmacol, 1976. **13**(4): pp. 635–47.
32. Bartus, R.T., et al., *Vivitrex, an injectable, extended-release formulation of naltrexone, provides pharmacokinetic and pharmacodynamic evidence of efficacy for 1 month in rats*. Neuropsychopharmacology, 2003. **28**(11): pp. 1973–82.
33. Woolfe, G. and A.D. MacDonald, *The evaluation of the analgesic action of pethidine hydrochloride (Demerol)*. J. Pharmacol Exp Ther, 1944. **133**: pp. 300–7.
34. Ankier, S.I., *New hot plate tests to quantify antinociceptive and narcotic antagonist activities*. Eur J Pharmacol, 1974. **27**(1): pp. 1–4.
35. Zukin, R.S., et al., *Naltrexone-induced opiate receptor supersensitivity*. Brain Res, 1982. **245**(2): pp. 285–92.
36. Tempel, A., R.S. Zukin, and E.L. Gardner, *Supersensitivity of brain opiate receptor subtypes after chronic naltrexone treatment*. Life Sci, 1982. **31**(12–13): pp. 1401–4.
37. Yoburn, B.C., V. Sierra, and K. Lutfy, *Chronic opioid antagonist treatment: assessment of receptor upregulation*. Eur J Pharmacol, 1989. **170**(3): pp. 193–200.
38. Yoburn, B.C., et al., *Pharmacokinetics and pharmacodynamics of subcutaneous morphine pellets in the rat*. J Pharmacol Exp Ther, 1985. **235**(2): pp. 282–6.
39. Morris, B.J., M.J. Millan, and A. Herz, *Antagonist-induced opioid receptor up-regulation. II. Regionally specific modulation of mu, delta and kappa binding sites in rat brain revealed by quantitative autoradiography*. J Pharmacol Exp Ther, 1988. **247**(2): pp. 729–36.
40. Unterwald, E.M., et al., *Quantitative immunolocalization of mu opioid receptors: regulation by naltrexone*. Neuroscience, 1998. **85**(3): pp. 897–905.
41. Goldstein, A. and A. Naidu, *Multiple opioid receptors: ligand selectivity profiles and binding site signatures*. Mol Pharmacol, 1989. **36**(2): pp. 265–72.
42. Dean, R.L., *The preclinical development of Medisorb Naltrexone, a once a month long acting injection, for the treatment of alcohol dependence*. Front Biosci, 2005. **10**: pp. 643–55.
43. Comer, S.D., et al., *Injectable, sustained-release naltrexone for the treatment of opioid dependence: a randomized, placebo-controlled trial*. Arch Gen Psychiatry, 2006. **63**(2): pp. 210–8.
44. Vickers, A.P. and A. Jolly, *Naltrexone and problems in pain management*. Bmj, 2006. **332**(7534): pp. 132–3.
45. O'Brien, B. and C. Cody, *Analgesia and sedation in the presence of a naltrexone implant: a novel pharmacological challenge*. Eur J Emerg Med, 2006. **13**(5): pp. 315–6.
46. Schug, S.A., D. Zech, and S. Grond, *Adverse effects of systemic opioid analgesics*. Drug Saf, 1992. **7**(3): pp. 200–13.

47. Shook, J.E., W.D. Watkins, and E.M. Camporesi, *Differential roles of opioid receptors in respiration, respiratory disease, and opiate-induced respiratory depression*. Am Rev Respir Dis, 1990. **142**(4): pp. 895–909.
48. Inturrisi, C.E., *Clinical pharmacology of opioids for pain*. Clin J Pain, 2002. **18**(Suppl. 4): pp. S3–13.
49. Borison, H.L., *Central nervous respiratory depressants - narcotic analgesics*. Pharmacol Ther [B], 1977. **3**(2): pp. 227–37.
50. Dayton, H.E. and C.E. Inturrisi, *The urinary excretion profiles of naltrexone in man, monkey, rabbit, and rat*. Drug Metab Dispos, 1976. **4**(5): pp. 474–8.
51. Ludden, T.M., et al., *Elimination of radioactivity following administration of [15,16–3H] naltrexone to rats and guinea pigs*. Drug Metab Dispos, 1978. **6**(3): pp. 321–8.
52. Pace, N.L., et al., *Pharmacokinetics of naloxone and naltrexone in the dog*. J Pharmacol Exp Ther, 1979. **208**(2): pp. 254–6.
53. Johnson, B.A., et al., *A pilot evaluation of the safety and tolerability of repeat dose administration of long-acting injectable naltrexone (Vivitrex) in patients with alcohol dependence*. Alcohol Clin Exp Res, 2004. **28**(9): pp. 1356–61.
54. Garbutt, J.C., et al., *Efficacy and tolerability of long-acting injectable naltrexone for alcohol dependence: a randomized controlled trial*. JAMA, 2005. **293**(13): pp. 1617–25.
55. Wall, M.E., D.R. Brine, and M. Perez-Reyes, *Metabolism and disposition of naltrexone in man after oral and intravenous administration*. Drug Metab Dispos, 1981. 9(4): pp. 369–75.

Chapter 36
The Development of Sustained-Release Naltrexone and Clinical Use in Treating Opiate Dependence

Gary K. Hulse, Sandra D. Comer, and Maria A. Sullivan

Abstract Heroin and related illicit opioid abuse continues to be a significant problem in the United States and globally, as measured by a variety of indicators. The ability of naltrexone to effectively antagonize heroin use is unequivocal. However, despite this pharmacological efficacy, noncompliance with oral naltrexone formulae has been a significant impediment to its adoption as a treatment. Noncompliance is often associated with a patient's withdrawal from treatment and return to heroin use, although several recent studies specifically aimed at improving medication compliance have yielded promising results. An alternative method of naltrexone maintenance delivery involves the injection or surgical insertion of a sustained release preparation of naltrexone. This approach removes the onus on patients to use daily oral naltrexone. To date, a number of sustained release preparation of naltrexone have been developed for intramuscular or subcutaneous injection, or surgical insertion. Optimally, these products should be easy to administer, have no "major" adverse tissue reaction (biocompatible), be biodegradable, provide therapeutically relevant blood naltrexone levels, and be clinically effective. This chapter reviews the history, development, and comments on the relative merits of different formulations.

Keywords: Heroin abuse; Oral naltrexone formulae; Medication compliance; Sustained release naltrexone

---

G.K. Hulse (✉), S.D. Comer, and M.A. Sullivan
Unit for Research and Education in Drugs and Alcohol,
School of Psychiatry and Clinical Neurosciences (MDP 521),
The University of Western Australia, 35 Stirling Highway, WA 6009
e-mail: ghulse@cyllene.uwa.edu.au

36.1 Introduction

36.1.1 Opioid Dependence and Consequences

36.1.1.1 Epidemiology

Heroin abuse continues to be a significant problem in the United States and globally, as measured by a variety of indicators. For example, treatment admission rates in the United States doubled between 1993 and 1999 in roughly half of the States, with a triple increase observed in the West and Northeast (DASIS 2002). In addition, emergency department (ED) mentions of heroin increased by ~50% between 1994 and 2001 (SAMHSA 2002a). In 1996, the economic costs of heroin abuse were estimated at $21.9 billion (Mark et al. 2001), highlighting the devastating costs of heroin abuse to both the individual and to society in general.

The nonmedical use and abuse of prescription opioids is also increasing (74), and at a much faster rate than heroin abuse. The 2001 report from the National Household Survey on Drug Abuse (NHSDA) revealed that ~2.0 million persons in the United States reported using a prescription opioid for a nonmedical reason for the first time in the year 2000, a number that has quintupled since the mid-1980s. In 2001, 0.2 million people were classified with heroin abuse/dependence, while 1.0 million people were classified with abuse/dependence on "pain relievers" (SAMHSA 2002c). In addition, among the 3.1 million people receiving treatment for alcohol or drug use in the past year, the number of individuals receiving treatment for abuse of pain relievers (0.32 million) was comparable to the number of patients receiving treatment for heroin abuse (0.30 million; SAMHSA 2002c). These epidemiological data show the scope and severity of the problem of heroin abuse and nonmedical use of prescription opioids, and they underscore the need for studies designed to evaluate potential medications for opioid abuse.

36.1.1.2 Treatment for Heroin Use

A number of pharmacotherapies are available as accepted treatments for heroin addiction. These include methadone (21, 22), buprenorphine (68), and naltrexone (63, 52). Of these, methadone, an orally administered opioid agonist, was one of the earliest and continues to be the most widely used form of pharmacotherapy maintenance treatment. Unlike methadone and buprenorphine, naltrexone is an opioid antagonist and hence detoxification of the heroin-dependent person is a prerequisite for naltrexone maintenance (29).

36.1.2 Oral Naltrexone

36.1.2.1 Pharmacology of Naltrexone

Naltrexone was one of many compounds synthesized after World War II in an effort to produce safer and more effective opiate analgesics. It consists of several simple modifications of the basic morphine molecular structure, similar to modifications that have been used to produce other opioid drugs, including buprenorphine and naloxone. Naltrexone is a potent long-acting competitive opioid antagonist at the μ-, κ-, and δ- opioid-receptors (65) that has been used as a maintenance pharmacotherapy with a recommended daily oral dose of 50 mg in persons who have detoxified completely from heroin (8, 3, 11, 40). The major therapeutic feature of naltrexone pharmacology that makes it useful for the treatment of opiate dependence is that when occupying receptors, it completely blocks the effects of opiate agonists that may be taken (63, 52).

36.1.2.2 Clinical Experience with Oral Naltrexone

Notwithstanding the unequivocal pharmacological efficacy of naltrexone to block the actions of heroin, early clinical trials of naltrexone in general populations of opioid-dependent patients were relatively discouraging. Dropout rates were high, and few patients completed more than 30–60 days of treatment (4, 9, 44). Even in patients who perform well on oral formulae, periodic relapse to heroin use is common (58, 34). A recent randomized clinical trial conducted in Iran (2) provides more contemporary evidence for the relative effectiveness of naltrexone versus agonist maintenance in a 24-week comparison between naltrexone (50 mg/day), sublingual buprenorphine (5 mg/day), and methadone (50 mg/day). The study enrolled 204 patients dependent on illicit intravenous (IV) buprenorphine. The rate of treatment completion was 21% in the group assigned to naltrexone compared to 59% on buprenorphine and 84% on methadone. Indeed, a recent review of the effectiveness of oral naltrexone maintenance for the treatment of opioid dependence concluded that there was "insufficient evidence to justify the use of naltrexone in maintenance treatment of opioid addicts" (43).

A major problem associated with oral naltrexone therapy is poor medication compliance. This may be attributed to several factors. For example, opioid users are accustomed to self-administering potent reinforcers and the complete absence of opioid-induced reinforcing effects may be unacceptable. In addition, unlike methadone, discontinuation of naltrexone maintenance has no adverse consequences, such as the emergence of opioid withdrawal effects. Furthermore, some studies suggest that naltrexone itself may induce adverse neuropsychiatric and gastrointestinal effects, such as dysphoria, nausea, and abdominal discomfort (17, 31, 54).

All of these factors may contribute to the poor medication compliance seen with oral naltrexone therapy. Thus, despite naltrexone's potent opioid antagonist properties, noncompliance with oral naltrexone formulae has been a significant impediment to its adoption as a major treatment for heroin dependence.

Despite this relatively discouraging outlook for oral naltrexone maintenance, clinical trials have suggested greater compliance and effectiveness in several subgroups including patients receiving family therapy (3), patients residing in a supportive family environment where naltrexone compliance is encouraged (11), patients who are professionals in jeopardy of losing their licenses (69) or patients in the parole and criminal justice systems at risk of returning to jail (16). Several recent studies specifically aimed at improving medication compliance have also yielded promising results (10, 23, 47, 55, 57). These studies show that inclusion of contingency management and/or family or partner involvement produces relatively good 6-month treatment retention rates ranging from 25% to 45%. These studies do suggest potential promise for oral naltrexone maintenance, depending on appropriate environmental circumstances or behavioral interventions.

36.1.2.3 Sustained-Release Naltrexone Preparations

One alternative to an oral naltrexone formula is the injection or surgical insertion of a sustained release preparation of naltrexone, which removes the onus on patients to use daily medication. Sustained release preparations have commonly involved using compressed naltrexone formulations (e.g., Wedgewood implant manufactured by Wedgewood Pharmacy, Sewell, NJ, USA), or by combining naltrexone with a polymer or copolymer base to allow for the more gradual release of naltrexone over elongated periods of time. Polymer or copolymer base have included, for example, a naltrexone-polylactic acid composite (73); naltrexone-copolymer (90% L-lactic acid and 10% glycolic acid) beads (13); 70% naltrexone base in poly(L-gactic-co-glycolic acid) (61); naltrexone pamoate linear poly (ortho esters) disk (49), and polylactide coglycolide microspheres (5).

The concept of a sustained-release preparation of naltrexone is not new. Beginning in the mid-1970s, depot formulations of naltrexone were developed and evaluated in laboratory animals (1, 30, 50, 56, 59, 62, 73). For the main part, these early formulations were abandoned because of wide between-subject variability in plasma concentrations of naltrexone, and lack of tissue compatibility.

In 1980, the US National Institute of Health published information on necessary/desirable characteristics for naltrexone-sustained release parenteral drug delivery systems. In addition to the ability to provide therapeutically relevant blood naltrexone levels, they noted that products should be clinically effective, biodegradable, have no adverse tissue reaction (biocompatible), and be easy to "implant" (53, 71).

36.1.2.4 Sustaining Therapeutic Levels

A number of clinical reports and studies have provided prima facie evidence on the efficacy of sustained preparations to antagonize the actions of heroin. These have reported serum naltrexone levels of 2.8 ng/ml delivered by implant naltrexone as being effective in blocking 500 mg of snorted pure pharmaceutical diamorphine (7), serum naltrexone levels ≤2 ng/ml (52, 28, 66, 51) as being effective in blocking the effects of 25 mg intravenously administered heroin, and others have reported plasma levels of less than 1 ng/ml as being capable of antagonizing the effects of 15 mg morphine (12). Most authorities now agree that the therapeutic blood level required to treat heroin dependence is above 2 ng/ml (6, 36, 15). To date, most sustained-release naltrexone formulations have been shown to maintain therapeutic blood levels of naltrexone for 4–8 weeks (13, 6, 15, 5).

36.1.2.5 Biodegradability

It has been known for more than two decades that polymers based on lactide isomers are biodegraded by hydrolysis and even when incorporated with other polymers are absorbed by the body without adverse reactions (48). In rats, D,L-lactide/glycolide copolymer microspheres have been shown to be biodegradable, with the vast majority of microsphere degradation occurring by day 150 (72). In humans poly(D,L) lactide in surgical sutures and screws is reabsorbed by the body through natural pathways (67). Similarly, following injection into the body, the poly-lactide co-glycolide hydrolyzes to lactic and glycolic acids, that are further metabolized into carbon dioxide and water (39). There is therefore a good in-principal case to suggest that polymers based on lactide isomers that have been and are being developed as part of naltrexone-sustained release preparations are likely to be biodegraded.

In vitro and in vivo studies indicate that total time to biodegradation might be commensurate with the size of implant mass used, with, for example, a large quantity of poly(D,L) lactide degrading over a longer time period than a smaller quantity (64, 27). The time to total biodegradation should not be an issue so long as good tissue compatibility is achieved.

36.1.2.6 Tissue Compatibility

A number of polymers or copolymers despite showing promising naltrexone release patterns, and being of "likely biodegradable materials," have shown varying therapeutic success. For example, Chiang et al. (13) conducted one of the early studies of sustained release naltrexone in normal, healthy volunteers implanted subcutaneously with naltrexone-copolymer (90% L-lactic acid and 10% glycolic acid) beads. Following an initial burst of release, this formulation yielded relatively constant plasma levels of naltrexone (0.3–0.5 ng/ml) for up to 1 month. However, when these investigators administered challenge doses of morphine (15 mg IV), the results were variable. In some participants, morphine was completely ineffective, while in others, morphine-like effects were observed. Perhaps more importantly however, data suggested that this naltrexone preparation had unacceptable levels of biocompatibility, with two of the three human subjects implanted with the naltrexone-copolymer (90% L-lactic acid and 10% glycolic acid) beads having them removed at ~3-4 weeks due to marked inflammatory reactions or other local tissue irritation. Chiang concluded that this result "may preclude the clinical use of this particular preparation of beads" (13).

Undoubtedly, comprehensive acceptability of sustained-release naltrexone products as a conventional treatment for opiate dependence is limited by studies showing an acceptable level of tissue reactivity in patients treated with sustained-release preparations.

36.1.2.7 Newer Formulations

Newer formulations of sustained-release naltrexone have provided more promising results. For example, injectable formulations of naltrexone, such as those produced by Biotek, Inc. (Depotrex®) (15, 45), Drug Abuse Sciences (Naltrel®) (24, 46, 41), and Alkermes, Inc. (Vivitrex®) (5), appear to produce both clinically relevant plasma concentrations of naltrexone, both within and between subjects, and a much lower and perhaps clinically acceptable incidence of tissue reactivity.

An injectable, depot formulation of naltrexone (Depotrex®), 192 mg, 384 mg naltrexone base antagonized the effects of intravenously administered heroin (0–25 mg) for 3–5 weeks, depending on naltrexone dose. This study demonstrated that Depotrex® was safe, effective, and well tolerated in opioid abusers who were not seeking treatment for their drug use. A subsequent "proof-of-concept" clinical trial of Depotrex® in treatment-seeking heroin abusers showed a robust, dose-related increase in treatment retention, supporting the use of depot naltrexone as a therapeutic strategy for opioid dependence (14).

Vivitrol, formerly known as Vivitrex, (Alkermes, Inc.) is an injectable [subcutaneous (SC) or intramuscular (IM)] formulation of depot of naltrexone encapsulated into polylactide coglycolide polymer microspheres (~100-µm diameter). Data from studies with rats administered a single (SC or IM) injection (50 mg/kg) indicate that it produces peak naltrexone plasma levels within 3 days (15 ± 1.4 and 19 ± 3.6 ng/ml, respectively), dropping to undetectable level (<1 ng/ml) by 35 days (5). Similar results have been reported in alcohol-dependent patients (IM 400 mg) with naltrexone maintained at presumed therapeutic levels for a full month (Alkermes, Inc., Press Release, November 21, 2000; December 11). In rats, these levels were capable of antagonizing the effects of morphine on a hot-plate test over a 4-week period (5). A sequential IM injection on day 34 produced a similar effect to the initial injection, suppressing morphine-induced analgesia up to day 68 (5). This polymer is known to readily hydrolyze to lactic and glycolic acid, which is further metabolized into carbon dioxide and water (39). Preliminary data indicate that in humans, IM Vivitrol (400 mg) is generally safe and well tolerated, and reported adverse effects are mild to moderate. Although over 10% of alcohol-dependent persons experienced some form of adverse event following Vivitrol treatment (nausea, headache, loss of appetite, and fatigue), less than 2% of patients discontinued treatment because of injection site reactions (in duration and angioedema)

(Alkermes, Inc., Press Release, April 22, 2004). With the exception of injection site reactions, reported common adverse effects with Vivitrol are similar to those seen with oral naltrexone formulations (25). A 12-month extension trial of alcohol-dependent persons found the most common adverse effects to be headache, nasopharyngitis, and respiratory tract infections (Alkermes, Inc., Press Release, May 23, 2005).

More recently, a poly-D,L-lactide implantable formulation of naltrexone has been developed which may provide even longer-lasting blockade of opioid receptors. The naltrexone implant (O'Neil Implant) developed by GoMedical Industries Pvt. Ltd. (Perth, Western Australia) has shown promise to deliver naltrexone at clinically relevant blood levels above 2 ng/ml for 5-6 months (32, 33). This implant is a diffusion-based delivery system, designed such that pockets of naltrexone are isolated by a polymer matrix (100-μm diameter poly-D,L-lactide) to ensure a more gradual release of the naltrexone as fluid enters the core. Human in vitro assessment of tissue samples (biopsies) from 54 subjects (34 males) at various periods of time postimplant showed an early phase (up to 12 months postimplant) of inflammation, foreign body reaction, and fibrosis, which gradually settled over the next 12 months until tissue returned to normal by 25+ months (37). Additional data from an ultrasound study on 71 heroin-dependent persons treated with this implant concluded that there was a total absence by an the poly(D,L-lactide) implant matrix by an average of 1,201 days.

The sustained release preparations described above are yet to be registered by regulatory authorities for therapeutic use in the management of opioid dependence, although Vivitrol® has now been approved for use in the United States by the US Food and Drug Administration (FDA) for the management of alcohol dependence.

36.2 Mode of Administration: Sustained-Release Preparation

Mode of administration and its acceptability to addiction practitioners and/or patients may prove to be a major consideration in selecting the type of sustained-release product to use in the treatment of heroin dependence. To date the rage of sustained release preparation of naltrexone have focused on IM or SC injection or surgical insertion.

Depot preparations have an advantage in that they are relatively easily administered by IM or SC injection (e.g., Vivitrex; Depotrex®), compared to implant (e.g., Wedgewood or O'Neil Implant), which are commonly inserted subcutaneously under local anesthesia through a small incision made on the side of the lower abdomen.

Clearly some additional physician training may be required to administer implant naltrexone compared to injectable depot preparations. In addition, patients may have a preference for a depot injection rather than being subjected to a more invasive procedure such as is required for implant treatment.

36.3 Other Considerations

There are, however, a number of additional clinical considerations that might outweigh this and favor implant treatment amongst community treatment programs for heroin dependence.

First, while tissue compatibility with recently produced naltrexone polymeric preparations is good, some significant events have been reported in a very small proportion of patients. In these isolated instances where removal of polymeric materials is deemed clinically desirable, this might be achieved more readily with an implant than an injectable depot preparation; the latter proving almost impossible to remove, short of excising a large area of tissue.

Second and perhaps more importantly, depot preparations only provide a period of coverage for 4–8 weeks compared to the O'Neil implant where prima-facie evidence suggests a clinical efficacy for several months.

Although no randomized clinical trials assessing the efficacy of this sustained-release preparations have been published, a recent study investigated heroin overdose requiring hospitalization in a large cohort of heroin-dependent persons treated with the long acting O'Neil sustained-release naltrexone implant. No opioid overdoses were reported in the 6-month period posttreatment, and a reduced number of opioid overdoses was found in the 6-2-month period postimplant treatment (38). This period of prophylaxis against opioid overdose was consistent with the reported pharmacokinetic data on this implant (33).

This finding is of considerable clinical significance not only because the mortality rates for regular IV heroin users are ~13 times greater than that for the general population, with accidental heroin overdose accounting for between 30% and 45% of all-cause mortality (35) but also because it suggests that patients are unlikely to relapse back to heroin use during the pharmacokinetic coverage period of 5–6 months, allowing a greater change of movement away from narcotic use and its associated lifestyle.

The clinical importance of preparations that provide a maximum elongated period of coverage can not be overstated. It is difficult to estimate the length of naltrexone antagonist treatment required to facilitate significant movement of a previously heroin-dependent person away from the narcotic network and back toward main-stream community involvement. Estimates might, however, start at 12 and extend up toward 60 months depending on an individual's entrenchment within the narcotic network. The provision of an enforced abstinence period of longer durations is likely to be a significant factor in assisting the formerly dependent heroin user to separate from heroin use, the narcotic network, and commence reintegration back into the broader community.

Additionally, despite addressing issues of daily noncompliance associated with oral naltrexone, sustained-release formulations still rely on the patient returning for a second implant. Given the propensity of the population toward relapse, it is more than likely that not all patients will return for a second procedure. Therefore, an important consideration in the ongoing management of the previously heroin-dependent person will involve encouraging retreatment before the pharmacokinetic efficacy of the preparation runs out. For a number of reasons, the initial use of a preparation that gives several rather than a single month of cover may be desirable. First, treatment with longer-acting preparations reduces the frequency of retreatments required over any given period. Second, a longer period of sustained naltrexone coverage is likely to produce a more stable patient who is more likely to return for retreatment. Third, the use of longer-acting preparations will create an elongated window of opportunity in which to perform a follow-up implant.

36.4 Merits of Depot Preparations

Having argued that the initial use of an implantable preparation that gives several rather than a single month of cover may be desirable, the more stable patients returning for retreatment may at this point opt for treatment with a depot preparation rather than once again undergoing the more invasive minor surgery associated with implant treatment. In this respect, different sustained-release preparations may be used sequentially as part of the same management program.

Additionally, there are some specific instances were the use of a more easily administered, shorter-acting depot preparation may have advantages over an implant administered by minor surgery. For example, relapse back to heroin use following release from prison is high, with significant morbidity and mortality observed in the weeks following release. Many reasons have been given for this. They include lack of social, economic, employment, and physical (i.e. housing) resources available to those recently released, which facilitates gravitation back to known networks and friends commonly with links to narcotic use. The provision of a period of opioid antagonism of 4–8 weeks while the newly released persons establish a level of stability in the new environment cannot be overrated. In such instances, the administration of a depot immediately prior to release might be more practical and appealing to the judicial authorities compared to a more invasive and time consuming implant procedure.

36.5 Polydrug Use

Polydrug use is an increasing part of heroin use (26, 18, 20). While naltrexone may provide antagonism against opioids, one concern is that other drug use may replace opioid use, posing a new risk situation for both dependence and risk of overdose. To date, clinical studies on depot (Comer 2004, #3188); (14) and implant naltrexone (38) have indicated that other drug use remained relatively low. This is consistent with findings from other studies reporting on patients entering oral naltrexone maintenance (42, 34, 58). Notwithstanding these issues, programs offering sustained-release antagonist treatment for opioid dependence should have an enhanced emphasis on preventing, detecting, and managing polysubstance use. This approach would also help to protect the small percentage of people who may either continue with or move to other drug use when implants block opioid use.

36.6 Accidental Opioid Overdose Following Treatment Cessation

It has been postulated from pharmacological studies that naltrexone exposure may increase opioid receptor sensitivity to heroin (70) [loss of tolerance to opioids and increased receptor sensitivity after chronic antagonist administration are two different phenomena] (19, 60). These assertions find some support from a study showing that the short (4-week)-acting depot preparation Vivitrex-induced changes in μ-opioid receptor density in many regions of the rat brain up to twofold following a single IM injection (50 mg/kg). Increased density of μ-opioid receptors seen in rats could potentially enhance hypersensitivity to opiates (5). Return to heroin use following use of a sustained-release product may therefore lead to an increased risk of fatal overdose and should also cite Jim Cornish's study showing a lack of support for supersensitivity in humans.

This may be especially problematic with single treatment shorter-acting sustained preparations where blood naltrexone levels fall away within days from therapeutic to nondetectable levels, and patients are likely to return to opioid use. This situation, however, may not be as prevalent with longer-acting preparations for two reasons. First, following a period of opioid antagonist coverage for several months, patients have a greater probability of remaining heroin free or not relapsing quickly. Second, the longer-acting O'Neil implant has been reported to keep plasma naltrexone levels above 1 ng/ml, a level shown to effectively antagonize the effects of 15 mg morphine (12). This suggests that while it might not block all the effects of heroin, it will likely provide a level of protection against respiratory suppression, thereby providing a prophylaxis against accidental overdose.

36.7 Pain Management: Antagonism of Opiates

I assume this will be dealt with in other parts of the book and reference should be made to this chapter and the management of patients.

36.8 Concluding Comments

The development of biocompatible, and biodegradable sustained-release naltrexone preparations that provide long-lasting coverage of naltrexone at therapeutic doses capable of providing resistance to opiate drugs in habituated users, thereby facilitating an opiate-abstinent lifestyle, is clearly desirable.

Despite the promise of sustained-release preparations to maintain therapeutic levels of naltrexone for significant periods, it should be emphasized that management with sustained-release formulations of naltrexone simply creates a window to facilitate movement of the previously opiate-dependent patient away from the narcotic network and back into the general community. The role of psychosocial auxiliary services as part of a treatment package to manage this transition should not be underestimated. Failure to provide adequate recourses to facilitate a heroin-free lifestyle after treatment with sustained-release naltrexone will undoubtable see a greater proportion of patients relapse back to dependent heroin use.

References

1. Abrahams, RA & Ronel, SH 1975. Biocompatible implants for the sustained zero-order release of narcotic antagonists. *Journal of Biomedical Materials Research*, **9,** 355–366.
2. Ahmadi, J 2003. Methadone versus buprenorphine maintenance for the treatment of heroin-dependent outpatients. *Journal of Substance Abuse Treatment*, **24,** 217–220.
3. Anton, RE, Hogan, I, Jalali, B, Riordan, CE & Kleber, HD 1981. Multiple family therapy and naltrexone in the treatment of opiate-dependence. *Drug and Alcohol Dependence*, **8,** 157–168.
4. Azarian, A, Papiasvilli, A & Joseph, H 1994. A study of the use of clonidine and naltrexone in the treatment of opiod addiction in the former USSR. *Journal of Addictive Diseases*, **13,** 35–52.
5. Bartus, RT, Emerich, DF, Hotz, J, Blaustein, M, Dean, RL, Perdomo, B & Basile, A 2003. Vivitrex, an injectable, extended-release formulation of naltrexone, provides pharmacokinetic and pharmacodynamic evidence of efficacy for 1 month in rats. *Neuropsychopharmacology*, **28,** 1973–1982.
6. Brewer, C 2001. Naltrexone implants for opiate addiction: new life for a middle aged drug. *The Pharmaceutical Journal*, **267,** 260.
7. Brewer, C 2002. Serum naltrexone and 6-beta-naltrexol levels from naltrexone implants can block very large amounts of heroin: a report of two cases. *Addiction Biology*, **7,** 321–323.
8. Callaghan, E, Rawson, R & McCleave, B 1980. The treatment of heroin addiction using naltrexone alone and with behaviour therapy. *International Journal of the Addiction*, **15,** 795–807.
9. Callahan, E, Rawson, R., Glazer, M., McCleave, B., & Arias, R 1980. In: Demetrios, J. & Renault, P. (Eds.). Comparison of two naltrexone treatment programs: naltrexone alone versus naltrexone plus behaviour therapy, pp. 150–157.
10. Carroll, KM, Ball, SA, Nich, C, O'Connor, PG, Eagan, DA, Frankforter, TL, Triffleman, EG, Shi, JM & Rounsaville, BJ 2001. Targeting behavioral therapies to enhance naltrexone treatment of opiod dependence: efficacy of contingency management and significant other involvement. *Archives in General Psychiatry*, **58,** 755–761.
11. Chan, KY 1996. The Singapore naltrexone community-based project for heroin addicts compared with drugfree community-based program: the first cohort. *Journal of Clinical Forensic Medicine*, **3,** 87–92.
12. Chiang, CN, Hollister, LE, Kishimoto, A & Barnett, G 1984. Kinetics of a naltrexone sustained-release preparation. *Clinical Pharmacology and Therapeutics*, **36,** 704–708.
13. Chiang, CN, Hollister, LE, Gillespie, HK & Foltz, RL 1985. Clinical evaluation of a naltrexone sustained-release preparation. *Drug and Alcohol Dependence*, **16,** 1–8.
14. Comer, S, Sullivan, MA, Yu, E, Rothenberg, JL, Kleber, HD, Kampman, K, Dackis, C & O'Brien, CP 2006. Injectable, sustained-release naltrexone for the treatment of opioid dependence: a randomized, placebo-controlled trial. *Archives of General Psychiatry*, **63,** 210–218.
15. Comer, SD, Collins, ED, Kleber, HD, Nuwayser, ES, Kerrigan, JH & Fischman, MW 2002. Depot naltrexone: long-lasting antagonism of the effects of heroin in humans. *Psychopharmacology (Berl)*, **159,** 351–360.

16. Cornish, JW, Metzger, D, Woody, GE, Wilson, D, McLellan, AT, Vandergrift, B & Obrien, CP 1997. Naltrexone pharmacotherapy for opioid dependent federal probationers. *Journal of Substance Abuse Treatment*, **14,** 529–534.
17. Crowley, TJ, Wagner, JE, Zerbe, G & Macdonald, MJ 1985. Naltrexone-induced dysphoria in former opioid addicts. *American Journal of Psychiatry*, **142,** 1081–1084.
18. Darke, S & Ross, J 1999. Heroin-related deaths in South Western Sydney, Australia, 1992–96. *Drug and Alcohol Review*, **18,** 39–45.
19. Darke, S, Sunjic, S, Zador, D & Prolov, T 1997. A comparison of blood toxicology of heroin-related deaths and current heroin users in Sydney, Australia. *Drug and Alcohol Dependence*, **47,** 45–53.
20. Darke, S, Ross, J, Zador, D & Sunjic, S 2000. Heroin-related deaths in New South Wales, Australia, 1992–1996. *Drug and Alcohol Dependence*, **60,** 141–150.
21. Dole, V, Nyswander, ME & Kreek, MJ 1966. Narcotic blockade. *Archives of Internal Medicine*, **118,** 304–309.
22. Faggiano, F, Versino, E, Vigna-Taglianti, F & Lemma, P. 2000. Methadone maintenance at different dosages for opioid dependence. Cochrane Database systemic reviews.
23. Fals-Stewart, W & O'Farrell, TJ 2003. Behavioral family counseling and naltrexone for male opiod-dependent patients. *Journal of Consulting and Clinical Psychology*, **71,** 432–442.
24. Galloway, GP, Koch, M, Gross, J & Smith, DE 2001. Safety, tolerability and pharmacokinetics of a sustained-release formulation of naltrexone in alcoholics. *Drug and Alcohol Dependence*, **63,** S52.
25. Garbutt, JC, Kranzler, HR, O'Malley, SS, Gastfriend, DR, Pettinati, HM, Silverman, BL, Loewy, JW, Ehrich, EW & Vivitrex Study Group 2005. Efficacy and tolerability of long-acting injectable naltrexone for alcohol dependence: a randomized controlled trial. *JAMA*, **293,** 1617–1625.
26. Gerostamoulos, J, Staikos, V & Drummer, OH 2001. Heroin-related deaths in Victoria: a review of cases for 1997 and 1998. *Drug and Alcohol Dependence*, **61,** 123–127.
27. Grizzi, I, Garreau, H, Li, S & Vert, M 1995. Hydrolytic degradation of devices based on poly(D-L-lactic acid) size-dependence. *Biomaterials*, **16,** 305–311.
28. Hamilton, RJ, Olmedo, RE, Shah, S, Hung, OL, Howland, MA, Perrone, J, Nelson, LS, Lewin, NL & Hoffman, RS 2002. Complications of ultrarapid opioid detoxification with subcutaneous naltrexone pellets. *Academic Emergency Medicine*, **9,** 63–68.
29. Hando, J, Hall, W, Rutter, S & Dolan, K. 1998. An information document on the current state of research on illicit drugs in Australia. Sydney: University of New South Wales.
30. Harrigan, SE & Downs, DA 1981. Pharmacological evaluation of narcotic antagonist delivery systems in rhesus monkeys. *NIDA Research Monograph*, **28,** 77–92.
31. Hollister, LE, Johnson, K, Boukhabza, D & Gillespie, HK 1981. Aversive effects of naltrexone in subjects not dependent on opiates. *Drug and Alcohol Dependence*, **8,** 37–41.
32. Hulse, GK & Basso, MR 2000. The association between naltrexone compliance and daily supervision. *Drug and Alcohol Review*, **19,** 41–48.
33. Hulse, GK & O'Neil, G 2002. A possible role for implantable naltrexone in the management of the "high risk" pregnant heroin user. *Australian and New Zealand Journal of Obstetrics and Gynaecology*, **42,** 93–94.
34. Hulse, GK, English, DR, Milne, E & Holman, CDJ 1999. The quantification of mortality resulting from the regular use of illicit opiates. *Addiction*, **94,** 221–229.
35. Hulse, GK, Arnold-Reed, DA, O'Neil, G, Chan, CT & Hansson, R 2004a. Achieving long-term continuous blood naltrexone and 6-β-naltrexol coverage following sequential naltrexone implants. *Addiction Biology*, **9,** 67–72.
36. Hulse, GK, Arnold-Reed, DE, O'Neil, G, Chan, CT, Hansson, R & O'Neil, P 2004b. Blood naltrexone and 6-β-naltrexol levels following naltrexone implant: comparing two naltrexone implants. *Addiction Biology*, **9,** 59–65.
37. Hulse, GK, Stalenberg, V, McCallum, D, Smit, W, O'Neil, G, Morris, N & Tait, RJ 2005a. Histological changes over time around the site of sustained release naltrexone-poly(D-L-Lactide) implants in humans. *Journal of Controlled Release*, **108,** 43–55.

38. Hulse, GK, Tait, RJ, Comer, SD, Sullivan, MA, Jacobs, IG & Arnold-Reed, DE 2005b. Reducing hospital presentations for opioid overdose in patients treated with sustained release naltrexone implants. *Drug and Alcohol Dependence*, **79,** 351–357.
39. Johnson, BA, Ait-Daoud, N, Aubin, H-J, van den Brink, W, Guzzetta, R, Loewy, J, Silverman, B & Ehrich, E 2004. A pilot evaluation of the safety and tolerability of repeat dose administration of long-acting injectable naltrexone [Vivitrex (R)] in patients with alcohol dependence. *Alcoholism: Clinical and Experimental Research*, **28,** 1356–1361.
40. Julius, D. 1976. NIDA's naltrexone research program. In: *Narcotic Antagonists: Naltrexone (NIDA Research Monograph No. 9)*, Julius, D. & Renault, P. (eds.), pp. 5–11. Rockville, MD: National Institute of Drug Abuse.
41. Kaplan, SA, Pouletty, P & Wesson, DR 2000. Pharmacokinetics of naltrexone from polylactide sustained-release naltrexone. *Drug and Alcohol Dependence*, **60,** S107.
42. Kirchmayer, U, Davoli, M, Verster, AD, Amato, L, Ferri, A & Perucci, CA 2002. A systematic review on the efficacy of naltrexone maintenance treatment in opiod dependence. *Addiction*, **97,** 1241–1249.
43. Kirchmayer, U, Davoli, M & Verster, A 2003. Naltrexone maintenance treatment for opioid dependence. *Cochrane Database of Systematic Reviews*, **Issue 2,** DOI: 10.1002/14651858.CD001333.
44. Kosten, TR & Kleber, HD 1984. Strategies to improve compliance with narcotic antagonists. *American Journal of Drug and Alcohol Abuse*, **10,** 249–266.
45. Kranzler, HR, Modesto-Lowe, V & Nuwayser, ES 1998. Sustained-release naltrexone for alcoholism treatment: a preliminary study. *Alcoholism: Clinical and Experimental Research*, **22,** 1074–1079.
46. Kranzler, HR, Wesson, DR, Billot, L and Drug Abuse Sciences Naltrexone Depot Study Group 2004. Naltrexone depot for treatment of alcohol dependence: a multicenter, randomized, placebo-controlled clinical trial. *Alcoholism: Clinical and Experimental Research*, **28,** 1051–1059.
47. Krupitsky, EM, Zvartau, EE, Masalov, DV, Tsoi, MV, Burakov, AM, Egorova, VY, Didenko, TY, Romanova, TM, Ivanova, EB, Bespalov, AY, Verbitskaya, EV, Neznanov, NG, Grinenko, AY, O'Brien, CP & Woody, GE in press. Naltrexone for heroin dependence treatment in St. Petersburg, Russia. *Journal of Substance Abuse Treatment*.
48. Lin, F-H, Chen, T-M, Lin, C-P & Lee, C-J 1999. The merit of sintered PDLLA/TCP composites in management of bone fracture internal fixation. *Artificial Organs*, **23,** 186–194.
49. Maa, YF & Heller, J 1990. Controlled release of naltrexone pamoate from linear poly(ortho esters). *Journal of Controlled Release*, **14,** 21–28.
50. Martin, WR & Sandquist, VL 1974. A sustained release depot for narcotic antagonists. *Archives of General Psychiatry*, **30,** 31–33.
51. Navaratnam, V, Jamaludin, A, Raman, N, Mohamed, M & Mansor, SM 1994. Determination of naltrexone dosage for narcotic agonist blockade in detoxified Asian addicts. *Drug and Alcohol Dependence*, **34,** 231–236.
52. Olmedo, R & Hoffman, RS 2000. Withdrawal syndromes. *Emergency Medicine Clinics of North America*, **18,** 273–288.
53. Olsen, JL & Kincl, FA 1980. A review of parental sustained-release naltrexone systems. In: *Naltrexone Research Monograph*, Willette, R. E. & Barnett, G. (eds.), pp. 187–264: National Institute on Drug Abuse.
54. Oncken, C, Van Kirk, J & Kranzler, HR 2001. Adverse effects of oral naltrexone: analysis of data from two clinical trials. *Psychopharmacology*, **154,** 397–402.
55. Preston, KL, Silverman, K, Umbricht, A, DeJesus, A, Montoya, ID & Schuster, CR 1999. Improvement in naltrexone treatment compliance with contingency management. *Drug and Alcohol Dependence*, **54,** 127–135.
56. Reuning, RH, Liao, SHT, Staubus, AE, Ashcraft, SB, Downs, DA, Harrigan, SE, Wiley, JN & Wise, DL 1983. Pharmacokinetic quantitation of naltrexone controlled release from a copolymer delivery system. *Journal of Pharmacokinetics and Biopharmaceutics*, **11,** 369–387.

57. Rothenberg, JL, Sullivan, MA, Church, SH, Seracini, A, Collins, E, Kleber, HD & Nunes, EV 2002. Behavioral naltrexone therapy: an integrated treatment for opiate dependence. *Journal of Substance Abuse Treatment*, **23,** 351–360.
58. San, L, Pomarol, G, Peri, JM, Olle, JM et al. 1991. Follow-up after a six-month maintenance period on naltrexone versus placebo in heroin addicts. *British Journal of Addiction*, **86,** 983–990.
59. Schwope, AD, Wise, DL & Howes, JF 1975. Lactic/glycolic acid polymers as narcotic antagonist delivery systems. *Life Sciences*, **17,** 1877–1886.
60. Seaman, SR, Brettle, RP & Gore, SM 1998. Mortality from overdose among injecting drug users recently released from prison: database linkage study. *British Medical Journal*, **316,** 426–428.
61. Sharon, AC & Wise, DL 1980. Development of drug delivery systems for use in treatment of narcotic addiction. *NIDA Research Monograph*, **28,** 194–213.
62. Sidman, CL, Bercovici, T & Gitler, C 1980. Membrane insertion of lymphocyte surface molecules. *Molecular Immunology*, **17,** 1575–1583.
63. Tennant, FS, Rawson, RA, Cohen, AJ & Mann, A 1984. Clinical experience with naltrexone in suburban opioid addicts. *Journal of Clinical Psychiatry*, **45,** 42–45.
64. Therin, M, Christel, P, Li, SM, Garreau, H & Vert, M 1992. In vivo degradation of massive poly(a-hydroxyacids): validation of in vitro findings. *Biomaterials*, **13,** 594–600.
65. Tucker, TK, Ritter, A, Maher, C & Jackson, H 2004. Natrexone maintenance for heroin dependence: uptake, attrition and retention. *Drug and Alcohol Review*, **23,** 299–300.
66. Vereby, K, Volavka, J, Mule, SJ & Resnick, RB 1976. Naltrexone: disposition, metabolism, and effects after acute and chronic dosing. *Clinical Pharmacology and Therapeutics*, **20,** 315–328.
67. Vert, M, Schwach, G, Engel, R & Coudane, J 1998. Something new in the field of PLA/GA bioresorbable polymers? *Journal of Controlled Release*, **53,** 85–92.
68. Walsh, SL, Preston, KL, Stitzer, ML et al. 1994. Clinical pharmacology of buprenorphine: ceiling effects at high doses. *Clinical Pharmacology and Therapeutics*, **55,** 569–580.
69. Washton, AM, Pottash, AC & Gold, MS 1984. Naltrexone in addicted business executives and physicians. *Journal of Clinical Psychiatry*, **45,** 39–41.
70. White, JM & Irvine, RJ 1999. Mechanisms of fatal opioid overdose. *Addiction*, **94,** 961–972.
71. Willette, RE 1982. Narcotic antagonists. An alternative for treating opioid dependence. *American Pharmacy*, **NS22,** 44–46.
72. Yamaguchi, K & Anderson, JM 1993. In vivo biocompatibility studies of medisorb 65/35 D,L-lactide/glycolide copolymer microspheres. *Journal of Controlled Release*, **24,** 81–93.
73. Yolles, S, Leafe, TD, Woodland, JHR & Meyer, FJ 1975. Long acting delivery systems for narcotic antagonists II: release rates of naltrexone from poly(lactic acid) composites. *Journal of Pharmacological Science*, **64,** 348–349.
74. Zacny, JP, Bigelow, GE, Compton, P, Foley, K, Iguchi, M & Sannerud, C 2003. College on Problems of Drug Dependence taskforce on prescription opioid non-medical use and abuse: position statement. *Drug and Alcohol Dependence*, **69,** 215–232.

Chapter 37
The Development of ProNeura Technology for the Treatment of Addictions

Lauren C. Costantini

Abstract The growing problem of addiction across the United States and globally, in particular to pain analgesics, has reached a level never seen before in history. Although treatments for addiction have advanced greatly in recent years, current pharmacotherapies are limited by patient compliance, medication blood levels, abuse and diversion, and adverse effects that limit clinical and patient acceptance. Even with treatment, chronic relapse is more common than abstinence. The ProNeura long-term delivery system discussed in this chapter has the potential to eliminate these limitations and improve existing pharmacotherapies. The ProNeura match-stick-sized implants are inserted subcutaneously, and maintain stable concentrations of medication for 6 months or longer. The system allows individually-tailored doses, and shows few adverse effects. The possibility of diversion and abuse is significantly reduced due to the physician-directed administration of the implants, and the difficulties involved in extracting the medication from the implants. By eliminating the need for frequent dosing, compliance to pharmacotherapy treatment is greatly improved. Patients will gain independence from frequent visits for medication, presenting an ideal opportunity to overcome the challenges associated with pharmacological treatment for addictions.

Keywords: Buprenorphine; Nalmefene; Opioid; Alcohol; Dependence; Alcoholism; Addiction; Long-term delivery; Sustained release; Ethylene vinyl acetate

37.1 Introduction

Addiction treatment research has advanced greatly in recent years, and the development of evidence-based guidelines for addiction treatment has been utilized with some success. While treatment methods are still closely tied to the craft

L.C. Costantini
Accera, Inc., Clinical Development, 380 Interlocken Crescent,
Suite 780, Broomfield, CO 80021
e-mail: lcostantini@accerapharma.com

of psychotherapy, dissemination of research findings regarding neurobiological mechanisms of addiction and the developments of pharmacotherapies to treat these addictions continues to add to the quality of care of patients. However, success with current pharmacotherapies for treatment of addictions is limited by a variety of factors, including poor patient compliance, fluctuations in drug blood levels, abuse and diversion of various formulations, and adverse effects at the doses required for clinical efficacy. These limitations often lead to a return to drug use and addictive behaviors within a short period of time, with chronic relapse more common than abstinence. A long-term delivery system could reduce these limitations and improve upon existing pharmacotherapies. The ProNeura long-term delivery system discussed in this chapter can be utilized for a variety of addiction disorders where compliance is problematic and where sustained blood levels of medication would provide more consistent exposure to medication and potentially improve outcome. These matchstick-sized implants are inserted subcutaneously (SC), and can maintain stable concentrations of medication for 6 months or longer. Individually-tailored doses can be achieved by implanting more than one ProNeura implant. These and other attributes of the ProNeura system present an ideal strategy to overcome the challenges associated with pharmacological treatment for addictions. The medications initially chosen for development include buprenorphine for treatment of opioid dependence and nalmefene for treatment of alcoholism.

37.2 Opioid Dependence

37.2.1 Overview of Opioid Dependence and Treatments

Opioid dependence is characterized by persistent drug use in spite of negative health, legal, social, and personal ramifications. Annual updates consistently report substantial levels of illicit drug use. Global estimates show 15.9 million people use opiates, of which 10.6 million are using heroin (1). Approximately 1.2 million heroin abusers were estimated in North America between 2002 and 2004 (1), and 4.7 million individuals were users of pain relievers for nonmedical purposes (2). In the United States (US) alone, 2.5 million individuals are prescription-opioid abusers, with 1.4 million becoming dependent in 2004 (3). Recent data from the Drug Abuse Warning Network (DAWN) showed that hydrocodone products were involved in 42,491 emergency room (ER) visits in 2004, oxycodone products in 36,559 ER visits, and methadone in 31,874 visits (4). Associated increases in the spread of infectious disease (i.e., HIV, hepatitis B and C) and overdose deaths have also been prevalent.

Addiction treatments that combine pharmacotherapy and behavioral interventions have been shown to significantly reduce drug use. Beyond reducing use, addiction treatments also ameliorate health problems, reduce mortality, improve employment, and reduce criminal involvement of patients (5–6). Unfortunately, only a small portion of addicted individuals who need treatment are receiving it for a variety of reasons, including the stigmatization of addiction patients which filters through society.

In addition, traditional treatments often require a considerable time commitment and impinge upon a patient's ability to work or perform other productive activities during the time that they are in treatment. Many addicted people are unwilling to forgo time now for the improved employment and income opportunities that addiction treatment affords.

Methadone maintenance treatment is one of the most commonly utilized pharmacotherapies for opioid dependence. However, methadone treatment has several characteristics which affect is widespread acceptance and potentially its effectiveness. Methadone is a full opioid agonist at the mu receptor, thus it has been termed "maintenance of dependency" or "opioid replacement" therapy. Detoxification from the medication can be a difficult and painful experience, and patients experience withdrawal if they miss a dose. Because of its full agonist activity, overdose can occur and is potentially fatal due to respiratory depression, and sedation and constipation are common. Daily dosing at federally-regulated methadone clinics is required, which can be inconvenient for the recovering opioid-dependent person, and exposes them to a negative environment on a daily basis. Naltrexone, naloxone, and levo-alpha-acetylmethadol (LAAM) are also utilized for treatment of opioid dependence [though LAAM was removed from the market due to cardiac-related adverse events (AEs)]. Most recently, buprenorphine has been approved in the US for treatment of opioid dependence.

37.2.2 Overview of Buprenorphine and Use in Opioid Dependence

Buprenorphine is a potent partial opioid agonist first approved for the management of pain, and is now widely available for the treatment of opioid dependence. Although buprenorphine has been shown to interact with multiple opioid receptors, its primary activity is partial agonist activity at the mu-opioid receptor and antagonist activity at the kappa receptor (7). As a partial agonist, a ceiling effect is observed whereby high doses of buprenorphine do not cause complications of overdose, and abuse potential is decreased due to the low degree of euphoria obtained with higher doses when compared with pure opioid agonists (8–9). Consequently, this results in a safety profile that is superior to methadone and LAAM, while efficacy of these three treatments is comparable (10).

Numerous outpatient, randomized, and controlled clinical trials have tested the efficacy of buprenorphine for the treatment of opioid dependence, both compared to placebo (11–13) and to methadone (14, 10, 15–22). In general, these studies have shown that buprenorphine can produce outcomes similar to moderate daily doses of methadone (~60 mg/day).

Treatment for opioid dependence made a leap forward when the Food and Drug Administration (FDA) approved buprenorphine and buprenorphine/naloxone as schedule III agents for such treatment in the US in October 2002. The approval and scheduling allowed qualified physicians to prescribe buprenorphine in their routine practice settings, although as of the writing of this chapter, the legislation limits each independent physician to be federally certified and to treat a maximum of 30 patients at any one time. A recent study showed that patients starting buprenorphine treatment were three times more likely to work full time and have fewer years of opioid dependence, suggesting that office-based treatment is associated with new types of patients entering into treatment (23).

Induction onto buprenorphine can occur within 2–7 days of treatment with increasing doses on each day (13, 24, 25). During this induction time, a dose is established for continued ("maintenance") treatment based upon control of withdrawal and cravings, tolerability, and decreases in patient self report of illicit opioid use during this period. Maintenance doses of buprenorphine vary, but generally fall within a range of 12–16 mg/day. Interventions during maintenance can include nonpharmacological interventions (such as counseling and psychotherapy), urine monitoring, and treatment of comorbid conditions.

In addition to the above-mentioned studies which predominantly included heroin-dependent patients, buprenorphine has also shown efficacy in patients addicted to prescription pain relievers, a quickly-growing population of opioid addicts in the US and other countries (3, 26).

37.2.3 Limitations of Current Delivery and the Need for Long-Term Release Formulations

Oral bioavailability of buprenorphine is low (~10%) due to extensive first-pass hepatic metabolism (27). Therefore, commercially available products include sublingual (SL) Subutex®, SL Suboxone® (buprenorphine and naloxone), SL and injectible Temgesic®, injectible Buprenex®, and 3-day transdermal Transtec®. SL buprenorphine is easily administered; however, long-term maintenance treatment via this route is problematic for various reasons. First, this route requires strict patient dosing compliance; one missed dose may allow cravings to increase to the point at which the patient seeks illicit drugs. Second, SL buprenorphine can be diverted for illicit use, or abused via crushing and intravenous injection (though the addition of naloxone in the formulation may reduce this form of abuse and diversion) (28, 29). Indeed, quarterly random surveys of physicians treating patients with buprenorphine in the US since 2003 have shown 15–30% of these physicians reporting knowledge of illegal sales of buprenorphine, and 10% reporting knowledge of prescription shopping (30). Third, plasma concentrations peak quickly and drop steeply with each SL dose, causing AEs at peak levels and withdrawal and craving symptoms at trough levels (31). Finally, SL buprenorphine requires frequent visits to the clinic for prescription refills that include daily supervised dosing in some countries, a factor negatively impacting compliance and overall treatment costs.

A long-term delivery formulation of buprenorphine could improve this treatment by ensuring compliance, reducing the likelihood of buprenorphine abuse and diversion, and maintaining stable plasma levels of medication for a longer duration of treatment time. Indeed, in a recent survey of physicians treating patients with buprenorphine, physicians treating patients for longer periods were more likely to report that the drug is effective, indicating that if one can remain in treatment longer (via utilization of a long-term delivery system), clinical outcome may improve (30).

37.2.4 Probuphine: Continuous, Long-Term Delivery of Buprenorphine

To achieve stable buprenorphine levels that may improve patient outcome, an implantable buprenorphine delivery system is in development and is targeted to provide bioavailable medication for 6 months. Probuphine is being developed for the treatment of opioid-dependent patients after they have completed induction on SL buprenorphine. Such a longer duration form of buprenorphine provides several improved features: compliance with daily or alternate-day administration is no longer needed, sustained and constant blood levels of medication are achieved (decreasing the risk of fluctuating symptoms such as craving or withdrawal that may occur during daily SL administration), lower overall medication levels decrease the likelihood of typical opioid AEs such as constipation and hormonal abnormalities, and the risk of diversion and abuse is significantly reduced since the treating physician directly administers the medication to the patient.

Probuphine is based on the ProNeura delivery system, a nonerodible implant consisting of drug-of-choice blended with ethylene vinyl acetate (EVA, a copolymer approved by the FDA for other applications). Buprenorphine is dry blended with EVA, then extruded to form a fiber 2.4 mm in diameter. The extruded fiber is cut into implants of 26 mm in length, with each Probuphine implant containing ~80 mg of drug (Fig. 37.1a). A scanning electron micrograph (SEM) of an implant in cross-section is shown in Fig. 37.1b, illustrating that EVA and buprenorphine are homogeneously distributed. Implants are then washed to remove surface drug, dried, placed in a foil pouch, and sterilized. Release from the implants is predominantly dependent on surface area, the rate of dissolution, and on passive diffusion through the polymer matrix.

Implants are inserted SC into the inner-upper arm of patients during a 15 minute office-based procedure under local anesthesia utilizing a trocar applicator. Long-term plasma buprenorphine levels can be maintained with one or multiple implants to achieve an individualized dose. Implants are readily removed at the end of treatment period via a similar 15 minute office-based procedure.

When compared with depot formulations of buprenorphine in development, which are irreversible once administered, the action of Probuphine can be rapidly terminated (e.g., in preparation for surgery under general anesthesia) by removal of the implants. Also, due to the solid matrix formulation of Probuphine, there is no possibility of a sudden release of medication or "drug dumping" from the implant as can occur with reservoir-system implants. While there is a risk that a patient may try to remove the implant, removal of buprenorphine from the implants for illicit use is not easily accomplished when compared with patch formulations of opioids and the SL version of buprenorphine.

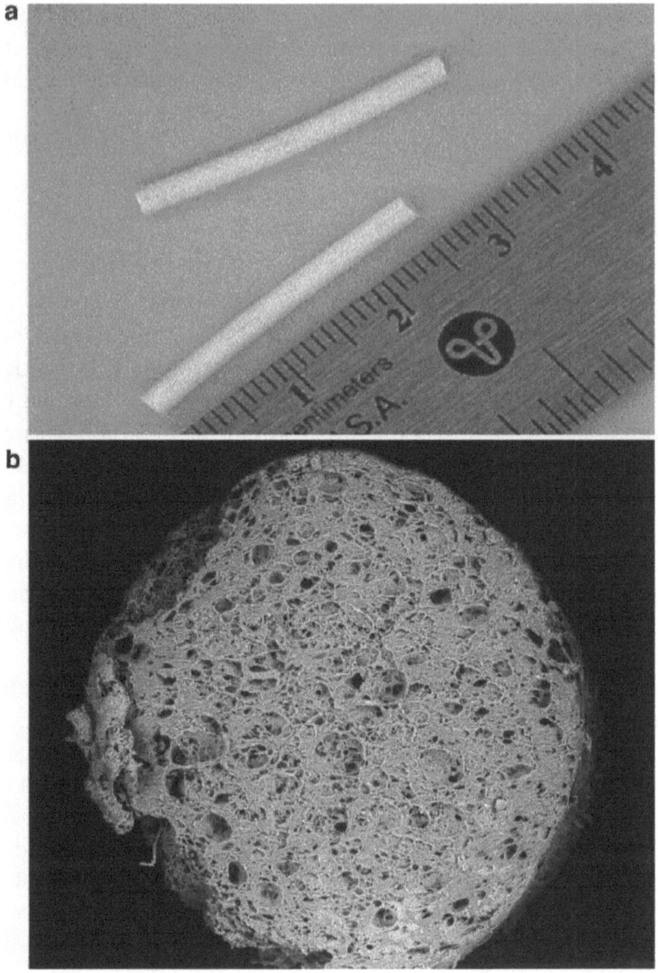

Fig. 37.1 Images of Probuphine implant. (**a**) Scale image, dimensions are 26 mm in length × 2.4-mm diameter ±10%. (**b**) SEM of cross-section of buprenorphine in ethylene vinyl acetate (*EVA*), showing a homogeneous mix of EVA and buprenorphine within the matrix

37.2.5 *Probuphine: Preclinical Studies*

In vitro testing of release from these implants showed steady-state release at ~0.5 mg/implant/day (32). In vivo pharmacokinetics and safety were examined for up to 1 year in beagle dogs receiving 8, 16, or 24 Probuphine or placebo implants. There were no test article-related AEs, and all animals tolerated the implant procedure well. No signs of toxicity or infection at the sites of implantation were observed in any dogs. Implants were easily removed at the end of treatment.

Minor adhesion to implants was observed; however, this was not enough to hinder explantation. No necrosis or visible vascularization was noted in the tissue adjacent to the implants after explantation. Microscopic examination of implant sites showed that tissues were within normal histomorphological limits (32).

Figure 37.2 illustrates plasma buprenorphine levels over time in dogs. Peak plasma levels were achieved within the first week in almost all animals, and then decreased in a nonmonotonic manner to a sustained-release phase at ~6-week post-implantation. Sustained release was maintained through the duration of the study period, and was dose proportional; animals receiving 16 and 24 implants maintained plasma levels 2.7- and 3.5-fold higher, respectively, than those receiving 8 implants. By week 36, plasma buprenorphine levels in the 24-implant animals reached ~80% of sustained release, the predetermined level at which supplemental implants were to be administered. Six additional Probuphine implants were inserted in these animals (as noted on Fig. 37.2 graph). Plasma levels increased within 2 h after implantation, sustained release was attained within 1 week, and was maintained through end of the study period in these animals.

Animals receiving 16 implants had implants removed at week 36 in order to determine off kinetics. Plasma samples showed that concentrations were quantifiable for 12 h after explantation, but dropped to below the limits of quantitation by 24 h. Animals with 8 and 24 implants had the implants removed at 10 or 12 months posttreatment, and a subset of implants was assayed for remaining drug content to

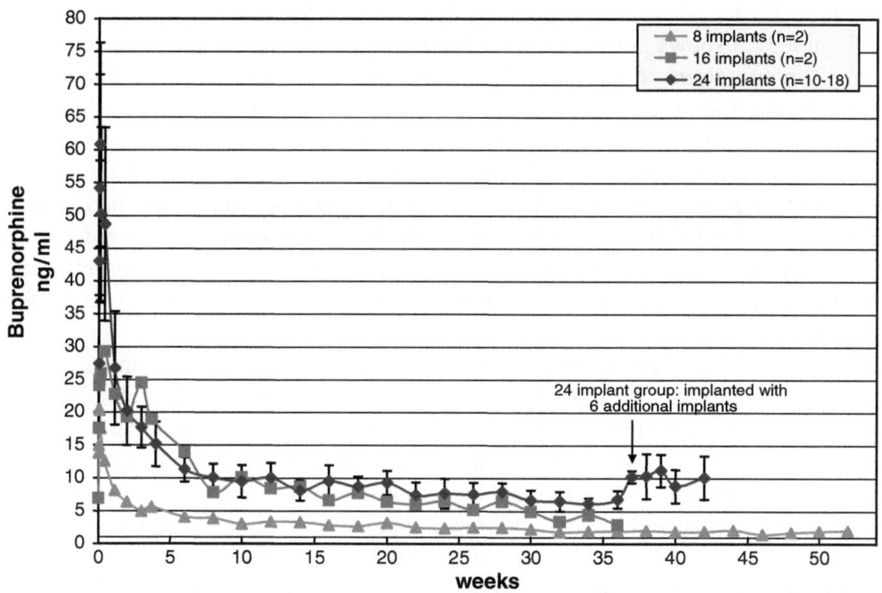

Fig. 37.2 Mean buprenorphine plasma levels in dogs maintained for up to a year with Probuphine. A subgroup of 24-implant animals was implanted with six additional implants at week 36. Animals receiving 16 implants were explanted at week 36 for off-kinetics (see text for details)

estimate the daily release rate per implant. The mean buprenorphine release rate was calculated to be 0.14 ± 0.04 mg/implant/day during the steady-state phase.

37.2.6 Probuphine: Clinical Studies

A phase I/II clinical study of Probuphine evaluated the safety, pharmacokinetics, and efficacy of Probuphine in 12 heroin-dependent volunteers diagnosed with heroin dependence by Diagnostic and Statistical Manual of Mental Disorders (DSM-IV) (33) criteria. Group A consisted of six patients who were maintained on 8 mg SL buprenorphine and were switched to two Probuphine implants. Group B consisted on six patients who were maintained on 16 mg SL buprenorphine and were switched to four Probuphine implants. Prior to SL buprenorphine treatment, the average heroin use was 2.3 times/day.

Safety measures showed Probuphine to be safe and well tolerated with no serious AEs. Minor, transient AEs at the time of insertion and removal were reported in seven patients and included bruising, itchiness, redness, swelling, hematoma, soreness, and pain. All resolved within 2 days and occurred evenly between the two treatment groups. Some AEs common to SL buprenorphine occurred, and no AEs required removal of Probuphine. No respiratory depression was detected by pulse oximetry or respiratory rate, oxygen saturation remained above 90%, and no sedation or behavioral impairments indicative of opioid overdose were observed. There was no evidence of attempted abuse or diversion of Probuphine.

Figure 37.3 shows plasma levels of buprenorphine in all patients after implantation. Buprenorphine levels showed an initially higher release immediately after implantation, followed by a plateau at 21 days and sustained buprenorphine levels lasting for 6 months. Plasma concentrations peaked at ~15–17 h posttreatment, with concentrations averaging ~2.0 ng/ml in the two implant group and ~3.2 ng/ml in the four implant group. The Probuphine peak concentrations were lower than concentrations measured 60 min after SL buprenorphine (~4.1 ng/ml for 8-mg dose, and ~4.6 ng/ml for 16 mg). Mean sustained-release concentration of buprenorphine after implantation was ~0.37 ng/ml for the two implant group and ~0.72 ng/ml for the four implant group.

Preliminary efficacy measures included opioid withdrawal symptoms (assessed by Subjective Opioid Withdrawal Scale, SOWS; Objective Opioid Withdrawal Scale, OOWS) as well as opioid cravings. SOWS scores remained low: on a scale of 0 (no symptoms) to 64 (most severe symptoms), the means during the treatment period for the 2-Probuphine and 4-Probuphine groups were 0.97 and 0.49, respectively. OOWS scores (assessed by study personnel) suggested minimal symptoms of opioid withdrawal: on a scale of 0 (no symptoms) to 13 (positive responses for 13 symptoms), the means during the treatment period for 2-Probuphine and 4-Probuphine groups were 0.49 for both groups. Cravings for opioids (0–100 visual analogue scale, VAS) remained low throughout Probuphine treatment: the mean 6-month scores were 1.77 and 2.25 for two-implant and four-implant groups, respectively.

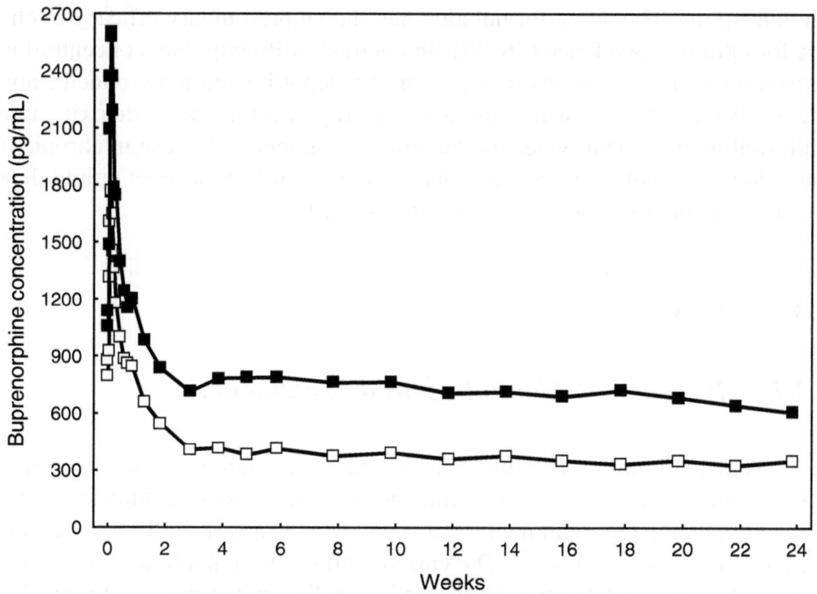

Fig. 37.3 Mean buprenorphine plasma levels after Probuphine insertion in patients with two implants (Group A, *open squares*) and four implants (Group B, *filled squares*)

Urine toxicology (which excluded buprenorphine and its metabolites) and patient self report were used to assess heroin use. Overall, 66% of all self-reports were negative, 28% indicated use of heroin, and 6% used other opioids. Cocaine, amphetamines, and cannabis use was similar between the two dose groups, 38% in the two-implant group and 27% in the four-implant group, and remained constant throughout the study. The overall rate of opioid-negative urines of 56% is within the range of historical published data treated with SL buprenorphine. Throughout Probuphine treatment, study subjects could receive SL buprenorphine at the investigators' discretion in order to help patients overcome temporary cravings or withdrawal symptoms. Out of 12 subjects, 5 were rescued with SL buprenorphine for an average of 4.8 days (out of 167 days of Probuphine treatment).

This study provides preliminary data regarding the safety, pharmacokinetics, and efficacy of Probuphine in the treatment of opioid-dependent patients for 6 months. Patients were safely and successfully transitioned from SL buprenorphine to Probuphine with no detectable increase in opioid effects or withdrawal. Site reactions were minor, resolved rapidly, and caused little discomfort. Buprenorphine plasma concentrations were maintained for 6 months at levels that controlled withdrawal and craving symptoms as well as heroin use with no significant side effects. Additional larger trials are planned to illustrate the clinical utility of these implants.

Additional formulations of buprenorphine under development include intranasal (34), buccal (35), depot (36, 37, 39), and 7-day transdermal (38) in an effort to enhance bioavailability and improve safety and efficacy outcomes in both addiction and pain indications. The depot formulation has shown preliminary efficacy in clinical trials for opioid dependence (36, 37). In contrast to Probuphine, concentrations of buprenorphine in the patients treated with the depot injection are undetectable by 6 weeks. This formulation may be more appropriate for use in detoxification or withdrawal management, whereas Probuphine is intended for use in chronic treatment. Biodegradeable naltrexone implants are also utilized to treat opioid dependence, and will be discussed in another chapter (40).

37.3 Alcoholism

37.3.1 Overview of Alcoholism and Treatments

The process of defining alcoholism is constantly changing, with socioeconomic forces yielding one or another predominant view. The dominant thinking about the cause will call for one treatment or another, which in turn will influence policy, programs, and professions (41). The current definition of alcoholism as defined by American Society of Addiction Medicine is as follows: "a primary, chronic disease with genetic, psychosocial, and environmental factors influencing its development and manifestations. The disease is often progressive and fatal. It is characterized by continuous or periodic impaired control over drinking, preoccupation with the drug alcohol, use of alcohol despite adverse consequences, and distortions in thinking, most notable denial."

In the US, 19 million people require treatment for an alcohol problem, and 16 million drink heavily (3). However, only 2.5 million have been diagnosed with the disease, and only 139,000 receive treatment. Chronic heavy drinking is the leading cause of cardiovascular illnesses and is the leading cause of illness and death from liver disease in the US (42). Many alcoholics initially achieve a period of sobriety with or without formal treatment. However, many return to drinking within a short period of time (43), with ~50% of treated patients relapse back to drinking within the first few months of treatment (44) and 75% relapse within the first year (45), illustrating the chronic and relapsing characteristics of this disorder.

Treatment for alcoholism has been significantly complicated by the multiple actions of ethanol at the neurotransmitter level, heterogeneity among patients, and the complexity of defining and measuring the phenomenon of craving (46). Alcohol is a central nervous system (CNS) depressant that acts on at least six different neurotransmitter systems. Acute intake leads to increased levels of dopamine, serotonin, and norepinephrine, and increased inhibitory systems such as gamma-aminobutyric acid (GABA) and *N*-methyl D-aspartate (NMDA) receptors. Chronic use leads to depletion of these systems and downregulation of GABA and NMDA receptors (46, 47).

Treatments for alcohol dependence include brief intervention, behavioral, and cognitive-behavioral approaches, psychosocial and motivation-enhancement treatments, and pharmacotherapies. Complete abstinence is the goal of treatment in some organizations; however, other organizations define treatment goals as relapse prevention once drinking has stopped. Scientific discoveries involving the imbalances of the CNS with alcohol use have given way to new pharmacotherapies. However, the various pharmacological treatments for alcoholism have shown modest effects.

Aversive therapy with disulfiram (Antabuse), developed over 55 years ago as an inhibitor of alcohol dehydrogenase, was the only pharmacological treatment for alcohol dependence available in the US for many years, despite high rates of severe adverse drug reactions, high rates of drinking relapse, medication noncompliance, and physicians reluctance to prescribe it due to the dangerous reactions (48). Its use is still quite limited as new pharmacotherapies began to move into the market.

Naltrexone (ReVia) is an opioid receptor antagonist, approved in 1994 as an oral nonaversive prescription drug for alcohol dependence on the basis of three trials (49–51), though benefits of oral naltrexone in recent studies are modest (52).

Interest in opioid antagonists for the treatment of alcoholism stem from studies in animal models showing: alkaloid compounds similar to morphine are formed when alcohol is metabolized (53); alcohol intake is increased in rats following treatment with low-dose morphine (54) but decreased when treated with moderate-to-high doses (55); opiate-receptor activity is increased in vitro in mouse cell membranes exposed to physiologic concentrations of ethanol (56). By blocking the mu-opioid receptors, naltrexone diminishes craving for alcohol and leads to a greater ability to resist urges to drink excessively. Reduced craving and risk of relapse to heavy drinking is observed among those who are highly compliant with naltrexone treatment (57–59). However, in addition to noncompliance, use of naltrexone has limitations including intolerable nausea (49) and dose-dependent hepatotoxic side effects [naltrexone is contraindicated in alcoholic patients with liver disease (60)]. Unfortunately, naltrexone is only prescribed for less than 13% of patients who are undergoing treatment for alcohol dependence and abuse (61). A 1-month depot formulation of naltrexone has been recently approved in the US, and will be described below.

Acamprosate (Campral®), available in 24 countries and recently approved in the US, is used in combination with psychosocial support for the maintenance of alcohol abstinence in patients who are abstinent at treatment initiation. Three positive trials showed significantly higher continuous abstinence when compared with placebo (62–64). One trial evaluated patients who were not required to be abstinent at baseline, and failed to demonstrate superiority over placebo (65). Common side effects include diarrhea, nausea, vomiting, and abdominal pain. Its mechanism of action is not understood; however, recent evidence suggests that acamprosate interacts with the glutamate system and modulates the excitatory system via NMDA receptors (66).

Combination studies of pharmacological and behavioral therapies show potentially synergistic effects (67). However, recent results from the Combined Pharmacotherapies and Behavioral Interventions (COMBINE) study did not show this synergism. COMBINE showed that patients receiving medical management with naltrexone, combined behavioral intervention (CBI), or both showed more improved drinking outcomes, whereas acamprosate showed no evidence of efficacy (with or without CBI). Naltrexone or CBI alone in the presence of medical management were equally effective (68).

A variety of other product candidates or already-approved drugs are being explored in clinical studies for the treatment of alcoholism, including but not limited to rimonabant, ondansetron, aripiprazole, baclofen, kudzu, sertraline, and topiramate.

37.3.2 Overview of Nalmefene and Use in Alcoholism

Nalmefene is a pure opioid antagonist structurally similar to naltrexone, and is approved in the US for reversal of effects of opioids and the management of opioid overdose (nalmefene hydrochloride injection; Revex®). Nalmefene has no agonist activity and thus no abuse potential (69), a long half-life (70), and no serious AEs such as respiratory depression or hepatotoxicity. Nalmefene acts on mu, lambda, and kappa receptors, providing more effective control of the non-mu receptor reinforcing effects of drinking when compared with naltrexone which blocks primarily mu receptors (56, 71). In addition, recent evidence suggests that nalmefene has partial agonist properties at kappa-opioid receptors, which theoretically would lower dopamine in brain regions important to the persistence of alcohol dependence, enhancing its therapeutic efficacy in addictive diseases (72).

Nalmefene is effective in animal models of alcoholism (73–75), and has progressed to clinical studies. Oral nalmefene has shown efficacy in several US studies for the treatment of alcohol dependence (76–78). In a US double blind, placebo-controlled study, alcoholic patients who had been abstinent for 2 weeks received 20 or 80 mg/day oral nalmefene along with weekly cognitive behavioral therapy. Fewer patients receiving nalmefene relapsed to heavy drinking over the 12-week study period versus placebo. One third of nalmefene patients did relapse, though they had significantly fewer heavy drinking episodes than relapsing patients receiving placebo. The number of abstinent days and self-reported craving was the same in treated and control groups. Transient nausea was observed in the nalmefene-treated patients, though no serious AEs occurred (77). An earlier pilot study also reported significantly lower rates of relapse, as well as a greater increase in the number of abstinent days per week, with 40 mg oral nalmefene when compared with placebo or 10 mg nalmefene in alcohol-dependent patients. Both 40 and 10 mg doses significantly decreased the number of drinks per drinking day (76).

A third study evaluated three doses of nalmefene (5, 20, or 40 mg) versus placebo in recently-abstinent outpatient alcohol-dependent patients. Four sessions of motivational enhancement therapy were administered throughout the 12 week study. AEs were mild albeit higher (though not statistically) in nalmefene-treated patients versus placebo and included insomnia, dizziness, and confusion and nausea. However, efficacy measures were also not statistically different between nalmefene and placebo (reduction in heavy drinking days, cravings, gamma glutamyl transferase, time to first heavy drinking) (78). Failure of this trial to show significant efficacy was attributed to type 2 error based on sample size considerations (the study was powered based on single-site studies, and did not take into account the variability observed in multisite studies). In addition, previous positive nalmefene studies utilized weekly behavioral therapy, whereas this trial provided less-frequent behavioral therapy. And finally, patients taking psychotropic medications were excluded from previous positive nalmefene studies but were included in this study.

Clinical laboratory paradigms have also shown effects of nalmefene in nontreatment-seeking alcoholics and social drinkers. One study showed reduced alcohol-induced cravings and stimulation with nalmefene among alcoholics, but less reductions in social drinkers (79).

A recent 16-week randomized, placebo-controlled study of nalmefene for the treatment of DSM-IV-diagnosed pathological gambling showed statistically significant reductions in severity of gambling (80), indicating its potential use for a variety of impulse-control disorders.

37.3.3 Limitations of Current Delivery and the Need for Long-Term Release Formulation

The first months following cessation of drinking show the highest risk for relapse and offer the greatest opportunity for pharmacological intervention. However, as discussed above, oral pharmacotherapies are limited by poor patient compliance (Campral must be dosed three times per day), variability in blood levels of the drug, and AEs at the doses required for clinical efficacy. A long-term delivery system would be an ideal formulation for these medications as it would improve compliance among patients, avoid first pass effects seen with oral formulations, increase duration of action, reduce the nausea associated with peak/trough blood levels, and increase total bioavailability.

The clinical benefits of a long-term delivery system for treatment of alcoholism are illustrated in the various developmental programs with implants and depots. Although SC implants of disulfiram appeared to be an attractive method to ensure compliance, the bioavailability of disulfiram was not demonstrated in therapeutic trials (81–85). Naltrexone implants have been utilized for analgesia and opioid detoxification (86–88), with excellent efficacy in patients; however, complications including pulmonary edema, prolonged withdrawal, drug toxicity, and the lack of formal regulatory approval for these implants limit their widespread utility (89).

A once-monthly injectible depot of naltrexone has been approved in the US. Vivitrol™ is used in combination with support from counseling or group therapy, and is indicated for alcohol-dependent patients who are able to abstain from drinking in an outpatient setting and who are not actively drinking when beginning the therapy (90). In studies utilizing a different naltrexone depot, active depot patients showed a significant advantage in time to first drinking day versus placebo depot when combined with motivational enhancement therapy (91). The black box warning to caution against liver toxicity associated with naltrexone itself is also applied to depots.

37.3.4 *ProNeura Nalmefene Implants: Continuous, Long-Term Delivery of Nalmefene*

A long-term delivery system would be an ideal formulation for nalmefene as it would improve compliance among patients, avoid first pass effects seen with oral formulations, increase duration of action, reduce the nausea associated with peak/trough blood levels, increase total bioavailability of nalmefene [40–50% bioavailable by oral administration (92)], and avoid the naltrexone black-box warning. The ProNeura-based nalmefene implants are also matchstick-sized implants for SC insertion, however, unlike Probuphine implants, the nalmefene implants are coated with a thin layer of EVA on the outside of the implant. The initial, uncoated in vitro release rate from nalmefene implants was approximately ten times that of the release rate from Probuphine implants, which was likely due to the high solubility of nalmefene (130 mg/ml vs buprenorphine 17 mg/ml, in water). Almost 100% of nalmefene was released in vitro within 21 days from uncoated implants. A variety of percentages of EVA coating were tested. A 25%-coated implant showed a steady release from approximately day 7 to day 56 of 0.36 mg/day (±0.05), a release rate that would allow long-term delivery in vivo. Therefore, implants with 25% coating were selected for further development (Fig. 37.4). The total percent of nalmefene released from these implants over 56 days was 30.4% (93).

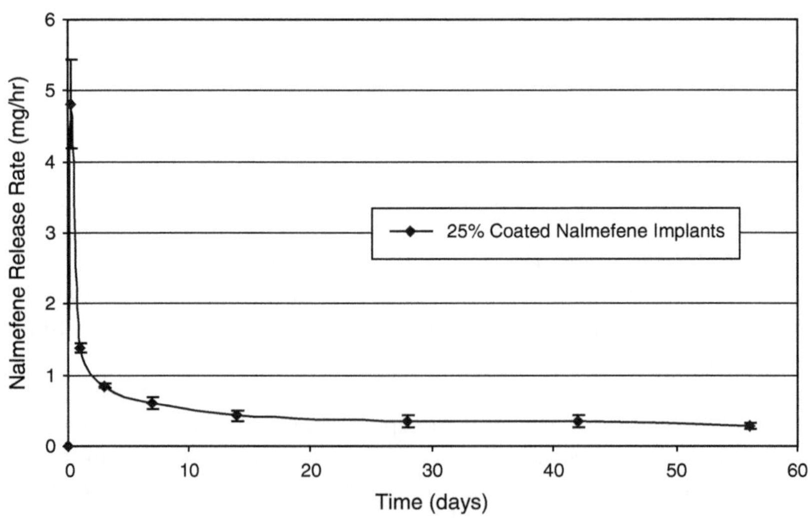

Fig. 37.4 In vitro release of nalmefene from ProNeura implants over time

To determine in vivo release from nalmefene implants, Wistar-derived rats were surgically implanted with either one or three implants containing 73 mg of nalmefene per implant. Implants were placed SC on the back of the animal parallel to the spine. Plasma samples were taken from the tail vein before implant, and at various times postimplant and postexplant. All animals tolerated the implant procedure well. Figure 37.5 shows the mean nalmefene plasma levels of each group. Plasma levels showed two phases, similar to the Probuphine implants: a phase of higher levels of drug that decreased by 3 weeks postimplant, followed by a sustained release phase from 3 weeks to 24 weeks. Plasma concentrations reached peak levels of 33 ng/ml for the one-implant group and 90 ng/ml for the three-implant group. Levels during the sustained-release period from 3 weeks to 24 weeks were ~3.2 ng/ml and 8.8 ng/ml for the one- and three-implant groups, respectively. Plasma nalmefene levels from the three-implant animals were ~three times higher than those of the one-implant animals at all time points. The elimination phase, monitored in four animals (two per group) postexplant, showed plasma nalmefene below quantifiable limits (0.05 ng/ml) by 6 h postexplant. Gross examination of implant sites revealed no vascularization or irritation at any time during study. Upon explantation, minimal fibrosis was encountered. Histological examination of tissues revealed no tissue responses, bacterial contamination, or other inflammatory processes (93).

Results from this study indicate that nalmefene implants can provide sustained release of drug for 6 months. The dose of nalmefene delivered from the current implants is slightly lower than required for clinical efficacy in humans. Previous clinical studies utilizing nalmefene for alcoholism have shown efficacy with oral doses of 20 mg. Studies are ongoing to increase the dimensions and drug loading of these implants to achieve a daily dose of 8 mg. In order to reduce the AEs associated with

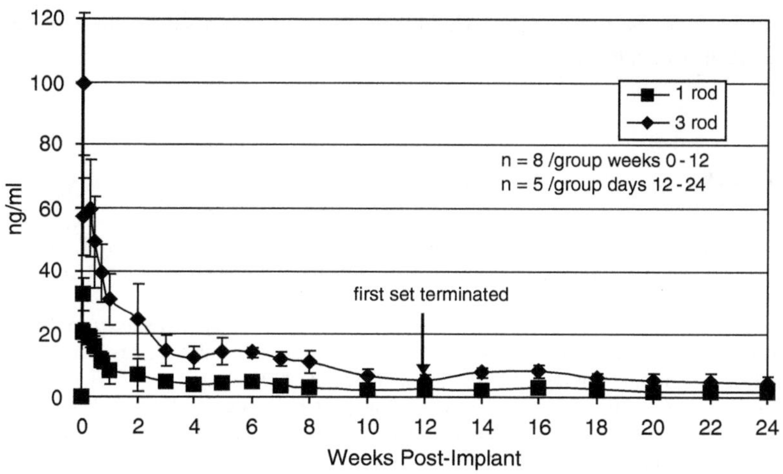

Fig. 37.5 Mean nalmefene plasma levels from animals implanted with one implant (*squares*), or three implants (*diamonds*)

peak levels of nalmefene, extrapolation of the peak levels from these animal studies to human levels (based on clearance and release rate) shows that peak levels would still be well within the safety range (92). In addition, as shown with the Probuphine implants and other ProNeura implants in development, washing implants prior to sterilization has been shown to eliminate this initially high release (94). The duration of treatment that these implants allow is seen by some physicians as advantageous for patients as they will not have to debate daily whether to take the drug as part of their treatment for a disease that impairs decision making.

37.4 Conclusions

Addictive disorders are common in the US and globally, and are associated with significant morbidity and mortality. Buprenorphine and nalmefene are opioid products shown to be effective for treatment of opioid dependence and alcoholism. However, adherence to daily oral pharmacotherapy can be problematic, and clinical acceptance and utility of these medications as well as alternate pharmacotherapies for these indications have been limited. The ProNeura delivery system produces sustained blood levels of these medications over 6 months of treatment with few AEs. By eliminating the need for frequent dosing, compliance to pharmacotherapy treatment is greatly improved, and patients will gain independence from frequent clinic visits for medication. Demands on staff time could also be reduced. ProNeura implants may reduce the potential risk of diversion and abuse due to the physician-directed administration of the medication and the difficulties involved in removing medication from the implants. In addition, the matrix design of ProNeura implants (rather than a reservoir design) eliminates the risk of drug dumping and decreases the likelihood of illicit abuse of medication. Overall, the sustained delivery of buprenorphine or nalmefene provided by ProNeura implants may allow advantages to other routes of administration.

References

1. World Drug Report 2005. Chawla S, Korenblik A, Kunnen S, Le Pichon T, Nathwana A, Pietschmann T et al. Volume 1: Analysis, pp. 1–82. 2005. Vienna International Centre, Vienna, Austria, United Nations Publication.
2. Office of Applied Studies. Overview of Findings from the 2003 National Survey on Drug Use and Health. 2004. Rockville, MD, Substance Abuse and Mental Health Services Administration.
3. SAHMSA. National Survey on Drug Use and Health. 2004.
4. DAWN - Drug Abuse Warning Network. National Estimates of Drug-Related Emergency Department Visits. 2004. Substance Abuse and Mental Health Services Administration, U.S. Department of Health and Human Services.
5. Fugelstad A, Agren G, Romelsjo A. Changes in mortality, arrests, and hospitalizations in non-voluntarily treated heroin addicts in relation to methadone treatment. Subst Use Misuse 1998; 33(14):2803–2817.

6. Hubbard RL, Craddock SG, Anderson J. Overview of 5-year followup outcomes in the drug abuse treatment outcome studies (DATOS). J Subst Abuse Treat 2003; 25(3):125–134.
7. Reisine T, Bell GI. Molecular biology of opioid receptors. Trends Neurosci 1993; 16(12): 506–510.
8. Lewis JW. Buprenorphine. Drug Alcohol Depend 1985; 14(3–4):363–372.
9. Walsh SL, Preston KL, Stitzer ML, Cone EJ, Bigelow GE. Clinical pharmacology of buprenorphine: ceiling effects at high doses. Clin Pharmacol Ther 1994; 55(5):569–580.
10. Johnson RE, Chutuape MA, Strain EC, Walsh SL, Stitzer ML, Bigelow GE. A comparison of levomethadyl acetate, buprenorphine, and methadone for opioid dependence. N Engl J Med 2000; 343(18):1290–1297.
11. Fudala PJ, Bridge TP, Chiang CN, Leiderman DB. A multi-site efficacy evaluation of a buprenorphine/naloxone product for opiate dependence treatment. NIDA Res Monogr 1998; 179(105).
12. Johnson RE, Eissenberg T, Stitzer ML, Strain EC, Liebson IA, Bigelow GE. A placebo controlled clinical trial of buprenorphine as a treatment for opioid dependence. Drug Alcohol Depend 1995; 40(1):17–25.
13. Ling W, Charuvastra C, Collins JF, Batki S, Brown LS, Jr., Kintaudi P et al. Buprenorphine maintenance treatment of opiate dependence: a multicenter, randomized clinical trial. Addiction 1998; 93(4):475–486.
14. Ahmadi J. Methadone versus buprenorphine maintenance for the treatment of heroin-dependent outpatients. J Subst Abuse Treat 2003; 24(3):217–220.
15. Johnson RE, Jaffe JH, Fudala PJ. A controlled trial of buprenorphine treatment for opioid dependence. JAMA 1992; 267(20):2750–2755.
16. Kosten TR, Schottenfeld R, Ziedonis D, Falcioni J. Buprenorphine versus methadone maintenance for opioid dependence. J Nerv Ment Dis 1993; 181(6):358–364.
17. Ling W, Wesson DR, Charuvastra C, Klett CJ. A controlled trial comparing buprenorphine and methadone maintenance in opioid dependence. Arch Gen Psychiatry 1996; 53(5):401–407.
18. Mattick RP, Ali R, White JM, O'Brien S, Wolk S, Danz C. Buprenorphine versus methadone maintenance therapy: a randomized double-blind trial with 405 opioid-dependent patients. Addiction 2003; 98(4):441–452.
19. Pani PP, Maremmani I, Pirastu R, Tagliamonte A, Gessa GL. Buprenorphine: a controlled clinical trial in the treatment of opioid dependence. Drug Alcohol Depend 2000; 60(1):39–50.
20. Petitjean S, Stohler R, Deglon JJ, Livoti S, Waldvogel D, Uehlinger C et al. Double-blind randomized trial of buprenorphine and methadone in opiate dependence. Drug Alcohol Depend 2001; 62(1):97–104.
21. Schottenfeld RS, Pakes JR, Oliveto A, Ziedonis D, Kosten TR. Buprenorphine vs methadone maintenance treatment for concurrent opioid dependence and cocaine abuse. Arch Gen Psychiatry 1997; 54(8):713–720.
22. Strain EC, Stitzer ML, Liebson IA, Bigelow GE. Comparison of buprenorphine and methadone in the treatment of opioid dependence. Am J Psychiatry 1994; 151(7):1025–1030.
23. Sullivan M, Ferrell B. Ethical challenges in the management of chronic nonmalignant pain: negotiating through the cloud of doubt. J Pain 2005; 6(1):2–9.
24. Johnson RE, Strain EC, Amass L. Buprenorphine: how to use it right. Drug Alcohol Depend 2003; 70(Suppl. 2):S59–S77.
25. McNicholas L. Clinical Guidelines for the Use of Buprenorphine in the Treatment of Opioid Addiction. A Treatment Improvement Protocol (TIP 40). 2004.
26. Chavez R, Amass L, Kamien JB, Prucha L. UCLA School of Medicine LAC, The Pain Institute at Little Company of Mary RBC, Friends Research Institute ILAC, editors. Buprenorphine Tablet Treatment for Opioid Dependence in Patients with Comorbid Chronic Severe Pain. 2004, June 14; CPDD 66th Annual Meeting, San Juan, PR.
27. Harris DS, Jones RT, Welm S, Upton RA, Lin E, Mendelson J. Buprenorphine and naloxone co-administration in opiate-dependent patients stabilized on sublingual buprenorphine. Drug Alcohol Depend 2000; 61(1):85–94.
28. Jenkinson RA, Clark NC, Fry CL, Dobbin M. Buprenorphine diversion and injection in Melbourne, Australia: an emerging issue? Addiction 2005; 100(2):197–205.

29. Auriacombe M, Fatseas M, Dubernet J, Daulouede JP, Tignol J. French field experience with buprenorphine. Am J Addict 2004; 13 Suppl. 1:S17–S28.
30. SAMHSA/CSAT's Evaluation of the Buprenorphine Waiver Program. In: Stanton A, McLeod C, Kissin WB, Sonnefeld J, Luckey JW, editors. Evaluation of the Buprenorphine Waiver Program: Results from SAMHSA/CSAT's Evaluation of the Buprenorphine Waiver Program. 2005. College on Problems of Drug Dependence.
31. Lopatko OV, White JM, Huber A, Ling W. Opioid effects and opioid withdrawal during a 24 h dosing interval in patients maintained on buprenorphine. Drug Alcohol Depend 2003; 69(3):317–322.
32. Kleppner SR, Patel R, McDonough J, Costantini LC. In-vitro and in-vivo characterization of a buprenorphine delivery system. J Pharm Pharmacol 2006; 58(3):295–302.
33. DSM-IV. American Psychiatric Association. Diagnostic and Statistical Manual of Mental Disorders. Fourth edn. Arlington, VA: American Psychiatric Association, 2005.
34. Eriksen J, Jensen NH, Kamp-Jensen M, Bjarno H, Friis P, Brewster D. The systemic availability of buprenorphine administered by nasal spray. J Pharm Pharmacol 1989; 41(11):803–805.
35. Kuhlman JJ, Jr., Lalani S, Magluilo J, Jr., Levine B, Darwin WD. Human pharmacokinetics of intravenous, sublingual, and buccal buprenorphine. J Anal Toxicol 1996; 20(6): 369–378.
36. Sigmon SC, Moody DE, Nuwayser ES, Bigelow GE. An injection depot formulation of buprenorphine: extended bio-delivery and effects. Addiction 2006; 101(3):420–432.
37. Sigmon SC, Wong CJ, Chausmer AL, Liebson IA, Bigelow GE. Evaluation of an injection depot formulation of buprenorphine: placebo comparison. Addiction 2004; 99(11):1439–1449.
38. Reidenberg B, Kennish L. A review of the effect of occlusive dressings on lamellar bodies in the stratum corneum and relevance to transdermal absorption. Dermatology Online Journal 11(3), 7. 2001.
39. Sobel BF, Sigmon SC, Walsh SL, Johnson RE, Liebson IA, Nuwayser ES et al. Open-label trial of an injection depot formulation of buprenorphine in opioid detoxification. Drug Alcohol Depend 2004; 73(1):11–22.
40. Hulse GK, Arnold-Reed DE, O'Neil G, Chan CT, Hansson R, O'Neil P. Blood naltrexone and 6-beta-naltrexol levels following naltrexone implant: comparing two naltrexone implants. Addict Biol 2004; 9(1):59–65.
41. Bierer MF. Alcoholism in America: From Reconstruction to Prohibition. In: Tracy SW, editor. N Engl J Med 354(4), pp. 426–427. 2006. Johns Hopkins University Press.
42. NIAAA. National Institute on Alcohol Abuse and Alcoholism. Tenth Special Report to the U.S. Congress on Alcohol and Health. 2000. NIH Publication No. 00-1583, Bethesda, MD.
43. Corrao G, Bagnardi V, Zambon A, Arico S, Dall'Aglio C, Addolorato G et al. Outcome variables in the evaluation of alcoholics' treatment: lessons from the Italian Assessment of Alcoholism Treatment (ASSALT) Project. Alcohol Alcohol 1999; 34(6):873–881.
44. Grant BF, Dawson DA, Stinson FS, Chou SP, Dufour MC, Pickering RP. The 12-month prevalence and trends in DSM-IV alcohol abuse and dependence: United States, 1991–1992 and 2001–2002. Drug Alcohol Depend 2004; 74(3):223–234.
45. Daley DC, Marlatt GA. Relapse prevention. In: Lowinson JH, Ruiz P, Millman RB, Langrod JG, editors. Substance Abuse: A Comprehensive Textbook. Philadelphia, PA: Wippincott Williams & Wilkins, 2005: 772–785.
46. Johnson BA, Ait-Daoud N, Aubin HJ, Van Den BW, Guzzetta R, Loewy J et al. A pilot evaluation of the safety and tolerability of repeat dose administration of long-acting injectable naltrexone [Vivitrex(R)] in patients with alcohol dependence. Alcohol Clin Exp Res 2004; 28(9):1356–1361.
47. Addolorato G, Leggio L, Abenavoli L, Gasbarrini G. Neurobiochemical and clinical aspects of craving in alcohol addiction: a review. Addict Behav 2005; 30(6):1209–1224.
48. Fuller RK, Branchey L, Brightwell DR, Derman RM, Emrick CD, Iber FL et al. Disulfiram treatment of alcoholism. A Veterans Administration cooperative study. JAMA 1986; 256(11):1449–1455.
49. Croop RS, Faulkner EB, Labriola DF. The safety profile of naltrexone in the treatment of alcoholism. Results from a multicenter usage study. The Naltrexone Usage Study Group. Arch Gen Psychiatry 1997; 54(12):1130–1135.

50. O'Malley SS, Jaffe AJ, Chang G, Schottenfeld RS, Meyer RE, Rounsaville B. Naltrexone and coping skills therapy for alcohol dependence. A controlled study. Arch Gen Psychiatry 1992; 49(11):881–887.
51. Volpicelli JR, Alterman AI, Hayashida M, O'Brien CP. Naltrexone in the treatment of alcohol dependence. Arch Gen Psychiatry 1992; 49(11):876–880.
52. Krystal JH, Cramer JA, Krol WF, Kirk GF, Rosenheck RA. Naltrexone in the treatment of alcohol dependence. N Engl J Med 2001; 345(24):1734–1739.
53. Davis VE, Walsh MJ. Alcohol, amines, and alkaloids: a possible biochemical basis for alcohol addiction. Science 1970; 167(920):1005–1007.
54. Reid LD, Delconte JD, Nichols ML, Bilsky EJ, Hubbell CL. Tests of opioid deficiency hypotheses of alcoholism. Alcohol 1991; 8(4):247–257.
55. Sinclair JD, Adkins J, Walker S. Morphine-induced suppression of voluntary alcohol drinking in rats. Nature 1973; 246(5,433):425–427.
56. Tabakoff B, Hoffman PL. Alcohol interactions with brain opiate receptors. Life Sci 1983; 32(3):197–204.
57. O'Malley SS, Jaffe AJ, Chang G, Rode S, Schottenfeld R, Meyer RE et al. Six-month follow-up of naltrexone and psychotherapy for alcohol dependence. Arch Gen Psychiatry 1996; 53(3):217–224.
58. Oslin D, Liberto JG, O'Brien J, Krois S, Norbeck J. Naltrexone as an adjunctive treatment for older patients with alcohol dependence. Am J Geriatr Psychiatry 1997; 5(4):324–332.
59. Volpicelli JR, Rhines KC, Rhines JS, Volpicelli LA, Alterman AI, O'Brien CP. Naltrexone and alcohol dependence. Role of subject compliance. Arch Gen Psychiatry 1997; 54(8):737–742.
60. Physicians' Desk Reference. PDR Staff. 51st edn. 1997; 957–959.
61. Mark TL, Kranzler HR, Poole VH, Hagen CA, McLeod C, Crosse S. Barriers to the use of medications to treat alcoholism. Am J Addict 2003; 12(4):281–294.
62. Pelc I, Verbanck P, Le Bon O, Gavrilovic M, Lion K, Lehert P. Efficacy and safety of acamprosate in the treatment of detoxified alcohol-dependent patients. A 90-day placebo-controlled dose-finding study. Br J Psychiatry 1997; 171:73–77.
63. Sass H, Soyka M, Mann K, Zieglgansberger W. Relapse prevention by acamprosate. Results from a placebo-controlled study on alcohol dependence. Arch Gen Psychiatry 1996; 53(8):673–680.
64. Paille FM, Guelfi JD, Perkins AC, Royer RJ, Steru L, Parot P. Double-blind randomized multicentre trial of acamprosate in maintaining abstinence from alcohol. Alcohol Alcohol 1995; 30(2):239–247.
65. Mason BJ, Goodman AM, Chabac S, Lehert P. Effect of oral acamprosate on abstinence in patients with alcohol dependence in a double-blind, placebo-controlled trial: The role of patient motivation. J Psychiatr Res 2006; 40(5):383–393.
66. De Witte P, Littleton J, Parot P, Koob G. Neuroprotective and abstinence-promoting effects of acamprosate: elucidating the mechanism of action. CNS Drugs 2005; 19(6):517–537.
67. Kiefer F, Jahn H, Tarnaske T, Helwig H, Briken P, Holzbach R et al. Comparing and combining naltrexone and acamprosate in relapse prevention of alcoholism: a double-blind, placebo-controlled study. Arch Gen Psychiatry 2003; 60(1):92–99.
68. Anton RF, O'Malley SS, Ciraulo DA, Cisler RA, Couper D, Donovan DM et al. Combined pharmacotherapies and behavioral interventions for alcohol dependence: the COMBINE study: a randomized controlled trial. JAMA 2006; 295(17):2003–2017.
69. Fudala PJ, Heishman SJ, Henningfield JE, Johnson RE. Human pharmacology and abuse potential of nalmefene. Clin Pharmacol Ther 1991; 49(3):300–306.
70. Dixon R, Howes J, Gentile J, Hsu HB, Hsiao J, Garg D et al. Nalmefene: intravenous safety and kinetics of a new opioid antagonist. Clin Pharmacol Ther 1986; 39(1):49–53.
71. Michel ME, Bolger G, Weissman BA. Binding of a new opiate antagonist, nalmefene, to rat brain membranes. Methods Find Exp Clin Pharmacol 1985; 7(4):175–177.
72. Bart G, Schluger JH, Borg L, Ho A, Bidlack JM, Kreek MJ. Nalmefene induced elevation in serum prolactin in normal human volunteers: partial kappa opioid agonist activity? Neuropsychopharmacology 2005; 30(12):2254–2262.

73. Chow BL, Sellers EM, Tomkins DM. Effect of naltrexone and its derivatives, nalmefene and naltrindole, on conditioned anticipatory behaviour and saccharin intake in rats. Behav Pharmacol 1997; 8(8):725–735.
74. Hubbell CL, Marglin SH, Spitalnic SJ, Abelson ML, Wild KD, Reid LD. Opioidergic, serotonergic, and dopaminergic manipulations and rats' intake of a sweetened alcoholic beverage. Alcohol 1991; 8(5):355–367.
75. June HL, Grey C, Warren-Reese C, Durr LF, Ricks-Cord A, Johnson A et al. The opioid receptor antagonist nalmefene reduces responding maintained by ethanol presentation: preclinical studies in ethanol-preferring and outbred Wistar rats. Alcohol Clin Exp Res 1998; 22(9):2174–2185.
76. Mason BJ, Ritvo EC, Morgan RO, Salvato FR, Goldberg G, Welch B et al. A double-blind, placebo-controlled pilot study to evaluate the efficacy and safety of oral nalmefene HCl for alcohol dependence. Alcohol Clin Exp Res 1994; 18(5):1162–1167.
77. Mason BJ, Salvato FR, Williams LD, Ritvo EC, Cutler RB. A double-blind, placebo-controlled study of oral nalmefene for alcohol dependence. Arch Gen Psychiatry 1999; 56(8):719–724.
78. Anton RF, Pettinati H, Zweben A, Kranzler HR, Johnson B, Bohn MJ et al. A multi-site dose ranging study of nalmefene in the treatment of alcohol dependence. J Clin Psychopharmacol 2004; 24(4):421–428.
79. Drobes DJ, Anton RF, Thomas SE, Voronin K. Effects of naltrexone and nalmefene on subjective response to alcohol among non-treatment-seeking alcoholics and social drinkers. Alcohol Clin Exp Res 2004; 28(9):1362–1370.
80. Grant JE, Potenza MN, Hollander E, Cunningham-Williams R, Nurminen T, Smits G et al. Multicenter investigation of the opioid antagonist nalmefene in the treatment of pathological gambling. Am J Psychiatry 2006; 163(2):303–312.
81. Johnsen J, Morland J. Disulfiram implant: a double-blind placebo controlled follow-up on treatment outcome. Alcohol Clin Exp Res 1991; 15(3):532–536.
82. Whyte CR, O'Brien PM. Disulfiram implant: a controlled trial. Br J Psychiatry 1974; 124(578): 42–44.
83. Wilson A, Davidson WJ, White J. Disulfiram implantation: placebo, psychological deterrent, and pharmacological deterrent effects. Br J Psychiatry 1976; 129:277–280.
84. Wilson A, Davidson WJ, Blanchard R, White J. Disulfiram implantation. A placebo-controlled trial with two-year follow-up. J Stud Alcohol 1978; 39(5):809–819.
85. Wilson A, Davidson WJ, Blanchard R. Disulfiram implantation: a trial using placebo implants and two types of controls. J Stud Alcohol 1980; 41(5):429–436.
86. Misra AL, Pontani RB. An improved long-acting delivery system for narcotic antagonists. NIDA Res Monogr 1981; 28:254–264.
87. Schwope AD, Wise DL, Howes JF. Development of polylactic/glycolic acid delivery systems for use in treatment of narcotic addiction. Natl Inst Drug Abuse Res Monogr Ser 1975; (4):13–18.
88. Yoburn BC, Cohen AH, Inturrisi CE. Pharmacokinetics and pharmacodynamics of subcutaneous naltrexone pellets in the rat. J Pharmacol Exp Ther 1986; 237(1):126–130.
89. Hamilton RJ, Olmedo RE, Shah S, Hung OL, Howland MA, Perrone J et al. Complications of ultrarapid opioid detoxification with subcutaneous naltrexone pellets. Acad Emerg Med 2002; 9(1):63–68.
90. Garbutt JC, Kranzler HR, O'Malley SS, Gastfriend DR, Pettinati HM, Silverman BL et al. Efficacy and tolerability of long-acting injectable naltrexone for alcohol dependence: a randomized controlled trial. JAMA 2005; 293(13):1617–1625.
91. Kranzler HR, Wesson DR, Billot L. Naltrexone depot for treatment of alcohol dependence: A multicenter, randomized, placebo-controlled clinical trial. Alcohol Clin Exp Res 2004; 28(7):1051–1059.
92. Dixon R, Gentile J, Hsu HB, Hsiao J, Howes J, Garg D et al. Nalmefene: safety and kinetics after single and multiple oral doses of a new opioid antagonist. J Clin Pharmacol 1987; 27(3):233–239.
93. Costantini LC, Kleppner SR, McDonough J, Azar MR, Patel R. Implantable technology for long-term delivery of nalmefene for treatment of alcoholism. Int J Pharm 2004; 283(1–2):35–44.
94. Bibbiani F, Costantini LC, Patel R, Chase TN. Continuous dopaminergic stimulation reduces risk of motor complications in parkinsonian primates. Exp Neurol 2005; 192(1):73–78.

Chapter 38
Development of Opioid Transdermal Delivery Systems

Kalpana S. Paudel, Stan L. Banks, Paul K. Kiptoo, Dana C. Hammell, R. Reddy Pinninti, Caroline Strasinger, and Audra L. Stinchcomb

Abstract Opioid therapies have been and will continue to be a vital part of opioid addiction and alcoholism treatments, as well as a vital part of chronic and acute pain management regimens. Transdermal delivery of opioid antagonists and agonists can be advantageous in order to help improve the quality of life of many patients. This mode of drug administration offers many advantages when compared to the traditional oral route of drug delivery, including avoidance of hepatic first-pass metabolism, the potential for long-term controlled release with smoothing of the typical peak-trough plasma drug concentration profiles associated with multiple dosing regimens, the ease of administration, and the possibility of immediate withdrawal of the treatment. Although the majority of the opioids used in clinical practice do not have ideal physicochemical properties that would allow them to reach therapeutic plasma levels by passive skin permeation, many advances have been made in the transdermal delivery of these agents with the advent of novel approaches including prodrugs, codrugs, microneedle (MN)-enhanced delivery, and other new formulation technologies. Many research and development avenues exist for the growth potential of the opioid transdermal drug delivery market in the next decade.

Keywords: Opioids; Transdermal drug delivery; Human skin; Guinea pig skin; Pharmacokinetics; In vitro–in vivo correlation

Opioids are useful for the treatment of various diseases; however, opioid antagonists are used primarily in the management of alcohol and opioid dependence. Investigational uses for opioid antagonists include decreasing opioid-induced constipation and pruritus (1) and attenuating the rewarding effects of cigarette smoking (2). Full and partial opioid agonists are used for the management of acute and chronic

K.S. Paudel, S.L. Banks, P.K. Kiptoo, D.C. Hammell, R.R. Pinninti, C. Strasinger, and A.L. Stinchcomb (✉)
Department of Pharmaceutical Sciences, University of Kentucky College of Pharmacy, Lexington, Kentucky 40536-0082
e-mail: astin2@email.uky.edu

pain conditions, and as adjuncts to anesthesia. Multiple dosage forms are available for these drugs, but recent research efforts have been to develop more transdermal delivery systems, as this would confer obvious advantages in the treatment of chronic conditions. The first transdermal patch was approved in 1981 by the FDA to prevent the nausea and vomiting associated with motion sickness. During the last 25 years, many transdermal products of various drug entities have emerged on the market, including one of the most successful transdermal products, the opioid agonist fentanyl. Most of the opioid antagonists or agonists do not have suitable physicochemical properties for required therapeutic skin absorption rates from reasonable-sized passive-delivery patches. However, several new drug delivery technologies have contributed significantly to the enhanced transdermal absorption of some of these drugs. This chapter contains a summary of the research undertaken in the process of transdermal delivery development for individual opioid antagonists and agonists.

38.1 Opioid Antagonists

Naloxone-hydrochloride (HCl) is available in 0.4 mg unit doses for injection and is used for the reversal of opioid overdose. Naloxone has a short half-life of about 64 min in humans (3). Because of this short half-life, it has been suggested that infusion may be preferred (4, 5). However, a regimen of frequent injections or intravenous infusion would not be desirable, and transdermal delivery might be more convenient. A few studies have been conducted both in vitro and in vivo in rats in an effort to evaluate the potential of a transdermal formulation of naloxone (6–8). After multiple applications of transdermal patches containing naloxone (10 mg/g of gel), maximum steady-state plasma concentrations of 1.56 ± 0.22 μg/ml were observed in rats. Steady-state levels were maintained from 4 to 48 h. Others have evaluated the enhancement of naloxone permeation through human skin in vitro using various vehicles and penetration enhancers. Studies by Aungst et al. revealed that addition of 10% lauric acid to propylene glycol gave the greatest naloxone flux estimated to be 235.2 ± 29.9 μg/cm^2/h (6).

Nalmefene, another nonselective opioid antagonist, has also been studied for the treatment of alcohol dependence (9, 10). In a 12-week study in which 105 alcohol-dependent patients were randomly assigned to placebo or nalmefene 20 mg/day, significantly fewer nalmefene-treated patients relapsed to heavy drinking compared with those treated with placebo (10). In comparison with naltrexone (NTX), nalmefene has a greater affinity for the δ- and κ-receptors, thus potentially providing effective control of non-μ receptor reinforcing effects of drinking (11). Additionally, nalmefene appears to be less hepatotoxic than NTX (12). However, in another study, nalmefene-treated subjects reported more insomnia, irritability, and trouble concentrating than NTX-treated subjects (13). To address compliance as well as adverse side effects associated with oral therapy, subcutaneous nalmefene implants have been studied in rats for long-term delivery (14). Results indicated that ethylene vinyl acetate-coated rods containing nalmefene (80.09 mg/rod) achieved estimated delivery rates of 0.29 ± 0.09 mg/day/rod over 6 months after administration of subcutaneous implants. However, the dose of nalmefene delivered from rods is slightly lower than required for clinical efficacy in humans. Moreover, implants require invasive surgical procedures and hence, transdermal delivery may be more suitable for long-term therapy in motivated patients. A formulation containing at least one fatty acid derivative has been described to enhance the transdermal penetration of nalmefene and other opioids (15). One patent describes a tamper-resistant transdermal dosage form with the first adhesive layer comprising 15 mg/cm^2 fentanyl free base and the second adhesive layer comprising 15 mg/cm^2 nalmefene-HCl (16).

NTX is one of the most extensively researched potent competitive opioid receptor antagonists (17, 18) which have been used in the treatment of opioid dependence and alcohol addiction (19, 20). NTX-HCl is presently available as 25, 50, and 100 mg film-coated oral tablets (ReVia® and generics) in USA. The drug has a high extraction ratio in the liver, and is subject to extensive first pass metabolism, resulting in a low bioavailability (5–40%) after oral administration (21, 22). The drug must be given regularly to maintain a minimum effective plasma drug concentration in maintenance therapy for alcohol abstinence. However, the oral administration of the drug may not be suitable for long-term therapy of opioid dependence and alcoholism because of patient compliance problems, hepatic and/or gastrointestinal side effects, and a wide interpatient variability in metabolism in compliant subjects (23). NTX was the second drug approved by the US FDA for the treatment of alcohol dependence (besides the relatively unpopular disulfiram, Antabuse), but due to the above-mentioned potential problems, the use of NTX for alcoholism treatment has been limited (22–27). Transdermal delivery of NTX would be preferable because it bypasses first pass metabolism, reduces the overall dose required in patients (which is especially important in patients with liver disease), minimizes the gastrointestinal side effects, increases patient compliance, and allows attainment of steady-state plasma concentrations for maintenance therapy in chronic opioid dependence or alcoholism. Transdermal patches are noninvasive as compared to many of the NTX implants that have been investigated (28–30). One of the injectable depot preparations of NTX (Vivitrol™) has been recently approved by the FDA for the treatment of alcoholism. Once-a-week patch treatments could be easily used at home by a motivated patient, without the physician visits that are required with implants or depot injections. However, the problem with NTX transdermal delivery is that the required therapeutic plasma level is not achieved due to the nonideal physicochemical properties of the drug (31). On the basis of the studies which have shown that the lowest effective plasma NTX concentration of 2 ng/ml provided an average of 86.5% blockade of 25 mg intravenous heroin effects, it is necessary to maintain a plasma level of NTX above 2 ng/ml in sustained or controlled release therapy for opiate antagonist activity (32). Considering an oral bioavailability range of 5–40% with a dosage of 50–100 mg/day, the daily dose range of NTX would be 7–118 μmol. Therefore, a required therapeutic transdermal delivery rate of NTX from a 25-cm^2 patch can be calculated to be in the range of 11–197 nmol/cm_2/h. Different approaches such as prodrugs, chemical enhancers, iontophoresis have been developed to improve skin permeation of drugs that do not have the ideal physicochemical properties for efficient skin permeation. The use of permeation enhancers has been investigated with the intention of reaching therapeutic NTX levels in humans with a transdermal patch (31), but these chemical enhancers can cause significant irritation due to alteration of the skin structure. Previous studies have described NTX prodrugs to increase the oral bioavailability and to mask the bitter taste for buccal delivery (33, 34), but no information existed about the use of these prodrugs transdermally prior to 1997.

Dr. Audra Stinchcomb's group has investigated a series of NTX prodrugs for transdermal delivery. The design, synthesis, and screening of prodrugs have helped to identify and quantify the important physicochemical properties that are responsible for improvement in NTX transdermal delivery rates as well as in the creation of more permeable NTX prodrugs to ultimately develop a successful transdermal dosage form of NTX. This would also help in the creation of a quantitative structure permeability relationship for future design of transdermal prodrugs for other poorly skin-permeable drugs.

The initial series of straight-chain 3-*O*-alkyl-ester prodrugs of NTX with two to seven carbons in chain length (Table 38.1) increased the NTX maximum flux rate across human skin in in vitro diffusion studies (35). The prodrugs increased the transdermal delivery rate of NTX across human skin by two- to sevenfold. Among the prodrugs, short-chain compounds, ACE-NTX, PROP-NTX, and HEX-NTX enhanced the NTX flux by factors of 6.2, 4.4, and 3.4, respectively (fluxes of NTX, ACE-NTX, PROP-NTX, and HEX-NTX were 2.5 ± 1.5, 15.6 ± 6.3, 11.1 ± 3.7, and 8.6 ± 2.2 nmol/cm_2/h, respectively). The melting points of prodrugs decreased as the alkyl chain was extended, by >100°C in the case of the HEX-NTX. Melting point is an important physicochemical property that is related to the solubility of drugs or prodrugs. A decrease in the melting points and heats of fusion of the prodrugs relative to the parent drug increases the calculated apparent thermodynamic activity coefficient which establishes the maximum practical driving force for permeation. These ester prodrugs have higher oil solubilities which provided a higher NTX flux across human skin rather than a change in permeability coefficient. Apart from oil solubility, aqueous solubility has been identified to be an important criterion in the design and success of the prodrugs. The prodrugs have much lower aqueous solubility than NTX, which corresponded with the increasing alkyl chain length. Ester prodrugs were almost completely hydrolyzed on passing through the skin and extensively converted to NTX in the viable skin layers, and this extent of bioconversion correlated with increased drug delivery rates. Therefore, as these prodrugs undergo rapid metabolic conversion in the skin, the more hydrophilic parent drug (NTX) diffuses with relative ease through the aqueous viable tissue. Overall, oil solubility and extent of prodrug bioconversion seemed to be critical in increasing the flux from this group of alkyl ester prodrugs.

The unique concept of a duplex "gemini" prodrug has been utilized to synthesize a novel prodrug of naltrexone, NTX-NTX (Fig. 38.1a), a prodrug which consists of two NTX molecules bonded together by a carbonate ester linkage (36). Previous papers have described the duplex prodrugs of naproxen (37), olsalazine (Dipentum™), and an antiviral drug in preclinical development (38). The prodrug equivalent flux was twice as high across human skin as compared to NTX base

Table 38.1 Structures of naltrexone prodrugs

Drug	Abbreviation	R-group	MW
Ester prodrugs – straight chain			
Naltrexone	NTX	H	341
Acetyl naltrexone	ACE-NTX	$–COCH_3$	383
Propanoyl naltrexone	PROP-NTX	$–COCH_2CH_3$	397
Butanoyl naltrexone	BUT-NTX	$–CO(CH_2)_2CH_3$	411
Valeryl naltrexone	VAL-NTX	$–CO(CH_2)_3CH_3$	425
Hexanoyl naltrexone	HEX-NTX	$–CO(CH_2)_4CH_3$	439
Heptanoyl naltrexone	HEP-NTX	$–CO(CH_2)_5CH_3$	453
Ester prodrugs – branched chain			
3-*O*-Pivalyl naltrexone	PIV-NTX	$–COC(CH_3)_3$	425
3-*O*-Isovaleryl naltrexone	ISOVAL-NTX	$–COCH_2CH(CH_3)_2$	425
3-*O*-(2-Ethylbutyryl) naltrexone	ETBUT-NTX	$–COCH(CH_2CH_3)_2$	439
3-*O*-Isobutyryl naltrexone	ISOBUTYRYL-NTX	$–COCH(CH_3)_2$	411
Carbonate prodrugs – straight chain			
Methyl carbonate naltrexone	ME-NTX	$–COOCH_3$	399
Ethyl carbonate naltrexone	ETH-NTX	$–COOCH_2CH_3$	413
Propyl carbonate naltrexone	PROP-NTX	$–COO(CH_2)_2CH_3$	427
Butyl carbonate naltrexone	BUTYL-NTX	$–COO(CH_2)_3CH_3$	441
Amyl carbonate naltrexone	PENTLY-NTX	$–COO(CH_2)_4CH_3$	455
Carbonate prodrugs – branched chain			
3-*O*-Isopropyloxycarbonyl naltrexone	ISOPROP-NTX	$–COOCH(CH_3)_2$	427
3-*O*-Tertiarybutyloxycarbonyl naltrexone	TERTBUTYL-NTX	$–COOC\ (CH_3)_3$	441
Carbamate prodrugs			
***N*-Monoalkyl**			
Ethyl carbamate naltrexone	ETHYL	$–CONHCH_2CH_3$	412
Propyl carbamate naltrexone	PROPYL	$–CONH(CH_2)_2CH_3$	425
Butyl carbamate naltrexone	BUTYL	$–CONH(CH_2)_3CH_3$	440
Pentyl carbamate naltrexone	PENTYL	$–CONH(CH_2)_4CH_3$	453
***N,N*-Dialkyl**			
N,N-Dimethylcarbamate naltrexone	DIMETHYL	$–CON(CH_3)_2$	412
N,N-Diethylcarbamate naltrexone	DIETHYL	$–CON(CH_2CH_3)_{max}2$	440
N,N-Diisopropylcarbamate naltrexone	DIISOPROPYL	$–CON(CH(CH_3)_2)_2$	468
Oxa-ester prodrugs			
3-*O*-(3-Methoxy)propionyl naltrexone	ETHOXY	$–CO(CH_2)_2OCH_3$	427
3-*O*-(3-Ethoxy) propionyl naltrexone	METHOXY	$–CO(CH_2)_2OCH_2CH_3$	441
3-*O*-(3-Isopropoxy)propionyl naltrexone	ISOPROPOXY	$–CO(CH_2)_2OCH(CH_3)_2$	455
3-*O*-(3-Cyclohexyloxy) propionyl naltrexone	CYCLOHEXYLOXY	$–CO(CH_2)_2OC_6H_{11}$	495

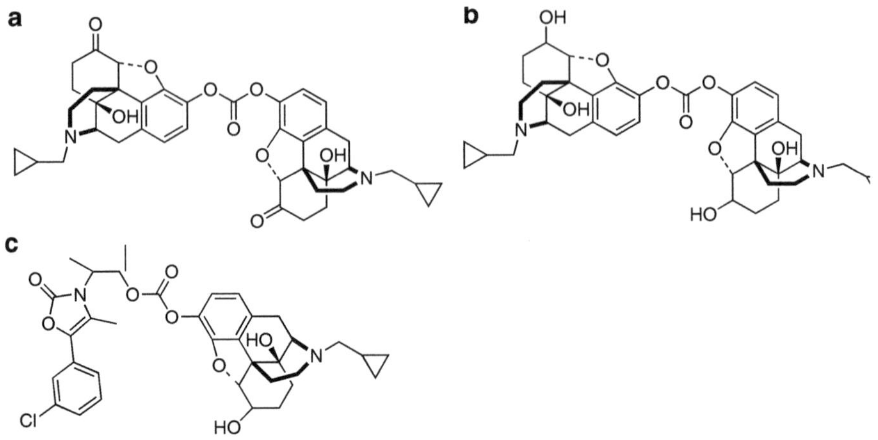

Fig. 38.1 Chemical structures of naltrexone duplex, NTX-NTX (**a**), 6-β-naltrexol duplex, NTXOL-NTXOL (**b**), and CB-NTXOL-BUPOH (**c**)

(3.0 ± 1.1 vs 6.2 ± 2.5 nmol/cm²/h). The NTX-NTX prodrug biotransformed into two NTX moieties via the skin enzymes after penetration into the skin layers and appeared mainly as NTX in the receiver solution in the in vitro diffusion experiments. The drug concentration in the skin after prodrug treatment was not significantly increased when compared to NTX. Since the NTX equivalent solubilities of NTX and the prodrug in the donor solution were similar, as well as the partition coefficients of the two drugs being similar, the increased flux from the NTX-NTX prodrug could be explained due to an increased concentration gradient in the skin as a result of rapid bioconversion of the prodrug and decreased hydrogen bonding.

Pillai et al. (39) evaluated the homologous series of straight-chain 3-*O*-alkyl carbonate prodrugs of NTX (Table 38.1) for the physicochemical properties, in vitro diffusion, and biotransformation across human skin. Within this prodrug series, the shortest chain prodrug, the ME-NTX, was the most skin-permeable compound. ME-NTX increased the flux of NTX from 2.9 ± 0.74 to 6.9 ± 0.5 nmol/cm²/h. Similar to the ester prodrugs, the carbonate prodrugs had decreased melting points relative to NTX. These decreased melting points led to increased oil solubilities and apparent thermodynamic activity coefficient, which was highest with ME-NTX and lowest with ISOPROP-NTX. The highest oil solubility did not result in the highest flux of the prodrugs and the drug that permeated the fastest had the highest aqueous solubility in this series. Aqueous solubility seems to play a significant role in the flux of this series of prodrugs compared with the ester prodrugs because of the slower metabolic bioconversion in the skin. All the carbonate prodrugs slowly hydrolyzed to NTX on passing through the skin with about 11–51% intact prodrug appearing in the receiver compartment. ME-NTX also had increased partitioning from the vehicle to the skin, a high apparent permeability coefficient, and the highest extent of bioconversion, which resulted in the highest flux of the series.

The shape (branching) of the side chain used in the design of transdermal prodrugs is important to the success of the compound. In one study, the branched-chain ester and carbonate prodrugs, PIV-NTX, ISOVAL-NTX, ETBUT-NTX, ISOBUTYRYL-NTX, ISOPROP-NTX, and TERTBUTYL-NTX (Table 38.1) were synthesized, and the in vitro human skin, permeation was compared with that of the straight-chain prodrugs with the same number of prodrug-moiety carbon atoms (40). Although the melting points of all the branched prodrugs were lower, and mineral oil solubilities higher than NTX, the branched prodrugs did not enhance the transdermal flux values as previously seen with the corresponding straight-chain prodrugs. Because of the presence of bulky prodrug moieties, the relative calculated thermodynamic activity coefficients, stratum corneum (SC)/vehicle partition coefficients, and skin permeability coefficients of the branched-chain ester and carbonate prodrugs were decreased compared to their straight-chain counterparts. These bulkier branched prodrugs did not convert to the parent molecule completely during the skin permeation process, and since their aqueous solubilities were lower than NTX, these prodrugs did not transport across viable aqueous tissue efficiently. The TERTBUTYL-NTX prodrug underwent the least amount of skin bioconversion to NTX, but it had the highest flux of the branched-chain prodrugs and also the highest aqueous solubility, correlating with its more efficient intact transport across the aqueous viable tissue.

Carbamate prodrugs of NTX (Table 38.1) have also been shown to enhance the skin permeation of NTX (unpublished results). However, *N*-monoalkyl substitution versus *N*,*N*-dialkyl substitution is critical to the design of a successful carbamate prodrug for skin permeation. Four *N*-monoalkyl carbamates, that is, ETHYL through PENTYL and a series of *N*,*N*-dialkyl carbamates, namely DIMETHYL, DIETHYL, and DIISOPROPYL were studied. The *N*-monoalkyl carbamate prodrugs significantly improved the skin permeation of NTX across human skin in vitro. Among the monoalkyl carbamates, ETHYL and PROPYL enhanced the NTX flux by 3.17- to 3.23-fold with flux values of 15.53 ± 11.26 and 17.44 ± 11.16 nmol/cm^2/h, respectively. The *N*-monoalkyl carbamate prodrugs had fast plasma hydrolysis rates, whereas the *N*,*N*-dialkyl carbamate prodrugs were unable to enhance NTX permeation, most likely due to the decreased partitioning and decreased enzymatic hydrolysis rates.

A study on the oxa-ester prodrugs of NTX (Table 38.1) showed that ISOPROPOXY and ETHOXY were the most promising prodrugs for NTX transdermal delivery (unpublished results). ISOPROPOXY, the only oil of the prodrug series (all others were solids), provided the highest NTX flux (10.16 ± 2.46 nmol/cm^2/h) followed by ETHOXY (8.02 ± 2.01 nmol/cm^2/h) which also exhibited the highest permeability coefficient. Addition of alkoxy groups to NTX decreased the melting points, enhanced the lipophilicity of the molecule, decreased the aqueous solubilities as compared to the parent drug, but resulted in higher fluxes for only two of the four prodrugs. Among the prodrugs, the more water-soluble compounds, ISOPROPOXY and ETHOXY, underwent the least bioconversion in the skin compared to the other prodrugs. The high aqueous solubilities of these successful prodrugs must have allowed efficient transport through the viable aqueous tissue layer and offset their decreased bioconversion rates. The aqueous solubility was the least for the CYCLOHEXYLOXY prodrug, which had the smallest permeability coefficient (and largest molecular weight), and was the most chemically and enzymatically labile prodrug. Thus, aqueous solubilities played an important role in the flux of this series of prodrugs in contrast to the straight-chain ester prodrugs, where aqueous solubilities have a negligible role because of rapid and complete bioconversion to NTX. However, if a molecule is too large to permeate the SC efficiently (e.g., CYCLOHEXYLOXY prodrug), this becomes the rate-limiting step to efficient drug transport. Obviously, the correct combination of the physicochemical parameters is critical to the overall flux improvement.

The studies discussed above showed that although the percutaneous penetration rate of NTX is at the borderline of therapeutic to subtherapeutic, straight-chain 3-*O*-alkyl ester, 3-*O*-alkyl carbonate, carbamate, oxa-ester, and duplex prodrugs of NTX improved human skin permeation. Among all the prodrugs, the highest flux was obtained from the short-chain ester prodrugs of NTX, ACE-NTX, and PROP-NTX, and the oxa-ester ISOPROPOXY which met the minimum necessary therapeutic delivery rate of 11 nmol/cm^2/h. HEX-NTX, VAL-NTX, HEP-NTX, NTX-NTX, ME-NTX, and ETHOXY did not meet the above criteria, but the required 25–40% increase in the flux may be possible with further formulation efforts. The skin permeation of these prodrugs correlated with the extent of bioconversion and the prodrug physicochemical properties. These studies also highlighted the importance for optimization of the relative oil and aqueous solubilities of the prodrugs, based on their relative skin bioconversion rates, to achieve a higher flux of NTX for therapeutic treatment.

Fresh human surgical waste skin provides a good estimate of clinical drug percutaneous absorption and biotransformation. However, human skin equivalent models can also be useful tools for assessing epidermal drug metabolism and topical/transdermal prodrug metabolic conversion. In a study with the EpiDerm™ skin model, a metabolically active human epidermal model, the prodrugs of NTX permeated in a rank-order comparison similar to the human skin (41). A branched-chain and straight-chain prodrug of NTX, ETBUT-NTX, and VAL-NTX with significantly different metabolic stabilities were compared. Similar to the human skin, VAL-NTX hydrolyzed rapidly in the EpiDerm™ and mainly (93 ± 4%) NTX was found in the receiver, whereas ETBUT permeated the skin mainly in intact form and only 15 ± 11% NTX was found in the receiver. The NTX flux enhancement with these prodrugs was similar to that observed in human skin diffusion studies. VAL-NTX has been a successful prodrug in human skin in vitro (33) as well as in the EpiDerm™ experiments. Similar prodrug bioconversion profiles were observed in the intact EpiDerm™ and human skin experiments. The extent of NTX metabolism to 6-β-naltrexol (NTXOL), the major active metabolite of NTX, in the skin was similar in EpiDerm™ and human tissue (NTX metabolized to 1 ± 0.5% NTXOL in the fresh human surgical waste skin vs. 3 ± 2% NTXOL in the intact EpiDerm™ human skin equivalent.)

It is desirable to have a good correlation between the in vitro and in vivo studies involving transdermal delivery as in any other route of drug delivery. In an in vivo pharmacokinetic study carried out in hairless guinea pigs with the application of transdermal patches of the 3-*O*-alkyl ester prodrugs, it was observed that the mean steady-state NTX plasma concentrations from NTX, ACE-NTX, PROP-NTX, and HEX-NTX were 4.2, 25.2, 16.0, and 8.3 ng/ml, respectively (Fig. 38.2) (42). ACE-NTX provided the highest maximum plasma concentration of NTX (34.8 ng/ml), when compared with NTX, PROP-NTX, and HEX-NTX (5.4, 20.1, and 11.0 ng/ml, respectively). These NTX plasma concentrations were maintained for 48 h and the levels declined after the removal of the patches indicating no reservoir effect of the drugs. The order of enhancement in the predicted steady-state NTX flux in the guinea pig with these prodrugs was similar to that obtained across human skin in vitro (35). Increased lipophilicity (alkyl chain length) did not result in increased plasma levels of NTX from the prodrugs, which reflected the results of human skin in vitro studies (35). This in vivo study confirmed that the ACE-NTX and PROP-NTX prodrugs of NTX were the most promising drug candidates for transdermal delivery.

In another study, four prodrugs of NTX: ETBUT-NTX, ME-NTX, ethyl-3-*O*-carbamate-NTX (ETHYL), and *N*,*N*-dimethyl-3-*O*-carbamate-NTX (DIMETHYL) were evaluated for the in vitro skin permeation across hairless guinea pig skin and in vivo skin permeation in hairless guinea pigs utilizing transdermal patches of the drugs (43). In in vitro studies, all the prodrugs hydrolyzed to NTX on passing through the guinea pig skin. ME-NTX and ETHYL underwent the highest extent of bioconversion to NTX as compared to ETBUT and DIMETHYL. ME-NTX provided the highest NTX flux with the highest apparent permeability coefficient as has been previously obtained with human skin (39). The flux values of these prodrugs were about 1.8 times higher than the flux values in the human skin. The results of the in vivo studies indicated that a significant amount of NTX was

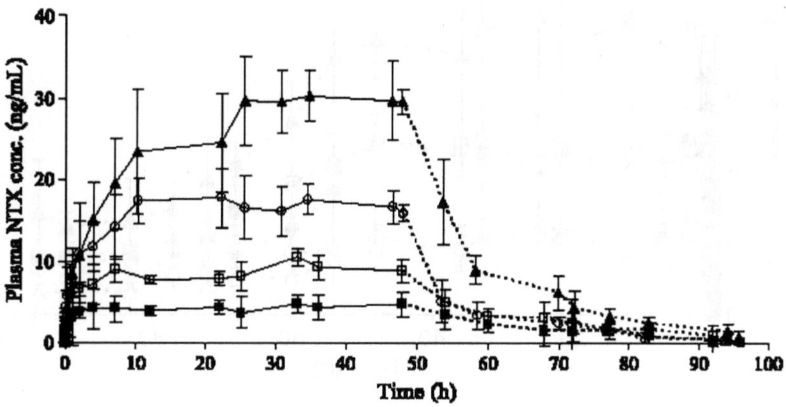

Fig. 38.2 Mean (±SD) plasma profiles of NTX in hairless guinea pigs ($n = 6$) after the application of transdermal patches containing NTX, ACE-NTX, PROP-NTX, or HEX-NTX. The *dotted line* (……) indicates the plasma concentration after the removal of patches (*closed square*, NTX from NTX base; *open square*, NTX from HEX-NTX; *open circle*, NTX from PROP-NTX; and *closed triangle*, NTX from ACE-NTX)

delivered after the application of transdermal patches of NTX prodrugs (Fig. 38.3). The 48-h mean steady-state NTX plasma concentrations from ETBUT, ME-NTX, ETHYL, and DIMETHYL were 3.5, 7.1, 3.1, and 2.7 ng/ml, respectively. The observed steady-state plasma levels were in good agreement with the predicted steady-state plasma levels from the in vitro data. Among these prodrugs, ME-NTX was found to be the most promising drug candidate for transdermal delivery. This study also validated the utility of the hairless guinea pig model for the transdermal development of NTX prodrugs.

Transdermal delivery systems need to be developed in order to move toward clinical testing of an optimized prodrug patch. One study aimed to develop a matrix type transdermal patch for the most successful prodrug, ACE-NTX which has the highest permeation rate of NTX (44). The prepared adhesive transdermal patches of NTX and its ACE-NTX prodrug showed good uniformity with regard to drug content and thickness. The DUROTAK® 87-2516 adhesive was found to be most suitable and compatible polymer for the transdermal delivery of NTX from the NTX and ACE-NTX patches. Increases in drug loading from 1% to 3% linearly increased the release flux and cumulative amount of NTX from the NTX and the ACE-NTX patches. Overall, the amounts of NTX released from the prodrug patches were significantly higher than from the NTX patches, at all three drug loading levels.

Microneedle (MN) treatment has become one of the most promising innovations under investigation for transdermal delivery. MN delivery is attractive because it is pain free, economical, and easy to use. MN technology was envisioned to deliver a diverse group of compounds, including large oligonucleotides, insulin, and highly

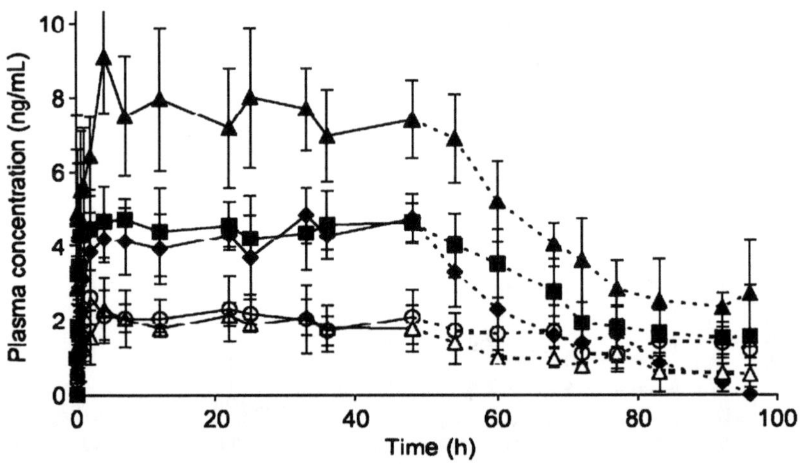

Fig. 38.3 Mean (±SD) plasma profiles of NTX in hairless guinea pigs ($n = 5$–6) after the application of transdermal patches containing NTX, *ETBUT-NTX, ME-NTX, ETHYL, or DIMETHYL. The *dotted line* (……) indicates the plasma concentration after the removal of patches (*closed diamond*, NTX from NTX base; *closed square*, NTX from ETHYL; *open triangle*, NTX from ETBUT-NTX; *closed triangle*, NTX from ME-NTX; and *open circle*, NTX from DIMETHYL). [*NTX profile reproduced from Valiveti et al. (42)]

water-soluble compounds. As compared with other methods of physically altering the SC to aid in improving transdermal transport, MN delivery is by far the simplest physical technique. MNs come in various forms, including biodegradable polymers, silicon, and stainless steel; all micromachined to increase permeability and decrease sensation.

Stinchcomb et al. are examining a novel approach to deliver the opioid antagonist NTX by MN delivery. As mentioned earlier, a host of prodrug moieties have been developed to enhance NTX's ability to permeate the skin, but further skin permeation enhancement could provide benefit to alcoholics and heroin addicts. By converting NTX base into a HCl salt, one expects even lower passive skin permeation rates as compared to NTX base, but in accompaniment with MN application, the enhancement of permeation of the highly water-soluble NTX-HCl should be great. A passive drug permeation comparison study of NTX base and HCl on hairless guinea pig skin in a PermeGear® flow through diffusion apparatus showed an elevated permeation rate of the more lipophilic NTX base (9.94 ± 2.75 nmol/cm^2/h) as compared to the salt form (2.71 ± 1.20 nmol/cm^2/h). Both forms of the compound had long lag times of 21.2–22.4 h with passive permeation (45). The flux values were greatly enhanced in MN-treated skin with NTX-HCl (27.16 ± 4.57 nmol/cm^2/h) as compared to NTX base without MN treatment. At 48 h, NTX-HCl levels were approximately 12 times as high as observed with passive NTX base permeation and a lag time change was observed from approximately 22 to 2.4 h, which suggests a change in permeation route (45). Conversely, NTX base (11.80 ± 5.02 nmol/cm^2/h) showed an approximate 1.2-fold flux enhancement with MN treatment and the lag time decreased by only a few hours from 21.2 to 18.9 h, suggesting that although the aqueous channels are easily accessible, the lipophilic base, with less solubility than the HCl salt, still predominantly diffused through the SC's lipid bilayers and not the MN pores. Finally, human full-thickness skin was tested with NTX-HCl with (18.11 ± 4.38 nmol/cm^2/h) and without (2.22 ± 0.72 nmol/cm^2/h) MNs, and no significant difference was observed between human and guinea pig skin data in vitro ($P > 0.05$) (45). This information tells us that we can use hairless guinea pig skin for modeling in vitro drug permeation profiles with MN application. Overall, the use of MN delivery, with NTX-HCl for increased aqueous solubility in order to deliver significantly higher amounts of NTX through aqueous MN channels, has been advantageous in delivering a poorly skin-permeable drug. MN delivery is still in its infancy and there are many questions to answer concerning pain, effectiveness, and safety, but many of these studies are already under way in humans. One important piece of information published recently was a pain study performed in humans by Kaushik et al., where it was determined that the sensation of MN application was that of a piece of tape applied to the skin (46). With a drug delivery application method that is minimally invasive and can be proven safe, MN delivery could be the most beneficial and cost effective of the modern physical methods of altering the SC, thus allowing low-maintenance patient compliance outside of a clinical setting.

Evaluation of the irritation and sensitization potential of a drug that is intended for transdermal delivery is very important at the preclinical stage. NTX produced mild transient skin irritation and no sensitization potential when tested in hairless guinea pigs according to the Buehler method (unpublished results). Hairless guinea pigs were treated for 24 h during the three induction phases, challenge and rechallenge phases with patches containing 24 mg/ml of saturated solution of NTX. A 14-day rest period followed between the last induction phase and the primary challenge. Skin irritation of the drug was measured by colorimeter and transepidermal water loss (TEWL) readings during the induction phases before and after patch removal. Sensitization potential of the drugs was evaluated by visual scoring on a scale of 0–3 at 24 and 48 h after patch removal during challenge and rechallenge phases. Colorimeter and TEWL readings were also taken at these time points. The method was validated with a known sensitizer, *p*-phenylenediamine. *p*-Phenylenediamine induced sensitization in 90% of the animals tested. NTX caused only mild temporary skin irritation during the first application of the patch. During subsequent applications, erythema was slightly increased but no skin damage was observed. This is consistent with the reaction from other transdermal opiate studies.

NTXOL, the major metabolite of NTX in humans (47) and in guinea pigs (48), is formed by rapid reduction of NTX. NTXOL may contribute to the therapeutic action of NTX in opioid and alcohol dependence due to its higher plasma concentration (21, 22, 47) and longer terminal half-life (22, 49, 50, 51) in humans compared to NTX. NTXOL, also an opioid receptor antagonist, has an affinity similar to NTX for the opioid receptor (52) but a lower potency than NTX in in vivo studies (53–55). However, the presence of a much higher plasma concentration of NTXOL may be expected to compensate for the lower potency, and thereby play a major role in the therapeutic efficacy of NTX. Low serum levels of NTX and NTXOL have been shown to block high doses of diamorphine in heroin addicts (56). Furthermore, NTXOL by itself is able to reduce alcohol consumption in rats in a dose-dependent manner (50, 57). In addition, higher serum concentrations of NTXOL have been associated with reductions in the number of drinks per month (58) and negative subjective effects of alcohol in humans (51). A major problem with NTX therapy has been a high relapse rate in subjects while on medication (19, 59). NTXOL may be useful in improving patient compliance as well. One clinical trial of NTX has shown that subjects with NTXOL levels of more than 40 ng/ml did not experience a relapse (58). NTXOL would also be a safer therapeutic agent in hepatocompromised patients since it is excreted mainly via the renal route. This combination of benefits indicates that NTXOL might be a useful therapy in alcoholism in the future.

The potential of transdermal delivery of NTXOL (60) across human and guinea pig skin in vitro and in hairless guinea pigs in vivo was examined in one study. The cumulative amount permeated, steady-state flux, and the skin drug disposition of NTXOL were 2.2–5.6 times lower than NTX in human skin and guinea pig skin in vitro. Similarly, the steady-state plasma concentration of NTXOL was about twofold lower than NTX (7.3 ± 1.3 vs 3.6 ± 0.5 ng/ml) in guinea pigs (Fig. 38.4). Although NTX and NTXOL have similar molecular weights and differ by only one hydroxyl group in their chemical structures, their permeation in in vitro and in vivo studies differed greatly. This emphasizes the difference that hydrogen-bonding

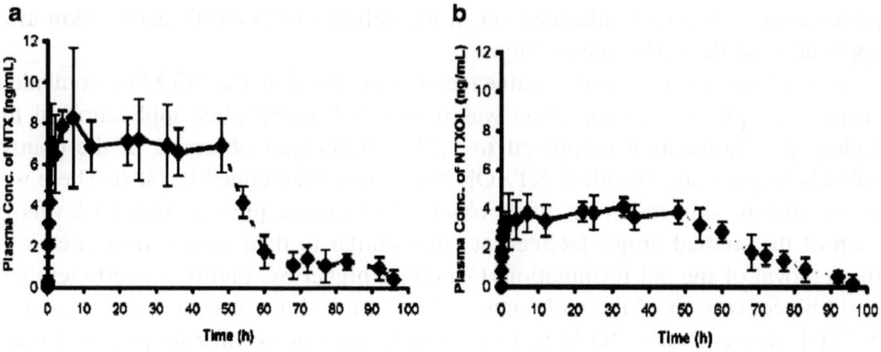

Fig. 38.4 Plasma concentration time profiles of NTX (**a**) and NTXOL (**b**) after application of transdermal patches in hairless guinea pigs. Data represent mean ± SD, n = 6 The dotted line (……) indicates the plasma concentration after the removal of patches

effects can make in skin transport. A good correlation existed between the in vitro and in vivo results. These results show that NTXOL can be delivered via the percutaneous route, although the permeation rates need to be further enhanced to be therapeutically effective.

The codrug approach has been shown to be successful in enhancing the permeability of NTXOL. A codrug or a mutual prodrug consists of two synergistic drugs chemically linked together in order to improve the drug delivery properties of one or both drugs. A novel duplex prodrug which consists of two NTXOL molecules bonded together by a carbonate ester linkage (Fig. 38.1b) underwent bioconversion back into two NTXOL molecules in skin by esterase enzymes (unpublished results). The maximum flux from the NTXOL-NTXOL duplex drug was 2.5-fold higher than the flux values from NTXOL alone. Another strategy was to link NTXOL to a molecule with better physicochemical properties necessary for transdermal delivery. Therefore, bupropion and its major active metabolite, hydroxybupropion, were chosen for linkage to NTXOL. Bupropion is used clinically as an antidepressant and in smoking cessation (61), and is extensively metabolized in humans with less than 10% of a bupropion dose being excreted unchanged (62). However, chemical synthesis procedures with bupropion gave unpredictable reaction products which were either difficult to isolate and/or too unstable. Simultaneous treatment of alcohol dependence and tobacco addiction would be beneficial because of the high prevalence of cigarette and alcohol coabuse. Pharmacological activity of bupropion might be due to, or receive significant contributions from, its major metabolite hydroxybupropion (62, 63). A carbonate codrug of NTXOL linked to hydroxybupropion, CB-NTXOL-BUPOH (Fig. 38.1c), was synthesized and evaluated (64). The carbonate codrug was hydrolyzed on passing through the skin and appeared as a combination of intact codrug and parent drugs, NTXOL and hydroxybupropion, in the receiver solution. The codrug provided a significantly higher NTXOL flux across human skin than NTXOL base. The maximum steady-state flux from the carbonate codrug in NTXOL equivalents was four times higher than that from NTXOL base alone (1.34 ± 0.35 nmol/cm^2/h vs 0.36 ± 0.15 nmol/cm^2/h), representing a fourfold enhancement in the delivery of NTXOL across skin after application of the carbonate codrug.

In vivo studies in hairless guinea pigs revealed that the NTXOL equivalent steady-state plasma concentration was 6.40 ± 0.93 ng/ml after application of the codrug gel formulation compared to 1.25 ± 0.51 ng/ml observed in the control animals (unpublished results). NTXOL levels were maintained for 48 h. There was no significant skin reservoir effect observed in guinea pigs, as plasma levels of each of the studied drugs declined at rates similar to their elimination rates after the removal of the gel formulation. Overall, a higher SC partition coefficient and rapid bioconversion of the carbonate codrug in the skin correlated with increased NTXOL delivery rates. NTXOL was found to have no sensitizing potential when tested in hairless guinea pigs by the Buehler method. NTXOL caused mild skin irritation comparable to NTX, but it was longer in duration.

38.2 Full and Partial Opioid Agonists

Morphine is the cornerstone of analgesia medications and the opioid agonist, to which all others are compared. Morphine induces analgesia with sedation, decreased concentration, apprehension, and euphoria (65). The normal routes of administration for morphine are orally, intramuscularly, or intravenously; however, an effective transdermal route for opioid therapeutics and long-term pain management would be highly desirable because the method provides constant plasma levels thereby reducing adverse side effects (66). An ideal passive delivery transdermal drug must be highly lipophilic, have a low molecular weight, and be highly potent (67). Therefore, morphine, codeine, and hydromorphone are not good candidates for passive transdermal administration. Because of this, various methods have been employed to optimize the delivery of morphine in vitro including the use of binary solvent systems as a vehicle for the drug (68), the use of ultrasound and chemical enhancers (69, 70), the development of morphine prodrug systems (71), delivery using iontophoretic technology both for human in vitro and in vivo studies (72–74), and deepithelialization of the skin in humans (75–76). Furthermore, several patents describing different morphine formulations to aid in transdermal delivery made use of monoglycerides (77), salts (78), chlorides and sulfates (79), and microemulsions (80). Despite the complexity of some of these methods for delivering morphine, the need for a transdermal route for chronic pain relief is evident. Using a more skin-permeable drug may alleviate some of the difficulty and variability that may arise when using intricate drug formulations and technologies. One such agonist is pethidine; however, while it has high transdermal permeability, it is a poor candidate for successful transdermal use because of low analgesic potency. Currently, fentanyl, sufentanil, and buprenorphine (a partial agonist) are the only proven suitable drugs for use in passive transdermal delivery systems (74).

Fentanyl is a synthetic opioid approximately 80 times more potent than morphine and was first introduced to the commercial foreign market in the 1960s. It is a μ-opioid agonist and its onset and duration is shortened because of its greater lipophilicity (65). Shorter onset and greater potency intensifies opioid receptor effects, which is needed in order for a transdermal system to produce comparable pain relief results of intravenous or oral routes of administration (65). Fentanyl is currently available by prescription for treatment of chronic pain as a transdermal patch called Duragesic®, and other generic manufacturers are also producing the popular blockbuster product (81). Clinical trials have shown that transdermal fentanyl has the advantages of ease of administration and patient acceptability, especially for patients who may have gastrointestinal problems or difficulty swallowing due to other therapies (82). It delivers controlled systemic amounts in a noninvasive fashion in 72 h increments. Additionally, patients experience reduced constipation, nausea, and drowsiness, a decreased use of rescue medication, and less guilt associated with using opioids as compared to its oral or parenterally administered morphine counterpart (82, 83).

Sufentanil, a drug that is 7.5 times more potent than fentanyl is also in the clinical trial stage for chronic cancer-pain treatment. It has a greater affinity for the opioid receptor than fentanyl, thereby intensifying the opioid effect and further decreasing the likelihood of side effects. Because of its potency, it offers greater diversity in dosing, and dramatically decreases the size of the patch which can be advantageous to the patient (65, 83). Transdermal sufentanil is under development in the Transdur® delivery system by the Durtec Corporation (84).

Buprenorphine is a synthetic agonist–antagonist opiate with 100 times higher potency than morphine (85). It is used as an analgesic by the parenteral route (86) and has also been found to be effective in drug abuse treatment when it is given sublingually at a high dose of 8 mg/day (87). However, these modes of administration give rise to immediately high levels of the drug in the blood, which may favor buprenorphine's illicit use. From this standpoint, a transdermal delivery system which administers the drug slowly into the body would be an ideal way to administer buprenorphine. Buprenorphine's high level of crystallinity, however, is likely to pose a problem to achieve a level required for opioid maintenance therapy. It was shown that straight-chain 3-alkyl ester prodrugs of buprenorphine decreased crystallinities and increased oil solubilities as compared to the parent compound (88), thus giving more favorable properties to the compound to improve its flux across a lipoidal barrier. In another study with full-thickness hairless mouse skin (89), it was found that among the three prodrug esters studied, the acetyl ester, butyl ester, and isobutyl ester, that the acetyl ester of buprenorphine enhanced the flux and permeation of buprenorphine. However, when tested in human skin in vitro, none of the 3-alkyl ester prodrugs enhanced the permeation of buprenorphine despite their decreased crystallinity (90). This may be due to the rate-limited diffusion of the prodrugs in the viable tissue as a result of their very high octanol/water partition coefficients. Recently, a transdermal matrix patch formulation of buprenorphine (Transtec®) has become available outside USA. This patch releases the drug at 35, 52.5, and 70 μg/h over a 72-h period (91). The minimum effective therapeutic plasma concentration of buprenorphine (100 pg/ml) after application of a single 35 or 70 μg/h patch was reached at 21 and 11 h, respectively.

38.3 Conclusion

Since transdermal products offer a variety of significant clinical benefits over other dosage forms, the transdermal drug delivery market for opioid agents is growing. Opportunities for improved transdermal drug delivery for opioid agents have been greatly expanding through various novel investigational techniques including prodrugs, codrugs, MNs, and other new formulation technologies.

References

1. Friedman JD, Dello Buono FA. Opioid antagonists in the treatment of opioid-induced constipation and pruritus. Ann Pharmacother 2001;35:85–91.
2. David S, Lancaster T, Stead LF. Opioid antagonists for smoking cessation. The Cochrane Database of Systematic Reviews 2001, Issue 3. Art. No.: CD003086. DOI: 10.1002/14651858.CD003086.
3. Ngai H, Berkowitz BA, Yang JC, Hempstead J, Spector S. Pharmacokinetics of naloxone in rats and in man: basis for its potency and short duration of action. Anesthesiology 1976;44:398–401.
4. Bradberryand JC, Raebel MA. Continuous infusion of naloxone in the treatment of narcotic overdose. Drug Intell Clin Pharm 1981;15:945–950.
5. Gourlayand K, Coulthard K. The role of naloxone infusions in the treatment of overdoses of long half-life narcotic agonists: application to nor-methadone. Br J Clin Pharmacol 1983; 15:269–271.
6. Aungst J, Rogers NJ, Shefter E. Enhancement of naloxone penetration through human skin in vitro using fatty acids, fatty alcohols, surfactants, sulfoxides and amides. Int J Pharm 1986; 33:225–234.
7. Aungst J, Blake JA, and Hussain MA. Contributions of drug solubilization, partitioning, barrier disruption, and solvent permeation to the enhancement of skin permeation of various compounds with fatty acids and amines. Pharm Res 1990;7:712–718.
8. Panchagnula R, Salve PS, Thomas NS, Jain AK, Ramarao P. Transdermal delivery of naloxone: effect of water, propylene glycol, ethanol and their binary combinations on permeation through rat skin. Int J Pharm 2001;219:95–105.
9. Mason J, Ritvo EC, Morgan RO, Salvato FR, Goldberg G, Welch B, Mantero-Atienza E. A double-blind, placebo-controlled pilot study to evaluate the efficacy and safety of oral nalmefene HCl for alcohol dependence. Alcohol Clin Exp Res 1994;18:1162–1167.
10. Mason J, Salvato FR, Williams LD, Ritvo EC, Cutler RB. A double-blind, placebo-controlled study of oral nalmefene for alcohol dependence. Arch Gen Psychiatry 1999;56:719–724.
11. Michel ME, Bolger G, Weissman BA. Binding of a new opiate antagonist, nalmefene, to rat brain membranes. Methods Find Exp Clin Pharmacol 1985;7:175–177.
12. Hamilton RJ, Olmedo RE, Shah S, Hung OL, Howland MA, Perrone J, Nelson LS, Lewin NL, Hoffman RS. Complications of ultrarapid opioid detoxification with subcutaneous naltrexone pellets. Acad Emerg Med 2002;9:63–68.
13. Drobes DJ, Anton RF, Thomas SE, Voronin K. A clinical laboratory paradigm for evaluating medication effects on alcohol consumption: naltrexone and nalmefene. Neuropsychopharmacology 2003;28:755–764.
14. Costantini LC, Kleppner SR, McDonough J, Azar MR, Patel R. Implantable technology for long-term delivery of nalmefene for treatment of alcoholism. Int J Pharm 2004;283:35–44.
15. Aungst B, Di Luccio, RC. Transdermal delivery of opioids. Eur Pat Appl. (1986), 25 pp.
16. Shevchuk I, Reidenberg, B. Transdermal dosage forms comprising a drug and a salt and free-base form of an adverse agent. PCT Int Appl 2004; 51.

17. Crabtree BL. Review of naltrexone, a long acting opiate antagonist. Clin Pharm 1984;3: 273–280.
18. Gonzalez JP, Brogden RN. Naltrexone: a review of its pharmacodynamic and pharmacokinetic properties and therapeutic efficacy in the management of opioid dependence. Drugs 1988;35: 192–213.
19. Volpicelli JR, Alterman AI, Hayashida M. NTX in the treatment of alcohol dependence. Arch Gen Psychiatry 1992;49:876–880.
20. Terenius L. Rational treatment of addiction. Curr Opin Chem Biol 1998;2:541–547.
21. Meyer MC, Straughn AB, Lo MW, Schary WL, Whitney CC. Bioequivalence, dose-proportionality, and pharmacokinetics of naltrexone after oral administration. J Clin Psychiatry 1984;45:15–19.
22. Wall M, Brine DR, Perez RM. Metabolism and disposition of naltrexone in man after oral and intravenous administration. Drug Metab Dispos 1981;9:369–375.
23. Kranzler HR, Lowe VM, Kirk JV. Naltrexone vs nefazodone for treatment of alcohol dependence. A placebo controlled trial. Neuropsychopharmacology 2000;22:493–503.
24. Volpicelli JR, Rhines KC, Rhines JS, Volpicelli LA, Alterman AL, O'Brien CP. Naltrexone and alcohol dependence. Role of subject compliance. Arch Gen Psychiatry 1997;54:737–742.
25. Verebey K. The clinical pharmacology of naltrexone: pharmacology and pharmacodynamics. NIDA Res Monogr 1980;28:147–158.
26. Croop RS, Faukner EB, and Labriola DF. The safety profile of naltrexone in the treatment of alcoholism. Results from the multicentre usage study. The naltrexone usage group study. Arch Gen Psychiatry 1997;54:1130–1135.
27. King AC, Volpicelli JR, Gunduz M, O'Brien CP, Kreek MJ. Naltrexone biotransformation and incidence of subjective side effects: a preliminary study. Alcohol Clin Exp Res 1997;21:906–909.
28. Comer SD, Sullivan MA, Yu E, Rothenberg JL, Kleber HD, Kampman K, Dackis C, O'Brien CP. Injectable, sustained-release naltrexone for the treatment of opioid dependence: a randomized, placebo-controlled trial. Arch Gen Psychiatry 2006;63:210–218.
29. Liu Y, Sunderland VB, O'Neil AG. In vitro and in vivo release of naltrexone from biodegradable depot systems. Drug Dev Ind Pharm 2006;32:85–94.
30. Galloway GP, Koch M, Cello R, Smith DE. Pharmacokinetics, safety, and tolerability of a depot formulation of naltrexone in alcoholics: an open-label trial. BMC Psychiatry 2005;5:18.
31. Chen YL, Chun LL, Enscore DJ. Transdermal therapeutic systems for the administration of naloxone, naltrexone, and nalbuphine. U.S. Patent No. 4,573,995 (March 4, 1986).
32. Vereby K, Volavka J, Mule SJ, Resnick RB. Naltrexone: disposition, metabolism and effects after acute and chronic dosing. Clin Pharmacol Ther 1976;20:315–328.
33. Hussain MA, Koval CA, Myers MJ, Shami EG, Shefter E. Improvement of the oral bioavailability of naltrexone in dogs. J Pharm Sci 1987;76:356–358.
34. Hussain MA, Aungst BJ, Koval CA, Shefter E. Improved buccal delivery of opioid analgesics and antagonists with bitterless prodrugs. Pharm Res 1988;5:615–618.
35. Stinchcomb AL, Swaan PW, Ekabo O, Harris KK, Browe J, Hammell DC, Cooperman TA, Pearsall M. Straight-chain naltrexone ester prodrugs: diffusion and concurrent esterase biotransformation in human skin. J Pharm Sci 2002;91:2571–2578.
36. Hammell DC, Hamad M, Vaddi HK, Crooks PA, Stinchcomb AL. A duplex "Gemini" prodrug of naltrexone for transdermal delivery. J Control Release 2004;97:283–290.
37. Rautio J, Nevalainen T, Taipale H, Vepsäläinen J, Gynther J, Pedersen T, Järvinen T, Synthesis and in vitro evaluation of aminoacyloxyalkyl esters of 2-(6-methoxy-2-naphthyl) propionic acid as novel naproxen prodrugs for dermal delivery. Pharm Res 1999;16:1172–1178.
38. Rossi L, Dominici S, Serafini S, Casabianca A, Cerasi A, Chiarantini L, Celeste AG, Cappellacci L, Franchetti P, Grifantini M, Magnani M. Pharmacokinetic and antiretroviral activity in mice of oral [P1,P2-bis[2-(adenin-9-yl)ethoxymethyl] phosphonate], a prodrug of 9-(2-phosphonylmethoxyethyl) adenine. J Antimicrob Chemother 2002;50:365–374.
39. Pillai O, Hamad MO, Crooks PA, Stinchcomb AL. Physicochemical evaluation, in vitro human skin diffusion, and concurrent biotransformation of 3-O-alkyl carbonate prodrugs of naltrexone. Pharm Res 2004;21:1146–1152.

40. Vaddi HK, Hamad MO, Chen J, Banks SL, Crooks PA, Stinchcomb AL. Human skin permeation of branched-chain 3–0-alkyl ester and carbonate prodrugs of naltrexone. Pharm Res 2005;22:758–765.
41. Hammell DC, Stolarczyk EI, Klausner M, Hamad MO, Crooks PA, Stinchcomb AL. Bioconversion of naltrexone and its 3-O-alkyl-ester prodrugs in a human skin equivalent. J Pharm Sci 2005;94:828–836.
42. Valiveti S, Hammell DC, Paudel KS, Hamad MO, Crooks PA, Stinchcomb AL. In vivo evaluation of 3-O-alkyl ester transdermal prodrugs of naltrexone in hairless guinea pigs. J Control Release 2005;102:509–520.
43. Valiveti S, Paudel KS, Hammell DC, Hamad MO, Chen J, Crooks PA, Stinchcomb AL. In vitro/in vivo correlation of transdermal naltrexone prodrugs in hairless guinea pigs. Pharm Res 2005;22:981–989.
44. Nalluri BN, Milligan C, Chen J, Crooks PA, Stinchcomb AL. In vitro release studies on matrix type transdermal drug delivery systems of naltrexone and its acetyl prodrug. Drug Dev Ind Pharm 2005;31:871–877.
45. Banks S, Pinninti RR, Gill HS, Prausnitz MR, Stinchcomb AL. In Vitro Permeation Studies of Naltrexone Base and Hydrochloride with Microneedle-Treated Hairless Guinea Pig Skin. Controlled Release Society. 2005: Miami, FL. USA.
46. Kaushik S, Hord AH, Denson DD, McAllister DV, Smitrs S, Allen MG, Prausnitz MR. Lack of pain associated with microfabricated microneedles. Anesth Analg 2001;92:502–504.
47. Cone EJ, Gorodetzky CW, Yeh SY. The urinary excretion profile of naltrexone and metabolites in man. Drug Metab Dispos 1974;2:506–512.
48. Reuning RH, Malspeis L, Frank S, Notari RE. Testing of drug delivery system for use in the treatment of narcotic addiction. Natl Inst Drug Abuse Res Monogr Ser 1975;4:43–45.
49. Ferrari A, Bertolotti M, Dell'Utri A, Avico U, Sternieri E. Serum time course of naltrexone and 6 beta-naltrexol levels during long-term treatment in drug addicts. Drug Alcohol Depend 1998;52:211–220.
50. Rukstalis M, Stromberg MF, O'Brien CP, Volpicelli JR. 6-b-Naltrexol reduces alcohol consumption in rats. Alcohol Clin Exp Res 2000;24:1593–1596.
51. McCaul ME, Wand GS, Rohde C, Lee SM. Serum 6-beta-naltrexol levels are related to alcohol responses in heavy drinkers. Alcohol Clin Exp Res 2000;24:1385–1391.
52. Davis RD, Nelson WL. Isothiocyanate-substituted benzyl ether opioid receptor ligands derived from 6-beta-naltrexol. J Med Chem 1995;38:570–579.
53. Fujimoto JM, Roerig S, Wang RI, Chatterjie N, Inturrisi CE. Narcotic antagonist activity of several metabolites of naloxone and naltrexone tested in morphine dependent mice (38558). Proc Soc Exp Biol Med 1975;148:443–448.
54. Blumberg H, Ikeda C. Comparison of naltrexone and 6-b-naltrexol for narcotic antagonist action in rats and mice. Fed Proc 1976;35:469.
55. Porter SJ, Somogyi AA, White JM. In vivo and in vitro potency studies of 6-b-naltrexol, the major human metabolite of naltrexone. Addict Biol 2002;7:219–225.
56. Brewer C. Serum naltrexone and 6-beta-naltrexol levels from naltrexone implants can block very large amounts of heroin: a report of two cases. Addict Biol 2002;7:321–323.
57. Stromberg MF, Rukstalis MR, Scott AM, Volpicelli JR,O'Brien CP. A comparison of the effects of 6-b-naltrexol and naltrexone on the consumption of ethanol or sucrose using a limited-access procedure in rats. Pharmacol Biochem Behav 2002;72:483–490.
58. McCaul M, Sullivan J, Mumford G, Quigley J. 6-beta-naltrexol level predicts alcohol relapse (abstract). Alcohol Clin Exp Res 1997;21:32A.
59. O'Malley SS, Jaffe AJ, Chang G, Schottenfeld RS, Meyer RE, Rounsaville B. Naltrexone and copying skills therapy for alcohol dependence. A controlled study. Arch Gen Psychiatry 1992;49:881–887.
60. Paudel KS, Nalluri BN, Hammell DC, Valiveti S, Kiptoo P, Hamad MO, Crooks PA, Stinchcomb AL. Transdermal delivery of naltrexone and its active metabolite 6-beta-naltrexol in human skin in vitro and guinea pigs in vivo. J Pharm Sci 2005;94:1965–75.

61. Johnston JA, Fiedler-Kelly J, Glover ED, Sachs DP, Grasela TH, DeVeaugh-Geiss J. Relationship between drug exposure and the efficacy and safety of bupropion sustained release for smoking cessation. Nicotine Tob Res 2001;3: 131–140.
62. Schroeder DH. Metabolism and kinetics of bupropion. J Clin Psychiatry 1983;44:79–81.
63. Belson MG, Kelley TR. Bupropion exposures: clinical manifestations and medical outcome. J Emerg Med 2002;23:223–230.
64. Kiptoo PK, Hamad MO, Crooks PA, Stinchcomb AL. Enhancement of transdermal delivery of 6-β-naltrexol via a codrug linked to hydroxybupropion. J Control Release 2006;113:137–145.
65. Barber D. The physiology and pharmacology of pain: a review of opioids. J Perianesth Nurs 1997;12:95–99.
66. Sittl R, Nuijten M, Nautrup BP. Changes in the prescribed daily doses of transdermal fentanyl and transdermal buprenorphine during treatment of patients with cancer and noncancer pain in Germany: results of a retrospective cohort study. Clin Ther 2005;27:1022–1031.
67. Johnson RE, Fudala PJ, Payne R. Buprenorphine: considerations for pain management. J Pain and Symptom Management 2005;29:297–326.
68. Rieg-Falson F, Huertas L, Blouquin P, Conrath G, Couarraze G. Characterization of the enhancing effect of a vehicle in a transdermal system. Drug Dev Ind Pharm 1989;15:2393–2406.
69. Monti D, Giannelli R, Chetoni P, Burgalassi S. Comparison of the effect of ultrasound and of chemical enhancers on transdermal permeation of caffeine and morphine through hairless mouse skin in vitro. Int J Pharm 2001;229:131–137.
70. Morimoto Y, Wada Y, Seki T, Sugibayashi K. In-vitro skin permeation of morphine hydrochloride during the finite application of penetration-enhancing system containing water, ethanol and l-menthol. Biol Pharm Bull 2002;25:134–136.
71. Bundgaard H, Christrup L, Drustrup J, Fullerton A, Nicklasson M. Transdermal delivery of prodrug derivatives of morphine. PCT Int Appl 1992;18 pp.
72. Maury P, Bevan B, Teillaud E, Herrenknecht C, Falson-Rieg F, Couarraze G. In-vitro model of the transdermal transport of morphine hydrochloride by iontophoresis. Congr Int Technol Pharm 1989;3:304–313.
73. Gentil C, Mikler C, Teillaud E. In-vitro evaluation of transdermal iontophoretic delivery of morphine hydrochloride across animal and human skin. Proceedings of the International Symposium on Controlled Release of Bioactive Materials 1994.
74. Grond S, Radbruch L, Lehmann KA. Clinical pharmacokinetics of transdermal opioids: focus on transdermal fentanyl. Clin Pharm 2000;38:59–89.
75. Ashburn MA, Stephen RL, Ackerman E, Petelenz TJ, Hare B, Pace NL, Hofman AA. Iontophoteric delivery of morphine for postoperative analgesia. J Pain Symptom Manage 1992; 7:27–33.
76. Westerling D, Hoglund P, Lundin S, Svedman P. Transdermal administration of morphine to healthy subjects. Br J Clin Pharmacol 1994;37:571–576.
77. Nishihara Y, Hirano K, Yamada H, Takehara M. Transdermal preparations containing morphines and monoglycerides. Jpn Kokai Tokkyo Koho 1990.
78. Shevchuk I, Reidenberg B. Transdermal dosage forms comprising a drug and a salt and free-base form of an adverse agent. PCT Int Appl 2004;51 pp.
79. Hashimoto M, Fukuda M, Azuma M. Transdermal preparations of morphine hydrochloride or sulfate. Jpn Kokai Tokkyo Koho 1994.
80. Nishimuro S, Hanyu H, Okada Y, Shindo C. Transdermal preparations containing basic drugs in microemulsions. Jpn Kokai Tokkyo Koho 2001.
81. Duragesic® (fentanyl transdermal system). ALZA Corp. Feb. (2005) <http://www.duragesic.com/active/janus/en_US/assets/common/company/pi/duragesic.pdf>.
82. Ross JR, Quigley C. Trasdermal fentanyl: informed prescribing is essential. Eur J Pain 2003; 7:481–483.
83. Reynolds L, Rauck R, Webster L, DuPen S, Heinze E, Portenoy R, Katz N, Charapata S, Wallace M, Fisher DM. Relative analgesic potency of fentanyl and sufentanil during intermediate-term infusions in patients after long-term opioid treatment for chronic pain. Pain 2004;110:182–188.

84. Transdermal sufentanil patch. *Durtec*. May. (2006) <http://www.durect.com/wt/durect/page_name/trans_sufentanil>.
85. Downing JW, Leary WP, White ES. Buprenorphine: a new potent long-acting synthetic analgesic. Comparison with morphine. Br J Anaesth 1977;49:251–255.
86. Gilman AG, Goodman LS, Rall TW, Murad F. In Goodman and Gilman's The pharmacological basis of Therapeutics, Gilman AG, Goodman LS (eds.), 1985, Macmillan Publishing Company, New York, pp. 523–524.
87. Johnson RE, Jaffe JH, Fudala PJ. A controlled trial of buprenorphine treatment for opioid dependence. JAMA 1992;267:2750–2755.
88. Stinchcomb AL, Dua R, Paliwal A, Woodard RW, Flynn GL. A solubility and related physicochemical property comparison of buprenorphine and its 3-alkyl esters. Pharm Res 1995;12:1526–1529.
89. Imoto H, Zhou Z, Stinchcomb AL, Flynn GL. Transdermal prodrug concepts: permeation of buprenorphine and its alkyl esters through hairless mouse skin and influence of vehicles. Biol Pharm Bull 1996;19:263–267.
90. Stinchcomb AL, Paliwal A, Dua R, Imoto H, Woodard RW, Flynn GL. Permeation of buprenorphine and its 3-alkyl-ester prodrugs through human skin. Pharm Res 1996;13:1519–1523.
91. Evans HC and Easthope SE. Transdermal Buprenorphine. Drugs 2003;63:1999–2010.

Chapter 39
Intranasal Naloxone for Treatment of Opioid Overdose

Anne-Maree Kelly, Debra Kerr, and Paul Dietze

Abstract In theory, intranasal (IN) naloxone should be effective and practical for the treatment of acute opioid overdose. To date, evaluation of its effectiveness has been limited, but what is known is promising with reports that it is effective and safe, can reduce the requirement for injected treatments and has comparable times to recovery with other routes of administration. Unfortunately, naloxone as it is currently manufactured is not ideal for IN administration, as effective doses require drug volumes in excess of recommended volumes for adequate nasal absorption. Further well-designed research is needed to confirm IN naloxone's effectiveness, adverse event profile and utility. If effectiveness and safety can be confirmed, wider distribution of naloxone treatment to community workers, family and peers may be feasible, with the potential to save lives.

Keywords: Naloxone; Opioid; Overdose; Intranasal

39.1 Introduction

Fatal and non-fatal opioid overdose have been widely studied in the context of heroin use. Heroin users are at significant risk of mortality and morbidity compared to other groups in the community – primarily from overdose, which is the leading cause of death among heroin users in most jurisdictions (1).

Primarily related to the injection of heroin (2, 3), overdose is typically characterized by loss of consciousness and respiratory suppression that ultimately leads to respiratory and subsequently cardiac arrest (4). Most heroin overdose deaths occur a considerable time after injection (5) meaning that there is opportunity for response and intervention. Full recovery is possible if hypoxia is reversed before organ damage has occurred. If treatment is delayed and hypoxia is prolonged a range of complications

A.-M. Kelly (✉), D. Kerr, and P. Dietze
Joseph Epstein Centre for Emergency Medicine Research, Sunshine Hospital, St Albans, Victoria 3021, Australia
e-mail: Anne-Maree.Kelly@wh.org.au

are possible, including hypoxic brain injury, rhabdomyolysis, cognitive impairment, pulmonary oedema and pulmonary aspiration (1). In severe cases, death may occur.

While the most widely recognized opioid overdose is of heroin associated with illicit drug-taking, other opioids such as morphine, fentanyl, oxycodone, methadone, buprenorphene and pethidine (whether prescribed or used illicitly) can also result in acute respiratory depression and death if taken in excess. However, popularity and availability of these opioid agents for illicit use are less common.

Risk factors for opioid overdose and adverse outcomes include poly-drug use (particularly combined use with benzodiazepines or alcohol) (6, 7), injecting as opposed to non-parenteral administration (2) and mental health issues (8). Recommencement of 'typical' use after conditions of reduced tolerance (e.g. as a result of imprisonment or detoxification), is known to result in increased overdose risk (9) and there is evidence of a dose–response effect of the amount of heroin used on overdose risk (10). Fatal outcome is more likely when the heroin user is alone (11).

Naloxone, as an adjunct and not as an alternative to support by oxygenation (usually in the form of rescue ventilation), has been used to reverse the effects of opioid overdose since the late 1960s. It is a pure opioid antagonist that challenges receptors of the central nervous system (12). When administered to patients who have not consumed opiates, it exerts little or no pharmacological effect (12). It is rapidly effective (within 1 to 2 min of intravenous [IV] administration) and has a half-life between 30 and 80 min (12). The rate of serious events (seizure, pulmonary oedema and asystole) has been reported as being between 0.3% and 1.6% (13–15). Patients are more likely to experience signs and symptoms of withdrawal, rather than adverse drug reaction, including confusion, headache, nausea or vomiting, aggressiveness, tachycardia, sweating and tremor (12, 13). Initially its use was parenteral (by intramuscular [IM] or IV injection) and confined to the hospital environment, but more recently availability and use has been extended within the community to ambulance officers/paramedics (16) and peers (17) with reported success.

Unfortunately, the parenteral routes of administration have some problems that must be weighed against naloxone's effectiveness. The IV route requires establishment of IV access that can be difficult in some client populations (in particular injecting drug users) and lead to delays to drug administration. Both the IV and IM routes require use of a needle and syringe. This carries a small, but real, risk of needlestick injury to the treating person that varies according to the level of training and clinician experience. As a significant proportion of heroin users are infected with blood-borne viruses (BBV) such as hepatitis C and HIV (18, 19), there is a risk of transmission of these viruses to the treating person. This latter risk may be a barrier to wide availability of these treatments in the community (20). Also, location in which treatment occurs can be less than ideal with limited space and lighting, increasing the complexity of cannula insertion.

To overcome these problems and, in particular, avoid the risk of BBV transmission, researchers have sought alternative routes for administration of naloxone. There is increasing evidence that the IN route may address these concerns while maintaining acceptable effectiveness.

39.2 Pharmacological Basis for IN Use

The IN route is an attractive one for administration of suitable drugs. The nose has a rich vascular plexus affording ready access to the bloodstream (21). It is also easy and convenient, painless and does not require the use of needles, thus obviating the risk of needlestick injury. This is a particularly important issue in cramped spaces where acute opioid overdoses often occur such as toilet cubicles, stairwells and other spaces hidden from public view (22).

Nasal absorption is dependent on drug factors (such as molecular size, pH, concentration/volume required and formulation vehicle), anatomical factors (such as nasal blockage and mucosal blood flow) and mechanical factors (such as site and method of administration) (23). Available evidence suggests that atomization of the drug for IN administration [e.g. using a commercial atomization device such as the Mucosal Atomizer Device (23)] is superior to administration using a spray or drops (23, 24).

The pharmacokinetics of naloxone make it suitable for IN administration; however, the commercially available formulations (made for IV and IM use) are of low concentrations [0.4–1 mg/ml (25–27)]. An initial dose of 1.6–2 mg, as directed in approved paramedic practice guidelines for suspected heroin overdose (28, 29), would result in volumes between 2 and 5 ml. The recommended maximum volume per nostril is 0.5–1 ml (23), and absorption and effectiveness are impaired by excess.

Initial investigation of naloxone administration by the IN route appeared in the literature in 1984 (30). Pharmacokinetics of naloxone were compared after IN and IV administration in rats. The IN route had 100% bioavailability, the same half life as the IV route (40–45 min) and achieved peak plasma concentrations within 3 min (30). In small studies from the field of drug addiction, IN naloxone was shown to be effective in identifying opioid dependence (31, 32).

39.3 The Evidence Regarding Use in Opioid Overdose Emergencies

39.3.1 Effectiveness

The first prehospital use of IN naloxone was reported in a case series by Barton et al. (33). The report describes findings of one month's experience using IN naloxone administered by paramedics in Denver, USA. Naloxone was administered as a 2-mg dose (half into each nostril, concentration 1 mg/mL) via a commercial mucosal atomization device. Of 30 patients treated for suspected opiate overdose in the month 11 (36.7%) responded to naloxone by any route (IV or IN). Of these, 91% (10/11) responded to IN naloxone alone with an average response time of 3.4 min (range: 2–6 min). Seven of the naloxone responders (7/11: 64%) did not require IV access in the prehospital setting. No comparison with alternative routes was attempted and the sample was small.

Hospital treatment of acute opioid overdose by IN naloxone was reported in a small case series (six patients) treated in an Australian emergency department (34). All patients had return of adequate spontaneous respiration within 2 min of IN naloxone administration, with a median response time of 50 s. Doses used ranged from 0.8 to 2 mg, were at the treating doctor's discretion and were administered as IN drops. IN administration was not compared with alternative modes and again the sample is small.

There has only been one randomized clinical trial comparing the effectiveness of IN naloxone to alternative administration routes (25). This prospective, unblinded study, conducted in the prehospital setting involved patients who required treatment with naloxone for suspected heroin overdose in Melbourne, Australia. To be eligible for entry patients had to have respirations less than ten per minute and be unrousable. Participants were randomized to receive 2 mg of naloxone by the IN or IM route, using a 0.4-mg/mL solution. The study enrolled 155 clients (71 received IM and 84 IN naloxone). Seventy-four per cent (62/84) of patients who received IN naloxone recovered without requiring a further dose of naloxone. Patients who received IM naloxone had slightly earlier achievement of adequate spontaneous ventilation (5 min [95% CI 4–6 min] vs 7 min [95% CI 6–8 min], $p = 0.006$). Time to adequate conscious state was not significantly different between the groups. A major limitation of this study was the preparation of naloxone that required applying 2.5 ml per nostril (2 mg in 5 mL), far exceeding recommendations of 0.5 to 1 mL per nostril for IN medication administration (23). In addition, the study was unblinded. Blinded treatment options would be more difficult to conduct for a comparison study with the additional complexities of prehospital emergency care.

These findings are supported by a case series of 95 patients who received IN naloxone over a 6-month period in the prehospital setting in Denver, Colorado (26). Participants were administered 2 mg IN naloxone prior to IV access followed by 2 mg IV naloxone. That study reported that 52 patients responded to naloxone by either IN or IV administration, of whom 43 (83%) responded to IN naloxone alone. Conclusions regarding the effectiveness of IN naloxone could be questioned however as all participants were administered IV naloxone as standard treatment after receiving IN naloxone. It is possible that IN naloxone may not have had time to take effect prior to IV naloxone administration.

Finally, the effectiveness of IN naloxone was also evaluated in a retrospective case review (35). This was a before-and-after study that evaluated the introduction of IN naloxone into prehospital protocols in California. One hundred fifty-four patients with suspected narcotic overdose were given naloxone in the field (104 IV [before] and 50 IN [after]). More patients who received IN naloxone received a subsequent dose of naloxone (18% IM vs 34% IN, $p = 0.05$), and time to adequate clinical response (GCS > 6 or increase in respiratory rate) was longer for the IN group (13 vs 8 min, $p = 0.02$). The time from initial patient contact to adequate response was however not different between the IN and IV groups (20.2 vs 20.7 min, $p = 0.9$), which probably reflects the difficulty of IV access in these patients. This study is limited by reliance on accurate documentation by paramedics in the field (particularly of times) and absence of reporting of IN naloxone dose, concentration and administration method.

In summary, while available data suggests that IN naloxone is effective, studies to date have failed to show superiority when compared with IM and IV routes and have been under-powered for equivalency. In addition, some of the endpoints examined have not been robust. Future studies should ensure samples have adequate power and that highly relevant endpoints such as total time from arrival at scene to recovery, adverse effects and proportion of cases where needles are avoided are reported. As previously noted, the preparation of naloxone available at present is less than ideal with volumes required far exceeding recommended amounts for IN administration. Future studies using more concentrated naloxone are needed.

39.3.2 Adverse Events

Adverse event profiling after IN naloxone administration has been limited to a single randomized clinical trial by Kelly et al. (25). In that study there were no reports of serious adverse events. Signs and symptoms experienced by study participants included agitation and/or irritation (2/84, 2.4%), nausea and/or vomiting (6/84, 7.1%), tremor (1/84, 1.2%) and sweating (1/84, 1.2%). Adverse events occurred more often in the group who received naloxone by injection (21% [IM] vs 12% [IN]), but this did not reach statistical significance.

39.3.3 Other Benefits

Non-client benefits from use of the IN route for naloxone administration can be divided into reduced risk of transmission of blood-borne infection to the person administering the drug, improved utility and reduction in aggressive behaviour after treatment.

Typically, clients treated for suspected opioid overdose are injecting drug users. The prevalence of BBV such as HIV and Hepatitis B and C are high in this population (18, 19). The treatment of such clients presents safety issues for those administering injected drugs because of the risk of needlestick injuries, particularly if treated in cramped environments. This increases the complexity of risk and exposure to needlestick injury. Even if viral transmission does not occur, needlestick injury of itself creates distress and turmoil for the affected person, families and work colleagues for months after the incident, as it takes months to establish if infection has occurred (36). In addition, medications for HIV prophylaxis are not well tolerated, resulting in considerable staff absence due to iatrogenic side effects (37). Administration by the IN route eliminates risk of needlestick injury.

Injected administration of naloxone (either IV or IM) requires training and specialized equipment. In particular, IV administration requires expert skills as many

IV drug users have damaged veins making cannula insertion quite difficult and time consuming. Regarding equipment, in addition to syringes and needles and training in appropriate techniques, the safe disposal of used syringes and needles is a major issue. These issues can limit the range of people who are able or willing to administer naloxone to suspected opioid overdose victims. IN administration is a simple treatment option that could be extended to non-healthcare settings.

An additional unexpected advantage of the IN route has been suggested by one of the research studies. Kelly et al. (25) reported that clients who received IN naloxone showed lower rates of aggression on emergence than those who received the drug intramuscularly (14% vs 2%). Post emergence aggression and violence is a significant issue and a risk to carers, so any reduction in this is welcome.

39.3.4 Gaps in the Evidence

Research investigating IN naloxone administration for opioid overdose has been limited, with few comparative studies evaluating alternative doses, drug formulations and delivery devices. Further well-designed research is needed to confirm effectiveness, adverse event profiling and clinical utility.

39.4 Discussion

39.4.1 Current Place in Treatment

Opioid overdose remains a significant cause of mortality and morbidity. Full recovery is possible if treatment is provided promptly. Conversely, delay can result in death or permanent disability. Fortunately, most heroin users report having witnessed and responded to others' heroin overdoses, highlighting again the possibility for intervention that could be peer-led (38).

The need for action has seen the development of initiatives aimed at heroin overdose prevention (39). These initiatives range from systemic approaches (e.g. supervised injecting facilities), the provision of overdose response services as a supplement to emergency treatment by acute health services and educative strategies designed to improve knowledge of overdose risk and appropriate response amongst heroin users and their immediate contacts (40).

In most places, access to naloxone is via health professionals, notably ambulance services and emergency departments. A recognized barrier to seeking assistance from emergency services is fear that police will be involved (11). Responding to this, some jurisdictions have implemented policy changes to ensure that police do not regularly attend overdoses (40). Nevertheless, the issue of police involvement is entirely dependent upon jurisdictional practice (41) and some jurisdictions continue to routinely send police to overdose situations in spite of the evidence that this may act as a barrier to calling for emergency services at witnessed overdoses.

It is generally accepted that the administration of injected naloxone in the out-of-hospital setting by ambulance paramedics is safe and effective. Indeed, with sufficient doses, heroin overdose can be treated by paramedics without the need for further treatment in hospital (3, 16, 42, 43). It is unclear where IN administration fits into current treatment practices. There are reports of naloxone administration by the IN route in some jurisdictions (26, 35), however use of this method is not widespread. We estimate that only a small proportion of all ambulance services are using IN naloxone as the preferred method of delivery at this time.

39.4.2 Potential Future Place in Treatment Systems

While naloxone for opioid overdose is typically administered by medically trained personnel, several other professional groups come into contact with heroin users in overdose situations as part of their day-to-day work. In addition, concerned others such as family and non-heroin-using friends may have the opportunity to administer life-saving measures such as resuscitation (with or without the addition of naloxone) in an effort to prevent overdose-related harm. Given its ease of use, lack of special equipment requirements and ease of disposal, an IN preparation of naloxone would be well suited for use by community outreach workers, non-medical emergency services personnel and family and friends.

Recently, in response to barriers to use of emergency services such as response time, fear of police involvement and fear of stigma, discrimination and identification that applies to the use of health services more broadly (44), programs have been developed in which naloxone is provided for peer administration (17). Such programs are typically implemented in combination with training on the recognition of overdose signs and symptoms and management strategies (45). Available data suggests that such programs would be well received among heroin users (46) as well as those who may be involved in the prescription of the drug in this context (47).

In some countries, injected naloxone has been made available to heroin users and community members. For example, in Italy naloxone is available from pharmacies over-the-counter, meaning that heroin users can be encouraged to purchase it for use in emergency situations (40). In other countries naloxone has been made available primarily to peers through distinct programs (45, 49). Case series data from some of these programs has shown that peers have been able to recognize heroin overdose, bring about successful resuscitation with naloxone and administer the drug in appropriate circumstances (17). One group claims that 'around 200 lives' have been saved by the naloxone distribution program operating in Chicago (49). Nevertheless, the evidence to date regarding peer programs is weak, as little is known about which client groups benefit for its availability, training and legal requirements, the extent of follow-up overall and any follow-up bias among cases of documented peer-based naloxone administration (17).

Work is being undertaken to address some of the evidence gaps. A UK pilot program has been established to distribute naloxone to heroin users during maintenance treatment or following discharge from inpatient detoxification, with negotiations underway to distribute the drug following residential rehabilitation (J. Strang, personal communication, 2006). Preliminary work has also been undertaken to establish a large randomized controlled trial of the efficacy of naloxone provision to heroin-using prisoners as part of an immediate post-release program (T. Butler, personal communication, 2005).

Notwithstanding the quality of the evidence to date, if effective, IN naloxone would be preferable to the injected form for peer use because of ease of training and use and lack of requirement for injecting equipment.

The utility of IN naloxone for non-medically-trained providers is currently limited by the available delivery devices and the absence of any clear evidence of equal effectiveness with injected forms. As noted above, the issues of absorption and naloxone concentration are yet to be resolved. Further, the devices currently available have a level of complexity that is not well suited to use in emergency situations by non-professionals. Clearly, while IN administration of naloxone has considerable promise, further work needs to be undertaken in order to establish appropriate dosage and concentration as well as a simpler delivery device (e.g. aerosol spray).

39.4.3 Unresolved Issues

The distribution of naloxone to peers and community members for administration to heroin users in overdose poses legal and practical challenges that have been well documented (17, 48). The main legal impediment concerns the provision of a drug for administration to a third party. However, this situation has been overcome with respect to other drugs used in life-threatening situations (e.g. epinephrine for anaphylaxis and glucagon for hypoglycaemia). The primary impediment to the wider distribution of naloxone appears to be reluctance on the part of policymakers to implement this strategy. A reason given is that wider availability of the antidote to heroin might promote heroin's use, although there is no evidence to support this view (17). An effective way of influencing this is to establish a more extensive evidence base on the effectiveness or otherwise of wider availability of naloxone. For this reason, Lenton and Hargreaves (50) detailed the requirements for a trial addressing this issue. In spite of this work, no formal trial of naloxone distribution has been undertaken in Australia or, to our knowledge, in any other jurisdiction.

The wider distribution of naloxone also poses practical challenges, in particular how the drug itself is managed. The shelf-life of naloxone is typically between 18 and 24 months (depending on preparation), meaning that program participants need to monitor the drug's expiry date. The mechanisms for drug delivery as well as the dose distributed are fundamental issues that need to be resolved.

Concerns have also been raised about the possibility for adverse outcomes subsequent to revival (i.e. a return of respiratory depression after the effects of naloxone have worn off) and the potential for additional risk taking among heroin users who may feel 'safer' given the increased opportunity for overdose management (17). These concerns are not supported by any evidence.

Importantly, at present naloxone is not licensed for use via the IN route. For IN naloxone to become standard treatment, legislative approvals from local authorities will be required.

References

1. Warner-Smith M, Darke S, Lynskey M, Hall W. Heroin overdose: causes and consequences. *Addiction* 2001;96:1113–1125.
2. Brugal MT, Barrio G, De LF, Regidor E, Royuela L, Suelves JM. Factors associated with non-fatal heroin overdose: assessing the effect of frequency and route of heroin administration. *Addiction* 2002;97:319–327.
3. Sporer KA. Acute heroin overdose. *Ann Internal Med* 1999;130:584–590.
4. White J, Irvine R. Mechanisms of fatal opioid overdose. *Addiction* 1999;94:961–972.
5. Zador D, Sunjic S, Darke S. Heroin-related deaths in New South Wales, 1992: toxicological findings and circumstances. *Med J Aust* 1996;164:204–207.
6. Martyres RF, Clode D, Burns JM. Seeking drugs or seeking help? Escalating "doctor shopping": by young heroin users before fatal overdose. *Med J Aust* 2004;180:211–214.
7. Ruttenber AJ, Luke JL. Heroin-related deaths: new epidemiologic insights. *Science* 1984;226:14–20.
8. Rossow I, Lauritzen G. Balancing on the edge of death: suicide attempts and life-threatening overdoses among drug addicts. *Addiction* 1999;94:209–219.
9. Seaman SR, Brettle RP, Gore SM. Mortality from overdose among injecting drug users recently released from prison: database linkage study. *BMJ* 1998;316:426–428.
10. Dietze P, Jolley D, Fry C, Bammer G. Transient changes in behaviour lead to heroin overdose: results from a case-crossover study of non-fatal overdose. *Addiction* 2005;100:636–642.
11. Davidson PJ, Ochoa KC, Hahn JA, Evans JL, Moss AR. Witnessing heroin-related overdoses: the experiences of young injectors in San Francisco. *Addiction* 2002;97:1511–1516.
12. MIMS on line. Retrieved June 23, 2006, from http://mims.hcn.net.au.
13. Buajordet I, Naess AC, Jacobsen D, Brors O. Adverse events after naloxone treatment of episodes of suspected acute opioid overdose. *Eur J Emerg Med* 2004;11:19–23.
14. Yealy DM, Paris PM, Kaplan RM, Heller MB, Marini SE. The safety of prehospital naloxone administration by paramedics. *Ann Emerg Med* 1990;19:902–905.
15. Osterwalder JJ. Naloxone – for intoxications with intravenous heroin and heroin mixtures – harmless or hazardous? A prospective clinical study. *J Toxicol Clin Toxicol* 1996;34:409–416.
16. Sporer KA, Firestone J, Isaacs SM. Out-of-hospital treatment of opioid overdoses in an urban setting. *Acad Emerg Med* 1996;3:660–667.
17. Baca C, Grant K. Take-home naloxone to reduce heroin death. *Addiction* 2005;100:1823–1831.
18. Davoli M, Perucci CA, Rapiti E, Bargagli AM, D'Ippoliti D, Forastiere F, Abeni D. A persistent rise in mortality among injection drug users in Rome, 1980 through 1992. *Am J Public Health* 1997;87:851–853.
19. Crofts N, Jolley D, Kaldor J, van Beek I, Wodak A. Epidemiology of hepatitis C virus infection among injecting drug users in Australia. *J Epidemiol Community Health* 1997;51:692–697.
20. Fry C, Dietze P, Crofts N. Naloxone distribution: remembering hepatitis C transmission as an issue. *Addiction* 2000;95:1865–1866.
21. Chien YW, Su KSE, Chang SF. Anatomy and physiology of the nose. In Nasal Systemic Drug Delivery (pp. 1–26), Dekker, New York, 1989.

22. Dovey K, Fitzgerald J, Choi Y. Safety becomes danger: dilemmas of drug-use in public space. *Health Place* 2001;7:319–331.
23. Wolfe TR, Bernstone T. Intranasal drug delivery: an alternative to intravenous administration in selected emergency cases. *J Emerg Nurs* 2004;30:141–147.
24. Henry RJ, Ruano N, Casto D, Wolf RH. A pharmacokinetic study of midazolam in dogs: nasal drop vs. atomizer administration. *Pediatr Dent* 1998;20:321–326.
25. Kelly AM, Kerr D, Dietze P, Patrick I, Walker T. A randomised trial of intranasal versus intramuscular naloxone in prehospital treatment for suspected opioid overdose. *Med J Aust* 2005;182:24–27.
26. Barton ED, Colwell CB, Wolfe T, Fosnocht D, Gravitz C, Bryan T, Dunn W, Benson J, Bailey J. Efficacy of intranasal naloxone as a needless alternative for treatment of opioid overdose in the prehospital setting. *J Emerg Med* 2005;29:265–271.
27. Ashton H, Hassan Z. Best evidence topic report. Intranasal naloxone in suspected opioid overdose. *Emerg Med J* 2006;23:221–223.
28. Metropolitan Ambulance Service, Rural Ambulance Service [Victoria]. Clinical Practice Guideline. CPG: AO806. Management of overdose. Metropolitan Ambulance Service 2001.
29. Central California Emergency Medical Services. Emergency Medical Technician – Treatment Protocols. Altered mental status, possible stroke, and syncope. Policy Number 520.18. Central california Emergency Medical Services 2005.
30. Hussain AA, Kimura R, Huang CH. Nasal absorption of naloxone and buprenorphine in rats. *Int J Pharm* 1984;21:233.
31. Loimer N, Hofmann P, Chaudhry HR. Nasal administration of naloxone for detection of opiate dependence. *J Psychiatr Res* 1992;26:39–43.
32. Loimer N, Hofmann P, Chaudhry HR. Nasal administration of naloxone is as effective as the intravenous route in opiate addicts. *Int J Addict* 1994;29:819–827.
33. Barton ED, Ramos J, Colwell C, Benson J, Baily J, Dunn W. Intranasal administration of naloxone by paramedics. *Prehosp Emerg Care* 2002;6:54–58.
34. Kelly AM, Koutsogiannis Z. Intranasal naloxone for life threatening opioid toxicity. *Emerg Med J* 2002;19:375.
35. Robertson T, Hendey GW, Stroh G, Shalit M. Prehospital intranasal versus intravenous administration of naloxone for narcotic overdose. *Acad Emerg Med* 2005;12(Suppl 1):166–167.
36. Howsepian AA. Post-traumatic stress disorder following needle-stick contaminated with suspected HIV-positive blood. *Gen Hosp Psychiatry* 1998;20:123–124.
37. Parkin JM, Murphy M, Anderson J, El-Gadi, Forster G, Pinching AJ. Tolerability and side-effects of post-exposure prophylaxis for HIV infection. *The Lancet* 2000;355:722.
38. Dietze P, Cantwell K, Burgess S. Bystander resuscitation attempts at heroin overdose: does it improve outcomes? *Drug Alcohol Depend* 2002;67:213–218.
39. Darke S, Hall W. Heroin overdose: research and evidence-based intervention. *J Urban Health* 2003;80:189–200.
40. Dietze P, Fry C, Rumbold G, Gerostamoulos J. The context, management and prevention of heroin overdose in Victoria, Australia: the promise of a diverse approach. *Addict Res Theory* 2001;9(5):437–458.
41. Williams P, Urbas G. *Heroin Overdoses and Duty of Care. Trends and Issues in Crime and Criminal Justice No. 188*. Canberra: Australian Institute of Criminology. 2001.
42. Dietze P, Jolley D, Cvetkovski S. Patterns and characteristics of ambulance attendance at heroin overdose at a local area level in Melbourne: implications for service provision. *J Urban Health* 2003;80:248–260.
43. Seidler D, Schmeiser-Rieder A, Schlarp O, Laggner AN. Heroin and opiate emergencies in Vienna: analysis at the municipal ambulance service. *J Clin Epidemiol* 2000;53:734–741.
44. Dietze P, Richards J, Rumbold G, Aitken C, Day C, McGregor C, et al. *Treatment Utilisation by Heroin Dependent Persons in Australia: Implications for Treatment Service Systems*. Melbourne: Turningpoint Alcohol and Drug Centre, Inc. 2003.

45. Dettmer K, Saunders B, Strang J. Take home naloxone and the prevention of deaths from opiate overdose: two pilot schemes. *BMJ* 2001;322:895–896.
46. Strang J, Powis B, Best D, Vingoe L, Briffiths P, Taylor C, et al. Preventing opiate overdose fatalities with take-home naloxone: pre-launch study of possible impact and acceptability. *Addiction* 1999;94:199–204.
47. Coffin PO, Fuller C, Vadnai L, Blaney S, Galea S, Vlahov D. Preliminary evidence of health care provider support for naloxone prescription as overdose fatality prevention strategy in New York City. *J Urban Health* 2003;80:288–290.
48. Hargreaves K, Lenton S. *The Naloxone Feasibility Study: A Study into the Provision of Naloxone Hydrochloride, for Peer Administration, As an Aid in the Prevention of Fatal Heroin-Related Overdose*. Perth, Western Australia: National Drug Research Institute. 2001.
49. Chicago Recovery Alliance 2005. *Opiate OD Prevention/Intervention Work in Chicago*. Retrieved May 3, 2005, from http://www.anypositivechange.org/OD1202.pdf.
50. Lenton SR, Hargreaves KM. Should we conduct a trial of distributing naloxone to heroin users for peer administration to prevent fatal overdose? *Med J Aust* 2000;173:260–263.

Index

E

P

MIX
Papier aus verantwortungsvollen Quellen
Paper from responsible sources
FSC® C105338

If you have any concerns about our products,
you can contact us on
ProductSafety@springernature.com

In case Publisher is established outside the EU,
the EU authorized representative is:
Springer Nature Customer Service Center GmbH
Europaplatz 3, 69115 Heidelberg, Germany

Printed by Libri Plureos GmbH
in Hamburg, Germany